OXFORD SPECIALTY TRAINING

Medicine for MRCP

OXFORD SPECIALTY TRAINING

Medicine for MRCP

SENIOR EDITOR

Rupa Bessant MBChB MSc (Dist) FRCP

Course Director, PassPACES, UK
www.passpaces.co.uk
(Formerly Consultant Rheumatologist, Guy's and St Thomas' NHS Foundation Trust, London, UK)

EDITORS

Jonathan Birns BSc MBBS PhD FRCP

Consultant in Stroke Medicine, Geriatrics and General Medicine, Guy's and St Thomas' NHS Foundation Trust, London, UK
Honorary Senior Lecturer, King's College London, UK
Deputy Head of School of Medicine, Health Education England, London, UK

Charlotte Ford BSc MBChB MRCP

Consultant Gastroenterologist, Western Sussex Hospitals NHS Foundation Trust, UK

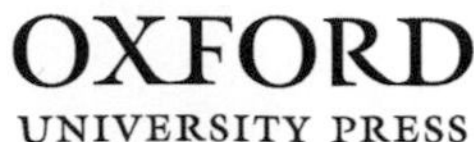

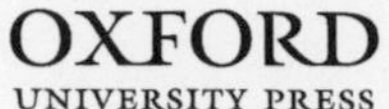

Great Clarendon Street, Oxford, OX2 6DP,
United Kingdom

Oxford University Press is a department of the University of Oxford. It furthers the University's objective of excellence in research, scholarship, and education by publishing worldwide. Oxford is a registered trade mark of Oxford University Press in the UK and in certain other countries

First Edition published in 2020

Published in the United States of America by Oxford University Press
198 Madison Avenue, New York, NY 10016, United States of America

British Library Cataloguing in Publication Data
Data available

Library of Congress Control Number: 2019939553

ISBN 978–0–19–877950–6

Printed in Great Britain by
CPI Group (UK) Ltd, Croydon CR0 4YY

For my daughters, Olivia and Serena,
who continue to inspire me each and every day,
and my parents, Ramola and Amiya,
for whose love and guidance I will always be grateful.
Rupa Bessant

For my sons Cassius, Jonah and Otto who
are my answers to everything.
Charlotte Ford

Foreword

Acquisition of the diploma of Membership of the Royal Colleges of Physicians is a crucial step in a physician's working life that enables them to pursue a career in one of the thirty medical specialties and two subspecialties that are recognised by the General Medical Council (GMC). The work and training that is required to pass the three parts of the examination should not be underestimated by anyone. Trying to learn the enormous extent of medicine so that the trainee has enough confidence to answer the questions that are posed is daunting and there are many theories about the best way to prepare. The changes that are occurring both in medical training and indeed the MRCP does not obviate the fact that studying medicine will require a sound grounding in knowledge. It is anticipated, however, that the provision of better training will aid in the acquisition of knowledge.

The main changes that are occurring in medical training in the UK have been driven by the Shape of Training report which recommended that all new curricula must better serve the patient need, have more generic skills to support the acute unselected take, provide continuity of care, improve care in the community, support credentialing and provide a more flexible approach to training. Furthermore, the GMC mandated that all postgraduate curricula must be based on higher level learning outcomes and incorporate the GMC defined Generic Professional Capabilities (GPCs). In response to this, stage 1 of The Joint Royal Colleges of Physicians Training Board (JRCPTB) designed Internal Medicine Training (IMT) programme was implemented in August 2019. This is an indicative three-year programme designed to better prepare doctors to become a medical registrar and provide them with the skills needed to manage patients presenting with a wide range of general medical symptoms and conditions. Experience in critical care medicine, geriatric medicine and outpatients is mandated and trainees will receive simulation training throughout the programme.

The use of all sources of information can only be assisted if there is an adequacy of time and the introduction by JRCPTB of quality standards for registrars in general internal medicine is now being augmented to cover the whole of internal medicine training.

The MRCP clinical examination is also changing and 2021 should see the introduction of the updated PACES exam to ensure it remains fair, relevant and fit for purpose. This has been the subject of a great deal of scrutiny, consultation and deliberation reflecting not only the place of the examination, but also the importance of the role of excellent clinical skills. Knowing how a disease presents and how and when to investigate such presentations is at the heart of what physicians do.

The editors for this book have enrolled an extensive field of authors who are experts in their fields to provide facts which may be assimilated rapidly and that will be helpful both in revising for the MRCP examinations and also in day to day practice. The consistency of editorship means that individual conditions are listed according to clinical features, diagnosis and management - a system that will serve anyone well at the bedside, whether in a clinical or exam setting. It covers aspects of medicine that have been ignored by the statutory definition of specialty but are enormously important in everyday presentations to the acute hospital, including obstetric medicine. The inclusion of critical care as a specific aspect for consideration complements well the ambition within the internal medicine training programme of generating doctors who are more able to manage the acutely ill patient. The editors have also ensured that there are chapters covering topics that traditionally are 'Cinderella areas' and yet are defined as being important in the new curriculum – these include Statistics and Medical Law and Ethics.

In summary, this work will help you in studying for the MRCP diploma but if used well will stand the reader in good stead for their future career.

Michael Jones
Medical Director, Training and Development
Joint Royal Colleges of Physicians Training Board
Federation of Royal Colleges of Physicians of the United Kingdom
Consultant Acute Physician
GIRFT National Clinical Lead for Acute and General Medicine

Preface

Medicine for MRCP aims to be a comprehensive guide to the MRCP Part 1 and Part 2 written examinations, and to provide the requisite theoretical knowledge in a user-friendly format. Each chapter has been written by highly experienced MRCP lecturers. The most relevant clinical information for the MRCP (UK) examinations is covered, incorporating the appropriate protocols, guidelines and treatment algorithms from NICE, UK, and European and American Colleges. An emphasis has been placed on a UK clinical setting. Latest developments and clinical treatments (e.g. biologic therapy) have been included throughout the text. Candidates who wish to read in greater depth are directed to relevant publications at the end of each section. Furthermore, the inclusion of links to carefully selected relevant websites (e.g. DVLA guidelines and current mental health legislation) are intended to provide up-to-date information to benefit doctors within their clinical setting and daily practice.

A well-structured and comprehensive approach to clinical medicine has been used to ensure that the text is an invaluable resource for candidates preparing for the MRCP Part 1 and Part 2, and PACES examinations, as well as the MRCPI, USMLE and PLAB examinations. Undergraduate students will also find this book beneficial and we believe that it will remain a valuable reference for trainees in acute medicine, accident and emergency medicine, anaesthetics, critical care and general practice.

Each chapter integrates the basic science required for the Part 1 written, with more clinically based information, concentrating on subjects that need to be covered for the Part 2 written and providing a solid foundation for candidates as they progress to the PACES examination. Where possible, the clinical implications of the theoretical knowledge covered in Part 1 are emphasised within the clinical context, thereby making this information easier to remember.

The text utilises a combination of flowcharts, tables and mnemonics to assist candidates in retaining and recalling the key relevant facts in both an examination setting and clinical practice. Multiple choice questions (MCQs) relevant to Part 1 and Part 2 written papers have been included at the end of each chapter, enabling candidates to build their confidence. The answers to these questions will help to consolidate the medical knowledge relevant to all three parts of the MRCP examination.

The editors and chapter authors have combined their extensive clinical knowledge and practical teaching experience to create a book that we believe will help to optimise the chances of examination success. We hope that candidates will both enjoy and benefit from this book during their revision and clinical practice.

Good luck to you all!

Rupa Bessant

Acknowledgements

Firstly, I wish to thank the whole editorial team at Oxford University Press for accepting the proposal for *Medicine for MRCP* and for giving me the privilege of editing this book. My particular thanks go to Geraldine Jeffers (Senior Commissioning Editor), Fiona Sutherland (Senior Assistant Commissioning Editor), Karen Moore (Senior Production Editor) and Susan Finlay (Copy Editor), for their ongoing support from commission to completion.

Secondly, I am grateful to all the contributors to this manuscript for their combined wisdom, and especially my co-editors, Jonathan Birns and Charlotte Ford, and to each of our families who have supported us all throughout this project.

I would especially like to thank my husband, David, whose continued patience and support, whilst editing these 27 chapters has, as always, been invaluable.

Finally, I wish to thank all my students whose intriguing questions continue to challenge me and to inspire my interest in medical education.

Rupa Bessant

Contents

Contributors

Please note that the start of each chapter lists the authors who have contributed to that chapter. Junior authors are listed before senior authors. Where there are more than one junior or senior author, they are listed in an order reflecting their contribution to the chapter; if two authors have contributed equally this is denoted with asterisks and a relevant footnote to this effect.

Robert Adam MA MBBS MRCP PhD FRACP

*Consultant Neurologist, Department of Neurology,
The Royal Brisbane and Women's Hospital, Brisbane, Australia*

Christine O. Ademokun MBBS BSc MRCP

*Specialist Registrar, Haematology Department, Hammersmith Hospital,
Imperial College NHS Trust, London, UK*

Behdad Afzali BSc MBBS PhD MRCP PGDip FHEA MAcadMEd

*Earl Stadtman Investigator and Consultant Nephrologist, Immunoregulation Section,
Kidney Diseases Branch, NIDDK, NIH Bethesda, MD, USA*

John Archer

*Consultant Physician and Clinical Toxicologist, Department of Clinical Toxicology,
Guy's and St Thomas' NHS Foundation Trust, London, UK*

Stephen R. Atkinson PhD MRCP

*Specialist Registrar in Gastroenterology and Hepatology,
Chelsea and Westminster NHS Foundation Trust;
Honorary Clinical Lecturer, Imperial College London, UK*

Chitrabhanu Ballav

*Consultant Physician and Endocrinologist, Diabetes and Endocrinology,
Buckinghamshire Healthcare NHS Trust, Aylesbury, UK*

David Bessant BSc MBChB MD FRCOphth

*Consultant Ophthalmologist, Clinical Director Moorfields Northwest,
Moorfields Eye Hospital, London, UK*

Rupa Bessant MBChB MSc (Dist) FRCP

*Course Director, PassPACES, UK (Formerly Consultant Rheumatologist,
Guy's and St Thomas' NHS Foundation Trust, London, UK)*

Jonathan Birns BSc MBBS PhD FRCP

*Consultant in Stroke Medicine, Geriatrics and General Medicine,
Guy's and St Thomas' NHS Foundation Trust, London, UK*

Anthony C. Brooms BSc MSc PhD FHEA

*Lecturer in Statistics, Department of Economics, Mathematics and Statistics,
Birkbeck, University of London, UK*

Anupam Chatterjee MBChB FRCSE Cert LRS (RCOphth)

Ophthalmologist, Brent Community Ophthalmology Service, Sudbury, Primary Care Centre, Wembley, London, UK

Danny Cheriyan MBBCh MD FRCPI

Consultant Gastroenterologist, Beaumont Hospital, Dublin, Ireland

Coziana Ciurtin MSc PhD FRCP

Consultant Rheumatologist, Associate Professor, Department of Rheumatology, University College London, UK

Rosemary E.J. Clarke MChem MBBS MSc PhD MRCP FRCPath

Consultant Medical Biochemist, NHS Highlands, UK

Sophie A. Clarke MBBS BSc PhD MRCP

Clinical Lecturer, Department of Endocrinology and Investigative Medicine, Imperial College London, UK

Cordelia E.M. Coltart MBBS BSc DTM&H MPH PhD MRCP FRCPath

Academic Clinical Lecturer, Institute for Global Health, University College London; Specialist Registrar in Infectious Diseases, University College London Hospitals NHS Foundation Trust, London, UK

Jennifer Crawley MBChB BSc MRCP

Consultant Dermatologist, Department of Dermatology, University College London Hospitals, London, UK

David Cunningham OBE MD FRCP FMedSci

Director of Clinical Research, Director of The Royal Marsden/Institute of Cancer Research NIHR Biomedical Research Centre, Royal Marsden NHS Foundation Trust, London, UK

Ameet Dhar PhD FRCP

Consultant Hepatologist and Honorary Senior Lecturer, Imperial College Healthcare NHS Trust, London, UK

Simon Edwards

Medical Director and Consultant Physician, Diggory Division, CNWL; Trustwide Quality Improvement Clinical Lead, CNWL; Honorary Associate Professor, University College London, UK

Michael Fertleman FRCP FFLM FHEA Barrister (NP)

Consultant Physician, St Mary's Hospital London; Visiting Professor, Department of Bioengineering, Imperial College, London, UK

Douglas Fink MRCP SCE(ID)

Registrar Infectious Diseases, Hospital for Tropical Diseases, University College London Hospitals NHS Foundation Trust, London, UK

Elisa Fontana

Medical Oncologist, The Institute of Cancer Research and The Royal Marsden Hospital, London, UK

Charlotte Ford BSc MBChB MRCP

Consultant Gastroenterologist, Western Sussex Hospitals NHS Foundation Trust, UK

Matthew C. Frise BM BCh DPhil MRCP FFICM

Consultant in Acute Medicine and Intensive Care, Royal Berkshire Hospital, Reading, UK

Nicholas Gall

Consultant Cardiologist, Department of Cardiology, King's College Hospital; Honorary Senior Lecturer, King's College London, UK

Benjamin Glickstein BSc MBBS MRCP

Consultant Geriatrician, Miramichi Regional Hospital, New Brunswick, Canada

Refik Gökmen MA PhD FRCP FHEA

Consultant Nephrologist, Guy's and St Thomas' NHS Foundation Trust, London, UK

Chris J. Harvey BSc MBBS MRCP FRCR

Consultant Radiologist, Hammersmith Hospital, London, UK

David Holdsworth MA, DPhil

Consultant Cardiologist, Oxford Heart Centre, John Radcliffe Hospital, Oxford, UK

Philip Howard MA GDipLaw LLM MA MD FRCP

Consultant Physician and Gastroenterologist, Department of Medicine, Epsom and St Helier University Hospitals NHS Trust; Honorary Senior Lecturer in Medicine, St George's Hospital Medical School, London, UK

Dev Kevat BMedSci MBBS LLB MSc FRACP

Consultant Endocrinologist, Western Health and Monash Health, Melbourne; Consultant Obstetric Physician, Royal Brisbane & Women's Hospital, Brisbane, Australia

Lucy Lamb PhD MRCP DTMH

Defence Senior Lecturer in Medicine, Honorary Clinical Associate Professor in the Division of Infection and Immunity UCL and Honorary Clinical Fellow, Imperial College, London, UK

Richard Lee MA MBBS MRCP PhD

Consultant Respiratory Physician with an Interest in Early Cancer Diagnosis, Royal Marsden Hospital, London, UK

Lucy Mackillop BMBCh MA FRCP

Consultant Obstetric Physician, Women's Centre, Oxford University Hospitals NHS Foundation Trust, Oxford, UK

Tim Mant

Visiting Professor, Clinical Pharmacology, King's College London, UK

Charles Marshall

Clinical Lecturer in Neurology, Preventive Neurology Unit, Wolfson Institute of Preventive Medicine, Queen Mary University of London, UK

Alan Maryon-Davis MBBChir MSc FFPH FRCP FFSEM FRCGP

Honorary Professor of Public Health, School of Public Health and Environmental Sciences, Kings College London, UK

Claire L. Meek MBChB PhD MRCP FRCPath

Senior Clinical Research Associate, Institute of Metabolic Science, University of Cambridge, UK; Consultant Chemical Pathologist and Metabolic Physician, Department of Chemistry, Peterborough City Hospital, Peterborough, UK

Nasir Saeed Mirza MBBS BSc MRCP FHEA

Senior Clinical Lecturer and Honorary Consultant Neurologist, Department of Molecular and Clinical Pharmacology, Institute of Translational Medicine, University of Liverpool, UK

Elena Nikiphorou MBBS BSc MD FRCP PGCME FHEA

Consultant Rheumatologist, Department of Rheumatology, King's College Hospital; Senior Clinical Research Fellow, Department of Inflammation Biology, King's College London, UK

Kingsley Norton MA MD FRCPsych

Medical Psychotherapist, DocHealth, BMA House, Tavistock Square, London, UK

Anna Nuttall BA MBBS MD MRCP MRCP

Rheumatology Consultant, Whittington Hospital, London, UK

Declan P. O'Regan FRCP FRCR PhD

Consultant Radiologist, Imperial College Healthcare NHS Trust, London, UK; Reader in Imaging Sciences, London Institute of Medical Sciences, Imperial College, London, UK

Donal O'Kane MBBCh BAO MRCP PhD

Consultant Dermatologist, Department of Dermatology, Royal Victoria Hospital, Belfast, UK

William L.G. Oldfield MSc PhD FRCP

Executive Medical Director, University Hospitals Bristol NHS Foundation Trust, Bristol, UK

Stephen Patchett

Consultant Gastroenterologist, Beaumont Hospital, Dublin; Clinical Associate Professor, Royal College of Surgeons of Ireland, Ireland

Munir Pirmohamed PhD FRCP FMedSci

David Weatherall Chair of Medicine, Department of Molecular and Clinical Pharmacology, The University of Liverpool, UK

Nita Prasannan MBBS MRCP FRCPath

Consultant Haematologist, Guy's and St Thomas' NHS Foundation Trust, London, UK

Deepti H. Radia BSc MSc (Med Ed) MRCPI FRCPath

Consultant Haematologist, Guy's and St Thomas' NHS Foundation Trust, London, UK

Brintha Selvarajah MA MBBS MRCP

Clinical Research Fellow, UCL Respiratory, University College London, UK

Gulshan Sethi MSc FRCP FHEA

Consultant Physician in Sexual Health and HIV, Guy's and St Thomas' NHS Foundation Trust; Honorary Senior Clinical Lecturer, King's College London, UK

Penelope Smith

Consultant Physician Acute Medicine and Infectious Diseases, Royal Free London NHS Foundation Trust, London, UK

Elizabeth Smyth MD

Consultant Medical Oncologist, Addenbrooke's Hospital, Cambridge, UK

Mike Stacey MD MRCP DTMH

Defence Senior Lecturer in Military Medicine and Consultant Physician, Chelsea & Westminster Hospital, London, UK

Rob Tandy MBBS MRCPsych

Consultant Psychiatrist, Tavistock Centre, London, UK

John Wass

Professor of Endocrinology, Department of Endocrinology, Churchill Hospital, Oxford, UK

Andrew Webb FRCP PhD

Senior Lecturer, King's College London; Guy's and St Thomas' NHS Foundation Trust, London, UK

Ingeborg Welters

Reader, University of Liverpool; Honorary Consultant in Intensive Care, Royal Liverpool University Hospital, Liverpool, UK; Professor of Anaesthesia, Justus-Liebig-Universität Gießen, Gießen, Germany

John Whitaker BMBCh PhD MRCP

Specialty Registrar in Cardiology, Guy's and St Thomas' NHS Foundation Trust; Clinical Research Fellow, King's College London, UK

Anthony S. Wierzbicki DM DPhil FRCPath

Professor and Consultant in Metabolic Medicine/Chemical Pathology, Department of Chemical Pathology, Guy's and St Thomas' NHS Foundation Trust, London, UK

Rupert P. Williams MBBS BSc PhD MRCP

Consultant Cardiologist, Kingston Hospital NHS Foundation Trust, Surrey, UK

Tom Wingfield MBChB PhD MRCP DTMH DipHIV PGCMedE

Senior Clinical Lecturer, Liverpool School of Tropical Medicine, Liverpool, UK and Karolinska Institutet, Stockholm, Sweden; Honorary Consultant Physician, Royal Liverpool and Broadgreen University Hospitals NHS Trust, Liverpool, UK

David R. Woods MD FRCP L/RAMC

Defence Professor of Military Medicine; Professor of Sport and Exercise Endocrinology, Carnegie Research Institute, Leeds Beckett University, Leeds, UK

Patrick Yong MBChB MSc PhD MRCP FRCPath

Consultant Immunologist, Department of Immunology, Frimley Park Hospital, Frimley, UK

Abbreviations

^{18}FDG	18-fluorodeoxy-D-glucose
21OH	21, hydroxylase
2,3-DPG	2,3- diphosphoglycerate
3-HMG CoA	3-hydroxy-3-methyl-glutaryl-CoA
5HIAA	5-hydroxyindoleacetic acid
5HT	5-hydroxytryptamine
6MWD	6-minute walk distance
αFP	alpha fetoprotein
βHCG	beta-human chorionic gonadotropin
A	adenine
AA	aplastic anaemia
AAFB	acid and alcohol-fast bacilli
AAV	ANCA-associated vasculitis
ABC	ATP-binding cassette transporter
ABG	arterial blood gas
ABPA	allergic bronchopulmonary aspergillosis
AC	activated charcoal; alternating current
ACA	anterior cerebral artery
ACE	angiotensin-converting enzyme
ACE-i	angiotensin-converting enzyme inhibitor
AChR	acetylcholine receptor
ACLE	acute cutaneous lupus erythematosus
ACR	albumin creatinine ratio
ACS	acute coronary syndrome
ACTH	adrenocorticotrophic hormone
AD	Alzheimer's disease; autosomal dominant
ADA	adenosine deaminase
ADCA	autosomal dominant cerebellar ataxia
ADCC	antibody-dependent cellular cytotoxicity
ADH	antidiuretic hormone
ADP	adenosine diphosphate
ADPKD	autosomal dominant polycystic kidney disease
ADR	adverse drug reaction
ADT	androgen-deprivation therapy
AE	adverse event; atopic eczema
AE1	anion exchanger
AF	atrial fibrillation
AFB	acid-fast bacilli
AFLP	acute fatty liver of pregnancy
AFP	alpha-fetoprotein
AG	anion gap
AGEP	acute generalised exanthematous pustulosis
aHUS	atypical haemolytic uraemic syndrome
AIDS	acquired immune deficiency syndrome
AIH	amiodarone-induced hypothyroidism
AIHA	autoimmune haemolytic anaemia
AIMSS	aromatase inhibitor-associated musculoskeletal syndrome
AIN	acute interstitial nephritis
AIP	acute intermittent porphyria
AIRE	autoimmune regulator
AIT	amiodarone-induced thyrotoxicosis
AJCC	American Joint Committee on Cancer
AKI	acute kidney injury
ALA	aminolaevulinic acid
ALARA	as low as reasonably achievable
ALD	alcoholic liver disease
ALF	acute liver failure
ALL	acute lymphoblastic leukaemia
ALP	alkaline phosphatase
ALS	amyotrophic lateral sclerosis
ALT	alanine aminotransferase
AML	acute myeloid leukaemia; angiomyolipoma
AMPA	α-amino-3-hydroxy-5-methyl-4-isoxazolepropionic acid
AMS	acute mountain sickness
ANA	antinuclear antibodies
ANCA	antineutrophil cytoplasmic antibody
ANOVA	analysis of variance
AP	accessory pathway
APB	atrial premature beat
APC	antigen-presenting cell
APD	automated peritoneal dialysis
APECED	autoimmune polyendocrinopathy, candidiasis, ectodermal dysplasia
APLA	antiphospholipid antibodies
APLS	antiphospholipid syndrome
APML	acute promyelocytic leukaemia
APO	apolipoprotein
APQ	Alcohol Problems Questionnaire
APTT	activated partial thromboplastin time
APUD	amine precursor uptake and decarboxylation
AR	autosomal recessive; aortic regurgitation
ARB	angiotensin receptor blocker
ARDS	acute respiratory distress syndrome
ARF	acute rheumatic fever
ARMD	age-related macular degeneration
ARPKD	autosomal recessive polycystic kidney disease
ART	antiretroviral therapy
ARVC	arrhythmogenic right ventricular cardiomyopathy
ARVD	arrhythmogenic right ventricular dysplasia
AS	Angelman syndrome; aortic stenosis; ankylosing spondylitis
ASD	atrial septal defect
AST	aspartate transaminase
AT	atrial tachycardia
ATG	anti-thymocyte globulin
ATLL	adult T cell leukaemia
ATN	acute tubular necrosis
ATP	adenosine triphosphate

ATRA	all-trans-retinoic acid
AUC	area under the curve
AUDIT	Alcohol Use Disorders Identification Test
AV	atrioventricular; arterio-venous
AVM	arterio-venous malformation
AVN	avascular necrosis
AVNRT	atrioventricular node re-entry tachycardia
AVRT	atrioventricular re-entry tachycardia
BAV	bicuspid aortic valve
BBB	blood-brain barrier; bundle branch block
BC	blood culture
BCG	Bacillus Calmette–Guérin
BCSP	bowel cancer screening programme
BD	twice daily
BG	blood glucose
B-hCG	B-human chorionic gonadotrophin
BHIVA	British HIV Association
BHR	bronchial hyper-responsiveness
BMD	bone mineral density
BMI	body mass index
BMT	bone marrow transplant
BNP	brain natriuretic peptide
BO	Barrett's oesophagus
BP	blood pressure; bullous pemphigoid
BRAF	B-rapidly accelerated fibrosarcoma
BRAO	branch retinal artery occlusion
BRVO	branch retinal vein occlusion
BSA	body surface area
BSR	British Society of Rheumatology
BTS	British Thoracic Society
C	cytosine
CA	cancer antigen
CABG	coronary artery bypass grafting
CAD	coronary artery disease
CADSIL	cerebral autosomal dominant arteriopathy with subcortical infarcts and leukoencephalopathy
CAH	congenital adrenal hyperplasia
cAMP	cyclic adenosine monophosphate
CAP	community acquired pneumonia
CAPD	continuous ambulatory peritoneal dialysis
CBD	common bile duct
CBT	cognitive behavioural therapy
CCB	calcium channel blocker
CCHF	Crimean–Congo haemorrhagic fever
CCK	cholecystokinin
CCP	cyclic citrullinated peptide
CD	Crohn's disease; cluster of differentiation
CDA	congenital dyserythropoietic anaemia
CDAD	*Clostridium difficile*-associated diarrhoea
CDI	*Clostridium difficile* infection
CDK	cyclin-dependent kinase
CDT	*Clostridium difficile* toxin
CEA	carcinoembryonic antigen
CETP	cholesterol ester transfer protein
CF	cystic fibrosis
cffDNA	cell-free fetal DNA
CFH	complement factor H
CFTR	cystic fibrosis transmembrane conductance regulator
CHART	continuous hyperfractionated accelerated radiotherapy
CHB	complete heart block
CHM	Commission on Human Medicines
CI	cardiac index
CIDP	chronic inflammatory demyelinating polyneuropathy
CK	creatine kinase
CKD	chronic kidney disease
CLE	cutaneous lupus erythematosus
CLL	chronic lymphocytic leukaemia
CM	chylomicron
CMC	carpometacarpal
CML	chronic myeloid leukaemia
CMML	chronic myelomonocytic leukaemia
CMR	cardiac magnetic resonance
CMT	Charcot–Marie–Tooth
CMV	cytomegalovirus
CN	cranial nerve
CNS	central nervous system
CO	carbon monoxide; cardiac output
COMT	catechol-o-methyl transferase
COPD	chronic obstructive pulmonary disease
COREC	Central Office for Research Ethics Committees
COX	cyclo-oxygenase
CPAP	continuous positive airway pressure
CPEO	chronic progressive external ophthalmoplegia
CPP	cerebral perfusion pressure
CPPD	calcium pyrophosphate dehydrate
CPR	cardiopulmonary resuscitation
CPVT	catecholaminergic polymorphic ventricular tachycardia
CRAO	central retinal artery occlusion
CRC	colorectal cancer
CRH	corticotropin-releasing hormone
CRP	C-reactive protein
CRT	cardiac resynchronisation therapy
CRT-D	cardiac resynchronisation therapy defibrillator
CRT-P	cardiac resynchronisation therapy pacemaker
CRVO	central retinal vein occlusion
CSC	cancer stem cells
csDMARDs	conventional synthetic DMARDs
CSF	cerebrospinal fluid; colony stimulating factor
CT	computed tomography
CTA	clinical trial authorisation
CTD	connective tissue disease
CTEPH	chronic thromboembolic pulmonary hypertension
CTI	cavo-tricuspid isthmus
CTIMP	clinical trials of investigational medicinal products

CTLA cytotoxic T-lymphocyte-associated
CT-NCAP CT neck, chest, abdomen, pelvis
CTPA computed tomography pulmonary angiography
CTX cross-linked C-telopeptide
CV cardiovascular; crystal violet
CVA cerebrovascular accident
CVC central venous catheter
CVD cardiovascular disease
CVP central venous pressure
CVVH continuous venovenous haemofiltration
CVVHD continuous venovenous haemodialysis
CVVHDF continuous venovenous haemodiafiltration
CXR chest X-ray
CYP450 cytochrome P450
DAH diffuse alveolar haemorrhage
DAS disease activity score
DAT direct antiglobulin test
DBA Diamond Blackfan anaemia
DBD donation after brain death
DBS deep brain stimulation
DC direct current; dyskeratosis congenita
DCCV DC cardioversion
DCD donation after circulatory death
DCM dilated cardiomyopathy
DCT distal convoluted tubule
DEXA dual energy X-ray absorptiometry
DHEA dehydroepiandrosterone
DHFR dihydrofolate reductase
DI diabetes insipidus
DIC disseminated intravascular coagulation
DILI drug-induced liver injury
DIP distal interphalangeal
DISH diffuse idiopathic skeletal hyperostosis
DKA diabetic ketoacidosis
DLB dementia with Lewy bodies
DLBCL diffuse large cell B-cell lymphoma
DLCO diffusion capacity
DLE discoid lupus erythematosus
DLQI Dermatology Life Quality Index
DM diabetes mellitus
DMARD disease-modifying anti-rheumatic drug
DMD Duchenne muscular dystrophy
DMPK dystrophia myotonica protein kinase
DNA deoxyribonucleic acid; double-stranded antibodies
DNACPR do not attempt cardiopulmonary resuscitation
DNAR do not attempt resuscitation
DRESS drug reaction with eosinophilia and systemic symptoms
DSM Diagnostic and Statistical Manual of Mental Disorders
DUSR Development Update Safety Report
DVT deep vein thrombosis
DWI diffusion weighted imaging
EASI Eczema Area and Severity Index
EBUS endobronchial ultrasound
EBV Epstein–Barr virus
ECG electrocardiogram
ECHO echocardiogram
ECMO extracorporeal membrane oxygenation
ECOG Eastern Cooperative Oncology Group
ECT electro-convulsive therapy
EDS Ehlers–Danlos syndrome
EDV end diastolic volume
EEG electroencephalogram
EGDT early goal-directed therapy
EGFR epidermal growth factor receptor
eGFR estimated glomerular filtration rate
EGFR epidermal growth factor receptor
EGPA eosinophilic granulomatosis with polyangiitis
EIA enzyme-linked immunoassay
EL elevated liver
ELISA enzyme-linked immunosorbent assay
EMA European Medicines Agency
EMG electromyogram
EMR endoscopic mucosal resection
EMT epithelial-mesenchymal transition
EN erythema nodosum
ENA extractable nuclear antigens
ENaC epithelial sodium channel
ENT ear, nose, and throat
EoE eosinophilic oesophagitis
EP electrophysiology
EPAP expiratory positive airway pressure
EPP exposure prone procedure
EPSP excitatory post-synaptic potential
ER endoplasmic reticulum
ERCP endoscopic retrograde cholangiopancreatogram
ESC European Society of Cardiology
ESKD end-stage kidney disease
ESQ Environmental Symptom Questionnaire
ESR erythrocyte sedimentation rate
ET essential tremor; essential thrombocythaemia
ETC electron transport chain
EU European Union
EUS endoscopic ultrasound
FAB French-American-British
FAERS FDA Adverse Event Reporting System
FasL Fas ligand
FASP fetal anomaly screening programme
FBC full blood count
FDA Food and Drug Administration
FDG fluorodeoxyglucose
FDP fibrin degradation product
FE fractional excretion [value]
FEV forced expiratory volume
FFP fresh frozen plasma
FFR fractional flow reserve
FGF fibroblast growth factor
FIA fluorescent immunoassay
FIGO International Federation of Gynaecology and Obstetrics

FISH	fluorescence in-situ hybridisation
FMD	fibromuscular dysplasia
FMF	familial Mediterranean fever
FNA	fine needle aspiration
FP	fetoprotein
FRAX	fracture risk assessment tool
FRAXA	fragile X type A syndrome
FRC	functional residual capacity
FRDA	Friedreich ataxia
FSGS	focal segmental glomerulosclerosis
FSH	follicle-stimulating hormone
FTD	frontotemporal dementia
FUS	fused in sarcoma
FVC	forced vital capacity
FVL	factor V Leiden mutation
G	guanine
G6PD	glucose-6-phosphate dehydrogenase
GABA	gamma-aminobutyric acid
GAD	glutamic acid decarboxylase
GAS	Group A Strep.
Gaβ-HS	Group A (beta haemolytic) *Streptococcus*
GBM	glomerular basement membrane
GBS	Group B Strep.
GCA	giant cell arteritis
GCP	good clinical practice
GCS	Glasgow Coma Score
GCSF	granulocyte-colony stimulating factor
GDH	glutamate dehydrogenase
GDM	gestational diabetes mellitus
GFR	glomerular filtration rate
GGT	gamma-glutamyl transferase
GH	gestational hypertension; growth hormone
GHRH	growth hormone-releasing hormone
GI	gastrointestinal
GIST	gastrointestinal stromal tumour
GMC	General Medical Council
GN	glomerulonephritis
GnRH	gonadotrophin-releasing hormone
GOJ	gastro-oesophageal junction
GORD	gastroesophageal reflux disease
Gp	glycoprotein
GPA	granulomatosis with polyangiitis
GPCR	G-protein coupled receptor
GPi	globus pallidus interna
GSD	glycogen storage disease
GTN	glyceryl trinitrate
GTP	guanosine triphosphate
GU	genitourinary
GUM	genitourinary medicine
GVHD	graft-versus-host disease
GWAS	genome-wide association study
H	haemolysis
H_1	histamine
HACE	high altitude cerebral oedema
HAP	hospital-acquired pneumonia
HAPE	high altitude pulmonary oedema
HAS	human albumin solution
Hb	haemoglobin
HbA1c	glycosylated haemoglobin
HBV	hepatitis B virus
HCAI	health care-associated infection
HCC	hepatocellular carcinoma
hCG	human chorionic gonadotrophin
HCHWA-D	hereditary cerebral haemorrhage with amyloidosis
HCM	hypertrophic cardiomyopathy
HCV	hepatitis C virus
HD	haemodialysis; Huntington disease
HDL	high-density lipoprotein
HDU	high dependency unit
HE	hepatic encephalopathy
HELLP	haemolysis, elevated liver enzymes and low platelets
HER	human epidermal growth factor receptor
HERNS	hereditary endotheliopathy with retinopathy, nephropathy and stroke
HF	haemofiltration; heart failure
HFpEF	heart failure with preserved ejection fraction
HFrEF	heart failure with reduced ejection fraction
HG	hyperemesis gravidarum
HGPRT	hypoxanthine guanine phosphoribosyltransferase
HHS	hyperglycaemic hyperosmolar state
HHT	hereditary haemorrhagic telangiectasia
HHV	human herpes virus
HIT	heparin-induced thrombocytopenia
HIV	human immunodeficiency virus
HIVAN	HIV-associated nephropathy
HL	Hodgkin's lymphoma
HLA	human leukocyte antigen
HMN	hereditary motor neuropathy
HNPCC	hereditary non-polyposis colon cancer
HNPP	hereditary neuropathy with liability to pressure palsies
HOA	hypertrophic osteoarthropathy
HP	*Helicobacter pylori*; hypersensitivity pneumonitis
HPV	human papillomavirus
HR	heart rate
HRA	Health Research Authority
HRCT	high-resolution CT
HRS	hepatorenal syndrome
HRT	hormone replacement therapy
HSAN	hereditary sensory-autonomic neuropathy
HSC	haematopoietic stem cell
HSE	Health and Safety Executive
HSIDU	high-security infectious disease unit
HSN	hereditary sensory neuropathy
HSV	herpes simplex virus
HT	hydroxytryptamine
HTLV	human T-cell lymphotropic virus
HU	Hounsfield unit

HUS haemolytic uraemic syndrome
HUV hypocomplementaemic urticarial vasculitis
IASLC International Association for the Study of Lung Cancer
IBA identification and brief advice
IBD inflammatory bowel disease
IBS irritable bowel syndrome
ICD implantable cardioverter defibrillator; International Classification of Diseases
ICD-O International Classification of Diseases for Oncology
ICP intracranial pressure
ICS Intensive Care Society
ICU intensive care unit
ID imprinting disorder
IDL intermediate-density lipoprotein
IDDM insulin-dependent diabetes mellitus
IE infective endocarditis
IFALD intestinal failure-related liver disease
IFG impaired fasting glucose
IFRT involved field radiation therapy
Ig immunoglobulin
IGF insulin-like growth factor
IGRA interferon gamma release assay
IGT impaired glucose tolerance
IHD ischaemic heart disease
IIP idiopathic interstitial pneumonia
IL interleukin
ILD interstitial lung disease
IM intramuscular
IMCA independent mental capacity advocate
IMD inherited metabolic disorder
IMP investigational medicinal product
IMRT intensity modulated radiotherapy
IMt intestinal metaplasia
INF interferon
INR international normalised ratio
IOL intraocular lens
IPAF interstitial pneumonia with autoimmune features
IPAH idiopathic pulmonary arterial hypertension
IPAP inspiratory positive airway pressure
IPEX immune dysfunction, polyendocrinopathy, and enteropathy, X-linked
IPF idiopathic pulmonary fibrosis
IPSP inhibitory post-synaptic potential
IPSS International Prognostic Scoring System
IR(ME)R Ionising Radiation (Medical Exposure) Regulations
IRMA intra-retinal microvascular abnormality
ITP immune thrombocytopenic purpura
ITT insulin tolerance test
IUGR intrauterine growth restriction
IV intravenous
IVC inferior vena cava
IVDU intravenous drug use
IVIG intravenous immunoglobulin
JAK Janus kinase
JIA juvenile idiopathic arthritis
JME juvenile myoclonic epilepsy
JVP jugular venous pulse
KCO transfer factor
LA left atrial; lupus anticoagulant
LABA long-acting inhaled β2 agonist
LAD left anterior descending
LAM lymphangioleiomyomatosis
LAP left atrial pressure
LBBB left bundle branch block
LCHAD long chain 3-hydroxyacetyl coenzyme-A dehydrogenase
LDH lactate dehydrogenase
LDL low-density lipoprotein
LFT liver function test
LGMD limb girdle muscular dystrophy
LGV lymphogranuloma venereum
LH luteinising hormone
LHC left heart catheterisation
LMF lipid maturation factor
LMS left main stem
LMWH low molecular weight heparin
LOS lower oesophageal sphincter
LP lichen planus; lumbar puncture
LPA Lasting Power of Attorney
LPL lipoprotein lipase
LPS lipopolysaccharide
LRP lipoprotein-related receptor
LRRK leucine-rich repeat kinase
LTBI latent tuberculosis infection
LTOT long-term oxygen therapy
LV left ventricle
LVEDP left ventricular end-diastolic pressure
LVEF left ventricular ejection fraction
LVOT left ventricular outflow tract
LVH left ventricular hypertrophy
MABP mean arterial blood pressure
MAC *Mycobacterium avium* complex
MACE major adverse cardiac events
MAGE melanoma-associated antigen
MALToma mucosa-associated lymphoid tissue
MAO monoamine oxidase
MAOI monoamine oxidase inhibitor
MAP mean arterial pressure
MAPK mitogen-activated protein kinase
MAPT microtubule-associated protein tau
MAS macrophage activation syndrome
MAU medical admissions unit
MC&S microscopy, culture and sensitivity
MCA Mental Capacity Ac; middle cerebral artery
MCD minimal change disease
MCGN mesangiocapillary glomerulonephritis
MCP metacarpophalangeal
MCR melanocortin receptor

MCTD	mixed connective tissue disease
MD	myotonic dystrophy
mDF	Maddrey's discriminant function
MDMA	3,4-methylenedioxymethamphetamine
MDR	multidrug resistance
MDS	myelodysplasia
MDT	multidisciplinary team
MELAS	mitochondrial encephalomyopathy with lactic acidosis and stroke-like episodes
MEN	multiple endocrine neoplasia
MEP	maximal expiratory pressure
MEPE	matrix extracellular phosphoglycoprotein
MERRF	myoclonus epilepsy with ragged red fibres
MERS	Middle East respiratory syndrome
MG	*Mycoplasma genitalium*
MGUS	monoclonal gammopathy of unknown significance
MHA	Mental Health Act
MHC	major histocompatibility complex
MHRA	Medicines and Healthcare products Regulatory Agency
MI	myocardial infarction
MIBG	meta iodobenzylguanidine
MIP	maximal inspiratory pressure
MLF	medial longitudinal fasciculus
MMF	mycophenolate mofetil
MMP	matrix metalloproteinase
MMR	mismatch repair
MMSE	mini-mental state examination
MN	membranous nephropathy
MND	motor neurone disease
MoCA	Montreal Cognitive Assessment
MODY	maturity onset diabetes of the young
MOG	myelin oligodendrocyte glycoprotein
MPA	microscopic polyangiitis
mPAP	mean pulmonary arterial pressure
MPL	myeloproliferative leukaemia
MPO	myeloperoxidase
MPS	myocardial perfusion scintigraphy
MR	mitral regurgitation
MRA	magnetic resonance angiography
MRCP	magnetic resonance cholangiopancreatogram
MRE	magnetic resonance enterography
MRI	magnetic resonance imaging
mRNA	messenger RNA
MRSA	meticillin-resistant *Staphylococcus aureus*
MS	mitral stenosis; multiple sclerosis
MSA	multiple system atrophy
MSCC	metastatic spinal cord compression
MSI	microsatellite instability
MSM	men who have sex with men
MSSA	meticillin-sensitive *Staphylococcus aureus*
MSU	mid-stream urine
mSv	milliSievert
MTB	mycobacterium tuberculosis
MTC	medullary thyroid cancer
MTCD	mixed connective tissue disease
MTP	metatarsophalangeal
MusK	muscle specific kinase
MVR	mitral valve replacement
MZ	monozygote
NA	noradrenaline
NAAT	nucleic acid amplification technique
NAC	N-acetylcysteine
NAD	nicotinamine adenine dinucleotide
NAFLD	non-alcoholic fatty liver disease
NAP	neutrophil alkaline phosphatase
NAPQI	N-acetyl-p-benzoquinone imine
NASH	non-alcoholic steatohepatitis
NBTE	non-bacterial thrombotic endocarditis
NCB1	sodium bicarbonate co-transporter
NCCT	sodium chloride co-transporter
NCS	nerve conduction studies
NDI	nephrogenic diabetes insipidus
NER	nucleotide excision repair
NET	neuroendocrine tumour
NF	neurofibromatosis; nuclear factor
NFCI	non-freezing cold injury
NG	nasogastric
NGT	nasogastric tube
NGU	non-gonococcal urethritis
NHL	non-Hodgkin's lymphoma
NHS	National Health Service
NICE	National Institute for Health and Care Excellence
NIPHS	non-insulinoma pancreatogenous hypoglycaemia syndrome
NIV	non-invasive ventilation
NJ	nasojejunal
NK	natural killer (cell)
NMDA	N-methyl-D-aspartate
NMJ	neuromuscular junction
NMO	neuromyelitis optica
NNRTI	non-nucleoside reverse transciptase inhibitor
NNT	number needed to treat
NO	nitric oxide
NOAC	novel oral anticoagulant
NOVAC	novel anticoagulant
NP	nasopharyngeal
NPH	neutral protamine Hagedorn
NPS	new psychoactive substance
NPSA	National Patient Safety Agency
NPV	negative predictive value
NRT	nicotine replacement therapy
NRTI	nucleoside reverse transcriptase inhibitor
NSAID	non-steroidal anti-inflammatory drug
NSC	National Screening Committee
NSCLC	non-small cell lung cancer
NSIP	non-specific interstitial pneumonia
NSR	normal sinus rhythm
NSTEMI	non-ST-segment elevation myocardial infarction
NSVT	non-sustained ventricular tachycardia

NT	nuchal translucency
nt-BNP	N-terminal brain natriuretic peptide
NTM	non-tuberculous mycobacteria
NTX	cross-linked N-telopeptide
NUV	normocomplementaemic urticarial vasculitis
NVP	nausea and vomiting of pregnancy
NYHA	New York Heart Association
OA	osteoarthritis
OAT	organic anion transporter
OC	obstetric cholestasis
OCT	organic cation transporter
OD	once daily
OGD	oesophagogastroduodenoscopy
OGTT	oral glucose tolerance test
OH	occupational health
OHS	obesity hypoventilation syndrome
OI	opportunistic infection
OMT	optimal medical therapy
ONJ	osteonecrosis of the jaw
OPAT	outpatient parenteral antibiotic therapy
OPG	osteoprotegenerin
OR	Odds ratio
OSA	obstructive sleep apnoea
OSAHS	obstructive sleep apnoea/hypoapnoea syndrome
OTC	ornithine transcarbamylase
PA	postero-anterior
PAC	pulmonary artery catheter
PAH	pulmonary arterial hypertension
PAI	plasminogen activator inhibitor
PALS	Patient Advice and Liaison Service
PAMP	pathogen associated molecular pattern
PAOP	pulmonary artery occlusion pressure
PAP	pulmonary artery pressure
PAPP-A	pregnancy-associated plasma protein-A
PARP	poly-ADP ribose polymerase
PASI	Psoriasis Area and Severity Index
PAVM	pulmonary arteriovenous malformation
PBC	primary biliary cirrhosis
PBF	peripheral blood film
PBG	porphobilinogen
PBP	progressive bulbar palsy
PCA	posterior cerebral artery
PCI	percutaneous coronary intervention
PCOS	polycystic ovarian syndrome
PCP	*Pneumocystis jirovecii* pneumonia (formerly *Pneumocystis carinii* pneumonia)
PCR	polymerase chain reaction
PCSK	proprotein convertase subtilisin/kexin
PCT	porphyria cutanea tarda; proximal convoluted tubule
PCWP	pulmonary capillary wedge pressure
PD	peritoneal dialysis; personality disorder; programmed death
PDA	patent ductus arteriosus
PDE	phosphodiesterase
PDF	probability density function
PE	pulmonary embolus
PEEP	positive-end-expiratory pressure
PEFR	peak expiratory flow rate
PEG	percutaneous endoscopic gastrostomy
PEM	protein-energy malnutrition
PEP	post-exposure prophylaxis
PERC	Pulmonary Embolism Rule out Criteria
PET	positron emission tomography; pre-eclamptic toxaemia
PEU	protein energy undernutrition
PFA	platelet function assay
PFT	pulmonary function test
PG	pyoderma gangrenosum
PGL	primary generalised lymphadenopathy
PH	pulmonary hypertension
PI	protease inhibitor
PICA	posterior inferior cerebellar artery
PICC	peripherally inserted central catheter
PiCCO	Pulse Contour Cardiac Output
PID	pelvic inflammatory disease; primary immunodeficiency
PIH	pregnancy-induced hypertension
PINK	phosphatase and tensin-holding homologue- induced putative kinase
PIP	proximal interphalangeal
PKC	protein kinase C
PIGF	placental growth factor
PLS	primary lateral sclerosis
PMA	progressive muscular atrophy
PMF	probability mass function
PMN	polymorphonuclear
PMNL	polymorphonuclear leukocytes
PO	by mouth
PO_2	partial pressure of oxygen
POEM	Patient-Orientated Eczema Measure; per-oral endoscopic myotomy
PON1	paraoxonase 1
POTS	postural orthostatic tachycardia syndrome
PPAR	peroxisome proliferator activated receptor
PPCI	primary percutaneous coronary intervention
PPCM	peri-partum cardiomyopathy
PPI	proton pump inhibitor
PPM	permanent pacemaker
PPMS	primary progressive multiple sclerosis
PPRF	paramedian pontine reticular formation
PPV	positive predictive value
PR3	proteinase 3
PRCA	pure red cell aplasia
PrEP	pre-exposure prophylaxis
PROMM	proximal myotonic myopathy
PRPP	5-phospho-alpha-d-ribosyl pyrophosphate
PRV	polycythaemia rubra vera
PS	performance status
PSA	prostate-specific antigen

PsA	psoriatic arthritis
PSC	primary sclerosing cholangitis
PSP	progressive supranuclear palsy
PT	prothrombin time
PTC	percutaneous transabdominal cholangiography
PTH	parathyroid hormone
PTHrp	parathyroid-related peptide
PTLD	post-transplant lymphoproliferative disorder
PTU	propylthiouracil
PUD	peptic ulcer disease
PUVA	psoralen plus ultraviolet A
PV	pemphigus vulgaris
PVE	prosthetic valve infective endocarditis
PWS	Prader–Willi syndrome
QDS	four times a day
QFT-GIT	QuantiFERON-TB Gold In-Tube
QoL	quality of life
QPPV	qualified person for pharmacovigilance
R&D	research and development
RA	rheumatoid arthritis; right atrium
RAI	radioactive iodine therapy
RAPD	relative afferent pupillary defect
RAS	renal artery stenosis; renin-angiotensin system
RAST	radioallergosorbent assay
RB	retinoblastoma
RBBB	right bundle branch block
RBC	red blood cell
RCAD	renal cysts and diabetes syndrome
RCOG	Royal College of Obstetricians and Gynaecologists
RCT	randomised controlled trial
RDT	rapid diagnostic test
ReA	reactive arthritis
REC	Research Ethics Committee
REM-BD	rapid eye movement (sleep) behavioural disorder
RET	re-arranged during transfection
RF	rheumatoid factor
RFA	radiofrequency ablation
RFCA	radiofrequency catheter ablation
RHC	right heart catheterisation
RIF	resistance to rifampicin
RIG	radiologically inserted gastrostomy
RNA	ribonucleic acid
ROC	receiver-operator characteristic
RP	relapsing polychrondritis; retinitis pigmentosa
RPF	renal plasma flow
RPR	rapid plasma regain
RR	respiratory rate
RRMS	relapsing-remitting multiple sclerosis
rRNA	ribosomal RNA
RRT	renal replacement therapy
RSV	respiratory syncytial virus
RTA	renal tubular acidosis
RUQ	right upper quadrant
RV	right ventricle
RVD	right ventricle dysfunction
RVEDP	right ventricular end-diastolic pressure
RVH	right ventricular hypertrophy
RVO	retinal vein occlusion
SA	sinoatrial
SAAG	serum albumin ascites gradient
SADQ	Severity of Alcohol Dependence Questionnaire
SAE	serious adverse event
SAH	subarachnoid haemorrhage
SARA	sexually acquired reactive arthritis
SARS	severe adult respiratory syndrome
SASSAD	six area six sign atopic dermatitis
SBP	spontaneous bacterial peritonitis
SBRT	stereotactic body radiotherapy
SC	subcutaneous
SCA	spinocerebellar ataxia
SCD	sickle cell disease; sudden cardiac death
SCF	stem cell factor
SCID	severe combined immunodeficiency
SCLC	small cell lung carcinoma
SCRA	synthetic cannabinoid receptor agonist
SCUF	slow continuous ultrafiltration
$ScvO_2$	central venous oxygen saturation
SD	standard deviation
SEGA	subependymal giant cell astrocytoma
SEN	subependymal nodule
SERM	selective oestrogen receptor modulator
SF	synovial fluid
sFlt1	fms-like tyrosine kinase 1
SHGB	sex hormone-binding globulin
SHO	senior house officer
SHOT	serious hazards of transfusion
SIADH	syndrome of inappropriate anti-diuretic hormone
SIBO	small intestinal bacterial overgrowth
SIJ	sacroiliac joint
SIRS	systemic inflammatory response syndrome
SJS	Stevens–Johnson syndrome
SLC	solute carrier
SLE	systemic lupus erythematosus
SLED	slow low-efficiency dialysis
SNMG	seronegative myasthenia gravis
SNRI	serotonin noradrenaline reuptake inhibitor
SOB	shortness of breath
SOD1	superoxide dismutase
SOFA	Sequential Organ Failure Score
SpA	spondyloarthropathy
SPECT	single-photon emission computed tomography
SPMS	secondary progressive multiple sclerosis
SpO_2	peripheral capillary oxygen saturation
SR	scavenger receptor
SSc	systemic sclerosis
SSRI	selective serotonin reuptake inhibitor
SSTI	skin and soft tissue infection

STEMI ST-segment elevation myocardial infarction
STI sexually transmitted disease
STIR short tau inversion recovery
SUDEP sudden unexpected death in epilepsy
SUSAR suspected unexpected serious adverse reaction
SV stroke volume
SVC superior vena cava
SVCO superior vena cava obstruction
SVD structural valve deterioration
SVR systemic vascular resistance
SVT supraventricular tachycardia
T thymine
T3 tri-iodothyronine
T4 thyroxine
TA Takayasu arteritis
TAA tumour-associated antigen
TACE transarterial chemoembolisation of tumour
TAL thick ascending loop of Henle
TAVI transcatheter aortic valve implantation
TB tuberculosis
TBG thyroid-binding globulin
Tc core temperature
TC total cholesterol
TCA tricyclic antidepressant
TCR T cell receptor
TDS three times daily
TED thromboembolic disease; dysthryoid eye disease
TEN toxic epidermal necrolysis
TENS transcutaneous electrical nerve stimulation
TFPI tissue factor pathway inhibitor
TFT thyroid function test
TG triglyceride
TGF tumour growth factor
THC Δ^9-tetrahydrocannabinol
TIA transient ischaemic attack
TIN tubulointerstitial nephritis
TINU tubulointerstitial nephritis and uveitis
TIPSS trans-jugular intrahepatic portosystemic shunt
TJ trans-jugular
TKI tyrosine kinase inhibitor
TLC total lung capacity
TLCO transfer factor for carbon monoxide
T-LOC transient loss of consciousness
TLR toll-like receptor
TLS tumour lysis syndrome
TNF tumour necrosis factor
TNM tumour, node, metastases
TOE transoesophageal echocardiogram
tPA tissue plasminogen activator
TPN total parenteral nutrition
TPO thyroid peroxidase
TPPA *Treponema pallidum* particle agglutination assay
TPR total peripheral resistance
TRH thyrotropin-releasing hormone
tRNA transfer RNA
TSA tumour-specific antigen
TSC tuberous sclerosis complex
tsDMARDs targeted synthetic DMARDs
TSH thyroid-stimulating hormone
TSP thrombospondin
TST tuberculin skin test
TTE transthoarcic echocardiogram
tTG anti-tissue transglutaminase
TTKG trans-tubular potassium gradient
TTP thrombotic thrombocytopenic purpura
TV *Trichomonas vaginalis*
U uracil
U&E urea & electrolytes
UC ulcerative colitis
UFH unfractionated heparin
UGI upper gastrointestinal
UICC Union for International Cancer Control
UIP usual interstitial pneumonitis
ULN upper limit of normal
UN United Nations
UPDRS unified PD rating scale
US ultrasound
UTI urinary tract infection
UV ultraviolet
VA alveolar volume
VAD ventricular assist device
VATS video-assisted thoracoscopic surgery
VCE video capsule endoscopy
VEGF vascular endothelial growth factor
VEP visual-evoked potential
VER visual-evoked response
VF ventricular fibrillation
VFA vertebral fracture analysis
VFR visiting friends and relatives
VGKC voltage-gated potassium channel
VHD valvular heart disease
VHF viral haemorrhagic fever
VL viral load
VLDL very low density lipoprotein
V/Q ventilation/perfusion
VRE vancomycin-resistant *Enterococci*
VRet venous return
VSD ventricular septal defect
VT ventricular tachycardia
VTE venous thromboembolism
vWF von Willebrand factor
VZIG varicella zoster immunoglobulin
VZV varicella zoster virus
WBCT whole-blood clotting test
WCC white cell count
WHO World Health Organization
WPW Wolff–Parkinson–White
XDR extensively drug resistant
XLD X-linked dominant
XP xeroderma pigmentosum
ZES Zollinger–Ellison syndrome
ZN Ziehl–Neelsen

Chapter 1 **Metabolic Medicine**

Rosemary E. J. Clarke, Claire L. Meek and Anthony S. Wierzbicki

Bone and calcium metabolism

Calcium: role and regulation

Role of calcium

In the body, calcium is required for:

- The structural role of the skeleton.
- Nervous transmission.
- Muscle contraction.
- Intracellular signalling in neuroendocrine secretion, cell metabolism and growth.

Physiology and regulation

Calcium is a divalent cation. 98% of calcium in the body is in bone:

- A small proportion of calcium in bone can be readily released into the extracellular fluid depending on metabolic circumstances and the hormonal milieu.

<1% total body calcium is present in the blood:

- half is free (ionised);
- the remainder is protein-bound (40%), mainly to albumin, or complexed to other ions (10%) such as lactate, bicarbonate and phosphates.

In the kidney, most calcium is passively reabsorbed. Some calcium is actively reabsorbed under the influence of parathyroid hormone (PTH), activated vitamin D, calcitonin, androgens and oestrogens.

In the gut, calcium is absorbed and secreted. Around 16 mmol/day is secreted in digestive juices and 3 mmol/day is excreted in faeces. Calcium is mostly absorbed in the duodenum and upper jejunum, and is enhanced by a high oral intake of calcium and an abundance of activated vitamin D.

Parathyroid hormone and 1,25(OH)$_2$ vitamin D (activated vitamin D)

The main hormones involved in calcium homeostasis are PTH and 1,25(OH)$_2$ vitamin D (Figure 1.1).

PTH is made in the parathyroid glands and is produced and released in response to a low extracellular calcium concentration or a high extracellular phosphate concentration. High calcium levels inhibit PTH secretion, and promote its metabolism and excretion. Hypomagnesaemia reduces PTH synthesis.

Actions of PTH include:

- Direct effect on bone:
  - PTH can stimulate bone resorption or bone formation depending on its concentration. Prolonged exposure to high concentrations of PTH favours bone resorption. 'High turnover' bone disease causes bone pain and increased fracture risk (osteitis fibrosa cystica). Adynamic or 'low turnover' bone disease is associated with low or normal PTH levels, which may be a result of treatment, and decreased bone resorption and formation.
- Direct effect on kidney:
  - increases the 1α-hydroxylation of vitamin D to create more activated $1,25(OH)_2$ vitamin D;
  - increases reabsorption of calcium in the distal convoluted tubule;
  - promotes excretion of phosphate by reducing reabsorption in the proximal tubule.
- Indirect effect on the gut by increasing the amount of active vitamin D.
- High PTH levels may also cause left ventricular hypertrophy, cardiac fibrosis and peripheral neuropathy.
- In chronic kidney disease, hyperparathyroidism, along with the poor control of serum phosphate and calcium-phosphate product, are associated with increased cardiovascular disease risk and vascular calcification. They are also risk factors for development of calcific uraemic arteriolopathy (calciphylaxis), a painful ulcerating skin condition which carries a high mortality.

$1,25(OH)_2$ vitamin D is made from vitamin D (D_2 [ergocalciferol] or D_3 [cholecalciferol] forms), which is made in the skin following exposure to UV-B sunlight (D_3 only) or obtained through the diet or supplementation (D_2 or D_3). Vitamin D is relatively inactive. Both vitamin D_2 and D_3 bind blood vitamin D-binding proteins and undergo 25-hydroxylation in the liver and 1α-hydroxylation in the kidney to produce the activated form $1,25(OH)_2$ vitamin D.

The rate-limiting step is the 1α-hydroxylation by the enzyme 1α-hydroxylase, the activity of which is subject to multiple homeostatic controls, and is:

- increased by PTH and hypophosphataemia, and indirectly by hypocalcaemia;
- decreased by hypercalcaemia, hyperphosphataemia, high levels of $1,25(OH)_2$ and fibroblast growth factor (FGF)-23. Vitamin D therefore reduces its own production via negative feedback.

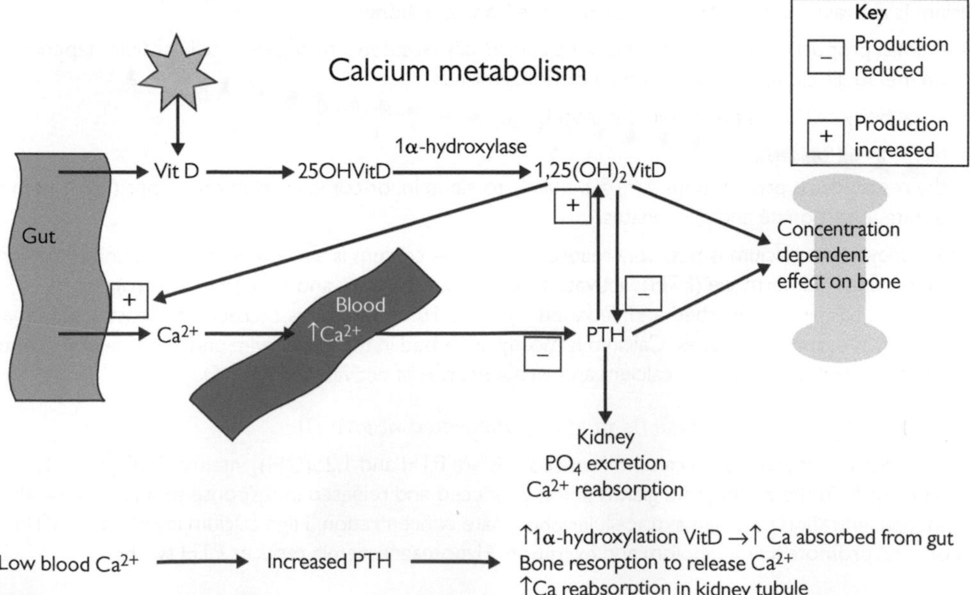

Figure 1.1 Flowchart showing summary of relationships between calcium, PTH and vitamin D.

25-OH vitamin D represents the total body vitamin D store.

1,25$(OH)_2$ vitamin D has direct action on:

- *Gut*: multiple actions on different proteins serve to increase absorption of calcium and phosphate.
- *Kidney*: inhibits its own synthesis by reduced 1α-hydroxylase activity.
- *Parathyroid glands*: inhibits PTH synthesis.
- *Bone*: at high concentrations, activated vitamin D increases osteoclastic activity, promoting bone resorption.

Hypercalcaemia

Measured calcium levels are corrected for albumin levels as follows:

Adjusted calcium concentration = Measured calcium + [(0.02 × (42-albumin level in g/L)].

A low adjusted calcium may be found in patients with severe hypoalbuminaemia, while true ionised calcium levels are normal. This reflects a non-linear relationship once the albumin levels fall below ~20–25 g/L (e.g. in patients with chronic liver disease, nephrotic syndrome, cardiac failure and malnutrition).

Hypercalcaemia (>2.6 mmol/L) is common.

- Adjusted calcium concentration 2.6–3.0 mmol/L, often asymptomatic.
- Adjusted calcium concentration >3.0 mmol/L, usually causes symptoms, including malaise, polyuria, polydipsia, nocturia, renal calculi, bone pain (due to osteitis fibrosa cystica), abdominal pain, nausea, constipation, dehydration, low mood and confusion.
- Adjusted calcium concentration >3.8 mmol/L carries risk of arrhythmias.

Causes

1. Primary and tertiary hyperparathyroidism
   - Primary hyperparathyroidism:
     - Increased PTH due to parathyroid adenoma(s) or hyperplasia.
     - 80% due to a benign solitary adenoma.
     - Multiple endocrine neoplasia (MEN) types 1 and 2A account for 2% of all cases. Patients presenting with hyperparathyroidism aged <40 years should, therefore, be screened for MEN (➲ see Multiple endocrine neoplasia, p. 700).
     - Characterised by high corrected serum and urine calcium, and low serum phosphate.
   - Tertiary hyperparathyroidism: autonomous secretion with high PTH despite hypercalcaemia.
   - (Secondary hyperparathyroidism does not cause hypercalcaemia but is characterised by increased PTH in response to hypocalcaemia with low active vitamin D levels because of renal disease or dietary deficiency.)
2. Malignancy
   - Hypercalcemia occurs in up to 30% of all cancers, with lung cancer, breast cancer and myeloma being the most frequent causes.
   - Two main mechanisms exist:
     - Cytokine release, which activates osteoclasts, e.g. osteolytic bony metastases in advanced breast carcinoma and haematological malignancies such as multiple myeloma.
     - Production of parathyroid-related peptide (PTHrp) or calcitriol by the tumour, e.g. squamous cell lung cancer, breast cancer, renal cell carcinoma.
3. Thyrotoxicosis: excessive production of thyroid hormones causes bone resorption, releasing calcium into the extracellular fluid.
4. Hypoadrenalism: glucocorticoid deficiency stimulates hypercalcaemia; although the mechanism is not fully known, it is probably due to reduced renal calcium excretion and increased calcium resorption from bone.
5. Thiazide diuretics: reduce calcium excretion from the kidneys.
6. Immobility: causes increased bone resorption.

7. Iatrogenic: usually due to high doses of calcium salts or excessive amounts of vitamin D.
8. Familial hypocalciuric hypercalcaemia: A rare autosomal dominant condition resulting from inactivating mutations affecting the calcium-sensing receptor gene (confirmed with genetic testing), leading to calcium hyposensitivity. It is characterised by low urinary calcium (<200 mg/day) and a urine calcium:creatinine ratio <0.01.
9. Sarcoidosis: involves extra-renal production of activated vitamin D.
10. Milk–alkali syndrome: excessive ingestion of calcium and alkali salts, for example, to control dyspepsia.

Investigation

- History: exclude iatrogenic causes and immobility; ask about symptoms of malignancy.
- Examination: look for signs of malignancy and investigate as appropriate.
- Blood tests for urea and electrolytes (to exclude renal impairment), calcium, PTH, vitamin D, phosphate and magnesium.
- Urine test for calcium (ideally a 24-hour collection) and calcium:creatinine ratio to exclude familial hypocalciuric hypercalcaemia.
- X-rays: look for characteristic sub-periosteal resorption of distal phalanges, tapering of distal clavicles, 'salt and pepper pot' skull lucencies and brown tumours of long bones.
- If PTH levels are appropriately suppressed in the face of a normal PTH axis, check thyroid stimulating hormone (TSH), protein electrophoresis, urinary Bence–Jones protein and consider a Synacthen® (tetracosactide) test.
- Parathyroid technetium (^{99m}Tc) sestamibi scan to identify parathyroid adenomas in primary hyperparathyroidism.
- If all aforementioned tests are negative, investigate further for malignancy.
- Dual energy X-ray absorptiometry (DEXA) scan for evidence of resulting osteoporosis.

Treatment

- Mild asymptomatic hypercalcaemia does not always need treatment. Affected patients should be monitored at intervals and advised to maintain hydration to reduce the risk of renal stones.
- Moderate or severe degrees of hypercalcaemia are often associated with significant dehydration. Prompt fluid resuscitation can cause a marked improvement in serum calcium concentration and should be a priority in all patients. Once fluid resuscitation is underway, a loop diuretic such as furosemide can be given to promote calcium excretion.
- Primary hyperparathyroidism has a long-term effect of osteoporosis and renal calculi. Surgical resection of the parathyroid lesion is indicated if an adenoma is identified in primary or tertiary hyperparathyroidism. Post-operative 'hungry bone syndrome' with prolonged hypocalcaemia is common. Watchful waiting may be adopted in an asymptomatic patient.
- Cinacalcet is a calcium sensing receptor agonist, which acts on the parathyroid cells, where it mimics the effect of hypercalcaemia, suppressing PTH synthesis and secretion. It may be prescribed in those with tertiary hyperparathyroidism due to chronic kidney disease, primary hyperparathyroidism unsuitable for surgery and hypercalcaemia from malignancy not responding to treatment. The combined use of vitamin D and calcimimetics has reduced the need for parathyroidectomy in the management of renal bone disease.
- Glucocorticoids can be useful in hypercalcaemia caused by malignancy, sarcoidosis and vitamin D toxicity.
- Bisphosphonates inhibit osteoclastic activity and prevent calcium release from bone. Intravenous pamidronate is commonly used in emergency situations. Patients with chronic severe hypercalcaemia may benefit from a bisphosphonate with a longer half-life (e.g. risedronate or zoledronic acid).

Further reading

1. Minisola S, Pepe J, Piemonte S, Cipriani C, 2015. The diagnosis and management of hypercalcaemia. *BMJ* 2015;350:2723.

Hypocalcaemia

Hypocalcaemia (<2.15 mmol/L) is common.

- Adjusted calcium concentration 2.0–2.15 mmol/L is often asymptomatic.
- Adjusted calcium concentration <2.0 mmol/L may cause symptoms of neuromuscular excitability, tetany and paraesthesiae of the extremities and perioral area, along with cramps and tetany. Trousseau and Chvostek signs may be demonstrated (Box 1.1) and an electrocardiogram (ECG) may show a prolonged QT_c interval.
- Adjusted calcium concentration <1.8 mmol/L may result in arrhythmias or seizures, especially with a rapid fall in serum calcium.

Box 1.1 Trousseau and Chvostek signs

Trousseau sign

A blood pressure cuff is placed around the arm, inflated to a pressure greater than the systolic blood pressure and held in place for 3 minutes. This occludes the brachial artery. In the absence of blood flow, the patient's hypocalcaemia and subsequent neuromuscular irritability induces spasm of the muscles of the hand and forearm. The wrist and metacarpophalangeal joints flex, the proximal and distal interphalanageal joints extend, and the fingers adduct.

Chvostek sign

On tapping the facial nerve at the angle of the jaw, the facial muscles on the same side of the face contract momentarily (typically a twitch of the nose or lips).

Causes

L Lysis syndromes, including rhabdomyolysis and tumour lysis syndrome, with widespread release of phosphate from damaged cells binding to calcium, lowering serum levels.

O Osteoblastic metastases with calcium uptake, e.g. from prostate, breast or bladder cancers.

W With infusion of citrate-containing blood products that can cause pronounced hypocalcaemia due to citrate complexing with calcium.

C Congenital disorders, e.g. DiGeorge syndrome, caused by the deletion of a small segment of chromosome 22.

A Acute pancreatitis where low calcium is a marker of severity.

L Longstanding inadequate dietary calcium or poor absorption of dietary calcium due to gut disorders.

C Chronic kidney disease with reduced renal hydroxylation of vitamin D leading to a lack of active $1,25(OH)_2$ vitamin D. Reduced renal phosphate excretion and hyperphosphataemia, leads to a further inhibition of 1α-hydroxylation of vitamin D.

I Iatrogenic causes including prolonged use of loop diuretics or bisphosphonates.

U Underactivity of PTH and vitamin D axes including:

- Hypoparathyroidism: associated with parathyroid damage, surgical removal (e.g. during thyroidectomy), autoimmune polyglandular endocrine syndromes and various mutations affecting the calcium sensing receptor.
- Pseudohypoparathyroidism (Albright's hereditary osteodystrophy): hypocalcaemia with measureable PTH, caused by end-organ resistance to the effects of PTH due to mutations.
- Vitamin D deficiency: causes rickets in children and osteomalacia in adults.
  - May be asymptomatic or cause myalgia, bone pain, proximal myopathy.
  - Causes include inadequate sunlight exposure or poor dietary intake, renal/liver disease, drugs (anticonvulsants, rifampicin), pregnancy/prolonged breast feeding, rare hereditary deficiency of 1α-hydroxylase or vitamin D receptor mutations.

M Magnesium deficiency causing impaired PTH secretion and promoting resistance to the actions of PTH.

Investigation

- History: ask about chronic kidney disease, longstanding hypertension, diabetes mellitus, malabsorption and family history.
- Review medication.
- Examination: look for signs of malignancy, malabsorption or gut disorders. Check for features of chronic kidney disease or Albright's hereditary osteodystrophy (short stature, characteristically shortened fourth and fifth metacarpals, rounded facies and often mild mental retardation).
- Blood tests: for calcium, PTH, vitamin D, phosphate, magnesium, urea and creatinine, liver function tests (LFTs), and creatine kinase (may be raised), ideally before treatment commences.
  - PTH levels should be increased if the PTH axis is working normally, e.g. when the primary defect is malabsorption, vitamin D deficiency or kidney disease.
  - If PTH levels are low or inappropriately normal, primary hypoparathyroidism should be considered.
- Urinary calcium and PO_4 excretion.
- Imaging: growth plate abnormalities in children, pseudofractures (Looser's zones), reduced bone mineral density (BMD) on DEXA.

Treatment

- Treat the underlying cause of hypocalcaemia where possible. Providing calcium supplementation with an uncorrected deficiency of magnesium and vitamin D will provide only short-term benefit.
- Mild hypocalcaemia does not always need treatment. Moderate hypocalcaemia (≤2.0 mmol/L) or mild symptomatic hypocalcaemia can be treated with oral calcium salts. More significant degrees of hypocalcaemia (<1.8 mmol/L) should be considered for intravenous calcium gluconate correction with ECG monitoring. Once serum calcium levels have normalised, patients may be switched to oral calcium and activated vitamin D.
- Vitamin D replacement:
  - <30 nmol/L: load with colecalciferol to provide a total of 300,000 IU vitamin D over 6–8 weeks followed by daily supplements.
  - 30–50 nmol/L: 1000–2000 IU colecalciferol daily. Additional calcium only required with malabsorption/inadequate oral intake. Plant-derived ergocalciferol can be used intramuscularly (IM) or by mouth (PO).
  - Active vitamin D most commonly with 1α-hydroxylated vitamin D, alfacalcidol, is used in chronic kidney disease. This corrects hypocalcaemia, and suppresses PTH synthesis and secretion.
  - Phosphate and calcitriol replacement in hypophosphataemic rickets.
  - Tumour resection in oncogenic osteomalacia.

Further reading

1. Society for Endocrinology Clinical Committee, 2013. Acute hypocalcaemia. https://www.endocrinology.org/clinical-practice/clinical-guidelines/

Magnesium and phosphate: role, regulation and pathology

Magnesium

Physiology and regulation

- Total body store is ~1 mol:
  - half is in bone; the remainder is intracellular (1–3 mmol/L).
- Plasma magnesium:
  - <1% total store; concentration 0.7–1.0 mmol/L.
  - 30% protein-bound, 15% anion-bound and the remainder ionic.
- Magnesium can be mobilised from bone; therefore, plasma levels do not reflect total body stores.

Magnesium is:

- an enzyme cofactor;
- bound to cyclic nucleotides made by G-protein receptors;
- involved in neuromuscular transmission.

To interpret magnesium physiology, consider calcium, phosphate, bicarbonate, vitamin D, PTH and creatinine levels.

Hypermagnesaemia

Hypermagnesaemia is rare.

- Levels >2 mmol/L result in decreased neuromuscular transmission and loss of deep tendon reflexes.
- Levels >4 mmol/L result in respiratory depression, hypotension, lethargy and reduced consciousness.

Causes include:

- Administration of oral (antacids), rectal (enemas) or intravenous magnesium, especially if renal function is impaired.
- Chronic kidney disease.
- Rhabdomyolysis.
- Familial hypocalciuric hypercalcaemia.

Hypomagnesaemia

Hypomagnesaemia is common and caused by:

- Enteric loss:
  - diarrhoea, fistulae, nasogastric suction, malabsorption.
- Renal loss:
  - exacerbated by hyperglycaemia, uraemia, hypercalcaemia, alcohol and loop diuretics;
  - glomerulonephritis, pyelonephritis, renal tubular acidosis.
- Metabolic acidosis.
- Low phosphate levels.

Hypomagnesaemia can lead to paraesthesiae, tetany, seizures and arrhythmias.

Phosphate

Physiology and regulation

Total body phosphate is ~20 mol, present as organic (e.g. phosphate esters, phospholipids) or inorganic forms (HPO_4^- and $H_2PO_4^-$). In the blood, 10% is protein-bound, 35% is cation-bound and the remainder is ionic.

Roles of phosphate

- Structural in bone as hydroxyapatite.
- A component of phospholipids, nucleotides, ATP (adenosine triphosphate) and creatine phosphate.
- A cofactor and intracellular signal, e.g. cAMP (cyclic adenosine monophosphate) and NADP (nicotinamide adenine dinucleotide phosphate).
- Involved in acid-base buffering.

To interpret phosphate physiology, consider calcium, magnesium, bicarbonate, vitamin D, PTH and creatinine levels.

Hyperphosphataemia

Hyperphosphataemia is common and may provoke symptomatic hypocalcaemia. Chronic hyperphosphataemia causes secondary hyperparathyroidism and soft tissue calcification. It can be caused by:

- Excessive consumption of phosphate.
- Impaired renal function.

- Cell lysis, e.g. rhabdomyolysis, haemolysis, cytotoxic therapy.
- Increased renal reabsorption of phosphate, e.g. hypoparathyroidism, acromegaly.
- Metabolic acidosis involving a phosphate shift.

Treating hyperphosphataemia involves identifying the cause. Reducing serum phosphate in chronic kidney disease includes dietary restriction to minimise intake of dairy products, eggs and certain cereals, and use of phosphate binders to reduce absorption of dietary phosphate. Phosphate binders are either calcium based (and therefore risk causing hypercalcaemia when co-administered with vitamin D) or non-calcium based. Non-calcium-based phosphate binders include the inorganic resin sevelamer and lanthanum carbonate; aluminium-based phosphate binders are now seldom used owing to concerns regarding aluminium toxicity.

Hypophosphataemia

Hypophosphataemia is common.

- Levels ~0.5 mmol/L are often asymptomatic.
- Levels <0.3 mmol/L cause muscle weakness, hypoxia, coma and damage to cells (haemolysis or rhabdomyolysis).

Causes include:

- Movement of phosphate into cells, due to the action of insulin.
- Reduced renal resorption of phosphate (e.g. hyperparathyroidism).
- Limited enteric uptake or increased loss of phosphate (e.g. phosphate binders, diarrhoea, malabsorption and vitamin D deficiency).
- Acidosis causing intracellular phosphate depletion.
- Fanconi syndrome (of inadequate reabsorption in the proximal renal tubules).
- Hereditary or acquired disorders of the *FGF23*/phosphate-regulating gene with homologies to endopeptidases on the X chromosome (PHEX)/matrix extracellular phosphoglycoprotein (MEPE) protein cascade that regulates systemic phosphate homeostasis and mineralisation, e.g. autosomal dominant hypophosphataemic rickets, X-linked hypophosphatemia and tumour-induced/oncogenic osteomalacia.

Further reading

1. Kidney Disease: Improving Global Outcomes (KDIGO) CKD-MBD Work Group. KDIGO clinical practice guideline for the diagnosis, evaluation, prevention, and treatment of Chronic Kidney Disease-Mineral and Bone Disorder (CKD-MBD). *Kidney Int Suppl*. 2009 Aug;(113):S1–130. https://kdigo.org/guidelines/ckd-mbd/
2. Ketteler M, Block GA, Evenepoel P, et al. Diagnosis, Evaluation, Prevention, and Treatment of Chronic Kidney Disease-Mineral and Bone Disorder: Synopsis of the Kidney Disease: Improving Global Outcomes 2017 Clinical Practice Guideline Update. *Ann Intern Med*. 2018 Mar;168(6):422–430.

Nutrition and total parenteral nutrition

Carbohydrate metabolism

Carbohydrate metabolism includes processes for metabolising glucose and producing lactate (glycolysis), synthesising glucose (gluconeogenesis), the pathway for metabolism of 2-carbon remnants (acetyl-CoA) derived from glucose or fatty acids (Krebs' cycle), production of energy storing ATP through oxidative phosphorylation, and pathways for synthesis of 5-carbon sugars for DNA metabolism (pentose phosphate pathway) (Figure 1.2).

Glycolysis

Glycolysis ('splitting glucose') involves the metabolism and splitting of glucose into two 3-carbon sugars, which are converted to pyruvate. In the presence of oxygen, the pyruvate is metabolised to acetyl-CoA for metabolism in the Krebs' cycle with production of ATP in the electron transport chain (ETC). In the

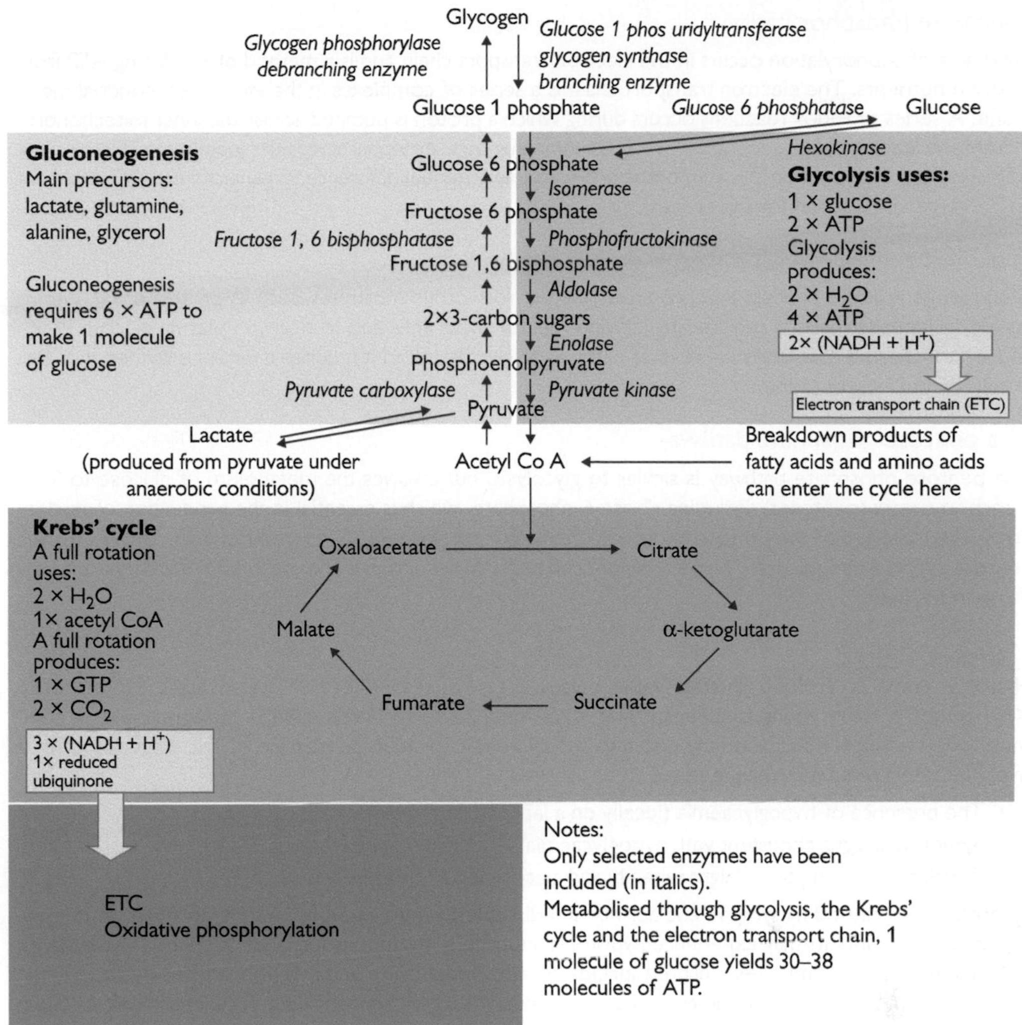

Figure 1.2 Key steps in carbohydrate metabolism: glycolysis, gluconeogenesis, Krebs' cycle, oxidative phosphorylation.

absence of oxygen, pyruvate is converted to lactate with a smaller net yield of ATP. Glycolysis takes place in the cytoplasm of cells, particularly in the liver. Many of the reactions of glycolysis occur spontaneously. The pathway is regulated at three main points by three enzymes: hexokinase, phosphofructokinase and pyruvate kinase. Glycolysis will proceed when cellular conditions favour it, i.e. when ATP is needed, precursors for biological processes are needed or when plasma glucose level is high. When the plasma glucose level is low, conditions favour gluconeogenesis instead (➲ see Gluconeogenesis, p. 10).

The Krebs' cycle

The Krebs' cycle is required for further processing of acetyl-CoA produced following glycolysis. The Krebs' cycle is also an important step in fat and protein metabolism. When food is scarce, fatty acids produced from beta-oxidation and certain amino acids can enter the cycle and be used to fuel oxidative phosphorylation. Thus, the Krebs' cycle facilitates energy production from carbohydrates, proteins and fats, and allows the interconversion of biological fuel substrates.

Oxidative phosphorylation

Oxidative phosphorylation occurs in the electron transport chain and is a method of producing ATP from oxidised nutrients. The electron transport chain is a series of complexes in the inner mitochondrial membrane. A series of redox reactions occurs during which a proton is pumped across the inner mitochondrial membrane leading to the generation of a gradient in electrical potential across the membrane. The enzyme ATP synthase is located on this membrane and uses this potential difference to generate new molecules of ATP. Oxygen is required for this process.

Gluconeogenesis

Gluconeogenesis is a process that produces glucose from other substrates, such as protein or fat. During fasting, gluconeogenesis is required to provide fuel for brain cells and to maintain plasma glucose levels. Gluconeogenesis is essentially the reverse pathway to glycolysis, but it requires different enzymes. It occurs in cells of the liver or kidney.

The pentose phosphate pathway

The pentose phosphate pathway is similar to glycolysis, but involves the metabolism of glucose to form 5-carbon sugars (pentoses), including ribose-6-phosphate, which is essential in the production of nucleotides. The main aim of the pentose phosphate pathway is to create NADPH (reduced form of NADP) and pentose sugars from glucose. The pentose phosphate pathway occurs in the cytoplasm of cells, particularly those in the liver.

Hypoglycaemia

Hypoglycaemia is a blood glucose value below a typical fasting level: <3.5 mmol/L for an adult, <2.6 mmol/L for a young child/infant and <2.2 mmol/L for a neonate. Mild hypoglycaemia is common, often asymptomatic and may not always require investigation or treatment. The diagnosis of true hypoglycaemia requires Whipple's triad to be satisfied:

- The presence of hypoglycaemia (ideally on a laboratory sample).
- Symptoms/signs consistent with hypoglycaemia.
- Resolution of symptoms/signs when blood glucose level normalises.

Symptoms are caused by sympathetic activity and disrupted central nervous system function due to inadequate glucose. Infants may experience hypotonia, jitteriness, seizures, poor feeding, apnoea and lethargy. Symptoms in adults and older children include tremor, sweating, nausea, light-headedness, hunger and disorientation. Severe hypoglycaemia can cause confusion, aggressive behaviour, focal neurological deficits and reduced consciousness.

Causes

1. Drug-treated diabetes mellitus is the most common cause, by insulin or oral hypoglycaemic drugs, particularly sulfonylureas.
   - There is a higher risk in type 1 diabetes due to hypoglycaemia unawareness and blunted glucagon response.
2. Variation of normal:
   - Mild hypoglycaemia is common during fasting, pregnancy and minor illness.
3. Non-diabetic drugs, e.g. quinine, indometacin.
4. Alcohol:
   - Inhibits gluconeogenesis; glycogen stores are often low.
5. Hepatic failure:
   - Impaired gluconeogenesis and glycogen storage.
6. Critical illness:
   - Often associated with abnormalities of glucose homeostasis.
7. Hormone deficiency, e.g. hypoadrenalism, growth hormone deficiency, glucagon deficiency, hypothyroidism.

8. Malignancy:
   - Some tumours use copious amounts of glucose and may produce insulin-like growth factor-2 (IGF-2) causing hypoglycaemia.
9. Insulinoma:
   - Excessive or inappropriate release of insulin from cells in the pancreas or elsewhere.
10. Non-insulinoma pancreatogenous hypoglycaemia syndrome (NIPHS):
    - Hypertrophy and new formation of pancreatic islets cause increased insulin production and typically post-prandial hypoglycaemia.
11. Bariatric surgery:
    - Altered gut physiology following bariatric surgery causes similar pathological changes to NIPHS.
12. Neonatal hypoglycaemia:
    - Particularly with prematurity, poor feeding or with mothers with diabetes, gestational diabetes or eclampsia.
13. Inherited metabolic disorders (IMDs) affecting enzymes involved in glucose and glycogen metabolism (➲ See Glucose and glycogen metabolism disorders, p. 30 and Figure 1.2).

Treatment

- Short-term treatments that aim to restore normal plasma glucose concentration:
  - oral glucose;
  - intravenous glucose;
  - IM glucagon injection.
- Long-term diagnosis-specific treatments that may prevent recurrence.

For an algorithm for differential diagnosis of acute hypoglycaemia, see Figure 1.3.

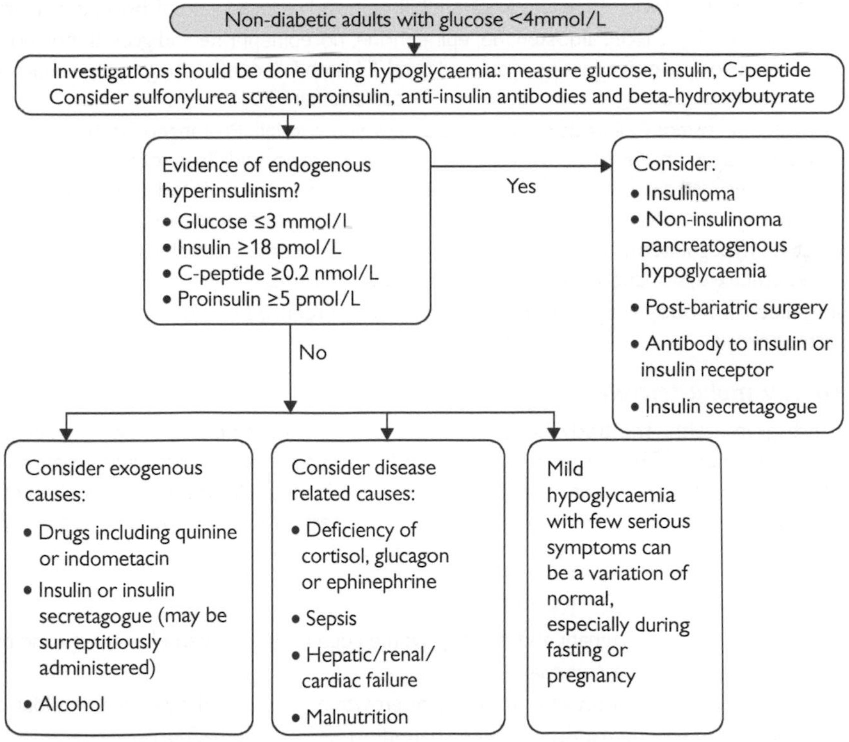

Figure 1.3 Algorithm for differential diagnosis of acute hypoglycaemia.

Starvation

Starvation involves a complete lack of nutrients. Causes include:

- Prolonged fasting.
- Anorexia nervosa and other eating disorders.
- Famine.

Metabolic priorities in starvation are:

- To maintain a fuel supply to the brain using glucose and ketoacids.
- To maintain a fuel supply to maintain essential body processes, such as the Na^+–K^+-ATPase pump required for cell health and membrane stability, and voluntary procedures such as movement.

Once calorie intake stops, glucose is released into the blood from the depletion of liver glycogen (this lasts ≤18 hours) and gluconeogenesis using fat or protein as a substrate. This is stimulated by falling levels of insulin and rising glucagon. Lipolysis of adipose tissue produces fatty acids. Hepatic processing of amino acids produces ketoacids (acetoacetic acid and beta-hydroxybutyric acid), which contribute further to a metabolic acidosis. The brain can use glucose or ketoacids as fuel. The main fuels used by muscle are fatty acids and ketoacids. The preferential preservation of body protein stores is key to preserving health during prolonged starvation.

Effects upon body systems:

- Renal: reduced glomerular filtration rate (GFR) with increased aldosterone secretion causes altered excretion of many solutes and electrolytes. There is increased urinary excretion of potassium, calcium, magnesium and phosphate. There is increased excretion of nitrogenous waste, but urate excretion is reduced due to competition with other solutes.
- Hepatic: reduced hepatic blood supply can result in areas of focal necrosis and transaminase release. Bile excretion is reduced with increases in serum bilirubin and reduced rate of bilirubin conjugation.
- Endocrine: increased glucagon, aldosterone, epinephrine, norepinephrine and growth hormone occur with reduced insulin production. Free and total T3 both fall, contributing to the reduced metabolic rate. With prolonged starvation, free T4 can also fall.
- Cardiovascular: an osmotic diuresis causes circulating volume to fall. Prolonged fasting causes reduced heart rate and reduced stroke volume. Release of amino acids from cardiac muscle contributes to reduced cardiac muscle bulk, electrical excitability and reduced contractility. Arrhythmias are common, especially with concomitant electrolyte disturbance.
- Reproductive: hypogonadotrophic hypogonadism occurs in males and females causing subfertility, impotence, erectile dysfunction, amenorrhoea and ovarian failure.
- Musculoskeletal: low body weight, vitamin D deficiency and reduced sex hormone production can cause osteoporosis.

Protein-energy malnutrition

In order to preserve health, the body needs adequate energy and protein to meet its requirements. Protein-energy malnutrition (PEM) or protein-energy undernutrition (PEU) occurs when a patient's intake is insufficient to meet the body's needs, either because intake is inadequate or because requirements have increased with no corresponding increase in intake. Severe undernutrition may be classified as <75% expected weight for age and body mass index (BMI) <16 kg/m^2.

Risk factors for protein-energy malnutrition

- Children, adolescents, and pregnant and lactating women due to high demand for energy and protein.
- Eating disorders, e.g. anorexia nervosa.
- Reduced food intake, physical activity, and levels of growth hormone and androgens in older people.
- Diseases with high energy demands, e.g. hyperthyroidism, sepsis, trauma, burns, cancer.
- Malabsorption.
- Alcohol or drug dependence with inadequate consumption of calories and protein.

- Dietary factors:
  - excluding food groups or dependence on a single type of food.

Clinical features

- General features such as apathy, malaise, irritability and impaired cognition.
- Jaundice.
- Anaemia.
- Oedema.
- Hypothermia.
- Changes to the hair (brittle changes) and skin (including pigmentation).
- Muscle weakness and reduced work capacity.
- Diarrhoea.
- Lost libido, amenorrhoea and atrophy of gonadal tissues.
- Wasting of fat and muscle, including cardiac muscle.
- Reduced cardiac output with reduction in pulse and blood pressure.
- Reduced respiratory function with reduced respiratory rate and vital capacity.

Investigations

- Haemoglobin, lymphocytes, glucose, Na^+, K^+, Ca^{2+}, Mg^{2+} and PO_4^- that are often low.
- Urea and creatinine that typically fall.
- Albumin levels that fall, but rise with inflammation.
- Blood culture, stool culture, urinalysis and chest X-ray to identify infection.

Concomitant vitamin and mineral deficiencies are common in PEM, and there is also a blunted inflammatory response to infection with no increase in C-reactive protein (CRP) and/or white cell count.

Treatment

The aim of treatment is to restore oral nutrition to provide adequate quantities of protein, energy and nutrients. However, aggressive feeding after a period of undernutrition can precipitate refeeding syndrome with insulin-induced movement of phosphate into cells, causing a dramatic hypophosphataemia, which may precipitate cardiac arrhythmias and death (➲ see Refeeding syndrome, p. 18).

Fluid or electrolyte abnormalities should be corrected. Infections should be identified and treated. Oral feeding should be initiated gradually, starting with small meals, with daily monitoring and daily assessment of K^+, Mg^{2+} and PO_4^-. Any precipitating factors, such as an unsafe swallow, poorly fitting dentures, and/or drugs affecting appetite or mood, should be appropriately managed.

Vitamins

Fat soluble

Vitamin A (retinol)

- Primarily required for the visual pigment system.
- Obtained from meat, fish or plant carotenes.
- Absorbed in the small intestine and processed in the liver.
- Deficiency (due to dietary lack, malabsorption or liver disease) causes night blindness, xerophthalmia, follicular hyperkeratosis and keratomalacia.
- Toxicity is possible and causes teratogenicity, liver disease, increased intracranial pressure, hypercalcaemia and renal insufficiency.

Vitamin E (tocopherol)

- An antioxidant obtained from vegetables, seed oils and nuts.
- Absorbed in the small intestine and transported bound to lipoproteins in the blood.

- Deficiency (due to fat malabsorption, total parenteral nutrition (TPN) and abetalipoproteinaemia) causes haemolytic anaemia, peripheral neuropathy, spinocerebellar syndrome, myopathy and retinopathy.

Vitamin K (phylloquinone)

- Required for clotting factors II, VII, IX and X, and osteocalcin.
- Obtained from bacteria in the gut and transported with lipoproteins.
- Deficiency (due to long-term broad spectrum antibiotics, chronic liver disease/biliary obstruction and fat malabsorption) causes clotting defects and low bone mineral density.

Water soluble

Vitamin B_1 (thiamine)

- Required for carbohydrate metabolism and neural function.
- Obtained from cereals (germinal layer) and meat.
- Absorbed in the small intestine.
- Deficiency (due to high alcohol intake [inhibits absorption], hyperemesis gravidarum, malnutrition, polished rice diet or renal dialysis) causes anorexia, low temperature, glossitis, dry beri-beri (peripheral neuropathy), wet beri-beri (high output cardiac failure), lactic acidosis and Wernicke-Korsakoff syndrome (➲ see Chapter 17, Ethanol, p. 640).

Vitamin B_2 (riboflavin)

- Obtained from milk, cheese, eggs, leafy vegetables, mushrooms and almonds.
- Required for the synthesis of flavin redox cofactors.
- Deficiency (ariboflavinosis) causes stomatitis, including painful red tongue with sore throat; chapped and fissured lips (cheilosis); inflammation of the corners of the mouth (angular stomatitis); seborrhoeic dermatitis; itchy, watery eyes that are sensitive to light; and normochromic normocytic anaemia.

Vitamin B_3 (niacin)

- Obtained from its precursor tryptophan or dietary yeast, lean meats and liver.
- Required for synthesis of the redox reaction coenzymes nicotinamine adenine dinucleotide (NAD) and NADP.
- Deficiency (due to lack of intake, carcinoid syndrome, isoniazid therapy or Hartnup disease) causes anorexia, lethargy, burning sensations, glossitis, headache, stupor, seizures and pellagra (pigmented dermatitis, dementia, diarrhoea).

Vitamin B_6 (pyridoxine)

- Dietary sources include fruit, vegetables and grain.
- Required in amino acid, glucose and lipid metabolism.
- Deficiency causes peripheral neuropathy, seborrhoeic dermatitis, glossitis, stomatitis, anaemia and seizures.

Vitamin B_{12} (cobalamin)

- Obtained from meat, dairy products, fish and cereals.
- Required as a cofactor for methionine synthesis from homocysteine (methylcobalamin) and succinyl-CoA synthesis from methylmalonyl-CoA (adenosylcobalamine).
- Forms a complex with intrinsic factor in the intestine. Intrinsic factor is produced by the gastric mucosal parietal cells. The vitamin B_{12}-intrinsic factor complex is absorbed in the terminal ileum. Vitamin B_{12} is then transported in the blood bound to transcobalamin II.

- Deficiency (due to pernicious anaemia [antibodies prevent binding to intrinsic factor], terminal ileum resection/malabsorption, metformin and proton pump inhibitors) causes glossitis, paraesthesia, macrocytic (megaloblastic) anaemia, subacute combined degeneration of the spinal cord, depression and diarrhoea.
- In deficiency, urinary and serum methylmalonic acid, plasma homocysteine and holotranscobalamin (the transporter protein without vitamin B_{12}) concentrations are increased.

Folic acid

- Obtained from green leafy vegetables, fruits, nuts, beans, dairy products, poultry and eggs.
- Deficiency (due to poor absorption, insufficient intake, excessive demands, and methotrexate and phenytoin therapy) causes glossitis, intestinal mucosal dysfunction, and a macrocytic (megaloblastic) anaemia and raised homocysteine concentration (as folate is another required cofactor for methionine synthesis).
- Deficiency is measured by either serum concentration (indicative of recent intake) or red blood cell concentration (more representative of stores).

Iron

Deficiency leads to symptoms related to anaemia (including fatigue and dyspnoea), glossitis and koilonychia (➲ see Chapter 9, Anaemia, p. 272, Figure 9.2 and Table 9.2).

Vitamin C (ascorbic acid)

- Obtained from fruit and vegetables.
- Absorbed in the stomach.
- Primarily required as a cofactor for collagen hydroxylase.
- Has a half-life in the body of 2 weeks.
- Deficiency (due to lack of intake) causes scurvy with poor wound healing, easy bruising, gingivitis, dental defects, anaemia and arthralgia.

Chronic trace element deficiencies

The trace elements (chromium, cobalt, copper, iodine, manganese, molybdenum, nickel, selenium, zinc) are essential for health but only required in minute quantities and can be harmful in excessive amounts (Table 1.1). They are obtained from the diet and so poor dietary intake, TPN without adequate supplementation, Roux-en-Y gastric bypass bariatric surgery, short gut or inflammatory bowel disease can all lead to deficiency.

Further reading

1. Supra-Regional Assay Service. Trace elements. http://www.sas-centre.org/assays/trace-elements for further information on trace element deficiency and toxicity, and appropriate testing

Principles of enteral and parenteral nutrition

Enteral feeding

Patients who are either unable to feed or take sufficient nutrition orally, but in whom the gastrointestinal tract is functioning, may be fed enterally by tube. Common underlying disease processes leading to enteral tube feeding include neurological disorders affecting swallowing, head and neck malignancy, and oesophagogastric diseases.

Nasogastric (NG)/nasojejunal (NJ) feeding

- Often used short term, e.g. in patients at high risk of aspiration.
- Not recommended for long-term feeding (>4–6 weeks) as it is prone to failure due to tube occlusion or dislodgement.

Table 1.1 Trace metal functions and deficiencies

Trace metal	Function	Specific causes of deficiency	Symptoms of deficiency	Important considerations
Chromium	Insulin cofactor.		Diabetes mellitus.	Toxicity observed with failing metal on metal hip joints.
Copper	Enzyme cofactor, e.g. cytochromes.	Menke's disease (X-linked recessive disorder involving mutation of the *ATP7A* gene that results in copper being poorly distributed to cells in the body). High zinc intake (competes for absorption).	Microcytic hypochromic anaemia. Neutropenia. Ineffective collagen synthesis. Menke's disease phenotype: growth failure, seizures, intellectual disability, blue sclera, osteoporosis and kinky, colourless or steel-coloured hair.	Levels increased in acute phase response and pregnancy.
Manganese	Enzyme cofactor, e.g. superoxide dismutase.			Toxicity causes parkinsonism.
Molybdenum	Enzyme cofactor, e.g. xanthine oxidase.		Tachycardia. Central scotomas.	
Selenium	Antioxidant, e.g. regulation of glutathione peroxidase.	Common in certain areas of China. May occur in patients with severely compromised intestinal function.	Keshan syndrome (cardiomyopathy). Kashin–Beck disease (osteoarthropathy).	
Zinc	Enzyme cofactor, e.g. alkaline phosphatase.	Acrodermatitis enteropathica (autosomal recessive disorder involving mutation of the *SLC39A4* gene on chromosome 8, which encodes a zinc uptake protein). High phytate diet.	Alopecia. Dermatitis. Poor wound healing.	Levels decreased in acute phase response.

Gastrostomy

- Placed endoscopically (percutaneous endoscopic gastrostomy [PEG]) or radiologically (radiologically inserted gastrostomy [RIG]).
- Complications may be:
  - Immediate: respiratory failure, bleeding, perforated viscus, peritonitis.
  - Early: pneumonia, infection, early tube displacement.
  - Late: aspiration pneumonia, infection, hypergranulation, leakage, fistula formation, small bowel ischaemia/obstruction, tumour seeding, tube malfunction/displacement.
    - A RIG may be preferable in patients with oesophageal stricturing, or head and neck malignancy where there is a perceived risk of tumour seeding.

Indications for total parenteral nutrition

TPN involves providing all nutritional needs via the intravenous route, usually via a 12-hour overnight infusion, and should only be considered for patients who are malnourished or at risk of malnutrition with either:

- inadequate or unsafe oral and/or enteral nutritional intake.
- a non-functioning, inaccessible or perforated gastrointestinal tract.

Before starting TPN, its potential duration, feasibility and effect upon quality of life and life expectancy should be considered.

Practicalities of total parenteral nutrition

Dedicated central venous access is preferred with insertion under strict aseptic technique. TPN must be prescribed according to individual nutritional requirements. Additions of electrolytes, vitamins and minerals should be performed in a sterile environment. TPN should start at <50% requirements for the first 24–48 hours and be titrated up to provide full nutritional requirements. Patients must be monitored daily initially (full blood count [FBC], urea & electrolytes [U&Es], LFTs, CRP) and regularly thereafter to identify complications. Some patients may require insulin to prevent hyperglycaemia. TPN should stop once requirements can be met orally/enterally.

Contents of total parenteral nutrition

- Water:
  - Volume determined by monitoring fluid output.
  - 30–40 mL/kg/day is often a reasonable starting point for patients without high outputs.
- Calories:
  - Calculated to allow maintenance of current weight and correct any undernutrition.
  - Extra calories given to patients with catabolic conditions or when there are high metabolic demands.
  - Energy is supplied in the form of:
    - Carbohydrate – provides 50–60% of energy requirements, mostly as dextrose.
    - Lipid – provides 20–30% of energy requirements.
    - Amino acids mixture – provides 10–20% of energy requirements; must include all essential amino acids.
- Electrolytes, vitamins and minerals to replace losses and provide daily requirements.

Complications of total parenteral nutrition

- Venous access-related complications, e.g. line infection, thrombosis or displacement.
- Adverse reactions to the lipid fraction of TPN causing rashes, dizziness, nausea, sweating and breathlessness.
- Hypoglycaemia and hyperglycaemia.
- Hypertriglyceridaemia.
- Gallbladder stasis causing stone formation and cholecystitis.
- Liver disease:
  - Elevated LFTs are common.
  - Intestinal failure-related liver disease (IFALD) with steatotic changes:
    - altering the composition of the TPN can help reduce progression.
  - Hyperammonaemia:
    - corrected by arginine supplements.
- Osteoporosis and/or osteomalacia.
- Fluid overload.

Further reading

1. National Institute of Health and Care Excellence. Nutrition support for adults: oral nutrition support, enteral tube feeding and parenteral nutrition. Clinical guideline CG32. https://www.nice.org.uk/guidance/cg32/chapter/1-guidance

Refeeding syndrome

Refeeding syndrome is defined as the potentially fatal shifts in fluids and electrolytes that may occur in malnourished patients on refeeding following a period of starvation. It is common in patients receiving artificial nutrition, but can also occur with oral refeeding, particularly if oral nutritional supplements are prescribed.

Pathogenesis

- A switch in metabolism from fat to carbohydrate results in insulin release.
- With carbohydrate repletion and increased insulin production there is an increased uptake of glucose, phosphorus, potassium and water into cells, and a stimulation of anabolic protein synthesis.
- The combined effect of depleted total body phosphorus during catabolic starvation and the movement of phosphorus into cells during refeeding leads to severe extracellular hypophosphataemia, often in association with hypokalaemia and hypomagnesaemia.

Presentation

- Neurological: delirium, seizures, ataxia, Wernicke's encephalopathy (➲ see Chapter 17, Ethanol, p. 640).
- Cardiac: arrhythmias, hypotension, cardiac failure, peripheral oedema.
- Metabolic: anaemia, uraemia, hypokalaemia, hypophosphataemia, hypomagnesaemia, hyperglycaemia, vitamin deficiency (e.g. vitamin B_{12}).
- Musculoskeletal: paraesthesiae, weakness, fasciculations.

Assessment of risk

A patient should be considered at risk of refeeding syndrome if they meet the following criteria:

- BMI <16 kg/m^2.
- Unintentional weight loss >15% in the past 3–6 months.
- Little or no nutritional intake for >10 days.
- Low levels of potassium, phosphate or magnesium before feeding.
- ≥2 of:
    - BMI <18.5 kg/m^2.
    - Unintentional weight loss >10% in the past 3–6 months.
    - Little or no nutritional intake for >5 days.
    - History of alcohol misuse or drugs, including insulin and diuretics.

For patients considered to be at high risk of refeeding syndrome, the following steps are advised:

- Nutrition support to commence at a maximum of 10 kcal/kg/day, increasing levels slowly to meet or exceed full needs by 4–7 days.
- Restoration of circulatory volume with close monitoring of fluid balance and overall clinical status.
- Oral supplementation with thiamine, vitamin B compound strong and a balanced multivitamin/trace element immediately before and during the first 10 days of feeding.
- Monitoring of potassium, calcium, magnesium and phosphate for the first 2 weeks and amendment of treatment as appropriate.

Further reading

1. Mehanna HM, Moledina J, Travis J. Refeeding syndrome: what it is, and how to prevent and treat it. *BMJ*. 2008 Jun 28;336(7659):1495–8.

Obesity

Obesity is currently defined on the basis of BMI (Table 1.2).

Table 1.2 Classification of body mass index (BMI)

BMI (kg/m^2)	Classification
<18.5	Underweight
18.5–25	Normal
25–30	Overweight
30–40	Obese
>40	Extreme obesity

Reprinted from World Health Organization. (2019). Body mass index - BMI. [online] Available at: http://www.euro.who.int/en/health-topics/disease-prevention/nutrition/a-healthy-lifestyle/body-mass-index-bmi [Accessed 1 Mar. 2019].

Obesity is common and usually secondary to long-term calorie excess. Genetic causes of obesity (melanocortin receptor [MCR]-4 mutation, Prader–Willi syndrome [males only], leptin deficiency, leptin receptor deficiency) are rare and should be suspected in patients with a history of severe neonatal/childhood obesity.

Many cases are associated with metabolic syndrome or other complications (➲ see Metabolic syndrome, p. 26). The necessity for intervention beyond calorie-reducing life-style measures is determined by the presence of metabolic co-morbidities.

The management of obesity depends on the co-existant co-morbidities:

- Metabolic:
  - Type 2 diabetes; insulin resistance syndrome (including polycystic ovary syndrome); renal failure/impairment.
- Cardiovascular:
  - Cardiovascular disease (CVD) event risk (secondarily adjusted for BMI); hyperlipidaemia, hypertension (especially resistant hypertension); atrial fibrillation; pulmonary hypertension; venous thrombosis.
- Respiratory:
  - Obstructive sleep apnoea; obesity hypoventilation; asthma; chronic obstructive pulmonary disease.
- Abdominal:
  - Non-alcoholic fatty liver disease (NAFLD) and non-alcoholic steatohepatitis; gallstones; endometriosis; previous abdominal surgery.
- Urogenital:
  - Urinary incontinence; erectile dysfunction.
- Neurological:
  - Benign intracranial hypertension; nerve compression syndromes.
- Osteological:
  - Osteoarthritis; spinal stenosis.
- Functional capacity for activities of daily living.
- Psychological:
  - Binge-eating; depression/anxiety; previous bulimia; psychosis.

Management

- Supervised calorie reduction programme for 6–12 months dependent on BMI and co-morbidities.
- Bariatric intervention if BMI >40 kg/m^2 or >35 kg/m^2 and other co-morbidities, e.g. type 2 diabetes mellitus. Options are gastric banding (15% total weight loss); sleeve gastrectomy (30% total weight loss); gastric bypass (Roux-en-Y) (40% total weight loss) and pancreatobiliary diversion (>50% total weight loss). Gastric bypass is a preferred option for rapid glycaemic correction in type 2 diabetes, which often precedes significant weight loss. Options such as intragastric balloon or endoscopic gastroplication placement exist for lower degrees of weight loss or for patients at too high risk for surgery, but have less evidence. An acute 'liver diet' (1000 kcal/day) is used acutely prior to surgery to reduce the amount of water, fat and glycogen in the liver, thereby to make the surgery technically easier.

Metabolic follow-up post-bariatric surgery

All patients should have regular quarterly, and then yearly, follow-up. Consequences of bariatric surgery include stress/reflux gastric/oesophageal ulceration and excess bile production. Doses of anti-hypertensive, lipid and especially hypoglycaemic therapies need regular monitoring and adjustment.

General vitamin supplementation with added vitamin D and iron is necessary post-surgery. In patients with post-gastric bypass surgery, higher dose supplementation is necessary allied with regular monitoring of HbA_{1c}, trace metals (iron, copper, zinc) and vitamins (cobalamin, folate, vitamin D). Patients with pancreatobiliary diversion require monitoring of all major trace elements (including selenium) and vitamins (A,B,D,E,K).

Further reading

1. National Institute of Health and Care Excellence. Obesity prevention. Clinical guideline CG43. http://www.nice.org.uk/guidance/CG43

Lipids and atherosclerosis

Lipid metabolism

Lipids is a term used to describe particles containing cholesterol, triglycerides and other components, such as phospholipids, sphingolipids, ceramides and free fatty acids. Their function is to transport fatty acids and cholesterol from the gut via the liver to peripheral tissues (exogenous gut and endogenous plasma pathways) and to recycle excess cholesterol back to the liver (reverse cholesterol transport). See Figure 1.4 for the major pathways of lipid metabolism.

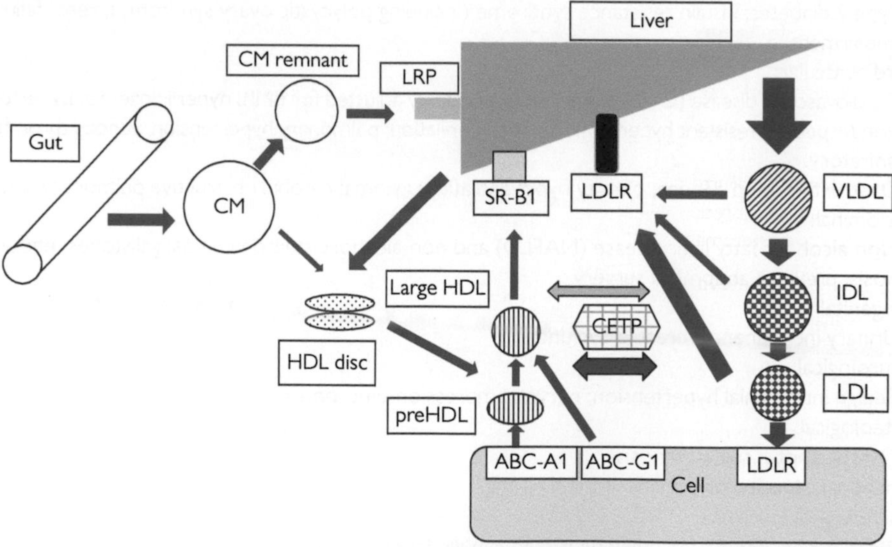

Figure 1.4 Chylomicrons (CMs) are secreted from the gut and delipidated by lipoprotein lipase (LPL). CM remnants are taken up by liver lipoprotein-related receptors (LRP). Very low density lipoprotein (VLDL) particles are secreted by the liver and delipidated by LPL to intermediate density lipoprotein (IDL) and low density lipoprotein (LDL) particles. LDL is taken up by/recycled by cellular LDL-receptors (LDLRs). High density lipoprotein (HDL) discs (containing apolipoprotein A1 (apoA-1)) are secreted from the liver or budded from CM and loaded with cholesterol by ATP-binding cassette transporter (ABC)-A1 and ABC-G1 to make high density lipoprotein (HDL). HDL is taken up by liver scavenger receptor B1 (SR-B1) and the apoA-1 is recycled. Cholesterol ester transfer protein (CETP) shuttles cholesterol in exchange for triglycerides from HDL to VLDL, IDL and LDL.

Lipid particles are classically subdivided by their size and density into chylomicrons (CM; 85% triglycerides, 4% cholesterol), very low density lipoproteins (VLDL; 50% triglycerides, 15% cholesterol), low density lipoproteins (LDL) and high density lipoproteins (HDL). They are usually measured using their cholesterol content, but can also be assayed by the protein concentration (e.g. apolipoprotein [apo] B-48 – chylomicrons; apoB-100 – VLDL and LDL; apoA-1 – HDL) or more detailed component analysis as part of the plasma lipidome. Intermediate density lipoprotein (IDL) and LDL contribute to atherosclerosis by entering the vascular wall, being oxidised and promoting the entry and then activation of macrophages. These then form foam cells and attempt to repair the vascular wall. Activation both induces foam cell apoptosis (death) and weakens the vessel structure, leading to exposure of wall collagen and coagulation, and/or embolism.

Epidemiological cross-sectional studies have established that the ratio of total cholesterol to HDL-cholesterol in plasma lipids may account for up to 55% of modifiable CVD risk. LDL particles are key to macrophage accumulation of lipids and thus raise the profile of LDL-cholesterol as a CVD risk factor. The ratio of apoB-100:apoA-1 particles/concentrations, or more simply expressed as the non-HDL-cholesterol (the difference between total and HDL cholesterol levels) (non-HDL-C), is a better predictor of CVD risk than LDL-cholesterol (LDL-C), as this incorporates the additional atherogenic risk due to triglyceride-rich particles.

Hyperlipidaemia

Cholesterol and triglycerides can be obtained from the diet or synthesised in the liver from acetyl-CoA, derived either from adipose tissue fatty acids or from glucose by the glycolysis pathway. The balance between glucose and fat-based metabolism is regulated by insulin and other hormones. Thus, plasma lipid profiles can reflect dietary conditions, gut function, liver, muscle or adipose tissue disease, or the effects of hormones on metabolism (e.g. thyroxine, glucocorticoids, glucagon, growth hormone), as well as defects of lipid metabolism. Primary hyperlipidaemia is the term used to describe specific defects of lipid metabolism, while secondary hyperlipidaemia refers to other genetic or hormonal causes of lipid abnormalities (Box 1.2).

Box 1.2 Secondary causes of hyperlipidaemia

Cholesterol elevated

- Diet rich in saturated fats.
- Hypothyroidism.
- Chronic renal failure.
- Renal transplant recipients.
- Nephrotic syndrome.

Triglycerides elevated

- Pregnancy.
- Obesity.
- Diabetes mellitus.
- Chronic renal failure.
- Renal transplant recipients.
- Chronic liver disease.
- Excess alcohol intake.
- Cushing's syndrome or other endocrine diseases.
- Drugs:
  - High dose thiazide diuretics.
  - High dose β-blockers.
  - High dose oral corticosteroids.
  - High dose oestrogens.
  - High dose progestogens.
  - Anabolic steroids.
  - Protease inhibitors.
  - Ciclosporin.

Cardiovascular risk assessment

Hyperlipidaemia is one of a number of CVD risk factors and is associated with increased risk of developing type 2 diabetes. Accepted abnormally high lipid levels are:

- Total cholesterol (TC) >5 mmol/L
- LDL-C >3 mmol/L
- Triglyceride (TG) >4.5 mmol/L (fasting)
- HDL-C <1 mmol/L (men) or <1.2 mmol/L (women)
- TC/HDL-C ratio >4.5.

Apart from at extreme levels, no individual CVD risk factor is sufficiently predictive of prognosis, so non-modifiable risk factors, such as age, gender, ethnicity and family history of CVD, are combined with modifiable risk factors, such as cigarette smoking, extent of hyperlipidaemia, blood pressure and diabetes, to allow calculation of prospective 10-year and lifetime CVD risks using risk calculators or tables (Figure 1.5). A CVD event risk >10% per decade (QRISK3; UK) warrants lipid-lowering drug therapy if lifestyle intervention has not worked. In patients with type 1 diabetes, statins are offered if any of the following is present: age >40 years, duration of diabetes >10 years, established nephropathy and any other risk factors for CVD. In patients with chronic kidney disease statins are offered for primary and/or secondary prevention. Risk assessment protocols (e.g. UK QRISK3, Europe SCORE, US ASCVD, GloboRISK [182 countries]) have been formalised into CVD screening programmes in various countries (Figures 1.5 and 1.6).

A 1 mmol/L reduction in LDL-C can result in a 21% reduction in CVD events and a 19% relative risk reduction of CVD death over 5 years. Statin therapy is maximised and LDL-C targets are lower for higher CVD risk categories. Treatment with high dose high intensity statin or to LDL-C <1.8 mmol/L or >50% LDL-C reduction is recommended for patients with established CVD or at highly increased risk (5–10%).

Genetic hyperlipidaemias

Familial hypercholesterolaemia

- Commonest genetic lipid disorder.
- Autosomal dominant disorder.
- Frequency of 1 in 250 to 1 in 500 for heterozygotes and 1 in 300,000–1,000,000 for homozygotes.
- Affects function of the LDL receptor pathway, resulting in reduced clearance of LDL from the circulation.
- Characterised by elevated plasma total and LDL-C levels >7.5 mmol/L and >4.7 mmol/L in heterozygotes and >13 mmol/L and >11 mmol/L in homozygotes, respectively.
- Associated with early onset CVD:
  - typically occurring prior to age 60 years with a strong family history of CVD with an autosomal dominant pattern and high penetrance.
  - very premature CVD-life expectancy of 33 years in homozygotes.
  - usual risk estimation tools underestimate risk of CVD.
- Deposition of cholesterol in extensor tendons (tendon xanthomata) and/or in the iris (arcus).
- Diagnosis confirmed by genetic analysis of mutations in the LDL receptor, apoB LDL-cholesterol binding domain or the LDL receptor controlling protein, proprotein convertase subtilisin kexin (PCSK)-9.
- Treated with statins and other LDL-cholesterol reducing therapies:
  - reducing LDL-C by >50% produces a 75% reduction in CVD mortality and normalises life span.

For an algorithm for diagnosis of familial hypercholesterolaemia, see Figure 1.7.

Polygenic hypercholesterolaemia

- Defective LDL clearance is the most common cause of isolated hypercholesterolaemia.
- Frequently picked up during screening or investigation of atherosclerosis.
- Patients do not display xanthomata or xanthelasmata.

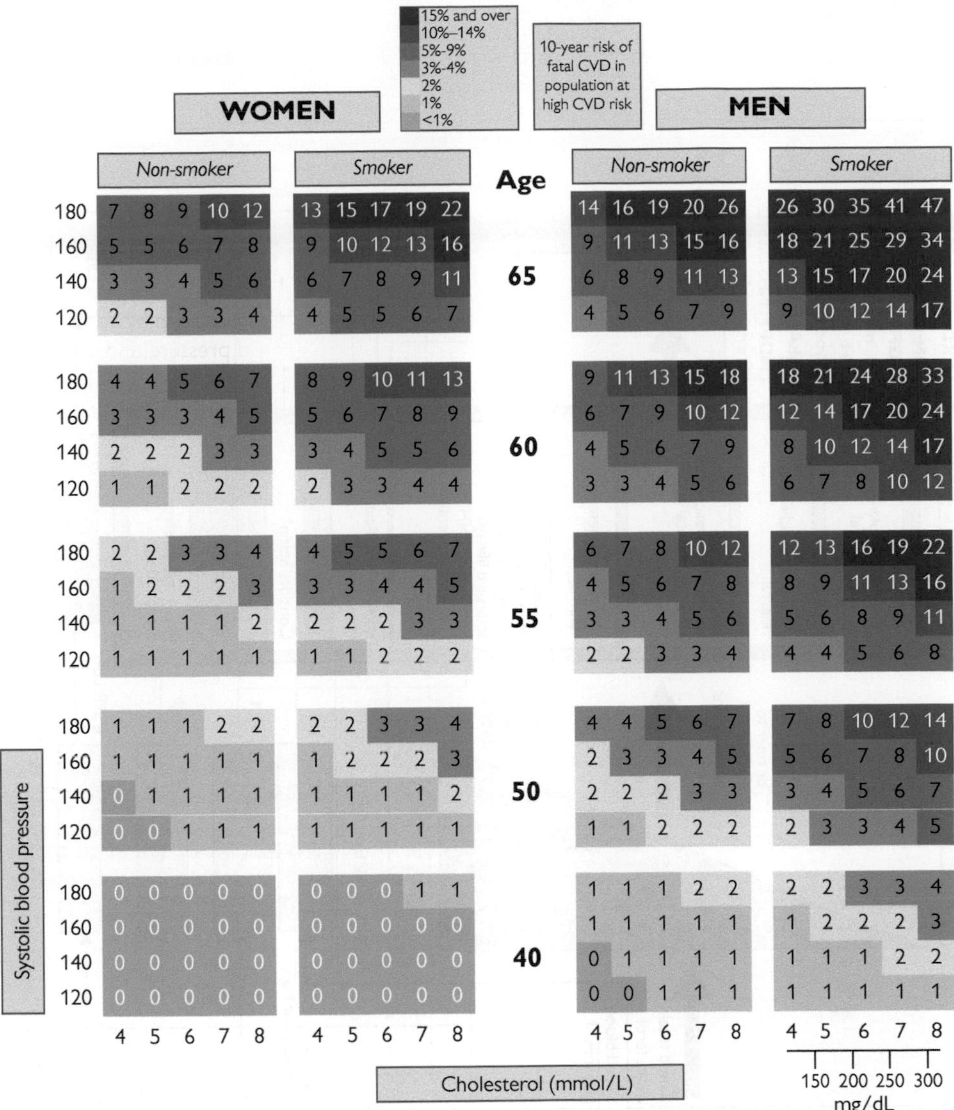

Figure 1.5 European 'SCORE' CVD risk calculator chart for estimation of 10-year risk of fatal CVD.

Reproduced with permission from Piepoli MF, et al. 2016 European Guidelines on cardiovascular disease prevention in clinical practice: The Sixth Joint Task Force of the European Society of Cardiology and Other Societies on Cardiovascular Disease Prevention in Clinical Practice (constituted by representatives of 10 societies and by invited experts). Developed with the special contribution of the European Association for Cardiovascular Prevention & Rehabilitation (EACPR). Eur Heart J. 37, 29, pp. 2315–81, by permission of European Society of Cardiology and Oxford University Press. Copyright © 2016, European Society of Cardiology. https://doi.org/10.1093/eurheartj/ehw106.

Familial combined hyperlipidaemia

- Associated with multiple genes at different loci.
- Frequency of 1 in 300.
- Characterised by:
  - hypercholesterolaemia and/or hypertriglyceridaemia in ≥2 members of the same family;
  - raised apoB;
  - increased risk of early onset CVD.

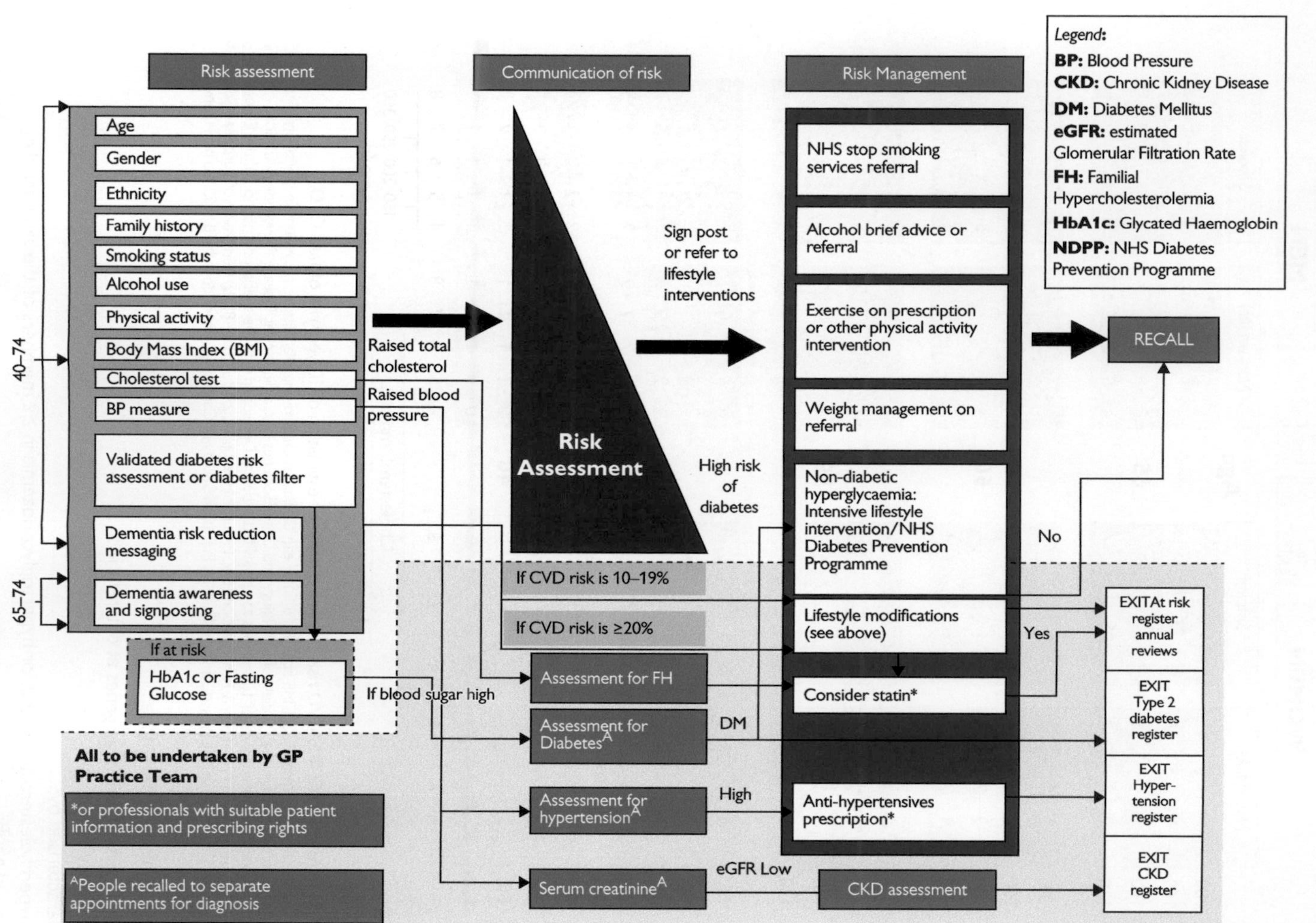

Figure 1.6 Chart of UK NHS Health Check screening protocol.

Reproduced with permission from Public Health England. NHS Health Check Best Practice Guidance. © 2017 Crown Copyright.

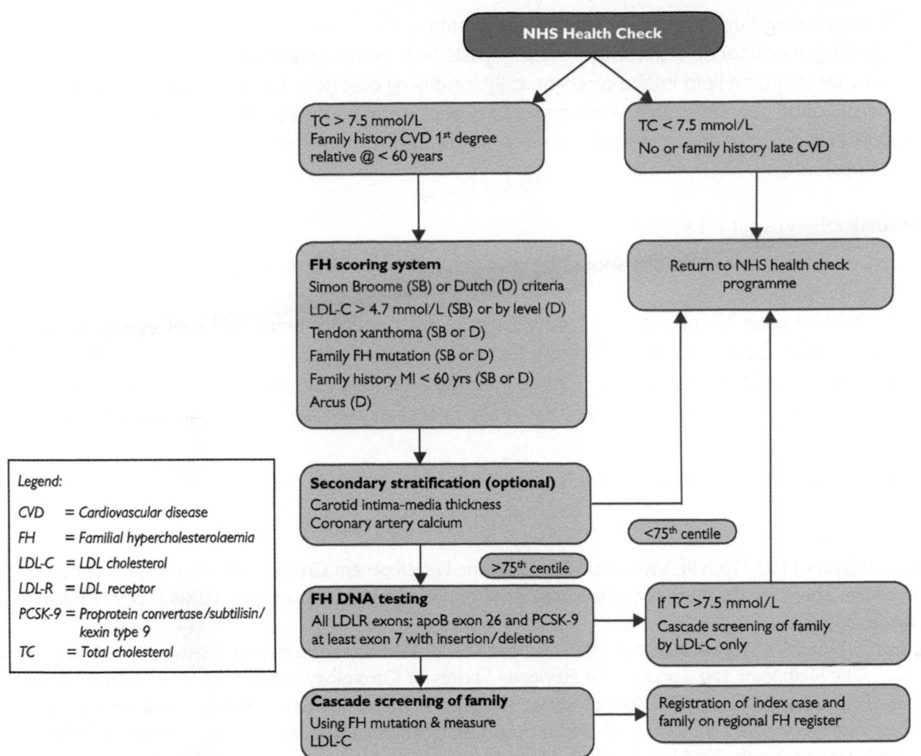

Figure 1.7 Algorithm for diagnosis of familial hypercholesterolaemia.

- Diagnosed using population-specific lipid normograms and a family history of CVD.
- Treated using statin therapy and, if residual hypertriglyceridaemia is present, by adding omega-3 fatty acids or fibrates.

Remnant hyperlipidaemia

- Occurs in 1 in 20,000.
- Associated with a mixed dyslipidaemia (elevated triglycerides and cholesterol), early onset coronary artery disease and aggressive pan-vascular bed atherosclerosis (especially peripheral arterial disease).
- Palmar striae xanthoma are characteristic and tuberous xanthomata may be seen at the elbows and knees.
- Hallmark is the presence of homozygosity for the apolipoprotein E2 or E4 genetic variants.
- Treated with a combination of fibrates and statins.

Familial hypertriglyceridaemia and familial chylomicronaemia syndromes

- Spectrum of TG disorders characterised by excess VLDL and/or chylomicrons.
- Occurs in 1 in 50,000.
- Most hypertriglyceridaemia is polygenic. Some severe cases caused by heterozygosity for mutations in lipoprotein lipase (LPL) and its related proteins (ApoC-2, ApoA-5, GPI-anchored HDL-binding protein 1 [GPI-HBP-1], lipid maturation factor-1 [LMF-1]) allied with secondary precipitants of mixed hyperlipidaemia. Extreme cases with onset in childhood are caused by homozygosity for defects in the 5 major genes for LPL metabolism.
- Severe hypertriglyceridaemia (>20 mmol/L) is associated with:
  - symptomatic and recurrent pancreatitis;
  - type 2 diabetes secondary to beta cell destruction;

- TG-containing skin rash and eruptive xanthomata;
- hypertriglyceridaemia visible within artery walls (e.g. retinal lipaemia).
- Treated by stopping lipid intake or chronically modifying diet (low fat diets), allied with tight glycaemic control and fibrates or omega-3 fatty acids to maximise clearance of TG-rich lipoproteins. Familial chylomicronaemia may be treated with antisense therapy to apolipoprotein C3 (volanesorsen).

Treatment of hyperlipidaemia

- Lifestyle/dietary interventions should be recommended for all patients with hyperlipidaemia (may reduce TC by up to 10%):
  - General: at least 30 minutes exercise per day with fat content being <35% of energy intake.
  - Reduce LDL-C and TC: reduce dietary fat and cholesterol, reduce weight, increase fibre.
  - Increase HDL-C: reduce weight, increase exercise, alcohol use in moderation, stop cigarette smoking.
  - Reduce TG: reduce weight and alcohol intake, increase exercise and fish oil/omega-3 fatty acid intake.

Drugs used in hyperlipidaemia are shown in Table 1.3.

Further reading

1. Rabar S, Harker M, O'Flynn N, Wierzbicki AS, Guideline Development Group. Lipid modification and cardiovascular risk assessment for the primary and secondary prevention of cardiovascular disease: summary of updated NICE guidance. *BMJ*. 2014 Jul 17;349:g4356.
2. Piepoli MF, Hoes AW, Agewall S, et al. 2016 European Guidelines on cardiovascular disease prevention in clinical practice: The Sixth Joint Task Force of the European Society of Cardiology and Other Societies on Cardiovascular Disease Prevention in Clinical Practice (constituted by representatives of 10 societies and by invited experts) Developed with the special contribution of the European Association for Cardiovascular Prevention & Rehabilitation (EACPR). *Atherosclerosis*. 2016 Sep;252:207–74.
3. Grundy SM, Stone NJ, Bailey AL, et al. AHA/ACC/AACVPR/AAPA/ABC/ACPM/ADA/AGS/APhA/ASPC/NLA/PCNA Guideline on the Management of Blood Cholesterol. Circulation. 2018 Nov 10:CIR0000000000000625.
4. Eckel RH, Jakicic JM, Ard JD, et al; American College of Cardiology/American Heart Association Task Force on Practice Guidelines. 2013 AHA/ACC guideline on lifestyle management to reduce cardiovascular risk: a report of the American College of Cardiology/American Heart Association Task Force on Practice Guidelines. *Circulation*. 2014 Jun 24;129(25 Suppl. 2):S76–99. Erratum in: *Circulation*. 2014 Jun 24;129(25 Suppl. 2):S100–1. *Circulation*. 2015 Jan 27;131(4):e326.
5. Gidding SS, Champagne MA, de Ferranti SD, et al.; American Heart Association Atherosclerosis, Hypertension, and Obesity in Young Committee of Council on Cardiovascular Disease in Young, Council on Cardiovascular and Stroke Nursing, Council on Functional Genomics and Translational Biology, and Council on Lifestyle and Cardiometabolic Health. The Agenda for Familial Hypercholesterolemia: a scientific statement from the American Heart Association. *Circulation*. 2015 Dec 1;132(22):2167–92.

Metabolic syndrome

Key features

- Waist circumference >94 cm (male); >80 cm (female):
  - Lower values apply to Asians (both Indian and Chinese).
- And two of the following four features:
  - Fasting triglycerides >1.7 mmol/L.
  - HDL-cholesterol < 1 mmol/L (male); <1.2 mmol/L (female).
  - Systolic blood pressure >130 mmHg.
  - Glucose >5.6 mmol/4L or HbA1c > 6% (≈40 mmol/mol).

The metabolic syndrome is associated with insulin resistance, pre-diabetes and a high chance of progression to frank type 2 diabetes. Presence of ≥4 features of the metabolic syndrome increases the risk of developing type 2 diabetes by 10–20-fold.

Table 1.3 Drugs used in hyperlipidaemia

Drugs with examples	Mechanisms of action	Clinical effects
3-HMG CoA reductase inhibitors (e.g. atorvastatin, simvastatin, rosuvastatin)	3-HMG CoA reductase is an enzyme involved in production of cholesterol from LDL. Competitive inhibition of the enzyme increases LDL receptor expression and internalisation of LDL cholesterol from blood.	↓LDL-C: 20–60% ↓TG: 10–33% Most commonly used and first-line lipid lowering agent. Classified into: • Low intensity (reduction in LDL 20–30%), e.g. simvastatin 10 mg/day. • Medium intensity (reduction in LDL 31–40%), e.g. atorvastatin at 10 mg/day and simvastatin 20–40 mg/day. • High intensity (reduction in LDL >40%), e.g. atorvastatin at ≥20 mg/day and simvastatin 80 mg/day. May cause myositis: indicated by muscle pain, high creatine kinase and liver transaminase levels. Simvastatin potentiates the effect of warfarin. Contraindicated with gemfibrozil due to interference with its metabolism.
Fibrates (e.g. bezafibrate, fenofibrate)	Works on PPAR-α in the liver increasing transcription of enzymes like lipoprotein lipase, which clears triglyceride rich lipoproteins (mainly VLDL) from the blood.	↓LDL-C: 6–20% ↓TG: 41–53% Preferred treatment in hypertriglyceridaemia. Potentiates the effect of warfarin.
PCSK-9 inhibitors (e.g. evolocumab, alirocumab)	Increases LDL receptors in the liver by inhibiting PCSK-9, the enzyme that destroys the LDL receptor after it has been internalised within the hepatocytes.	↓LDL-C: 60% Fortnightly injections. Expensive.
Nicotinic acid derivatives (e.g. niacin)	Inhibits lipolysis in adipocytes, in turn reducing VLDL.	Modest effect on LDL-C and TG. Side effects include flushing, headache and myositis.
Bile acid sequestrants (e.g. colestyramine, colesevelam)	Resins that bind to bile acids and form an insoluble complex excreted in faeces. There is compensatory increase in hepatic bile acid synthesis using up cholesterol.	Modest effect on LDL-C. Little effect on TG. Side effects include abdominal cramps, nausea, myositis and acanthosis nigricans.
Ezetimibe	Inhibits gut cholesterol absorption.	Modest effect on lipids. Well tolerated and often the second agent to be added to statins or used when statins are not tolerated. Side effects include myalgia and voice changes.
Omega 3 fatty acid (e.g. Omacor®)	Inhibits secretion of VLDL from the liver by increasing destruction of intracellular Apo B100.	Modest effect on TG levels. Nausea and bloating are common side effects.
Lomitapide	Inhibits the microsomal triglyceride transfer protein necessary for VLDL assembly and secretion.	Adjunct to dietary measures and other lipid-regulating drugs with or without LDL apheresis used in homozygous familial hypercholesterolaemia.

3-HMG CoA: 3-hydroxy-3-methyl-glutaryl-CoA; LDL: low density lipoprotein; LDL-C: low density lipoprotein cholesterol; PPAR: peroxisome proliferator activated receptors; PCSK-9: proprotein convertase subtilisin/kexin type 9; TG: triglyceride; VLDL: very low density lipoprotein.

Non-alcoholic fatty liver disease and liver fat/glucose disorders

Metabolic syndrome is associated with deposition of fat in many visceral tissues. The increased free fatty acid flux from adipose tissue to the liver in insulin resistance leads to TG synthesis and NAFLD (➔ see Chapter 15, Non-alcoholic fatty liver disease and non-alcoholic steatohepatitis, p. 538). As plasma lipids are derived from hepatic export of lipoproteins, NAFLD is often associated with mixed hyperlipidaemia. Given the strong associations of plasma triglycerides with insulin resistance, NAFLD is also associated with pre-diabetes and poorly controlled diabetes.

Disorders of TG metabolism are also a feature of alcoholic liver disease (increased carbohydrate supply and alcohol-related liver damage) or disorders of carbohydrate metabolism (e.g. glycogen storage diseases). Lysosomes play a key role in cholesterol metabolism; so lysosomal storage disorders are associated with hepatic steatosis and hypercholesterolaemia.

Muscle, fat and lipids

Muscle contains fat globules and is actively involved in using triglycerides and cholesterol. Both primary and secondary myopathies can be associated with hyperlipidaemia. Mitochondrial myopathies are associated with severe hypercholesterolaemia and if type 2 diabetes is present mixed hyperlipidaemia can occur. Similarly, primary disorders of muscle carbohydrate metabolism, such as McArdle's disease or Pompe's disease, may be associated with mixed hyperlipidaemia. Patients with primary muscle disease are far more likely to develop myalgia or myopathy with lipid-lowering drugs, especially statins.

Adipose tissue disorders are often associated with insulin resistance and, thus, with mixed hyperlipidaemias. Both primary and secondary lipodystrophy syndromes are commonly associated with mixed hyperlipidaemia. Minimising insulin resistance is a key feature of treatment of these disorders.

Drugs and lipids

A number of commonly used drugs have secondary effects on lipids, usually as a result of changing rates of metabolism (e.g. thyroxine), through their effects on glucose metabolism (hypoglycaemics, glucagon, growth hormone, glucocorticoids) or through their actions on modifying the fatty acid ligand pathways mediated through receptors allied to the retinoid-X receptor (e.g. thiazolidinediones) (Figure 1.8).

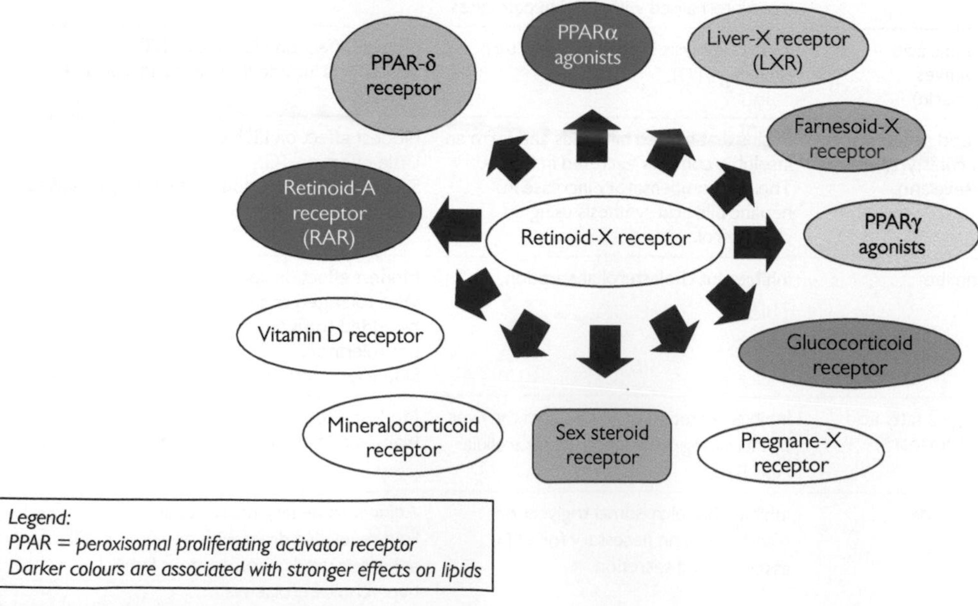

Figure 1.8 Pathways associated with lipid metabolism linked to the retinoid-X receptor.

Further reading

1. Alberti KG, Eckel RH, Grundy SM, et al.; International Diabetes Federation Task Force on Epidemiology and Prevention; National Heart, Lung, and Blood Institute; American Heart Association; World Heart Federation; International Atherosclerosis Society; International Association for the Study of Obesity. Harmonizing the metabolic syndrome: a joint interim statement of the International Diabetes Federation Task Force on Epidemiology and Prevention; National Heart, Lung, and Blood Institute; American Heart Association; World Heart Federation; International Atherosclerosis Society; and International Association for the Study of Obesity. *Circulation*. 2009 Oct 20;120(16):1640–5.

Inherited metabolic disorders

IMDs occur in 1 in 784 live births in the UK, although each individual disease is rare. They are monogenic disorders that result from a deficiency or malfunction of an enzyme, usually inherited in an autosomal recessive manner (unless otherwise stated in the text). Pathology occurs either due to build-up of a toxic metabolite or absence of an essential metabolite.

Amino acid disorders

Phenylketonuria

- Due to a deficiency of phenylalanine hydroxylase, which converts phenylalanine to tyrosine.
- Resultant deficiency of dopamine-related neurotransmitters and accumulation of toxic phenylalanine metabolites results in severe neurological damage.
- Usually detected on neonatal screening by an elevated phenylalanine and normal or decreased tyrosine concentration.
- Natural protein-restricted diet with adequate phenylalanine-free protein supplementation can allow normal brain development.
- Sapropterin is a new drug that activates residual phenylalanine hydroxylase, leading to improvement of phenylalanine metabolism and decreasing phenylalanine concentrations (➲ see Table 3.4).

Alkaptonuria

- Due to a deficiency of homogentisate dioxygenase (which is also part of the phenylalanine/tyrosine breakdown pathway).
- Results in accumulation of homogentisic acid in cartilage and other tissues (ochronosis):
  - blue/black discolouration of ear cartilage and sclera;
  - spine and large joint arthritis;
  - cardiac valve disease;
  - renal calculi.
- Diagnosed by elevated homogentisic acid in urine; homogentisic acid also causes urine to turn red/black on standing.
- Treatment is with a low phenylalanine and tyrosine diet.
- Nitisinone, which blocks an upstream pathway in phenylalanine/tyrosine breakdown, is currently being evaluated for treatment.

Homocystinuria

- Due to a deficiency of cystathionine beta-synthase, a vitamin B_6-dependent enzyme, involved in the breakdown of homocysteine to cysteine.
- Symptoms are ocular, skeletal, neurological or vascular, and include downward lens dislocation, cataract, progressive myopia, 'Marfanoid' long bone appearance, osteoporosis, mental retardation, seizures, dyspraxia and thromboembolism.
- Diagnosed by elevated methionine and homocysteine (reduced sulphydryl monomer form) concentrations in plasma and increased homocystine (oxidised disulphide) concentration in urine.
- Depending on the exact genetic mutation, patients may respond to high dose vitamin B_6, vitamin B_{12}, folic acid, betaine or a methionine-restricted diet.

Glucose and glycogen metabolism disorders

Hereditary fructose intolerance

- Due to deficiency of aldolase B.
- Manifests when sucrose, fructose or sorbitol is introduced into the diet.
- Pathology is due to the accumulation of fructose-1-phosphate, which inhibits gluconeogenesis and sequesters phosphate from ATP.
- Symptoms include hypoglycaemia, hypophosphataemia, vomiting, renal dysfunction and hepatic failure.
- Diagnosed by enzyme/genetic studies.
- Strict fructose-restricted diet must be followed.

Galactosaemia

Three IMDs associated with an inability to breakdown galactose exist, with galactose-1-phosphate uridyltransferase deficiency being the most common. Since galactose cannot be metabolised fully, intermediate metabolites such as galactitol and galactose-1-phosphate accumulate. Galactosaemia manifests shortly after birth and the initiation of milk feeds, with vomiting, liver dysfunction (including jaundice), bilateral cataracts and Gram-negative sepsis. Diagnosis is by enzyme studies and treatment is with a lactose-free diet. Even if patients follow the diet, due to endogenous galactose production, long-term sequelae are seen including ovarian dysfunction, osteoporosis and psychomotor delay.

Glycogen storage diseases

Glycogen storage diseases (GSDs) are a group of enzyme disorders affecting glycogen breakdown and synthesis which can cause symptoms relating to the liver, muscle or both. They are diagnosed by enzyme or genetic studies. Important types include:

- Type I (von Gierke):
  - glucose-6-phosphatase deficiency;
  - affects glycogenolysis and gluconeogenesis;
  - causes hypoglycaemia 3–4 hours post-prandially, hepatomegaly and elevated lactate, triglycerides and urate;
  - treated with continuous slow-release glucose polymers;
  - long-term sequelae include hepatomas, gout, osteoporosis and renal failure.
- Type II (Pompe):
  - α-1,4-glucosidase deficiency;
  - causes glycogen accumulation in lysosomes;
  - slowly progressive skeletal muscle weakness; vacuolated lymphocytes;
  - treated with physiotherapy, high protein diet and enzyme replacement.
- Type III (Forbes-Cori):
  - deficiency in debranching enzyme amylo-1,6-glucosidase;
  - causes milder phenotype of Type I (von Gierke).
- Type V (McArdles's):
  - muscle phosphorylase deficiency;
  - causes exercise intolerance and muscle cramps;
  - patients may have myoglobinuria and a positive standardised non-ischaemic forearm test (measures concentration of lactic acid in the blood before and after local exertion of a muscle group).

Lipid storage diseases

- Classified into:
  - Sphingolipidoses (as they relate to sphingolipid metabolism):
    - Incidence of approximately 1 in 10,000.
    - Include Niemann–Pick disease, Krabbe disease, Gaucher disease, Tay–Sachs disease, metachromatic leukodystrophy, multiple sulfatase deficiency and Farber disease.
    - Includes Fabry disease inherited in an X-linked fashion (➲ see Chapter 16, Fabry disease, p. 581).
    - Fabry disease and Gaucher disease are treated with enzyme replacement therapy, allowing patients to survive to adulthood.

- ◆ Non-sphingolipidoses, including fucosidosis, Schindler disease and Wolman disease.
- Diagnosis may be achieved through clinical assessment, muscle biopsy, genetic testing, molecular analysis of cells or tissues, and enzyme assays.

Urea cycle disorders

The urea cycle converts the neurotoxin ammonia (produced by the deamination of amino acids, gut bacteria, and muscle and renal metabolism) to urea, which can be safely excreted (Figure 1.9). Urea cycle IMDs cause hyperammonaemia, symptoms of which include encephalopathy and lethargy. Normal adult venous ammonia concentration should be <40 μmol/L. Examples of urea cycle IMDs include the X-linked recessive condition, ornithine transcarbamylase (OTC) deficiency (diagnosed by low plasma citrulline, high urinary orotic acid [produced from excess carbamylphosphate] and mutation analysis) and citrullinaemia, caused by argininosuccinic acid synthetase deficiency with raised plasma citrulline and urine orotic acid.

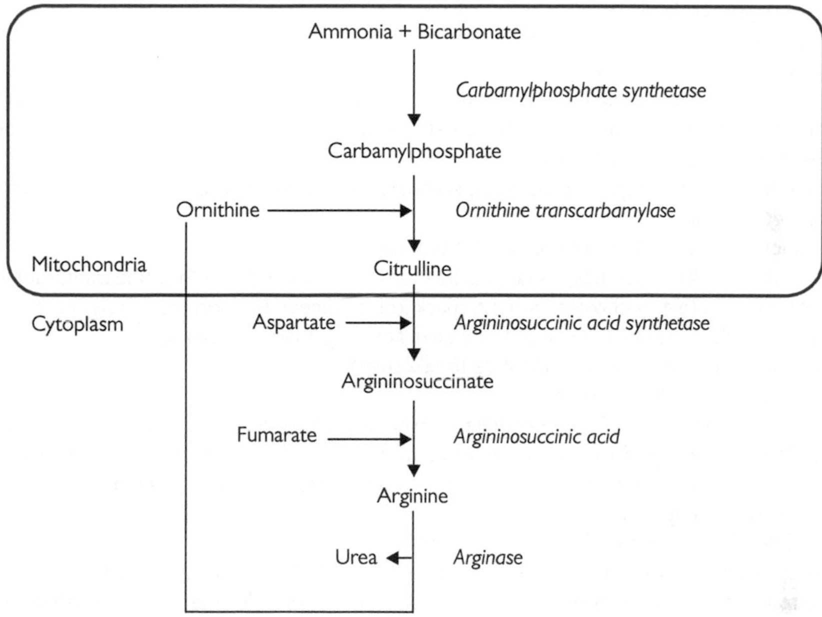

Figure 1.9 Diagram of urea cycle showing major enzymes.

Differential diagnosis of hyperammonaemia

- Urea cycle disorders.
- Organic acidurias (send urine for organic acid analysis).
- Very long chain fatty acid oxidation defects (send blood for carnitine profile).
- Severe liver failure.
- Increased muscle activity.
- Poor phlebotomy technique and delay in the sample reaching the laboratory.

Management of acute hyperammonaemia

- Stop/minimise protein intake (but do not stop for >48 hours).
- Promote anabolism by providing sufficient carbohydrates, e.g. intravenous 10% glucose.
- Correct dehydration, electrolyte and acid-base disturbances.
- Treat any infections/constipation/known precipitants.
- Consider haemofiltration if ammonia level >500 μmol/L.

- Sodium phenylbutyrate and sodium benzoate to help ammonia elimination by encouraging other metabolism routes.
- Arginine and/or citrulline supplementation.

Purine disorders

The purines adenine and guanine are constituents of DNA and RNA, and are both synthesised endogenously and obtained exogenously from the diet. Excretion is via conversion to uric acid (urate). (Males have a slightly lower excretion than females of urate.) Urate has a poor solubility and in excess precipitates out in joints (gout), subcutaneous tissues (gouty tophi, e.g. ears) and the renal system causing calculi. (For the clinical manifestation and management of gout, ➲ see Chapter 20, Gout, p. 713.)

Causes of hyperuricaemia

- Under-excretion (most common):
  - Decreased glomerular filtration:
    - in hypothyroidism and lead toxicity.
  - Decreased renal tubular secretion:
    - in patients with acidosis, e.g. diabetic ketoacidosis, ethanol or salicylate intoxication, starvation ketosis;
      - organic acids accumulating in these conditions compete with urate for tubular secretion.
  - Increased renal tubular reabsorption:
    - with anti-uricosuric drugs, e.g. diuretics, salicylate, ciclosporin, pyrazinamide, ethambutol;
    - in diabetes insipidus.
- Overproduction (accounts for a minority of patients):
  - Exogenous (diet rich in purines): offal (e.g. liver, kidneys, heart); game (e.g. pheasant, rabbit, venison); oily fish (e.g. anchovies, herring, mackerel, sardines); seafood (especially mussels, crab, shrimps and other shellfish); meat and yeast extracts (e.g. Marmite, Bovril).
  - Endogenous (increased purine nucleotide breakdown):
    - Due to enzymatic defects such as:
      - Complete deficiency of hypoxanthine guanine phosphoribosyltransferase (HGPRT) (which facilitates recycling of hypoxanthine into purine nucleotides) in Lesch–Nyhan syndrome (X-linked recessive condition with gout, renal calculi, motor retardation, self-mutilation, spasticity and choreoathetosis).
    - Partial deficiency of HGPRT in Kelley–Seegmiller syndrome.
    - Increased 5-phospho-alpha-d-ribosyl pyrophosphate (PRPP) synthetase activity.
    - Due to rapid cell proliferation and turnover, e.g. blast crisis of leukaemia; cell death in rhabdomyolysis and after cytotoxic therapy (tumour lysis syndrome), severe exfoliative psoriasis.
- Combined mechanisms (under-excretion and overproduction):
  - Most commonly alcohol consumption that results in accelerated hepatic breakdown of ATP and the generation of organic acids that compete with urate for tubular secretion.
  - Enzymatic defects such as glucose-6-phosphatase deficiency (Type I [von Gierke] GSD).

Metalloprotein disorders

Wilson's disease

Wilson's disease is caused by mutations in the ATPase-dependent copper transporter ATP7B that causes reduced biliary excretion of copper and impaired incorporation of copper into caeruloplasmin. Copper accumulates in tissues causing a variety of symptoms, including hepatic dysfunction, Kayser–Fleischer rings at the edge of the cornea, psychosis and basal ganglia degeneration. The clinical features, diagnosis and management of Wilson's disease are discussed in Chapter 15 (➲ see Wilson's disease, p. 540).

Porphyrias

The porphyrias are a group of disorders caused by disorders of haem synthesis (Figure 1.10). Acute intermittent porphyria, hereditary coproporphyria and variegate porphyria are all characterised by episodes of acute symptoms due to elevated aminolaevulinic acid and porphobilinogen concentrations, and have autosomal dominant inheritance with incomplete penetrance (Table 1.4). Of porphyria cutanea tarda cases,

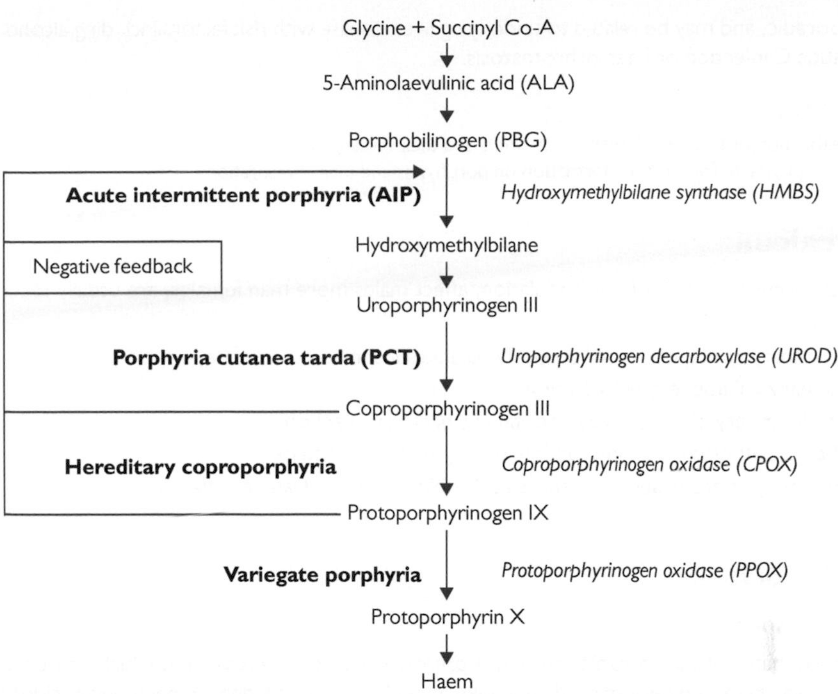

Figure 1.10 Diagram of porphyrin synthesis showing major enzymes.

Table 1.4 Porphyrias: symptoms, investigation and treatment

	Symptoms	Investigation	Treatment
Acute intermittent porphyria (AIP)	Polyneuropathy. Autonomic dysfunction. Abdominal pain. Neuropsychiatric symptoms. Hyponatraemia/syndrome of inappropriate of antidiuretic hormone.	Elevated urinary aminolaevulinic acid (ALA) and porphobilinogen (PBG). Erythrocyte enzyme studies.	Stop precipitating drugs. Haem arginine to suppress haem synthesis. Manage symptoms.
Porphyria cutanea tarda	Photosensitive rash with bullae. Chronic changes include scarring, pigmentary change and milia (small white papules). Hypertrichosis (especially cheeks and forearms).	Urinary and faecal analysis for characteristic porphyrins.	Treat precipitants, e.g. oestrogens, alcohol, iron. Sun cream. Low-dose antimalarials.
Hereditary coproporphyria	Acute symptoms ± photosensitive rash with bullae.	Acutely raised ALA and PBG. Increased faecal coproporphyrin.	As for AIP + sun avoidance.
Variegate porphyria	Acute symptoms ± photosensitive rash with bullae.	Acutely raised ALA and PBG. Increased faecal protoporphyrin.	As for AIP + sun avoidance.

75% are sporadic, and may be related to underlying liver disease with risk factors including alcohol, oestrogens, hepatitis C infection or haemochromatosis.

Further reading

1. www.metbio.net for further information on IMDs and their investigation.
2. https://porphyria.eu for further information on porphyrias and their investigation.

Renal calculi

Renal calculi occur in 5–10% of the population, affect males more than females, are usually recurrent and arise due to:

- A high urinary concentration of a poorly soluble substance, e.g. oxalate, urate.
- Low urinary volume, e.g. dehydration.
- Change in urinary pH, e.g. urease-containing bacterial infection.
- Renal tract pathology, e.g. obstruction, polycystic kidney disease.
- A low urinary concentration of renal calculi inhibitors, e.g. citrate, magnesium.
- IMDs.

Types of renal stones

Calcium phosphate

Calcium phosphate calculi are radiodense and primarily due to hypercalciuria, which can occur due to hypercalcaemia, increased calcium/sodium intake, medullary sponge kidney, renal tubular acidosis, steroid use/Cushing's syndrome, prolonged immobilisation, Paget's disease, excessive vitamin D supplementation and furosemide. Thiazide diuretics can help reduce urinary calcium concentration.

Calcium oxalate

Calcium oxalate calculi are also radiodense and are due to hypercalciuria and/or increased urinary oxalate concentration. Causes of a raised urinary oxalate concentration include high dietary intake (rhubarb, spinach, tea), high absorption (low calcium intake, inflammatory bowel disease) and primary hyperoxaluria. Reducing dietary oxalate, animal protein and salt intake, and increasing calcium intake will reduce urinary oxalate concentration.

Primary hyperoxlauria type I is autosomal recessive and due to an alanine:glyoxalate aminotransferase mutation, which causes excessive oxalate synthesis and hence excretion, causing renal failure and oxalosis (deposition of oxalate in the body tissues). Treatment is by kidney and liver transplantation.

Triple phosphate

Triple (magnesium; ammonium; calcium) phosphate calculi are associated with chronic urinary tract infections with organisms capable of splitting urea, e.g. *Proteus*, which elevate the urinary pH >7.

Uric acid

Uric acid calculi are radiolucent and can be associated with gout or hyperuricaemia. Urinary pH is usually low as this promotes the formation of uric acid stones. Treatment is therefore to alkalinise the urine and provide the xanthine oxidase inhibitor, allopurinol, to reduce uric acid production (➲ see Chapter 20, Gout, p. 713).

Cystine

Cystine calculi are due to cystinuria (➲ see Chapter 16, Cystinuria, p. 563).

Xanthine

Xanthine stones occur in patients with xanthine oxidase deficiency and are a known side effect of allopurinol therapy.

Drug-related stones

Drug-related stones, e.g. with the HIV protease inhibitor, indinavir.

Investigation and management of renal stones

Initial radiological investigation is by plain X-ray, intravenous urogram or spiral CT scan. Acute management is analgesia and hydration. Calculi <5 mm usually pass spontaneously; ultrasonic extracorporeal shock wave lithotripsy is suitable for calculi between 5 mm and 2 cm. Any stone or fragments obtained should be sent for analysis to determine the type of calculi. Basic investigations should be undertaken at least 6 weeks after the episode of renal colic to help prevent recurrence and assign a cause, and include:

- 24-hour urine collection for creatinine, protein, calcium, oxalate, sodium and citrate;
- urine pH;
- microbiology;
- renal stone analysis;
- plasma bone profile, renal profile and urate.

Chronic management to prevent recurrence may include:

- Potassium citrate if urinary citrate concentration is low:
    - causes of decreased citrate include distal renal tubular acidosis, chronic diarrhoea, renal failure, urinary tract infection and thiazide diuretic use.
- Increasing urinary volume.
- Treating the underlying cause, e.g. infection, inflammatory bowel disease.

Further reading

1. Qaseem A, Dallas P, Forciea MA, Starkey M, Denberg TD; Clinical Guidelines Committee of the American College of Physicians. Dietary and pharmacologic management to prevent recurrent nephrolithiasis in adults: a clinical practice guideline from the American College of Physicians. *Ann Intern Med*. 2014 Nov 4;161(9):659–67.

Multiple choice questions

Questions

1. Which of the following is not a feature of parathyroid hormone?
    A. To increase calcium excretion in the urine.
    B. To increase the activation of vitamin D.
    C. To be released in response to a low extracellular calcium concentration.
    D. To be released in response to or a high extracellular phosphate concentration.
    E. To increase phosphate excretion in the urine.
2. What condition can cause hyperphosphataemia?
    A. Diarrhoea.
    B. Hyperparathyroidism.
    C. Malabsorption.
    D. Metabolic acidosis.
    E. Rhabdomyolysis.
3. Which metabolic process is responsible for maintaining blood glucose levels during fasting?
    A. Glycolysis.
    B. Gluconeogenesis.
    C. Krebs' cycle.

D. Oxidative phosphorylation.
E. Urea cycle.

4. What is the most common cause of hypoglycaemia in adults?
A. Hepatic failure.
B. Hypoadrenalism.
C. Indometacin.
D. Insulinoma.
E. Treated diabetes mellitus.

5. Malnutrition is a common and devastating condition. What electrolyte disturbance is common in malnourished people?
A. Hypercalcaemia.
B. Hyperkalaemia.
C. Hypernatraemia.
D. Hyperphosphataemia.
E. Hypokalaemia.

6. A patient presents with abdominal pain and is found to have triglycerides of 45 mmol/L and a glucose level of 10 mmol/L. What is the most effective lipid management strategy for chronic treatment?
A. Statin.
B. Niacin.
C. Ezetimibe.
D. Fibrate.
E. Omega-3 fatty acids.

7. Which of the following is not appropriate management for a patient with recurrent calcium oxalate stones?
A. Reduce dietary sodium intake.
B. Increase fluid intake.
C. Reduce dietary oxalate intake.
D. Reduce dietary calcium intake.
E. Reduce animal protein intake.

Answers

1. A. Parathyroid hormone increases reabsorption of calcium in the distal convoluted tubule. (➲ See Parathyroid hormone and 1,25$(OH)_2$ vitamin D [activated vitamin D], p. 1.)
2. E. Muscle cell lysis causes release of intracellular phosphate; all the other answers are causes of hypophosphataemia. (➲ See Hyperphosphataemia, p. 7 and Hypophosphataemia, p. 8.)
3. B. Gluconeogenesis is the process by which glucose is produced from proteins and fats. (➲ See Carbohydrate metabolism, p. 8.).
4. E. Overtreatment of diabetes mellitus by insulin or sulphonylureas is the most common cause of hypoglycaemia. (➲ See Hypoglycaemia, p.10.)
5. E. Low concentrations of potassium, sodium, magnesium, phosphate and calcium are seen due to diminished intake. (➲ See Protein-energy malnutrition, p. 12.)
6. D. Fibrates show a baseline dependent reduction in triglycerides up to 70% in extreme hypertriglyceridaemia. (➲ See Drugs used in hyperlipidaemia, Table 1.3.)
7. D. Reducing dietary calcium intake will increase oxalate uptake from the gut. (➲ See Renal calculi, p. 34.)

Chapter 2 **Molecular Medicine and Genetics**

Nasir Saeed Mirza and Munir Pirmohamed

Chromosomes: structure, function and analysis

Chromosomes are the physical carriers of genes, consisting of deoxyribonucleic acid (DNA) and associated proteins. They serve two distinct and vital functions:

1. They facilitate and help to regulate the transcription of genes into messenger ribonucleic acid (mRNA), which is then translated into protein.
2. They enable DNA to be replicated and transmitted during cell division to daughter cells.

Human somatic (body) cells are diploid, having two sets of 23 chromosomes, one set derived from the mother and one from the father. Chromosomes are categorised into autosomes and sex chromosomes. Females have two of the same kind of sex chromosome (XX) in their diploid cells, while males have two distinct sex chromosomes (XY). The normal female and male karyotypes are denoted 46,XX and 46,XY, respectively. Gametes (sperm and ovum) are haploid, having one set of 23 chromosomes.

Meiosis

Meiosis produces gametes from a diploid germline cell. Prior to meiosis chromosomes are replicated. This process creates two exact copies from each chromosome, known as sister chromatids, attached at the

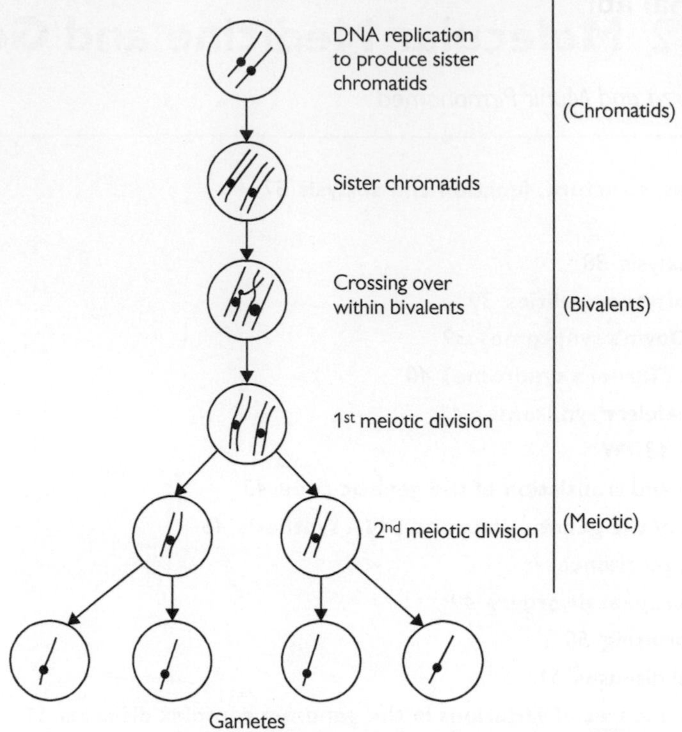

Figure 2.1 The process of genetic recombination and segregation during meiosis.
Reproduced with permission from Wilkins R. *Oxford Handbook of Medical Sciences*, 2nd edn, Oxford, UK: OUP. Copyright © 2011, Oxford University Press. DOI: 10.1093/med/9780199588442.001.0001. Reproduced with permission of the Licensor through PLSclear.

centromere region. During meiosis, each cell undergoes two divisions in sequence to create four gametes (Figure 2.1):

- First division (meiosis I): homologous maternal and paternal chromosomes undergo 'crossing over' (synapsis) to create recombinant chromosomes, which contain a mixture of maternal and paternal DNA. These chromosomes are subsequently separated from each other and segregate randomly into daughter cells.
- Second division (meiosis II): the sister chromatids are separated from each other and, again, segregate randomly into daughter cells (the haploid gametes).

Failure of the maternal and paternal chromosomes or of the sister chromatids to separate from each other during this process may lead to chromosomal abnormalities.

Further reading

1. Cohen PE, Holloway K. 2014. Mammalian Meiosis. In: Plant TM, Zeleznik AJ (Eds) *Knobil and Neill's Physiology of Reproduction*. Cambridge: Academic Press, pp. 5–57.

Karyotype analysis

During karyotype analysis, cells from the patient are examined under a light microscope after applying a stain that creates a characteristic and reproducible light-and-dark band pattern across each chromosome.

- This allows numerical and large structural chromosomal abnormalities to be identified for diagnosis of chromosomal abnormalities, e.g. Down's syndrome.

Chromosomal abnormalities

Chromosomal abnormalities may be numerical or structural.

- Aneuploidy: loss or gain of one chromosome.
- Polyploidy: the addition of a complete haploid.
- Microdeletion: a chromosomal deletion too short to be identified under the light microscope.
- Duplication: a chromosomal anomaly in which more than one copy of a particular chromosomal segment is present within a chromosome set.
- Translocation: a change in position of a chromosomal segment within the genome without leading to a change in the total number of genes present.
- Inversion: a chromosomal anomaly in which a chromosome segment has been turned through 180°.
- Mosaicism: presence of two or more cell lines of different genetic or chromosomal material within one individual.

Trisomy 21 (Down's syndrome)

Down's syndrome affects 1 in 700 live births. It most commonly results from sporadic non-disjunction, resulting in trisomy 21 (three copies of chromosome 21 instead of two copies).

Antenatal screening

Down's syndrome may be detected during antenatal screening (see Box 2.1), but is more commonly diagnosed following clinical observations postnatally and requires confirmatory genetic analysis. Investigations to identify congenital abnormalities are completed in the neonatal period and early childhood.

Box 2.1 Screening for Down's syndrome in pregnancy

All pregnant women in England are offered the first trimester combined screening test for Down's, Edwards' and Patau's syndromes as part of the NHS fetal anomaly screening programme (FASP).

The screening process for these three trisomy abnormalities includes a dating scan at 8–14 weeks of pregnancy, and a blood test (pregnancy-associated plasma protein-A [PAPP-A] and free B-human chorionic gonadotrophin [B-hCG]) and a nuchal translucency (NT) ultrasound scan in the first trimester of pregnancy (normally at 12 weeks). If the first trimester screening was not undertaken, then the second trimester quadruple blood test (alpha-fetoprotein [AFP], B-hCG, inhibin-A, oestriol) is offered between 14 and 20 weeks. It is not as accurate as the combined test. A second trimester ultrasound scan can also check for abnormalities.

The combined test generates two risk scores, one for Down's syndrome, and one for both Edwards' and Patau's syndromes. Pregnant women who are shown to be at a higher risk (>1:150 chance) of carrying a fetus with one of these conditions are offered follow-up diagnostic tests (chorionic villus sampling or amniocentesis). These tests are accurate but invasive and, therefore, carry a small (1:100) risk of miscarriage.

Cell-free fetal DNA testing

This test detects DNA fragments in a maternal blood sample. Most of the DNA fragments are maternal, but some fragments, called cell-free fetal DNA (cffDNA), are from the unborn baby. cffDNA is detectable from around 7 weeks of pregnancy, and the level rises as the pregnancy continues.

cffDNA is a highly sensitive test for Down's syndrome, but it gives rise to false positive results, which may, therefore, incorrectly identify pregnancies as high risk of Down's syndrome. cffDNA testing has not therefore replaced the current diagnostic test used in the FASP.

Data from https://www.gov.uk/guidance/fetal-anomaly-screening-programme-overview

Clinical features

Characteristic craniofacial findings

These include flat facies, hypertelorism, up-slanting palpebral fissure, medial epicanthal folds, hypoplastic nasal bone, depressed nasal bridge, small low-set ears with an overfolded helix, a small mouth with a tendency for tongue protrusion, high-arched palate, dental abnormalities, and a short and broad neck.

General physical features

Physical features include short stature and obesity, short limbs, broad, short hands, feet and digits, short fifth middle phalanx, simian palmar creases, a wide gap between the first and second toes, hypotonia, and joint hyperflexibility.

Other associated conditions

- Nervous system: moderate-to-severe intellectual disability, seizure disorders and Alzheimer's disease.
- Cardiorespiratory: ventricular septal defects and other cardiac defects (see Table 13.52), tracheal stenosis, tracheoesophageal fistula, pulmonary hypertension.
- Other: duodenal atresia, renal malformations, cryptorchidism and hypospadias, refractive errors, strabismus, nystagmus, cataracts, hearing loss (mostly conductive), atlantoaxial instability, scoliosis, atopic or seborrhoeic dermatitis, premature ageing (decreased skin tone, early greying or loss of hair), macrocytosis, leukaemias, hypothyroidism, diabetes, coeliac disease and systemic lupus erythematosus (SLE).

Management

People with Down's syndrome are often well integrated into society and may live largely independently. Specific manifestations should be medically and surgically managed as necessary. Other therapies include physical, occupational and speech therapy.

- Lifestyle and dietary modification may reduce the risk of obesity and diabetes.
- Surgical repair of congenital anomalies (cardiac and gastrointestinal), atlantoaxial subluxation or cataracts may become necessary at different points in life.
- There is earlier onset of age-related health issues; a third have Alzheimer-like dementia after the age of 35 years and patients have a shortened life expectancy with median age of death of 49 years.

Monosomy X (Turner's syndrome)

Turner's syndrome affects 1 in 2500 live-born females. The majority of patients have a 45,X karyotype, secondary to sporadic non-disjunction, a minority are found to have a partial second sex chromosome, X or Y, affected by a translocation or deletion.

Presentation may be:

- In childhood with short stature, or following discovery of an incidental cardiac murmur.
- In adolescence with primary or secondary amenorrhoea or lack of secondary sex characteristics.
- The majority of patients with Turner's syndrome are infertile.

Clinical features include:

- General: excessive numbers of naevi, webbed neck, shield chest (broad chest with widely spaced nipples), cubitus valgus, short fourth and fifth metacarpals and metatarsals, hypoplastic or hyperconvex nails, a low or indistinct hairline, scoliosis, high-arched palate, ptosis, strabismus, amblyopia and cataracts.
- Cardiovascular: hypoplastic left heart, coarctation of the aorta, bicuspid aortic valve, increased risk of aortic dissection and hypertension (➔ see Chapter 5, Case 5, p. 124, and Table 13.52).

- Other: renal anomalies, e.g. horseshoe kidney, hypothyroidism, otosclerosis, lymphoedema, obesity, diabetes mellitus and hyperlipidaemia.
- Reproductive: elevated levels of luteinising hormone (LH) and follicle-stimulating hormone (FSH) confirm ovarian failure.

Monitoring

Tests looking for associated medical conditions should be repeated on a regular basis:

- Four-limb blood pressures (looking for evidence of coarctation).
- Blood tests: urea and creatinine, fasting glucose and lipid levels, thyroid function.
- Scoliosis screening (before reaching adulthood).
- Bone mineral density (after reaching adulthood).
- Renal ultrasonography.
- Cardiac and aortic imaging.
- Audiology.

Management

- Standard medical treatment includes growth hormone therapy and oestrogen replacement.
- Lifestyle and dietary modification may reduce the risk of osteoporosis, hypertension, diabetes and hyperlipidaemia.

Prognosis

- Most women with Turner's syndrome are able to lead normal lives.
- Overall mortality is increased and some deaths can be prevented by management of associated conditions.
- Turner's syndrome is not an inherited disorder. However, rarely, Turner's syndrome caused by an X chromosome deletion may be stable enough to be passed down through the generations and, thus, also allows fertility.

47,XXY (Klinefelter syndrome)

Klinefelter syndrome results from maternal meiotic sporadic non-disjunction. It affects 1 in 700 male births. Patients present in adolescence and early adult life with pubertal delay, gynaecomastia, micro orchidism and infertility.

Clinical features include:

- Musculoskeletal: fifth digit clinodactyly, genu valgum, pes planus, tall stature (with disproportionately long arms and legs), narrowed shoulders, mild hypotonia and decreased muscle mass and strength.
- Sexual: eunuchoid body habitus, a high-pitched voice, sparse or absent facial, axillary, pubic or body hair, erectile dysfunction and decreased libido.
- Cognitive: language impairment and academic difficulty (although most patients have normal intelligence), psychosocial problems.

Other associated conditions

Affected adult men are at higher risk of tumours (breast and germ cells), osteoporosis, diabetes, hypothyroidism and other autoimmune diseases (including SLE, rheumatoid arthritis and Sjögren syndrome), venous insufficiency leading to recurrent leg ulcers, mitral and aortic valve disease, and thromboembolic disease.

Investigation

- Diagnosis is by karyotype analysis.
- Hormonal profile is variable, but may reveal low blood testosterone levels, and elevated blood FSH and LH and urinary gonadotropin levels. The increase in testosterone levels in response to administration of human chorionic gonadotropin is diminished.

- Tests to identify associated medical conditions include fasting glucose levels, bone mineral density test, echocardiography and hypercoagulability screening.

Management

- Testosterone: life-long replacement is required. Testosterone is titrated to symptoms, aiming to maintain age-appropriate blood testosterone levels.
- Lifestyle and dietary modification may reduce the risk of osteoporosis and diabetes.
- Regular breast self-examination is advised due to the increased risk of breast cancer.
- Speech and behavioural therapy may be indicated for language impairment and psychosocial problems, and physical and occupational therapy for motor difficulties.
- Surgical mastectomy can be performed to correct gynaecomastia, which may be a cause of psychological distress in addition to increasing the risk of breast cancer.

Prognosis

- Life expectancy is normal.
- Infertility is almost universal in men affected by Klinefelter syndrome. For parents with a child affected by Klinefelter syndrome, risk of recurrence in a future pregnancy is no greater than in the general population.

For indications for referral to a clinical genetics service, see Box 2.2.

Box 2.2 Indications for referral to a clinical genetics service

Congenital anomalies

- Multiple congenital anomalies.
- Isolated congenital anomaly in conjunction with dysmorphic features, developmental delay, abnormal growth parameters or a family history.

Dysmorphic features

- Especially in conjunction with developmental delay, learning disability, congenital anomaly, abnormal growth parameters.
- A family history suggestive of a recurrent abnormality.

Developmental delay/learning disability

- Unexplained severe developmental delay or learning disability.
- Developmental delay or learning disability in conjunction with dysmorphic features, congenital anomaly, abnormal growth parameters or a family history.

Multiple problems and no diagnosis

- Child with multiple problems and under the care of many specialists with no unifying diagnosis.

New diagnosis of a genetic disorder

- Enables explanation of the genetic basis of the condition.
- Essential if the diagnosis may have implications for other relatives.
- Important if parents would like advice regarding future pregnancies.

Teenager with a genetic disorder

- Patients diagnosed with a genetic disorder in infancy/early childhood should be reviewed by a clinical geneticist in their mid-teens to ensure that they understand the genetic basis of their condition and the risks to any future offspring.

Data from Firth HV, Hurst JA, Hall JG. (2005). *Oxford Desk Reference Clinical Genetics*. Oxford, UK: Oxford University Press.

Further reading

1. Tyler C, Edman JC. Down syndrome, Turner syndrome, and Klinefelter syndrome: primary care throughout the life span. *Prim Care*. 2004; 31(3):627–48, x–xi. https://www.ncbi.nlm.nih.gov/pubmed/15331252. An overview of the healthcare needs for people with the most common chromosomal abnormalities.

Nucleic acids

Nucleic acids are organic compounds that store, transcribe, translate and transmit the genetic code. Nucleic acids are of two types: DNA and RNA.

DNA and the genetic code

Human somatic cells contain two sets of 23 chromosomes. Each chromosome consists of one macromolecule of DNA (and ancillary proteins). Each macromolecule of DNA consists of two polynucleotide chains. Each nucleotide consists of a phosphate group, a sugar residue and a nitrogenous base. In DNA, the sugar is deoxyribose. The nitrogenous bases are of two types – purines and pyrimidines. In DNA, the purine bases are adenine (A) and guanine (G), and the pyrimidine bases are thymine (T) and cytosine (C). The order of the bases determines the genetic code, each sequence (triplet) of three bases coding for one amino acid.

The structure of DNA

- DNA strands have a 5′ to 3′ orientation: each nucleotide added to the strand is attached by the formation of a covalent bond between the 5′ phosphate group of the new nucleotide and the 3′-OH group of the nucleotide to which it is being attached.
- The two strands comprising a molecule of DNA are coiled clockwise around one another to form a double helix.
- The double helix is held together by the hydrogen bonds formed between 'complementary base pairs' facing each other on the two helical DNA chains.
- Base pairing between the chains is specific: bonding occurs between A and T, or between G and C. Due to this strict specificity, the parallel strands must be complementary to one another. Thus, if one strand reads 5′-ATGC-3′, the complementary strand must read 5′-GCAT-3′.

Two anti-parallel strands of DNA are shown in Figure 2.2 and the backbone arrangements of the DNA double helix showing base pairs are shown in Figure 2.3.

RNA

In RNA, the sugar is ribose. RNA contains A, G and C, but contains uracil (U) in place of T.

See Table 2.1 for the key differences between DNA and RNA.

Transcription and translation of the genetic code

- *Transcription* is the first step in the manufacture of proteins in cells. Transcription is the synthesis of RNA on a template of DNA. It is the process by which the information contained in the genetic code is transferred from DNA to messenger RNA (mRNA).
- *Translation* is the process through which the genetic information encoded in mRNA is read or 'translated' into a sequence of amino acids in a polypeptide chain.

Codons

The genetic code in DNA takes the form of a series of triplets of bases. Each triplet of bases codes for one amino acid. The complementary nucleotide triplets in mRNA are termed codons.

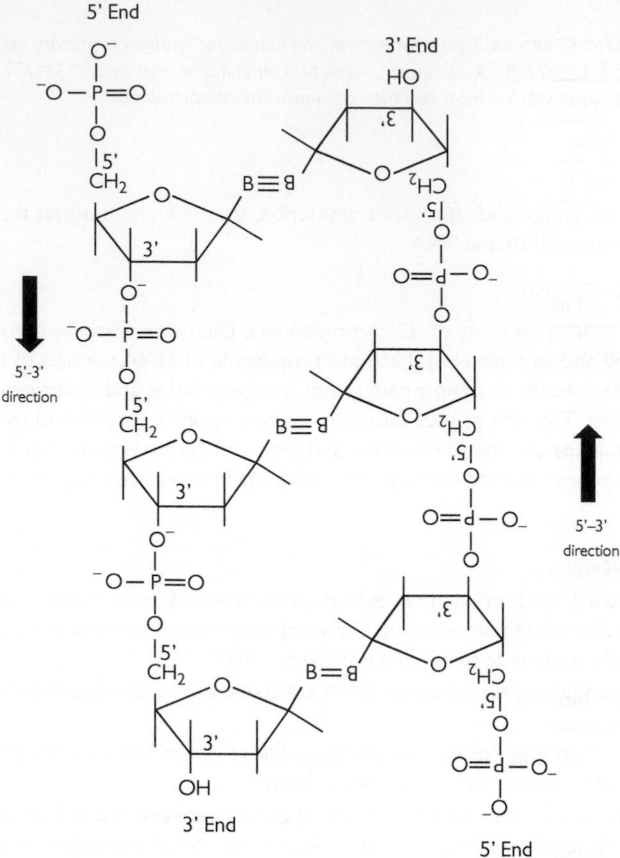

Figure 2.2 Two anti-parallel strands of DNA. B = base.

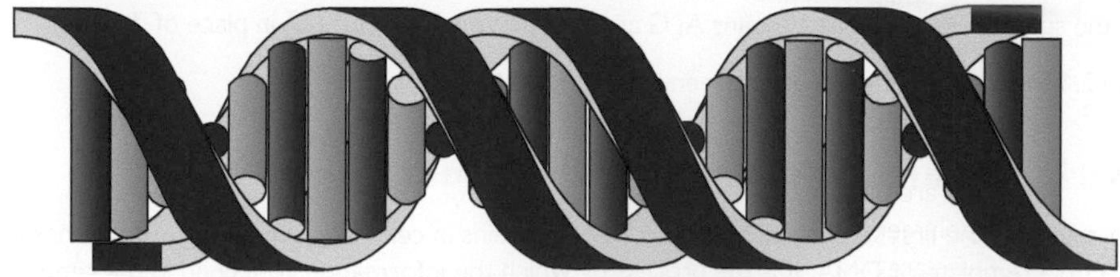

Figure 2.3 Backbone arrangements of DNA double helix showing base pairs in the centre of the helix.

The sequence of these codons is translated into a sequence of amino acids during protein synthesis. Although there are only 20 amino acids, there are 64 ($=4^3$) possible triplet combinations of the four bases present in nucleic acids. Hence, some of the amino acids are coded by more than one codon.

In addition, some codons have other functions. For example, stop codons (UGA, UAA and UAG) signal the termination of the process of translation of an mRNA in protein. Analogously, the start codon, AUG, is the triplet of nucleotides on a messenger RNA molecule at which the process of translation is initiated.

Table 2.1 Key differences between DNA and RNA

DNA	RNA
Found in nucleus (and in small amounts in mitochondria).	Found in nucleus and cytoplasm.
Sugar residue is deoxyribose.	Sugar residue is ribose.
Pyrimidine bases are C and T.	Pyrimidine bases are C and U.
Double-stranded macromolecule.	Single-stranded macromolecule.
Functionally of one type only.	Different types exist: mRNA, tRNA, rRNA, etc.
Responsible for storage and transmission of genetic information.	Responsible for control of translation into protein.

mRNA: messenger RNA; tRNA: transfer RNA; rRNA: ribosomal RNA.

Transcription

During transcription, the RNA is formed on a template comprising only one of the DNA strands: the 'antisense' strand (Figure 2.4).

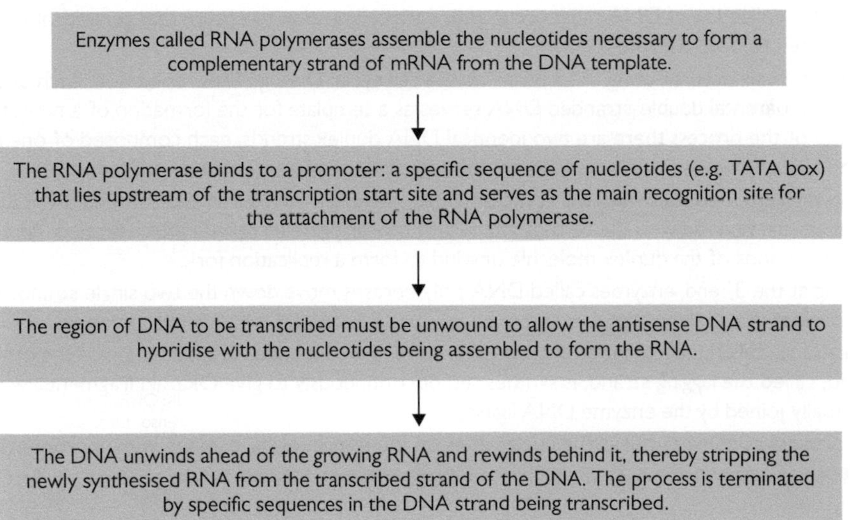

Figure 2.4 Transcription.

Transcription factors are proteins that control the rate of transcription by promoting or blocking the recruitment of RNA polymerases.

In eukaryotes, there are three main types of *RNA polymerase*:

- RNA polymerase II synthesises mRNA (and heterogenous nuclear RNA) and, hence, mediates the transcription process described in Figure 2.4.
- RNA polymerases I and III synthesise ribosomal RNA (rRNA) and transfer RNA (tRNA).

Pre-messenger RNA and post-transcriptional modification

- The primary RNA transcript transcribed from DNA is termed the pre-messenger RNA. It must undergo post-transcriptional modification in the nucleus in order to become a mature mRNA.
- One of the most important of these modifications is RNA splicing: a process in which introns (which are initially transcribed into RNA) are removed and the nucleotide sequences transcribed from non-adjacent DNA segments are then joined together.

Introns are part of the DNA of genes that is not expressed in the polypeptide chains. The process of splicing takes place within a spliceosome.

- The number and size of introns within genes varies greatly; their function is still a matter of debate.
- Other post-transcriptional processing steps include addition of a methylated cap to the 5′ end of the primary transcript, and a poly-A tail to the 3′ end.
- After post-transcriptional modifications are complete, mature mRNA leaves the nucleus.

Translation

Translation is the next stage of protein synthesis. Translation occurs in the cytoplasm and is accomplished in three steps:

1. Initiation: an initiation complex comprising mRNA, ribosome and tRNA is formed.
2. Elongation: the ribosome moves along the mRNA reading each codon in turn. Each codon is recognised by a matching tRNA, which contributes its amino acid to the end of a growing polypeptide chain.
3. Termination: protein synthesis ceases when a stop codon is reached.

Transmission of the genetic code and DNA synthesis

- Accurate replication of DNA must occur with each cell division to ensure that genetic information is transmitted to both daughter cells.
- DNA synthesis occurs during the S phase of the cell cycle. During DNA replication, each of the strands in parental double-stranded DNA serves as a template for the formation of a new strand. At the end of the process there are two identical DNA duplex strands, each composed of one parental strand and one newly synthesised strand; this is termed semi-conservative replication.
- The hydrogen bonds between the complementary bases on the two strands of the parent DNA molecule are severed with the help of a family of motor proteins called DNA helicases. As a result, the two strands of the duplex molecule unwind to form a replication fork.
- Starting at the 3′ end, enzymes called DNA polymerases move down the two single strands linking free nucleotides to their complementary bases on the templates with hydrogen bonds.
- One strand, called the leading strand, is synthesised in a continuous fashion, whereas the other strand, called the lagging strand, is synthesised discontinuously to give Okazaki fragments, which are eventually joined by the enzyme DNA ligase.
- The process continues until all the nucleotides on the templates have joined with appropriate free nucleotides and two identical molecules of DNA have been formed.

Further reading

1. Alberts B, et al. How cells read the genome: from DNA to protein. In: Alberts B (Ed.) *Molecular Biology of the Cell*, 6th edn, pp. 299–369. Garland Science, 2014.
2. Earlier editions of *Molecular Biology of the Cell* can be accessed online:
   - From DNA to RNA https://www.ncbi.nlm.nih.gov/books/NBK26887/
   - From RNA to Protein https://www.ncbi.nlm.nih.gov/books/NBK26829/

Principles of inheritance

Single-gene disorders

- Single-gene disorders occur due to mutations in one or both members of a pair of autosomal genes, or genes on the X or Y chromosomes.
- These disorders exhibit characteristic 'Mendelian' patterns of inheritance: autosomal dominant, autosomal recessive or sex-linked.

For the key terms used to describe patterns of inheritance, see Box 2.3.

Box 2.3 Key terms used to describe patterns of inheritance

Autosomal: the affected gene is on one of the autosomes.
X-linked: the affected gene is on the X chromosome. Females have two copies of the gene, but males only have one.
Y-linked: the affected gene is on the Y chromosome. Males have one copy of the gene; females have none.
Homozygous: the alleles at a given locus on homologous chromosomes are identical.
Heterozygous: the alleles at a given locus on homologous chromosomes are different.
Dominant mutation: a heterozygous individual will exhibit the disease.
Recessive mutation: an individual will only exhibit the disease if both of their alleles contain disease-causing mutations. In consanguineous pedigrees these mutations will typically be homozygous.

Autosomal dominant disorders

Autosomal dominant (AD) disorders are expressed in individuals homozygous or heterozygous for the mutation. AD inheritance typically exhibits the following features:

- Affected individuals have at least one affected parent. The rare exception to this rule is that some affected individuals will possess de novo mutations.
- Males and females are affected in a 1:1 ratio.
- The trait can be passed through either the male or female germline.
- An individual who is homozygous for the mutation is usually more severely affected than an individual who is heterozygous for the mutation.
- Each child that results from the mating between a heterozygous affected individual and an unaffected individual has a 50% probability of being affected.

Penetrance

Penetrance is the proportion of individuals of a specified genotype that show the expected phenotype. A number of clinically significant AD disorders exhibit incomplete penetrance.

An example of a highly penetrant disorder is neurofibromatosis (NF) type 1 – almost all individuals with an *NF1* gene mutation have some phenotypic traits of the syndrome (➲ see Chapter 17, Neurocutaneous syndromes, p. 637).

In contrast, familial breast cancer due to mutations in the *BRCA1* gene is an example of an AD condition showing incomplete penetrance. Females with a mutation in this gene have an approximately 80% lifetime risk of developing breast cancer (➲ see Chapter 10, Factors enabling development of cancer, p. 317).

Expressivity

Variable expressivity refers to the range of signs and symptoms that can occur in different people with the same genetic condition. Even highly penetrant diseases can exhibit variable expressivity. For example, NF type 1 is characterised by highly variable clinical expressivity with marked variation in the number of clinical features (➲ see Chapter 17, Neurocutaneous syndromes, p. 637).

Anticipation

Certain AD disorders exhibit anticipation – the earlier onset and more severe manifestation of the disease in successive generations.

Anticipation occurs in trinucleotide repeat expansion disorders, e.g. Huntington's disease. Although trinucleotide repeat sequences are normally transmitted stably, they can become unstable and expand to pathological lengths. Once the normal length has expanded, the number of repeats tends to increase with each successive generation resulting in anticipation.

For autosomal dominant and X-linked disorders, see Table 2.2.

Table 2.2 Autosomal dominant and X-linked disorders

Disease	Inheritance	Gene
Familial hypercholesterolaemia	Autosomal dominant	*LDLR*, etc.
Familial hypertrophic cardiomyopathy	Autosomal dominant	*MYH7*, etc.
Von Willebrand disease	Autosomal dominant	*VWF*
Adult polycystic kidney disease	Autosomal dominant	*PKD1*
Neurofibromatosis type 1	Autosomal dominant	*NF1*
Marfan syndrome	Autosomal dominant	*FBN1*
Tuberous sclerosis	Autosomal dominant	*TSC1, TSC2*
Myotonic dystrophy	Autosomal dominant	**MD1*
Huntington's disease	Autosomal dominant	**HTT*
Haemophilia A	X-linked recessive	*F8*
Haemophilia B	X-linked recessive	*F9*
Becker muscular dystrophy	X-linked recessive	*DMD*
Duchenne muscular dystrophy	X-linked recessive	*DMD*
Fragile X syndrome	X-linked recessive	*FMR1*
Red–green colour blindness	X-linked recessive	*OPN1LW*
Vitamin D-resistant rickets	X-linked dominant	*PHEX*
Charcot–Marie–Tooth disease, X-linked dominant, 1	X-linked dominant	*GJB1*
Rett syndrome	X-linked dominant	*MECP2*

*Trinucleotide repeat disorder genes.

Autosomal recessive disorders

Autosomal recessive (AR) disorders are only expressed in individuals if both of their alleles contain disease-causing mutations. In the absence of parental consanguinity or being part of a genetically isolated population, the risk to offspring of an affected individual is relatively low.

The probability that the offspring of an affected individual or unaffected carrier will exhibit an AR disorder is dependent on the carrier frequency of the mutation, assuming that the other parent has no family history of the disease.

AR inheritance typically exhibits the following features:

- Affects only one generation of a family. An AR condition will only recur in a successive generation if mating occurs with another affected individual or a gene carrier.
- When both parents are affected, all their offspring will be affected.
- When both parents are heterozygous unaffected carriers of the mutation, each of their children has a 25% probability of being affected (and a 50% probability of being an unaffected carrier).
- The parents of an affected individual may be either affected or unaffected carriers.
- Males and females are affected in a 1:1 ratio.
- The trait can be passed through either the male or the female germline.

Generally, AR disorders are less likely than AD disorders to exhibit incomplete penetrance or variable expressivity.

Table 2.3 shows the AR disorders and carrier frequencies of their respective mutations in Caucasian populations.

Table 2.3 Autosomal recessive disorders and carrier frequencies of their respective mutations in Caucasian populations

Disease	**Gene**	**Carrier frequency**
Cystic fibrosis	*CFTR*	1/25
Haemochromatosis	*HFE*	1/10
α-1 antitrypsin deficiency	*SERPINA1*	1/50
Spinal muscular atrophy	*SM1*	1/50

Sex-linked diseases

Sex-linked diseases are caused by mutations in genes found on one of the sex chromosomes. Since the human Y chromosome contains a small number of genes that are related to sex determination and spermatogenesis, Y-linked diseases of clinical significance are rare.

X-linked recessive disorders typically exhibit the following features:

- Males are predominantly affected.
- There is no male-to-male transmission.
- Affected males inherit the mutant allele from their mother.
- If a carrier female mates with an unaffected male, each son has a 50% chance of being affected, and each daughter has a 50% chance of being a carrier and a 50% chance of being mutation-free.
- Mating between an affected male and a mutation-free female produces no affected offspring, but all daughters are carriers.
- If a carrier female mates with an affected male, 50% of both male and female offspring will be affected.

X-linked dominant (XLD) diseases are rare. They typically exhibit the following features:

- Both males and females are affected, but males are often more severely affected than females, as females possess a normal copy of the gene on the other X chromosome.
- There is no male-to-male transmission.
- If a heterozygous affected female mates with an unaffected male, each child has a 50% probability of being affected.

Further reading

1. A historic perspective on the experiments performed by Gregor Mendel (1822–1884) that established Mendelian patterns of inheritance described above. Griffiths AJF, Miller JH, Suzuki DT (Eds). *An Introduction to Genetic Analysis*. New York: W.H. Freeman, 2000. https://www.ncbi.nlm.nih.gov/books/NBK22098/
2. Online Mendelian Inheritance in Man (OMIM)®, An Online Catalog of Human Genes and Genetic Disorders, a database of genetic disorders, and the relevant genes and patterns of inheritance. https://www.omim.org/

Trinucleotide repeat disorders

Although polymorphic trinucleotide repeat sequences are abundant in the human genome, only a subset is associated with disease.

Expansion of trinucleotide repeat sequences lead to a number of disorders, including fragile X type A syndrome (FRAXA), Friedreich ataxia (FRDA), Huntington disease (HD), myotonic dystrophy (MD), and several spinocerebellar ataxias (SCA) (Table 2.4).

Key points

- Expanded trinucleotide repeats are unstable, changing in size when transmitted to successive generations. Disease severity correlates with the repeat length.

- The diseases frequently exhibit anticipation.
- Parent-of-origin effects are also common. For example, with maternal transmission, the trinucleotide repeat sequence expansion is greater, resulting in more severe anticipation in MD and fragile X syndrome.

Trinucleotide repeat diseases fall into two broad groups:

1. Degenerative disorders of the nervous system caused by *CAG repeat expansions* that encode polyglutamine tracts in the disease gene protein. This leads to a gain of function that is particularly deleterious to neurons. Diseases within this first group include HD and SCA1.
2. Multisystem disorders (with neurological features) caused by *non-CAG repeats outside the protein-coding region*, which alter expression of the gene. These include MD and FRAXA.

Table 2.4 Features of trinucleotide repeat disorders

Disorder	Inheritance	Gene	Repeat	Normal repeat number	Mutation range
Fragile X syndrome	XLD	FMR1	CGG	6–52	60–200
Friedreich ataxia	AR	FRDA1	GAA	6–34	112– >1700
Huntington disease	AD	HD	CAG	11–34	36–121
Myotonic dystrophy	AD	DMPK	CTG	5–37	50– >3000
Spinocerebellar ataxia type 1	AD	SCA1	CAG	6–39	41–81

Although the majority of dynamic mutations are expansions of trinucleotide repeats, some involve other sequences such as tetranucleotide repeats (CCTG) in MD type 2, pentanucleotide repeats (ATTCT) in SCA10, and dodecamer repeats (C4GC4GCG) in progressive myoclonus epilepsy 1.

Further reading

1. Zoghbi HY. Trinucleotide repeat disorders. In: Runge MS, Patterson C. (Eds) *Principles of Molecular Medicine*. Totowa, NJ: Humana Press, 2006, pp 1114–22. https://link.springer.com/chapter/10.1007%2F978-1-59259-963-9_116

Genomic imprinting

- Genomic imprinting is a form of epigenetic control of gene expression in which one allele of a gene is preferentially expressed according to the parent-of-origin of the allele.
- Some imprinted genes are expressed from the paternally inherited allele and others from the maternally inherited allele. Although imprinted genes represent a small fraction of the human genome, they are vital for normal development and function.
- The normal expression of imprinted genes can be disrupted by different types of mutations and epimutations: uniparental disomy (the inheritance of both chromosomal homologues from the same parent), chromosomal rearrangements (deletions, duplications, translocations), intragenic point mutations in imprinted genes, and epimutations (aberrant methylation without alteration of the genomic DNA sequence).
- Disruption of imprinting can result in a number of human imprinting disorders, the most prominent being Prader–Willi syndrome (PWS) and Angelman syndrome (AS). Both diseases are caused by (epi)mutations in 15q11–13.
- Loss of expression of paternally inherited genes within the 15q11–13 region causes PWS, while altered maternal expression of a gene within the 15q11–13 region causes AS. Both disorders are associated with mental retardation, but further clinical features differ. Features of PWS include hyperphagia, obesity, hypogonadism, short stature and behavioural problems. Features of AS include microcephaly, ataxia and seizures.

Further reading

1. Carlberg C, Molnár F. Genomic Imprinting. In: Carlberg C, Molnár F. (Eds) *Mechanisms of Gene Regulation*, 2016, pp. 147–58. Dordrecht: Springer.

Mitochondrial diseases

- Mitochondrial function is under dual genetic control by:
  - mitochondrial DNA contained within mitochondria encoding 37 proteins;
  - nuclear DNA contained within the nucleus encoding the remaining ~1300 proteins of the mitoproteome.
- Mitochondrial dysfunction can arise from defects in either mitochondrial DNA or nuclear DNA-encoded genes. As with nuclear DNA, mitochondrial DNA mutations can be inherited or occur de novo during embryonic development (somatic mutations).
- Point mutations and large-scale deletions are the two most common kinds of mitochondrial DNA mutations, the former usually being maternally inherited and the latter typically occurring de novo.
- Unlike nuclear DNA, which is diploid and follows Mendelian laws of inheritance, mitochondrial DNA is exclusively maternally transmitted.
- Clinical manifestations can arise in childhood or adulthood, and can affect one organ in isolation or be multisystemic.
- Owing to its high energy requirements, muscle is frequently affected; neurological symptoms are also particularly common. Examples of diseases caused by mitochondrial DNA deletions include chronic progressive external ophthalmoplegia and Kearns Sayre syndrome (see Table 18.4).

Further reading

1. Schapira AH. Mitochondrial diseases. *Lancet* 2012; 379(9828): 1825–34.

Clinical consequences of variations in the genome: complex diseases

Estimating the genetic contribution to complex diseases

Most common disorders (for example, cancer, cardiovascular disease, diabetes and Alzheimer's disease) are complex genetic diseases: while they do not exhibit Mendelian patterns of inheritance, genetic factors do play an important role in determining an individual's susceptibility.

Evidence of a genetic contribution to these diseases comes from the observation of an increased risk of the disorders in relatives of those affected. However, some of the increased risk in relatives is also likely to reflect shared environmental factors.

Concordance for complex genetic diseases is ~60% in monozygotic twins and ~10% in dizygotic twins, highlighting the role of both environmental and genetic factors in the development of these disorders.

Heritability

Heritability quantifies the proportion of variance of liability to disease attributable to inherited genetic factors. The risks of disease to relatives are used to estimate heritability. Unlike single-gene Mendelian disorders, each individual susceptibility allele makes a small contribution to the individual's overall risk of developing a complex disorder. Each affected individual possesses hundreds, perhaps thousands, of such disease-risk variants, which additively contribute to risk for the disease.

Candidate-gene and genome-wide association studies

Candidate gene approach

Historically, association studies for detecting alleles conferring increased risk of a complex genetic disease have adopted the 'candidate gene' approach. This involves examining polymorphisms in genes thought to be involved in the pathogenesis of the disease.

Polymorphisms to be tested are selected on the basis of:

- Being effective proxies for unselected (potentially, as yet, unidentified) disease-causing polymorphisms because of linkage disequilibrium. Linkage disequilibrium occurs when two or more sections of DNA tend to segregate and be inherited together due to close proximity within the genome.
- Their ability to effect levels of mRNA expression or the structure of the protein product.

Finally, the polymorphisms are tested for disease association by comparing their frequency of occurrence in patients with the disease and in control subjects without the disease.

Advantages and disadvantages of candidate gene studies

The advantages of candidate gene studies are that they are relatively cheap and quick to perform. The major disadvantage of the candidate gene approach is that *a priori* knowledge of the pathogenesis of the disease is required. If the molecular mechanism is poorly understood, the wrong genes can be selected for study, leading to negative or spurious results.

Genome-wide association study

The genome-wide association study (GWAS) is a comprehensive unbiased hypothesis-generating strategy in which common genetic variants across the entire genome are simultaneously analysed using high-throughput genotyping platforms, and then tested for association with the disease.

Advantages and disadvantages of GWAS

In contrast to candidate gene studies, no prior knowledge of disease pathogenesis is required. Hence, GWAS provides the potential of identifying genes not previously suspected of causing the disease and has provided novel insights into the aetiology of numerous diseases. One drawback of GWAS is that it carries a very high 'multiple testing burden' due to the large number of statistical tests conducted (at least 500,000 genetic variants are tested for association). To overcome this multiple-testing burden, very large sample sizes are required for GWAS in most complex genetic phenotypes.

Although candidate gene and GWAS analyses have been performed in numerous clinical phenotypes, most results that have been translated into clinical practice to date have been in the area of pharmacogenetics (see Table 3.17).

Further reading

1. Schork NJ, Murray SS, Frazer KA, Topol EJ. Common vs. rare allele hypotheses for complex diseases. *Curr Opin Genet Dev*. 2009; 19(3):212–19.
2. Bush WS, Moore JH. (2012). Chapter 11: Genome-wide association studies. *PLoS Comput Biol*. 2012; 8(12):e1002822.
3. A curated collection of all published genome-wide association studies: The NHGRI-EBI GWAS Catalog. https://www.ebi.ac.uk/gwas/

Cancer genetics

Oncogenes and tumour suppressor genes

- An oncogene is a type of cancer gene that is a mutated form of a normal cellular gene called a proto-oncogene.
- Proto-oncogenes encode proteins that promote cell proliferation, for example, growth factors, growth-factor receptors, nuclear factors regulating gene expression proteins and protein kinases.

- Proteins encoded by oncogenes characteristically exhibit a higher level of activity than the protein products of the corresponding non-mutated proto-oncogene. In turn, increased activity of these protein products leads to accelerated cell proliferation characteristic of cancer.
- Examples of oncogenes include *Myc*, which is implicated in some cases of Burkitt's lymphoma, and *BCL2*, which is implicated in some cases of follicular lymphoma.
- Tumour suppressor genes encode proteins that suppress uncontrolled cell proliferation. In contrast to proto-oncogenes, where mutations causing increased activity promote carcinogenesis, loss-of-function mutations in tumour suppressor genes increase cancer susceptibility. Examples of tumour suppressor genes include *RB1*, which is implicated in some cases of retinoblastoma, and the *TP53* gene, which is associated with a number of cancers.

Genetic cancer syndromes and screening

- Most cancers result from the accumulation of somatic mutations of small effect in multiple genes. However, ~5% of cancers are attributable to single-gene germline mutations of major effect that follow a Mendelian pattern of inheritance that, in most cases, is autosomal dominant with incomplete penetrance.
- In such cases, there is a substantial risk of cancer occurrence in relatives. Unaffected members of these families should be considered for specialist genetic counselling followed by genetic testing, which, if positive, prompts clinical surveillance and, in some cases, prophylactic treatment.

For important hereditary cancer syndromes, see Table 2.5.

Table 2.5 Important hereditary cancer syndromes

Syndrome	Associated genes	Related cancer types
Hereditary breast cancer and ovarian cancer	*BRCA1*, *BRCA2*	Female breast and ovarian cancers, male breast and prostate cancers (see Tables 10.2 and 10.5).
Li–Fraumeni syndrome	*TP53*	Multiple cancers including breast cancer, soft tissue sarcoma, osteosarcoma, leukaemia, brain tumours, adrenocortical carcinoma (➲ see Chapter 10, Hallmarks of cancer, p. 315).
Cowden syndrome	*PTEN*	Hamartomas and multiple cancers, including breast, thyroid and endometrial.
Lynch syndrome	*MSH2*, *MLH1*, *MSH6*, *PMS2*, *EPCAM*	Colorectal, endometrial, ovarian, renal pelvis, pancreatic, small intestine, liver and biliary tract, stomach, brain and breast cancers (see Table 10.2).
Familial adenomatous polyposis	*APC*	Multiple non-malignant colon polyps and cancers of the colon and rectum and, less frequently, of small intestine, brain, stomach, bone, skin and other tissues.
Retinoblastoma	*RB1*	Retinoblastoma, pinealoma, osteosarcoma, melanoma and soft tissue sarcoma (➲ see Chapter 10, Hallmarks of cancer, p. 315).
Multiple endocrine neoplasia type 1	*MEN1*	Usually benign pancreatic endocrine, parathyroid and pituitary gland tumours (➲ see Chapter 19, MEN1, p. 700).
Multiple endocrine neoplasia type 2	*RET*	Medullary thyroid carcinoma, pheochromocytoma, parathyroid adenoma (➲ see Chapter 19, MEN2, p. 701).
Von Hippel–Lindau syndrome	*VHL*	Multiple malignant and benign neoplasms, most frequently retinal, cerebellar and spinal haemangioblastoma, renal cell carcinoma, phaeochromocytoma and pancreatic tumours (➲ see Chapter 17, Neurocutaneous syndromes, p. 637).

Further reading

1. Ruddon RW. 2003. What makes a cancer cell a cancer cell? In: Kufe DW, Pollock RE, Weichselbaum RR, et al. (Eds), *Holland-Frei Cancer Medicine*, 2003. Hamilton (ON), BC: Decker. https://www.ncbi.nlm.nih.gov/books/NBK12516/

Principles of pharmacogenetics

- Genetic factors contribute to the large variability in drug response (both efficacy and toxicity) between different patients treated with the same drugs for the same disease.
- Adverse drug reactions (ADRs) represent a huge burden on the health-care system, costing £1 billion per year in the United Kingdom. It is estimated that up to 10–20% of adverse drug reactions may be wholly or partly due to genetic factors.
- To improve the personalisation of medicine, it will be important to identify these genetic variables to ensure that each patient receives the right drug at the right time at the right dose for the right disease. Some genetic factors have been identified and incorporated into clinical practice.
- The genetic contribution to the variation in the efficacy of the same drug from patient-to-patient is typified by asthma and the response to β2 agonists. Up to 50% of patients may not benefit optimally from these agents, with approximately 60% of the variability in treatment response being heritable.
- Genetic factors can affect both drug pharmacokinetics (absorption, bioavailability, distribution, metabolism and excretion) and drug pharmacodynamics (function of the drug target).
- Progress in pharmacogenetics has focused largely on pharmacokinetic sources of variation. Twin studies have shown that genetic factors are the main determinants of the inter-individual variation in the metabolism of a number of drugs, for example, phenytoin and phenylbutazone. One of the most extensively studied pharmacogenes is the cytochrome P450 enzyme CYP2D6, which is responsible for the metabolism of 25% of drugs. Allelic variants in the *CYP2D6* gene can cause complete loss of enzyme activity or, conversely, can lead to an increase in enzyme activity.

Further reading

1. Alfirevic A, Pirmohamed M. Genomics of adverse drug reactions. *Trends Pharmacol Sci*. 2017; 38(1):100–9.
2. Collins SL, Carr DF, Piromohamed M. Advances in the pharmacogenomics of adverse drug reactions. *Drug Saf.* 2016; 39(1):15–27.
3. Lonergan M, Senn SJ, et al. Defining drug response for stratified medicine. *Drug Discov Today* 2017; 22(1):173–9.

Immunogenetics and HLA-associated diseases

➲ See Chapter 6, Aetiology of autoimmunity, p. 165 and HLA molecules, p. 171.

Further reading (for Chapter 2)

1. Passarge E. *Color Atlas of Genetics*. Stuttgart: Thieme, 2013.
2. Rimoin DL, Pyeritz PE, Korf BR, Emery AEH. *Emery and Rimoin's Essential Medical Genetics*. Amsterdam: Elsevier/Academic Press, 2013.
3. Sweet KM, Michaelis RC. *The Busy Physician's Guide to Genetics, Genomics and Personalized Medicine*. Dordrecht: Springer, 2011.

Multiple choice questions

Questions

1. Which of the following gene and cancer syndrome associations is incorrect:
   A. *MEN1* and multiple endocrine neoplasia type 1.
   B. *MEN2* and multiple endocrine neoplasia type 2.

C. *VHL* and von Hippel–Lindau syndrome.
D. *TP53* and Li–Fraumeni syndrome.
E. *PTEN* and Cowden syndrome.

2. Which of the following disorders is caused by monosomy X:
   A. Down's syndrome.
   B. Klinefelter syndrome.
   C. Turner's syndrome.
   D. Angelman syndrome.
   E. Williams syndrome.
3. The following is incorrect in relation to X-linked recessive disorders:
   A. Males are predominantly affected.
   B. There is no male-to-male transmission.
   C. Affected males inherit the mutant allele from the mother only.
   D. If a carrier female mates with an unaffected male, each son has a 25% chance of being affected.
   E. A mating between an affected male and a mutation-free female produces no affected offspring, but all daughters are carriers.
4. Which of the following enzymes is required for transcription in human cells:
   A. Reverse transcriptase.
   B. DNA helicase.
   C. DNA ligase.
   D. DNA polymerase.
   E. RNA polymerase II.
5. In the DNA double helix, if a sequence of bases on one strand is 5′-ATGC-3′, the complementary sequence on the other stand must read:
   A. 5′-GCAT-3′.
   B. 5′-ATGC-3′.
   C. 5′-CGTA-3′.
   D. 5′-TACG-3′.
   E. 5′-GCTA-3′.

Answers

1. B. MEN2 is associated with the *RET* gene (➲ see Table 2.5).
2. C. The majority of patients with Turner's syndrome have a 45,X karyotype (➲ see Monosomy X (Turner's syndrome), p. 40).
3. D. The risk is 50% as half of her offspring will inherit her affected X chromosome (➲ see Sex-linked diseases, p. 49).
4. E. RNA polymerase II synthesises mRNA and mediates the transcription process (➲ see Transcription, p. 45).
5. A. Complementary DNA strands are coded in opposing directions, i.e. the 5′ end of one strand is paired with the 3′ end of the complementary strand (➲ see DNA and the genetic code, p. 43, and Figures 2.2 and 2.3).

Chapter 3 **Clinical Pharmacology and Toxicology**

Andrew Webb and John Archer**

Clinical pharmacology

Clinical pharmacology is about the **DRUG** (**D**evelopment, **R**egulation, **U**se and **G**eneration [of new drugs])[1] and the patient/population (and the interactions between them). A framework for prescribing principles is '**BRAINS** & **AIMS**' (**B**enefits, **R**isks, **A**dverse effects, **I**nteractions, **N**ecessary prophylaxis, **S**usceptibilities; **A**dministering, **I**nforming, **M**onitoring and **S**topping)'.[2] Thus, the clinical pharmacology section of this chapter has been organised under these headings.

Benefits

A drug should not be prescribed unless the patient is likely to benefit, taking into account the evidence base/ guidelines available (Tables 3.1 and 3.2) (➲ see Chapter 4, Preclinical and clinical phases of drug development, p. 102). Indeed, one should select the most **A**ppropriate **D**rugs **A**nd **P**atient-**T**ailor them (**ADAPT**).[3]

Table 3.1 Levels of evidence for benefits of drugs

Level of evidence	Multiple RCTs/meta-analyses			Single RCT/controlled non-randomised or observational studies		Uncontrolled clinical observations (e.g. case series)
	Design and execution	**Representative of population**	**Estimate of effect**	**Design and execution**	**Estimate of effect**	**Estimate of effect**
A: High	Good	Yes	High certainty			
B: Moderate	Minor limitations	Minor limitations	Moderate certainty	Good	Moderate certainty	
C: Low	Major limitations	Major limitations	Low certainty	Major limitations	Low certainty	Low certainty

RCT = randomised controlled trial.
Data from 'Grading of Recommendations Assessment, Development and Evaluation (GRADE) toolbox' developed by the international GRADE working group (http://www.gradeworkinggroup.org/).

* Andrew Webb wrote the Clinical Pharmacology section and John Archer wrote the Toxicology section.

[1] © Andrew Webb 2008 (original mnemonic).

[2] © Andrew Webb and Sabih Huq 2005 (original mnemonic).

[3] © Andrew Webb 2014 (original mnemonic).

Table 3.2 Classes of recommendations for committees developing clinical practice guidelines

Class of recommendation	Definition	Suggested wording to use
Class I	Evidence and/or general agreement that a given treatment or procedure is beneficial, useful and effective.	Is recommended/is indicated.
Class IIa	Weight of evidence/opinion is in favour of usefulness/efficacy.	Is reasonable to administer treatment.
Class IIb	Usefulness/efficacy is less well established by evidence/opinion.	May be considered.
Class III	Evidence or general agreement that the given treatment or procedure is not useful/effective, and in some cases may be harmful.	Is not recommended.

Adapted from 'Recommendations for Guidelines Production, A document for Task Force Members Responsible for the Production and Updating of ESC Guidelines, Committee for Practice Guidelines (CPG) of the European Society of Cardiology (ESC)' Copyright © 2010 European Society of Cardiology. https://www.escardio.org/static_file/Escardio/Guidelines/ESC%20Guidelines%20for%20Guidelines%20Update%202010.pdf

Mechanisms of drug action

Drugs may act at many sites:

- Outside the cell:
  - chemical, e.g. antacids;
  - osmosis, e.g. purgatives.
- On the cell membrane:
  - receptors, e.g. β-blockers;
  - ion channels, e.g. calcium channel blockers (CCBs);
  - enzymes and pumps, e.g. digoxin, selective serotonin re-uptake inhibitors (SSRIs);
  - physicochemical, e.g. anaesthetic agents.
- Within the cell:
  - enzyme inhibition, e.g. monoamine oxidase inhibitors (MAOIs);
  - transport, e.g. probenecid;
  - substitution, e.g. 5-fluorouracil;
  - metabolism, e.g. trimethoprim.

It is also important to 'think beyond the receptor' and consider a whole body/systems biology approach. The body often tries to react with counter-regulatory mechanisms to maintain homeostasis, e.g. increasing renin (and thus the activity of the renin-angiotensin-aldosterone system) in response to a diuretic used for hypertension, which limits the effectiveness of the diuretic. In addition, the acute and chronic effects of drugs may be opposite (paradoxical pharmacology), e.g. β-blockers acutely have negative inotropic effects, but by starting carefully with low doses, they result in a chronic effect that is opposite, with improved cardiac ejection fraction. Some drugs also lose their effect with prolonged or repeated exposure, e.g. downregulation/internalisation of β_2-adrenoceptors (by β-arrestin) with overuse of salbutamol leading to a loss of effect; tolerance to nitrovasodilators (with loss of anti-anginal/antihypertensive effects) due in part to a supersensitivity to vasoconstrictors secondary to a tonic activation of protein kinase C (PKC) and inhibition of the bioactivation of nitrates.

Drug targets

Receptors

For receptor types, see Table 3.3 and for G-protein coupled receptor (GPCR) signalling, see Figure 3.1.

Table 3.3 Receptor types

Receptor	Description/mechanism	Examples
Type 1: Ligand-gated ion channel	Ion channel coupled to a membrane receptor – direct signalling.	Nicotinic ACh receptor; $GABA_A$ receptor.
Type 2: GPCR	7-transmembrane helix. Activated by a ligand that creates a conformational change that is transmitted to the bound Gα subunit of the coupled heterotrimeric G protein (containing α, β and γ subunits) via protein domain dynamics. The activated Gα subunit exchanges GTP in place of GDP which in turn triggers the dissociation of the Gα subunit from the Gβγ dimer and from the receptor. The dissociated Gα and Gβγ subunits interact with other intracellular proteins to continue the signal transduction cascade, while the freed GPCR is able to rebind to another heterotrimeric G protein to form a new complex that is ready to initiate another round of signal transduction. (GPCR coupling to G proteins is blocked by arrestin proteins that bind to the cytoplasmic face of the receptor [occluding the binding site for the heterotrimeric G-protein preventing its activation] and promote receptor internalisation). Signal via second messengers: α-subunit: adenylate cyclase-cAMP-PKA (Figure 3.1); phospholipase C-inositol tri-phosphate-↑Ca^{2+}/ diacylglycerol-↑PKC. βγ-subunit: K^+-channels; voltage-gated Ca^{2+} channels; GRKs; MAPKs.	Group A: rhodopsin-like, e.g. muscarinic ACh receptor; β-adrenoceptor. Group B: secretin receptor family, e.g. glucagon receptor. Group C: metabotropic glutamate receptor.
Type 3: Kinase-linked receptor	Single transmembrane helix. Directly links extracellular receptor to intracellular kinase domain/cascade: e.g. Ras/Raf/MAP kinase pathway; Jak/Stat pathway.	Receptor tyrosine kinase, e.g. epidermal growth factor receptor; nerve growth factor receptor. Receptor serine/threonine kinase, e.g. insulin receptor, TGF receptor.
Type 4: Nuclear receptors	Type I: cytosolic – ligand binds and translocates to the nucleus where it binds to HREs resulting in transactivation or transrepression of genes. Type II: nuclear – ligand forms a heterodimer with a receptor to effect gene transcription.	Type I: Steroid hormone receptor, e.g. cortisol receptor (glucocorticoid), spironolactone receptor (mineralcorticoid), oestrogen receptor, progesterone receptor; constitutive androstane receptor; pregnane X receptor. Type II: Retinoic acid receptor, PPAR for pioglitazone and fibrates.

ACh = acetylcholine; cAMP = cyclic adenosine monophosphate; GABA = gamma-aminobutyric acid; GDP = guanosine diphosphate; GPCR = G-protein coupled receptor; GRK = G-protein coupled receptor kinase; GTP = guanosine triphosphate; HREs = hormone response elements; Jak = janus kinase; MAPK = mitogen-activated protein kinase; PKA = protein kinase A; PPAR = peroxisome proliferator-activated receptor; Raf = rapidly accelerated fibrosarcoma; Ras = rat sarcoma; Stat = signal transducer and activator of transcription; TGF = transforming growth factor.
Data from *Rang and Dale's Pharmacology*, Seventh Edition, Elsevier, Section 1, Chapter 3.

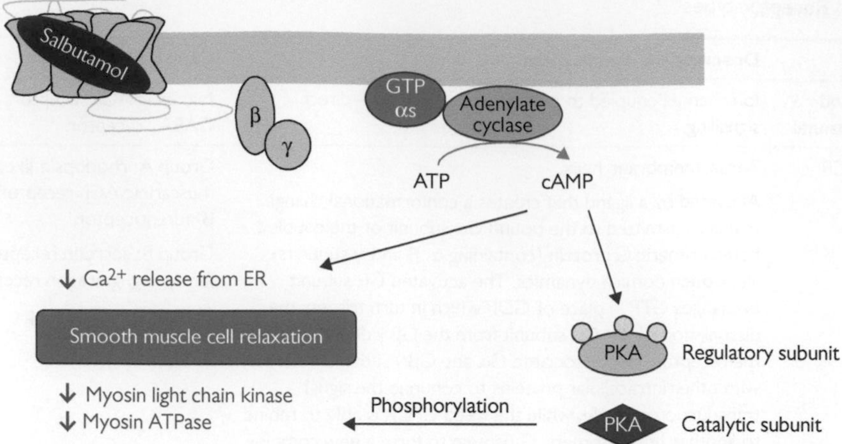

Figure 3.1 G-protein coupled receptor signalling (using lung β2-adrenoceptor as an example). Salbutamol binds to its domain within the GPCR and causes dissociation of the stimulatory G protein (Gs). The αs subunit activates adenylyl cyclase, increasing conversion of adenosine triphosphate (ATP) to the second messenger cAMP. cAMP binds to the regulatory subunit of PKA, resulting in the dissociation/activation of the catalytic subunit, which results in the phosphorylation of key regulatory proteins involved in the control of muscle tone, such as myosin light chain kinase. cAMP also results in inhibition of calcium ion (Ca^{2+}) release from intracellular stores (endoplasmic reticulum [ER]), reduction of membrane Ca^{2+} entry, and sequestration of intracellular Ca^{2+}, leading to relaxation of airway smooth muscle.

Nomenclature

- Affinity refers to the tendency of a drug to bind to a receptor that determines the occupancy of the receptor at a given concentration of the drug:
  - Affinity constant is the ratio of rate of association of the drug to the receptor (k_{+1}):rate of dissociation of the drug from receptor (k_{-1}).
- Intrinsic efficacy (receptor activation):
  - Most GPCRs have constitutive activity (at any one moment ~10% are spontaneously active in the absence of an agonist) and agonists bind preferentially to a GPCR in the active state (R*) shifting the equilibrium so that more receptors are in the active state.
  - Full agonists produce a maximal response with <100% receptor occupancy (e.g. adrenaline at adrenoceptors).
  - Most antagonists are inverse agonists (e.g. β-blockers at β adrenoceptors) and bind to a GPCR in the inactive state (R) shifting the equilibrium so that more receptors are in the inactive state.
  - Neutral antagonists (e.g. bucindolol at β adrenoceptors in patients with a particular genotype) bind to GPCRs in either the active (R*) or inactive state (R) and do not change overall activity but block agonist binding.
  - Partial agonists (e.g. salbutamol at β_2 adrenoceptors) will preferentially bind to R* as opposed to R, but to a lesser degree than a full agonist.
- Irreversible competitive antagonism:
  - An antagonist binds to the same site as the agonist on the receptor, but dissociates very slowly and is not displaced by the agonist, preventing full occupancy by the agonist, e.g. phenoxybenzamine, which binds covalently and irreversibly to the α-adrenoceptor (causing alkylation); hence, its use in phaeochromocytoma to provide constant protection against intermittent surges in catecholamines, particularly during adrenalectomy.
- Biased agonism:
  - Different agonists binding to the same receptor may preferentially activate different downstream signalling pathways, resulting in different responses.
- Potency refers to weight-for-weight activity, e.g. bumetanide 1 mg has a much greater effect than furosemide 1 mg.

- Clinical efficacy:
  - e.g. maximum effect of bumetanide is similar to that of furosemide, but with 1 mg bumetanide equating to 30–40 mg furosemide.
- Selectivity:
  - e.g. propranolol is non-selective for β1 and β2 receptors, while nebivolol is highly β1-selective.

As well as binding to the main site on the receptor, drugs may bind to other, allosteric binding sites and can modify the responses to drugs, e.g. sulfonylureas at K_{ATP} channels and benzodiazepines at $GABA_A$ receptors.

Ion channels

- In addition to activating type 1 receptor ligand-gated ion channels directly (Table 3.3), drugs may alter the ability of ion channels to open and close; the main cation channels having selective permeability for Na^+, K^+ and Ca^{2+}, and the major anion channel having selective permeability for Cl^-:
  - e.g. CCBs that reduce the opening of voltage-gated calcium channels;
  - e.g. dantrolene that binds to the ryanodine receptor on the sarcoplasmic reticulum, decreasing free intracellular calcium concentration to depress excitation-contraction coupling in skeletal muscle.

Enzymes

Examples of enzymes being drug targets include:

- Angiotensin-converting enzyme (ACE):
  - competitive inhibitors, e.g. ramipril.
- Cyclo-oxygenase (COX):
  - acetylation of the serine residue in the enzyme by acetylsalicylic acid results in irreversible/non-competitive inhibition.

Transporters

➲ See Excretion, p. 69 and Table 3.14.

Examples of transporters being drug targets include:

- ATP-binding cassette (ABC) transporters (that utilise the energy of ATP binding and hydrolysis to energise the translocation of various substrates across membranes), e.g. Na^+/K^+ ATPase in cardiac myocytes inhibited by digoxin.
- Solute carrier (SLC) transporters that facilitate passive movement down an electrochemical gradient:
  - Organic cation transporters (OCTs), e.g. SLC family 22 member 3 protein transporting histamine, dopamine and serotonin inhibited by cocaine.
  - Organic anion transporters (OATs), e.g. OATs in the kidney that bind probenecid in preference to uric acid, preventing uric acid reabsorption.

Mechanism of action of recently developed drugs

For mechanism of action of recently developed drugs, see Table 3.4.

Risks

'First do no harm' is an important principle in clinical pharmacology. Risks of harm to patients are not limited to adverse reactions (➲ see Specific adverse reactions, p. 65 and Tables 3.6–3.10.), but also may arise from:

- Dosing errors.
- Ignoring drug allergies, contraindications and/or interactions.
- Prescription via the incorrect route.
- Continuation after an adverse drug reaction (ADR).
- Premature discontinuation.
- Lack of dose alteration when drug levels are out of range.

Table 3.4 Mechanism of action of recently developed drugs

Drug	Mechanism	Indications
Abatacept	Fusion protein of the extracellular domain of CTLA-4 linked to a modified IgG1 Fc portion that binds to CD80 and CD86 on antigen presenting cells blocking their activation of CD28 on T cells and cytokine production.	Moderate to severe rheumatoid arthritis unresponsive to other DMARDs including at least one TNFα blocker, or where patients have been intolerant of such drugs (➲ see Chapter 20, Biologic disease-modifying anti-rheumatic drugs, p. 709).
Bedaquiline	Selectively inhibits mycobacterial ATP synthase, causing cell death in both replicating and non-replicating mycobacteria.	As part of a combination regimen to treat pulmonary multidrug-resistant tuberculosis when alternative treatments are not available.
Denosumab	Human monoclonal IgG2 antibody that binds to RANKL on osteoblasts preventing interaction with, and activation of RANKL on osteoclasts, inhibiting bone resorption.	Osteoporosis in post-menopausal women at increased risk of fracture and men receiving hormonal therapy for prostate cancer (➲ see Chapter 20, Antiresorptive, p. 725).
Eculizumab	Long-acting humanised monoclonal antibody against complement C5 that inhibits its cleavage into C5a and C5b, thus inhibiting deployment of the terminal complement system (C5b-8)/formation of the MAC (C5b-9) and haemolysis.	Paroxysmal nocturnal haemoglobinuria and atypical haemolytic uraemic syndrome (life-threatening, progressive disease characterised by systemic thrombotic microangiopathy caused by chronic, uncontrolled activation of the complement system [➲ see Chapter 16, Atypical haemolytic uraemic syndrome, p. 578).
Icatibant	Selective, competitive bradykinin B2 receptor antagonist.	Acute attacks of hereditary angioedema in patients with C1-esterase inhibitor deficiency.
Lomitapide	Inhibits the microsomal triglyceride transfer protein necessary for very low-density lipoprotein assembly and secretion.	Adjunct to dietary measures and other lipid-regulating drugs with or without low-density lipoprotein apheresis in homozygous familial hypercholesterolaemia.
Maraviroc	Negative allosteric modulator of the CCR5 receptor on the surface of white blood cells thereby blocking the HIV protein gp120 from associating with the receptor and preventing HIV from being able to enter macrophages and T-cells.	CCR5-tropic HIV infection in combination with other antiretroviral drugs in patients previously treated with antiretrovirals.
Mirabegron	Selective β3-adrenoreceptor agonist that relaxes detrusor muscle and promotes contraction of the urethra.	Symptoms associated with overactive bladder (urgency, urge incontinence, and increased frequency of micturition).
Panitumumab	Monoclonal antibody specific to the epidermal growth factor receptor that binds to its extracellular domain and prevents its activation, leading ultimately to increased apoptosis, reduced proliferation of tumour cells and reduced angiogenesis.	Treatment of non-mutated Ras metastatic colorectal cancer.
Raltegravir	Inhibits the HIV integrase enzyme preventing insertion of viral DNA into the host cell genome, DNA transcription, viral replication and propagation.	HIV infection in combination with other antiretroviral drugs.
Ranolazine	Inhibits late inward sodium current in cardiac myocytes, preventing reverse mode sodium-calcium exchange and diastolic accumulation of intracellular calcium.	Adjunctive therapy in the treatment of stable angina in patients inadequately controlled or intolerant of first-line anti-anginal therapies.

Table 3.4 *continued*

Drug	Mechanism	Indications
Retapamulin	Pleuromutilin antibiotic that binds to the 50S subunit of bacterial ribosomes with high affinity, inhibiting ribosomal peptidyl transferase activity and partially inhibiting the binding of the initiator transfer RNA substrate to the ribosomal P-site.	Superficial bacterial skin infection caused by *Staphylococcus aureus* and *Streptococcus pyogenes* (if resistant to first line topical antibacterials).
Sapropterin	Synthetic form of the cofactor tetrahydrobiopterin that activates residual phenylalanine hydroxylase, improving phenylalanine metabolism and decreasing phenylalanine concentrations.	Hyperphenylalaninaemia in patients with phenylketonuria (or tetrahydrobiopterin deficiency).
Tolvaptan	Vasopressin-2 receptor antagonist that decreases expression of aquaporin channels, increasing free water clearance, decreasing urine osmolality and increasing serum sodium concentration.	Hyponatremia secondary to syndrome of inappropriate antidiuretic hormone secretion.

BRCA = breast cancer susceptibility protein; CCR5 = C-C chemokine receptor type 5; CD = cluster of differentiation; CTLA-4 = cytotoxic T-lymphocyte-associated antigen; DMARDs = disease-modifying anti-rheumatic drugs; Fc = fragment crystallisable; Ig = immunoglobulin; MAC = membrane attack complex; RANKL = receptor activator of nuclear factor kappa B ligand); TNF = tumour necrosis factor.
Data from 'New Drug Mechanisms' series in the *British Journal of Clinical Pharmacology*, Wiley.

Risks of harm may also be to people looking after, or in close contact with, the patient, through toxic effects of the drug (e.g. radioactive or chemotherapeutic agents), or to the wider population, such as by spread of antibiotic resistance from the over-use of antibiotics.

Adverse effects

ADRs are defined as 'an appreciably harmful or unpleasant reaction resulting from an intervention related to the use of a medicinal product'. ADRs usually predict hazard from future administration, and warrant prevention, or specific treatment, or alteration of the dosage regimen or withdrawal of the product.

Prevention

ADR prevention is by careful consideration of prescribing principles (BRAINS and AIMS) that facilitate weighing up risk:benefit ratios, avoiding or minimising harm from interactions, considering whether other medications are needed to minimise adverse reactions (necessary prophylaxis [➲ see Chapter 1, Treatment, p. 6]), identifying which patients are likely to be susceptible to adverse effects, and considering components of drug administration and patient information.

Classification

Dose dependency

- Supra-therapeutic doses of drugs typically result in toxic effects, e.g. hepatoxicity with paracetamol overdose; cardiac arrhythmias with digoxin.
- Side (or collateral) effects occurring at normal therapeutic doses, e.g. renal failure with non-steroidal anti-inflammatory drugs (NSAIDS); cough with ACE-inhibitors.
- Sub-therapeutic doses may result in adverse reactions in patients who are hyper-susceptible, e.g. penicillin anaphylaxis.

Phenytoin is an example of a drug that exhibits clear, predictable, dose-dependent side effects (Figure 3.2). As the phenytoin concentration exceeds its narrow therapeutic range (40–80 μmol/L), the following adverse effects are likely to be observed:

- Nystagmus (concentrations ~80–120 μmol/L).
- Ataxia (concentrations ~120–160 μmol/L).
- Confusion and coma (concentrations >160 μmol/L).

Time-dependent reactions

- Immediate reactions occurring within seconds or minutes, e.g. red man syndrome due to massive histamine release from rapid intravenous (IV) vancomycin infusion (prevented by slow infusion); acute anaphylaxis due to type I immediate hypersensitivity to penicillin (➲ see Table 3.5 and Chapter 6, Type I hypersensitivity, p. 160).
- Rapid, first-dose hypotension within hours of a first dose of an ACE inhibitor (prevented by a recommendation to take the first dose in the evening, with a reasonably large glass of water, then to lay down for several hours).
- Intermediate duration reactions, e.g. agranulocytosis with use of carbimazole and 5-aminosalicylic acid (mesalazine) and its derivatives, with the highest risk during the first 3 months of treatment and reduced risk subsequent to this.
- Delayed type hypersensitivity reactions (Table 3.5) (➲ see Chapter 6, Type IV hypersensitivity, p. 162).
- Late reactions with risk increasing with time, e.g. osteoporosis with prolonged use of corticosteroids (prevention may involve 'necessary prophylaxis' with bone protection [e.g. bisphosphonates; ➲ see Chapter 20, Treatment of glucocorticoid-induced osteoporosis, p. 726]).
- Withdrawal syndromes, e.g. withdrawal from benzodiazepines (anxiety and insomnia); withdrawal from centrally acting antihypertensives such as clonidine, methyldopa and moxonidine (rebound hypertension); withdrawal from β-blockers (exacerbation of angina).

Table 3.5 Allergic drug reactions

Type	Examples
Type I	Urticaria and anaphylaxis with penicillins by production of reaginic IgE antibody to penicilloyl moiety.
Type II	Direct antiglobulin test positive warm autoimmune haemolytic anaemia with methyldopa Thrombocytopenia with quinine.
Type III	Interstitial nephritis with penicillins. Amiodarone lung. Hydralazine-induced systemic lupus syndrome.
Type IV	Stevens–Johnson syndrome with carbamazepine use. Contact dermatitis with topical penicillin or neomycin.

- Delayed reactions occurring years later, e.g. carcinogenesis following immunosuppression with ciclosporin or chemotherapeutic agents.

Time-independent reactions

- Pharmacokinetic changes:
  - Change in formulation of medicine that alters the systemic bioavailability of the drug, e.g. modified release formulations of theophylline and lithium.
  - Change in pharmacokinetic handling and resultant change in drug concentration, e.g. decreased clearance of digoxin (with digoxin toxicity) in patients with deteriorating renal function.
- Pharmacodynamic changes:
  - Increased sensitivity of effector organs, e.g. increased sensitivity of the myocardium to digoxin in the face of hypokalaemia, hypomagnesaemia, hypoxia, acidaemia, hypothyroidism and/or hypercalcaemia.

Diagnosis

- Type A:
  - dose-dependent;
  - common;
  - usually less severe.
- Type B:
  - idiosyncratic;
  - rarer (~1:1000 – 1:10,000);
  - usually more severe.

A careful drug history is essential, paying attention to the timing (onset, offset, reappearance on re-challenge) of the ADR. Provocation testing, such as skin testing, by patch or intradermal injection, may be helpful, but is not commonly used for drugs other than penicillin. Serological testing may be misleading as circulating antibodies to the drug may not be the cause of the symptoms. In the case of patients on multiple medications, it may not be clear which drug(s) is/are contributory, and stopping all drugs and then reintroducing essential, chemically unrelated alternative drugs, if available, in turn, can be considered.

Treatment

- Withdrawal and avoidance of the drug is usually adequate (with supportive measures such as correcting electrolyte or fluid imbalances).
- Examples of specific antidotes include:
  - Idarucizumab – a humanised monoclonal antibody fragment to reverse direct oral thrombin inhibition by dabigatran.
  - Icatibant – a selective bradykinin B2 receptor antagonist to treat life-threatening angioedema with ACE inhibitors.
  - IV lipid emulsion (Intralipid®) to treat/prevent cardiotoxicity of excessive local anaesthetic administration or absorption.

Reporting

➲ See Chapter 4, Adverse event reporting, p. 105; and Yellow Card and other systems, p. 105.

Specific adverse reactions

- Gingival hyperplasia with:
  - calcium antagonists (associated with MDR1 G2677T/A polymorphism);
  - ciclosporin;
  - phenytoin.
- Gynaecomastia with:
  - cimetidine;
  - digoxin;
  - metronidazole;
  - methyldopa;
  - spironolactone.

For hepatotoxic ADRs, see Table 3.6; for nephrotoxic ADRs, see Table 3.7; for pulmonary fibrotic ADRs, see Table 3.8; for important ADRs of specific drugs, see Table 3.9; and for important ADRs of specific cytotoxic drugs, see Table 3.10.

Table 3.6 Hepatotoxic adverse drug reactions

Hepatotoxicity	Features	Examples
Hepatitis	Hepatocellular necrosis with initial rise in ALT.	Dose dependent: paracetamol, aspirin. Dose independent: isoniazid, pyrazinamide, valproate, methyldopa, NSAIDs, phenytoin, statins.
Cholestasis	Initial rise in ALP and bilirubin (but often associated with a secondary hepatitis due to impaired bile excretion from hepatocellular canaliculi).	Dose dependent: rifampicin, oestrogens, anabolic steroids. Dose independent: chlorpromazine, clarythromycin, chlorpropamide, carbimazole, cimetidine, co-amoxiclav, flucloxacillin.
Microvesicular steatosis	Characterised by accumulation of small intracytoplasmic fat vacuoles (liposomes).	Aspirin, valproate, tetracyclines.
Macrovesicular steatosis	Abnormal intracellular retention of lipid in vesicles large enough to displace the cytoplasm and distort the nucleus.	Amiodarone, methotrexate.

ALP = alkaline phosphatase; ALT = alanine aminotransferase.

Table 3.7 Nephrotoxic adverse drug reactions

Mechanism	Examples
Glomerulonephritis	Gold salts, penicillamine, NSAIDs*
Acute tubular necrosis	Gentamicin, NSAIDs*
Type I (distal) renal tubular acidosis	Amphotericin, quinolones
Type II (proximal) renal tubular acidosis	Acetazolamide
Interstitial nephritis	Vancomycin, NSAIDs*
Nephrogenic diabetes insipidus	Lithium, amphotericin

*NSAIDs inhibit vasodilatory prostaglandin production resulting in reduced renal blood flow, especially in patients with endothelial dysfunction and diminished nitric oxide production who are dependent on the vasodilatory prostaglandins. NSAIDs may also cause injury at several sites along the nephron (glomerulonephritis; acute tubular necrosis; interstitial nephritis; papillary necrosis).

Table 3.8 Pulmonary fibrotic adverse drug reactions

Drug class	Examples
Antibiotic	Nitrofurantoin
Anti-arrhythmic agent	Amiodarone
Chemotherapy agent	Bleomycin, busulfan, carmustine, chlorambucil, cyclophosphamide, melphalan, methotrexate, mitomycin
DMARD	Gold, penicillamine, sulfasalazine

Table 3.9 Important ADRs of specific drugs

Drug	ADRs
ACE inhibitors	**C**ough **A**ngioedema/anaphylaxis **P**alpitations **T**aste disturbance **O**rthostatic hypotension **P**otassium elevation **R**enal impairment **I**mpotence **L**eukocytosis
Amisulpiride	Akathisia, amenorrhoea, galactorrhoea, insomnia, QT prolongation, weight gain
Amiodarone	**S**late grey skin discolouration (and photosensitivity) **L**iver damage (steato-hepatitis) **A**taxia/arrhythmias **T**hyroid dysfunction (hyper and hypothyroidism) **E**ye/corneal reversible microdeposits **T**aste disturbance/tremor **A**lveolitis (may progress to fibrosis) **N**europathy (peripheral)
Carbamazepine	Dizziness, diarrhoea, ataxia, nausea, syndrome of inappropriate antidiuretic hormone secretion.
Clozapine	Cardiomyopathy, constipation, agranulocytosis, seizures, hypotension.
Corticosteroids	**A**cne **M**yopathy (proximal) **C**ushingoid facies/cataracts **U**lcers (with impaired healing) **S**triae/skin thinning **H**ypertension/hypokalaemia **I**mmunosuppression/infections **N**ecrosis (avascular necrosis of femoral head) **G**lycosuria **O**besity/osteoporosis **I**nsomnia **D**epression
Lamotrigine	Depression, influenza-like symptoms, maculopapular rash, Stevens–Johnson syndrome.
Lithium	Leucocytosis, diabetes insipidus, tremor, teratogenicity, hypothyroidism, interstitial nephritis, nausea/vomiting, acne, weight gain, T wave flattening/inversion on ECG.
Methotrexate	Mucositis, myelosuppression, liver fibrosis, pneumonitis.
Valproate	**V**omiting/vasculitis **A**taxia **L**iver dysfunction (hepatitis) **P**ancreatitis/pancytopenia **R**ash **O**edema/obesity **A**lopecia (transient with curly regrowth) **T**remor **E**osinophila (➲ 'DRESS' – drug reaction with eosinophilia and systemic symptoms [see Chapter 21, Drug reaction with eosinophilia and systemic symptoms, p. 772])
Warfarin	Cholesterol microembolisation, hair loss, mouth ulcers, skin necrosis.

By permission from Mannan I, Cheung V, Grout C, Mullish M; *MRCP Part 1: 400 BOFs* Second Edition; JP Medical Ltd 2016. Data from Dykewicz, M.S. Cough and angioedema from angiotensin-converting enzyme inhibitors: new insights into mechanisms and management. *Curr Opin Allergy Clin Immunol* 4(4):267. Copyright © 2004 Lippincott Williams and Reardon LC. Macpherson DS. *Arch Intern Med* 1998; 158(1):26; and *Clin Chest Med.* 2004 Sep;25(3):479–519, vi. Drug-induced and iatrogenic infiltrative lung disease.

Table 3.10 Important ADRs of specific cytotoxic drugs

Drug	ADRs
Bleomycin	Lung fibrosis
Capecitabine	Hand-foot syndrome (desquamating rash)
Cisplatin	Interstitial nephritis, ototoxicity, peripheral neuropathy
Cyclophosphamide	Bone marrow suppression, haemorrhagic cystitis, secondary acute myeloid leukaemia
Doxorubicin	Cardiomyopathy, rash
Etoposide	Bone marrow suppression, hypotension
Vincristine	Peripheral neuropathy

Adapted from Mannan I, Cheung V, Grout C, Mullish M; *MRCP Part 1: 400 BOFs* Second Edition; JP Medical Ltd 2016.

Interactions

Drug interactions may involve pharmacokinetic ('ADME': absorption, distribution, metabolism, excretion) and/or pharmacodynamic processes. Interactions may be beneficial or adverse through synergistic or antagonistic processes: some examples are given in Table 3.11; note these are pharmacodynamic interactions.

Table 3.11 Drug interactions

	Beneficial	Adverse
Synergistic	E.g. combination of antihypertensives to control blood pressure.	E.g. combination of antihypertensives causing hypotension and acute kidney injury.
Antagonistic	E.g. reversal of heroin with naloxone.	E.g. NSAIDs blocking the natriuretic/ antihypertensive effects of diuretics.

Pharmacokinetic interactions

Absorption

The extent of drug absorption may be reduced by the drug binding to another drug, e.g. binding of colestyramine to digoxin and warfarin; chelation by antacids (containing aluminium, magnesium and/or calcium) to tetracyclines. Alteration of gut motility also affects the rate of absorption of many drugs:

- Reduced gut motility by opioids and antimuscarinic tricyclic antidepressants (TCAs) slows absorption, e.g. morphine use is associated with a delayed onset of action of prasugrel and ticagrelor.
- Increased gut motility by metoclopramide (with increased tone of the lower oesophageal sphincter and relaxation of the pylorus) increases the rate of absorption of paracetamol to achieve a more rapid relief of a headache.

Distribution

Redistribution of drugs occurs following displacement from binding sites, freeing them to exert their effect. A 'free' drug is, however, also free to be metabolised and be excreted, and so unless these clearance processes are saturated (➲ see First and zero order kinetics, p. 79), the equilibrium is rapidly restored with a minimal change in drug action and without a clinically significant interaction. Therefore, a second mechanism is usually needed to result in a clinically significant interaction (usually an inhibition of metabolism or excretion). Examples include:

- Sodium valproate displaces phenytoin from plasma proteins in the circulation and inhibits its metabolism.
- Aspirin and NSAIDs displace methotrexate from plasma proteins in the circulation and reduce its secretion, risking methotrexate toxicity.
- Amiodarone displaces digoxin from tissue-binding sites and may impair its excretion; this approximately doubles digoxin levels.
- Dipyridamole blocks adenosine uptake via the equilibrative nucleoside transporter, which increases adenosine levels and greatly potentiates its effect.

Metabolism

The majority of drug metabolism occurs via cytochrome P450 (CYP450) enzymes. The combination of a precipitant drug, which is a strong enzyme inhibitor, with an object drug possessing a narrow therapeutic range will result in inhibition of the breakdown or metabolism of the object drug, resulting in an increase in its concentration, risking a toxic effect. An enzyme inducer will increase the breakdown or metabolism of the object drug, resulting in a decrease in its concentration and loss of effect. The opposite effect exists for inactive pro-drugs, which require metabolism to their active form, which will be blocked by an enzyme inhibitor. Table 3.12 shows the CYP450 isoenzymes and the clinically important inhibitors, substrates and inducers.

For interactions involving inhibitors of other 'extra-microsomal' enzymes, see Table 3.13.

The following are 'inactive pro-drug → active metabolite' combinations:

- Azathioprine → mercaptopurine.
- Clopidogrel -*CYP2C19, CYP2B6, CYP1A2*→ 2-oxo-clopidogrel -*CYP2C19, CYP2C9,CYP2B6, CYP3A4*→ $\text{clopidogrel}_{\text{active metabolite}}$:
  - the majority (~85%) of absorbed clopidogrel is hydrolysed by esterases into an inactive form leaving ~15% to be converted by the CYP450 family of enzymes, and paraoxonase 1 (PON1), to the active metabolite required for inhibition of the platelet adenosine diphosphate receptor P2Y12.
    - CYP2C19 contributes to 40% of the hepatic conversion of clopidogrel into the short half-life active metabolite that irreversibly binds to the platelet P2Y12 receptor.
    - In addition to pharmacogenetic differences due to polymorphisms in CYP2C19 and PON1, variability of anti-platelet effect also exists through enzyme induction due to smoking and inhibition of CYP2C19 through drug interactions with proton pump inhibitors (e.g. omeprazole and lansoprazole, and to a lesser extent, pantoprazole) and statins.

Excretion

A range of transporters involved in renal drug excretion/reabsorption may be inhibited by other drugs. Examples include:

- Inhibition of penicillin secretion via OAT3 by probenecid, blocking renal clearance of penicillin by ~80%.
- Inhibition of methotrexate secretion via OAT3 by salicylates and some NSAIDs such as indometacin.
- Inhibition of urate reabsorption by SLC22A12 by probenecid, sulfinpyrazone, losartan and fenofibrate.
- Competition between hydrochlorothiazide and uric acid for transport via OAT1, resulting in increased plasma uric acid levels with increasing hydrochlorthiazide dosing.

Transporters exist in organs other than the kidney and are similarly involved in drug interactions (Table 3.14).

Table 3.12 CYP450 isoenzymes and clinically important inhibitors, substrates and inducers

CYP isoenzyme	**2C9**	**2C19**	**3A4**	**2D6**	**1A2**	**2E1**
Strong inhibitors (↑AUC of substrate > 5-fold or ↓ clearance >80%)		Fluconazole, fluvoxamine, ticlopidine.	Clarithromycin, grapefruit juice, indinavir, itraconazole, ketoconazole, nefazodone, nelfinavir, posaconazole, ritonavir, saquinavir, telaprevir, telithromycin, voriconazole.	Bupropion, fluoxetine, paroxetine, quinidine.	Ciprofloxacin, fluvoxamine.	Disulfiram.
Moderate inhibitors (↑ AUC of substrate 2–5-fold or ↓ clearance 50–80%)	Amiodarone, fluconazole, miconazole.	Esomeprazole, fluoxetine, moclobemide, omeprazole, voriconazole.	Aprepitant, atazanavir, ciprofloxacin, diltiazem, erythromycin, fluconazole, fosamprenavir, imatinib, verapamil.	Cinacalcet, duloxetine, terbinafine.	Mexiletine, oral contraceptives, thiabendazole.	Ethanol.
Substrates	Warfarin, phenytoin, celecoxib.	Lansoprazole, omeprazole, S-mephenytoin.	Alfentanil, ciclosporin, ergotamine, fentanyl, pimozide, quinidine, simvastatin, sirolimus, tacrolimus, codeine, tramadol.	Atomoxetine, desipramine, dextromethorphan, metoprolol, nebivolol, perphenazine, tolterodine, venlafaxine.	Theophylline, alosetron, caffeine, duloxetine, melatonin, ramelteon, tacrine, tizanidine.	Paracetamol, ethanol.
Strong inducers (≥80% ↓ in AUC)			Carbamazepine, phenytoin, rifampicin, St. John's wort.			
Moderate inducers (50–80% ↓ in AUC)	Carbamazepine, rifampicin.	Rifampicin.	Bosentan, efavirenz, etravirine, modafinil.		Montelukast, phenytoin, cigarette smoking.	Ethanol.

AUC = area under the curve in a plot of plasma drug concentration against time; typically, the area is computed starting at the time the drug is administered and ending when the concentration in plasma is negligible (➲ see Absorption, p. 76).
Adapted from the FDA's Drug Development and Drug Interactions: Table of Substrates, Inhibitors and Inducers http://www.fda.gov/Drugs/DevelopmentApprovalProcess/DevelopmentResources/DrugInteractionsLabeling/ucm093664.htm#classInhibit

Table 3.13 Interactions involving inhibitors of other 'extra-microsomal' enzymes

Precipitant	Enzyme	Object
Allopurinol	Xanthine oxidase	Azathioprine
Carbidopa	Dopa decarboxylase	Levodopa
Metronidazole. disulfiram	Aldehyde dehydrogenase	Alcohol
MAOIs	Monoamine oxidase	Tyramine; amphetamine

Table 3.14 Transporter-mediated clinically significant drug interactions

Gene	Aliases	Tissue	Function	Interacting drug	Substrate (affected drug)	Changes in substrate plasma AUC (AUC ratios)
ABC transporters of clinical importance in the absorption, disposition and excretion of drugs						
ABCB1	P-gp, MDR1	Intestinal enterocyte, kidney proximal tubule, hepatocyte (canalicular), brain endothelia	Efflux	Dronedarone	Digoxin	2.6-fold
				Ranolazine	Digoxin	1.6-fold
				Tipranavir/ritonavir	Loperamide	0.5-fold
				Tipranavir/ritonavir	Saquinavir/ Ritonavir	0.2-fold
SLC transporters of clinical importance in the disposition and excretion of drugs						
SLCO1B1	OATP1B1 OATP-C OATP2 LST-1	Hepatocyte (sinusoidal)	Uptake	Lopinavir/ritonavir	Bosentan	5-48-fold
				Ciclosporin	Pravastatin	9.9-fold
SLCO1B3	OATP1B3, OATP-8	Hepatocyte (sinusoidal)	Uptake	Ciclosporin	Rosuvastatin	7.1-fold
				Ciclosporin	Pitavastatin	4.6-fold
				Lopinavir/ritonavir	Rosuvastatin	2.1-fold
SLC22A2	OCT2	Kidney proximal tubule	Uptake	Cimetidine	Dofetilide	1.5-fold
				Cimetidine	Pindolol	1.5-fold
				Cimetidine	Metformin	1.4-fold
SLC22A6	OAT1	Kidney proximal tubule, placenta	Uptake	Probenecid	Cefradine	3.6-fold
				Probenecid	Cidofovir	1.5-fold
				Probenecid	Aciclovir	1.4-fold
SLC22A8	OAT3	Kidney proximal tubule, choroid plexus, brain endothelia	Uptake	Probenecid	Furosemide	2.9-fold

P-gp = p-glycoprotein; MDR = multidrug resistance; LST = liver-specific transporter.
Adapted from Drug Development and Drug Interactions: Table of Substrates, Inhibitors and Inducers http://www.fda.gov/Drugs/DevelopmentApprovalProcess/DevelopmentResources/DrugInteractionsLabeling/ucm093664.htm#classInhibit

The reabsorption of weak acids such as acetylsalicylic acid (aspirin) are inhibited in alkaline urine as they are more ionised (alkaline diuresis).

Pharmacodynamic interactions

- Actions on receptors:
  - Antagonistic, e.g. naloxone for morphine overdose.
  - Non-selective, e.g. β-blockers and salbutamol.
- Actions on body systems:
  - Antagonistic, e.g. NSAIDs (salt retention) and diuretics (natriuresis).
  - Synergistic:
    - Verapamil and β-blockers resulting in asystole.
    - Theophylline and β-agonists potentiating arrhythmias as both cause tachycardia and hypokalaemia.
    - Loop diuretics and aminoglycosides both being ototoxic.
    - Sedation with amitriptyline and diazepam.

Necessary prophylaxis

For a few drugs, co-prescription with another drug to reduce the incidence of side effects is recommended; this potentially is also dependent on the susceptibilities of the individual patient. Examples include:

- Use of a proton pump inhibitor in combination with dual anti-platelet therapy in patients at high risk of gastrointestinal bleeding (e.g. history of gastrointestinal ulcer/haemorrhage, chronic NSAID/corticosteroid use).
- Use of laxatives and anti-emetics with opioids to minimise constipation, and nausea and vomiting, respectively.
- Use of 'bone prophylaxis' with bisphosphonates in patients likely to take ≥7.5 mg prednisolone daily for 3 or more months.
- Use of pyridoxine with isoniazid to reduce the risk of peripheral neuropathy, optic atrophy, convulsions and psychosis.
- Use of mesna with cyclophosphamide to reduce the risk of haemorrhagic cystitis.
- Use of rasburicase (and allopurinol) for the prophylaxis and treatment of acute hyperuricaemia with initial chemotherapy for haematological malignancy.

Susceptible patients

Allergy

The risk of allergic responses is increased in patients with:

- Infectious mononucleosis:
  - associated with an increased likelihood of cutaneous reactions to penicillins and other antimicrobials.
- HIV infection:
  - e.g. hypersensitivity to trimethoprim-sulfamethoxazole occurs in 20–80% (compared with 1–3% in the general population).
- Cystic fibrosis:
  - e.g. ~30% of patients develop allergy to one or more antibiotics (e.g. piperacillin, ceftazidime and ticarcillin).

Sex

Men are more susceptible to cholestasis with co-amoxiclav. Women have been considered to have increased susceptibility to:

- Effects of alcohol.
- Neuropsychiatric effects of mefloquine.
- ACE-inhibitor cough.

- Drug-induced systemic lupus erythematosus.
- Hepatitis due to methyldopa.
- Cholestasis with flucloxacillin.

Age

The elderly are particularly susceptible to the effects of commonly prescribed drugs (Table 3.15), therefore it is important to avoid such drugs if possible. If they need to be used, the lowest possible dose should be prescribed and the patient should be monitored carefully.

Table 3.15 Common ADRs in elderly patients

Drug class	Effect
Diuretics	Hypokalaemia, hyponatraemia, dehydration, acute kidney injury, hypotension.
Antihypertensives	Postural hypotension.
NSAIDs	Kidney injury, salt and water retention, cardiac failure, hypertension.
Tricyclic antidepressants	Anticholinergic side effects, including postural hypotension and confusion.
Benzodiazepines	Sedation.
H_1 antihistamines and H_2-receptor antagonists	Confusion, drowsiness.
Opioids	Delirium, constipation, respiratory depression.

Patients with renal and hepatic impairment

In patients with renal impairment, accumulation of renally cleared drugs with a narrow therapeutic range leads to toxicity; for several of these, therapeutic drug monitoring is performed to reduce the risk (➲ see Monitoring, p. 79). In patients with hepatic impairment, a number of processes impact on drug pharmacodynamics and pharmacokinetics (Table 3.16).

Table 3.16 Processes impacting on drug pharmacodynamics and pharmacokinetics in patients with hepatic impairment

Process altered	Drugs affected
Impaired synthesis of clotting factors	Increased bleeding risk with anticoagulants, anti-platelets and NSAIDs.
Impaired synthesis of albumin	Increased free/active drug of highly protein bound drugs, such as phenytoin and prednisolone.
Increased salt and water retention due to hypoalbuminaemia, secondary hyperaldosteronism and renal impairment	Impaired response to diuretics.
Reduced activity of CYP450 enzymes	Increased sedative effects with chlormethiazole and morphine; increased hypotension with calcium blockers.
Encephalopathy	Increased risk of ADRs to sedatives and opioids.
Hepato-renal syndrome	Reduced clearance of lithium and gentamicin; increased nephrotoxicity of NSAIDs.
Portal hypertension (with relative systemic hypotension)	Hypotension/cardiovascular collapse with antihypertensive/vasoactive agents.

Patients with myasthenia gravis

Myasthenic symptoms may be exacerbated by:

- Antibiotics, e.g. aminoglycosides, fluoroquinolones, macrolides, tetracyclines.
- Cardiovascular drugs, e.g. β-blockers, lidocaine, verapamil.
- Anti-epileptics, e.g. gabapentin, phenytoin.
- Psychoactive drugs, e.g. chlorpromazine, lithium.
- Disease modifying antirheumatic drugs (DMARDs), e.g. chloroquine, penicillamine.

Pharmacogenetics

For the effects of pharmacogenetic polymorphisms, see Table 3.17.

Table 3.17 Effects of pharmacogenetic polymorphisms

Pharmacogenetic polymorphism	Increased effect of:	Decreased effect of:
Under-expression		
CYP2D6	Metoprolol: with risk of bradycardia and hypotension. Flecainide: with risk of arrhythmias. Amitriptyline: with risk of confusion.	Codeine
CYP2C9	Tolbutamide: causing hypoglycaemia. Warfarin: causing haemorrhage.	
TPMT (thiopurine methyl transferase)	Azathioprine: putting patients at risk of bone marrow suppression.	
SLC01B1	Statin-induced rhabdomyolysis (4- and 16-fold greater risk with 1 and 2 defective alleles, respectively).	
N-acetyl transferase 2	Hydralazine. Isoniazid. Procainamide. Sulfonamides. These 4 drugs are associated with drug-induced lupus.	
Pseudocholinesterase	Suxamethonium – resulting in prolonged paralysis.	
Over-expression		
CYP3A5		Tacrolimus
HER (human epidermal growth factor receptor) 2	Trastuzumab: improving disease-free and overall survival.	

Malignant hyperthermia

Malignant hyperthermia (or malignant hyperpyrexia) is an autosomal dominant disorder for which there are at least six genetic loci of interest, most prominently a defect affecting the ryanodine receptor gene. Patients have few or no symptoms unless they are exposed to a triggering agent, the most common being volatile anaesthetic gases, such as halothane, sevoflurane, desflurane, isoflurane and enflurane, or the depolarising muscle relaxants suxamethonium and decamethonium. In susceptible individuals, these drugs can predispose to excessive release of sarcoplasmic calcium resulting in a hypermetabolic state with high temperature, tachycardia, increased carbon dioxide production and oxygen consumption, acidosis, muscle contraction and rigidity, and rhabdomyolysis (Table 3.18). Treatments include dantrolene, cooling, oxygen and fluids.

Table 3.18 Common toxidromes and their causes

Toxidrome	Clinical features	Examples
Anticholinergic	Agitation, hallucinations, delirium, mydriasis, dry flushed skin, dry mucous membranes, decreased bowel sounds, urinary retention, choreoathetosis, seizures.	TCAs, antihistamines, atropine, anti-Parkinsonian agents, phenothiazine.
Cholinergic	Confusion, miosis, bradycardia, hypertension, salivation, urinary and faecal incontinence, diaphoresis, lacrimation, weakness, seizures.	Organophosphate and carbamate insecticides, nicotine, physostigmine.
Neuroleptic malignant syndrome	Agitation, mydriasis or normal pupil size, tachycardia, hypertension, hyperthermia, diaphoresis, lead-pipe rigidity, hyporeflexia.	Antipsychotics, e.g. chlorpromazine.
Malignant hyperthermia	Normal pupil size, tachycardia, hypertension, hyperthermia, diaphoresis, generalised rigidity, hyporeflexia.	Inhalational anaesthetics.
Serotonin syndrome	Agitated delirium, coma, mydriasis, limb clonus, diaphoresis, tachycardia, hypertension, tremor, hyperreflexia, rigidity, hyperthermia; sometimes leading to multi-organ failure with rhabdomyolysis and DIC.	SSRIs, MAOIs, TCAs, amphetamines, cocaine, tramadol.
Opioid	CNS depression, pinpoint pupils, hypotension, hypothermia, respiratory depression, bradycardia, hyporeflexia.	Opioids.
Sedative-hypnotic	CNS depression, confusion, coma, variable pupil response, hypothermia, bradycardia, apnoea, hyporeflexia.	Benzodiazepines, barbiturates, GHB, alcohols, zopiclone.
Sympathomimetic	Agitation, delirium, hallucinations, paranoia, hyperthermia, mydriasis, tachycardia, hypertension, sweating, seizures, hyperreflexia.	Cocaine, amphetamines, NPS, e.g. cathinones.
Hallucinogenic	Hallucinations, perceptual distortions, agitations, mydriasis, hyperthermia, tachycardia, hypertension.	Phencyclidine, LSD, psilocybin.

CNS = central nervous system; DIC = disseminated intravascular coagulation ; GHB = gamma-hydroxybutyrate; LSD = lysergic acid; NPS = new psychoactive substance.

Glucose-6-phosphate dehydrogenase deficiency

- Glucose-6-phosphate dehydrogenase (G6PD) deficiency results from variations in the *G6PD* gene.
- Haemolysis occurs 2–3 days after ingesting an oxidant substance (due to decreased levels of reduced glutathione in the red cell membrane, rendering the red cell susceptible to oxidant stress).
- Drugs causing haemolysis (oxidising agents) include:
  - dapsone;
  - nitrofurantoin;
  - primaquine;
  - quinolones;
  - sulfonamides.

Methaemoglobinaemia

- Haem iron is oxidised from the Fe^{2+} state to the met/Fe^{3+} state, either spontaneously in congenital methaemoglobinaemia (often due to hereditary deficiency of methaemoglobin reductase, which would normally reduce Fe^{3+} to Fe^{2+}) or in response to an oxidising agent.
- Drugs with oxidising potential to precipitate methaemoglobinaemia include:
  - nitrates, e.g. glyceryl trinitrate;

  - nitroprusside;
  - nitrofurantoin.
- Congenital methaemoglobinaemia often responds to the reducing agent ascorbic acid, whereas reactions to substances associated with significant methaemoglobinaemia require IV methylene blue.

Acute intermittent porphyria

➲ See Chapter 1, Porphyrias, p. 32.

- Drugs that risk precipitating an acute crisis in acute porphyrias include:
  - A – alcohol, amphetamines, antidepressants, antihistamines.
  - B – barbiturates.
  - C – cephalosporins.
  - D – diuretics.
  - S – sulfonamides, sulfonylureas, sex steroids (oral contraceptive).

Other examples utilising pharmacogenetics

- Hypersensitivity to abacavir (including rash and fever, respiratory and gastrointestinal effects) is associated with the *HLA-B*5701* allele (5% of population).
- Hypersensitivity to carbamazepine (rash; Stevens–Johnson syndrome; toxic epidermal necrolysis) is associated with the *HLA-B*1502* allele, particularly in South East Asians.
- Pharmacogenetic variation of vitamin K epoxide reductase complex 1 (that recycles reduced vitamin K) is associated with resistance to warfarin.

Pregnancy

Pharmacological risks in pregnancy include:

- NSAIDs: premature closure of ductus arteriosus.
- Thiazide diuretics: neonatal thrombocytopenia.
- β-blockers: intra-uterine growth retardation, hypoglycaemia, bradycardia.
- ACE inhibitors: hypotension, oligohydramnios.
- Sulfonamides and aspirin: kernicterus.
- Dihydrofolate reductase inhibitors (e.g. methotrexate, sulfasalazine, pyrimethamine, triamterene and trimethoprim): neural tube defects, cardiovascular defects, oral clefts, urinary tract defects.

Many drugs pose teratogenic risks including:

- Thalidomide: stunted limb growth.
- Phenytoin: growth restriction, dysmorphism.
- Carbamazepine: microcephaly.
- Valproate: neural tube defects.
- Lithium: cretinism, Ebstein's anomaly.
- Warfarin: chondrodysplasia punctata.

In pregnancy, renal clearance is increased potentiating reduction in levels of penicillins, digoxin and lithium, with loss of effect.

Administering

Absorption

The extent to which a drug is absorbed via a given route (e.g. oral or transdermal) is termed the bioavailability. The bioavailability is calculated from the ratio of the area under the curve (AUC) following, for example, oral administration versus the AUC following IV administration, the latter having 100% bioavailability, i.e.

$$Bioavailability = \frac{AUC\,plasma[drug](following\ PO\ administration)}{AUC\,plasma[drug](following\ IV\ administration)}$$

The bioavailability of a drug determines whether it can be effectively administered via a given route (e.g. oral) and the dose that is needed to achieve a therapeutic concentration. A notable exception is vancomycin, which has an oral bioavailability of ~10–20%, meaning it can usually be used 'locally' and safely for its antibacterial activity within the gut lumen against *Clostridium difficile*. However, over time, clinically significant absorption resulting in toxicity can occur, especially in patients with inflamed bowel (bioavailability >33% reported), and therapeutic drug monitoring should be considered during prolonged administration.

Understanding the site of absorption of drugs is important. Specific examples include nifedipine that is administered sublingually but that has most of its absorption, when it is swallowed, in the upper gastrointestinal tract, and timolol that is administered topically to the eye but that has much of its absorption, via the nasolacrimal duct, directly into the systemic circulation. The rate of absorption determines the onset of action of a drug; this is quantified by the time, Tmax, to the maximum concentration achieved, Cmax.

Distribution

The plasma concentration (C) (often in mg/L) of a drug is calculated by the amount measured (A) divided by the volume of plasma sampled (V), i.e.

$$C = A / V$$

Dose = C × V but drugs do not remain in the circulation (the 'central compartment'); rather they are rapidly taken up by the tissues (the 'peripheral compartment'). This is particularly the case with lipid-soluble drugs, which distribute rapidly and widely in body fat stores, as opposed to water-soluble/highly plasma protein-bound drugs that may remain mainly in the circulation. Therefore, to obtain a rapid therapeutic effect, a loading dose is needed to fill the peripheral compartment and achieve an adequate plasma concentration. To calculate a loading dose, one needs to know what plasma volume the drug would take up if the whole dose was present in a single compartment at the same concentration as that measured in the plasma (C) – this is the 'apparent' volume of distribution (Vd). If the dose of a drug (D) is known and the plasma concentration (C) is measured over time, (assuming uniform distribution of the drug throughout the body) the linear component of the concentration-time graph may be extrapolated back towards a theoretical concentration at time zero (when the drug was administered) to calculate C_0.

$$Vd = D / C_0$$

$$\text{Loading dose} = C \times Vd$$

If an entire drug remained in the plasma, Vd = V. Since plasma volume is ~5% or 0.05 L/kg of body weight, this is ~3.5 L in a 70 kg person; so Vd is ~3.5 L/70 kg.

- Warfarin is very highly bound (~99%) to plasma proteins, with a Vd ~8 L/70 kg. Heparin is >95% bound to plasma proteins and is too large to readily cross the capillary wall, and has a Vd of 0.05–0.1 L/kg (3.5–7 L/70 kg).
- Phenytoin is ~92% protein bound, but is relatively lipid-soluble and is distributed throughout the total body water (~10-fold greater than the plasma ~0.55 L/kg); hence phenytoin has a Vd ~0.7 L/kg (or 49 L/70 kg).
- Lipid-soluble (lipophilic) drugs distribute widely, being concentrated in body fat stores, and have large Vds, e.g. morphine ~250 L/70 kg, propranolol ~300 L/70 kg.
- While digoxin is not widely distributed/concentrated in fat stores, it is only 20–30% bound to plasma proteins, and is widely taken up by tissues (cardiac and skeletal muscle, kidneys and intestine) and has a very large Vd ~400 L/70 kg. The loading dose of digoxin for rapid digitalisation for atrial fibrillation or flutter is 0.75–1.5 mg given over 24 hours in divided doses, that is much larger than the usual maintenance dose of 125–250 micrograms daily (according to renal function).

The reason to give a loading dose is to achieve a steady state concentration of the drug sooner if an acute effect is desired. Therefore most drugs given as a loading dose have long half-lives (➲ see Excretion, p. 78). Loading doses are also used for drugs with short half-lives if an immediate effect is needed e.g. IV lidocaine (with a half-life of ~1 hour).

Metabolism

- Phase I metabolism – modification:
  - Comprises oxidisation, reduction and hydrolysis.
  - Reactions catalysed mainly by the cytochrome P450 dependent mixed function oxidases (➲ see Metabolism, p. 69 and Table 3.12).
  - Affects drug detoxification or conversion of an inactive pro-drug to an active drug.
- Phase II metabolism – conjugation:
  - Comprises conjugation with sulphate and glucuronide, for example.
  - Renders lipid soluble drugs water soluble for renal and biliary excretion.
- Phase III metabolism – further modification:
  - Reactions include reduction by glutathione.

The majority of drug metabolism occurs in the liver, but important metabolic activity also takes place at other sites including the gut wall (e.g. Phase II sulphation/activation of minoxidil and chlorpromazine) and red blood cells (e.g. red cell esterases that metabolise the short-acting β-blocker esmolol).

First pass metabolism

If the majority of a drug (>60%) is metabolically altered following enteral administration before it reaches the systemic circulation, this is described as first pass metabolism. This affects the bioavailability of the drug, which influences the route of administration and is important for determining the dose. In patients with liver cirrhosis, the fibrotic/sclerotic process results in diversion of blood from its normal route through the hepatic sinusoids so that it bypasses the liver enzyme-containing hepatocytes and instead is shunted directly from the portal to the systemic circulation. As a result of this portosystemic shunting, more unaltered drug reaches the systemic circulation and its bioavailability increases.

Excretion

There are many routes through which drugs are excreted/secreted, all of which require them to be rendered water soluble (e.g. via Phase II metabolic pathways):

- enterohepatic circulation;
- enterosalivary circulation;
- exhalation;
- sweat;
- semen;
- tears;
- urine.

With regards to enterohepatic circulation, it is important to remember to inform a woman of child-bearing age taking the oral contraceptive pill of the risk of pregnancy (and to take alternative contraception) when prescribing a broad spectrum antibiotic, as removal of the bowel flora means that conjugated oestrogens secreted in the bile will not be deconjugated by the bowel flora, and thus will not be reabsorbed via the enterohepatic circulation, leading to increased oestrogen clearance, lower oestrogen levels and loss of the contraceptive effect of the pill. This is an acute effect with recolonisation occurring with chronic ingestion of broad spectrum antibiotics beyond 3 weeks.

The half-life of a drug, which is related to its clearance (via metabolism and excretion), determines the daily maintenance dose, dosing frequency, and the time to reach steady state. The time to reach steady state equates to ~5 half-lives of the drug (after 1st, 2nd, 3rd, 4th and 5th half-life, the drug will have achieved 50%, 75%, 87.5%, 93.75% and 96.875%, respectively). Depending on renal function, the half-life of digoxin is ~40 hours and so a steady state will be achieved at 5 × 40 hours, i.e. 200 hours or ~8 days. Therefore, it would take over a week to reach steady state and control ventricular rate if the patient were initiated on the daily maintenance dose alone, as opposed to hours with a loading dose. The relatively long half-life means that once daily dosing is adequate.

Informing

- Discuss and document key points of 'BRAINS & AIMS' with patients, ensuring they consent to the prescribed treatment.

Monitoring

Monitoring of the beneficial and adverse effects of drugs is needed, e.g. pain relief from analgesics (subjective assessment), elevated blood glucose with corticosteroids, renal impairment with ACE inhibitors, raised creatinine kinase (CK) and liver function tests (LFTs) with statins (objective assessment).

The therapeutic range of a drug is the concentration range required for a therapeutic effect. The therapeutic index (also known as therapeutic ratio) is the ratio of the concentration associated with a therapeutic effect to that causing a toxic effect, and is calculated as LD_{50}/ED_{50}, where LD_{50} is the lethal dose of a drug for 50% of an animal population in preclinical studies and ED_{50} is the minimum effective dose for 50% of that population. In drugs with a wide therapeutic range (e.g. penicillin) precise dosing is less critical, but in drugs with a narrow therapeutic range (e.g. phenytoin) great care with dosing and monitoring is needed to avoid toxic or sub-therapeutic effects. If a drug with a narrow therapeutic range displays a good relationship between its concentration in the blood and its therapeutic effects, it may be suitable for therapeutic drug monitoring, e.g. the renally excreted drugs gentamicin, vancomycin, digoxin and lithium, and the hepatically metabolised drugs phenytoin and ciclosporin.

First and zero order kinetics

For most drugs, the relationship between the dose of the drug administered and the plasma concentration in their therapeutic range is linear and therefore predictable: this is first order kinetics. This is because the rate of clearance of the drug is directly proportional to the dose administered. If, however, the clearance mechanisms of the drug become saturated, the relationship between the dose and the concentration will no longer be linear; the concentration of the drug will begin to rise exponentially so that a much greater, unpredictable increase in concentration will occur for a given increase in dose: this is zero order kinetics. For the majority of drugs this only occurs in the supratherapeutic or toxic range and explains the delayed recovery of high levels of drugs such as aspirin and theophylline. However, in the case of alcohol, saturation of clearance mechanisms (mainly hepatic metabolism) may occur with ~2/3 unit. Consumption of further alcohol will result in a disproportionate, exponential elevation in alcohol levels (zero order kinetics) with the risk of unpredictable and toxic effects. A similar issue arises with phenytoin. Whilst phenytoin displays first order kinetics in the sub-therapeutic range, as the concentration increases into the therapeutic range, the hepatic metabolism of phenytoin becomes saturated and its relationship with the dose becomes non-linear, predisposing to toxicity (saturation kinetics [➔ see Phenytoin, p. 89]; Figure 3.2A). Different patients will respond differently, dependent on their metabolic capacity and co-prescription of enzyme-inhibiting or enzyme-inducing drugs (Figure 3.2B).

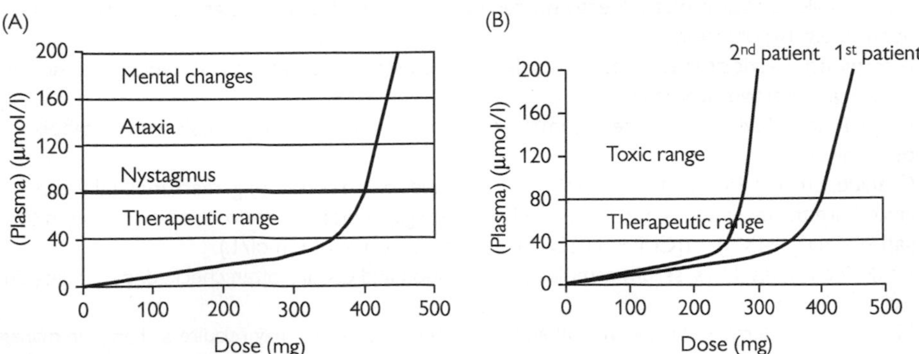

Figure 3.2 Pharmacokinetics of phenytoin.

Adapted with permission from Chapter 3: Drug Interactions, Figure 3.5, p.22. In *Oxford Textbook of Clinical Pharmacology and Therapeutics and Drug Therapy*, Second Edition, D.G. Grahame-Smith and J.K. Aronson, Oxford, UK: OUP. © 1992 Oxford University Press. Reproduced with permission of the Licensor through PLSclear.

Stopping

It is important to identify the appropriate duration of treatment (e.g. antibiotic stewardship), reasons for stopping (e.g. toxic effects) or not stopping medications, and special precautions for stopping/withdrawing drugs including:

- Corticosteroids: withdrawal should be gradual (i.e. reduced rapidly down to physiological doses [equivalent to prednisolone 7.5 mg daily] and then reduced more slowly).
- Opiates, benzodiazepines: withdrawal syndromes occur with abrupt withdrawal.
- β-blockers: abrupt withdrawal, especially in patients with ischaemic heart disease can cause a rebound worsening of myocardial ischaemia.

Toxicology

Acute poisoning accounts for up to 5–10% of hospital admissions. Most cases are due to intentional drug ingestion, for which mortality is low (<0.5%).

Principles of management

Clinical assessment

- History from patient, family, friends, emergency services and/or bystanders.
- Emergency assessment:
  - 'Airway, breathing, circulation' approach as acutely poisoned patients may present with a reduced conscious level.
  - Airway obstruction (e.g. dentures, vomit) must be removed.
  - Definitive airway protection (e.g. intubation) and ventilation may be required in those at risk of aspiration and is especially important when methods of gut decontamination are appropriate.
  - Circulatory monitoring (blood pressure [BP], heart rate [HR] and rhythm, urine output and peripheral perfusion) is often required.
- Examination:
  - Pupil size, body temperature, HR, BP, respiratory rate and agitation level may help to narrow down the potential toxin responsible. Specific groups of clinical signs/symptoms may be characteristic for the effects associated with exposure to certain agents (toxidromes; Table 3.18). However, they are of less benefit when used in isolation or confounded when multiple drugs have been co-ingested as they may have opposing effects leading to an overlap or suppression of clinical signs.

Investigations

- Blood gas analysis:
  - A metabolic acidosis is often directly related to the drug itself or occurs as a secondary consequence, e.g. hypotension.
  - A respiratory acidosis may be due to inadequate ventilation in a patient with reduced consciousness, e.g. a sedative overdose.
  - In significant salicylate overdose, a combined picture of a respiratory alkalosis with metabolic acidosis may occur.
  - Cyanide, ethanol, isoniazid, metformin, salicylate and toxic alcohols (e.g. methanol, ethylene glycol) are the most frequent causes of a high anion gap metabolic acidosis in poisoning (anion gap = $([Na^+] + [K^+]) - ([Cl^-] + [HCO_3^-])$: normal range 10–14 mmol/L).
- Urea & electrolytes, LFTs, serum osmolality, coagulation and CK are often checked, depending on the clinical indication.
  - Many drugs undergo renal elimination and significant renal failure may require a change in management.
  - An osmolar gap suggests the presence of unmeasured osmotically active compounds (e.g. methanol, ethylene glycol) and is the difference between laboratory-measured serum osmolality (O_m)

and the calculated serum osmolality (O_c) (2[Na^+ + K^+] + urea + glucose) which is normally <10 mmol/L. Early after ingestion of methanol or ethylene glycol, the anion gap is normal and osmolar gap elevated. However, as they are metabolised to formic acid and glycolic acid, respectively (toxic metabolites), the osmolar gap begins to fall, a metabolic acidosis ensues and the anion gap steadily rises as the metabolites accumulate.

- Chest X-ray:
  - Aspiration is not uncommon in patients presenting with a reduced consciousness.
- Drug levels:
  - Specific poisonings that require serum levels include digoxin, lithium, paracetamol and salicylate.
- Urinalysis:
  - Rapid reaction dipstix to screen for common drugs of abuse and recreational drugs by immunoassay are available, but not used routinely owing to false-positive results, detection of metabolites rather than the parent drug (which may be positive for several days post-ingestion), and cross-reactivity with other drugs, including prescription and over-the-counter medicines.

Gut decontamination

- Activated charcoal (AC):
  - Viscous black liquid that may be difficult to tolerate.
  - Porous structure with an extremely large surface area.
  - Highly effective at absorbing toxins from the gastrointestinal tract (although not strong acids and alkalis, alcohols, cyanide, elemental metals and pesticides).
  - Given usually as a 50g once only dose.
  - Commonly causes vomiting and prior administration of an anti-emetic should be considered.
  - Should be avoided in patients at risk of aspiration unless given via a nasogastric tube (NGT) in those with a protected airway.
  - Given to all patients who present within 1 hour of ingesting a potentially toxic amount of drug(s).
  - Toxicity of certain drugs (e.g. opioids, anticholinergics, TCAs) can slow gastric emptying and so the use of AC may still be effective longer than 1 hour post-overdose.
  - Repeat doses should also be considered in the following overdoses and given every 4 hours until clinically indicated to stop:
    - Carbamazepine, dapsone, digoxin, phenobarbital, quinine and theophylline; AC enhances drug elimination by interrupting the enteroenteric/enterohepatic circulation or by leaching drugs from the intestinal circulation into the gut lumen down a diffusion gradient.
    - Modified or sustained release preparations or significant salicylate ingestions where drug absorption is prolonged from the gastrointestinal tract; AC reduces drug absorption.
  - Repeat doses may lead to constipation and so patients requiring repeat doses should be given laxatives.
- Whole bowel irrigation:
  - Oral administration of a non-absorbable gut cleansing agent (high molecular weight polyethylene glycols, e.g. Klean-Prep® or MoviPrep®), which causes a liquid stool and reduces drug absorption by physically forcing contents rapidly through the gastrointestinal tract.
  - Can be given orally or via NGT.
  - Should only be considered when the airway is protected.
  - Usual dose for an adult is 1.5–2 L/hour and should be continued until rectal effluent is clear.
  - Role in treating large overdoses that are not absorbed by AC (e.g. lithium, iron) or where the drug may have prolonged absorption from the gastrointestinal tract, e.g. sustained release or enteric-coated preparations (e.g. CCBs, theophylline).
- Ipecacuanha-induced emesis and gastric lavage are no longer routinely recommended because they are ineffective at removing significant amounts of poison, increase the risk of aspiration, and delay or limit the use of AC.

Enhancing drug elimination

- Urinary alkalinisation (previously known as forced alkaline diuresis):
  - Treatment of choice for moderate to severe salicylate poisoning (➲ see Salicylates (aspirin), p. 85 and Figure 3.4).
  - Potentially useful for poisoning with phenobarbital and methotrexate.
  - May be combined with multiple doses of AC.
  - Involves the IV administration of 8.4% sodium bicarbonate solution (recommended dose of 225 mL over 1 hour in adults) to achieve a urine pH of 7.5–8.5 (checked every 30 minutes).
  - Hypokalaemia must be corrected or prevented for effective alkalinisation to be achieved.
- Extracorporeal techniques:
  - Include plasmapheresis, haemodialysis, haemofiltration, haemodiafiltration and haemoperfusion.
  - Worthwhile only if total body clearance is increased by at least 30%.

Antidotes and therapies for poisoning

Antidotes are available for only a small number of poisons (Table 3.19). Indiscriminate use of some antidotes/therapies can potentially increase morbidity, e.g. administration of flumazenil (a competitive benzodiazepine antagonist) may precipitate convulsions or arrhythmias, particularly if the patient has a history of underlying epilepsy or has ingested pro-convulsants or pro-arrhythmic drugs, and as such, is only recommended for reversal of conscious sedation from benzodiazepine toxicity.

Table 3.19 Antidotes and specific therapies for common overdoses and poisonings

Poisoning	Antidotes and specific therapies
Benzodiazepines	Flumazenil
β-blockers	Glucagon, high dose insulin-glucose combination
Calcium channel blockers	Calcium chloride, high dose insulin-glucose combination
Digoxin	Digoxin specific antibodies
Heparins	Protamine
Iron	Desferrioxamine
Local anaesthetics	Intralipid®
Methaemoglobinaemia	Methylthioninium chloride
Opioids	Naloxone
Paracetamol	N-acetylcysteine
Serotonin syndrome	Cyproheptadine
Toxic alcohols (e.g. methanol, ethylene glycol)	Fomepizole/4-methylpyrazole
TCAs	Sodium bicarbonate
Valproate	Levocarnitine

Supportive care and monitoring

Morbidity in the poisoned patient usually results from the acute effects of a drug/poison on the cardiovascular, respiratory and central nervous systems. Therefore, good supportive care of the acutely poisoned patient should be maintained, including monitoring of fluid balance, correction of electrolytes and provision of organ support if required. Management plans for agitated delirium and a psychosocial risk assessment (in cases of deliberate self-harm) should be made. The duration of monitoring/observation required is dependent on the drug(s) taken and the route of administration, formulation (e.g. standard release versus sustained release), half-life and any delays to drug elimination that can be predicted, e.g. renal failure for drugs that undergo renal excretion.

Poisons information centres

Clinical toxicology remains an experienced-based specialty, with recommendations often based on a literature of case reports and case series, rather than controlled clinic trials. Specialist poisons information centres exist worldwide, to advise on, and assist with, the prevention, diagnosis and management of poisoning. In the UK an internet-based information service is available to clinicians (https://www.toxbase.org) as well as a 24-hour national telephone poisons information service.

Analgesics

Paracetamol

Paracetamol overdose remains the most common drug overdose that presents to Emergency Departments in the UK. In overdose, there is increased Phase I oxidative metabolism of paracetamol by CYP450 enzymes (predominantly CYP2E1) to its toxic metabolite N-acetyl-p-benzoquinone imine (NAPQI) as normal Phase II hepatic conjugation pathways (with glucuronide and sulphate) are saturated (zero order kinetics). Endogenous glutathione (a tripeptide sequence of glutamine/cysteine/glutamate) will detoxify NAPQI to cysteine and mercaptate conjugates that are excreted in the urine. However, once depleted, NAPQI is left to bind covalently and irreversibly to hepatocytes leading to cell death, necrosis and the release of inflammatory mediators, perpetuating hepatocyte cell death (➲ see Chapter 15, Paracetamol poisoning and drug-induced liver injury, p. 533).

The antidote for paracetamol poisoning is N-acetylcysteine (NAC), which is administered IV. NAC acts as a thiol donor and acts as a glutathione precursor (or substitute) leading to an increase in glutathione. Maximal protective effect is time-dependent with the best results occurring in those who receive NAC within 8 hours of ingestion. Administration of NAC >16 hours from overdose may not prevent severe liver damage, but should still be used since the outcome from paracetamol-induced fulminant liver failure (that has a 10% mortality rate) is improved.

Presentation

Patients often present with very few clinical signs of toxicity in the early stages (24–48 hours post-overdose). Those with significant poisoning who present late to hospital, may complain of nausea, vomiting, right upper quadrant (RUQ) tenderness or have signs of fulminant liver failure. Early presentations in those with massive paracetamol overdose (initial 4-hour paracetamol concentration >800 mg/L) may present in coma with a lactic acidosis (a direct effect of the paracetamol on mitochondrial metabolism).

Management

- Patients presenting with ingestion >150 mg/kg within 1 hour should be considered for AC.
- NAC treatment guidelines are based on the 'paracetamol overdose treatment nomogram' with a treatment line starting at a 4-hour paracetamol concentration of 100 mg/L (Figure 3.3).
- In patients who have taken an overdose at a known time, serum paracetamol levels should be taken 4 hours after ingestion and patients with values above the treatment line should be treated with NAC. If levels are unknown at/after 8 hours from ingestion, NAC should be commenced in patients who are thought to have ingested ≥150 mg/kg. Paracetamol levels are then taken and NAC discontinued if they fall below the treatment line.
- In patients who have taken an overdose at an unknown time, NAC should be given if the dose ingested is >75 mg/kg in the last 24-hour period. Treatment is essential if the dose is >150 mg/kg. Patients with clinical features of hepatic injury (e.g. jaundice, RUQ tenderness) should be treated. Interpretation of paracetamol levels (if detected) cannot be made without a reliable time of ingestion and should not therefore be relied upon.
- In patients who have taken a staggered overdose (defined as the dose taken over >1 hour) or a supratherapeutic excess (defined as more than a licensed dose for that individual), with the total

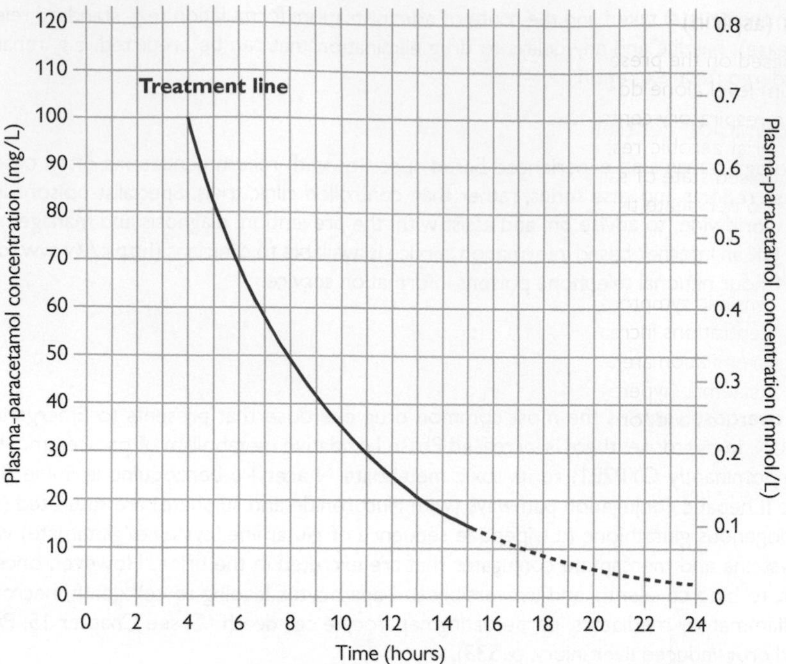

Figure 3.3 Paracetamol overdose treatment nomogram.

Reproduced with permission from Royal College of Emergency Medicine. *Paracetamol overdose: new guidance on the use of intravenous acetylcysteine*. London, UK: RCEM. Copyright © The Royal College of Emergency Medicine. https://www.rcem.ac.uk/RCEM/Quality-Policy/Clinical_Standards_Guidance/RCEM_Guidance.aspx?WebsiteKey=b3d6bb2a-abba-44ed-b758-467776a958cd&hkey=862bd964-0363-4f7f-bdab-89e4a68c9de4&RCEM_Guidance=6

dose taken <75 mg/kg in the last 24 hours, treatment with NAC is not recommended as toxicity is very unlikely. Treatment is, however, recommended if the total dose taken is >75 mg/kg and must be given if the dose is >150 mg/kg. Patients with clinical features of hepatic injury should be treated. Paracetamol levels are not helpful in staggered overdoses and supratherapeutic excess, while paracetamol may be detected, the level can provide no guidance in relation to the nomogram treatment line.

- The NAC treatment regimen is as follows:
  - 150 mg/kg in 200 mL 5% glucose infused over 1 hour, followed by:
  - 50 mg/kg in 500 mL 5% glucose infused over 4 hours, followed by:
  - 100 mg/kg in 1l 5% glucose over 16 hours.
- At the end of treatment, patients with evidence of liver injury (international normalised ratio [INR] >1.3 and/or ALT ≥ twice the upper limit of normal), a further dose of NAC (100 mg/kg in 1L 5% dextrose over 16 hours) should be administered until the patient's condition and liver function improves.
- Expert opinion should be sorted early from a regional centre if liver failure progresses as liver transplantation may be necessary.
- Anaphylactoid reactions to NAC occur in up to 20% of patients treated, usually during or soon after the first infusion. They are more likely when paracetamol concentrations are low or absent, in women and in those with a family history of allergies. The reactions commonly cause nausea, vomiting, flushing, urticarial rash, angioedema, tachycardia and bronchospasm. More severe reactions are rare. Management includes stopping the infusion, and if needed, an antihistamine, e.g. chlorphenamine. Bronchodilators may be helpful. Steroids are not indicated as the reaction is not IgE-mediated. Once the reaction has settled, NAC can be recommenced at a slower rate.

Salicylates (aspirin)

Toxicity is based on the presence of clinical features in relation to serum salicylate concentrations (Figure 3.4). A serum level alone does not determine prognosis. Salicylate initially triggers ventilation as a direct effect via the respiratory centre leading to a respiratory alkalosis. In more significant overdoses, inhibition of mitochondrial aerobic respiration (uncoupling oxidative phosphorylation) results in a lactic acidosis. Due to the ionised state of salicylate, small reductions in pH produce large increases in non-ionised drug, which is able to permeate tissues particularly the central nervous system (CNS).

Presentation

The earliest signs and symptoms of salicylate toxicity are nausea, vomiting, diaphoresis and tinnitus. As CNS salicylate concentrations increase, tinnitus is followed by diminished auditory acuity or even deafness. Vertigo and hyperventilation are also common in mild to moderate poisoning. Other findings include hypoglycaemia, hypokalaemia, hyperpyrexia and rarely haematemesis. Coma, pulmonary oedema, severe acidosis, renal failure, seizures and/or salicylate levels >700 mg/L are all signs that toxicity is severe.

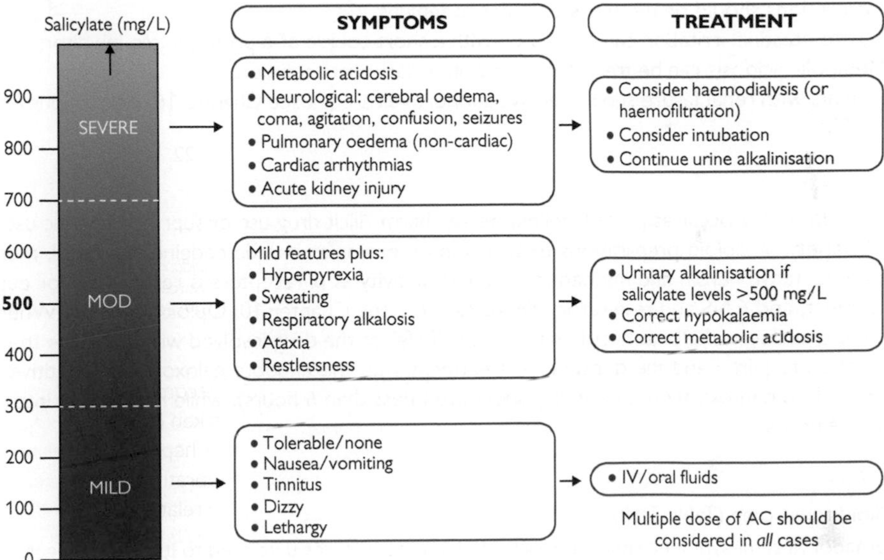

Figure 3.4 Symptoms and treatment of salicylate poisoning in adult patients.

Management

- The benefit of gastric decontamination is uncertain, but it is generally accepted that repeat doses of AC are recommended for use with large ingestions. In overdose, salicylate tends to form concretions in the stomach, which delay absorption, hence increasing its half-life from 4 hours up to 20 hours. Salicylate levels should therefore be taken every 2–4 hours in those who are symptomatic until concentrations are shown to be falling. AC should be given within 1 hour of ingestion of >125 mg/kg and a further dose given if salicylate levels continue to rise.
- IV fluid is given to replace fluid losses and for resuscitation.
- Hypokalaemia and hypoglycaemia should be corrected on an urgent basis.
- Urinary alkalinisation decreases the amount of non-ionised salicylate available to enter tissues and 'traps' salicylate within the renal tubule for excretion in the urine. By raising the urine pH suitably, a greater than five-fold increase in total salicylate excretion can be achieved. It should be considered

in moderate toxicity and when levels are >500 mg/kg. Hypokalaemia must be corrected in order to achieve effective alkalinisation.

- Haemodialysis (or haemofiltration) is the treatment of choice for severe poisoning.

Other NSAIDS

Presentation

Symptoms of NSAID overdose tend to be mild and consistent with irritant effects such as gastrointestinal symptoms. In acute overdose, gastrointestinal haemorrhage is not common unless it occurs as a secondary effect from a Mallory–Weiss tear. Large overdoses (e.g. >400 mg/kg of ibuprofen) can be associated with a metabolic acidosis and/or renal impairment. Overdoses of mefenamic acid are associated with convulsions in up to 15% of patients.

Management

- AC can be given for large ingestions within 1 hour of the overdose.
- Supportive care and symptom control:
  - Convulsions should be treated with benzodiazepines.
  - Gastrointestinal irritation can be treated with a short course of a proton pump inhibitor.
  - Metabolic acidosis can be treated with sodium bicarbonate solution.
  - Patients with renal failure should receive supportive care (➲ see Chapter 16, Acute kidney injury, p. 583).

Opioids

Opioid overdose may occur as part of deliberate self-harm, illicit drug use or supratherapeutic use of analgesia. A variety of opioid preparations exist; common examples include codeine, tramadol, morphine, oxycodone, fentanyl, heroin and methadone. Agonist activity at μ-receptors is responsible for euphoria, analgesic effect, and CNS and respiratory depression (➲ see Chapter 10, Opioids, p. 339). When managing opioid overdoses, the pharmacokinetics (i.e. half-life) of the drug involved will determine the period of observation required and the duration of treatment with the antidote naloxone (competitive opioid antagonist). Heroin intoxication is relatively short lived (less than 6 hours), while methadone intoxication may last >24 hours.

Presentation

- Opioid toxidrome (Table 3.18).
- Tramadol (a semi-synthetic opioid) toxicity can exhibit features unrelated to its opioid effect, including agitation, tachycardia, seizures and rarely a serotonin syndrome through inhibition of 5-hydroxytryptamine (HT) re-uptake.
- In toxicity, opioids may induce hypotension and depress cardiac myocyte isometric force of contraction, leading to reduced cardiac output, which may be ameliorated with naloxone.

Management

- AC may be effective for oral presentations.
- Due to the availability of combination paracetamol/codeine preparations, all patients with opiate toxicity should be suspected of a paracetamol overdose with paracetamol levels being checked.
- Naloxone in 200–400-microgram boluses should be given IV and titrated to clinical response. Intramuscular (IM) naloxone should be avoided where possible due to a slow and unpredictable absorption.
- In patients who fail to respond to doses of up to 2 mg naloxone, an alternative diagnosis should be considered, e.g. pontine haemorrhage, encephalitis.
- Patients should be observed for up to 6 hours from the last dose of naloxone. Repeated doses may be required, particularly in those who have ingested long-acting (e.g. methadone) or sustained/modified-release opiate preparations. In these patients, a naloxone infusion may be appropriate.

- A 12-lead electrocardiogram (ECG) should be completed in patients who have taken a methadone overdose as it can block cardiac potassium channels leading to a delay in cardiac repolarisation, prolonging the QTc interval and so increasing the risk of torsade de pointes.
- Intubation and mechanical ventilation may be required if respiratory depression is not rapidly reversed with naloxone or if complicated by aspiration.

Anti-depressants and mood stabilisers

Lithium

Once ingested and absorbed, lithium substitutes for sodium and potassium ions, and modulates intracellular secondary messenger systems. It has a large volume of distribution, including the CNS, where in overdose it acts as a neurotoxin. Its elimination is almost entirely by the kidneys and clearance is therefore dependent on glomerular filtration rate (GFR), and will be reduced in water- and sodium-depleted states.

Presentation

A single acute overdose in naive individuals usually caries low risk and leads to only mild symptoms independent of serum lithium concentrations. In a patient maintained on long-term lithium treatment, acute overdoses can lead to severe toxicity. Lithium toxicity may also occur through chronic accumulation related to factors such as incorrect dosing, dehydration or an interaction with other drugs (e.g. NSAIDs, thiazide diuretics, ACE-inhibitors). Symptoms of toxicity can be divided into:

- Mild: nausea, vomiting, diarrhoea, fine tremor, polyuria, weakness.
- Moderate: increasing confusion, myoclonic jerks and twitches, hyperreflexia, initial restlessness then stupor, hypernatraemia.
- Severe: coma, convulsions, arrhythmias, renal failure.

Management

- Acute overdose: lithium concentration measured at 6 hours from ingestion and then every 4–6 hours.
- Chronic overdose/accumulation: lithium concentration measured at arrival to hospital and then every 4–6 hours.
- Lithium is not absorbed by AC and whole bowel irrigation should be considered in those who have ingested a potentially toxic amount of lithium (>4 g).
- Careful IV correction of any fluid and sodium deficits, and restoration of renal function are essential to maximise lithium excretion.
- Extracorporeal elimination should be considered in patients with features of severe toxicity or if serum lithium concentrations are >5 mmol/L (or >4 mmol/L in those with renal impairment).

Selective serotonin reuptake inhibitors

Presentation

Many patients with SSRI (e.g. citalopram, fluoxetine, fluvoxamine, sertraline) overdose remain asymptomatic. Symptoms may develop within 4 hours of ingestion and are a result of serotonin 'excess', commonly featuring anxiety, tremor, tachycardia, mydriasis and mild hypertension. A full serotonin syndrome may develop including convulsions and coma (Table 3.18). Cardiac arrhythmias have been reported including wide complex bradycardia and torsade de pointes (due to SSRI inhibition of inwardly rectifying potassium channels leading to a dose-dependent prolongation of the QTc interval). Citalopram appears to be the most potent in overdose and with its active metabolite, didesmethylcitalopram, has an increased half-life of up to 33–59 hours.

Serotonin syndrome occurs as a consequence of excess serotonergic neurotransmission, both peripherally and centrally, resulting in a triad of CNS, autonomic and neuromuscular dysfunction. It most commonly occurs after co-ingestion of several serotonergic drugs (therapeutically and/or in overdose [including non-SSRI drugs such as venlafaxine and tramadol]), but may also occur after the introduction or increase in dose of a single serotonergic drug, or as an interaction between a prescribed drug and an illicit drug e.g. cocaine, 3,4-methylenedioxymethamphetamine (MDMA).

Management

- General principles:
  - AC should be considered up to 1 hour after significant ingestions.
  - Benzodiazepines are effective as first-line agents for agitation, hyperthermia and seizures.
  - Cardiac monitoring is recommended in those who are tachycardic and/or have a prolonged QTc interval.
- Management of serotonin syndrome:
  - Meticulous supportive cardiorespiratory care with organ support where indicated.
  - Review and cessation of medication that may be attributable, e.g. SSRIs, serotonin noradrenaline reuptake inhibitors (SNRIs), TCAs, MAOIs, tramadol, fentanyl, metoclopramide, ondansetron, valproate.
  - Benzodiazepines are useful for agitated delirium and reducing tachycardia, hypertension, hyperpyrexia and seizures.
  - α-adrenergic antagonists, e.g. doxazosin, or direct vasodilators, e.g. glyceryl trinitrate (GTN) infusion, may be used to treat hypertension that is refractory to initial treatment.
  - If body temperature is >38.5°C, continuous body temperature monitoring, and internal and external cooling measures are indicated, e.g. administration of cold IV fluid and ice packs, as well as benzodiazepines.
  - If body temperature remains >39°C, the 5-HT_{2A} antagonist cyproheptadine is also given orally or via a NGT.
  - Neuromuscular paralysis, intubation and ventilation may be required in an effort to control muscle-generated heat and/or control refractory seizures, coma and agitation.

Tricyclic antidepressants

TCAs remain one of the leading causes of death from drug overdose. Toxic effects are mediated via inhibition of a number of receptor types including muscarinic (M_1), histamine (H_1) and peripheral post-synaptic α_1-adrenergic receptors. Cardiac toxicity is predominantly through blockade of inactivated fast sodium channels, slowing the rate of rise of the action potential, leading to QRS prolongation and, also, negative dromotropic and inotropic effects. TCAs are rapidly absorbed following oral administration with peak levels occurring within 2 hours, leading to rapid clinical deterioration. Toxicity is worsened by acidaemia, hypotension and hyperthermia.

Presentation

- Ingestion of >10 mg/kg is likely to lead to significant toxicity.
- Features tend to include anticholinergic features (Table 3.18).
- In severe toxicity there are depressed respiratory and conscious levels, convulsions, hypotension (α-adrenergic antagonist effects) and cardiac arrhythmias. Neurological findings include brisk reflexes with extensor plantars.
- ECGs may indicate:
  - a progressive widening of the QRS interval. QRS intervals >100 msec are predictive of seizures and QRS intervals >160 msec are associated with an increased risk of arrhythmias.
  - QT prolongation (through inhibition of cardiac delayed rectifier potassium channels).
  - A broad complex tachyarrhythmia – often associated with toxicity, but all forms of rhythm and conduction disturbance have been described.

Management

- Repeated doses of AC should be considered due to delayed gastric emptying from TCA toxicity.
- If agitation occurs, benzodiazepines should be used first line for sedation.

- Continuous cardiac monitoring should be provided.
- Reversing an acidosis with sodium bicarbonate aiming for a serum pH 7.45–7.55 significantly reduces the availability of free drug, while 'sodium loading' (increasing the extracellular concentration of sodium) may overcome effective blockade of sodium channels through gradient effects. Therefore, 8.4% sodium bicarbonate (in 50 mL boluses) should be given IV to patients (even in the absence of a metabolic acidosis) with QRS prolongation, arrhythmia or hypotension. It should also be considered in those with convulsions. If a patient requires ventilatory support, hyperventilation inducing a respiratory alkalosis can also help to reverse an acidosis and improve outcome.
- If arrhythmias are recurrent, Class 1a anti-arrhythmic agents (e.g. disopyramide) should be avoided as they may lead to worsening arrhythmia. Cardioversion and defibrillation are unlikely to be successful and lidocaine is second-line therapy.

Anti-epileptics

Carbamazepine

Carbamazepine is slowly and unpredictably absorbed from the gastrointestinal tract and undergoes hepatic metabolism to form an active metabolite. Enterohepatic recirculation of carbamazepine leads to a prolonged half-life. In overdose it results in dose-dependent CNS and anticholinergic effects. Ileus secondary to muscarinic antagonism may also result in prolonged absorption for several days. Serum carbamazepine levels do not correlate well with toxicity, but can aid diagnosis and allow for a more accurate assessment of the clinical course in more severe toxicity. Levels >20 mg/L (85 μmol/L) are often associated with CNS and anticholinergic effects, while levels >40 mg/L (140 μmol/L) typically cause life-threatening toxicity.

Presentation

CNS effects including nystagmus, ataxia, tremor, dysarthria, convulsions and delirium are common. In severe toxicity, fluctuating coma and cardiovascular toxicity (including hypotension and arrhythmias) may occur.

Management

- Multiple doses of AC are indicated after large ingestions. If CNS features are present, the patient must have a protected airway due to the risk of vomiting and aspiration. If bowel sounds are diminished/ absent, further doses of AC should be withheld in case of intestinal obstruction from an ileus.
- Benzodiazepines are beneficial for agitated delirium.

Phenytoin

Phenytoin is slowly and unpredictably absorbed from the gastrointestinal tract and peak serum concentrations may be delayed for 24–48 hours. As phenytoin metabolism is saturable within the liver, plasma concentrations and elimination half-life may rise dramatically with small increases in daily doses (see Figure 3.2). Toxicity therefore results from both supratherapeutic dosing and acute overdose.

Presentation

Supratherapeutic or chronic intoxication usually results in gradual onset ataxia. Nausea and vomiting usually occur early in acute overdose followed by neurological symptoms including ataxia, dysarthria, tremor, vertical or slow horizontal nystagmus, and drowsiness. In severe cases, toxicity may lead to seizures and coma. Cardiovascular toxicity is unusual, but is associated with IV administration of phenytoin.

Management

The majority of patients require good supportive care only. Multiple doses of AC can increase elimination of phenytoin, but there is no evidence that this improves outcome.

Valproate

Presentation

Valproate increases levels of GABA that can act as a central inhibitory neurotransmitter. Following overdose, most patients experience CNS depression and drowsiness, which correlates with rising serum levels.

In more severe toxicity (levels >850 mg/L) coma is accompanied by myoclonic movements, convulsions, cerebral oedema, and respiratory and cardiac failure. Metabolic derangements may occur, including a metabolic acidosis, hyperammonaemia (resulting from carnitine depletion leading to suppression of hepatic ammonia metabolism), hypoglycaemia, hypocalcaemia and hypernatraemia.

Management

- Supportive management is generally all that is required.
- Serum valproate levels are not measured routinely, but may be helpful if the diagnosis is in doubt in a mixed overdose or if haemodialysis is being considered.
- In massive overdose or when patients have hyperammonaemia or hepatotoxicity, administration of levocarnitine should be considered. This may have benefit as an antidote for valproate-induced mitochondrial effects.
- Valproate is highly protein bound at therapeutic concentrations, but in overdose, protein binding may become saturated with a subsequent increase in free valproate concentrations. Its low volume of distribution and low molecular weight, renders extracorporeal techniques (preferably intermittent haemodialysis) helpful in enhancing valproate clearance.

Cardiovascular drugs

β-blockers

β-blockers (e.g. atenolol, bisoprolol, carvedilol, esmolol, metoprolol, pindolol, propranolol and sotalol) are competitive antagonists of β_1 and β_2 adrenoceptors that are rapidly absorbed from the gastrointestinal tract, with serum concentrations peaking within 3 hours of ingestion.

β-adrenergic antagonism leads to a reduced activity of adenylate cyclase and a reduction in intracellular cAMP. This, in turn, leads to a down-regulation of protein kinase A-mediated phosphorylation of myocyte proteins, including L-type voltage sensitive calcium channels, resulting in a blunting of chronotropic and inotropic effects of endogenous catecholamines.

Presentation

The individual response to β-blocker toxicity is variable, but the common clinical features are hypotension and bradycardia that may be refractory to standard treatment. Varying degrees of heart block may also occur from QT prolongation (sotalol overdose blocks delayed rectifier potassium channels and so lengthens myocyte repolarisation) to complete heart block and asystole. Propranolol may lead to QRS prolongation, and ventricular arrhythmias (as it can block sodium channels) and CNS effects (as it is lipophilic) including drowsiness, confusion, convulsions and coma.

Management

- AC should be considered in patients presenting within 1 hour of overdose. Multiple doses of AC may be required in those who have taken a sustained-release preparation.
- Atropine and IV fluids are commonly used for bradycardia and hypotension, respectively, but are only likely to be effective in mild poisoning.
- If toxicity worsens, IV glucagon is the next step (5–10 mg bolus over 1–2 minutes). Glucagon increases adenylate cyclase activity, independent of β- adrenoceptors, leading to a dose-dependent increase in cAMP. If beneficial, the initial bolus can be repeated or an infusion commenced. Glucagon can cause vomiting with a risk of aspiration that may limit further administration. Hyperglycaemia and hypocalcaemia may also occur.
- High-dose insulin, which is effective in the treatment of CCB toxicity, is also beneficial in β-blocker toxicity (➲ see Calcium channel blockers, p. 91).
- Inotropes (e.g. β-adrenoceptor agonists such as isoprenaline and dobutamine) and cardiac pacing can be considered, based on the patient's clinical condition.
- Mechanical methods such as intra-aortic balloon pumping and extracorporeal membrane oxygenation may be considered.

Calcium channel blockers

CCBs prevent the opening of voltage-sensitive L-type calcium channels found in vascular smooth muscle and cardiac myocytes. This blockade results in a decrease in calcium influx leading to muscle relaxation, slowing of cardiac conduction and reduced force of cardiac contractility. CCB classes bind different receptor regions on the α_1 subunit of the calcium channel, which determines their therapeutic roles. The dihydropyridines (e.g. amlodipine and nifedipine) act selectively on calcium channels in peripheral vascular smooth muscle and reduce peripheral vascular resistance. The phenylalkylamines (e.g. verapamil) and benothiazepines (e.g. diltiazem) inhibit sinoatrial (SA) and atrioventricular (AV) nodal tissue, and therefore predominantly affect cardiac conduction.

Presentation

The therapeutic selectivity of CBBs is less apparent in overdose with the main effect being hypotension. This is caused by a combination of peripheral vasodilation, bradycardia and decreased contractility. Cardiac shock may be refractory and lead to death. Secondary metabolic effects include a metabolic lactic acidosis and hyperglycaemia. Hyperglycaemia is an indicator of severe poisoning resulting from reduced insulin secretion (as pancreatic β cells require effective calcium signalling mediated via L-type calcium channels for insulin release) and insulin resistance.

Management

- AC is advisable up to 1 hour after ingestion. For sustained-release preparations toxicity may be delayed >16 hours and multiple doses of AC are recommended.
- In symptomatic patients, meticulous supportive care is required, including monitoring of cardiac rhythm and blood glucose, early invasive haemodynamic monitoring and airway support, if needed.
- If hypotension continues after an appropriate IV fluid challenge, the next step is IV calcium chloride (10 mL of 10% solution) or calcium gluconate (20–30 mL of 10% solution). Calcium chloride has three times more ionised calcium compared with calcium gluconate and may lead to an improvement in BP and HR. If beneficial, repeated doses or an infusion can be administered, with monitoring of serum calcium level to ensure it remains <3 mmol/L, above which there is a risk of inducing myocardial depression.
- Atropine may be used for symptomatic bradycardia, although this is unlikely to have a sustained effect. Cardiac pacing may be used to increase HR, but capture may not improve cardiac output, possibly due to impaired ventricular relaxation and contractility.
- If hypotension is refractory to the above measures, high-dose insulin-glucose is indicated. An initial bolus of 1 unit/kg of short-acting insulin is administered followed by an infusion of 0.5–2 units/kg/hour of short-acting insulin. Higher doses may be given to patients who do not respond. Euglycaemia is maintained with 10% or 20% glucose infusions and blood glucose monitoring every 30 minutes. The use of high-dose insulin in CCB toxicity facilitates carbohydrate dependence within the myocardium, providing greater myocardial energy and oxygen supply, and improving calcium signalling. At the doses used in this regimen, insulin is also positively inotropic.
- Inotropes and vasopressors are often commenced in tandem with high-dose insulin-glucose, the choice of which is guided through invasive haemodynamic monitoring and/or echocardiography.
- Other measures may be tried as 'salvage' therapy if patients continue to deteriorate, including glucagon, Intralipid®, methylthioninium chloride, levosimendan, vasopressin and metaraminol. The evidence for these is predominantly based on case reports and the benefits remain unclear.
- Mechanical methods such as intra-aortic balloon pumping and extracorporeal membrane oxygenation may be considered.

Digoxin

Digoxin is a cardiac glycoside that inhibits the Na^+-K^+ ATPase transporter, causing a shift of intracellular potassium to the extracellular space, and subsequent increases in intracellular calcium, enhancing automaticity and inotropicity. It also enhances vagal tone, resulting in decreased SA and AV node conduction velocity.

Presentation

Toxicity either occurs from an acute ingestion or, more commonly, in a patient who is on chronic therapy. This may develop in patients taking a supratherapeutic dose or in patients with acute renal failure; digoxin is excreted in the urine unchanged and will accumulate in renal failure. Commonly, toxicity is associated with nausea, vomiting, abdominal pains and weakness. Cardiovascular instability may develop, often related to a cardiac arrhythmia. Any bradyarrhythmia or tachyarrhythmia from increased automaticity is possible. Severe poisoning may lead to hyperkalaemia. Blurred vision or altered colour perception (classically xanthopsia) is a rare feature.

Management

- AC is given up to 1 hour post-ingestion and repeated doses are effective in interrupting enterohepatic recirculation.
- Serum digoxin levels are helpful, but do not equate to total body burden or correlate well with features of toxicity. They should be measured 6 hours post-ingestion or more urgently in severe poisoning, when they can be used to calculate treatment with digoxin-specific antibody fragments.
- Hyperkalaemia should be treated with insulin-glucose.
- Persistent hyperkalaemia (>6.5 mmol/L) and arrhythmia associated with hypotension should be treated with digoxin-specific antibody fragments, which are effective within 15–30 minutes. Atropine may be used as a holding measure while the antibodies are being obtained.

Recreational drugs

Recreational drugs can be broadly categorised into established recreational drugs and new psychoactive substance (NPSs), which can be further subdivided into drugs that are stimulants, hallucinogens and depressants (sedatives) (Table 3.20).

Table 3.20 Classification of recreational drugs

Classification	Established recreational drugs: • Widely available for many years. • Internationally controlled. • Risks and acute toxicity well documented.	NPSs • Relatively recent phenomenon of substances. • Produced to mimic the effect of more established illegal drugs and circumvent loop holes in recreational drug legislation. • Mistakenly known as 'legal highs'.
Stimulants	Amphetamines. Cocaine. MDMA (Ecstasy).	Benzofurans. Cathinones (e.g. mephedrone). Indanes. N-methoxybenzyl (NBOMe; N bomb). Piperazines. Pipradols.
Hallucinogens	Ketamine. LSD. Psilocybin (magic mushrooms).	Glaucine. Ketamine analogues. Salvia. Synthetic cannabinoids. Trifluoromethylphenylpiperazine (TFMPP). Tryptamines.
Depressants	Benzodiazepines. GHB. Heroin and opioids.	Gammabutyrolactone (GBL). 1,4-butanediol. Novel opioids.

Established recreational drugs

Amphetamines

Numerous derivatives of amphetamine exist (e.g. MDMA) based on various side chain substitutions on the basic amphetamine structure. Amphetamines enhance catecholamine (e.g. noradrenaline, dopamine, serotonin) release and block their reuptake leading to CNS and peripheral vascular stimulation.

Presentation

Patients with amphetamine toxicity commonly present with a sympathomimetic toxidrome (Table 3.18) and in severe cases may develop paranoid psychosis, arrhythmias (commonly supraventricular), serotonin syndrome and convulsions. Medical complications may include rhabdomyolysis, renal failure and haemorrhagic stroke. In MDMA toxicity, patients may present with hyponatraemia and cerebral oedema secondary to syndrome of inappropriate antidiuretic hormone secretion and/or increased water ingestion (➲ see Chapter 19, Hyponatraemia, p. 691 and Syndrome of inappropriate antidiuretic hormone, p. 692).

Management

- Benzodiazepines are the first line treatment for agitated or psychotic patients and may have a central effect in reducing tachycardia, hypertension, convulsions and hyperpyrexia.
- Second line agents for hypertension include α-blockers or direct vasodilators, e.g. nitrates.
- Serotonin syndrome management (➲ see Management, p. 88).
- Supportive management in a critical care environment is likely to be required for those patients with prolonged hyperthermia leading to rhabdomyolysis, metabolic acidosis, disseminated intravascular coagulation (DIC) and multiple organ failure.

Cocaine

Cocaine blocks presynaptic catecholamine re-uptake, resulting in sympathomimetic toxicity. It also has anaesthetic effects through sodium channel blockage.

Presentation

Patients with acute cocaine toxicity present with symptoms and signs of sympathomimetic and stimulant toxicity similar to that of amphetamines. However, there is an additional risk of cocaine-related vasospasm, which can result in vascular dissection, intracranial haemorrhage and acute cardiomyopathy. Myocardial ischaemia related to cocaine may also occur due to increased myocardial oxygen demand from tachycardia, and cocaine-induced platelet aggregability, and stimulation of endothelin release and inhibition of nitric oxide production, potentiating vasoconstriction. Blockage of myocardial-fast sodium channels by cocaine may result in ventricular arrhythmias.

Management

- Management is similar to that for amphetamine toxicity and in both scenarios, β-blockers are contraindicated due to a risk of unopposed α-adrenoceptor stimulation leading to worsening hypertension.
- Patients presenting with chest pain should be treated for acute coronary syndrome, including antiplatelet therapy, but with some important exceptions. Benzodiazepines should be given early to reduce sympathetic drive, reducing myocardial oxygen demand, as well as to facilitate coronary artery vasodilatation via benzodiazepine receptors. For continuing chest pain, sublingual followed by IV nitrates should be administered in an attempt to reverse potential vasospasm. In those who fail to respond, conventional management should then be followed including thrombolysis or primary angiography (➲ see Chapter 13, Invasive management (revascularisation), p. 427 and Acute medical management, p. 428).

Heroin

➲ See Opioids, p. 86 and Table 3.18.

New psychoactive substances

Many NPSs are synthetic amphetamine-like psychostimulants and share a number of the well-documented adverse effects. In comparison to more established recreational drugs, patients with acute NPS toxicity frequently present with overlapping stimulant and hallucinogenic toxidromes. Clinical management in toxicity is generally orientated towards providing symptomatic care.

Cathinones

Cathinones are β-ketone amphetamine analogues, which block the re-uptake of dopamine, norepinephrine and serotonin, as well as stimulate the release of dopamine. Synthetic cathinones are related to the parent compound cathinone, which is one of the psychoactive substances found in khat (*Catha edulis*) or synthesised from pseudoephedrine. One of the commonly available cathinones sold on the recreational market is mephedrone (4-methylmethcathinone). Acute toxicity of mephedrone and many of the other related NPSs resembles that of amphetamines, although the duration of effect may be prolonged due to increased elimination half-life. Treatment is similar to that of amphetamines and predominantly requires supportive care.

Synthetic cannabinoid receptor agonists

Synthetic cannabinoid receptor agonists (SCRAs) are synthetic compounds that are sprayed or soaked on to a plant-based material, which when smoked are intended to mimic the effects of the natural psychoactive substances found in cannabis (e.g. Δ^9-tetrahydrocannabinol [THC]). They often have considerably higher affinity for CB_1 cannabinoid receptors than THC and are therefore significantly more potent. Early SCRAs detected in herbal smoking mixtures were commonly known as 'spice'. It is now believed that around 150–200 SCRAs exist with a wide variety of product names, many of which contain different compositions. Little is known about the detailed pharmacology and toxicology of these compounds. In acute toxicity they may present with pronounced psychoactive effects, but they are also reported to lead to stimulant effects, including agitated delirium, tachycardia, hypertension, chest pain, convulsions and renal failure. As with other recreational drugs, treatment is based on supportive care and symptom control.

Acknowledgements

The editors would like to thank Satnam Lidder for his input on this chapter.

Further reading

1. 'New Drug Mechanisms' series in *British Journal of Clinical Pharmacology*.
2. National Poisons Information Service primary clinical toxicology database: https://www.toxbase.org
3. European Monitoring Centre for Drugs and Drug Addiction: http://www.emcdda.europa.eu
4. Dargan P, Wood D. *Novel Psychoactive Substances: Classification, Pharmacology and Toxicology*. London: Academic Press, 2013.

Multiple choice questions

Questions

1. Which of the following statements is true?
   A. Warfarin is highly bound to plasma proteins.
   B. Human epidermal growth factor receptor-2 overexpression decreases the effect of trastuzumab.
   C. Malignant hyperthermia is most commonly an autosomal recessive disorder.
   D. Cytochrome P450 3A5 isoenzyme over-expression increases the effect of tacrolimus.
   E. Hydrochlorothiazide has no interaction with organic anion transporters.

2. Where C = the plasma concentration of a drug and Vd = the apparent volume of distribution of the drug, the loading dose of that drug equals:
   A. C + Vd
   B. C/Vd
   C. C – Vd
   D. Vd/C
   E. C × Vd

3. The neuroleptic malignant syndrome toxidrome is characterised by:
   A. Meiosis.
   B. Hyper-reflexia.
   C. Hypotension.
   D. Diaphoresis.
   E. Bradycardia.

4. Which of the following statements about amphetamines is not true?
   A. Amphetamines block noradrenaline re-uptake.
   B. Amphetamines block dopamine re-uptake.
   C. Amphetamines block serotonin re-uptake.
   D. Amphetamine overdose predisposes to hypothermia.
   E. Amphetamine overdose predisposes to rhabdomyolysis.

5. Which of the following statements is true?
   A. β-blockers are slowly absorbed from the gastrointestinal tract.
   B. β-blockade leads to a reduced activity of adenylate cyclase.
   C. β-blockade improves detrusor hyperactivity.
   D. β-blockade upregulates protein kinase A-mediated phosphorylation of myocyte proteins.
   E. β-blockade increases intracellular cAMP.

6. Which of the following statements about activated charcoal treatment for poisoning is true?
   A. It has an important role to play in the management of lithium toxicity.
   B. It has no role in the management of digoxin toxicity.
   C. It is not associated with vomiting.
   D. Repeat doses normally cause diarrhoea.
   E. It may be helpful in cases of large salicylate overdose.

7. Tacrolimus metabolism is inhibited by:
   A. Clarithromycin.
   B. Carbamazepine.
   C. St John's wort.
   D. Phenytoin.
   E. Rifampicin.

Answers

1. A. Warfarin is very highly bound (99%) to plasma proteins. Trastuzumab is a monoclonal antibody to human epidermal growth factor receptor-2 (HER2). It is more effective in, and licensed for, the treatment of HER2-positive breast cancer, i.e. which overexpresses HER2. Malignant hyperthermia (or malignant hyperpyrexia) is an autosomal dominant disorder for which there are at least six genetic loci of interest, most prominently a defect affecting the ryanodine receptor gene. Tacrolimus is metabolised/inactivated by cytochrome P450 enzymes 3A4 and 3A5, and is characterised by high pharmacokinetic variability. CYP3A5 expressers have higher apparent clearance of tacrolimus (decreasing its effect) compared with CYP3A5 non-expressers. Competition between

hydrochlorothiazide and uric acid for transport via OAT1 in the proximal tubule results in increased plasma uric acid levels with increasing hydrochlorothiazide dosing (with a risk of precipitating gout). (➲ See Pharmacokinetic interaction, p. 68, Pharmacogenetics, p. 74, and Administering, p. 76).

2. E. The plasma concentration (C) of a drug is calculated by the amount measured (A) divided by the volume of plasma sampled (V), i.e. C = A/V. Dose = C × V, but drugs do not remain in the circulation (the 'central compartment'); rather they are rapidly taken up by the tissues (the 'peripheral compartment'). This is particularly the case with lipid-soluble drugs, which distribute rapidly and widely in body fat stores, as opposed to water-soluble/highly plasma protein-bound drugs that may remain mainly in the circulation. Therefore, to obtain a rapid therapeutic effect, a loading dose is needed to fill the peripheral compartment and achieve an adequate plasma concentration. To calculate a loading dose, one needs to know what plasma volume the drug would take up if the whole dose was present in a single compartment at the same concentration as that measured in the plasma (C) – this is the 'apparent' volume of distribution (Vd). If the dose of a drug (D) is known and the plasma concentration (C) is measured over time (assuming uniform distribution of the drug throughout the body), the linear component of the concentration-time graph may be extrapolated back towards a theoretical concentration at time zero (when the drug was administered) to calculate C_0. Vd = D/C_0 and the loading dose of a drug = C × Vd (➲ see Distribution, p. 77).
3. D. Toxidromes refer to specific clinical signs/symptoms that are characteristic for the effects associated with exposure to certain agents (➲ see Table 3.18).
4. D. Amphetamines enhance catecholamine (e.g. noradrenaline, dopamine, serotonin) release and block their re-uptake, leading to CNS and peripheral vascular stimulation. Patients with amphetamine toxicity commonly present with a sympathomimetic toxidrome (with hyperthermia, mydriasis, tachycardia and hypertension). Medical complications may include rhabdomyolysis, renal failure and haemorrhagic stroke (➲ see Amphetamines, p. 93).
5. B. β-blockers are generally absorbed over a few hours and do not reduce gut motility. β-adrenergic antagonism leads to a reduced activity of adenylate cyclase and a reduction in intracellular cAMP. This in turns leads to a downregulation of protein kinase A-mediated phosphorylation of myocyte proteins, including L-type voltage-sensitive calcium channels, resulting in a blunting of chronotropic and inotropic effects of endogenous catecholamines. Mirabegron is a selective β3-adrenoreceptor agonist that relaxes detrusor muscle and promotes contraction of the urethra (➲ see Mechanisms of drug action, p. 58, Drug targets, p. 58 and Table 3.4).
6. E. Activated charcoal is highly effective at absorbing toxins from the gastrointestinal tract. Lithium is not absorbed by activated charcoal and whole bowel irrigation should be considered in those who have ingested a potentially toxic amount of lithium. Repeat doses of activated charcoal should be considered in the overdoses of carbamazepine, dapsone, digoxin, phenobarbital, quinine and theophylline, and significant salicylate ingestions. Activated charcoal commonly causes vomiting and prior administration of an anti-emetic should be considered. Repeat doses may lead to constipation and so patients requiring repeat doses should be given laxatives (➲ see Gut decontamination, p. 81).
7. A. Tacrolimus is metabolised by cytochrome P450 enzymes 3A4 and 3A5, and is characterised by high pharmacokinetic variability. Clarithromycin is a strong inhibitor of CYP 3A4 and therefore inhibits tacrolimus metabolism. Carbamazepine, St John's wort, phenytoin and rifampicin are cytochrome P450 enzyme inducers that result in an increase of drug metabolism (➲ see Pharmacokinetic interactions, p. 68 and Table 3.12).

Chapter 4 **Drug Development and Clinical Trials Translational Medicine**

Coziana Ciurtin and Tim Mant

Background

Throughout history, medical discoveries have changed society and the way we live our lives. Patients suffering from currently incurable conditions hope that, one day, medical advances will enable them to have a healthy, symptom-free, life. Beyond each individual patient's needs, new therapies can benefit the whole of society by reducing the cost of healthcare and the negative impact of reduced productivity.

Ethical pharmaceutical companies share the same goal of developing new medicines that can prevent diseases, improve patients' health, and save lives. When used appropriately, medicines can halt or slow disease progression, limit complications, improve quality of life, prevent hospitalisation and invasive therapies, and avert debilitating diseases.

Citizens in an ageing population are at greater risk of cognitive impairment, multiple pathologies, frailty and social exclusion, with considerable negative consequences for their quality of life, and the sustainability of health and care systems. Any negative consequences of changing environment and demographics in the modern era could be reduced by earlier detection of risks associated with ageing, combined with the understanding of complex factors contributing to health preservation, and the delivery of timely and targeted treatments.

Molecular biology

Progress made in molecular biology research enables a better understanding of disease pathogenesis and facilitates the discovery of new effective therapies targeting disease-specific abnormalities. Modern molecular biology started with the discovery of the double helix structure of DNA and its significance for information transfer in living material.

The following molecular biology technologies are used for more rapid generation of information and more efficient identification of therapeutic targets:

- *Polymerase chain reaction (PCR)*: enabling the amplification of a single copy or a few copies of a fragment of DNA and generation of thousands to millions of copies of a particular DNA sequence.
- *Representational difference analysis*: a sensitive technique that identifies differences between DNA samples based on PCR and used for the identification of unknown pathogens, genetic changes in cancer and polymorphic markers linked to a trait, as well as the identification of different gene expression patterns.
- *Transgenic/gene knockout technology*: a method that disrupts an existing gene's expression before birth or in an early embryo to induce a stable gene expression in an organism.
- *Gene therapy*: a method that enables gene delivery to cells and tissues for therapeutic purposes.

Understanding of pathophysiology

There is a need to address the current knowledge gaps in understanding causes and mechanisms of disease in order to support innovation in the development of evidence-based treatments. In this context, a better understanding of the mechanisms that are common to several diseases, in particular of those leading to co-morbidities, constitutes an important challenge.

The understanding of pathophysiology has important therapeutic implications when designing new therapies:

- Effective treatments often require combination therapy to correct multiple pathophysiological defects and/or tackle the development of tachyphylaxis/resistance.
- Treatments should be based upon correction of established pathogenic abnormalities to prevent or alleviate symptoms and disabilities with objective improvement in quality of life.
- Therapy must generally be initiated early in the natural history of disease to prevent irreversible pathology.
- Benefits must outweigh any unwanted risk of acute, chronic or delayed adverse effects.

Pharmacogenomics

Pharmacogenomics uses information about a person's genetic make-up, or genome, to choose the drugs and drug doses that are likely to work best for that particular person. Much research is currently directed into understanding how genomic information can be used to develop more personalised and cost-effective strategies for drug selection to improve human health.

There are numerous examples of the use of pharmacogenomics in current practice, such as:

- Selection of patients with breast cancer based on their particular genetic profile, as it is recognised that patients with overproduction of a specific human epidermal growth factor 2 (HER2) protein are responsive to trastuzumab.
- Genetic testing before starting treatment with mercaptopurine in patients with acute lymphoblastic leukaemia and inflammatory bowel disease to exclude those with a genetic variant affecting the enzyme thiopurine S-methyltransferase, which results in altered metabolism of the drug, potentially leading to severe myelosuppression.
- Identification of genetic variations that influence the response of depressed people to citalopram, which belongs to a widely used class of antidepressant drugs called selective serotonin re-uptake inhibitors (SSRIs).
- Using a patient's CYP2C9 (an important cytochrome P450 enzyme with a major role in the oxidation of both xenobiotic and endogenous compounds) and VKORC1 (Vitamin K epoxide reductase complex subunit 1) genotype to determine the initial warfarin dose.

Genome research can help decide the way in which both existing drugs are used and new drugs are developed. Instead of developing drugs with broad action against a disease, researchers are frequently using genomic information to identify targets and design drugs aimed at subgroups of patients with specific genetic profiles. In addition, researchers are using pharmacogenomic tools to search for drugs that target specific molecular and cellular pathways involved in disease.

Other 'omics', epigenetics and informatics

'Omic' technologies are aimed at the universal detection of genes (genomics), mRNA (transcriptomics), proteins (proteomics) and metabolites (metabolomics) in a specific biological sample, providing a comprehensive way of analysing complex systems (Figure 4.1). A major challenge of the modern era is to apply usefully the information generated by 'omics' for the development of personalised and stratified approaches in health promotion, disease prevention and treatment. The integration of these technologies is called 'systems biology'.

Transcriptomics

Transcriptomics is the study of mRNA within a cell or organism, and reflects the genes that are actively expressed at a given moment in time (the transcriptome). The transcriptome is measured by gene expres-

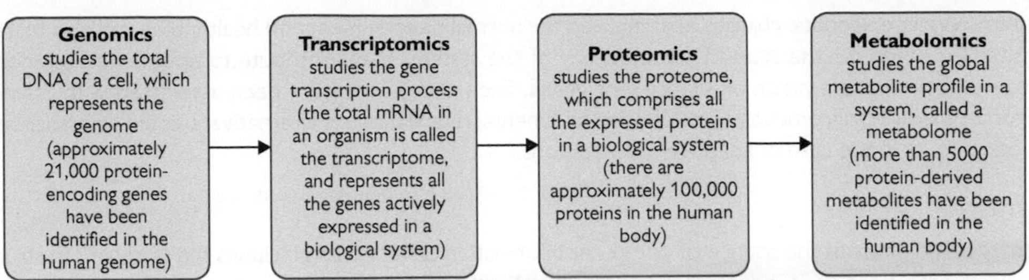

Figure 4.1 The interaction of 'omics' sciences enables the study of a disease as an 'integrated system' by identifying pathological abnormalities associated with different molecular and cellular processes.
Data from *Cross-over trials in clinical research*. Chichester: John Wiley, 1993.

sion microarrays, which identify the packaged mRNA (mRNA with the introns spliced out) as a summary of gene activity.

Proteomics

Proteomics defines the study of protein biochemistry on a genome-wide scale, including information on protein concentration, variation and modification, along with interacting partners and networks, in order to understand cellular processes. The complex understanding of the molecular basis associated with disease onset and progression has the potential to facilitate the discovery of effective treatments based on the identification of biomarkers.

There are a few general principles governing the synthesis and function of proteins in a living cell, which are studied by transcriptomics and proteomics:

- *One gene can encode more than one protein*:
  - There are about 21,000 protein-encoding genes identified in human genome studies and the total number of proteins in human cells is estimated to be between 250,000 and 1 million.
- *Proteins are dynamic*:
  - Proteins undergo continuous changes, such as cell membrane binding, coupling with other proteins to form complexes, or ongoing synthesis and degradation.
- *Proteins are co- and post-translationally modified*:
  - This results in considerable variability between the types of proteins measured under different environmental conditions, or even within the same person at different ages or states of health.
- *Proteins have a wide range of concentrations in the body*:
  - This makes identification of low abundance proteins in a complex biological matrix (such as blood) difficult.

Metabolomics

Metabolomics is defined as the study of global metabolite profile in a biological system (cell, tissue or organism) under a given set of conditions. The metabolome comprises the final downstream product of gene transcription, being at the same time the closest to the phenotype of the biological system studied, therefore having major implications in the study of disease pathogenesis and drug development.

Epigenetics

Epigenetics is the study of dynamic alterations in the cellular transcription potential of a cell, generating cellular and physiological trait variations that are not caused by changes in the DNA sequence. Unlike genetics, which describes changes to the DNA sequence (the genotype), epigenetics studies the changes in gene expression or cellular phenotype caused by environmental stimuli. Examples of mechanisms that produce such changes are DNA methylation, histone modification and RNA-associated silencing, each of which alters how genes are expressed without altering the underlying DNA sequence.

Epigenetic changes may last through cell divisions for the duration of the cell's life and may also last for multiple generations even though they do not involve changes in the underlying DNA sequence of the organism. While epigenetic changes are required for normal development and health, they can also be responsible for some disease states. Disrupting any of the systems that contribute to epigenetic alterations can cause abnormal activation or silencing of genes. Such disruptions have been associated with cancer, syndromes involving chromosomal instabilities and mental retardation or, alternatively, could be associated with benefits, as in the case of adaptive modifications.

Informatics

Informatics is defined as the science of computer information systems. This includes the study of the structure, algorithms, behaviour and interactions of natural and artificial systems that store, process, access and communicate information. Drug discovery involves the processing of a large amount of information, which is generated by innovative technologies. The role of informatics is to generate information from the large amount of data collected through clinical research and to generate knowledge through the processing of this information.

Health informatics, particularly with advances in technology, also has the potential to facilitate patient-centred care by enabling patients to share critical information with their physician, family, friends and other patients, and ultimately to exert a greater control over their own care. Clinicians may also use information systems, such as electronic medical records, to coordinate care and share information with other clinicians, contributing in this way to the dissemination of medical knowledge. It is essential that any use of such data complies with the Data Protection Act (1998).

Process of developing a new medicine

The principal goal of biomedical research is to identify modifiable risk factors and to develop new medicines, which ultimately lead to public health improvement. Translational research programmes aim at creating a link between basic science and clinical benefit, emphasising the need to redefine the interface between preclinical and clinical research for identifying ways of translating basic biomedical discoveries into practical applications. Translational medicine ultimately aims to discover diagnostic and therapeutic solutions for the benefit of public health. Translational medicine (also named 'discovery medicine' or 'experimental medicine') brings together pharmaceutical research and clinical pharmacology, when applied to drug discovery. The process of developing a new medicine comprises a primary translation from target discovery to clinical evaluation, followed by a secondary translation from market authorisation to real-life patient care, both with potential major impact on the optimal utilisation of research resources and patient care provision.

The main purposes of translational medicine are to:

- Investigate and validate therapeutic targets in humans.
- Investigate and validate biomarkers (characteristics that are objectively measured and evaluated as indicators of normal biological processes, pathogenic processes, or pharmacologic responses to therapeutic intervention).
- Evaluate the safety and efficacy of stimulating or blocking identified targets in humans using biomarkers.
- Use the intact living human as the ultimate screening test system for the proposed therapeutic targets.

Target identification/screening

The large and vast datasets generated through 'omics' technology revealed aspects of biological function that were not available to the traditional methods of biomedical research, easing the process of identification of potential targets. This approach was named 'discovery-based research'. Large portions of genomes or proteomes may be examined for the purpose of identifying biomarkers with diagnostic and prognostic utility.

The process of drug discovery is usually triggered by an unmet clinical need and initiated by preliminary research, often performed in academia, generating hypotheses linked to the inhibition or activation of a protein or pathway, which can result in therapeutic benefit. Following the hypothesis generation and multiple testing, a potentially suitable target is selected, which will require further validation prior to being developed into the lead discovery phase if the selection justifies a drug discovery effort. During this process of lead discovery, the research is directed at identifying a drug-like small molecule or biological therapeutic, usually defined as a 'development candidate', which will hopefully progress into preclinical and further into clinical development, if predicted to be safe and effective for a particular clinical application (Figure 4.2).

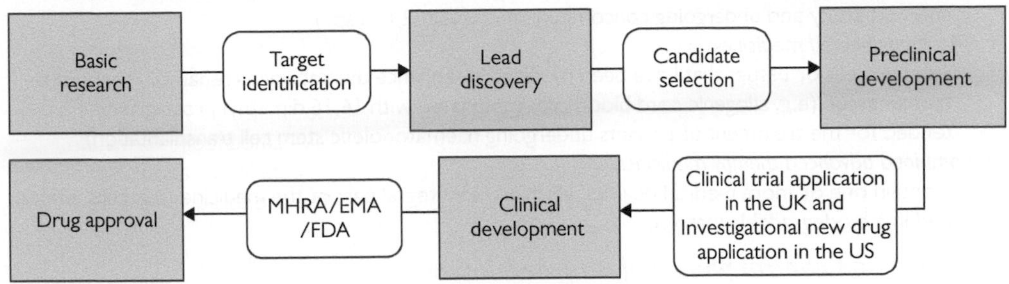

Figure 4.2 The phases of drug development.
MHRA, Medicines and Healthcare products Regulatory Agency (MHRA); EMA, European Medicines Agency; FDA, Food and Drug Administration.
Data from *Cross-over trials in clinical research*. Chichester: John Wiley, 1993.

Target identification and validation are the most important steps in developing new medicines. A target is a generic term, which can refer to a broad range of biological entities, such as proteins, genes and RNA. A suitable target needs to be accessible to the investigational medicinal product. Upon binding, a biological effect should be produced, both *in vitro* and *in vivo*. The reasons for failing to develop a drug from a suitable target include inadequate desired therapeutic effect and poor safety. Good target identification and validation are supported by suitable research data proving a functional link between target and disease, which usually proves that the modulation of the specific target is associated with mechanism-based effects.

Small molecules and biologics

Traditionally, drugs were small, chemically manufactured, active-substance molecules that were easily absorbed into the blood stream and exerted their effect by reaching virtually any desired destination within the body. They are often able to penetrate cell membranes due to their small molecular weight (less than 900 Daltons) and are characterised by lipophilicity. Advances in biotechnology have enabled the discovery of many new biologics, which include protein-based drugs (monoclonal antibodies, therapeutic protein hormones, cytokines and growth factors), vaccines, and cell or gene therapies. In comparison with small molecules, most biologics are large protein-based molecules, which can be optimised versions of human proteins obtained by genetic engineering. Over 200 monoclonal antibodies are now either licensed or tested in clinical trials. Monoclonal antibodies bind to designated cell receptors or molecules, which are associated with a particular disease process. Antibody–drug conjugates act as carrier molecules for 'toxic' substances, enabling their delivery to their exact site of action, which improves efficacy and minimises toxicity. Therapeutic vaccines act by stimulating the immune system to target specific antigens associated with the disease. Cytokines are used for enhancing the immune response to cancer or for anti-inflammatory properties in chronic inflammatory conditions.

Advanced therapies

Unlike small molecules and biologics, advanced therapies are not made from chemicals or proteins, but are classified into four groups, according to their mechanism of action:

- *Gene-therapy medicines*:
  - Use recombinant genes created in the laboratory by combining DNA from different sources. A major challenge is delivery to the site of action.
  - Aim to treat a variety of diseases, including genetic disorders, cancer or chronic diseases, e.g. Strimvelis®, an *ex vivo* stem cell gene therapy approved to treat ADA-SCID (severe combined immunodeficiency due to adenosine deaminase deficiency) and T-Vec, a genetically modified form of Herpes virus to treat advanced melanoma.

- *Somatic-cell therapy medicines*:
  - Contain cells or tissues, which are manipulated genetically to change their biological characteristics, so that they can be used for a different function than that of the original cells or tissues.
  - Can be used to cure, diagnose or prevent diseases (e.g. living, autologous, melanoma-derived lymphocytes [CD3+] for treatment of metastatic melanoma in patients pre-conditioned with chemotherapy and undergoing concomitant interleukin-2 therapy).
- *Tissue-engineered medicines*:
  - Contain cells or tissues that have been modified to enhance their ability to repair or regenerate human tissue (e.g. allogenic cord blood cells modulated with 16,16 dimethyl prostaglandin E2 intended for the treatment of patients undergoing haematopoietic stem cell transplantation).
- *Combined advanced-therapy medicines*:
  - Contain one or more medical devices which are an integral part of the medicine (e.g. cells embedded in a biodegradable matrix).

Preclinical and clinical phases of drug development

Once a lead small molecule drug candidate is confirmed (which may be based on preliminary chemistry, pharmacology, toxicology, basic pharmacokinetics, bio-availability and *in vivo* model studies), and following detailed preclinical characterisation (including stability testing, purity analysis and assay development) the new medicine is subjected to the formalised preclinical phases of drug development required before an investigational medicinal product can be administered to humans. These are highly regulated, and in most countries follow the International Conference on Harmonisation guidelines, which facilitate both the preclinical and clinical development of new medicines:

1. 14–28-day repeat dose toxicity studies in two species.
2. Pharmacokinetic and toxicokinetic studies.
3. Genotoxicity (to assess the likelihood of a drug to be mutagenic or carcinogenic).
4. Drug metabolism.
5. Immunotoxicity.
6. Reproductive toxicity.
7. Juvenile toxicity.
8. Carcinogenicity.

The timing of some of the studies (5–8) in relation to first administration to humans may vary depending on the nature of the molecule and the target population. Longer duration studies in animals, primarily to determine toxicity associated with chronic dosing, are usually conducted after the initial human studies.

The preclinical development of biologics, although following similar basic principles, is adapted to take into account that:

1. Toxicity is more likely to be related to exaggerated pharmacology and 'downstream' effects, rather than 'off target' effects (as a result of modulation of other targets related or unrelated biologically).
2. Interspecies variation is much more likely and the target may not be expressed in any species other than humans.

The insertion of a part or all of a human gene or gene sequence to create 'humanised' mouse models can facilitate the *in vivo* assessment of biologics. Following the regulatory approval of the investigational new drug/clinical trial application, the new medicine enters the phases of clinical development. Based on the clinical research objectives, the clinical studies are grouped traditionally into three phases before application for a product license to market the medicine. All protocols involving clinical trials of investigational medicinal products (CTIMPs) require regulatory and Research Ethics' Committee approval in the UK.

Phase I clinical trials (human pharmacology)

Phase I clinical trials evaluate the tolerability, pharmacokinetics and, when possible, the pharmacodynamics of the investigational medicinal product (IMP). Phase I studies are commonly run in healthy volunteers. The trials are usually double-blind and placebo controlled. They include the administration of initial single ascending doses and short-term repeated doses, in order to determine a practical, potentially effective and well-tolerated dose range for Phase II studies, and identify some possible side effects of the new medicine. Increasingly, pharmacodynamic biomarkers and, in some indications, patients, are included in Phase I studies to provide evidence of 'proof of mechanism' or 'proof of concept', although these studies are not expected to produce direct therapeutic benefit to the participants.

Phase II clinical trials (therapeutic exploratory)

Phase II clinical trials are usually small-scale exploratory trials, including approximately 100–300 patients (but numbers can vary considerably), aiming to evaluate the drug's preliminary efficacy and safety profile in the target population. Additional clinical pharmacology studies in patients may be included in this category. Usually, in a Phase II trial, a new treatment is compared with another treatment already in use (considered standard of care), or with placebo (if ethical) in a randomised and, if possible, double-blind design. If the results of Phase II trials show that a new treatment may be as effective as existing treatments, or better, it then moves into Phase III. One important objective of Phase II is to determine the appropriate dose or doses to be investigated in the 'confirmatory' Phase III studies, which involve larger numbers of patients, longer duration and increased expense.

Phase III clinical trials (therapeutic confirmatory)

Phase III clinical trials look at the safety and efficacy of a medication in larger patient populations (often hundreds or even thousands of patients) at many sites in different countries. These trials usually compare the new treatment with the standard treatment and help determine the overall benefit:risk ratio of the new treatment. Most Phase III trials are double-blind and randomised.

Phase IV clinical trials

Phase IV trials are undertaken after a drug has been shown to be effective with an acceptable safety profile and has been granted a license for use as a treatment for a certain indication(s). They may include different formulations, doses, durations of treatment and drug interactions. Their scope is to provide additional information about the tolerability and safety of the drug in wider, more varied populations, as well as the long-term risks and benefits.

Regulatory and ethics requirements

The process of developing new drugs is highly regulated to ensure the protection of public health. Preclinical studies of new treatments that are submitted to the regulatory authorities have to be conducted to the high standards of Good Laboratory Practice. The key principle of toxicology is to identify the potential side effects of a given compound and assess the likelihood of humans to experience such hazards under the given circumstances of a clinical trial or therapeutic use. The following steps are usually taken to assess the potential risk of an investigational drug in the preclinical phase of development:

- Identification of principal side effects in two animal species (one rodent, one non-rodent).
- Mechanistic and quantitative evaluation of the risk of such adverse events (AEs) occurring in humans.
- Assessment of the potential risk against the expected benefit.
- Removing the compound from the clinical development programme or redefining its conditions of use, as necessary.

Regulatory toxicity testing in animal models, employed to ensure an independent evaluation of medicinal products, includes three different phases according to the stages of drug development:

1. *Preclinical testing: in vitro* and *in vivo* studies – to screen for potential side effects before the new medicine is tested for the first time in humans.
2. *Testing during Phases I and II of drug development*: collection of toxicity data and information about effects on fertility and embryo-fetal development following medium- and long-term administration of the new treatment in animal models prior to clinical trials.
3. *Testing during Phase III of drug development*: carcinogenicity and reproductive toxicity (peri- and post-natal development) studies to enable the registration of the drug as intended for human use.

The preclinical animal and *in vitro* studies aim at identifying, predicting and quantifying risks for healthy volunteers and patients. The toxicology requirements needed for new drug approval are regulated by different agencies, as detailed in ➲ Regulatory and ethical approval, p. 108.

Post-marketing pharmacovigilance

The need

Medicines and medical devices become available to the general population once they are approved for use, and after leaving the protected scientific environment of clinical trials. In the majority of cases, new drugs will only have been tested in humans for a relatively short period of time, on small and carefully selected populations, before being licensed for a specific medical indication. Once released, it is crucial that new treatments and medical devices are monitored for their effectiveness and safety under real-life conditions. Continuous and rigorous monitoring is essential long after release, since it is recognised that many drug interactions and side effects may become apparent only many years later.

The post-marketing surveillance gives the possibility to study:

- Low frequency reactions (not always identified in clinical trials).
- High-risk population groups (usually not included in clinical trials).
- Long-term effects.
- Drug–drug/food interactions.
- Increased severity or frequency of known AEs (previously reported by clinical trials).

Pharmacovigilance is defined as the science and activities relating to the detection, assessment, understanding and prevention of adverse effects, or other problems related to the use of drugs. Pharmacovigilance programmes are designed to:

- Improve patient care and safety in relation to the use of medicines, and other medical and non-medical interventions.
- Improve public health and safety in relation to the use of medicines.
- Contribute to the assessment of benefit, harm, effectiveness and risk of medicines (encouraging their safe, rational and effective use).

Safety monitoring of medicines in common use should be an integral part of clinical practice and has a huge impact on the quality of healthcare. In the European Union (EU), the holder of an authorisation for a medicinal product (usually a pharmaceutical company) must have an appointed qualified person for pharmacovigilance (QPPV) who not only ensures a robust system for pharmacovigilance is established and maintained, but also must provide reports as requested by health authorities and acts as a single contact point for health authorities on a 24-hour basis. However, responsibility for pharmacovigilance should not be restricted solely to health professionals but should be redefined to address the changing patterns in drug use in modern society, where non-prescription medicines are widely available. The key partners in monitoring the safety of medicines are the following:

- Government and industry.
- Hospitals and academia.
- Medical and pharmaceutical associations.
- Poison and medicine information centres.
- Health professionals.
- Patients.
- Consumers.
- The media.
- World Health Organization (WHO).

The WHO has a Programme for International Drug Monitoring. National governments are responsible for the provision of good quality, safe and effective medicines, and their appropriate use. However, expert-only satisfaction with the level of safety of a given medicine or medical device is not sufficient; public perception of the risk associated with its use is equally important. Healthcare providers, the pharmaceutical industry and governments have a duty to communicate accurately and effectively available data regarding the level of benefit and safety associated with the use of medicines.

Adverse event reporting

AEs to drugs are usually reported in the context of clinical trials or during the post-marketing surveillance period. An AE is defined as 'any untoward medical occurrence in a patient or clinical investigation subject administered a pharmaceutical product and which does not necessarily have to have a causal relationship with this treatment'. In clinical trials, a clear distinction is made between non-serious AEs and serious adverse events (SAEs). By most definitions, any event which causes death, permanent damage, birth defects or requires hospitalisation is considered an SAE. It is crucial that unexpected health problems caused by an investigational new drug used in a clinical trial are identified as soon as possible. Mechanisms through regulatory authorities are in place to ensure AEs are reported and participant risk is minimised during a clinical trial:

1. Each site investigator is required, by law, to notify the study sponsor if one of the study participants at their site has an SAE.
   If the reported SAE is considered unexpected (i.e. not previously associated with the investigational new drug or reported in the investigator brochure) and has a possible causal association with the investigational drug, it is reported as a suspected unexpected serious adverse reaction (SUSAR). Once aware of the event, the sponsor must notify the SUSAR to the Medicines and Healthcare products Regulatory Agency (MHRA) and all other investigators involved in the clinical trial:
   - within 24 hours if the SUSAR is fatal or life-threatening;
   - within 15 days if neither fatal nor life-threatening.

   SUSAR reports should be submitted to the Research Ethics Committee (REC) within 15 days of the chief investigator becoming aware of the event. Reports of related and unexpected SAEs in double-blind trials should be unblinded.
2. In order to ensure that investigators uphold their obligations of care for study participants (and notify their institutional review board of unanticipated side effects), they should be continuously informed about the developing risk profile of the investigated drug.
3. Annual Development Update Safety Reports (DUSRs), which concisely describe all new safety information, must be submitted to the MHRA and the REC.

Furthermore, the results of clinical trials (including reported AEs) are often included in the labelling of the medication to provide information both for patients and the prescribing physicians. The AEs, especially when previously unknown, should also be analysed and their significance should be communicated effectively to an audience that has the knowledge to interpret the information, ensuring that the right decision about the further use of the medicine is taken.

Virtually anyone can report drug-related AEs to appropriate regulatory bodies using different reporting schemes, as detailed below. Factors affecting the voluntary reporting of AEs outside the clinical trials environment include:

- Media attention.
- Litigation (class action lawsuits).
- Nature of the AE (the more severe ones are usually reported).
- Type of drug product and indication.
- Length of time on market.
- Extent and quality of manufacturer's surveillance system.
- Prescription or 'over the counter' product status.
- Reporting regulations.

Yellow Card and other systems

The Yellow Card Scheme is a UK initiative run by the MHRA and the Commission on Human Medicines (CHM) aiming to gather information on AEs to medicines. This includes all licensed medicines, from medicines prescribed by physicians to medicines bought over the counter. The scheme also includes vaccines, blood factors and immunoglobulins, herbal medicines and homeopathic remedies, unlicensed medicines found in cosmetic treatments, and all medical devices available on the UK market. The scheme gives healthcare professionals, including physicians, pharmacists and nurses, as well as patients, the opportunity to report side effects to regulatory authorities associated with the use of these products.

In addition to monitoring the safety of all healthcare products in the UK, and ensuring the proper regulation of their use, the scheme collects information on suspected problems or incidents involving defective and counterfeit medicines and devices. It is crucial that problems experienced with medicines or medical devices are reported in order to determine previously unidentified issues. The MHRA will review the product if necessary and take action to minimise risk and maximise benefit to patients. The MHRA will also investigate counterfeit, or fake, medicines or devices, and take appropriate action to protect public health. The Yellow Card Scheme plays a central role in public health protection in the UK.

The Food and Drug Administration (FDA) Adverse Event Reporting System (FAERS) in the USA is the equivalent of the Yellow Card Scheme in the UK. This is a computerised database, including spontaneous reports of side effects to medicines. There are two major sources of reporting:

1. Voluntary reports of patients, consumers and health professionals via the FDA MedWatch website – 5% of FAERS database.
2. Manufacturer reports via the FDA (regulatory requirement) – 95% of FAERS database.

Clinical trials

Clinical trials are key to advances in medical knowledge and improvement in the quality of healthcare. This is achieved by comparing the value and effectiveness of various intervention(s) against a control in humans. Typical interventions include, but are not restricted to, drugs, vaccines, cells and other biological products, surgical and radiological procedures, devices, physiotherapy, psychological interventions, and changes in lifestyle, such as diet and exercise.

Although review of historical data is important, prospective randomised controlled clinical trials (RCTs) are considered 'the gold standard' to determine the effects of an intervention. As physicians, we should base our decisions and actions on the best possible evidence to improve patient outcomes and minimise the risk of harm. Without such evidence, there is a risk that people could be given treatments that have no benefit, waste health system resources and cause harm.

The ability to appraise critically medical information for validity and utility, while incorporating the growing body of evidence into clinical practice, has been termed 'evidence-based medicine'. Clinical trials, if properly designed and conducted, provide the best available data for healthcare decision-making.

Design

A good clinical trial design is one that is feasible, ethical and able to answer a research question with relevant clinical, public health and/or other scientific value. An ideal clinical trial is one that is prospective, randomised, controlled and double-blinded. RCTs are comparative studies with an intervention group and a control group; the assignment of the subject to a group is determined by the process of randomisation (➔ see Randomisation, p. 107). In some clinical trials, deviation from this standard is unavoidable, although major potential drawbacks can be prevented by adhering to the fundamental rules of design, conduct and analysis (as imposed by appropriately reviewed and approved clinical trial protocols). Poor study design might expose participants to unnecessary risk from intervention, or lead to failure to identify a beneficial intervention and/or might also affect the quality of data generated by the study.

Control

Control is a research strategy used to test the effect of an intervention, where one group of subjects receive the study intervention, e.g. the novel drug, and a second group of subjects (the control) receive either an alternative licensed therapy or a placebo (a substance with no pharmacological effect). Often a new intervention is added to usual care or standard care and compared against that care plus placebo. The clinical trial must not cause any harm by preventing the placebo group to be treated, if suitable therapies are available.

Blinding

Blinding refers to the concealment of group allocation from one or more individuals involved in a clinical trial. The optimal strategy to minimise the likelihood of a subject involved in a clinical trial receiving preferential treatment or influence the way he/she is assessed is to 'blind' the study participants and clinicians. If neither the patient nor the researcher knows who is receiving the study intervention or control medication/placebo, the process is called double-blinding. If participants are not blinded, knowledge of group assignment may affect their behaviour during the trial, and their responses to subjective outcome measures. Blinded clinicians are much less likely to transfer influence to the participants or to provide differential treatment to the active and placebo groups. Since bias may also be introduced during the statistical analysis of the trial through the selective use and reporting of statistical tests, data managers and statisticians should also be blinded. It is not unusual to have a non-blinded clinician on a safety monitoring committee. If the risk:benefit ratio is clearly in favour of one treatment over another, or if there are concerns about the efficacy or toxicity of the trialled medication, the safety monitoring committee can recommend cessation of the study. Occasionally, double-blinding is not practical: e.g. intrathecal placebo would be unethical, although a sham intrathecal injection, which poses no risk, may be considered; in other cases, invasive surgery could be compared with non-surgical treatment.

Inclusion/exclusion criteria

Inclusion criteria are defined as attributes of subjects that are essential for selection to participate in a clinical trial. Inclusion criteria are meant to reduce the influence of specific confounding variables and ensure a homogenous study population. Exclusion criteria are a set of predefined definitions used to identify subjects who will not be included, or who will have to withdraw from a research study after having been included. Together with inclusion criteria, exclusion criteria represent the eligibility criteria that assess the suitability of potential participants to take part in a research study. Similar to inclusion criteria, exclusion criteria are established according to the scientific objective of the study, and have important implications for the scientific rigour and ethical principles of a study. Commonly used exclusion criteria seek to exclude subjects unable to comply with follow-up visits, those who are not able to provide biological specimens and data, and those whose safety and ethical protection cannot be assured if involved in the study.

Randomisation

Randomisation is a process ensuring the baseline characteristics of participants are equally likely to be assigned to either the treatment/intervention group or the control/placebo group in a clinical trial, according to a random mechanism (i.e. a process analogous to the flipping of a coin).

Parallel and cross-over trial design

A parallel designed clinical trial compares two separate groups of participants, one on intervention, the other the control. A cross-over design allows each participant to serve as his own control, as every participant will receive either intervention or control in the first period of the study and the alternative in the succeeding period. For a comparison of the two designs, see Figure 4.3.

The duration of a parallel-group trial may be shorter because only one treatment period is involved, although this may be offset by the larger number of patients needed to be recruited and the time required to complete patient recruitment. Apart from studies in healthy volunteers, parallel-group trials usually require a multicentre design to enable appropriate recruitment, with the inevitable logistic problems involved in coordinating research activities in several centres and/or countries to minimise confounding factors that may affect data interpretation.

The cross-over design requires a smaller number of patients for a similar statistical power because patients act as their own controls; a particular advantage when the type or severity of a medical condition varies widely among the patients recruited. As a result, the financial cost of the trial is smaller and fewer patients are exposed to the study intervention. On the other hand, there is a theoretical risk that effects from the first treatment period might carry over into the second treatment period, and thereby confound the detection of treatment effects. In addition, the time of an individual's participation in a cross-over study is longer. Cross-over is not possible in some indications, e.g. antibiotics in bacterial meningitis.

For general rules for the design and conduct of clinical trials, see Box 4.1.

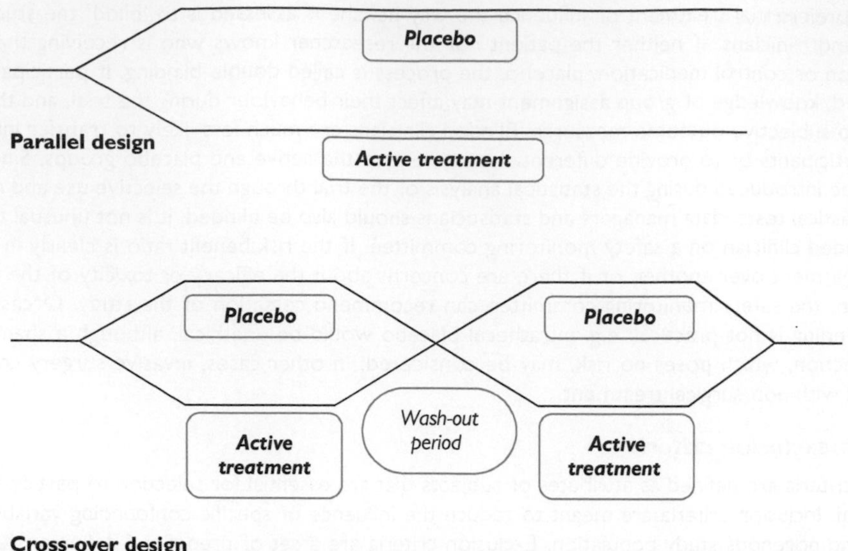

Figure 4.3 Parallel and cross-over trial design.
Data from *Cross-over trials in clinical research.* Chichester: John Wiley, 1993.

Box 4.1 General rules for the design and conduct of clinical trials

1. Clinical trial design should contain a control group, against which the intervention group is compared.
2. Randomisation is the preferred way of assigning participants to control and intervention groups.
3. Ideally, investigators would have no interests other than the well-being of the study participants, and all the participants in the study should be blinded to the study interventions, assessments and data allocation.
4. Proper, voluntary informed consent must be sought before involving any potential participant in a clinical trial.

Data from RP Horgan and LC Kenny, 'SAC review 'Omic' technologies: genomics, transcriptomics, proteomics, and metabolomics,' *The Obstetrician and Gynaecologist*, 2001;13:189–195.

Regulatory and ethical approval

In addition to ethical approval, CTIMPs conducted in the UK require clinical trial authorisation (CTA) from the MHRA. Researchers wishing to conduct research within the NHS should seek NHS management permission (also known as research and development [R&D] approval). Clinical trials using medical devices also require MHRA approval, except where devices are to be used within their intended purpose, or where the device has been manufactured for 'in house' use. NHS permission is also required if the medical device is tested within the NHS. Non-CTIMPs (studies involving no investigational medicinal products) require only NHS permission and ethical approval.

International multicentre clinical trials provide a greater number of potential participants and access to broader populations, offering advantages for generalisation of the results. All clinical trials performed in the EU must be conducted in accordance with the Clinical Trials Regulation EU No 536/2014. This enables a uniform application of the legislation in Europe, ensuring that the rules for conducting clinical trials are identical throughout the EU, and the application procedure for gaining approval is streamlined. It also aims to increase levels of legal certainty, safety and transparency of EU research projects.

Ethical review and approval are needed to ensure that clinical trials protect the health, safety and dignity of the people taking part in research. In order to ensure that all research activities involving humans are covered by the same regulations, the medical community generated the first set of ethical rules in 1964, when the Declaration of Helsinki was endorsed by the World Medical Association. Compliance with ethical standards included in this Declaration is needed to provide public assurance that the rights, safety and well-being of trial participants are protected, and that the data generated by clinical trials are credible. The Declaration defines the ethical principles of research in humans, without being a legally binding document in international law since it cannot overrule local legislations and laws. Its purpose is to provide guidance regarding human research, which must comply with the code of Good Clinical Practice (GCP). GCP is defined as 'an international ethical and scientific quality standard for designing, conducting, recording and reporting trials that involve human participants'. The main objective of the GCP code of regulations is to offer an operational guideline for the conduct of clinical trials, which also details the responsibilities surrounding clinical trials. GCP has had a significant impact on the globalisation of industry-sponsored clinical research, since clinical trial data collected in concordance with GCP regulation can be used for drug indication approval across the world.

A favourable opinion on clinical research involving humans granted by institutional review board/independent RECs (as set out in the GCP guideline for international use) is required by legislation together with authorisation from a competent authority (the MHRA in the UK) before a clinical trial can commence. The UK Central Office for Research Ethics Committees (COREC) is the main source for information on ethical issues related to clinical trials, and its guidelines are in concordance with the GCP guidelines and the Declaration of Helsinki.

RECs review and subsequently approve or reject research protocols submitted by investigators/researchers. There are different types of RECs; some review protocols for animal studies, some for human studies in social sciences (such as psychology and education), and others for clinical trials in patients or healthy volunteers. Many countries require and legally enforce approval by a REC before clinical trials can be initiated for testing new drugs or vaccines, medical devices, diagnostics and medical procedures. The following principles should be kept in mind when completing an application form for REC review:

- RECs include lay members; therefore, it is essential to use non-technical language.
- All the abbreviations used in the application should be explained.
- The information included should be sufficient to enable a thorough ethics review (e.g. final version of the study protocol, patient information sheet [failure to use language that can be understood by a layman is a common cause of delay] and consent form, clinical trial advertising materials, letter to the GP, scientific review of the research proposal, sponsor letter, etc.).

The Health Research Authority (HRA) approval of clinical trials is the new process for the NHS in England that brings together an assessment of governance and legal compliance, undertaken by dedicated HRA staff, with an independent REC opinion provided through the UK research ethics service. It replaces the need for local checks of legal compliance and related matters by each participating organisation in England; therefore aiming at streamlining the research approval process.

Further reading

1. Biomarkers Definitions Working Group. Biomarkers and surrogate endpoints: preferred definitions and conceptual framework. *Clin Pharmacol Ther.* 2001; 69:89–95.

Multiple choice questions

Questions

1. Which of the following statements is not correct?
   A. Genomics defines the study of the genome.
   B. One gene usually encodes one protein.
   C. Epigenetics is the study of transcriptional variations that are not caused by changes in the DNA.
   D. Proteomics includes information about interactions of proteins in cellular processes.
   E. Transcriptomics reflects only the genes actively expressed at a given moment in time.

2. Which of the following is an advanced therapy?
   A. Monoclonal antibodies.
   B. Small molecules.
   C. Gene therapy.
   D. Therapeutic vaccines.
   E. Cytokines.
3. Who is responsible for reporting drug side effects?
   A. Pharmaceutical companies.
   B. Patients.
   C. Investigators/doctors.
   D. Media.
   E. All the above.
4. Which of the following is not always required for a clinical trial ethical approval?
   A. Evidence that the investigational product was tested and it is safe for use in humans.
   B. A complete clinical trial protocol.
   C. Consent form.
   D. Clinical trial advertising material.
   E. Patient information letter.
5. For a typical IgG monoclonal antibody, such as adalimumab, in comparison with a small molecule drug, such as ibuprofen, which of the following is not correct:
   A. Oral bioavailability is poor.
   B. Drug distribution is target-mediated.
   C. The pharmacokinetics are more likely to be non-linear.
   D. Elimination is predominantly renal.
   E. The elimination half-life is long.

Answers

1. B. (➲ See Other 'omics', epigenetics and informatics, p. 98 and Figure 4.1 for more detail.) The information carried by our genome in the form of DNA goes through various processes before it can be translated into proteins. Therefore, depending on the segments that are removed, several mRNAs can result from the same pre-mRNA sequence and different proteins are generated from the same DNA sequence. It is estimated that 70% of our genes code for at least four proteins each.
2. C. (➲ See Advanced therapies, p. 101.) Gene therapy uses recombinant genes created in the laboratory by combining DNA from different sources, which are inserted into the body, for the scope of treating a variety of diseases. Small molecules are chemical compounds used for therapeutic purposes, and antibodies, cytokines and vaccines are all protein-based drugs.
3. E. (➲ See Adverse event reporting, p. 105.) All the above are responsible to protect the safety associated with the use of medicines by ensuring the timely reporting of side effects.
4. A. (➲ See Regulatory and ethics requirements p. 103; Preclinical and clinical phases of drug development, p. 102.) In some cases (Phase I clinical trials), the information regarding the safety of the investigational product in humans is not available, but will be generated by the clinical trial seeking ethical approval.
5. D. (➲ See Small molecules and biologics, p. 101.) Degradation in, and poor absorption through, the gastrointestinal tract prevents oral bioavailability of monoclonal antibodies. IgG is too large to be filtered at the glomerulus. Monoclonal antibodies often demonstrate target-mediated distribution and elimination. Target-mediated elimination is capacity limited (saturable) because of finite expression of the target.

Chapter 5 **Radiological Investigations and Applications**

Chris J. Harvey and Declan P. O'Regan**

Introduction and guide to imaging modalities

Imaging has a central role in the management of patients with new technologies bringing rapid advances in both diagnosis and therapy. There are a range of imaging modalities that include plain radiography, fluoroscopy, interventional radiology, ultrasound (US), computed tomography (CT), magnetic resonance imaging (MRI) and nuclear medicine. The fundamentals of each of these techniques is described in this chapter and illustrated with clinical cases.

Plain film radiography

X-rays are ionising radiation, which are absorbed or scattered by human tissues. Plain films are often the first-line imaging investigation of patients. The area to be imaged is placed between an X-ray source and a flat-panel detector. Four densities can be resolved on plain radiographs – air, fat, soft tissue and calcification:

- Bones contain calcium, with a high atomic number, which efficiently attenuate X-rays. Bones and other calcifications therefore appear white on the radiograph.

* Joint first authors.

- Air causes almost no attenuation of X-rays, so air-filled structures, such as the lungs and bowel, appear black.
- Fat weakly attenuates X-rays, thus adipose tissue in the abdomen and around joints appears relatively dark.
- Soft tissue is of intermediate density compared to fat and bone.

A large difference in either density or atomic number between two adjacent organs allows the contours of these structures to be clearly visualised on a radiograph because of the high inherent natural contrast (e.g. heart and lungs, bone and soft tissue). On a normal chest radiograph (CXR) the heart and mediastinal interface is clearly visualised against the black lungs. However, in the presence of adjacent lung collapse or consolidation, X-rays are absorbed by the diseased lung, rendering it more opaque and of similar density to the adjacent mediastinum. The contour of adjacent structures is therefore lost, resulting in the 'loss of the silhouette sign', e.g. loss of the adjacent right heart border in right middle lobe collapse/consolidation.

Interpretation of the chest radiograph

- Technical factors: a postero-anterior (PA) CXR is taken with the X-ray tube behind the patient and the detector against the anterior chest. The medial ends of the clavicles should be equidistant from the spinous processes in a correctly centred film.
  - In a good inspiratory film the right hemidiaphragm should reach the anterior aspect of the sixth rib.
  - A poor inspiration may simulate the appearance of basal collapse and cause spurious cardiomegaly.
- Trachea: this should normally be central. It may be deviated away from a superior mediastinal mass, e.g. thyroid goitre, or pulled by any process that causes volume loss, e.g. lung fibrosis.
- Heart: the normal cardiothoracic ratio (ratio of transverse cardiac diameter to transverse inner thoracic diameter) is <50%.
- Mediastinal contour: the entire border of the heart and mediastinum should be clearly visualised.
- Hilar regions: these are made up of the pulmonary arteries and veins (predominantly the upper lobe pulmonary vein and the lower lobe pulmonary artery). They have a concave lateral margin. They are of equal density and the right hilum is lower than the left.
- Lungs: these should be equal in density. When there is asymmetry, the side of decreased vascularity is usually the abnormal side. Inspect for focal lesions. The right horizontal fissure can be seen on the frontal view, whereas the oblique fissures are only usually visualised on the lateral views.
- Diaphragm: on full inspiration, the right hemidiaphragm is at the level of the sixth rib anteriorly. Inspect for free subdiaphragmatic gas due to perforation of a viscus (unless there is a known iatrogenic cause, such as a recent laparotomy or continuous ambulatory peritoneal dialysis. Also look for subphrenic abscesses, calcified liver lesions, gallstones and dilated bowel loops.
- Review areas: check that both breasts are present, look for lesions behind the heart silhouette and lung apices, and at the hila. Check the bones for focal abnormalities and density. Check the skin for surgical emphysema, soft tissue lumps (e.g. neurofibroma) or calcified parasites.

Interpretation of the abdominal radiograph

- Bowel gas pattern:
  - Gas is normally seen in the stomach and colon. Small amounts may be seen in the small bowel.
  - Gas in the small bowel and colon can be differentiated by the presence of valvulae conniventes, which cross the whole small bowel loop, and haustral folds, which usually extend only across part of the large bowel lumen, and are thicker and farther apart than valvulae conniventes.
  - Small bowel loops should not exceed 2.5–3 cm in diameter. The colonic calibre is variable, but dilatation occurs when the diameter is >5 cm, e.g. in obstruction, paralytic ileus, ischaemia and inflammation.
  - Look for free intraperitoneal gas, which may be recognised as Rigler's sign, with visualisation of both the inner and outer bowel walls.

  - Inspect for intramural gas. Linear intramural gas is seen in ischaemic bowel, whereas cystic intramural gas is a feature of the benign condition pneumatosis intestinalis.
- Calcifications: inspect for renal tract calculi (>90% are radio-opaque), gallstones (10% are radio-opaque), pancreatic calcification, appendoliths and calcified aortic aneurysms. Renal tract calcification may be due to calculi, nephrocalcinosis, prostatic calcification and tumours. Most calcifications are not significant (phleboliths, lymph nodes, arterial walls, fibroids and costal cartilage).
- Ectopic gas: look for aerobilia, portal venous gas (due to bowel ischaemia or infection) and gas in the genitourinary tract (secondary to infection or instrumentation).
- Viscera: the liver, spleen, kidneys and psoas silhouettes may be normally seen.
- Pelvic masses: may be bladder or gynaecological lesions.

Computed tomography

CT uses X-rays to produce axial images of the body of excellent anatomical spatial resolution. Modern multi-detector CT scanners are extremely fast, allowing the whole body to be scanned in 30–40 seconds. Fast imaging also enables angiographic images to be acquired, as well as cardiac-gated imaging of the heart. The CT X-ray tube rotates around the patient as they move on a table so that a volume of data is acquired via multiple rows of detectors; these data can be reconstructed to produce multiplanar and three-dimensional images.

- Lesions of high attenuation are white (fresh haemorrhage, calcification) while low attenuation lesions are black (air, fat).
- The amount of absorption, with reference to water, is measured in Hounsfield units (HU) (after Sir Godfrey Hounsfield, the inventor of CT). Thus, water has a HU of 0, air –1000 HU, soft tissues +40 to +60 HU, and calcium +400 to +1000 HU, approximately.
- Applications of CT include:
  - Body imaging (chest/abdomen/pelvis, e.g. oncology), coronary/cerebral/abdominal/peripheral angiography, CT colon and brain imaging).
  - Cardiac-gated CT coronary angiography is widely used for the investigation of suspected angina coronary artery stenosis.

CT is the modality of choice in the acute assessment of trauma patients as it quickly and accurately allows the detection of brain, spine, solid organ, bowel, skeletal, urological and vascular injury. Contusions, lacerations, perforation, dissections and active bleeding may be identified on CT, facilitating early intervention.

The disadvantages of CT are that patients receive a considerable dose of ionising radiation (Table 5.1), the potential side effects of intravenous (IV) contrast agents (nephrotoxicity, allergic reaction) and the relative high cost. CT has a higher spatial resolution than MRI, while MRI has a higher contrast resolution than CT. CT is not as sensitive as MRI in imaging of the central nervous system (CNS), spine, myocardium, musculoskeletal and gynaecological conditions, but is better than MRI for imaging the pulmonary system and renal tract (especially calculi).

Radiation dosage

X-rays ionise atoms, resulting in the liberation of electrons and ion pairs, which can lead to harmful biological effects, including the production of free radicals, which potentially may lead to both carcinogenesis and mutagenesis.

It is very important that the radiation dose both to patients and to medical personnel is minimised. X-ray exposure should be avoided unless there is a net benefit to the patient, and that exposure should be kept **as low as reasonably achievable** (the ALARA principle). The Ionising Radiation (Medical Exposure) Regulations (IR[ME]R), introduced by the Department of Health in May 2000, require that all medical exposures to ionising radiation are clinically justified and authorised.

The biological damage produced by a given exposure can be estimated by weighting the dose by the radiation sensitivity of different tissues. This value (the effective dose equivalent) is measured in milliSieverts (mSv), and gives an estimate of the adverse effects of different types of radiological procedure. The average background radiation exposure in the UK is 2.5–3 mSv/year. The dose from a CXR is very low

Table 5.1 Effective dose from radiological procedures (approximate figures)

	Effective dose (mSV)	Relative dose	Equivalent period of background dose
Chest X-ray (single film)	0.02	1	2.5 days
Abdominal film (single)	0.4	30	2 months
Lumbar spine series	0.6	40	3 months
Intravenous urography	2.1	140	11.5 months
Barium swallow	1.5	100	8 months
Barium enema	2.2	150	1 year
CT chest	6.6	440	3 years
CT chest/abdomen/pelvis	10	670	4.5 years
CT colon	10	670	4.5 years
CT KUB	5.5	370	2.5 years
CT brain	1.4	90	7.5 months
Bone scan	3	200	1.5 years
V/Q (ventilation/perfusion) scan	1.4	90	7.5 months
Sestamibi cardiac stress scan	6	400	2.7 years
PETCT (positron emission tomography CT)	18	1200	8.1 years

(0.02 mSv), while the dose from procedures such as CT may be hundreds of times higher (Table 5.1). For comparison the radiation dose from a transatlantic flight is approximately 0.07 mSv.

Ultrasound

US produces real-time images of body structures using high-frequency (1–20 MHz) sound waves, is non-invasive, quick and inexpensive, and avoids the use of ionising radiation. It has the disadvantages of being operator-dependent and is reflected by bone and air, so preventing imaging deep to these structures. Fluid, in all forms (ascites, bile, urine, blood), is black (anechoic) as it transmits sound well. Solid organs are depicted in various shades of grey, hence the term grey-scale or B-mode (B for brightness). The higher the frequency employed, the better the resolution with a penalty of more attenuation, so the lower the depth of insonation possible. Hence, high frequency applications (7–14 MHz) include superficial structures, such as peripheral arteries and veins, scrotum, breast, neck and musculoskeletal tissue. The lower frequency applications (3–6 MHz) include abdominal and transabdominal pelvic studies.

The real-time nature of ultrasonography is highly suited to biopsy and to other interventional procedures.

Doppler US is based on the fact that when incident sound waves are reflected by a moving structure, the frequency is shifted by an amount proportional to the velocity of the reflector (e.g. a red blood cell flowing in a vessel); this shift can be quantified and displayed as a colour overlay (colour Doppler) or a spectral Doppler scan. Colour Doppler can be used to assess vessel patency and direction of flow. Spectral Doppler examination of a vessel gives velocities to assess and grade vascular stenoses.

Magnetic resonance imaging

MRI uses strong magnetic fields to provide imaging of the body with excellent tissue contrast and resolution. The patient is positioned within the bore of a super-conducting magnet, which enables protons (mainly in fat and water molecules) to absorb energy when an oscillating magnetic field is briefly applied at a precise resonant frequency. The protons then emit this energy as a radiofrequency signal, which can be detected by coils in the scanner. Contrast between tissues is determined by the rate at which hydrogen atoms return to their equilibrium energy state.

There are several basic sequences that allow imaging of different tissues/pathologies by varying scanning parameters and input signals:

- Common sequences are T1, T2, proton density, fat suppression (short tau inversion recovery [STIR]) and diffusion weighted imaging (DWI).
- On a T1-weighted image fat typically gives a high signal and on T2 images water (urine, bile, cerebrospinal fluid [CSF]) is bright (white). The addition of fat suppression (removing the signal from fat) causes the fat to become black.
- MRI does not use ionising radiation, but is expensive and scanning times (20–40 minutes) are much longer than those with CT. Claustrophobia may be a problem for patients.
- There are no known biological hazards of MRI, but most pacemakers and implantable defibrillators, cochlear implants and certain metal clips and stents are contraindicated in MRI scanners because of their potential movement or heating effects.

Nuclear medicine

Nuclear medicine provides functional, rather than anatomical, information, unlike the other imaging modalities. It is based on the imaging of radionuclide-labelled physiologically active molecules that may be taken up by different body tissues. The most widely used radioisotope is technetium^{99m}, which emits gamma rays that are detected by gamma cameras. Disadvantages of this modality include that it has a radiation penalty (Table 5.1), is time-consuming and has a low spatial resolution.

Positron emission tomography (PET)-computed tomography combines the functional information of nuclear medicine with the excellent anatomical spatial resolution of CT. PET uses cyclotron-produced iso topes (particularly the glucose analogue, 18-fluorodeoxy-D-glucose [^{18} FDG]) of extremely short half-life that emit positrons.

PET can be used to document the increased uptake of glucose in tumours so is predominantly used in oncology (➲ see Chapter 10, Positron emission tomography, p. 321).

- PET-CT is used to stage tumours, assess response to therapy, distinguish benign from malignant lymphadenopathy, look for recurrence and differentiate tumour from scarring, e.g. post-radiotherapy.
- Increased uptake in areas of inflammation or high metabolic activity can cause diagnostic problems.
- Disadvantages include its high radiation burden (Table 5.1) and that it requires the patient to lie still for a long period of time.

Imaging contrast agents

Contrast agents have a vital use in clinical radiology as they offer greater diagnostic confidence, improve the discrimination between healthy and diseased tissue, and also provide useful information on the haemodynamic characteristics of many lesions. When there is no natural contrast, contrast agents are used to artificially alter X-ray attenuation locally (e.g. blood vessels in an organ).

Contrast media may be divided into 'positive' contrast agents of high radiodensity, which block X-rays and appear white (e.g. iodine, barium), and 'negative' agents of low density, which appear black (e.g. air, carbon dioxide).

- Double contrast combinations of air and barium can also be used in many situations to opacify body compartments. Most contrast agents are specific for a particular imaging modality.
- Radiographic contrast agents are the most widely used media and have applications in CT, catheter angiography and fluoroscopy. These agents exploit the physical properties of high atomic number iodine and barium to attenuate the energy of X-rays used in diagnostic radiography.

- MRI uses mainly gadolinium-based contrast media, as these have a specific effect on magnetisation within tissues.
- Contrast-enhanced microbubble US is increasingly available for assessment of liver lesions.

Iodine-based contrast agents

- These contrast media are commonly used in CT and angiography, as well as IV urography, hysterosalpingography, dacrocystography, retrograde cysto-urethrography and interventional procedures.
- In CT, large-bore peripheral cannulas are required for high flow rate injections. Tunnelled central venous catheters can rupture if excessive pressure is used.
- In rare cases, an idiosyncratic anaphylactoid reaction may occur. These do not require previous sensitisation and may not consistently recur. Symptoms range from urticaria and vomiting to laryngeal oedema, hypotension, arrhythmias and death. Risk factors include a history of allergic reactions and asthma. There is no specific cross-sensitivity with shellfish or iodine tincture. Premedication with steroids is of uncertain benefit.
- Predictable non-idiosyncratic reactions are more commonly observed and include a metallic taste, nausea, sensation of warmth and vasovagal response.
- Contrast-related nephropathy is controversial as patients often have multifactorial causes of renal impairment. If it occurs, renal impairment is usually mild and transient, but can lead to sustained oliguria.
- There is no need to stop metformin after contrast medium in patients with normal renal function. If the serum creatinine is above normal or the estimated glomerular filtration rate (eGFR) is below 60 mL/min, any decision to withhold metformin for 48 hours should be made in consultation with the team managing the patient's diabetes.
- In exceptional circumstances iodinated contrast may be used in pregnancy. Due to a small risk of neonatal thyroid suppression, thyroid function tests should be performed in the first week after birth.
- Extravasation of contrast medium is usually treated with aspiration, elevation and ice. Rarely compartment syndrome may develop, requiring surgical intervention.
- Oral or rectal preparations may be used to assess anastomotic leaks, suspected bowel obstruction and gastrointestinal (GI) fistulae on plain radiographs or fluoroscopy. A dilute preparation is sometimes used to provide bowel contrast for abdominal CT.

Barium-based contrast agents

- Barium sulphate is widely used in a variety of preparations to demonstrate pathology of the GI tract.
- 'Double contrast' is provided by air in the lumen with barium coating the mucosa.
- Barium swallow is used to assess the anatomy and function of deglutition, the oesophageal mucosa and the gastro-oesophageal junction. The patient is asked to swallow the barium suspension, while multiple images are taken as the bolus passes down the upper GI tract.
- Video fluoroscopy is used to evaluate disorders of swallowing.
- Barium swallow has a role in diagnosing oesophageal cancer and strictures, achalasia, gastro-oesophageal reflux, pharyngoesophageal (Zenker's) diverticula and tracheoesophageal fistulae.
- Barium meal has largely been replaced by oesophagogastroduodenoscopy (OGD), although it still has a role in the diagnosis of stomach cancer, especially linitis plastica. Iodine-based contrast media are used to evaluate post-surgical anastomotic leaks as barium peritonitis has a high mortality.
- Barium enema. A tube is passed per rectum and the bowel is coated in barium and then insufflated with gas to produce a double contrast study. This has now largely been replaced by colonoscopy or CT virtual colonography.
- A barium flow-through allows images to be taken of the small bowel over a period of a few hours. This can be useful for evaluating small bowel strictures, dysmotility and inflammatory bowel

disease. Improved distension can be achieved by instilling the barium through a nasojejunal tube (enteroclysis). Alternatives include capsule endoscopy and MR enterography.

Gadolinium-based contrast agents

- Contrast agents containing the rare earth metal gadolinium are used in MRI. These nuclei have paramagnetic properties, which shorten the T1 relaxation of water.
- Low-toxicity gadolinium chelate preparations are used. Most agents are hydrophilic and do not cross the intact blood–brain barrier. The contrast medium is rapidly distributed into the extracellular compartment, where it causes an increase in signal intensity on T1-weighted images. Image contrast may be further improved by using fat suppression sequences. The effect on T2-weighted images is variable and usually non-diagnostic.
- Hepatobiliary agents, which are taken up and excreted by hepatocytes, are also available.
- Blood pool agents and iron oxide contrast media are not currently available for clinical use.
- Gadolinium is usually administered IV and has similar applications to iodine-based media in CT for lesion characterisation, angiography and perfusion assessment.
- It is generally well tolerated and the incidence of serious acute reactions is lower than for iodine contrast media.
- Nephrogenic sclerosing fibrosis is a potentially fatal disease of the skin and internal organs, which has been associated with high doses of gadolinium contrast medium in patients with severe renal impairment. The evaluation of renal function prior to scanning and the use of non-ionic cyclic compounds have reduced the incidence of this complication.
- Dilute preparations of gadolinium are used for MR arthrography to assess muscle and tendon tears of the shoulder and hip.

Microbubble contrast-enhanced ultrasound

- Microbubble agents are used as echo enhancers in US and can be imaged simultaneously alongside a co-registered greyscale US image.
- They are composed of a gas-filled lipid shell about the same size as a red blood cell. In an US field they resonate and emit harmonic signals, which can be imaged using microbubble-specific software available on all commercial US systems.
- The microbubbles are administered IV and are small enough to pass through the pulmonary vasculature to reach the systemic circulation.
- Microbubbles are predominantly used for liver lesion characterisation where they offer real-time arterial, portal venous and delayed phase imaging.
- The high temporal and spatial resolution of contrast-enhanced US allows accurate characterisation of focal liver lesions with a sensitivity and specificity rivalling CT and MRI.
- The agents are generally very well tolerated with only rare instances of allergy. Concerns were raised about safety in patients with severe underlying cardiac conditions, but the evidence for this is weak.

Further reading

1. iRefer. *Making the best use of clinical radiology*, 8th edn. London: Royal College of Radiologists, 2017. http://www.rcr.ac.uk/iRefer.
2. The Royal College of Radiologists. *Standards for intravascular contrast agent administration to adult patients*, 3rd edn. London: The Royal College of Radiologists, 2015.
3. Thomsen HS, Webb JAW. *Contrast media: safety issues and ESUR Guidelines (Medical Radiology/Diagnostic Imaging)*, 3rd edn. Berlin: Springer, 2014.

Case 1

History

A 52-year-old smoker with known bronchiectasis presented acutely with a torrential haemoptysis. See Figure 5.1A for a CXR of an aspergilloma, and Figure 5.1B for a CT scan of an aspergilloma.

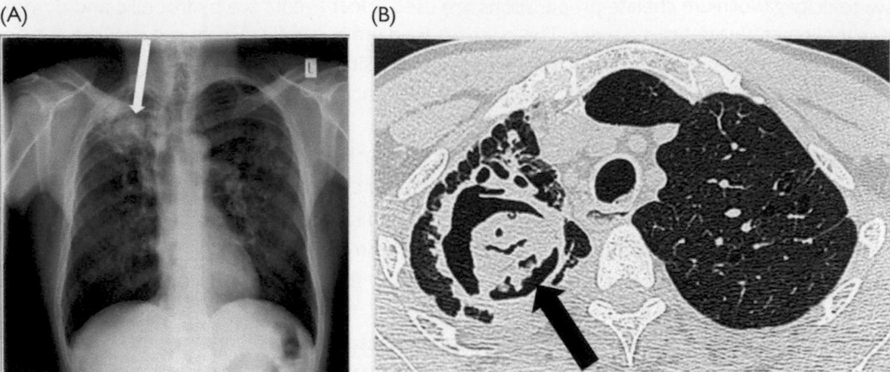

Figure 5.1 (A) Chest radiograph demonstrating an aspergilloma (arrow) in a right upper lobe cavity. There is bilateral widespread bronchiectasis seen as bronchial wall thickening and dilatation. (B) Computed tomography shows the aspergilloma (black arrow) lying centrally positioned in a thick-walled cavity in contact with the wall.

Differential diagnosis

The differential diagnosis is that of a focal mass lesion:

- *Primary bronchogenic carcinoma*: this may form a cavitating mass, particularly in squamous cell cancer. However, the findings of a separate mass in a cavity would be atypical for a cancer.
- *Pneumonia*: superimposed infections are common on a background of bronchiectasis and may present with haemoptysis. Consolidation with air bronchograms are the hallmark of infection. A cavitating pneumonia would usually be multifocal. The finding of an air crescent around a mass lesion in a cavity is not consistent with this diagnosis.
- *Pulmonary arteriovenous malformation*: this lesion is seen as a curvilinear opacity with feeding and draining vessels. The CXR and CT findings are not consistent with this condition.
- *Aspergilloma (mycetoma)*: the CXR finding of a mass within a cavity are classic of this condition.

Diagnosis: aspergilloma (mycetoma)

Key features

Clinical

- *Aspergillus fumigatus* is a ubiquitous soil fungus. It may be isolated in the sputum of healthy people.
- Aspergillus fungi colonise pre-existing cavities/cysts that occur in fibrotic cavity-forming conditions, such as old tuberculosis (TB), ankylosing spondylitis, previous radiotherapy, sarcoidosis, as well as bronchiectasis.
- An aspergilloma is composed of tangled hyphae forming a matted ball.
- Patients are usually immunocompetent, compared with invasive aspergillosis when the patient is immunosuppressed. Allergic bronchopulmonary aspergillosis (ABPA) is a type III hypersensitivity pneumonitis in patients with long-standing asthma, characterised by central proximal bronchiectasis and eosinophilia. Aspergillomas are unusual in ABPA.
- Patients present with haemoptysis, which may be life-threatening, as the fungal ball erodes blood vessels in the wall of the cavity.

- Management consists of surgical resection or radiological embolisation. Antifungals are ineffective as these agents cannot penetrate into the fungal ball.

Radiological

- On CXR aspergillomas are seen in cavities with a crescent of air separating the fungal ball from the cavity wall. This is known as the 'moon sign'.
- On CT the aspergilloma has a sponge-like structure. It lies within a thick walled cavity.
- The aspergilloma may move with a change in patient position.

Further reading

1. Passera E, Rizzi A, Robustellini M, et al. Pulmonary aspergilloma: clinical aspects and surgical treatment outcome. *Thorac Surg Clin*. 2012;22:345–61.
2. Kousha M, Tadi R, Soubani AO. Pulmonary aspergillosis: a clinical review. *Eur Respir Rev*. 2011;20:156–74.

Case 2

History

A 24-year-old patient with recurrent chest infections since childhood.
A CXR showing hyperinflated lungs in an adult patient with cystic fibrosis (CF) is shown in Figure 5.2A.
A coronal CT chest scan of varicose bronchiectasis is shown in Figure 5.2B.

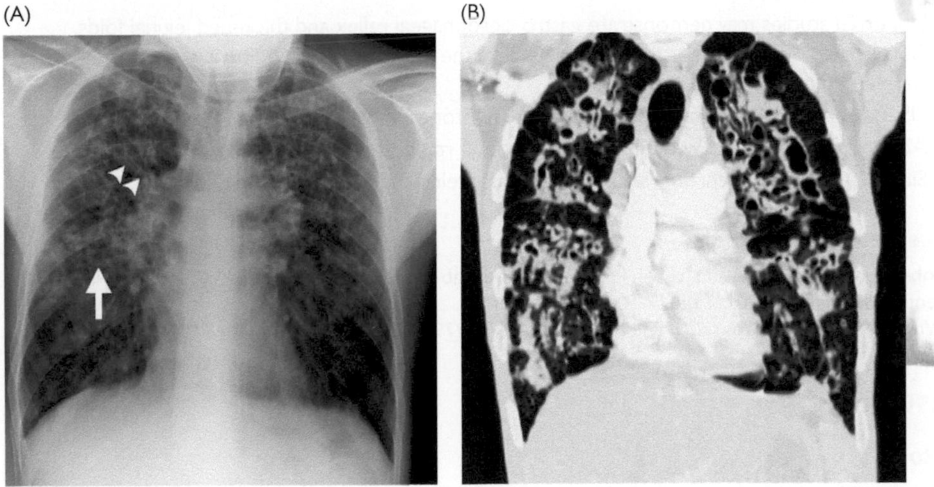

Figure 5.2 (A) Chest X-ray revealing hyperinflated lungs, ring shadows (arrow) and parallel tramlines (arrowheads) of bronchiectatic airways in an adult patient with CF. (B)
Coronal CT of the chest showing varicose bronchiectasis in the lungs.

Differential diagnosis

The differential is that of ring shadows in a young adult:

- *Alpha-1-antitrypsin deficiency*: lower lobe emphysema causing hyperinflated radiolucent lungs with thin-walled bullae.
- *Pulmonary abscess*: often a single necrotic cavity as a consequence of aspiration or airway obstruction, or multiple abscesses from haematogenous infection.
- *Pneumocystis pneumonia*: subpleural pneumatocoeles with perihilar opacities on CXR. Ground-glass opacity on high-resolution CT (HRCT) with septal thickening.
- *Cystic fibrosis*: hyperinflated lungs with bronchiectasis and mucus plugging.

- *Lymphangioleiomyomatosis (LAM)*: typically occurs in premenopausal women. Associated with hyperinflated lungs containing multiple thin-walled cysts of varying size.

Diagnosis: bronchiectasis in cystic fibrosis

Key features

Pathogenesis and clinical features; ➲ see Chapter 11, Cystic fibrosis, p. 358.

Radiological

- Bronchiectasis is recognised by tram-track parallel lines and ring shadows due to varicose dilatation of the airways.
- Air-trapping causes hyperinflated lungs with flattened diaphragms.
- Cor pulmonale may develop with pulmonary artery dilatation and right ventricular enlargement.
- Intercurrent infection and airway plugging may lead to lobar collapse, pneumonia and abscess formation.
- Patients may have a port-a-cath for IV antibiotics.
- CT shows varicose and cystic bronchiectasis, with peribronchial wall thickening and lung cysts. There is branching mucus-plugging of small airways with consolidation and sub-segmental collapse.
- In babies meconium ileus results in multiple dilated segments of small bowel, often without air-fluid levels due to viscous meconium. Intestines may have frothy 'soap-bubble' appearance on plain films. Antenatal perforation may lead to meconium peritonitis causing intra-abdominal calcifications and pseudocysts.
- Upper GI studies may demonstrate gastro-oesophageal reflux and thickened jejunal folds. Fibrosing colonopathy may cause a stricture of the ascending colon following long-term lipase supplementation.
- US may be used to detect hepatic steatosis, gallstones, biliary cirrhosis and portal hypertension.
- Abdominal CT may show diffuse pancreatic fatty replacement.
- Sinus CT may reveal chronic sinusitis with mucoceles and nasal polyps.

Further reading

1. Robertson MB, Choe KA and Joseph PM. Review of the abdominal manifestations of cystic fibrosis in the adult patient. *Radiographics* 2006;26(3):679–90.
2. Whittaker A. Cystic fibrosis. *Clin Chest Med*. 2007;28(2):279–478.

Case 3

History

A 26-year-old patient with haemoptysis and nose bleeds.
Figure 5.3A shows a CXR of a large pulmonary arteriovenous malformation (PAVM) in the right lower lung lobe; Figure 5.3B shows an axial CT scan of a PAVM.

Differential diagnosis

- *Primary bronchogenic carcinoma*: the presence of a serpiginous structure with supplying vessels emanating from the hilum goes against this diagnosis.
- *Pulmonary arteriovenous malformation*: The presence of a lobulated serpiginous mass with large feeding and draining vessels is characteristic of this condition.
- *Benign nodules*: granulomas, hamartomas and carcinoid. Granulomas are well defined and may be calcified; hamartomas tend to be peripheral and may contain popcorn calcification and fat; carcinoids tend to be endobronchial with calcification. None of them have large supplying vessels. Rim calcification may be seen in PAVMs.

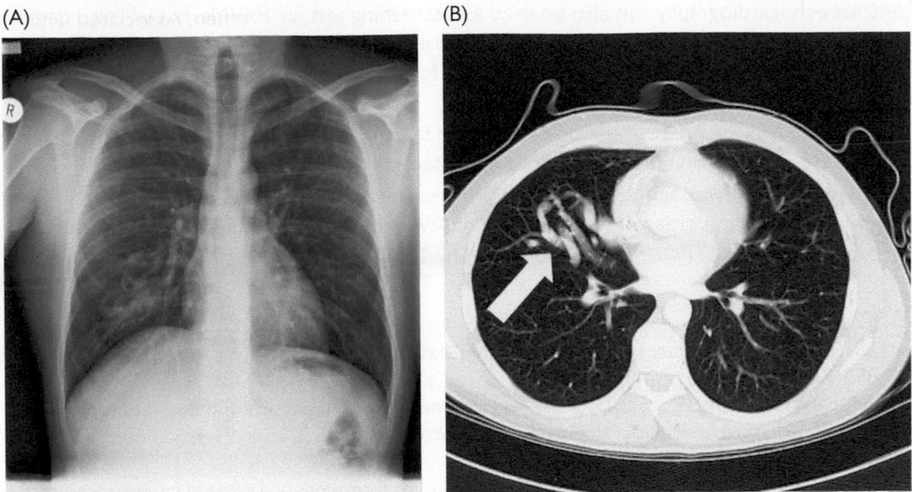

Figure 5.3 (A) Chest radiograph showing a large PAVM in the right lower lobe with feeding and draining vessels seen. (B) Axial CT showing a PAVM characterised by multiple serpiginous vessels (arrow).

- *Infection*: the pattern of lung involvement is not one of lobar consolidation/collapse (➔ see Plain film radiography, p. 111 and Case 1, Differential diagnosis, p. 118), nodularity or cavitation.
- *Metastatic disease*: these may be multifocal and are not usually this large. The presence of vessels is against this diagnosis. Arterial feeding vessels may be seen on CT but they are not usually this large. Draining veins are not seen associated with metastases.

Diagnosis: pulmonary arteriovenous malformation

Key features

Clinical

- Hereditary haemorrhagic telangiectasia (HHT) or Osler–Weber–Rendu syndrome is a autosomal dominant condition where there are telangiectasiae (arteriovenous malformations) of the lungs, lips, mouth, nose, GI, urinary tract and skin, which can lead to haemoptysis, recurrent epistaxis, and occult GI bleeding and chronic iron deficiency anaemia. Complications include cerebrovascular accidents or abscesses due to paradoxical embolism.
- The presence of multiple PAVMs is associated with HHT in 90% of cases, but only 10% of patients with HHT have PAVMs.
- PAVMs cause right to left shunting of deoxygenated blood through the lungs to the systemic circulation.

Radiological

- 70% of PAVMs are in the lower lobes and are characterised by a lobulated serpiginous mass with a large feeding and draining vessel.
- CT is the most sensitive modality for detecting PAVMs and for assessing suitability for embolisation.
- ^{99m}Tc-labelled macroaggregates can estimate the size of the right to left shunt by measuring the activity in the kidney following an IV injection of microbubbles (normally undetectable). Macroaggregates are too big to pass through the normal pulmonary capillary bed, but contrast echocardiography reveals their presence on the left side of the circulation in the presence of a right to left shunt. CT cannot be used to quantify the right to left pulmonary shunt.

- Contrast echocardiography can also be used as a screening test for PAVMs, but will also detect intracardiac shunts (patent foramen ovale, and atrial and ventricular septal defects). Therefore, CT is performed to confirm and characterise PAVMs, following a positive contrast echocardiography shunt study.
- The presence of a significant shunt or PAVMs with feeding arteries >3 mm diameter are indications for intravascular embolisation, usually done with steel coils.
- Postural oximetry: hypoxaemia caused by PAVMs is exaggerated in the upright position (orthodeoxia) due to increased shunting through AVMs in the lower lobes (70% of PAVMs).
- Hypoxaemia caused by PAVMs is not corrected by 100% oxygen rebreathing.

Further reading

1. Govani FS, Shovlin CL. Hereditary haemorrhagic telangiectasia: a clinical and scientific review. *Eur J Hum Genet.* 2009;7:860–71.
2. Lacombe P, Lacout A, Marcy PY, et al. Diagnosis and treatment of pulmonary arteriovenous malformations in hereditary hemorrhagic telangiectasia: an overview. *Diagn Interv Imaging*. 2013 Sep;94(9):835-48. doi: 10.1016/j.diii.2013.03.014. Epub 2013 Jun 12.
3. Shovlin C, Wilmshurst P, Jackson J. Pulmonary arteriovenous malformations and other pulmonary aspects of Hereditary haemorrhagic telangiectasia. *Eur Resp Mon*. 2011;54:218–45.

Case 4

History

A 68-year-old woman presenting with a 6-month history of increasing breathlessness.
Figure 5.4A shows a CXR of bilateral peripheral interstitial shadowing.

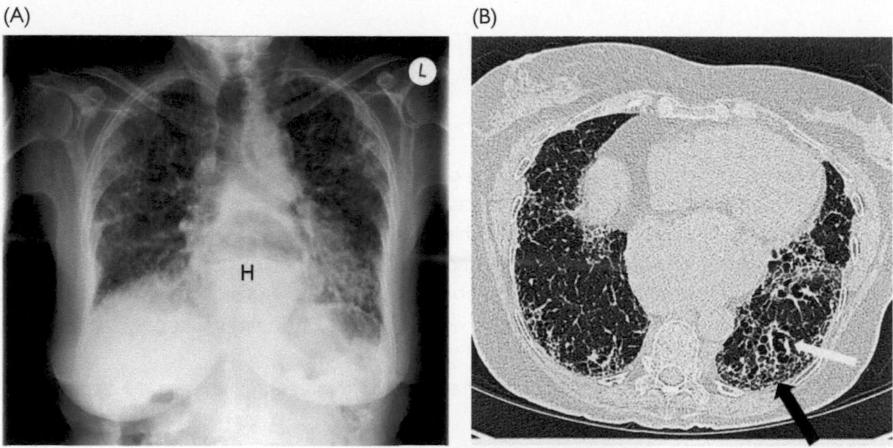

Figure 5.4 (A) Chest radiograph showing bilateral peripheral interstitial shadowing. Note the incidental large hiatus hernia (H). (B) High resolution CT showing subpleural honeycombing (black arrow), thickening of the interlobular septi and traction bronchiectasis (white arrow).

Differential diagnosis

- *Infection*: this is unlikely as the shadowing is not airspace consolidation and does not fit a lobar pattern.
- *Pulmonary oedema*: the shadowing is usually bilateral perihilar airspace shadowing giving a 'bat's wing' appearance. The pattern in this patient is bilateral peripheral interstitial shadowing, which may be

seen in early interstitial pulmonary oedema, but the history would usually be acute. Also the heart size is normal in this patient.

- *Usual interstitial pneumonitis*: the finding of bilateral peripheral interstitial shadowing on CXR along with subpleural honeycombing, thickening of the interlobular septi and traction bronchiectasis on CT makes this the most likely diagnosis.
- *Interstitial lung disease associated with connective tissue*: the appearances may be indistinguishable from usual interstitial pneumonitis (UIP), although in rheumatoid arthritis there may be pleural effusions, shoulder arthropathy or erosion of the distal clavicles, and in scleroderma a dilated oesophagus or soft tissue calcification.
- *Asbestosis*: this condition may have an identical appearance, but pleural plaques and effusions may also be seen in asbestos exposure.
- *Chronic silicosis*: typically shows calcified hilar lymphadenopathy (eggshell calcification) and pleural thickening.
- *Beryllium*: reticulonodular appearances are seen throughout the lungs ± macular lesions.
- *Drug-induced interstitial lung disease*: appearances may be identical, typically causing a peripheral distribution of fibrosis, and can only be distinguished by history.
- *Hypersensitivity pneumonitis*: this usually produces fibrosis of the upper two-thirds of the lungs with the presence of nodules in the acute setting.
- *Sarcoidosis*: nodules and bilateral hilar lymphadenopathy are usually seen in this condition with an upper zone predilection for fibrosis.

Diagnosis: usual interstitial pneumonitis

Key features

➲ See Chapter 11, Interstitial lung disease, p. 348 and Table 11.1.

Radiological

- The CXR shows peripheral and bibasal reticulonodular interstitial shadowing with volume loss.
- The diagnosis is usually confirmed by high-resolution CT, which shows subpleural honeycombing, thickening of the interlobular septi and traction bronchiectasis. The presence of ground glass shadowing may indicate a more favourable response to steroids.

Causes of fibrosis

Upper zone

TB, histoplasmosis, ankylosing spondylitis (➲ see Chapter 20, Ankylosing spondylitis, p. 720 and Table 20.5), post-radiotherapy (maybe unilateral or paramediastinal), sarcoidosis, hypersensitivity pneumonitis (also known as chronic extrinsic allergic alveolitis), pneumoconiosis, silicosis, progressive massive fibrosis.

Lower zone

Connective tissue diseases (systemic sclerosis, rheumatoid arthritis, systemic lupus erythematosus (SLE), interstitial pneumonias (cryptogenic), drugs (cytotoxics, amiodarone, methotrexate, nitrofurantoin), asbestosis and chronic aspiration with fibrosis.

Further reading

1. Jawad H, Chung JH, Lynch DA, Newell JD Jr. Radiological approach to interstitial lung disease: a guide for the nonradiologist. *Clin Chest Med*. 2012; 33(1):11–26.
2. Behr J. Approach to the diagnosis of interstitial lung disease. *Clin Chest Med*. 2012;33(1):1–10.

Case 5

History

A 36-year-old patient with a thoracotomy scar presents to the cardiology clinic with increasing shortness of breath and worsening hypertension.

Bilateral inferior rib notching was visible on a CXR (Figure 5.5A). Figure 5.5B shows a volume-rendered MR angiogram showing re-coarctation of the thoracic aorta.

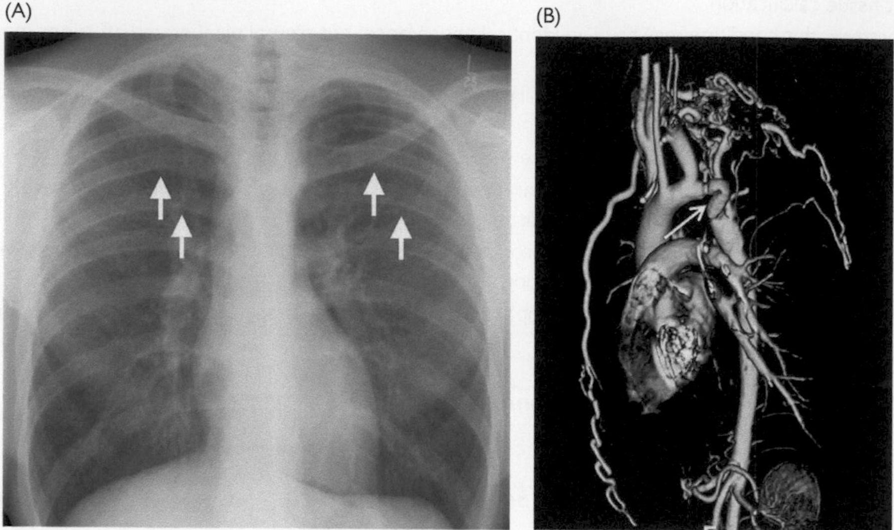

Figure 5.5 (A) A plain frontal chest radiograph showing bilateral inferior rib-notching (arrows). (B) A volume-rendered MR angiogram showing re-coarctation of the thoracic aorta (arrow) following a graft repair in childhood.

Differential diagnosis

Rib notching on a chest X-ray

- *Superior vena caval obstruction*: dilated venous collateral vessels.
- *Aortic coarctation*: congenital narrowing of a segment of thoracic aorta causing dilated intercostal arteries.
- *Nerve sheath tumours*: local pressure on rib due to adjacent tumour.
- *Hyperparathyroidism*: pseudo-rib notching due to periosteal changes.

Diagnosis: re-coarctation of the aorta following surgical repair

Key features

Clinical

- Coarctation of the aorta is due to a congenital narrowing of the thoracic aorta, most commonly just distal to the origin of the left subclavian artery.
- The pathophysiology is uncertain and may be due to haemodynamic effects in the fetal circulation or inappropriate migration of smooth muscle cells around the aorta.
- Findings on clinical examination include a blood pressure differential between upper and lower limbs with radio-femoral delay.

- Half of patients have associated congenital cardiac defects, most commonly bicuspid aortic valve and ventricular septal defects.
- As a result of chronic aortic obstruction, a collateral blood supply develops from the pre-stenotic subclavian arteries (from the axillary, internal thoracic and external thoracic arteries) and supplies the post-stenotic aorta via a network of intercostal anastomoses.
- 10–12% of patients with Turner's syndrome have an associated coarctation of the aorta. A female patient presenting with coarctation should undergo karyotyping.
- Surgical intervention may be undertaken:
  - to prevent the development of systemic hypertension; normotension is not necessarily restored in patients with established hypertension;
  - if there is significant aortic stenosis;
  - urgently for heart failure secondary to coarctation of the aorta.
- Surgical procedures include interposition grafts, patch aortoplasty and end-to-end anastomosis. Balloon dilatation and endovascular stenting are increasingly performed. Repair should be considered prior to pregnancy.

Radiological

- The collateral blood supply is demonstrated on a plain CXR as rib notching (inferior costal erosions) due to dilated intercostal arteries, typically between the third and eighth ribs. The first two spaces may be spared as they are supplied by the highest intercostal artery, which is a branch of the costocervical trunk of the subclavian arteries.
- Unilateral rib notching may occur on the left side only when the coarctation is proximal to an aberrant right subclavian artery, and on the right side only when the coarctation is proximal to the origin of the left subclavian artery.
- The '3' sign describes the appearance of the focal aortic stenosis on a plain CXR below the aortic arch. However, in the absence of heart failure, the CXR is usually normal.
- An upper GI series (barium swallow) may show the 'E sign' due to indentation of the pre- and post-stenotic aortic segments.
- Contrast-enhanced CT angiography will demonstrate the anatomy of the coarctation and the distribution of the collateral blood supply.
- Cardiac MRI also allows:
  - detailed visualisation of the cardiothoracic vasculature, including any associated congenital cardiac defects;
  - assessment of any post-surgical complications, such as re-coarctation and aneurysm formation;
  - measurement of the cross-sectional area of the stenosis, flow deceleration in the post-stenotic aorta and the collateral shunt volume.
- Echocardiography provides a non-invasive assessment of the coarctation, including Doppler flow measurements across the stenosis.
- Cardiac catheterisation provides invasive measurement of the pressure gradient across the coarctation. Intervention may be required if the gradient >20 mmHg.

Further reading

1. Darabian S, Zeb I, Rezaeian P, Razipour A, Budoff M. Use of noninvasive imaging in the evaluation of coarctation of aorta. *J Comput Assist Tomogr*. 2013;37(1):75–8.
2. Shih MC, Tholpady A, Kramer CM, Sydnor MK, Hagspiel KD. Surgical and endovascular repair of aortic coarctation: normal findings and appearance of complications on CT angiography and MR angiography. *Am J Roentgenol*. 2006;187(3):W302–12.
3. Bondy CA. Congenital cardiovascular disease in Turner syndrome. *Congen Heart Dis*. 2008;3:2–15.

Case 6

History

A 58-year-old patient presents to the emergency department with chest pain and a left hemiparesis. The mediastinum appeared widened on a portable CXR (Figure 5.6A) and the patient proceeded to a CT aortogram. Figure 5.6B is an unenhanced CT showing a crescent intramural haemorrhage in the ascending aortic wall. Figure 5.6C shows a contrast-enhanced CT aortogram.

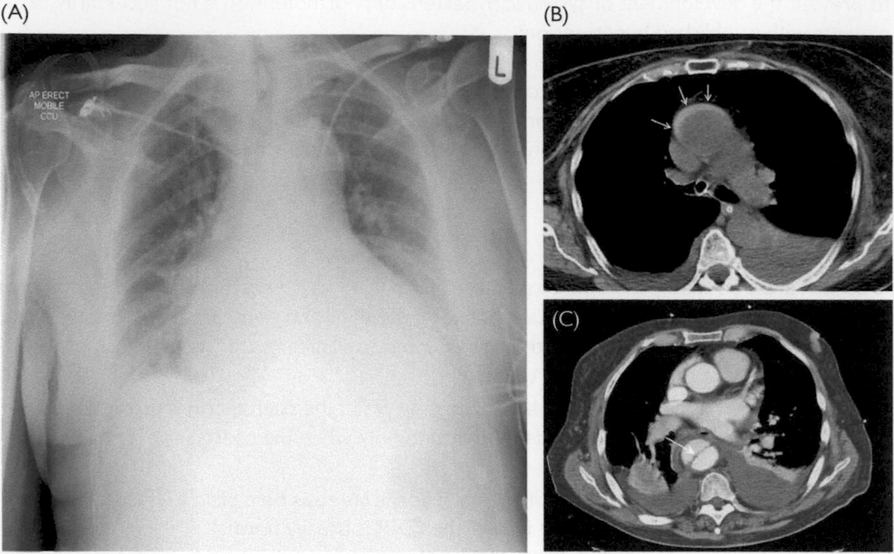

Figure 5.6 (A) Portable CXR showing a widened mediastinum and pleural effusions. (B) Unenhanced CT showing a crescent of intramural haemorrhage in the ascending aortic wall (arrow). (C) Contrast-enhanced CT aortogram revealing a dissection flap (arrow) in a Stanford Type B dissection.

Differential diagnosis

Suspected dissection on CT aorta:

- *Penetrating atherosclerotic ulcer*: an ulcerated atherosclerotic lesion penetrating the elastic lamina, and leading to haemorrhage and haematoma formation within the media of the aortic wall.
- *Dissecting thoracic aortic aneurysm*: a dissection flap separating a true and false lumen within the aorta.
- *Motion artefact mimicking a dissection flap*: cardiac motion artefact in the root of the aorta, which may be visible when electrocardiogram (ECG)-gating is not used.

Diagnosis: Stanford type A aortic dissection

Key features of aortic dissection

Clinical

See Table 13.49.

- The most common site of dissection is the right lateral wall of the aortic root with 90% occurring within 10 cm of the aortic valve. The next most frequent location is just distal to the origin of the left subclavian artery. The remainder do not have an obvious intimal tear and are attributed to rupture of the aortic vasa vasorum.
- There are two major classifications of aortic dissection:

- The DeBakey classification[1]:
  - Type I: occurs in the ascending aorta and extends into the descending aorta.
  - Type II: only involves the ascending aorta.
  - Type III: only involves the descending aorta:
    - Type IIIA begins distal to the left subclavian artery and extends to the diaphragm.
    - Type IIIB involves the descending aorta below the diaphragm.
- The Stanford classification[2] has only two types:
  - Type A: The ascending aorta is involved (equivalent to DeBakey types I and II).
  - Type B: The descending aorta is involved (equivalent to DeBakey type III).

Radiological

- CXR findings include widened mediastinum (59%), an abnormal aortic contour (50%) and pleural effusion (20%). Radiography is only helpful when evaluating those without high-risk features.
- A PA radiograph gives better diagnostic accuracy than an anteroposterior (AP) radiograph, as the AP projection may magnify structures in the anterior chest. A mediastinal width of >8 cm on an AP radiograph has moderate diagnostic accuracy for a dissection.
- Stable patients with suspected aortic dissection should be investigated with a CT aortogram:
  - A non-contrast study may show a crescent of high density intra-mural haematoma.
  - A timed bolus of IV contrast medium is then used to show the whole aorta to below the bifurcation.
- A dissection flap is visible on CT dividing the true and false lumens. It is easiest to start upstream of the dissection flap to identify the true lumen. Pericardial, pleural and mediastinal haemorrhage may also accompany aortic rupture.
- A dissection flap may be visible within the coronaries, great vessels, mesenteric and renal arteries.
- In selected patients MRI may be used to assess flowing blood and thrombus within the aorta.
- Trans-oesophageal echocardiography is particularly useful for assessment of aortic regurgitation in unstable patients.

Further reading

1. Chiu KW, Lakshminarayan R, Ettles DF. Acute aortic syndrome: CT findings. *Clin Radiol.* 2013; 68(7):741–8.

Case 7

History

A 58-year-old man presents with chest discomfort, which was worsened by lying flat.
Figure 5.7A shows a CXR revealing globular dilatation of the cardiac outline. Figure 5.7B shows a cardiac MRI of a large pericardial effusion.

Differential diagnosis

The differential of an enlarged cardiac outline on a CXR include:

- *Left ventricular aneurysm*: focal dilatation at the left ventricle apex often with curvilinear calcification.
- *Pericardial effusion*: globular enlargement of the cardiac silhouette.
- *Pulmonary hypertension*: dilatation of the pulmonary arteries and right ventricle.
- *Congestive cardiac failure*: increased cardiothoracic ratio with septal (Kerley B) lines and pleural effusions.

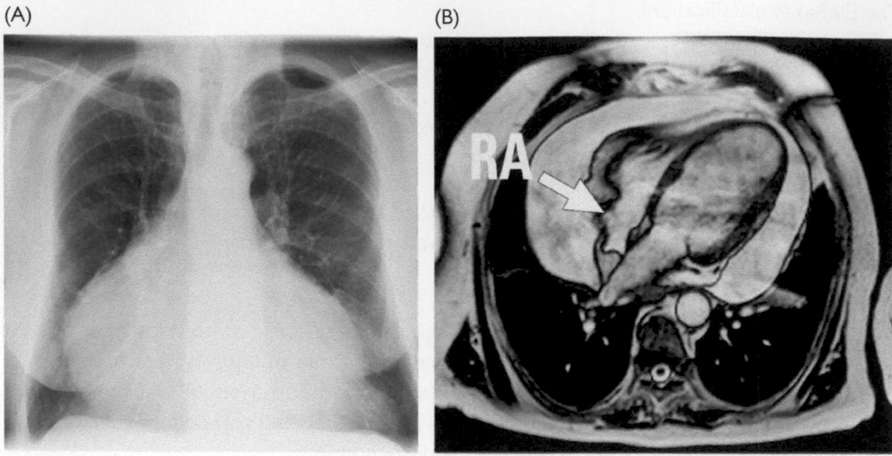

Figure 5.7 (A) CXR revealing globular dilatation of the cardiac outline. (B) Cardiac magnetic resonance imaging showing a large pericardial effusion with collapse of the right atrium.

Diagnosis: pericardial effusion

Key features

➲ See Chapter 13, Pericardial disease, p. 458 and Table 13.46.

Radiological

- A CXR may demonstrate an enlarged cardiac silhouette, but is insensitive to smaller pericardial effusions. The heart is typically globular in shape and described as a 'water bottle heart'. Around one-third of patients have a coexistent pleural effusion.
- Echocardiography is the preferred imaging modality to distinguish a dilated heart from a pericardial effusion:
  - Fluid appears as an anechoic space within the pericardial sac and often begins near the right atrium.
  - Echocardiography may reveal cardiac compromise, including collapse of the right atrium and right ventricle (initially diastolic collapse).
  - A haemorrhagic effusion due to aortic dissection may have fibrinous strands or blood clot(s) visible.
- Cardiac MRI may identify a haemorrhagic effusion which is bright on T1-weighted imaging. Pericardial thickening and constrictive pericarditis, and biventricular function can also be assessed. Gadolinium enhancement is used to visualise pericardial tumours or metastases. T2-weighted imaging is helpful to characterise associated myopericarditis.
- CT scanning reveals the presence of the effusion, calcified pericardium and may help determine the underlying cause, e.g. malignancy.

Further reading

1. Peebles CR, Shambrook JS, Harden SP. Pericardial disease--anatomy and function. *Br J Radiol*. 2011; 84(Spec No 3):S324–37.

Case 8

History

A 32-year-old female patient presented with symptoms of malaise and visual disturbance. She had a carotid bruit on examination and was referred for vascular imaging investigations.

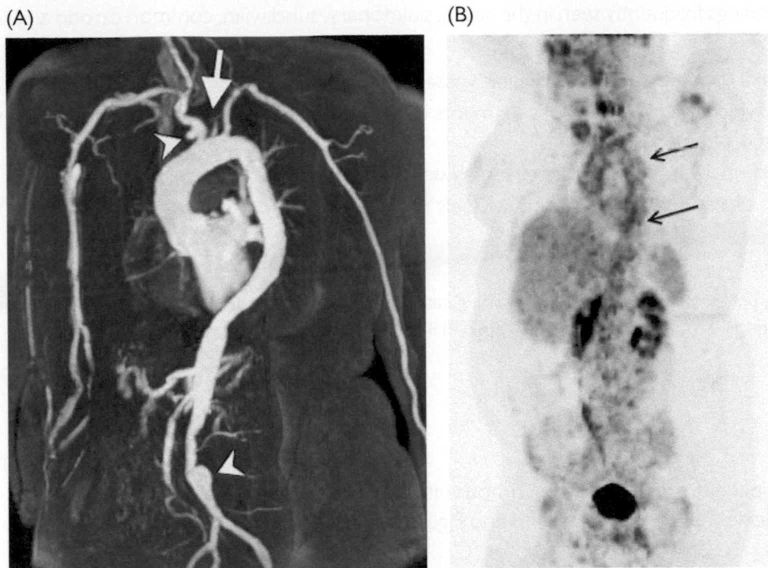

Figure 5.8 (A) Contrast-enhanced MR aortogram shows an occluded left common carotid artery (arrow) and saccular aneurysms (arrowheads). (B) A whole body ^{18}FDG-PET study showing increased metabolic activity in the aorta (arrows).

MR angiogram showed multiple stenoses affecting the origins of the great vessels (Figure 5.8A). Figure 5.8B shows a whole body ^{18}FDG-PET study showing increased metabolic activity in the aorta.

Differential diagnosis

- *Fibromuscular dysplasia*: angiopathy affecting medium-sized arteries predominantly in young women of childbearing age.
- *Takayasu's arteritis*: a relapsing and remitting inflammatory vasculitis causing occlusion and stenoses of the aorta and its major branches.
- *Atherosclerotic disease*: calcified and non-calcified plaques causing stenoses and end-organ ischaemia.
- *Aortic coarctation*: congenital abnormality of the aorta causing a focal narrowing and collateral vessel formation.
- *Buerger disease*: non-atherosclerotic vaso-occlusive disease. Strongly associated with tobacco use.

Diagnosis: Takayasu arteritis

Key features

➲ See Chapter 20, Takayasu arteritis, p. 741.

Radiological

Radiological investigations in patients with Takayasu arteritis include:

- Contrast-enhanced MR angiography for monitoring disease activity. Vessel wall imaging may also have a role in assessing response to treatment.
- CT angiography is suitable for patients who cannot tolerate MRI.
- PET scanning with ^{18}FDG for detecting active inflammation and in monitoring response to immunosuppressive agents.
- US for assessing the vessel wall and flow waveforms of the carotid and subclavian arteries.

Radiological findings frequently seen in the aorta, pulmonary, subclavian, common carotid and renal arteries include:

- Aneurysmal dilatation with an irregular vessel contour.
- Stenoses which may involve short segments of artery or cause diffuse disease. Increased vessel tortuosity is often present.
- Circumferential vessel wall thickening may occur, especially involving the carotid arteries.
- In chronic disease multiple collateral vessels may develop.

Further reading

1. Mavrogeni S, Dimitroulas T, Chatziioannou SN, Kitas G. The role of multimodality imaging in the evaluation of Takayasu arteritis. *Sem Arthrit Rheumat*. 2013;42(4):401–12.

Case 9

History

A 68-year-old patient presented with a 6-hour history of increasing abdominal pain.
Figure 5.9A shows a plain abdominal film and Figure 5.9B shows a coronal CT scan.

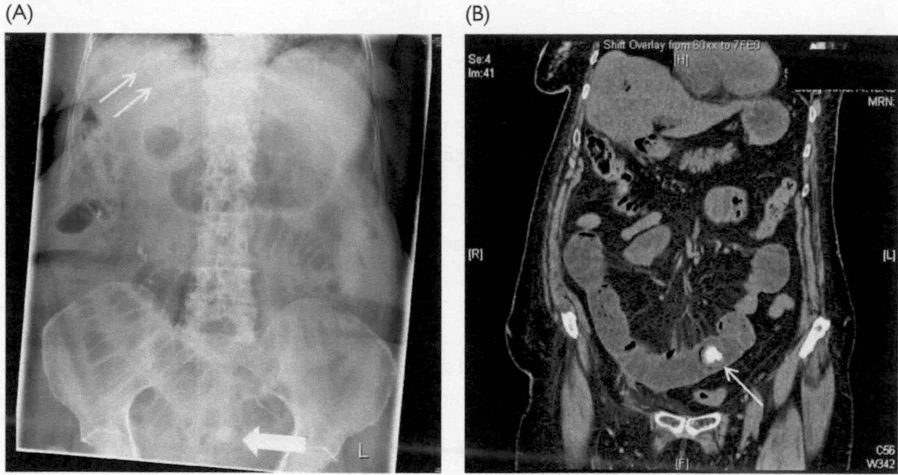

Figure 5.9 (A) Plain abdominal film showing dilated small bowel loops of obstruction, aerobilia (thin arrows) and an obstructing ectopic calcified gallstone in the distal small bowel (thick arrow). (B) Coronal CT showing dilated loops of small bowel and an ectopic obstructing gallstone (arrow) in the distal small bowel.

Differential diagnosis

- *Small bowel obstruction secondary to a hernia*: there are dilated small loops consistent with small bowel obstruction, but the hernial orifices have not been imaged on the abdominal film.
- *Small bowel obstruction secondary to adhesions*: while adhesions and hernia are the commonest causes of small bowel obstruction, these entities would not account for the presence of aerobilia seen on the abdominal film.
- *Perforation of a viscus*: there is no free intraperitoneal gas to support this diagnosis. Dilated loops of both large and small bowel due to an ileus may accompany the peritonitis associated with perforation.
- *Gallstone ileus*: aerobilia, small bowel obstruction and an ectopic gallstone in the distal small bowel is seen on the abdominal X-ray.

Diagnosis: gallstone ileus

Key features

Clinical

- Gallstone ileus is a rare cause of small bowel obstruction (1%) and is commoner in females.
- There is usually a past history of gallbladder disease as inflammation is the cause of formation of a fistula between the gallbladder and duodenum (60%) or colon.
- The gallstone enters the bowel via the fistula and most commonly impacts at the ileocaecal junction (60–70%). The stone has to be >2 cm to cause obstruction. The condition has a high mortality and warrants surgical decompression.

Radiological

- An abdominal film shows the classical Rigler's triad of aerobilia, small bowel obstruction and an ectopic calcified gallstone in the distal small bowel, found in 25% of patients with gallstone ileus.
- CT is the modality of choice to confirm the diagnosis depicting the fistula, ectopic stone and level of obstruction, as well as complications such as perforation. However, CT may not show the gallstone as only 10% are calcified.

Case 10

History

This 40-year-old male with a long-standing bowel condition presented with itching, intermittent jaundice and right upper quadrant pain. An endoscopic retrograde cholangiopancreatogram (ERCP) and plain abdominal film were performed (Figure 5.10A and B).

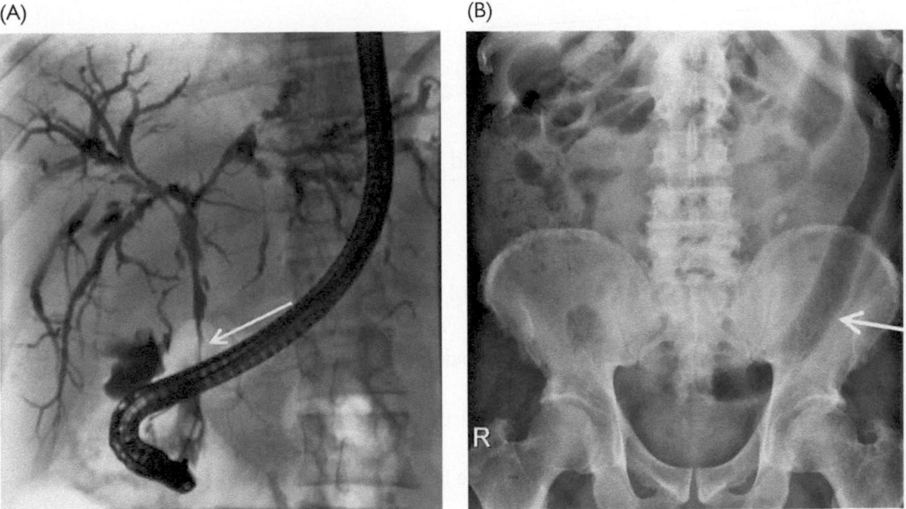

Figure 5.10 (A) Endoscopic retrograde cholangiopancreatogram (ERCP) showing intrahepatic multifocal stricturing and dilatation, giving a 'beaded' appearance with a stricture of the common bile duct (arrow). (B) Plain abdominal radiograph showing the classic lead pipe sign of chronic ulcerative colitis with complete loss of haustra in the diseased segment (arrow).

Differential diagnosis

- *Chronic ulcerative colitis*: the abdominal film shows the classic lead pipe sign of chronic ulcerative colitis (UC) with complete loss of haustra in the diseased segment, which is smooth walled.

- *Primary sclerosing cholangitis*: there is a stricture in the common bile duct (CBD) with stricturing and dilatation of the intrahepatic biliary tree. In the context of ulcerative colitis the diagnosis is most likely to be primary sclerosing cholangitis (PSC).
- *Cholangicarcinoma*: causes of a CBD stricture in PSC may be inflammatory or a cholangicarcinoma.
- *Secondary sclerosing cholangitis*: a differential due to pyogenic cholangitis in the context of gallstones or previous obstruction.
- *Bile duct injury*: if there is a history of previous surgery.
- *Primary biliary cirrhosis*: the disease is usually limited to the intrahepatic biliary tree and strictures are less pronounced. Typically, middle-aged women with high titres of antimitochondrial antibodies.

Diagnosis: primary sclerosing cholangitis with an inflammatory common bile duct stricture associated with ulcerative colitis

No evidence of malignancy was found and the stricture was successfully balloon-dilated (cholangioplasty).

Key features of primary sclerosing cholangitis

Clinical

➲ See Table 15.10.

Radiological

- ERCP and magnetic resonance cholangiopancreatogram (MRCP) are the most sensitive and specific modalities.
- Areas of ductal normality existing between the ductal strictures, along with dilatation of the ducts gives rise to the 'beaded' appearance typical of PSC. As the process progresses, peripheral ducts become obliterated and the appearance of the biliary tree is that of a 'pruned tree'. There may be 'diverticula' up to 10 mm (25%).

Case 11

History

A 68-year-old man presented with bone pain around the wrist and ankles. A bone scan and CXR were performed (Figure 5.11A–C).

Differential diagnosis

The differential of a symmetrical periosteal reaction is:

- *Thyroid acropathy*:
  - Occurs in 0.5–10% of patients following thyroidectomy for thyrotoxicosis irrespective of thyroid status.
  - The periosteal reaction is seen as solid and spiculated (lace-like), and not smooth as in hypertrophic osteoarthropathy (HOA).
  - Typically affects the upper limbs more than the lower limbs, especially the diaphysis of the metacarpals and phalanges of the hands.
- *Vascular insufficiency*:
  - The periosteal reaction usually affects the lower limbs.
  - Is seen as a solid undulating periosteal reaction with overlying soft tissue swelling.
  - Periosteal reaction is not related to ulceration.
  - May be seen in arterial, venous or lymphatic insufficiency.
- HOA: this is the most likely diagnosis. The periosteal reaction occurs in the diaphysis and metaphysis of the radius, ulna, tibia and fibula, and less commonly the humerus and femur.

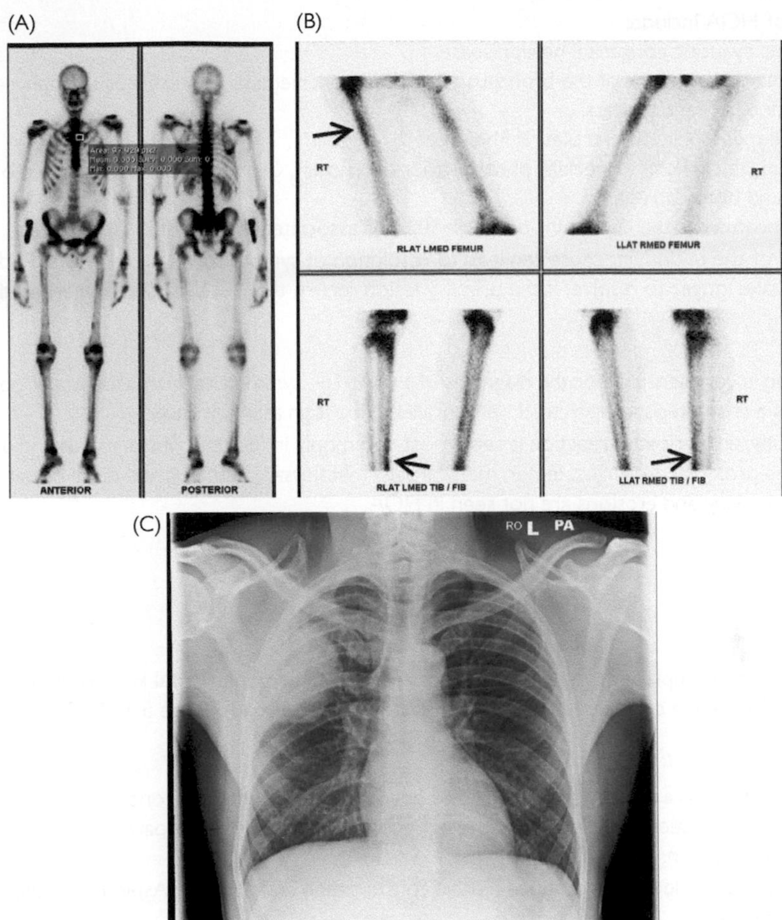

Figure 5.11 (A) Whole body bone scan showing increased tracer uptake along the cortices of the femora and both distal radii/ulna and distal tibia. (B) Magnified view of the legs from the bone scan confirming that the increased tracer uptake is sited along the periosteum of both femora and distal tibia (arrows). No abnormality of the underlying bone is seen. (C) Chest radiograph showing a large right upper lobe bronchogenic carcinoma.

- Pachydermoperiostitis: this is a familial condition that affects boys at puberty and is more common in coloured people. It is associated with clubbing and is painless. The periosteal reaction is thick, shaggy, irregular and involves the epiphyses, as well as the diaphyses and metaphyses.
- Fluorosis: this is a rare chronic metabolic bone disease due to ingestion of large amounts of fluoride. It is characterised by dense bones and ligamentous/tendinous ossification. The periosteal reaction is solid and undulating.

Diagnosis: hypertrophic osteoarthropathy associated with primary bronchogenic carcinoma

Key features

- HOA is accompanied by digital clubbing and causes painful swelling of the wrists, elbows, ankles and knees. Peri-articular osteoporosis and joint effusions may be present. The thickness of the periosteal reaction correlates with duration of disease activity.

- Causes of HOA include:
  - Cardiac: cyanotic congenital heart disease.
  - Pulmonary: carcinoma of the bronchus (1–10%), bronchiectasis/cystic fibrosis, emphysema, metastatic deposits and abscess.
  - Pleural: mesothelioma and pleural fibroma.
  - Abdominal: cirrhosis (especially primary biliary cirrhosis), Crohn's disease, ulcerative colitis, neoplasia and biliary atresia.
- Pleural fibroma has the highest incidence (>30%) of associated HOA, but is itself rare.
- Removal of the underlying cause can lead to resolution of symptoms within 24 hours. Radiographic changes take longer to resolve. If the primary lesion recurs, the HOA may be exacerbated.

Radiological

- Bone scan is very sensitive for the diagnosis of HOA. The symmetrical increased tracer uptake produces a characteristic 'tram track' or 'parallel stripe' sign as in this case.
- Metadiaphyseal periosteal reaction is seen most commonly in the tibia, fibula, radius and ulna, but also in the proximal phalanges, femur, metacarpals/metatarsals, humerus and distal phalanges. Joint space narrowing and erosions are not seen in HOA.

Case 12

History

A 64-year-old man complained of acute dyspnoea. He had undergone a total knee replacement 1 week previously. A CXR and a contrast-enhanced CT chest were performed (Figure 5.12A–C).

Differential diagnosis

- *Pneumonia*: there are bilateral pleurally based opacities, with right lower zone collapse/consolidation and blunting of the right costophrenic angle. This pattern would be unusual for infection.
- *Aspiration*: this would usually produce bibasal consolidation and collapse. Aspiration usually occurs peri-operatively.
- *Pleurally based lesions*: the differential includes pleural metastases (thymona, breast, bronchus), pleural fibroma, mesothelioma (usually circumferential pleural thickening of the hemithorax), empyema (usually seen as a loculated pleural collection), folded lung (may be associated with asbestos exposure and typically a single lesion with an adjacent 'comet's tail' appearance due to parenchymal distortion), pleural plaques (due to asbestos exposure; these may be calcified and have a 'holly-leaf' appearance *en face*).
- *Acute pulmonary embolism*: this is the most likely diagnosis given the history and peripheral sites of the lesions, which represent areas of pulmonary infarction. Comparison with a pre-operative CXR would confirm their new development. In the majority (>90%) of patients with a pulmonary embolus (PE), the thrombus originates in the leg veins, but may arise from the pelvic veins or catheters/devices (e.g. caval filters). PEs are a well-recognised complication of surgery, especially knee and hip surgery, and most commonly occur in the lower lobes (>50%).

Diagnosis: acute pulmonary embolism with pulmonary infarcts

Key features

Clinical features and management

➲ See Chapter 11, Pulmonary embolism, p. 365 and Tables 11.4 and 11.5.

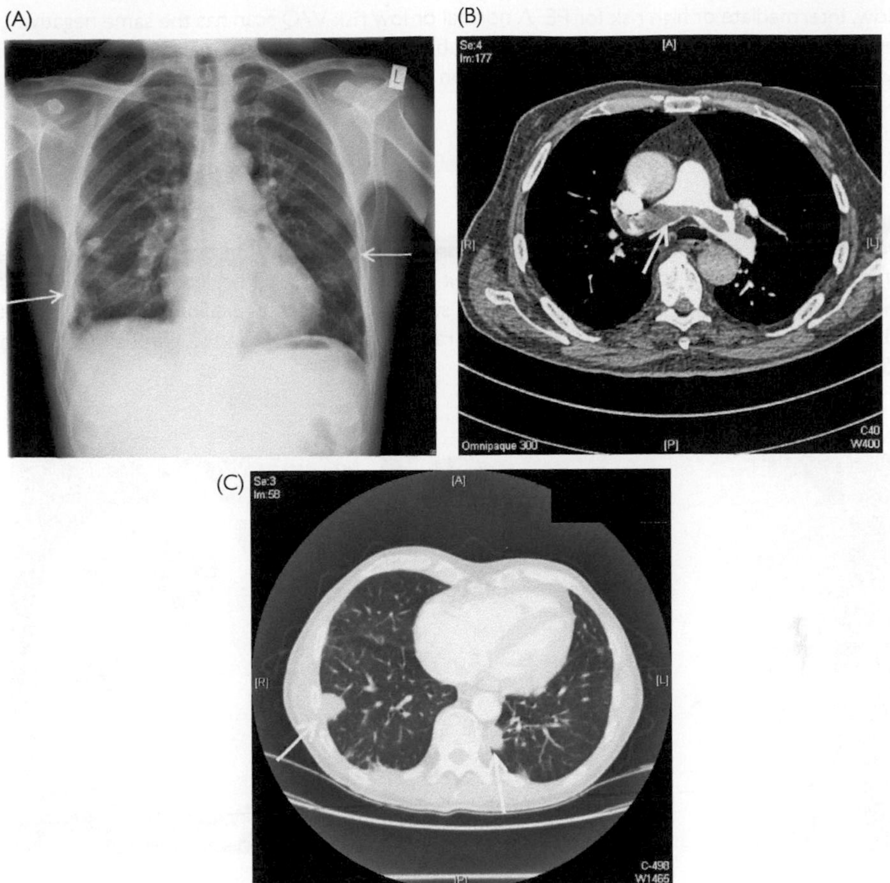

Figure 5.12 (A) Chest radiograph showing bilateral peripheral opacities (arrows) (Hampton's humps) consistent with infarctions after correlation with CT. There is also a small right pleural effusion, with a right lower zone collapse/consolidation and elevation of the right hemidiaphragm. (B) CTPA showing a saddle pulmonary embolus (arrow). (C) CTPA (viewed on lung windows) showing two Hampton's humps (pulmonary infarcts) (arrows).

Radiological

- The CXR is usually the first line of radiological investigation, but may be normal (>30%). There are several signs associated with PE, including subsegmental atelectasis (small volumes of collapse seen as linear densities), consolidation, infarction and pleural effusion. Some other well-recognised, although infrequently occurring signs include:
  - The Westermark sign: focal area of oligaemia distal to an embolus; present in 2% of cases.
  - The Fleischner sign: dilatation of the pulmonary artery proximal to an embolus.
  - Hamptons humps: pleurally based opacity due to infarction.
- Computed tomography pulmonary angiography (CTPA) is the modality of choice. Both sensitivity and specificity are >90%. CTPA demonstrates PEs as intraluminal filling defects or as contrast surrounding the thrombus ('polo mint' sign). Those with an abnormal CXR or significant cardiopulmonary disease should have a CTPA.
- Patients with a normal or near normal CXR should have a ventilation/perfusion (V/Q) scan. PEs are seen as a mismatch between perfusion and ventilation on a V/Q scan. V/Q scans are reported

as low, intermediate or high risk for PE. A normal or low risk V/Q scan has the same negative predictive value as a normal CTPA. A high probability result may, however, be a false positive. The advantages of a V/Q scan are the lower radiation dose and no exposure to IV contrast.

Case 13

History

An 18-year-old man presented with progressive hearing loss and tinnitus. On examination, he had several subcutaneous nodules on the torso, but no *café au lait* patches or axillary freckles.

Figure 5.13A shows an abdominal radiograph with several cutaneous neurofibromas. The patient was referred for MRI of the brain, which revealed bilateral enhancing masses in the cerebellopontine angles (Figure 5.13B).

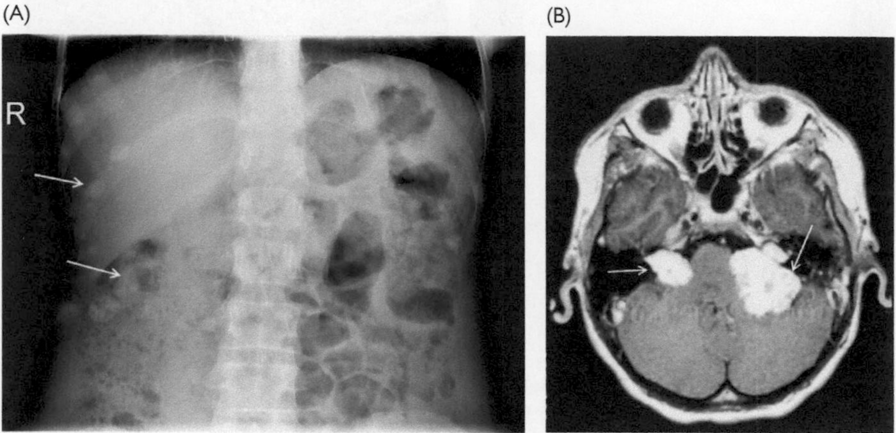

Figure 5.13 (A) Abdominal radiograph showing several cutaneous neurofibromas (arrows) in a patient with NF2. (B) Axial T1-weighted contrast enhanced MR image of the cerebellopontine angles. Bilateral enhancing vestibular schwannomas (arrows) are present, which are diagnostic of NF2.

Differential diagnosis

The differential is of a disease predisposing to intracranial tumour development (➲ see Chapter 17, Neurocutaneous syndromes, p. 637):

- *Tuberous sclerosis*: autosomal dominant disorder associated with giant cell astrocytomas, cortical tubers and subependymal nodules, as well as cutaneous, renal, pulmonary and cardiac manifestations.
- *Neurofibromatosis type 2 (NF2)*: autosomal dominant disease predisposing to vestibular schwannomas, meningiomas and ependymomas.
- *Von Hippel–Lindau syndrome*: autosomal dominant disease associated with haemangioblastomas, retinal angiomatosis, phaeochromocytoma and renal cell carcinoma.

Diagnosis: neurofibromatosis type 2

Key features

Clinical

- NF2 is an inherited autosomal dominant disease due to a mutation of the *NF2* gene, which is located on the long arm of chromosome 22. Mutations lead to truncations of the tumour-suppressing protein called 'merlin'. Half of all mutations occur sporadically, of which 25% show somatic mosaicism.
- NF2 is associated with bilateral vestibular schwannomas, spinal cord schwannomas, gliomas, meningiomas and juvenile cataracts. The mnemonic MISME can be used to remember the main

features (Multiple Inherited Schwannomas, Meningiomas and Ependymomas). Cutaneous lesions are less pronounced than in NF1, with schwannomas more commonly present than neurofibromas.

Radiological

- MRI has a key role in the diagnosis of CNS tumours in NF2. Post-contrast T1-weighted imaging is accurate at detecting cerebellopontine angle lesions and meningiomas. Vestibular schwannomas occur at the internal auditory canal, usually affecting the inferior vestibular division of the VIII cranial nerve; larger lesions may cause local mass effect. CT is indicated only when MRI is contraindicated.
- Meningiomas typically show homogenous enhancement and a may have a broad-based dural tail.
- Ependymomas in NF2 usually occur within the cervical cord or cervicomedullary junction, with evidence on imaging in 33–53% of patients with NF2. They often have high signal on T2-weighted imaging, show signs of enhancement, and may cause expansion of the cord. Tumours usually exhibit an indolent growth pattern with progression limited to a minority of patients. Spinal ependymomas are the most common intramedullary neoplasm in adults, comprising 60% of all glial spinal cord tumours.
- Cutaneous nodules may be visible on plain radiographs as well-defined opacities within the superficial soft tissues. They can be misinterpreted as lung nodules, which have a similar appearance. Neural foraminal widening can sometimes result from a schwannomas. Scoliosis may also be present.

Further reading

1. Yohay K. Neurofibromatosis types 1 and 2. *Neurologist*. 2006;12:86–93.

Case 14

History

A 21-year-old man with Down's syndrome presented with a 3-week history of neck pain, bilateral leg weakness and a gait disturbance. Spinal MRI was performed initially, followed by CT (Figure 5.14A and B).

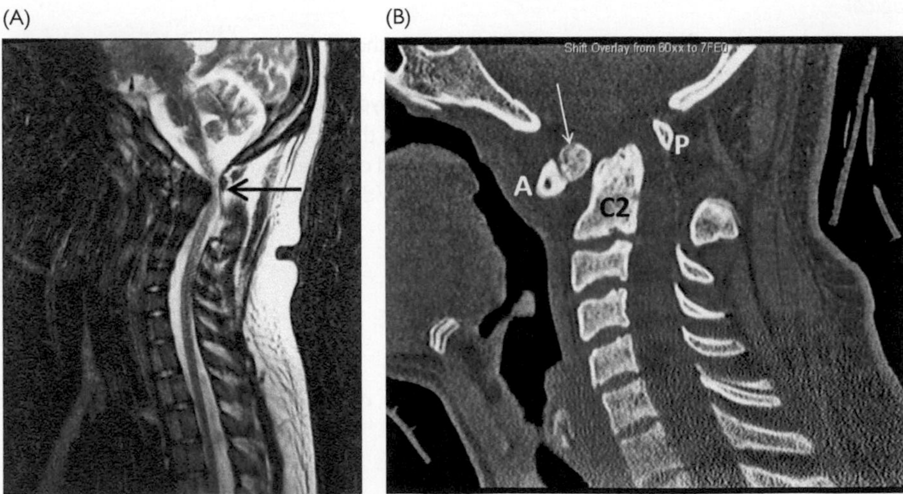

Figure 5.14 (A) Sagittal T2-weighted MR image of the cervical spine showing severe cord compression (arrow) just inferior to the craniocervical junction. The cause is difficult to establish. High signal is seen in the cord consistent with oedema. (B) CT sagittal reformat of the cervical spine showing a fracture of the tip of the odontoid peg (arrow) of C2. The fractured odontoid peg tip has dislocated anteriorly with the anterior arch (A) of C1. The atlantoaxial joint is intact. The spinal canal is severely compromised just inferior to the craniocervical junction. The resultant cord compression is not as well depicted as on MR. P: posterior arch of C1.

Differential diagnosis

- *Cord compression secondary to a tumour*: The upper cervical cord is compressed, but no definite bony or soft tissue mass is seen on the initial MRI.
- *Cord compression secondary to a prolapsed disc*: The upper cervical cord is compressed, maximally just below the craniocervical junction, but there is no discal material seen in the spinal canal.
- *Cord compression due to fracture/dislocation of the odontoid peg*: The tip of the fractured odontoid peg has dislocated anteriorly with the anterior arch of C1.

Diagnosis: cord compression due to fracture/dislocation of the odontoid peg

Key features

Clinical

Suspected cord compression is an emergency.

- Cord compression is a clinical diagnosis. The diagnosis is more difficult in the presence of decreased consciousness, and in patients with a poor history (as in this case).
- Cord compression typically presents with a predominantly motor pyramidal weakness, spasticity and a sensory level. Urinary and bowel sphincter disturbance should always be sought in the history. Lesions above T1 may cause upper limb signs and high cervical lesions may result in respiratory problems.
- Causes of cord compression are:
  - Space occupying lesions (majority of cases):
    - metastases;
    - primary intramedullary lesions: ependymona, astrocytoma, glioblastoma;
    - primary extramedullary lesions: meningioma, neurofibroma, schwannoma.
  - Other causes, including trauma, infection (epidural abscess, vertebral osteomyelitis), prolapsed discs, atlantoaxial subluxation and spinal canal stenosis (e,g. congenital such as Klippel–Feil syndrome).

Radiological

- The imaging modality of choice in the spine is MRI as it shows the spinal cord, spinal canal, bone marrow signal changes, nerve roots and discs better than CT. However, CT is better at depicting cortical bone (which appears as low signal on MRI and hyper-dense on CT) and hence fractures.
- The acquisition time of MRI scans is longer than CT and therefore is more susceptible to movement artefact, as illustrated in this scan. MRI revealed the cord compression although it did not establish the cause (Figure 5.14A). CT clearly shows the fracture/dislocation of the odontoid peg (Figure 5.14B).

Case 15

History

A 45-year-old lady gave a 6-month history of abdominal pain, diarrhoea and flushing. A contrast-enhanced CT image of the pelvis is shown (Figure 5.15).

Differential diagnosis

- *Colon cancer*: the mass is centred in the mesentery outside bowel loops, which goes against colon cancer.
- *Carcinoid*: this is the most likely diagnosis of a soft tissue mass in the small bowel mesentery with associated desmoplastic reaction. This diagnosis is in keeping with the history of flushing and diarrhoea.
- *Crohn's disease*: while Crohn's disease could produce an inflammatory mesenteric mass or abscess, the adjacent small bowel loops are normal, which is against this diagnosis.

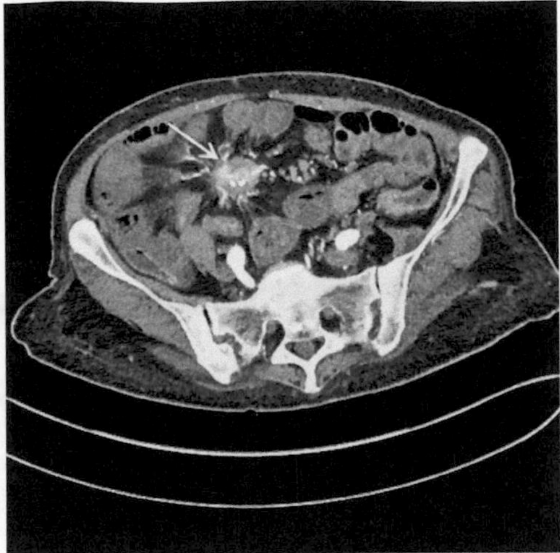

Figure 5.15 Axial CT at the level of the pelvis showing a partially calcified mass (arrow) centred on the mesentery with fibrotic desmoplastic reaction which is characteristic of a carcinoid tumour.

- *Metastases*: these may be sited on the serosal or peritoneal surface (e.g. ovarian, pancreatic, stomach and colon). The surrounding desmoplastic reaction is not typical of a metastasis.

Diagnosis: carcinoid tumour

Key features

➲ See Chapter 19, Neuroendocrine tumours, p. 700.

- Carcinoid is a neuroendocrine tumour, which arises from the amine precursor uptake and decarboxylation (APUD) system and are found in the GI tract, as well as the lung. They are slow growing tumours, but can metastasise.
- Carcinoid tumours are the most common tumour of the small bowel and appendix:
  - 85% of carcinoid tumours occur in the GI tract; ~2% of GI tract tumours are carcinoid tumours.
  - One-third occur in the small bowel, of which ~50% occur in the appendix. They are more common in the terminal ileum than jejunum.
  - One-third have metastases, one-third are multifocal, and one-third have a second malignancy.

Radiological

- Carcinoid tumour is typically seen on CT as a partially calcified soft tissue mass in the small bowel mesentery with associated classic desmoplastic reaction (surrounding distortion and fibrotic stranding reaction in the surrounding fat).
- Carcinoid tumour can be diagnosed by barium studies, CT, MRI or nuclear medicine.
- Metaiodobenzylguanidine, (I^{123} MIBG) and octreotide scintigraphy are taken up by carcinoid tumours and are useful in monitoring disease.
- The liver metastases are typically hypervascular on CT and MRI in the arterial phase, and may be hypointense or isointense in the portal venous phase.

Further reading

1. Ganeshan D, Bhosale P, Yang T, Kundra V. Imaging features of carcinoid tumors of the gastrointestinal tract. *Am J Roentgenol*. 2013;201:773–86.

Case 16

History

A 38-year-old female patient with sickle cell disease developed progressive pain in her right hip that did not respond to simple analgesia. A pelvic X-ray showed sclerosis in the head of the right femur and she was referred for an MRI (Figure 5.16A and B).

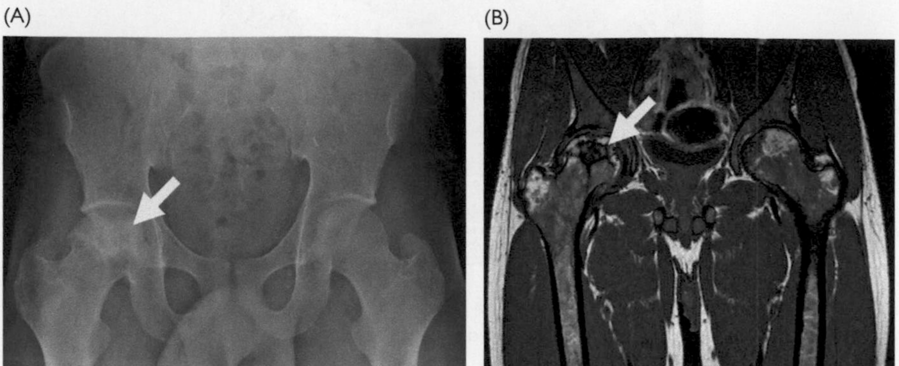

Figure 5.16 (A) A frontal pelvic X-ray shows sclerosis in the right femoral head (arrow). (B) A coronal T1-weighted MRI of the pelvis shows corresponding abnormal subchondral signal (arrow) with marrow hyperplasia.

Differential diagnosis

The differential is that of hip complications in sickle cell disease:

- *Avascular necrosis*: osteopenia, sclerosis and cortical fragmentation.
- *Osteomyelitis*: periostitis and osteopenia.
- *Septic arthritis*: diffuse marrow oedema, bone destruction in acetabulum and femoral head, joint effusion.
- *Osteoporosis*: overall reduction in bone density due to marrow hyperplasia.
- *Growth impairment*: delayed skeletal maturation.

Diagnosis: avascular necrosis

Key features

➲ See Chapter 9, Sickling disorders, p. 277, and Figure 9.5.

- Sickle cell disease (SCD) is a genetic haemoglobinopathy mostly affecting people of African and Mediterranean descent.
- The sickling process occurs when HbS is exposed to tissue hypoxia or acidosis, and forms an insoluble polymer.
- Vaso-occlusive crises may also be provoked by infection, pregnancy and exertion.
- SCD is a chronic multisystem disorder with varied complications that occur both chronically and acutely.
- Avascular necrosis (AVN) of the femoral head develops by adulthood in around one-third of patients with SCD.
- Treatment is controversial and may involve conservative measures initially. Removal of necrotic material may be performed with core decompression; an arthroplasty is an option if other measures are unsuccessful.

Radiological

- The Ficat staging system covers a range of multimodality imaging appearances for AVN.
- In deciding on treatment, the extent of cortical involvement and compression should be assessed, as well as the presence of secondary osteoarthritis.
- Plain radiographs may initially be normal; the earliest signs are mild osteopenia. More advanced disease may show mixed area of subchondral sclerosis and lucency (rim sign). Cortical fragmentation and degenerative joint disease eventually occurs.
- MRI is the most sensitive imaging modality for AVN and may be used for screening the asymptomatic hip for AVN as well. T1-weighted imaging shows low signal oedema bordered by high signal haemorrhage. T2-weighted may show the specific 'double line sign' between normal and ischaemic bone marrow.
- Infarction and infection can be difficult to distinguish. Cortical defects, fluid collections and marrow enhancement are suggestive of sepsis.

Further reading

1. Ejindu VC, Hine AL, Mashayekhi M, Shorvon PJ, Misra RR. Musculoskeletal manifestations of sickle cell disease. *Radiographics*. 2007;27(4):1005–21.

Case 17

History

A 42-year-old patient developed syncope during exercise with increasing dyspnoea. An echocardiogram showed suspected left ventricular hypertrophy and he was referred for a cardiac MRI (Figure 5.17).

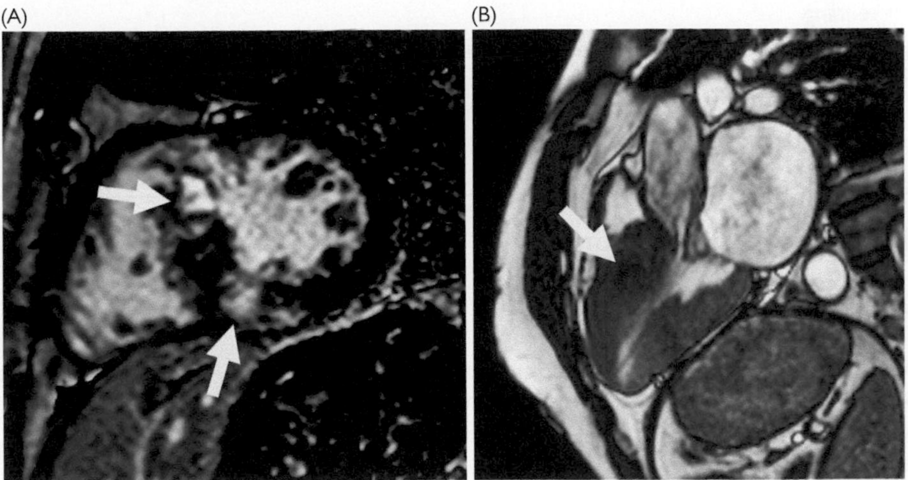

Figure 5.17 A cardiac MR in a patient with HCM. (A) A late enhancement sequence with typical patchy enhancement (arrows) in the thickened interventricular septum. (B) A long axis view of the left ventricle showing basal septal hypertrophy (arrow) and outflow tract obstruction.

Differential diagnosis

The differential is that of left ventricular hypertrophy:

- *Aortic stenosis*: symmetric hypertrophy (<15 mm) with calcified and stenotic aortic valve.
- *Hypertensive heart disease*: symmetric hypertrophy (<15 mm) in known hypertensive.

- *Hypertrophic cardiomyopathy (HCM)*: asymmetric septal hypertrophy (>15 mm) with myocardial fibrosis and outflow tract obstruction.
- *Athletic heart syndrome*: symmetric hypertrophy (<15 mm), often with biventricular dilatation.
- *Amyloid*: global hypertrophy with functional impairment and diffuse contrast enhancement.
- *Fabry's disease*: alpha-galactosidase deficiency leading to aberrant accumulation of Gb3 glycolipid in myocardium (and other tissues) (➲ see Chapter 16, Fabry disease, p. 581).

Diagnosis: hypertrophic cardiomyopathy

Key features

➲ See Chapter 13, Hypertrophic cardiomyopathy, p. 445 and Tables 13.25–13.28.

Radiological

- Conventional 2D echocardiography is usually sufficient to make a diagnosis, but in equivocal cases cardiac MRI is useful and also determines if there is myocardial fibrosis.
- Adenosine-stress perfusion scan may exclude obstructive coronary disease and detect microvascular ischaemia.
- Late gadolinium enhancement may reveal areas of patchy enhancement and provides additional information for assessing sudden cardiac death risk.
- HCM may be evident on CT, but caution should be used in measuring wall thickness on studies that are not cardiac gated.
- Cardiac CT may also show myocardial bridging which are short-tunnelled segments of coronary arteries.

Further reading

1. Bogaert J, Olivotto I. MR Imaging in hypertrophic cardiomyopathy: from magnet to bedside. *Radiology*. 2014;273(2):329–48.

Multiple choice questions

Questions

1. A 33-year-old man presents with recurrent chest infections and asthma. A CXR shows widespread bronchiectasis and situs inversus. What is the most likely diagnosis?
   A. Allergic bronchopulmonary aspergillosis.
   B. Cystic fibrosis.
   C. Kartagener's syndrome.
   D. Hypogammaglobulinaemia.
   E. Swyer–James syndrome.
2. A 38-year-old male smoker presents to the respiratory clinic with increasing shortness of breath and decreased exercise tolerance. A CXR reveals bilateral lower lobe emphysema. A HRCT of the chest shows parenchymal destruction and bronchial wall thickening, predominantly at the lung bases. What is the likely diagnosis?
   A. Pneumocystis pneumonia.
   B. Cystic fibrosis.
   C. Alpha 1 antitrypsin deficiency.

D. Lymphangioleiomyomatosis.
E. Bronchial atresia.

3. A 36-year-old man presents with a 6-month history of increasing breathlessness, shoulder, hip and back pain. His CXR shows bilateral upper lobe fibrosis. What is the most likely diagnosis?
   A. Systemic sclerosis.
   B. Rheumatoid arthritis.
   C. Ankylosing spondylitis.
   D. Asbestosis with hypertrophic pulmonary osteoarthropathy.
   E. Systemic lupus erythematosus (SLE).

4. A 67-year-old hypertensive man presents to the emergency department complaining of acute headache on the left and is found to have ipsilateral Horner's syndrome. His ECG shows a sinus tachycardia, but no signs of ST elevation. What is the likely diagnosis?
   A. Skull base tumour.
   B. Lateral medullary syndrome.
   C. Apical lung neoplasm.
   D. Demyelination.
   E. Left internal carotid artery dissection.

5. A 28-year-old man presents with atypical chest pain and an elevated serum troponin level. His CXR and ECG are normal, and coronary angiography does not show any obstructive disease. A cardiac MR was performed, which revealed subepicardial late enhancement and oedema in the lateral wall of the left ventricle. What is the most likely diagnosis?
   A. Tuberculous pericarditis.
   B. Non-ST elevation myocardial infarction.
   C. Acute myocarditis.
   D. Pericardial effusion.
   E. Coronary vasculitis.

6. A 44-year-old woman with known adult polycystic kidney disease presents with intermittent jaundice and right upper quadrant pain. Ultrasound and MRCP showed widespread saccular dilatation of the intrahepatic ducts. No dilatation or abnormalities of the extrahepatic ducts is seen and there are no gallstones.

   What is the most likely diagnosis?
   A. Polycystic liver disease.
   B. Primary sclerosing cholangitis.
   C. Caroli's disease.
   D. Primary biliary cirrhosis.
   E. Cholangiocarcinoma (Klatskin type).

7. A 66-year-old male, ex-smoker, presents with painful ankles and wrists and is noted to have digital clubbing. A CXR shows a smooth well-defined mass, which has an obtuse angle with the chest wall (suggesting it is pleurally based). CT shows a homogeneously enhancing pedunculated pleural mass with no cavitation, calcification or rib erosion. Wrist and ankle radiographs show symmetrical periosteal thickening along the distal radii and tibia.

   What is the most likely diagnosis?
   A. Malignant mesothelioma with hypertrophic osteoarthropathy.
   B. Pleural fibroma with hypertrophic osteoarthropathy.
   C. Bronchogenic carcinoma with hypertrophic osteoarthropathy.
   D. Empyema with hypertrophic osteoarthropathy.
   E. Pleural lipoma with hypertrophic osteoarthropathy.

8. A 24-year-old 30 weeks pregnant woman presents with breathlessness and pleuritic chest pain. What is the most accurate lowest radiation dose technique to diagnose pulmonary embolus?
   A. CTPA.
   B. Ventilation/perfusion scintigraphy.
   C. Perfusion scintigraphy.
   D. CXR.
   E. D-dimer assay.

9. A 34-year-old man with a history of renal cell cancer and cysts presents with back pain and altered sensation. An MR spine shows an intramedullary lesion at the level of T8. The lesion consists of a cystic component with a 1-cm enhancing mural nodule with feeding and draining vessels. What is the most likely diagnosis?
   A. Angioma associated with Sturge–Weber syndrome.
   B. Spinal ependymomas associated with neurofibromatosis type 2.
   C. Meningioma associated with neurofibromatosis type 2.
   D. Haemangioblastoma associated with Von Hippel–Lindau disease.
   E. Ependymal nodule of tuberous sclerosis.

10. CT abdomen and pelvis reveals dilated small bowel loops down to a mass related to the terminal ileum. The mass enhances, and has distortion and scarring of the surrounding fat with adjacent angulated thickened small bowel loops. What is the most likely diagnosis?
   A. Meckel's diverticulum.
   B. Lymphoma.
   C. Crohn's disease.
   D. Carcinoid tumour.
   E. Internal hernia.

11. A 16-year-old child with SCD presents with worsening pain in the thigh for the last 10 days. There is localised bone pain and soft tissue swelling. A plain X-ray of the leg shows cortical destruction and a periosteal reaction in the distal femur. What is the most likely complication?
   A. Avascular necrosis.
   B. Osteomyelitis.
   C. Non-accidental injury.
   D. Marrow hyperplasia.
   E. Secondary osteoarthritis.

12. An elderly man presents with signs of right heart failure. His ECG shows complete heart block, with low-amplitude QRS complexes. His CXR shows cardiac enlargement with prominent vascular markings. A cardiac MRI showed left ventricular hypertrophy with severe biventricular impairment and massive biatrial dilatation. Following contrast administration, the left ventricle demonstrated global diffuse enhancement. What is the likely diagnosis?
   A. Fabry's disease.
   B. Sarcoidosis.
   C. Hypertrophic cardiomyopathy.
   D. Cardiac amyloidosis.
   E. Thalassaemia.

Answers

1. C. Kartagener's syndrome. Kartagener's syndrome is a familial condition characterised by immotile cilia (due to generalised deficiency of dynein arms of cilia), situs inversus/dextrocardia, bronchiectasis, sinusitis, deafness, infertility due to immotile sperm and fallopian tube dysmotility. The combination of generalised bronchiectasis and situs inversus makes this the most likely diagnosis. Aetiology of bronchiectasis (➲ see Chapter 11, Aetiology, p. 356).

2. C. Alpha 1 antitrypsin deficiency often presents in the 4th decade of life. The most common type of severe deficiency occurs in individuals who are homozygous for the Z-type protein (*PIZZ*). The emphysema has a lower lobe predominance and bullae are present in a third of cases. Bronchial wall thickening and dilatation may sometimes also be present. (➲ See Chapter 11, Bronchiectasis, p. 356.)
3. C. Patients with ankylosing spondylitis may develop upper lobe fibrosis with cavitation (1%) which can become colonised with aspergillus forming an aspergilloma. While 70–80% of patients have axial skeletal involvement initially, 10–20% may have appendicular involvement at presentation, eventually rising to 50%. (➲ See Case 4, p. 122.)
4. E. Patients presenting with an acutely painful Horner's syndrome (➲ see Chapter 18, Pupils, p. 650 and Horner's syndrome: interruption of the sympathetic pathway, p. 651; also Table 18.2 and Figure 18.4) should be considered to have an internal carotid artery dissection unless there is evidence to the contrary. Carotid artery dissection causes a post ganglionic interruption of the sympathetic pathway and may be assessed with MRI of the head with contrast, and MR or CT angiography of the head and neck.
5. C. Acute myocarditis often presents as chest pain, which is atypical for ischaemic heart disease. The subepicardial inflammation seen within the inferior or lateral wall of the left ventricle on MR imaging is a typical finding of myocarditis which may also involve the mid-wall. Dilated non-ischaemic cardiomyopathies can also have a similar myocardial scar distribution on late gadolinium enhancement, but typically do not show oedema (on T2 imaging). Conversely, an ischaemic scar (on late enhancement) starts in the subendocardial layer, with increasing degrees of transmurality depending on the total coronary occlusion time. This degree of transmurality, alongside the extent of myocardium involved, predicts myocardial viability and the likely response to revascularisation. Other typical late enhancement patterns include HCM (focal myocardial scar at superior and inferior right ventricle [RV] insertion points onto the left ventricle [LV], seen best on short axis images) and sarcoid (multiple discrete patches of subepicardial or transmural myocardial scar). (➲ See Case 7, p. 127.)
6. C. (➲ See Case 10, p. 131.) Cholangiocarcinoma (Klatskin type) causes dilatation of the intrahepatic tree, which occurs distal to the hilar tumour. Polycystic liver disease in autosomal dominant polycystic kidney disease (ADPKD) has multiple cysts, which do not connect with the biliary tree. In primary biliary cirrhosis there is no intrahepatic biliary dilatation.

   Caroli's disease:
   - A rare autosomal recessive disorder consisting of multifocal saccular dilatation of segmental intrahepatic bile ducts. It is also classified as a type V choledochal cyst.
   - Belongs to the spectrum of fibropolycystic liver disease and is associated with fibrocystic anomalies of the kidneys, sharing the same gene defect. It is associated with periportal fibrosis (in children) as well as a medullary sponge kidney, ADPKD and autosomal recessive polycystic kidney disease (ARPKD).
   - Caroli's disease may be diffuse, lobar or segmental. Dilatation is usually saccular, rather than fusiform, which helps to differentiate it from the fusiform dilatation and multifocal strictures of primary sclerosing cholangitis.
   - Complications include intrahepatic stone formation, recurrent cholangitis, hepatic abscesses and cirrhosis, and portal hypertension. There is an increased risk of cholangiocarcinoma. Prognosis is generally poor. If the disease is localised, segmentectomy or lobectomy is an option, and liver transplantation is indicated in diffuse disease.
7. B. (➲ See Case 11, p. 132.)
   - Pleural fibromas are usually a benign pleural tumour (20% malignant), which is typically large, pedunculated and peripheral. It is not associated with asbestos exposure.
   - Bronchogenic carcinoma is the commonest cause of HOA but the CT features in this case are consistent with a benign pleural tumour.
   - Malignant mesothelioma is associated with HOA, but is typically seen as an irregular pleural mass/thickening encasing the hemithorax with rib destruction.

- An empyema is seen as a loculated pleural effusion with enhancing thickened pleura.
- A pleural lipoma is seen as fat density on CT and is not associated with HOA.

8. C. (➲ See Table 5.1.)
   - A normal perfusion scintigram excludes significant pulmonary emboli in pregnancy.
   - A CTPA has a higher sensitivity and specificity than a perfusion scintigram, however it carries a significantly higher radiation dose than a perfusion scintigram (6–7 mSv). Although the fetal dose from a CTPA is lower than a perfusion scintigram, the dose to the breasts is very high.
   - A ventilation/perfusion scan is more sensitive than a perfusion scintigram alone but has a higher radiation burden (1.4 mSv).
   - A CXR is non-specific. Major pulmonary embolism can be present with a normal CXR.
   - D-dimer assay is non-specific as this is elevated in pregnancy and in inflammatory and infectious conditions.
   - The investigation of choice should involve discussion between the Radiologists and Obstetric Medicine teams, weighing up the radiation risk to both mother and fetus, against the potentially life-threatening risk of incorrect diagnosis of an underlying PE. Radiation risk to the fetus in the third trimester is significantly reduced compared with the first trimester.
9. D. (➲ See Chapter 17, Neurocutaneous syndromes, p. 637; and Case 13, p. 136 and Case 14, p. 137.) Haemangioblastomas have characteristic features with an enhancing mural nodule within a cyst with feeding vessels. 90% occur in the posterior cranial fossa with 5–10% in the spinal cord. Large tumours may haemorrhage. Management is resection, embolisation or palliative radiotherapy. They do not calcify unlike the subependymal nodules of tuberous sclerosis, which are found in the brain. Meningiomas are seen as focal, enhancing, durally based lesions. Sturge–Weber syndrome is characterised by a cerebral pial-based venous angioma, which calcifies. They also occur in the spine. Spinal ependymomas do not have large feeding and draining vessels.
10. D. (➲ See Case 9, p. 130 and Case 15, p. 138.)
    - Carcinoid tumour is a rare cause of small bowel obstruction.
    - The commonest cause of small bowel obstruction are adhesions and hernias in adults.
    - Lymphoma (usually non-Hodgkins lymphoma) is seen as a focal small bowel mass with adjacent lymphadenopathy and possibly splenomegaly.
    - Crohn's is an uncommon cause of small bowel obstruction due to an inflammatory/fibrous stricture or complicating cancer.
    - Meckel's diverticulum is seen as a diverticulum arising from the distal small bowel and may present with obstruction due to intussusception, abdominal pain, bleeding or perforation.
11. B. (➲ See Case 16, p. 140, and Chapter 8, Osteomyelitis, p. 258 and Tables 8.23 and 8.24.) Sickling crises are far more common than osteomyelitis in patients, but osteomyelitis is important to recognise and treat appropriately. Initially plain radiographs will be normal, but after 10–14 days, bone destruction and a periosteal reaction may be evident. MRI may be more sensitive and specific at diagnosing osteomyelitis and differentiating it from infarction. The pathogen is frequently bacterial in SCD, most commonly *Staphylococcus aureus*, salmonella and enterobacter.
12. D. Cardiac amyloidosis is usually part of a primary systemic amyloidosis (AL) (➲ see Chapter 9, Amyloidosis, p. 304) and is caused by extracellular deposition of insoluble fibrils. It leads to arrhythmias and congestive heart failure. On MRI, the left ventricle is hypertrophied and shows both systolic and diastolic impairment. A diagnosis can usually be made using T1-mapping or by the distinctive diffuse pattern of myocardial enhancement.

Chapter 6 **Immunology**

Patrick Yong

Basic science of the immune system

Innate and adaptive immune systems, molecules (mediators and receptors) and cells

The immune system has primarily evolved to provide defence against infectious organisms; to do this it must possess the ability to discriminate between self and non-self. Untreated individuals with significantly defective immune systems will be overwhelmed by and succumb to infection early in life. Conversely, the immune system can fail to distinguish appropriately between self and non-self, and generate an inappropriate response to host cells or innocuous foreign material. This forms the basis of either autoimmune diseases, including Type I diabetes, Grave's disease and systemic lupus erythematosus (SLE), or allergy.

Physical barriers

Physical barriers act as a non-specific first line of defence against invading pathogens. In order for an invading pathogen to gain access to the host, it must first cross epithelial layers, e.g. dead cells like the skin or living cells, which line the respiratory and gastrointestinal tracts. These surfaces also have additional defences including:

- Mucus secreted by mucosal epithelial cells.
- Mucociliary clearance, where the cilia in respiratory epithelial cells beat upwards to remove microbes.
- Various antimicrobial substances secreted at epithelial surfaces that directly kill pathogens including:
  - lysozyme which digests bacterial walls;
  - IgA antibodies in tears and saliva, which prevent microbial attachment;
  - small peptides, e.g. defensins;
  - digestive enzymes in the stomach.
- Non-pathogenic commensal bacteria preventing pathogenic bacteria from colonising the same site.

Innate and adaptive immune system

Broadly, the immune system can be divided into the innate and the adaptive immune systems, although these do not function as discrete entities and have significant interactions. The main features and differences between the two are summarised in Table 6.1.

Both the innate and adaptive immune system are made up of cellular and humoral mediators.

Cells of the innate immune system

The cells of the innate immune system comprise phagocytes, natural killer (NK) cells, eosinophils, mast cells and basophils.

- Phagocytes are specialised 'eating cells' (from the Greek word 'to eat', phagein), and are made up of neutrophils and monocytes, which migrate to tissue and transform into macrophages.

Table 6.1 Characteristics of the innate and adaptive immune systems

	Innate immune system	Adaptive immune system
Speed of response	Rapid: responses occurring immediately, but lasting several days (giving sufficient time for the adaptive immune response to develop).	Slower: requiring days to mount an initial response, but with more rapid response on second and subsequent encounters of the same pathogen.
Specificity	Limited specificity.	Highly specific.
Memory	No memory (subsequent responses to same pathogen of similar magnitude).	Highly specific memory for individual pathogens.
Humoral components	Complement proteins. Acute phase proteins. Cytokines.	Antibodies (immunoglobulin molecules). Cytokines.
Cellular components	Myeloid cells (e.g. neutrophils, macrophages, monocytes, basophils, eosinophils). Natural Killer (NK) cells. Mast cells.	Lymphocytes (T cells, B cells).
Molecules recognised	Recognition of patterns generally conserved and shared by different pathogens (pathogen associated molecular patterns [PAMPs]); these patterns are often repeating structures like glycoproteins.	Recognition of a variety of molecular patterns specific to individual pathogens.
Nature of recognition	Limited number of recognition receptors encoded in germline DNA.	Almost unlimited number of recognition receptors possible by molecular processes that alter germline encoded DNA by variable, diverse and joining somatic recombination and somatic hypermutation).

- Eosinophils are responsible for immune defence against parasites and function by releasing multiple toxic compounds after binding to their target.
- Basophils (in the circulation) and mast cells (present in connective tissue) are similar in morphology and contain granules with similar chemicals. They play a role in allergic reactions, although their exact physiological role is less clear.
- NK cells are lymphocytic cells, but are larger and contain more granules. Their main role is in killing virally infected cells and certain tumours.
- Erythrocytes and platelets also play a role in innate immunity. Activated platelets release factors that initiate the complement cascade, and erythrocytes are able to bind immune complexes and clear them from the circulation.

Immune receptors expressed by innate immune cells

Innate immune cells recognise pathogens by means of a variety of invariant receptors. These receptors recognise pathogen associated molecular patterns (PAMPs) expressed in pathogens but not the host. Some examples of these receptors include:

- Mannose receptors.
- The family of toll-like receptors (TLRs).

- CD14 (expressed on monocytes, which recognises lipopolysaccharide (LPS) in conjunction with TLR4).
- Fc receptors (which bind immunoglobulin molecules, produced by the adaptive immune system).
- Complement binding receptors.
- Killer immunoglobulin receptors (KIRs) expressed by NK cells, which recognise major histocompatibility complex (MHC) molecules and can have inhibitory or activating functions.

Humoral mediators of the innate immune system

The main humoral mediators of the innate immune system are the complement molecules, acute phase proteins and cytokines.

The complement system is a family of plasma proteins made by hepatocytes. It has several pathways of activation (the classical, alternative and mannose binding pathways) and a final common pathway (➲ see Complement, p. 150 and Figure 6.1).

Acute phase proteins produced in response to inflammation (e.g. C-reactive protein [CRP], serum amyloid A, mannose binding protein, fibrinogen) also play roles in innate defence, as well as tissue repair. They can:

- Bind to microbes.
- Activate the complement system.
- Bind metal ions necessary for microbial growth.
- Enhance the process of opsonisation (that targets microbes for destruction by phagocytosis).

The innate immune system secretes a variety of cytokines in response to infection. Cytokines are small molecules that mediate cell signalling. Chemokines are a group of cytokines, which have chemoattractant properties and are responsible for directing immune cells. Interleukins (IL) refer to a group of cytokines that were first discovered to be expressed in leukocytes (hence inter- to signify communication between, and -leukin referring to white cells). Some of the more important cytokines are IL-1, IL-6 and tumour necrosis factor (TNF)-α secreted by monocytes, which activate inflammatory processes, and the interferons (IFN) which are particularly important in viral defence.

Dendritic cells

Dendritic cells provide an interface between the innate and adaptive immune systems. They function as 'professional' antigen-presenting cells (APC) as they initiate and determine the nature of primary immune responses. They possess multiple innate immune receptors that recognise microbial particles. Dendritic cells process microbes and, along with the appropriate co-receptor and cytokine signals, are able to 'present' them to T cells to generate the adaptive immune response required.

Cells and receptors of the adaptive immune system

The cells of the adaptive immune system are lymphocytes, which are made up of T and B cells. These cells are indistinguishable morphologically, but are very different functionally. T cells can be sub-divided as helper T (CD4+) cells, cytotoxic T (CD8+) cells or regulatory T cells. T cells distinguish different antigen specificities by having a unique T cell receptor (TCR) that is generated through a process of recombining different DNA segments. The receptor recognises short peptides presented on MHC molecules in conjunction with the CD4 or CD8 molecules.

The MHC (known as HLA, human leukocyte antigens in humans) is a group of highly polymorphic molecules that allow interaction with cells of the immune system. They are divided into several classes. Class I MHC are expressed on all nucleated cells and serve to present mainly self-peptides to CD8+ T cells (known as the endogenous pathway of antigen presentation). Class II MHC are expressed on antigen presenting cells (i.e. dendritic cells, macrophages, B cells) and serve to present peptides (mostly from ingested microbes) to CD4+ T cells (known as the exogenous pathway of antigen presentation).

CD4 is required for TCR recognition of peptides presented on MHC II, and CD8 is required for recognition of peptides presented on MHC I (a process known as MHC restriction).

Principal roles of T and B cells

- *Helper T cells* provide 'help' for other immune cells to perform their function:
  - enable B cells to produce antibody;
  - activate and enable the killing function of cytotoxic T cells;
  - enable macrophages to kill ingested microbes.
- *Cytotoxic T cells* are responsible for killing off virally infected or cancer cells and achieve this mainly by release of toxic granules on recognition of target antigens.
- *Regulatory T cells* serve to modulate immune responses, promote tolerance to self-molecules and prevent autoimmune disease.
- The main role of *B cells* is the production of antibodies, which they do after differentiation into plasma cells.

Humoral mediators of the adaptive immune system

Antibodies, also known as immunoglobulins, bind to antigens, and are the main humoral mediator in the adaptive immune system.

- Antibodies are proteins that have a highly variable binding region generated by a process known as somatic hypermutation. This process is similar to the generation of the TCR, but with the potential for further mutation.
- Antibodies recognise targets known as antigens, derived from '*ant*ibody *gen*erator'
  - Antigens may have several *epitopes* (or antigenic determinants), and each epitope can bind an individual antibody; hence, each antigen can potentially bind many different antibodies.
  - *Haptens* are low molecular weight molecules that can only generate an antibody response when bound to a larger carrier molecule.
- Antibodies exist in soluble form, as well as on the surface of B cells.
- Antibodies serve a variety of protective functions:
  - Neutralisation of pathogens and toxins by binding to them.
  - Activation of the classical complement system.
  - Enable activation of effector cells that have receptors for antibodies.
- Antibodies are made up of five different isotypes, which have different functions:
  - IgG is the most common antibody in plasma and performs all of the functions necessary to protect against invading pathogens.
  - IgM is the first antibody produced in response to infection and may exist as a pentamer resulting in high avidity.
  - IgA is the antibody most commonly found in secretions and provides mucosal immunity.
  - IgE is associated with allergy and protection against parasites.
  - IgD is found on naïve B cells as an antigen receptor and is involved in B cell activation, although its exact function is not well understood.
- Antibody bound to antigen forms an *immune complex* (also known as an antigen–antibody complex)

Effector and regulatory processes, and functions

Complement

The complement cascade (Figure 6.1) is one of the more important effector mechanisms in the innate immune system and may be activated through several pathways:

- Classical pathway: triggered by antibody (of the IgM or IgG isotype) binding to antigen, activating the C1q component, which then activates C4, followed by C2, resulting in activation of the common component C3.
  - C1q is also activated by binding directly to some bacterial surface components, and by CRP bound to phosphocholine residues in bacterial polysaccharides.
- Alternative pathway: triggered by component C3 binding to bacterial surfaces.

- Lectin pathway: triggered by mannose binding lectin binding to microbes and activating C4, similar to C1q.

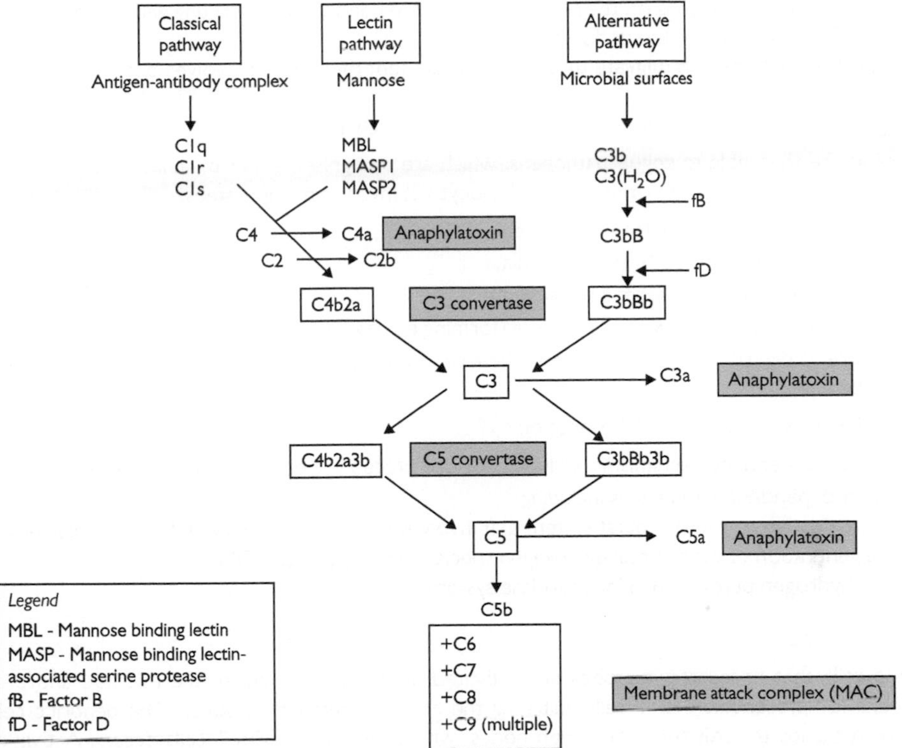

Figure 6.1 The complement cascade

Activation of complement components results in:

- Cleavage of a downstream component, leading to an activation cascade with a rapid amplification of the inflammatory response.
- Small molecules (resulting from the cleavage), which have chemoattractant properties and can act as opsonins (making pathogens easier to phagocytose) and anaphylatoxins, which can activate mast cells, directly resulting in local inflammation.
- C3 on the surface of microbes sequentially activating components C5–C9 to form a structure known as the membrane attack complex that punches holes in cell membranes resulting in microbe lysis.

There are also several regulatory mechanisms that prevent the destructive effect of the complement cascade on host cells:

- Several soluble proteins bind activated complement components, resulting in inactivation, e.g. C1 esterase inhibitor, C4 binding protein, Factor H and Factor I.
- Host cells express proteins on their surface that inactivate complement and prevent formation of the membrane attack complex, e.g. DAF and CD59.

Neutrophil response

Various chemoattractant molecules (e.g. CXCL8 previously known as IL-8, complement components C3a and C5a) result in migration of neutrophils or monocytes to the site of inflammation. This process known as chemotaxis consists of four steps:

1. Rolling adhesion: this occurs along vessel walls and is mediated by molecules called selectins on the vessel wall, which interact with glycoproteins on the neutrophil or monocyte.
2. Tight binding: the leukocyte becomes firmly attached to the endothelium and stops rolling, a process mediated by integrins on the leukocyte (e.g. LFA-1 and CR3) interacting with molecules such as ICAM-1 and ICAM-2 on the endothelium.
3. Diapedesis: where cells migrate through the basement membrane; involves both integrins and CD31.
4. Migration through tissues: occurring in the direction of chemokines.

Neutrophils are then able to engulf pathogens, which are recognised either by innate receptors or have been opsonised by complement or antibody. Phagocytosis involves multiple steps:

- Phagocyte migration towards the microbe.
- Engulfment of the microbe by pseudopodia.
- Fusion of pseudopodia to form a phagosome.
- Fusion of the phagosome with a lysosome (forming a phagolysosome).
- Exposure to digestive enzymes and toxic chemicals in the lysosome, that can kill and break down the microbe.

Killing mechanisms in the neutrophil consist of:

- Oxygen-independent mechanisms, including various proteolytic enzymes and anti-microbial peptides.
- Oxygen-dependent mechanisms including:
  - The oxidative respiratory burst system that involves the use of the enzyme NAPDH resulting in the generation of various reactive oxygen species (e.g. O_2^-, H_2O_2, $^{\cdot}OH$).
  - The hydrogen peroxide-myeloperoxidase system.

T cell response

Dendritic cells that encounter microbes are activated, and will phagocytose the microbe and process its antigens for presentation to T cells, initiating the adaptive immune response. The dendritic cell migrates from tissues towards the local lymph nodes, where interaction with T cells occurs. Activation of the dendritic cell results in a change in its morphology, surface molecules (with up-regulation of HLA and co-stimulatory molecules) and function (from sensing the local environment to antigen presentation). Dendritic cells activate T cells through three sets of signals:

- Signal 1: antigen presentation on the HLA molecule.
- Signal 2: co-stimulatory molecules (e.g. CD80 and CD86).
- Signal 3: secreted cytokines.

There is a subsequent clonal expansion of the activated T cell to deal with the specific microbe.

CD4+ helper T cells can be subdivided according to their profile of cytokine secretion. Initially, two main groups were identified: T helper 1 (Th1) and T helper 2 (Th2) subsets. A third subset of highly pro-inflammatory T helper cells, Th17 has also been described.

- *Th1 cells* develop after exposure to IL-12 and secrete the signature cytokine interferon (IFN)-γ. Th1 cells promote cell-mediated inflammatory responses, by activating monocytes/macrophages to kill intracellular bacteria and up-regulating their antigen presenting capabilities, promoting production of IgG1 and IgG3 antibodies and directing CD8+ cytotoxic T cells.
- *Th2 cells* develop after exposure to IL-4, and secrete IL-4, IL-5, IL-10 and IL-13. Th2 cells promote antibody responses. The cytokines produced by Th2 cells result in production of IgG2, IgA and IgE, recruitment of eosinophils for parasite killing, and are also important for B cell growth and differentiation.
- *Th17 cells* are characterised by secretion of IL-17. These cells are less well understood and probably develop under the influence of IL-1β and IL-6. They play a role in immune defence against fungi and staphylococci, as well as in the development of some autoimmune diseases, like rheumatoid arthritis.

Most immune responses involve a mixture of the T helper subsets, the predominance depending on the nature of the immune response required for pathogen clearance. Some T cells remain as memory T cells, which are long-lived and respond more quickly to subsequent infection with the same microbe. T helper cells also provide help for B cells by interaction of surface molecules, e.g. the interaction of CD40L (also known as CD154) on T cells with CD40 on B cells, which promotes antibody class switching to different isotypes.

CD8+ cytotoxic T cells are primarily responsible for killing of cells infected with viruses and certain tumour cells. Killing is initiated after recognition of a target cell through interaction of the T cell receptor with class I MHC on the target and is mediated via 3 main mechanisms:

1. *Cytotoxic granule* release on to the target cell surface including:
   - perforin – forms pores in the cell membrane, similar to the membrane attack complex in the complement cascade;
   - granzymes – activate a protein called caspase-3 that initiates cell apoptosis.
2. *Toxic cytokines*, e.g. INF-γ and TNF-α.
3. Interaction between *death-inducing surface molecules* on the cytotoxic cell and receptors on the target cell induced by viral infection. One of the most well-known molecules is Fas ligand (FasL) that interacts with Fas on the target cell, activating caspase, that results in apoptosis.

NK cells kill in a similar way to cytotoxic T cells, although their recognition mechanisms are different.

B cell response

B cells are primarily responsible for antibody production and humoral immunity. They are also able to present antigen to T helper cells, although not as potently as dendritic cells. Clonal expansion of the activated B cell results in amplification of response to the microbe. Naïve B cells initially express IgM and IgD, and are activated in the lymph nodes. With help from T cells, they can then switch to expressing the other immunoglobulin isotypes, IgG, IgA and IgE. After antigenic exposure, somatic hypermutation, which further mutates the binding regions of the immunoglobulin molecule, enables the development of antibodies of very high affinity and specificity to the target antigen. Activated B cells differentiate into plasma cells and memory B cells. Plasma cells are end-stage differentiated B cells; they do not express surface immunoglobulin and produce large amounts of soluble immunoglobulin. Plasma cells are long-lived and reside in the bone marrow, spleen and lamina propria of the gut. Memory B cells are capable of responding more quickly to subsequent infection. Typically, a primary immune response results in the production of IgM after 5–10 days, followed by IgG after a further 2–3 days; a secondary response occurs within 3–5 days and results in larger amounts of production of IgG.

Regulatory processes

In addition to activation of the immune response, regulation is as important to prevent excessive damage to the host once the microbe has been contained. Multiple regulatory mechanisms exist:

- In the innate immune system:
  - Multiple soluble and cell membrane proteins limit complement activation on host tissues.
  - Cells recognise molecular patterns present on microbes that are not present on host cells.
- In the adaptive immune system:
  - T cells and B cells undergo a process of deletion during their development that removes autoreactive cells from the circulating pool.
  - There are subsets of different types of regulatory CD4+ T cells (Treg) that regulate the immune system. One of the better described subsets is characterised by expression of CD4 and CD25 and a transcription factor called Foxp3. Regulatory T cells are thought to mediate their actions through direct cell-to-cell contact, expression of receptors that bind co-stimulatory molecules (e.g. CTLA-4 which binds to CD80 and CD86, displacing CD28, which activates T cells), and secretion of cytokines like IL-10 and TGF-β. Tregs activated by recognition of their cognate antigen can also regulate nearby cells (a process known as bystander suppression).

Key developmental aspects

Most cells of the immune system originate from common pluripotent haematopoietic stem cells (HSCs) that are replicating, self-renewing cells found in bone marrow and in the fetal liver. HSCs differentiate into the common myeloid precursor and the common lymphoid precursor. The common myeloid precursor gives rise to neutrophils, basophils, eosinophils, monocytes and dendritic cells; the common lymphoid precursor gives rise to T cells, B cells and NK cells.

- *Granulocytes*: most granulocytes (neutrophils, basophils and eosinophils) circulate in blood and can migrate into tissues in response to inflammation. The exception to this is mast cells that are resident in tissues.
- *Monocytes* spend about 24 hours in the circulation and then migrate into tissue and transform into *macrophages*. Different tissues have different forms of macrophages, e.g. alveolar macrophages in the lung, Kupffer cells in the liver, osteoclasts in bone and microglial cells in the brain.
- *T lymphocytes* undergo maturation in the thymus (hence 'T' cells). Within the thymus, critical development of a functional repertoire of T cells and elimination of self-reactive clones takes place. Naïve T cells that have not yet encountered antigen emerge at the end of this process. The thymus is proportionately at its largest at birth and declines in size with age.
- *B lymphocytes* undergo a similar maturation process in the bone marrow. An organ called the bursa of Fabricius in birds was shown to be crucial for their development (hence 'B' cells).

The type or lineage of cell into which HSC differentiates is determined by the microenvironment.

- *Stromal cells* (e.g. epithelial cells, endothelial cells, fibroblasts) influence HSC differentiation by creating distinct foci and structures, as well as engaging receptors on the HSC via cell to cell contact (e.g. through adhesion molecules and other receptors).
- *Cytokines* are important for HSC differentiation and homing of immune cells to the appropriate tissues:
  - HSC regeneration is dependent on stem cell factor (SCF), IL-1 and IL-3.
  - Development of granulocytes and monocytes is dependent on colony stimulating factors (GCSF and MCSF, respectively, and GMCSF for both).
  - Differentiation of T and B cells is dependent on a variety of other cytokines, as described elsewhere in this chapter.

Clinical immunology

Infectious disease immunology

Viral infection

There are multiple components in the initial response to a primary viral infection:

- Viral replication results in cell death, which leads to the release of:
  - Viral components (e.g. single-stranded RNA) that are recognised by innate immune receptors and can activate dendritic cells and other antigen-presenting cells.
  - Cytokines and chemokines that attract other immune cells.
- Type I INFs (α and β), which inhibit viral replication and increase MHC I presentation of viral peptides.
- Early killing of virally infected cells is mediated by NK cells. At a later stage, the NK cells can also be activated by Th1 cells.

Subsequently, the adaptive immune response comes into play:

- Activated dendritic cells initiate the adaptive immune response by presentation of viral particles to helper T cells in the germinal centres of lymph nodes.
- Activated T helper cells then help B cells generate antibody specific to the virus and activate cytotoxic T cells to kill virally infected T cells.
- Cytotoxic T cells recognise the virally infected cells by viral peptides presented on MHC I molecules.
- Antibodies produced can bind to:
  - Circulating virus preventing attachment and entry of virus into host cells.
  - Viral particles expressed on cell surfaces allowing clearance by Fc receptor expressing cells.

- For viruses inside cells that cannot be reached by antibodies, cytotoxic T cells (and NK cells) are required for eradication.
- Long-lasting memory T and B cells, and circulating antibody provide future immunity against the same virus.

Bacterial infection

The mechanisms for bacterial immunity vary depending on whether the bacterium is extracellular or intracellular.

Extracellular bacteria

- Activation of the complement pathway results in:
  - Lysis of bacteria.
  - Migration of phagocytes to the site of infection (induced by the chemotactic effect of complement components and bacterial products).
  - Neutrophil migration to the site of infection.
  - Dendritic cells that phagocytose bacteria migrate to lymph nodes where they can encounter T cells and initiate the adaptive immune process.
- Local mast cell degranulation results in further cytokine and chemokine release, which increases vascular permeability and blood flow.
- The antibodies produced against bacteria can also act as opsonins for Fc-bearing cells (which include neutrophils, dendritic cells and macrophages), activate complement and interfere with bacterial function. Early antibodies tend to be of the IgM isotype, which has high avidity. These switch to the IgG and IgA isotypes later in infection.

Intracellular bacteria

Some bacteria (e.g. *Listeria monocytogenes, Salmonella typhi* and *Mycobacterium tuberculosis* [TB]) invade and replicate inside host cells and thus avoid extracellular defence mechanisms (like complement and antibodies). To counter this, the immune system mounts a cell-mediated immune response.

Fungal, protozoal and worm infections

Fungal immunity is problematic in immunocompromised individuals. Neutrophils and cellular immunity are likely to play the most important roles as patients with these deficiencies are more likely to suffer invasive fungal infection. IL-17 (produced by Th17 cells) is involved in neutrophil function and plays an important role in fungal immunity.

Immunity to protozoa and worms is more difficult to achieve. These organisms are complex and often possess multiple stages in their life cycles. Both humoral and cellular immunity are likely to be required for protozoal immunity; eosinophils and mast cells are likely to be the most important components in anti-helminthic immunity.

Opportunistic infections

Opportunistic infections are infections by organisms that typically affect individuals with a compromised immune system. Organisms associated with opportunistic infection include pneumocystis jirovecii, toxoplasma, human herpes virus (HHV)-8 resulting in Kaposi's sarcoma and cytomegalovirus (CMV).

Pathogen strategies to evade the immune system

Most virulent pathogens have developed means to overcome immune defence mechanisms usually by avoiding recognition by the immune system or by inactivating immune effector mechanisms.
Pathogens can avoid recognition by several means:

- Intracellular pathogens avoid direct recognition by the innate and adaptive immune systems (e.g. obligate intracellular organisms like viruses, mycobacteria, plasmodium).

- Microbes can change the expression of cell surface antigens by mutation in several ways:
  - Antigenic *drift* refers to the accumulation of mutations affecting antigenic sites, preventing recognition by previously acquired immunity.
  - Antigenic *shift* refers to the process when two or more viral strains combine to form a virus with a new phenotype, with a mixture of antigens from the two strains, e.g. influenza virus.
  - Some pathogens are able to change their antigenic structure continuously to avoid detection, e.g. trypanosomes.
- Mimicking host structures ('molecular mimicry').

Pathogens are able to inactivate almost every component of the host immune system including:

- Prevention of phagocytosis by encapsulated bacteria.
- Inhibition of the respiratory burst required for killing by bacterial enzymes.
- Inhibition of cytokine production, e.g. INF-α by virally infected cells.
- Destruction of antibodies by proteases.
- Neutralisation of antibodies by release of large amounts of soluble antigen.
- Production of proteins that bind the antibody Fc region.
- Inhibition of the terminal complement pathway by inclusion of complement regulatory proteins into the cell membrane by some viruses.
- Killing of cells involved in the immune response, e.g. HIV killing CD4+ T cells.
- Inhibition of antigen processing and presentation.
- Skewing of immune responses towards a non-protective immune response, e.g. endotoxins produced by salmonella promote a Th2 response predisposing to a humoral response, rather than the cellular immunity required.

Immunodeficiency states

Primary immunodeficiency

Pathogenesis and epidemiology

Primary immunodeficiency (PID) diseases arise from a genetic origin, with estimates of prevalence ranging between 1 in 1000 to 1 in 10,000 people. Defects in >300 single genes have been identified, although the exact gene responsible for a large number of PIDs remain unidentified. It is likely that some PIDs are polygenic disorders, with susceptibility genes and some form of environmental trigger.

Presentation and classification

PIDs can first present at any age and the nature of the presentation depends on the component of the immune system affected (Table 6.2).

There is an average diagnostic delay of 5–7 years from onset of symptoms to identification of PID, which can result in significant morbidity and mortality. The possibility of PID should be considered if there is a family history of PID or if the patient has:

S severe infections.

P persistent infections.

U unusual infections.

R recurrent infections.

A set of 10 warning signs was also developed by the Jeffrey Modell Foundation to help with earlier identification of PID (Box 6.1).

Investigations and diagnosis

Investigations for diagnosis of a PID start from relatively simple tests (e.g. measurement of FBC, immunoglobulin levels and lymphocyte subsets) to more complicated ones (e.g. assessment of lymphocyte proliferation, phagocyte function, and family or genetic studies). The tests required should be guided by the history, which should indicate the likely defect in the immune system.

Table 6.2 Types of primary immunodeficiency

Cells/immune components affected	Key features	Infection susceptibility/clinical phenotype	Management
Combined T and B cell deficiency	*Severe combined immunodeficiency (SCID)*: - Most severe form of combined T and B cell deficiency, severe infections, failure to thrive, paediatric emergency, fatal if not treated. - Should be suspected in any baby <6 months old with a low lymphocyte count. *Wiskott–Aldrich syndrome*: - Mutations in WASp. - Thrombocytopenia, small platelets, eczema, recurrent bacterial infections. *Ataxia telangiectasia*: - Cerebellar ataxia, progressive neurological deterioration, radiosensitivity, telangiectasia. *DiGeorge syndrome*: - 22q11 deletion syndrome. - Variable immunodeficiency due to thymic absence/ reduction, hypoparathyroidism, convulsions, tetany, cardiovascular abnormalities, dysmorphic facies.	Opportunistic infections, bacterial and fungal infections.	HSC transplantation (HSCT). Immunoglobulin replacement. Antibiotics. Cytokines and gene therapy as appropriate.
T cell deficiency	Some previous classifications had T cell deficiencies as a separate category (e.g. including DiGeorge syndrome). Defects affecting T cells also affect B cells as T cell help is required for B cells to be fully functional. The most up to date international classification scheme classifies these under combined immunodeficiencies.	As above.	As above.
B cell deficiency	Most common form of PID. Failure of immunoglobulin production. Examples include: X-linked agammaglobulinaemia (Bruton's agammaglobulinaemia), common variable immunodeficiency (CVID).	Encapsulated bacteria, recurrent sinopulmonary infection.	IV immunoglobulin. Antibiotics.
Complement deficiency	Deficiency of early components (C1, C2, C4).	Immune complex disease or SLE-like syndrome.	Treatment of autoimmune disease with standard therapies.
	Deficiency of common component (C3).	Serious infections with pyogenic bacteria.	Antibiotics.

continued

Table 6.2 *continued*

Cells/immune components affected	Key features	Infection susceptibility/clinical phenotype	Management
	Deficiency of membrane attack complex (C5–C9).	Susceptibility to neisserial infections and recurrent meningitis.	Prophylactic antibiotics. Vaccination.
	C1 esterase inhibitor deficiency results in *hereditary angioedema* and patients present with recurrent angioedema (without urticaria). Acquired C1 inhibitor deficiency is associated with lymphoid malignancy. Complement C4 is used as a screening test – if levels are low, then C1 inhibitor levels are tested.	No increased risk of infections.	Anabolic steroids (e.g. danazol or stanozolol). Tranexamic acid. C1 inhibitor replacement (FFP as alternative). Icatibant (selective and specific antagonist of bradykinin receptors; ➲ see Chapter 3, Table 3.4).
Phagocyte deficiency	Reduction in numbers. Examples include: Severe congenital neutropenia. Cyclic neutropenia. Deficiency in function. Examples include: Defective respiratory burst in chronic granulomatous disease (CGD) and deficiency in the IL-12/IFN-γ pathway. Deficiency in adhesion molecules (e.g. CD18) resulting in leukocyte adhesion defects. Abnormal granulocyte chemotaxis and phagolysosome formation in Chediak–Higashi syndrome.	Variable depending on severity of phagocyte defect. Neutropenia associated with fungal and bacterial infections. Milder neutropenic disorders may predispose to viral infections only. Additional features dependent on syndrome associated with phagocyte deficiency, e.g. deficiency in the IL-12/IFN-γ pathway results in susceptibility to atypical mycobacteria.	Dependent on underlying disorder, but includes: Antibiotics. Cytokine supplementation (particularly GCSF for neutropenias). HSCT.

Prognosis

Prognosis in PID is variable, depending both on the nature of the PID and the delay in diagnosis. Good therapies are available for some of the PIDs and if detected early, can result in very good outcomes.

Secondary immunodeficiency

For causes of secondary immunodeficiency, see Table 6.3.

Secondary immunodeficiency states are far more common than PIDs. A large proportion of secondary immunodeficiencies are iatrogenic in nature, mostly as a side effect of immunosuppressive treatment or cytotoxic agents given for chemotherapy. Patients on these treatments need careful monitoring, particularly those receiving highly specific monoclonal antibodies that target the immune system (e.g. TNF inhibitors predispose to TB infection).

Box 6.1 Ten warning signs of a primary immunodeficiency

For children

1. Four or more new ear infections within 1 year.
2. Two or more serious sinus infections within 1 year.
3. Two or more months on antibiotics with little effect.
4. Two or more pneumonias within 1 year.
5. Failure of an infant to gain weight or grow normally.
6. Recurrent, deep skin or organ abscesses.
7. Persistent thrush in mouth or fungal infection on skin.
8. Need for intravenous antibiotics to clear infections.
9. Two or more deep-seated infections including septicaemia.
10. A family history of primary immunodeficiency.

For adults

1. Two or more new ear infections within 1 year.
2. Two or more new sinus infections within 1 year, in the absence of allergy.
3. One pneumonia per year, for more than 1 year.
4. Chronic diarrhoea with weight loss.
5. Recurrent viral infections.
6. Recurrent need for IV antibiotics to clear infections.
7. Recurrent, deep abscesses of the skin or internal organs.
8. Persistent thrush or fungal infection on skin or elsewhere.
9. Infection with normally harmless tuberculosis-like bacteria.
10. A family history of primary immunodeficiency.

These warning signs were developed by the Jeffrey Modell Foundation Medical Advisory Board. Consultation with Primary Immunodeficiency experts is strongly suggested.

Table 6.3 Causes of secondary immunodeficiency

Malignancy	Tumours can directly invade tissues responsible for producing immune cells and can also express and secrete immunosuppressive molecules e.g. IL-10, transforming growth factor beta (TGF-β).
Drugs	Cytotoxic drugs used for chemotherapy. Immunosuppressive agents. Carbimazole – causes agranulocytosis. Carbamazepine – can cause hypogammaglobulinaemia.
Immunosuppression by microbial pathogens	HIV. Malaria. TB. Measles.
Malnutrition	Most common cause of secondary immunodeficiency worldwide.
Trauma or major surgery	Increased susceptibility to infection probably secondary to release of immunosuppressive stress hormones like glucocorticoids.
Protein loss	Loss of immunoglobulins, e.g. in nephrotic syndrome.
Extremes of age	The immune system is relatively immature in infants and declines variably with senescence.
Other diseases	Metabolic diseases like diabetes and renal failure are associated with increased susceptibility to infection.

In general, treatment of secondary immunodeficiency involves:

- Treatment or removal of the underlying cause.
- The use of treatments used in PID (e.g. antibiotics and immunoglobulin) if the secondary immunodeficiency state is likely to persist and there are significant infective complications.

Hypersensitivity disorders

The immune system is meant to respond to microbial pathogens. Immune responses can be over-exaggerated for the stimulus, for example, in response to microbes, or inappropriate against innocuous substances or host tissues. Hypersensitivity reactions refer to these excessive reactions, which can cause damage to the host. There are five main types of hypersensitivity reactions (Table 6.4).

Table 6.4 Gell and Coombs classification of hypersensitivity reactions

Reaction type	Immune mechanism
I	IgE mediated; immediate
II	Antibody-mediated cytotoxicity
III	Antibody-antigen complexes
IV	T cell-mediated; delayed
V	Stimulatory; antibody-mediated*

* Gell and Coombs originally classified Types I-IV; Type V subsequently described.
Adapted with permission of Wiley, from *Clinical Aspects of Immunology*, Gell PGH and Coombs RRA (eds.), 1st ed. Oxford, England: Blackwell; 1963. Section IV, Chapter 1; permission conveyed through Copyright Clearance Center, Inc.

Type I hypersensitivity

Type I hypersensitivity is the mechanism underlying the group of disorders termed as 'allergic'. Allergic disease is increasing, particularly in Westernised countries, with estimates of between 10 and 30% of the population having some form of allergic disease. The main diseases considered to have an allergic origin are:

- Asthma (➲ see Chapter 11, Asthma, p. 345 and Figure 11.1).
- Eczema (➲ see Chapter 21, Eczema, p. 761 and Tables 21.5 and 21.6).
- Allergic rhinitis/rhinoconjunctivitis.
- Food allergy.
- Insect venom allergy.
- Drug allergy.

Pathogenesis

Type I reactions are mediated by interaction of antigen with IgE antibodies bound to the surface of mast cells through the high-affinity IgE receptor. Immediate degranulation of the mast cell and release of various chemical mediators cause vasodilation, capillary leak and inflammation, resulting in the symptoms present in an allergic reaction. The propensity for an individual to form IgE antibodies against allergens is termed *atopy*.

Presentation

Allergic reactions can result in localised inflammatory symptoms, as well as more dangerous generalised reactions. The resulting symptoms depend on the site affected by the reaction:

- Nasal allergy: nasal congestion, rhinorrhoea and itching.
- Ocular allergy: redness and itching of the conjunctiva.
- Allergic reactions in the airways: bronchoconstriction, wheezing, breathlessness or laryngeal swelling.

- Skin allergy: eczema or urticaria.
- Gastrointestinal tract: oral itching, vomiting, diarrhoea and abdominal pain.

Anaphylaxis refers to a severe systemic allergic reaction with skin reactions, airway and laryngeal constriction and hypotension, and can be potentially fatal (➲ See Chapter 12, Anaphylactic shock, p. 394).

The pathophysiology of eczema and asthma is more complex than just Type I hypersensitivity, and includes other immune and non-immune mechanisms. In addition, eczema and asthma can both occur in patients who are not atopic.

Investigations and diagnosis

Specific IgE antibodies to different allergens can be identified on skin prick testing (with a small amount of allergen with observation for the presence of a weal) or blood testing. Skin prick testing provides results similar to specific IgE testing and is quicker to perform, but can give false negatives if the patient is on medication like antihistamines. Modern techniques to measure specific IgE in blood no longer use the radioallergosorbent assay (RAST). Some commonly tested allergens include aero-allergens (e.g. house dust mite, grass pollen, tree pollen, cat and dog dander), food allergens (e.g. peanuts and tree nuts, cow's milk, egg, seafood) and insect venoms (e.g. bee and wasp). Both methods of testing identify the presence of atopy, although a positive result does not necessarily indicate that clinical allergy is present, and needs to be correlated with the history. Challenge testing (i.e. exposing a patient to increasing amounts of a potential allergen, e.g. food or medication) can be undertaken if the results of the skin prick testing/specific IgE and history are unclear, or if trying to confirm that there is no allergy. In view of the risk of provoking significant allergic reactions, challenge testing should be undertaken where facilities for resuscitation are immediately available.

Total IgE levels can also be measured and are elevated in atopic individuals. However, these are not helpful in identifying specific allergens. If anaphylaxis is suspected, serum tryptase levels should be measured to confirm that mast cell degranulation has occurred. Serial tryptase measurements as soon as possible after emergency treatment has started, and then within 1–2 (but no later than 4) hours, and 24 hours (to determine baseline) are recommended. Mast cell degranulation can occur due to non-IgE-mediated causes and an elevated tryptase level does not necessarily mean that the reaction is due to allergy.

Management

Treatment for the symptoms of allergic disease depends on the individual manifestations of the disease.

The management of severe anaphylaxis is covered in ➲ Chapter 12, Anaphylactic shock, p. 394.

For milder systemic reaction with only skin or mucosal changes, oral prednisolone 40 mg and chlorphenamine 8 mg can be given.

Allergic rhinitis is treated with *antihistamines* and *intranasal steroids*. Severe allergic rhinitis may be treated by *immunotherapy* or desensitisation, a process by which the patient is exposed to gradually increasing amounts of allergen. Patients are treated for 3 years and there are long-lasting effects after the course of treatment is completed. For tree and grass pollen, it may be administered subcutaneously or sublingually; uncontrolled asthma is a contraindication; for venom allergy resulting in anaphylaxis, it may be administered subcutaneously. *Allergen avoidance* is also recommended, particularly in drug and food allergy. Avoidance is less easy to implement for aero-allergens (e.g. house dust mite and pollens) and the clinical benefit is less evident.

For treatment of asthma (➲ see Chapter 11, Acute management, Long-term management and Further treatment for chronic asthma, pp. 347–8) and eczema (➲ see Chapter 21, Management, p. 763.).

Type II hypersensitivity

Type II hypersensitivity reactions occur when antibodies (of IgM or IgG isotype) bind to cellular antigens. This results in destruction of the cell through cell lysis by complement activation, opsonisation and antibody-dependent cellular cytotoxicity (ADCC). The target antigens can be autoantigens or foreign antigens. Examples of autoantigen-induced disease are:

- Autoimmune haemolytic anaemia where host red cells are destroyed.
- Goodpasture's syndrome where autoantibody is directed against glomerular basement membrane resulting in pulmonary haemorrhage and renal failure.

Examples of disease caused by foreign antigens are:

- Transfusion reactions, where natural antibodies known as isohaemagluttinins target incompatible red blood cells resulting in their destruction.
- Rhesus incompatibility where pregnant mothers who are Rhesus D negative can develop antibodies against the Rhesus D antigen in their babies resulting in haemolytic disease of the newborn (➲ see Chapter 9, Blood groups, p. 282).

Type V reactions are a special version of Type II reactions, where antibody binds to receptor on cells, resulting in activation of that cell rather than its destruction (e.g. thyroid stimulating antibodies in Graves' disease [➲ see Chapter 19, Graves' disease, p. 680]).

Type III hypersensitivity

Type III hypersensitivity reactions occur when antibody binds to soluble antigen. This results in the formation of immune complexes that can activate complement and attract neutrophils, which then degranulate and release lytic enzymes, resulting in tissue destruction.

- Local deposition of immune complexes in the subcutaneous tissue results in the so-called *Arthus reaction*, originally described in experiments where horse serum was injected subcutaneously into rabbits. This has been reported to occur with diphtheria and tetanus vaccination.
- Localised deposition can also occur in the lung, resulting in extrinsic allergic alveolitis, farmer's lung (reaction against fungal antigens in mouldy hay) and bird fancier's disease (reaction against various avian antigens) (➲ see Chapter 11, Interstitial lung disease, p. 348).
- Immune complexes can occur systemically and result in a variety of symptoms including fever, lassitude, vasculitis, arthritis and glomerulonephritis due to deposition in various organs. An example of this is *serum sickness*, in which antibodies develop against foreign proteins present in sera or antitoxins, derived from a non-human animal source, generally administered to prevent or treat an infection or envenomation, e.g. horse anti-tetanus toxin to protect against tetanus.

Type IV hypersensitivity

Type IV hypersensitivity reactions are delayed reactions mediated by T cells and macrophages, and begin to occur 24 hours after contact with the antigen. One of the best known examples is the tuberculin (Mantoux) test, in response to mycobacterial antigens, which tests the subject's 'recall' for mycobacterial antigens. Granuloma formation occurs if there is persistence of the antigen (e.g. when a microbe like TB is able to evade elimination). In a granuloma, macrophages fuse to form giant cells and there is proliferation of local fibroblasts resulting in containment of the offending antigen. This occurs with infectious diseases (e.g. TB and leprosy) and other conditions where the antigen is unknown (e.g. sarcoidosis [➲ see Chapter 11, Sarcoidosis, p. 351] and Crohn's disease [➲ see Chapter 14, Inflammatory bowel disease, Crohn's disease and ulcerative colitis, p. 510]). In contact dermatitis (➲ see Chapter 21, Exogenous, p. 762) small molecules (e.g. nickel and hair dyes) penetrate the skin resulting in sensitisation and a subsequent type IV eczematous reaction. Patch testing can be undertaken to identify the offending substances.

Systemic autoimmune and autoinflammatory disorders

Principles of autoimmunity

Autoimmunity is defined as the production of immune responses against self. Responses can involve both the humoral and cellular arms of the immune system, with formation of auto-antibodies and auto-reactive T cells. Autoimmune disease occurs when autoimmune responses result in tissue damage and pathology.

In theory, the immune system possesses the capability of generating a response towards virtually any molecule or cell. Auto-reactive antibodies and T cells can be present in healthy individuals. The majority of these individuals will not develop overt autoimmune disease, indicating that protective mechanisms must exist to prevent this from occurring. These include:

- Deletion of auto-reactive T and B cells during their development.
- Suppression of auto-reactive T and B cells by other cells or cytokines.

- Idiotype/anti-idiotype responses.
- Immunosuppressive adrenal hormones.

The development of autoimmune disease occurs when these suppressive responses fail.

Autoimmune diseases may be:

- Systemic:
  - Affecting multiple organ systems:
    - Typically, the target auto-antigen is expressed in multiple tissues.
- Organ-specific:
  - Limited to a single organ:
    - Immune recognition is usually limited to a tissue specific auto-antigen.

Autoimmune diseases have a familial tendency and individuals affected are more likely to develop other autoimmune diseases, suggesting either a common genetic tendency or pathological basis. Although immune responses involve the entire immune system, the pathology can be mediated by individual components, e.g. in Goodpasture's disease, pathology is primarily antibody-mediated; in multiple sclerosis, T-cells are more significant; and in rheumatoid arthritis, both T and B cells play an important role. Examples of various systemic and organ-specific autoimmune diseases are listed in Table 6.5. A fuller description of each condition is covered in the relevant chapter.

Table 6.5 Systemic and organ-specific autoimmune diseases

Autoimmune diseases	Autoantibodies present on laboratory testing
Systemic	
Systemic lupus erythematosus (SLE)	ANA (sensitive, but not specific). Double stranded DNA antibodies. Anti-Ro antibodies (can cause neonatal lupus and congenital heart block due to passive transfer from mother to fetus). Anti-La antibodies. Anti-Sm antibodies.
Rheumatoid arthritis	Rheumatoid factor. Anti-CCP antibodies.
Systemic sclerosis	Anti-Scl70 antibodies. Anti-centromere antibodies.
Sjogren's syndrome	Anti-Ro antibodies. Anti-La antibodies.
ANCA-associated vasculitides	The associations for ANCA associated vasculitides are not absolute and can be reversed (i.e. C-ANCA can be found with MPO specificity); the disease association is also not absolute (e.g. Wegener's granulomatosis can be associated with P-ANCA). Although the main target for C-ANCA is PR3 and for P-ANCA is MPO, other ANCA specificities exist e.g. BPI, cathepsin G, elastase, lactoferrin and lysozyme, but the clinical significance of these is less clear.
Wegener's granulomatosis (granulomatosis with polyangiitis)	C-ANCA antibodies. PR3-ANCA antibodies.
Microscopic polyangiitis	P-ANCA antibodies. MPO-ANCA antibodies.
Churg—Strauss syndrome	P-ANCA antibodies. MPO-ANCA antibodies.
Goodpasture's syndrome	Anti-GBM antibodies.

continued

Table 6.5 *continued*

Autoimmune diseases	Autoantibodies present on laboratory testing
Systemic	
Antiphospholipid syndrome	Anti-cardiolipin antibodies. Lupus anticoagulant (test does not detect antibodies per se, but forms part of the diagnostic criteria). Anti-β2GP1 antibodies. Both IgG and IgM isotypes are tested.
Organ-specific	
Endocrine	
Type 1 diabetes	Islet cell antibodies including: GAD antibodies. IA2 antibodies. Insulin antibodies.
Addison's disease	Adrenal antibodies: 21 hydroxylase is one of the major antigens.
Graves' disease	TSHR antibodies.
Hashimoto's thyroiditis	TPO antibodies.
Cutaneous	
Pemphigus vulgaris	Antibodies against intracellular cement in epidermis: specific antigens include desmoglein 1 and desmoglein 3.
Bullous pemphigoid	Basement membrane antibodies: target antigens are hemidesmosomal proteins BP180 and BP230.
Haematological	
Pernicious anaemia	Gastric parietal cell antibodies. Intrinsic factor antibodies.
Immune thrombocytopenic purpura (ITP)	Platelet antibodies (although diagnosis does not usually rely on their presence).
Autoimmune haemolytic anaemia (AIHA)	Antibodies to red blood cell surface membrane antigens. *Direct Coombs (direct antiglobulin) test* is used to detect these antibodies or complement proteins that may subsequently bind to the surface of the red blood cells.
Gastrointestinal	
Coeliac disease	tTG antibodies. Endomysial antibodies. Gliadin antibodies (no longer recommended for testing in current guidelines due to lower sensitivity and specificity). Coeliac disease antibodies are typically of the IgA isotype, but in patients with coeliac disease who have IgA deficiency, testing for the IgG isotype is indicated.
Hepatic	
Primary biliary cirrhosis	Anti-mitochondrial antibodies (particularly the M2 subtype directed against pyruvate dehydrogenase).
Autoimmune hepatitis	ANA. Anti-smooth muscle antibodies. Anti-LKM antibodies.
Neurological	
Myasthenia gravis	Acetylcholine receptor antibodies.
Guillain–Barré syndrome	Ganglioside antibodies.

Most pathological antibodies in clinical practice are of the IgG isotype, although there are some exceptions as noted.
ANA, Anti-nuclear antibody; ANCA, anti-neutrophil cytoplasmic antibody; B2GP1, beta 2 glycoprotein 1; BPI, bactericidal/permeability increasing protein; CCP, cyclic citrullinated peptide; GAD, glutamic acid decarboxylase; GBM, glomerular basement membrane; IA2, Islet antigen 2 (or insulinoma antigen 2); LKM, liver kidney microsomal; MPO, myeloperoxidase; PR3, proteinase 3; TPO, thyroid peroxidase; TSHR, thyroid stimulating hormone receptor; tTG, tissue transglutaminase.

Aetiology of autoimmunity

It is estimated that between 3.2 and 9.4% of the general population have some form of autoimmune disease. Multiple autoimmune diseases are more likely to occur within the same individual and within families. Factors related to the development of autoimmunity include:

- Age: autoantibodies are more prevalent in older people, and most autoimmune diseases tend to occur in adulthood, rather than childhood.
- Gender: many autoimmune diseases (with a few exceptions, e.g. ankylosing spondylitis) show a significant female bias e.g. SLE has a 10:1 female:male ratio.
- Genetics: autoimmune diseases tend to co-segregate in families suggesting a genetic component; in particular, certain HLA types have been associated with certain autoimmune diseases. Polymorphisms in genes relating to lymphocyte activation and regulation have been linked to autoimmunity.
  - Single gene defects can also result in autoimmune disease:
    - e.g. Autoimmune polyendocrinopathy, candidiasis, ectodermal dysplasia (APECED) due to mutations in autoimmune regulator (AIRE); this gene is expressed in the thymus and thought to be involved in the development of central tolerance to non-thymic self-proteins.
    - Immune dysfunction, polyendocrinopathy, and enteropathy, X-linked (IPEX) due to mutations in *FOXP3;* this gene is required for development of regulatory T cells.
- Infections: various common microbes (e.g. mycoplasma, streptococci, EBV) have been linked to autoimmune diseases. Some examples include rheumatic fever and streptococcal infection, and type 1 diabetes and coxsackie B virus.
- Drugs: certain medications can induce autoimmunity, e.g. procainamide and hydralazine may result in SLE.
- Immunodeficiency: this could be due to the persistence of infection or failure of regulation of the immune system associated with immunodeficiency.

Disease mechanisms of systemic autoimmunity

Multiple mechanisms are thought to contribute to the breakdown of tolerance and development of autoimmunity. These include:

- Molecular mimicry:
  - Some micro-organisms express antigenic epitopes that are very similar to host tissues. Hence, activation of the immune system to eliminate the pathogen may result in a sustained response directed against the similar host tissue. Breakdown of tolerance to a single peptide can result in inflammation leading to presentation of other peptides and widening of the immune response – a process known as epitope spreading. An example of this is rheumatic fever – the immune response to Group A streptococci targets an epitope very similar to that found in cardiac muscle.
- Polyclonal activation due to microbial antigens:
  - Certain microbes or microbial products are able to activate lymphocytes independent of their antigenic specificity. Examples include lipopolysaccharide (LPS), staphylococcal enterotoxin (SEB) and Epstein–Barr virus (EBV).
  - Polyclonal activation of lymphocytes can result in activation of auto-reactive lymphocytes, e.g. polyclonal B cell activation by leishmaniansis can result in laboratory and clinical features of autoimmunity. In addition, polyclonal lymphocyte activation by EBV may contribute to the development of rheumatoid arthritis.
- Release of sequestered self-antigen:
  - Infection and trauma can result in the release of antigens that had previously been sequestered. (Immunological tolerance occurs mostly during embryonic development and consequently, the immune system would not previously have been exposed to sequestered antigens and would not subsequently recognise them as self.) An example of this is sympathetic ophthalmia, where trauma to one eye can result in uveitis affecting both the affected and unaffected eyes.

- Modification of cells by drugs and microbes:
  - Viruses may alter the cell surface by expression of viral epitopes and drugs may be adsorbed to cells resulting in a hapten effect. A transient immune response usually removes these cells, but sometimes the immune response can be sustained beyond the initial stimulus resulting in significant immunological disease.

The effector mechanisms that mediate autoimmune damage are the same as those that are directed against infectious pathogens. However, unlike pathogens, autoantigens remain within the body resulting in an ongoing immune process. Some of the effector mechanisms include:

- Autoantibody mediated cellular destruction either by activation of complement or phagocytosis of cells, e.g. destruction of cells in immune thrombocytopenic purpura (ITP) or autoimmune haemolytic anaemia (AIHA).
- Interference of cellular function by autoantibody binding, e.g. acetylcholine receptor antibodies preventing function in myasthenia gravis.
- Activation of cellular function: e.g. thyrotropin-stimulating hormone (TSH) receptor antibodies causing overstimulation of the thyroid gland in Graves' disease.
- Immune complex deposition resulting in glomerulonephritis or vasculitis,
- T cell infiltration of cellular tissue, e.g. in type 1 diabetes.

Diagnosis of autoimmune diseases is made from the clinical assessment with appropriate laboratory investigations to confirm evidence of autoimmunity. Treatment of autoimmune disease can consist of:

- Replacement therapy, e.g. thyroxine for autoimmune hypothyroidism and insulin for type 1 diabetes.
- Immunosuppressive medication to suppress the autoimmune process.

Autoinflammatory syndromes

Autoinflammatory syndromes are a collection of disorders characterised by inflammation and an acute phase response, without any evidence of specific autoimmunity (see Table 6.6). In contrast to autoimmune disorders, which result from inappropriate activation of the adaptive immune system, the autoinflammatory syndromes are due to abnormal activation of the innate immune system. Although many of these diseases are the result of single gene defects, some are due to more complex polygenic disorders or can be acquired. Most have a common final pathway, which results in activation of caspase 1 and subsequent production of active IL-1β, a potent pro-inflammatory cytokine. Clinically, this leads to recurrent inflammation, which can present as episodes of fever, rash, lymphadenopathy, arthritis and serositis. With long-term inflammation, amyloid deposition can occur. Many of these conditions respond to treatments that antagonise the action of IL-1, including anakinra (an IL-1R antagonist) and canakinumab (an anti-IL-1 monoclonal antibody). Colchicine is effective in the treatment of familial Mediterranean fever (FMF). Some of the other autoinflammatory syndromes respond to corticosteroid therapy.

The immune system and malignancy: principles of immune surveillance and malignancy of the immune system

It is generally thought that the immune system is engaged in surveillance and eradication of neoplastic cells. Patients (and animals) that are immunodeficient or immunosuppressed are more likely to develop tumours (see Table 6.7). In some of these patients, it is failure of the immune system to control viruses (that result in virally driven tumours), rather than failure to eradicate tumour cells per se.

Specific immune responses can be detected against various tumours suggesting that the immune system does recognise these tissues as abnormal and is attempting to remove them. Manipulation of the immune system (immunotherapy) in addition to surgery, chemotherapy and radiotherapy has also been used as a means to treat tumours.

Tumour antigens

Although tumours are derived from host cells, they can express various abnormal antigens, which can result in the generation of an immune response. Tumour antigens may be defined as tumour-specific antigens (TSA) or tumour-associated antigens (TAA). TAA can also be found on normal cells, although their expression in tumour cells may be aberrant or excessive. Another method of classifying antigens is as:

Table 6.6 Autoinflammatory syndromes

	Inheritance pattern	Gene/protein defect	Clinical features
Hereditary periodic fevers			
FMF	Autosomal recessive	*MEVF*/pyrin	Affects Armenian, Arab, Jewish, Turkish populations. Onset at <20 years. Fever attacks last 1–4 days. Pleuritis, monoarthritis, sterile peritonitis, pericarditis, rarely rash. Renal amyloid common if untreated.
Mevalonate kinase deficiency/hyper-IgD syndrome (MVK/HIDS)	Autosomal recessive	*MVK*/mevalonate kinase	Affects Dutch, French populations. Onset in childhood. Attacks last 3–7 days. Cervical adenopathy, abdominal pain, arthralgia, rash, hepatosplenomegaly, aphthous ulcers.
Cryopyrin-associated periodic syndromes (CAPS)	Autosomal dominant	*CIAS1*/cryopyrin	Affects all ethnic groups. Three different phenotypes (in order of increasing severity): • Familial cold autoinflammatory syndrome (FCAS) – fever, rash, arthralgia after cold exposure. • Muckle Wells syndrome (MWS) – fever, urticaria, arthritis, hearing loss, eye inflammation. • Neonatal onset multisystem inflammatory disease (NOMID)/chronic infantile neurological cutaneous and articular syndrome (CINCA) – continuous inflammation, fever and rash, uveitis, bone deformities, aseptic meningitis and mental retardation.
TNF-receptor associated periodic syndromes (TRAPS)	Autosomal dominant	*TNFRSF1A*/TNF receptor 1	Affects mainly Northern Europeans. Fever episodes last 1–3 weeks. Adenopathy, chest and abdominal pain, peri-orbital oedema, monocytic fasciitis.
Familial cold autoinflammatory syndrome 2 (FCAS2)	Autosomal dominant	*NLRP12*/NLRP12	Clinical features resemble FCAS. Fever attacks last 2–10 days. Triggered by cold. Urticaria, abdominal pain, adenopathy, hearing loss.
Diseases with pyogenic lesions			
Deficiency of IL-1 receptor antagonist (DIRA)	Autosomal recessive	*IL-1RN*/IL-1 receptor antagonist	Onset in neonatal period. Multifocal osteomyelitis, periostitis, pustular skin lesions.
Pyogenic arthiritis, pyoderma gangrenosum and acne (PAPA) syndrome	Autosomal dominant	*CD2BP1*/PSTPIP1	Presents in early childhood. Pyogenic arthritis, pyoderma gangrenosum, cystic acne.

continued

Table 6.6 *continued*

	Inheritance pattern	Gene/protein defect	Clinical features
Majeed syndrome	Autosomal recessive	*LPIN2*/Lipin 2	Bone and skin inflammation, recurrent fever, dyserythropoeitic anaemia, autosomal recessive form of CRMO.
Chronic recurrent multifocal osteomyelitis (CRMO)	Sporadic	Probably polygenic	Recurrent episodes of multifocal osteomyelitis.
Diseases with granulomatous lesions			
Blau syndrome (familial juvenile systemic granulomatosis)	Autosomal dominant	*NOD2*/Nod2	Onset before 3–4 years. Dermatitis, granulomatous uveitis, arthritis.
Diseases with psoriasis			
Deficiency of IL-36 receptor antagonist (DITRA)	Autosomal recessive	*IL36RN*/IL-36	Present in adults and children. Flares of generalised psoriasis.
Diseases with panniculitis-induced lipodystrophy			
JMP (joint contractures, muscle atrophy and panniculitis-induced lipodystrophy) syndrome	Autosomal recessive	*PSMB8*/Inducible β5 subunit of the immunoproteasome	Presents in adults with joint contractures, muscle atrophy and panniculitis-induced lipodystrophy.
CANDLE (chronic atypical neutrophilic dermatosis with lipodystrophy and elevated temperature) syndrome	Autosomal recessive	*PSMB8*/Inducible β5 subunit of the immunoproteasome	Presents in childhood. Fever, neutrophilic dermatosis, purpura, swollen eyelids, arthralgia, progressive lipodystrophy, anaemia, delayed physical development.
Nakajo-Nishimura syndrome (NNS)	Autosomal recessive	*PSMB8*/Inducible β5 subunit of the immunoproteasome	Presents in early infancy. Periodic fever, rash, lipomuscular atrophy, joint contractures.
Other autoinflammatory syndromes			
Early onset inflammatory bowel disease	Autosomal recessive	*ILIL10RA*/IL-10 receptor *IL-10RB*/IL-10 receptor and part of IL-22, -26, -28, -29 receptors	Continuous fever pattern. Colitis, fistula formation, folliculitis.
PFAPA (periodic fever, aphthous stomatitis and pharyngitis) syndrome	Sporadic	Probably polygenic	Presents in childhood. Fever attacks lasting 3–6 days associated with pharyngitis, adenitis and aphthae. Occurs every 2–6 weeks.
Behçet's disease	Sporadic	Probably polygenic HLA-B51 is associated	Common in 'silk road' countries in Far East, Mediterranean and Middle East. Oro-genital ulceration, skin lesions, eye inflammation, pathergy.
Acquired autoinflammatory syndromes			
Schnitzler syndrome	Acquired	N/A	Chronic urticarial-like rash, monoclonal IgM gammopathy and systemic inflammation usually presenting as fever.

Table 6.7 Immunodeficiency and malignancy

Immunodeficiency state	Associated tumours
HIV infection	Kaposi's sarcoma (human herpes virus 8-associated). Lymphoma (often EBV-associated). Cervical cancer (human papilloma virus-associated). Anal cancer. Liver cancer. Lung cancer.
Common variable immunodeficiency	Lymphoma. Gastric cancer.
Immunosuppressive medication and chemotherapy (e.g. for transplants, autoimmune disease)	Multiple cancer types (including lymphoma, lung, liver, kidney, skin cancers).

- Virally or chemically induced antigens:
  - Viruses infecting a host cell can result in expression of viral proteins.
  - DNA mutation due to chemical or radiation damage can result in abnormal protein expression unique to the individual tumour.
- Oncofetal antigens:
  - Typically found on cells during normal development and found in low levels in serum.
  - Expressed in high amounts by certain tumours.
  - Not necessarily tumour specific or necessarily diagnostic of tumour.
  - Can be used for monitoring tumour burden.
  - Examples include carcinoembryonic antigen (CEA) or α-fetoprotein (α-FP).
- Differentiation antigens:
  - Expressed at different stages of normal cell development.
  - Can be expressed on tumour cells depending on the stage at which tumour cell differentiation is arrested.
  - Can be used to determine what stage of differentiation the malignant event occurred, particularly in myeloid and lymphoid malignancies.

Immune effector mechanisms directed against tumours

NK cells are most likely responsible for surveillance and elimination of tumours. In established tumours, specific anti-tumour responses, similar to those directed against bacterial or viral pathogens, result in anti-tumour antibodies and T cells. These mechanisms include:

- Natural killer cell cytotoxicity:
  - NK cells express FCγRIII receptor, which binds IgG, are activated by production of IFN-γ and IL-2, and can kill antibody-coated tumour cells.
  - Some tumours have reduced expression of MHC to avoid detection by cytotoxic T cells. Tumour cells with lower or absent MHC expression are more susceptible to NK cell killing. NK cells detect MHC expression. Reduction or absence of MHC results in NK cell activation and killing of the target cell. This phenomenon is known as the 'missing self' hypothesis.
- Specific cytotoxic T cells killing cells bearing tumour specific or tumour associated antigens.
- Induction of apoptosis by antibody.
- Antibody-mediated complement activation.
- Antibody dependent cell-mediated cytotoxicity (by neutrophils, macrophages and lymphocytes with Fc receptors).
- Phagocytosis by macrophages.

Immune evasion by tumours

Malignant tumours are able to survive and grow despite expression of aberrant antigens, which can activate the immune system. The immune evasion and survival mechanisms employed by tumours include:

- Tolerance to tumour antigens:
  - Some tumour associated antigens are naturally occurring self-molecules (although abnormally expressed in tumours). Consequently, there is a degree of self-tolerance to them, which renders the immune system unresponsive.
- Selection for less immunogenic tumour variants:
  - Tumour cells expressing highly antigenic molecules would be eliminated by the immune system. The selection of the remaining tumour clones would be more similar to non-tumour cells, that are less antigenic and able to avoid immune detection (not be recognised as 'foreign').
- Tumours have low immunogenicity:
  - Tumours can avoid detection by T cells by reducing their expression of MHC molecules. Although this renders them more susceptible to NK cell killing, NK cells do not possess memory and will not expand sufficiently to cope with tumour burden.
- Modulation of tumour antigen expression:
  - Antibodies that bind to tumour antigens can be internalised resulting in removal of that antigen from the tumour cell surface and resistance to detection by the same antibody.
- Tumour secretion of immunosuppressive factors:
  - Some tumours secrete cytokines like IL-10 and TGF-β, which have immunosuppressive properties.
  - Tumours can shed antigen, which can interfere with antibody binding and T cell recognition of tumour.
- Expression of Fas ligand:
  - Some tumours express FasL. This allows the tumour cells to induce apoptosis in infiltrating lymphocytes which express Fas.

Tumours of the immune system

In addition to providing protection against malignancy, tumours can also develop from both myeloid and lymphoid cells. Chronic inflammation or infection can increase the risk of some immune system tumours, which may be due to prolonged immune stimulation. The commonest types of tumours (covered in more detail in ➲ Chapter 9, Haematological malignancy, p. 293, Boxes 9.1 and 9.2, Figures 9.7, 9.8 and 9.9.) are:

- Leukaemias:
  - Can be divided into acute and chronic, and myeloid or lymphocytic depending on the lineage of tumour cell.
  - Originate in bone marrow.
- Lymphomas:
  - Divided into Hodgkin's and non-Hodgkin's lymphomas, both of which have multiple subtypes.
  - Originate in lymph nodes, but can infiltrate other organs.
- Myeloma:
  - A tumour of plasma cells present in bone marrow.

A malignant event can occur at any stage of development of the immune cell and this results in different subtypes of malignancy. Cells express different cell surface molecules ('differentiation antigens'), which can be used to identify the type of tumour and guide treatment and prognosis.

Transplantation immunology

Basic concepts

Transplantation of tissues and cells for the management of failing organs is now part of routine clinical practice. Organs that are more commonly transplanted include kidneys, liver, pancreas, heart, lung, skin, cornea, blood and stem cells/bone marrow. Small bowel, limbs and facial transplants have also been carried out. Stem cell/bone marrow transplantation is used in the treatment of some haematological malignancies, aplastic anaemia, severe immunodeficiencies and some inborn errors of metabolism. The major challenge to any successful transplant is the risk of rejection as the immune system mounts a response against the foreign transplanted organs. Graft-versus-host disease (GVHD) represents a special instance of rejection where the recipient has received an allogeneic bone marrow or stem cell transplant. Lymphocytes that are present in the graft can recognise host tissue as foreign and mount an immune response. The typical organs involved include skin, gut and lung.

The organs and tissues used in transplants can originate from several different sources:

- Autografts:
  - Grafting of the individual's own tissue.
  - Examples include skin transplants from one part of the body to another and bone marrow, which is removed prior to high dose chemotherapy, and replaced afterwards.
  - No risk of rejection.
- Allografts:
  - Grafting of tissue between two genetically dissimilar individuals.
  - Risk of rejection depends on the closeness of the 'match' of the tissue, i.e. how genetically similar the donor and recipient tissues are.
  - Most common form of organ transplant.
- Xenografts:
  - Grafting across different species.
  - High risk of rejection as there are species differences.
  - Of research interest in view of the shortage of organs required for transplantation.

Transplantation antigens

The main antigens that are recognised as foreign include the ABO blood group system on red blood cells and the HLA molecules. There are also 'minor transplantation antigens' that usually provoke a weaker immune response. These include the non-ABO blood groups and antigens associated with the sex chromosome.

ABO blood groups

ABO blood groups are the major antigens present on red blood cells. Incompatibility can lead to transfusion reactions (➲ see Chapter 9, Blood groups, p. 282). These antigens are important in transplantation as they are expressed on vascular endothelium.

Human leukocyte antigen molecules

- The HLA system is a set of genes encoding the MHC in humans.
- The MHC comprises cell surface proteins essential for the adaptive immune system to recognise foreign molecules. The human MHC genomic region, at chromosomal position 6p21, contains the densest distribution of genes sequenced in the human genome.
- HLA alleles from each parent are co-dominantly expressed.
- Human MHC genes are categorised into three groups: class I, class II and class III.
- Class I HLA encoded proteins are present on all nucleated cells:
  - The genes are found in three different loci (positions): A, B and C.
  - They present self-peptides to CD8+ T cells.
- Class II HLA molecules are present on antigen presenting cells:
  - Found in DP, DQ and DR loci.
  - Responsible for presenting foreign peptide to CD4+ T cells.
- Class I and II HLA are highly polymorphic molecules:
  - There are many possible variants of each HLA molecule in the human population, so the probability of two individuals having an identical HLA type is very small.
- Class III HLA encodes for complement proteins: these are non-polymorphic and do not show the variation found in Class I and II HLA.

- Differences in HLA type can result in rejection of a transplanted organ or GVHD with a higher probability of rejection with greater mismatch.
- The HLA loci are very close to each other, and therefore tend to be inherited together, giving a 'HLA haplotype'. One haplotype is inherited from each parent giving a 25% chance that a sibling will be HLA identical.

In organ transplantation, the degree of mismatch between donor and recipient is typically described for HLA-A, HLA-B and HLA-DR. As each individual expresses two alleles at each locus, this results in a maximum of six mismatches, expressed as 0-0-0 through to 2-2-2. The amount of matching required depends to some extent on what organ is transplanted:

- Bone marrow/stem cell transplant: a complete match of the HLA region gives the best outcomes.
- Renal transplant: Class II HLA matching is more important than Class I for survival. ABO matching is also important as ABO antigens are expressed on vascular endothelial cells.
- Liver and heart transplants: HLA matching not routinely performed due to urgency of procedure.
- Corneal transplants: HLA matching not routinely done. Risk of rejection occurs if the graft becomes vascularised.

Mechanisms of rejection

Rejection of a transplanted organ can be classified by its speed of onset:

- Hyperacute rejection:
  - Occurs within minutes to hours of graft revascularization.
  - Due to pre-formed circulating antibody present in the donor.
  - Antibody usually directed against ABO antigens (present in vascular endothelial cells) or can be anti-HLA antibodies (if there has been a previous sensitising event, e.g. blood transfusion, previous transplantation or women who have been exposed to paternal HLA present in the fetus).
- Acute rejection:
  - Occurs within days to months after transplant.
  - Rejection mediated by T cells and monocytes/macrophages.
  - Graft histology shows infiltrating lymphocytes and monocytes with increased HLA expression.
  - Important to diagnose as should be treated promptly with increased immunosuppression.
- Chronic rejection:
  - Occurs months to years after the transplant.
  - Results in gradual loss of graft function.
  - Mechanism of rejection is unclear, but possibly due to development of immunity against HLA antigens (which can take time due to only a small amount of HLA mismatch and immunosuppression).
  - T cells are thought to play an important role and antibody responses may also be involved.

The immunopathological response to a transplanted graft is similar to that directed against infectious microorganisms, consisting of a sensitisation (or recognition) phase and an effector phase. Recognition of the foreign graft ('allorecognition') can occur both in the transplanted graft and in the regional lymph nodes. At least two pathways of allorecognition are thought to exist:

- Direct allorecognition:
  - Occurs when host T cells recognise intact HLA molecules on donor cells.
  - Donor HLA and donor peptide on donor cells is 'seen' by host immune cells as self HLA and foreign peptide, the combination of which results in activation.
  - Probably the most important pathway in the early immune response.
- Indirect allorecognition:
  - Occurs when host T cells recognise donor peptides presented on host APCs.
  - Probably the more important mechanism in late or chronic rejection.

The effector phase results in activation of the immune system and utilises all the effector components present in the response to infectious pathogens, including complement, NK cells, T cells and antibodies.

GVHD occurs only:

(i) In the presence of immunocompetent cells in the graft.
(ii) In the presence of alloantigens: usually due to HLA mismatching, but other antigens can play a role as well.
(iii) If the host is in a state of profound cellular immune deficiency: typically occurs due to the chemotherapy used prior to the bone marrow/stem cell transplant, but also in individuals with an inherited immunodeficiency (e.g. SCID).

GVHD can be divided into:

- Acute GVHD:
  - Occurs within 100 days of the transplant.
  - Presents with skin rash, fever, liver involvement (with pruritus and abnormal LFTs, and more rarely hepatic failure), diarrhoea due to gut involvement; other organs may also be involved.
- Chronic GVHD:
  - Occurs >100 days after transplant.
  - Can be an extension of acute GVHD, but may occur without previous GVHD or after acute GVHD has gone into remission.
  - Presents with more diverse features.
  - Ocular, oral, gastrointestinal, lung, neuromuscular involvement.

Grafts depleted of T cells prior to transplantation have a reduced incidence of GVHD, but an increased rate of relapse of leukaemia. This suggests a graft-versus-leukaemia effect provided by the transplanted immunocompetent T cells.

Prevention of graft rejection and complications of transplantation

The main measures undertaken to improve graft survival are to obtain the best tissue match and the use of immunosuppressive medication. The risks of transplantation include rejection in solid organ transplant and failure of engraftment, or GVHD in bone marrow/stem cell transplantation. There is also the increased risk of infection (with both conventional and opportunistic pathogens) and malignancy due to immunosuppression or cytotoxic drugs used as part of the transplantation process. Other factors can also influence graft survival, e.g. duration of kidney ischaemia and donor age.

Several steps can be undertaken to ensure that matching between donor and recipient is optimal:

- Transplantation from a family member:
  - The HLA molecules tend to be inherited as a whole locus, meaning that any sibling has a 1 in 4 chance of being an identical match.
- Tissue typing:
  - Undertaken to determine the HLA type of donor and recipient.
  - Molecular PCR based and serological techniques used.
  - Donor and recipient HLA types are compared to determine how similar their HLA alleles are.
  - For stem cell/bone marrow transplant, aim is for 10/10 allele match (HLA-A, B, C, DR and DQ).
    - International bone marrow registries are available to assist with finding the best match.
  - For renal transplants, aim is to match 6/6 alleles (HLA-A, B and DR) with HLA-DR matching the most important for reducing the risk of graft rejection, followed by HLA-B and A).
    - ABO compatibility is also important, i.e. the ABO type doesn't have to be identical, just compatible, e.g. an O donor can be given to an AB recipient (➔ see Chapter 9, Blood groups, p. 282).
- Antibody screening – primarily for solid organ transplants:
  - Patients awaiting a transplant should be regularly screened to identify HLA antibodies.
  - Particularly important after any potential sensitising events, e.g. blood transfusion, pregnancy.

- Cross matching – primarily for solid organ transplants:
  - Anti-donor antibodies are detected by mixing donor lymphocytes with recipient serum; their presence being detected by lysis of the cells (complement-dependent cytotoxicity) or by fluorescent staining and flow cytometry.
    - Presence of anti-donor antibody indicates higher risk of rejection.

In addition to the use of immunosuppressive drugs to reduce the risk of rejection of solid organ transplants, the following are used.

For prevention of acute rejection (induction therapy at the time of transplantation):

- anti-CD25 monoclonal antibodies (basiliximab; daclizumab no longer in use);
- anti-thymocyte globulin (ATG);
- anti-CD52 (alemtuzumab);
- anti-CD3 (OKT3): no longer in use.

For the treatment of certain forms of rejection:

- ATG;
- terminal complement inhibitor (eculizumab);
- ivIG;
- plasma exchange.

Although the preference is for a well-matched organ, high-risk antibody incompatible transplants (due to ABO and HLA mismatch) are performed, usually with more intensive immunosuppressive regimens for antibody removal. These include the use of plasma exchange, high dose IV immunoglobulin, rituximab and immunoabsorption.

Measures taken to reduce the occurrence of GVHD are similar to prevention of solid organ rejection. These include:

- HLA matching.
- Prophylaxis with immunosuppressants, typically ciclosporin for 6 months.
- T cell depletion.

The treatment of GVHD depends on the severity:

- For mild skin GVHD, topical steroids alone may be sufficient.
- For more severe systemic GVHD, immunosuppressive medications used include ciclosporin, corticosteroids, mycophenolate, anti-CD3 monoclonal antibodies and ATG.

Fetal tolerance

The fetus is a physiological example of immune tolerance to a transplant. The fetus possesses HLA alleles from both parents and, hence, is actually an allograft in close contact with the maternal tissues. Some of the potential mechanisms that prevent the fetus from being rejected include:

- A skewing towards a Th2 response in pregnancy, resulting in a shift from cell-mediated immunity to humoral immunity.
- The placenta acts as an immunological barrier between mother and fetus through several means:
  - Production of complement regulatory proteins by cytotrophoblast.
  - Production of IL-10, which is an immunosuppressive cytokine, by cytotrophoblast.
  - Expression of HLA-G on cytotrophoblast, which immunosuppresses NK cells.
  - Syncytiotrophoblast does not express conventional HLA molecules, which are needed for cytotoxic T cell responses.
  - Production of indole-amine 2,3-dioxygenase, which degrades tryptophan that is necessary for T cell activation.

Immunopharmacology: overview of vaccines, immunoglobulin therapy, anti-inflammatory and immunosuppressive treatment, and biologics

Vaccines

Immunisation has been one of the most effective means of controlling many infectious diseases including smallpox, measles, tetanus and polio. Immunity can be divided into active and passive immunity, both of which can be acquired naturally or artificially.

- Active immunity:
  - Protection generated by the individual's own immune system.
  - Can be lifelong.
  - Normally mediated by both antibody and cell-mediated immunity.
  - Generated by natural exposure to infection or artificially by vaccination.
- Passive immunity:
  - Passive protection provided by transfer of products produced by another individual or animal.
  - Normally delivered by injecting product, e.g. anti-tetanus immunoglobulin after a contaminated wound.
  - Occurs naturally in pregnancy when the mother's antibodies are transferred to the fetus.
  - Effective, but effects are temporary and wane with time.
  - Normally mediated by antibodies.

Vaccination refers to the process of administering antigenic material to an individual to generate a protective adaptive immune response. Vaccines can be delivered by different routes – typically through IM or subcutaneous (SC) injection, but also through oral, intranasal and intradermal routes. Several different types of vaccines are available:

- Live attenuated:
  - Made of low virulence live organisms.
  - Attenuation (i.e. the process of making the pathogen less virulent or harmless while keeping it alive) is done by different methods including:
    - multiple passage – the pathogen is grown repeatedly in unfavourable conditions and non-virulent organisms are selected;
    - targeted mutations – the pathogen is altered to remove virulence genes.
  - Examples – BCG, measles, mumps, rubella, oral polio vaccine.
  - Generally provides better immunity.
  - Small risk of infection or reversion to wild type.
  - Contraindicated in immunosuppressed or immunodeficient individuals.
- Whole inactivated (killed) organisms:
  - Made by growing whole organisms and killing them (e.g. with heat or formaldehyde).
  - Generally induce weaker immune responses and require higher doses, but no risk of contracting disease from vaccine.
  - Examples – Salk vaccine for polio, vaccines for influenza, pertussis and typhoid.
- Fractional vaccines:
  - Made by purifying components from whole organisms or by recombinant DNA technology.
  - Some of these include:
    - Toxoids (inactivated toxins) – tetanus, diphtheria.
    - Capsular polysaccharides – pneumococcus, meningococcus, haemophilus.
    - Recombinant viral particles – hepatitis BsAg, human papillomavirus (HPV).

The efficacy of vaccines (particularly poorly immunogenic ones) can be enhanced by:

- administering them with an *adjuvant* that enhances the immune response by:
  - acting as depots for antigens;

- ◆ prolonging release of antigens;
- ◆ acting as chemical irritants to enhance the immune response.

  Most adjuvants in common clinical use are aluminium compounds, e.g. alum (potassium aluminium sulphate), aluminium hydroxide, aluminium phosphate.
- conjugating weakly immunogenic polysaccharide vaccines to more immunogenic carrier proteins (e.g. tetanus or diphtheria toxoid). *Conjugated vaccines* have been developed for pneumococcus, haemophilus and meningococcus.

Routine childhood vaccination programmes exist in many countries and play a major role in reducing the burden of infectious disease. In addition to protecting the individual, vaccination provides *herd immunity* if sufficient numbers of individuals are vaccinated, limiting spread of the infection.

Routine vaccination is recommended for several groups of patients including those with:

- Splenectomy and hyposplenism/asplenia:
  - ◆ Patients are at risk of overwhelming sepsis as splenic function is required to generate antibodies against polysaccharide antigens.
  - ◆ Vaccination is advised against encapsulated organisms (pneumococcus, haemophilus and meningococcus) and influenza.
  - ◆ Vaccination should be started at least 2 weeks before an elective splenectomy.
  - ◆ Prophylactic antibiotic treatment is also recommended (typically phenoxymethylpenicillin).
- Cochlear implants: vaccination advised against pneumococcus.
- Complement deficiency: vaccination advised against pneumococcus, haemophilus and meningococcus.
- Ongoing haemodialysis: vaccination advised against influenza, pneumococcus and hepatitis B.
- Haemophilia: vaccination advised against hepatitis A and B.
- Chronic medical conditions (respiratory, cardiac, renal, neurological and liver disease, diabetes and patients who are immunosuppressed).

Up-to-date vaccine recommendations for the UK are available online in Immunisation against Infectious Disease (also known as the Green Book [produced by Public Health England]). Effective vaccines remain to be developed for diseases like HIV and malaria, which have a significant burden in the developing world. TB remains a significant global burden where the current vaccine (Bacillus Calmette-Guerin [BCG]) is not completely adequate as it provides variable protection.

Cancer vaccination

Strategies to manipulate the immune system against cancer are challenging as many of the antigens expressed by cancer cells are also naturally expressed. Approaches have targeted antigens over-expressed or expressed only in cancer cells (e.g. melanoma-associated antigen in melanoma) although efficacy so far has been limited.

Vaccination against infective organisms associated with the development of cancer is one way of preventing the subsequent development of cancer. The HPV vaccine, directed against the HPV types that are associated with the development of cervical cancer, is given to prevent cervical cancer.

Immunoglobulin therapy

Human immunoglobulin can be extracted from plasma and purified for use as a therapeutic product. Each immunoglobulin batch is pooled from several thousand individuals. The products contain mainly IgG with a subclass distribution similar to normal blood. As immunoglobulins cannot yet be manufactured, supplies are potentially limited.

Immunoglobulin therapy is normally given at a dose of 0.3 to 0.6 g/kg every 3 to 4 weeks to treat primary and secondary immunodeficiency states (immunoglobulin has a half-life of 3 weeks), and at high doses (usually 2g/kg every 4 to 8 weeks) for immunomodulatory effects in the treatment of autoimmune diseases (Box 6.2). The mode of action for its immunomodulatory properties is unclear but one of the main mechanisms is thought to be its binding to Fc receptors. Anti-cytokine and anti-idiotype antibodies may also play a role. Specific antibodies can be used to prevent sensitisation e.g. the administration of anti-D to Rhesus D negative mothers.

Box 6.2 Approved conditions for use of immunoglobulin

Primary and secondary antibody deficiency states

- Primary immunodeficiencies.
- Thymoma with immunodeficiency.
- Haematopoeitic stem cell transplant in primary immunodeficiencies.
- Specific antibody deficiency.
- Secondary antibody deficiency (any cause).

Haematological disorders

- Acquired red cell aplasia.
- Alloimmune thrombocytopenia (feto-maternal/neonatal).
- Autoimmune haemolytic anaemia.
- Coagulation factor inhibitors (alloantibodies and autoantibodies).
- Haemolytic disease of the newborn.
- Haemophagocytic syndrome.
- ITP (acute and persistent, excluding chronic*).
- Post-transfusion purpura.

Neurological disorders

- Chronic inflammatory demyelinating polyradiculoneuropathy.
- Guillain–Barré syndrome.
- Inflammatory myopathies (dermatomyositis, polymyositis, inclusion body myositis).
- Myasthenia gravis.
- Lambert–Eaton myasthenic syndrome.
- Multifocal motor neuropathy.
- Paraprotein-associated demyelinating neuropathy (IgM, IgG or IgA).
- Rasmussen syndrome (chronic focal encephalitis).
- Stiff person syndrome.

Others

- Autoimmune congenital heart block.
- Autoimmune uveitis.
- Immunobullous diseases.
- Kawasaki disease.
- Necrotising (Panton–Valentine Leukocidin-associated) staphylococcal sepsis.
- Severe or recurrent *Clostridium difficile* colitis.
- Staphylococcal or streptococcal toxic shock syndrome.
- Toxic epidermal necrolysis, Stevens–Johnson syndrome.
- Transplantation (solid organ).

*The Department of Health recommends immunoglobulin treatment is appropriate in some circumstances when ITP is newly diagnosed (acute) or persistent (3 to 12 months duration). For chronic (≥12 months duration) ITP, use of immunoglobulin would be exceptional and alternative approaches should be considered.

Reproduced from *Clinical Guidelines for Immunoglobulin Use*, Second Edition, 2011, Department of Health.

Anti-inflammatory/immunosuppressive therapy

Immunosuppressive drugs have been developed to prevent rejection of organ transplantation and for treatment of autoimmune disease. Some of these drugs are also used for treating cancers (e.g. methotrexate and cyclophosphamide). These drugs mediate their action by targeting specific cellular function or by inhibiting general cellular replication. Immunosuppressive drugs predispose to an increased risk of infection in addition to their specific side effects. For commonly used immunosuppressive medications and their mechanisms of action, see Table 6.8.

Biologics

Biologics refer to medicinal products developed using biological processes. The number of biologic products being developed in recent years has increased significantly in line with advances in recombinant DNA technology (Table 6.9). Broadly, most biologics are one of:

- Monoclonal antibodies directed against a specific target.
- Fusion proteins, usually with a receptor combined with part of the immunoglobulin molecule.
- Biosynthetic molecules, e.g. recombinant insulin or growth hormone.

Table 6.8 Commonly used immunosuppressive medications and their mechanism of action

Class of medication	Medication	Mechanism of action/effect
Corticosteroids		• Binds to glucocorticoid receptor and translocates to nucleus. • Activates transcription of anti-inflammatory genes and inhibits expression of inflammatory genes. • Reduces lymphocyte numbers and functions. • Reduces antibody formation. • Increases blood neutrophils due to (i) reduced margination (adherence to endothelial walls) due to reduction in adhesion molecules on neutrophils and endothelial cells, (ii) reduced migration into tissues (also due to reduction in adhesion molecules), (iii) decreased neutrophil apoptosis (mechanism unknown) and (iv) increased release from bone marrow. • Reduces macrophage function. • Reduces prostaglandin synthesis. • Also has effects on metabolism, cognition, fluid homeostasis and development. • Excess resulting in Cushing's syndrome (➲ see Chapter 19, Cushing's syndrome, p. 687).
Calcineurin inhibitors	Ciclosporin	• Macrolide antibiotic derived from fungal metabolite. • Interacts with cyclophilin, a cytosolic protein, forming a complex that inhibits the action of calcineurin (which normally dephospohrylates NFAT [nuclear factor of activated T-cells, which migrates to the cell nucleus and increases transcription of genes encoding IL-2]) that is required for T cell (and NK cell) activation. • Inhibits T cell function.
	Tacrolimus (FK506)	• Fungal metabolite. • Interacts with FK-BP12 (FK binding protein 12) which then inhibits calcineurin. • Similar effects to ciclosporin.
mTOR (mammalian target of rapamycin) inhibitor	Sirolimus (rapamycin)	• Fungal metabolite. • Binds to FK-BP12, but the complex inhibits mTOR (instead of cyclophilin). • Prevents the response to IL-2. • Similar effects to ciclosporin.

Table 6.8 *continued*

Class of medication	Medication	Mechanism of action/effect
Anti-metabolites	Azathioprine	• Interferes with purine synthesis. • Converted to 6-mercaptopurine and inhibits synthesis of inosinic acid (which is a precursor of purines). • Results in inhibition of DNA synthesis and reduction in cell replication. • Profound bone marrow suppression can result from deficiency in TPMT (thiopurine methyltransferase); patients should be routinely screened for TPMT deficiency prior to commencing treatment.
	Mycophenolate mofetil	• Interferes with purine synthesis. • Inhibits inosine monophosphate dehydrogenase which is required by T and B lymphocytes for de novo synthesis of purines. • Little effect on non-lymphoid cells.
	Methotrexate	• Interferes with tetrahydrofolate synthesis from folic acid by inhibiting the enzyme dihydrofolate reductase. • Interferes with DNA synthesis because folic acid is required for thymidine synthesis.
Alkylating agents	Cyclophosphamide	• Binds and cross-links DNA (and possibly RNA). • Interferes with nucleic acid replication and transcription. • Results in lymphopenia and reduced antibody production. • Side effects include bone marrow suppression, infertility, secondary malignancy and haemorrhagic cystitis (due to acrolein, a metabolite of cyclophosphamide). • In patients where a high dose of cyclophosphamide is given or who are at risk of haemorrhagic cystitis (e.g. those who have had pelvic irradiation) mesna is given prophylactically to reduce the risk of this complication. • Regular blood tests should be carried out while on treatment (with FBC checked prior to and 10 days post-infusion; subsequent infusion dose may need adjusting if leucocyte/neutrophil nadir count too low).

The commonly used immunosuppressive agents in transplantation (specifically related to renal transplantation) are discussed in ➲ Chapter 16, Table 16.14, p. 589).

Immunodiagnostics: principles of protein, cellular and molecular diagnosis in immunology

The principles and main applications of some of the commonly used diagnostic tests in immunology are described below.

Protein investigations

Nephelometry and turbidimetry

- Main methods used in automated measurement of proteins.
- Very rapid.
- Based on measuring the formation of immune complexes in the fluid phase that occurs when specific antisera against the protein of interest are added to serum; immune complex formation alters the optical properties of the fluid medium and this allows absorbed or scattered light to be measured (turbidimetry and nephelopmetry, respectively).

Table 6.9 Commonly used biologic products

Biologic therapy	Type of product	Usage
Abatacept	CTLA-4 (Cytotoxic T-lymphocyte-associated protein 4) immunoglobulin fusion protein.	Rheumatoid arthritis.
Abciximab	Anti-glycoprotein IIb/IIIa monoclonal antibody.	Platelet aggregation inhibitor used in coronary artery procedures.
Adalimumab	Anti-TNF monoclonal antibody.	Rheumatoid arthritis. Crohn's disease, ulcerative colitis. Psoriasis. Psoriatic arthritis. Ankylosing spondylitis.
Anakinra	IL-1 receptor antagonist.	Rheumatoid arthritis. Periodic fever syndromes.
Etanercept	TNF receptor fusion protein.	Rheumatoid arthritis. Psoriasis. Psoriatic arthritis. Ankylosing spondylitis.
Infliximab	Anti-TNF monoclonal antibody.	Rheumatoid arthritis. Crohn's disease, ulcerative colitis. Psoriasis. Psoriatic arthritis. Ankylosing spondylitis.
Natalizumab	Anti-$\alpha 4$ intergrin monoclonal antibody.	Multiple sclerosis.
Omalizumab	Anti-IgE monoclonal antibody.	Allergic asthma.
Rituximab	Anti-CD20 monoclonal antibody.	B cell lymphoma. Autoimmune diseases including rheumatoid arthritis and SLE.
Tocilizumab	Anti-IL6 monoclonal antibody.	Rheumatoid arthritis.
Trastuzumab	Anti-HER2 (human epidermal growth factor receptor 2)/*neu* monoclonal antibody.	Breast cancer.
Ustekinumab	Monoclonal antibody directed against IL-12 and IL-23.	Crohn's disease. Psoriasis. Psoriatic arthritis
Vedolizumab	Monoclonal antibody binding $\alpha 4\beta 7$ integrin.	Crohn's disease, ulcerative colitis.

Protein electrophoresis

- One of the most basic techniques to evaluate serum or urine proteins.
- Used mainly for detection and quantitation of paraprotein bands.
- Serum is applied to an agarose gel and an electric current applied across the gel.
- Proteins migrate based on their size and charge and are visualised by using a protein-binding dye.
- The amount of protein present is proportional to the amount of dye bound, allowing quantitation of protein bands.
- More modern technology allows the same process of protein separation by an electric current to occur in sub-millimetre capillaries, rather than using the more traditional agarose gel.

Immunofixation

- Used to identify the type of proteins separated in electrophoresis.
- Mainly used for identification of monoclonal proteins.

- Antisera is applied to the electrophoretic strip.
- Unreacted proteins are washed out before staining.

Isoelectric focusing

- Used to detect proteins in CSF as concentration of IgG is lower.
- Electrophoretic separation is done in a gel containing ampholytes, which set up a pH gradient.
- Proteins migrate in the gel until they reach the point where they are electrically neutral.
- Immunofixation is then done with antisera against IgG.

Radial immunodiffusion

- Simple, but slow method for protein measurement.
- Antiserum is mixed in an agarose gel and allowed to set.
- Regular holes are cut in the gel and serum added to the holes.
- The serum diffuses out and forms a white halo due to immunoprecipitation between the protein of interest and the antisera in the gel.
- The size of the halo is proportional to the log (concentration) of the protein.

Ouchterlony double immunodiffusion

- Used for non-quantitative identification of proteins.
- Holes are cut in an agarose gel and serum and the antisera are placed in adjacent wells and allowed to diffuse towards each other.
- Lines of precipitation form when the protein of interest is present in the serum.
- When multiple samples are tested, lines of identity and partial identity may form.
- An electric current can be applied across the gel to speed up the process – this is referred to as countercurrent immunoelectrophoresis.

Investigations for autoantibodies

Multiple techniques can be used to measure individual autoantibodies. Different techniques do not necessarily provide the same result when measuring the same sample, and results can differ between different laboratories. Although used mostly for detection of autoantibodies, these techniques can also be used for measurement of other analytes, e.g. enzyme immunoassays are used for hormone measurements as well.

Indirect immunofluorescence

- Widely used technique for the detection of autoantibodies.
- Tissue or cell suspensions are applied to slides.
- Slides are incubated with dilutions of test and control sera.
- Serum is washed off and the slide is incubated with anti-human immunoglobulin (isotype specific) antisera conjugated to a fluorescent probe.
- Unbound antisera is then washed off.
- Slides can be fixed or counterstained if required.
- Slides are viewed under a fluorescent microscope to detect the presence of autoantibodies.
- Alternatives to using a fluorescent probe include using enzymes that give a colour reaction – the slide can be viewed under a normal light microscope.

Direct immunofluorescence

- Technique is similar to indirect immunofluorescence.
- Tissue obtained from patient is snap frozen and applied to slide.
- Conjugated antisera is added and the slide visualised under the microscope.
- Antibody bound to tissues in the patient is detected using this method.
- Other proteins including complement and fibrinogen can also be detected.

Immunoprecipitation assays

- Ouchterlony double diffusion, countercurrent immunoelectrophoresis and nephelometry/turbidimetry (➔ see Nephelometry and turbidimetry, p. 179) can all be used to detect autoantibodies.

Enzyme-linked immunosorbent assay, enzyme-linked immunoassay and fluorescent immunoassays

- Antigen is bound to a solid phase (plate or bead) and then incubated with serum.
- Serum is then washed off and human immunoglobulin antisera is added.
- The antisera is conjugated to either an enzyme or fluorescent label.
- In an enzyme-linked immunosorbent assay (ELISA) or enzyme-linked immunoassay (EIA), the enzyme is then incubated with a substrate, which gives a colour reaction that can be measured using a spectrophotometer.
- In fluorescent immunoassays (FIA), the fluorescence is measured by using an appropriate exciting light source.

Radioimmunoassay

- Radioactive isotopes are used to assess binding of various autoantibodies.
- Considered the 'gold standard' for several assays including double-stranded DNA antibodies (the Farr assay) and acetylcholine receptor (AChR) antibodies.
- Less used in most laboratories due to the radioactivity.

Immunoblotting

- Antigens are applied to or electrophoresed in a matrix, which is then incubated in serum.
- If antibodies are present, they will bind to antigen.
- The matrix is then washed and processed with conjugated antisera and substrate.
- If antibody is bound to antigen, this gives a coloured band.

Cellular investigations

Cellular investigations are used to:

- Enumerate various cell types.
- Identify intracellular constituents.
- Assess cellular function and activation status.
- Identify secreted products, e.g. cytokines and chemokines.
- Phenotype lymphoma and leukaemia cells.

These tests are performed to:

- Enumerate lymphocyte subsets, in particular CD4 and CD8 T cells in the context of HIV.
- Phenotype lymphoma/leukaemia and enumerate B and NK cells.
- Many of the rest of these tests are primarily done in a research context.

The main techniques used include:

- Flow cytometry:
    - Involves the measurement of fluorescently labelled cells passing through an exciting laser.
    - Requires single cell suspensions.
    - Is the principal method used for CD4 and CD8 T cell enumeration.
    - Can evaluate other cell types and intracellular antigens and cytokines.
- Tissue culture and functional assays:
    - Can be used to assess:
        - Lymphocyte proliferation.
        - Lymphocyte function – cytokine production, apoptosis.

    - Neutrophil oxidative burst, phagocytosis and migration.
    - NK cell function.
  - Have little standardisation and some are purely research tools.

Molecular investigations

Molecular techniques have become increasingly used as advances in technology have resulted in a significant drop in cost, more rapid processing of samples, and more powerful bioinformatics tools to analyse the vast amounts of data generated. It is likely that as time progresses, more of these techniques will become routine investigations.

Clinical applications using molecular techniques include:

- DNA analysis: for identification of gene defects and genetic mutations.
- HLA typing.
- Gene rearrangement studies: for assessment of malignancy.
- DNA microarrays: can be used for studying gene expression, assessing genome content as well as investigating disease mechanisms, biomarkers and therapeutic targets.

Further reading

1. Murphy K. *Janeway's Immunobiology*, 8th edn. Abingdon: Garland Science, 2012.
2. Spicket G. *Oxford Handbook of Clinical Immunology*, 3rd edn. Oxford: Oxford University Press, 2013.
3. Chapel H, Haeney M, Misbah S, Nowden N. *Essentials of Clinical Immunology*, 6th edn. Oxford: Wiley-Blackwell, 2013.
4. Sompayrac L. *How the Immune System Works*, 4th edn. Oxford: Wiley-Blackwell, 2011.

Multiple choice questions

Questions

1. Which one of the following immunoglobulins are present in the greatest amounts at mucosal surfaces?
   A. IgA.
   B. IgE.
   C. IgG.
   D. IgM.
   E. IgD.
2. What are the typical cytokines secreted by T helper 2 (Th2) cells?
   A. IFN-beta, IL-4, IL-8.
   B. IL-4, IL-5, IL-10, IL-13.
   C. IFN-gamma, IL-2, IL-3.
   D. IL-17.
   E. IL-1, IL-6, TNF-alpha.
3. Which one of the following primary immunodeficiency disorders is due to a defect in neutrophil function?
   A. Bruton's agammaglobulinaemia.
   B. Wiskott–Aldrich syndrome.
   C. Common variable immunodeficiency.
   D. Chronic granulomatous disease.
   E. DiGeorge syndrome.

4. Deficiency in which complement component is likely to predispose to recurrent episodes of meningococcal meningitis.
   A. C1.
   B. C2.
   C. C3.
   D. C4.
   E. C5.
5. In the Gell and Coombs classification, what type of hypersensitivity reaction occurs in autoimmune haemolytic anaemia?
   A. Type I reaction.
   B. Type II reaction.
   C. Type III reaction.
   D. Type IV reaction.
   E. Type V reaction.
6. A 29-year-old man required a splenectomy as a result of a road traffic accident. Which of the following is not standard treatment as a result of the splenectomy?
   A. Pneumococcal vaccination.
   B. Meningococcal vaccination.
   C. Tetanus vaccination.
   D. Haemophilus vaccination.
   E. Prophylactic antibiotics.
7. Which of the following is not an indication for immunoglobulin therapy?
   A. Idiopathic thrombocytopenic purpura.
   B. Dermatomyositis.
   C. Guillain-Barre syndrome.
   D. Thrombotic thrombocytopenic purpura.
   E. Kawasaki disease.

Answers

1. A. IgA provides mucosal immunity and is predominantly found in secretions at mucosal surfaces. ➲ See Humoral mediators of the adaptive immune system, p. 150, for the function of the other immunoglobulin isotypes.
2. B. IL-4, IL-5, IL-10 and IL-13 are produced by Th2 cells. Th1 cells typically produce IFN-gamma and Th17 cells produce IL-17. IL-1, IL-6 and TNF-alpha are secreted by macrophages. ➲ See T cell response, p. 152, for further information on the actions of T cells.
3. D. Bruton's agammaglobulinaemia (X-linked agammaglobulinaemia) and common variable immunodeficiency are due to B cell/antibody defects. Wiskott–Aldrich syndrome and DiGeorge syndrome affect T cells (and B cells by extension as T cell help is required for B cells to function properly). ➲ See Primary immunodeficiency, p. 156 and Table 6.2.
4. E. Deficiency in any of the complement components making up the membrane attack complex (i.e. C5, C6, C7, C8 and C9) result in susceptibility to neisserial infections and recurrent meningococcal meningitis. Deficiency in C1, C2 or C4 result in autoimmune disease or an SLE-like syndrome. Deficiency in C3 results in serious pyogenic bacterial infections. ➲ See Primary immunodeficiency, p. 156 and Table 6.2.
5. B. Autoimmune haemolytic anaemia is a type II reaction where antibodies bind to cellular antigens (i.e. red cells in this instance) resulting in their destruction. ➲ See Hypersensitivity disorders, p. 160 (specifically section on Type II hypersensitivity, p. 161).

6. C. Patients with hyposplenism or asplenia are recommended to have vaccinations for encapsulated organisms (pneumococcus, haemophilus and meningococcus) and influenza, as well as prophylactic antibiotics to reduce the risk of infection. ➲ See Vaccines, p. 175–6 (specifically bullet point starting: Splenectomy and hyposplenism/asplenia).
7. D. The first-line treatment of thrombotic thrombocytopenic purpura is plasma exchange. Immunoglobulin therapy is *not* a recognised treatment for this condition. The Department of Health has published guidance on which conditions should be treated with immunoglobulin, which includes the other 4 conditions in the question. ➲ See Immunoglobulin therapy, p. 176 and Box 6.2.

Chapter 7 **Genitourinary Medicine and HIV**

Tom Wingfield, Gulshan Sethi and Simon Edwards

Genitourinary medicine service provision and sexually transmitted infection epidemiology in the UK

Many different providers contribute to the provision of sexual health care including general practice, family planning and third sector organisations (such as Brook centres for those aged under 25). Since 1917 specialist open access genitourinary medicine (GUM) services have been established for the management of sexually transmitted diseases (STIs). GUM clinics provide treatment of conditions and, if indicated, notify the partners of those affected. They also have some responsibility for recording epidemiological data.

Confidentiality and communication with other health-care professionals

The Venereal Diseases Regulations was first established in 1916 and provided specific legal obligations on patient confidentiality in GUM departments. These strict regulations apply to all GUM services in the UK and ensure that identifiable information is not shared beyond the clinic without specific patient consent. With the advent of electronic patient records careful consideration should be given to ensuring confidentiality is protected as a much wider group of staff may have access to a patient's notes.

Sexually transmitted infection epidemiology in the UK

For decades information on STI diagnoses has been collected through GUM clinics. The major advantage of the current system is that, in addition to diagnoses, information may be collected on a patient's place of residence, which enables rates of disease and testing to be calculated for different geographical areas/ local authorities.

Principles of treatment

Due to the infectious nature of STIs, people with infection are advised to abstain from sex until the infection has been treated, and partner notification and treatment is discussed at the time of diagnosis. A test of cure of infection post-treatment may be advised where antibiotic resistance is known.

Partner notification

A central tenet in the treatment of people with STIs is treatment of their sexual partners/contacts. This is known as 'partner notification'. The primary aim of partner notification is finding and treating new cases of STIs and providing epidemiological treatment to individuals exposed to STIs. This can be performed by the index case themselves (patient referral) or by the provider (provider referral).

For GUM epidemiology key points, see Box 7.1.

Box 7.1 GUM epidemiology key points

- In recent year, STI diagnoses have risen. There were 7137 diagnoses of syphilis reported in 2017, a 20% increase relative to the year prior and a 148% increase relative to 2008 There were 44,676 diagnoses of gonorrhoea reported in 2017, a 22% increase relative to the year prior.
- Large increases in STI diagnoses were seen in men who have sex with men (MSM), although partly due to increased testing in this population; high levels of condomless sex probably contributed to the rise.
- MSM are a group at increased risk of specific sexually transmitted infections (STIs) such as gonorrhoea, syphilis and lymphogranuloma venereum (LGV).
- Young adults (aged 16–24 years) account for >50% of all STI diagnoses, despite making up only 12% of the population. Factors contributing to this increased risk in young adults are thought to include higher rates of sexual partner change and higher numbers of concurrent partnerships than in older age groups.

Data from: Alcabes P, Muñoz A, Vlahov D, Friedland GH. Incubation period of human immunodeficiency virus. *Epidemiological Review*, 1993; 15:303-308; Cohen MS, Gay C, Busch M, et al. The detection of acute HIV infection. *Journal of Infectious Diseases*, 2010;202: S270-S277

Genitourinary tract anatomy and physiology

Figures 7.1 and 7.2 show the male and female reproductive organs respectively. Tables 7.1 and 7.2 show the function and structure of the respective reproductive systems.

Non-gonoccocal urethritis

Pathogenesis

Urethritis (inflammation of the urethra) in men is a multifactorial condition, which can be sexually acquired. The organisms most commonly associated with non-gonoccocal urethritis (NGU) are:

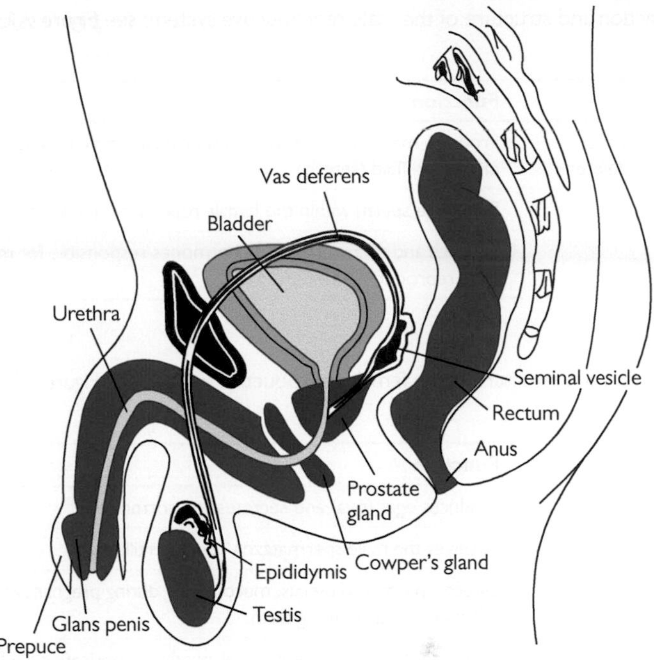

Figure 7.1 Male reproductive organs.

Reproduced with permission from Handy P. MBE. The standard clinic process and sexual health in primary care. In *Oxford Handbook of Genitourinary Medicine, HIV, and Sexual Health*, 2nd edn, Pattman R. et al. (eds). Oxford: OUP. Copyright © 2010 Oxford University Press. DOI: 10.1093/med/9780199571666.001.1. Reproduced with permission of the Licensor through PLSclear.

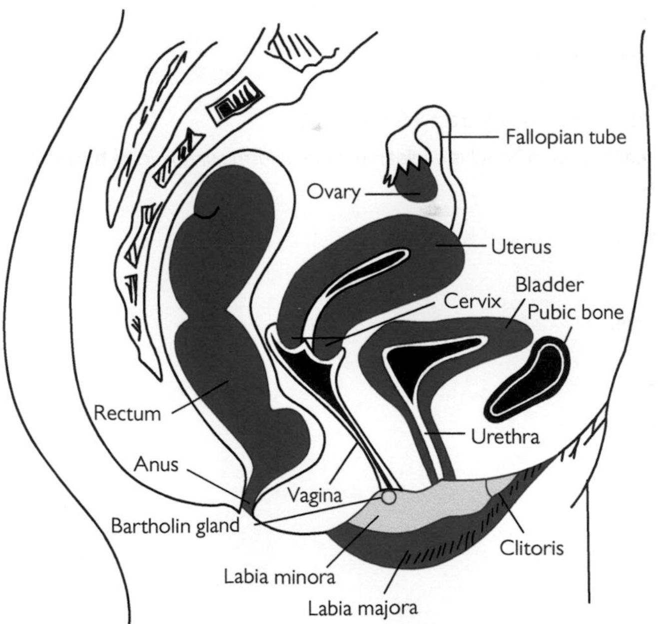

Figure 7.2 Female reproductive organs.

Reproduced with permission from Handy P. MBE. The standard clinic process and sexual health in primary care. In *Oxford Handbook of Genitourinary Medicine, HIV, and Sexual Health*, 2nd edn, Pattman R. et al. (eds). Oxford: OUP. Copyright © 2010 Oxford University Press. DOI: 10.1093/med/9780199571666.001.1. Reproduced with permission of the Licensor through PLSclear.

Table 7.1 The function and structure of the male reproductive system; see Figure 7.1 for male genital anatomy

Structure	Function
Prostate, bulbourethral gland, seminal vesicles, ductus deferens.	Produce, maintain and transport sperm (the male reproductive cells) and protective fluid (semen).
Ejaculatory ducts, penis.	Discharge sperm within the female reproductive tract during sex.
Testes.	Produce and secrete male sex hormones responsible for maintaining the male reproductive system.

Table 7.2 The function and structure of the female reproductive system; see Figure 7.2 for female genital anatomy

Structure	Function
Ovaries.	Produces eggs (ova) and secretes sex hormones.
Oviduct.	Receives the male spermatazoa during fertilisation.
Cervix.	Directs sperm into uterus, mucous plug during pregnancy prevents infections, dilates during birth.
Vagina.	Delivers fetus through birth canal, produces lubricating fluids.
Uterus.	Site of embryo development.

- *Chlamydia trachomatis* (11–43%).
- *Mycoplasma genitalium* (9–25%).
- Adenoviruses 2–4%.
- *Trichomonas vaginalis* (1–20%).
- *Herpes simplex* virus (2–3%).
- Other organisms causing urinary tract infection (6%).

The exact role of ureaplasmas in NGU is unclear, but *Ureaplasma urealyticum* biovar 2 is thought to account for 5–10% of NGUs.

Clinical presentation

Symptoms

- Urethral discharge.
- Dysuria.
- Penile irritation.
- May be asymptomatic.

Signs

- Urethral discharge.
- Examination may be normal.

Diagnosis

The diagnosis of NGU is made by confirming the presence of polymorphonuclear leukocytes (PMNLs) in the anterior urethra. This can be done in two ways:

- A Gram-stained urethral smear (which for diagnosis should contain ≥5 PMNL per high power microscopic field, averaged over five fields with greatest concentration of PMNLs); and/or
- a Gram-stained preparation from a centrifuged sample of a first passed urine specimen (which for diagnosis should contain ≥10 PMNL per high power microscopic field, averaged over five fields with greatest concentration of PMNLs).

A mid-stream urine (MSU) should also be taken if a urinary tract pathogen is suspected. As part of the diagnostic work-up, full STI screen should be performed to test for human immunodeficiency virus (HIV), *Treponema pallidum, Neisseria gonorrhoeae* and *Chlamydia trachomati.*

Additional screening for *Mycoplasma genitalium* (MG) and *Trichomonas vaginalis* (TV) should be undertaken in men presenting as a contact of people with these infections or with recurrent or persistent urethritis. It is likely that as availability of testing for these infections becomes more widespread that testing will be become part of initial screening and assessment.

Management

First line treatment:

- Doxycycline 100 mg twice a day (BD) orally for 7 days.

Alternatives:

- Azithromycin 1 g stat orally followed by 500 mg (OD) for 2 days or ofloxacin 200 mg BD or 400 mg once daily (OD) for 7 days.

Complications

- Persistent/recurrent NGU that is defined as persistent or recurrent symptomatic urethritis occurring 30-90 days following treatment of acute NGU:
  - Occurs in 10-20% of patients, the aetiology being unknown.
  - May be treated with a prolonged course of macrolides/doxycycline plus metronidazole depending on the first line treatment.
- Acute epididymo-orchitis (➲ see Epididymo-orchitis, p. 202 and Table 7.9).

Sexually acquired reactive arthritis/Reiter's syndrome

Reactive arthritis (ReA) is a sterile inflammation of the synovial membrane, tendons and fascia triggered by a remote infection, typically GI or sexually transmitted. ReA activated by an STI is referred to as sexually acquired reactive arthritis (SARA). In addition to the classical triad of urethritis, arthritis and conjunctivitis in Reiter's syndrome, cutaneous or mucous membrane lesions, such as keratoderma blennorrhagica, circinate balanitis/vulvitis, uveitis and oral ulceration, and cardiac or neurological involvement may occur (➲ see Chapter 20, Reactive arthritis, p. 716 and Box 20.3).

Vulvovaginitis

Pathogenesis

The causative agents/ organisms are:

- *Candida albicans* 80–92%.
- Non-albicans species, e.g. *Candida glabrata, Candida tropicalis, Candida krusei, Candida parapsilosis* and *Saccharomyces cerevisiae*.

Clinical features

Symptoms

- Vulval itch.
- Vulval soreness.

- Vaginal discharge.
- Superficial dispareunia.
- External disuria.

Signs

- Erythema.
- Fissuring.
- Discharge, non-offensive and typically curdy.
- Oedema.
- Satellite lesions.
- Excoriation.

Diagnosis

Budding hyphae/spores in wet slide (sensitivity 40–60%) or Gram-stained film of vaginal secretions (sensitivity 65–80%). Positive *Candida* culture on Sabouraud's selective medium.

Management

20% of women during reproductive years may be colonized with *Candida* sp., but have no clinical signs or symptoms. These patients do not require treatment.

First-line treatment

- Fluconazole 450 mg OD orally and clotrimazole 1% cream BD topically for 7 days to the vulva. Oral fluconazole is of equal efficacy to intravaginal treatments, but is significantly less expensive. Oral fluconazole is not licensed in pregnancy.

Second-line treatments

- Clotrimazole pessary 500 mg vaginally nocte as a single dose and clotrimazole 1% cream BD topically for 7 days.
- Clotrimazole 10% vaginal cream 5 g vaginally nocte as a single dose and clotrimazole 1% cream BD topically for 7 days.

Complications

Recurrent vulvovaginal candidiasis

- This is defined as >4 confirmed episodes of vulvovaginal candidiasis in a 12-month period.
- Consider the presence of any predisposing factors, including recent use of antibiotics and immunosuppression (e.g. long-term steroid dependence, HIV, diabetes).
- Consider the presence of non-albicans species, the majority of which are *Candida glabrata*. While most non-albicans species have higher minimum inhibitory concentrations (MICs) to -azoles, *Candida krusei* is intrinsically resistant to fluconazole. Speciation and resistance testing may be required. Treatment is with fluconazole 150 mg every 72 hours for three doses, followed by maintenance therapy with fluconazole 150 mg once each week for (up to) 6 months.

Balanitis

Pathogenesis

Balanitis is inflammation of the glans penis, often involving the prepuce (balanoposthitis) and affects approximately 10% of men attending a GUM clinic. For causes of balanitis, see Table 7.3.

Table 7.3 Causes of balanitis

	Common	Uncommon
Infectious	*Candidia albicans.* Anaerobes. HPV. Syphilis. *Herpes simplex.* *Staphylococcus aureus.* Streptococci (Group A and B).	Follman balanitis due to syphilis. *Entamoeba histolytica.* Mycobacteria. *Trichomonas vaginalis.*
Skin disorders	Lichen sclerosus. Psoriasis. Zoon's balantitis.	Stevens–Johnson syndrome. Lichen planus. Fixed drug eruption. Circinate balanitis.
Miscellaneous	Trauma. Irritant. Poor hygiene.	Contact allergy. Premalignant condition (Bowen's disease, Bowenoid papulosis, erythroplasia of Queyrat).

Clinical presentation

Presenting symptoms

- Local rash.
- Soreness.
- Itch.
- Odour.
- Inability to retract foreskin.
- Discharge from glans/behind foreskin.

Associated symptoms

- Rash elsewhere on the body.
- Sore mouth.
- Joint pains.
- Swollen/painful lymphadenopathy locally or distally.

For signs associated with balanitis, see Table 7.4.

Table 7.4 Signs associated with balanitis

Genital signs	Erythema, scaling, ulceration, fissuring, crusting, exudate, oedema, leukoplakia, sclerosis, purpurae, odour, phimosis.
General signs/systemic manifestations	Lymphadenopathy, non-genital rash, oral ulceration, arthritis.

Complications

- Phimosis (inability to retract prepuce over glans penis).
- Meatal stenosis.
- Malignant transformation.

Investigations

It is paramount that a full STI screen is performed in all cases of balanitis. Other investigations include:

- Subpreputial (under the foreskin) swab for *Candida* and bacterial culture.
- Urine analysis for glucose.
- Consider swab for *Chlamydia trachomatis* to exclude lymphogranuloma venereum (LGV).
- Herpes simplex/*Treponema pallidum* PCR if ulcer present.
- Dark ground microscopy to exclude syphilis if ulcer present.
- A biopsy may be indicated in persistent cases.

Management

The following treatments should be considered:

- Combined topical antifungal/steroid (such as Canesten HC® OD) if candidal balanitis is suspected (continued until symptoms have resolved).
- If an anaerobic infection is diagnosed (such as *Bacteroides* spp.) treatment is with metronidazole 400 mg BD for 7 days.
- Moisturising soap substitutes such as emulsifying ointment is advisable as soaps can be irritant to inflamed skin.
- Ongoing symptoms may require a specialist dermatology opinion with view to a diagnostic biopsy.

Chlamydia and lymphogranuloma venereum

Chlamydia

Pathogenesis

Chlamydia trachomatis (serovars D to K) is the most common STI in the UK. Recent data confirm that 5–10% of sexually active men and women under 24 years of age are currently infected with chlamydia. As chlamydia is often asymptomatic and it can have serious health consequences (including pelvic inflammatory disease [PID]), opportunistic screening through the National Chlamydia Screening Programme remains an essential element of good quality sexual health services for young adults.

Clinical presentation

- In women:
  - Asymptomatic in approximately 70%.
  - Post-coital or intermenstrual bleeding.
  - Lower abdominal pain.
  - Purulent vaginal discharge.
  - Mucopurulent cervicitis and/or contact bleeding.
  - Dysuria.
- In men:
  - Asymptomatic in >50% in a community setting.
  - Urethral discharge.
  - Dysuria.
- *Rectal infections:* Usually asymptomatic, but may cause anal discharge and anorectal discomfort (proctitis).
- *Pharyngeal infections:* These are uncommon and usually asymptomatic.
- *Conjunctival infections*:
  - Chlamydia can cause an inclusion conjunctivis, which may present with a red eye and associated mucopurulent conjunctival discharge.
  - *Chlamydia trachomatis* (serovars A–C), can cause trachoma, predominantly in the developing world. Worldwide, it is the leading cause of preventable blindness of infectious origin.

Complications

- PID:
  - occurs in 10–40% of patients;
  - risk increases with each recurrence of chlamydia;
  - can result in tubal factor infertility, ectopic pregnancy and chronic pelvic pain.
- Fitz-Hugh–Curtis syndrome (perihepatitis).
- Neonatal transmission (neonatal conjunctivitis, pneumonia).
- Epididymo-orchitis.
- Adult conjunctivitis.
- SARA/Reiter's syndrome (commoner in men).

Diagnosis

Testing using nucleic acid amplification technique (NAAT) is the standard of care with NAATs being 90–95% sensitive and 99–100% specific.

Management

- First line treatment (regardless of site): doxycycline 100 mg oral BD for 7 days.
- Second line treatment: azithromycin 1 g stat orally followed by 500 mg OD for 2 days.
- Alternative treatments: erythromycin 500 mg oral BD for 14 days *or* ofloxacin 200 mg BD or 400 mg OD for 7 days.

Lymphogranuloma venereum

Pathogenesis

LGV is a systemic disease caused by one of three invasive serovars L1, L2 or L3 of *Chlamydia trachomatis*. It has an incubation period of between 1 and 6 weeks. LGV is endemic in some parts of Africa, Asia, South America and the Caribbean, and may cause outbreaks of mostly proctitis in MSM.

Clinical presentation

Primary stage

- Anogenital ulcer:
  - non-specific appearance;
  - may be tender ± induration;
  - often transient and goes unnoticed;
  - resolves spontaneously.
- Primary proctitis can occur following direct rectal inoculation of the organism in MSM. This usually presents as a severe haemorrhagic proctitis with pain, bleeding and purulent anal discharge.

Secondary stage

- Usually inguinal lymphadenitis ± suppuration and bubo formation
  - may be bilateral ± 'groove sign' (nodes above and below inguinal ligament; Figure 7.3);
  - buboes may rupture and cause chronic discharging sinuses.
- Proctitis may occur at a secondary stage in heterosexual LGV with associated pelvic lymphadenitis.

Tertiary stage

- Lymphatic obstruction.
- Fibrosis and scarring.
- Lymphoedema and elephantiasis including esthiomene (elephantiasis of the female genitals).
- Rectal stricture.

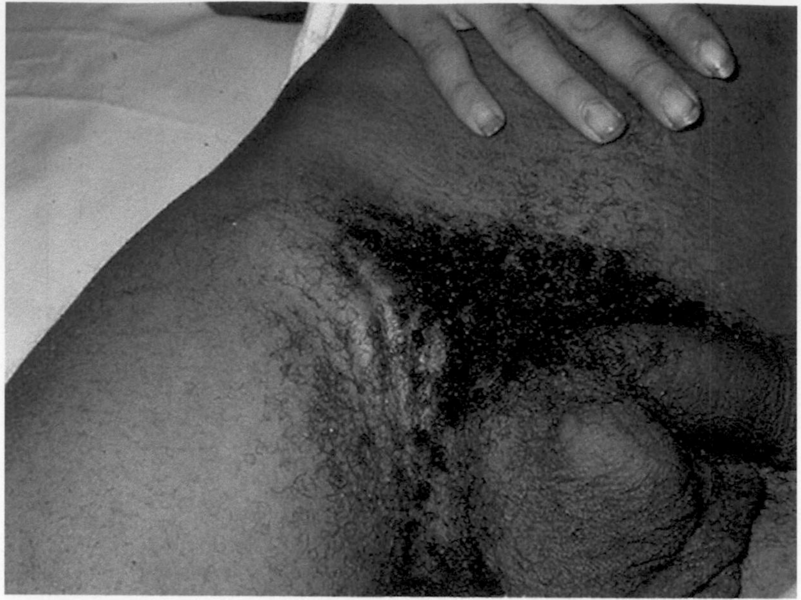

Figure 7.3 (see colour plate section) Groove sign in lymphogranuloma venereum.
Reproduced with permission from Edson, R.S. Sexually Transmitted Diseases. In *Mayo Clinic Infectious Diseases Board Review*. Temesgen Z (Ed.). Oxford, UK: OUP. Copyright © 2012 Mayo Foundation for Medical Education and Research. DOI: 10.1093/med/9780199827626.001.0001. Reproduced with permission of the Licensor through PLSclear.

Diagnosis

- Testing for *Chlamydia trachomatis* using NAAT is the standard of care.
- Alternatively, or in addition, a swab may be taken from an ulcer, the rectum, urethra, cervix or any other site that shows features of infection.
- Buboes should be aspirated using a lateral approach through unaffected skin and the aspirated pus can be transferred to a swab.
- LGV is confirmed when DNA from the L-serovars are detected.

Management

- First-line treatment: doxycycline 100 mg BD for 21 days.
- Second-line treatment: erythromycin 500 mg QDS orally for 21 days. Azithromycin may be considered in exceptional circumstances (such as intolerance or allergy to doxycycline), and at an increased dose of 1 g weekly for 21 days or 500 mg daily for 10–14 days.

Gonorrhoea

Pathogenesis

The Gram-negative intracellular diplococcus *Neisseria gonorrhoeae* is spread by sexual contact, including vaginal, anal and oral sex. Infection can occur from contact with asymptomatic individuals. The transmission rate during one episode of vaginal sex is likely to be:

- 20–40% risk from infected woman to male partner.
- 60–90% risk from infected man to female partner.

The incubation period for gonorrhoea has a wide range with a median in males of about 6 days.

Clinical presentation

Women

- Asymptomatic in approximately 50%.
- Post-coital or intermenstrual bleeding.
- Lower abdominal pain.
- Purulent vaginal discharge.
- Mucopurulent cervicitis and/or contact bleeding.
- Dysuria.

Men

- Urethral discharge.
- Dysuria.
- Asymptomatic in 10%.

Rectal infection is usually asymptomatic, but may cause anal discharge and anorectal discomfort (proctitis). Pharyngeal infection is commonly asymptomatic.

Diagnosis

- *Neisseria gonorrhoeae* can be diagnosed by detection of amplified nucleic acid and by culture.
- Microscopy of Gram-stained specimens from the ano-genital mucosae can facilitate rapid diagnosis of *Neisseria gonorrhoeae* in symptomatic patients.

Microscopy

- A direct smear for Gram-staining of urethral discharge in men or endocervical discharge in women demonstrates intracellular Gram-negative kidney-shaped diplococci in polymorphonuclear leukocytes (Figure 7.4)

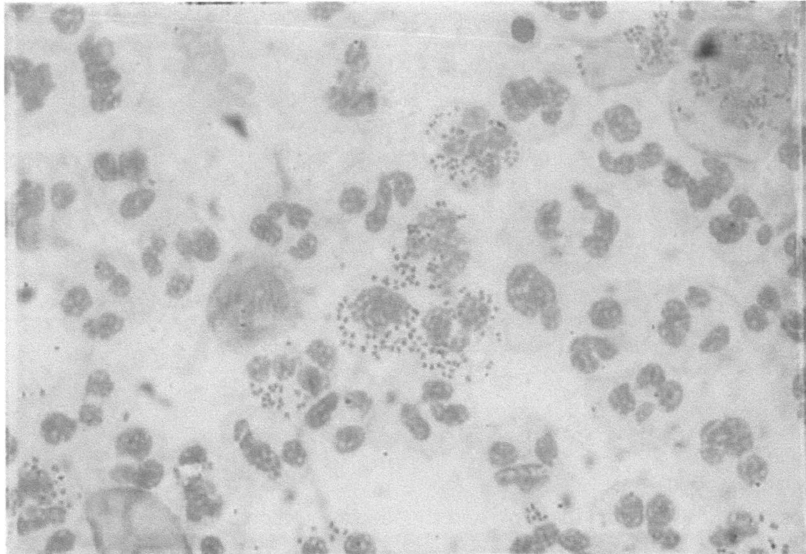

Figure 7.4 Gram-stained urethral discharge showing Gram-negative intracellular diplococci.

Reproduced with permission from Barlow D. et al. Neisseria gonorrhoeae. In *Oxford Textbook of Medicine*, Fifth Edition, Warrell D.A. et al. (Eds.). Oxford, UK: OUP. Copyright © 2010 Oxford University Press. DOI: 10.1093/med/9780199204854.001.1. Reproduced with permission of the Licensor through PLSclear.

- May be used as a near patient test (to provide an immediate presumptive diagnosis of gonorrhoea).
- Culture is essential to determine antimicrobial susceptibility in cases of treatment failure and for monitoring emerging resistance to therapy.
- Microscopy has poor sensitivity for detecting rectal and pharyngeal infection.

NAATs for Neisseria gonorrhoeae:

- Have become the most popular screening test in the UK and are generally more sensitive than culture.
- Show high sensitivity (>96%) in both symptomatic and asymptomatic infection.
- Provide testing on a wider range of specimen types and are less demanding in specimen quality, transportation and storage.

Management

Antimicrobial treatment eradicates 95% of uncomplicated gonococcal infections within the community. Recommended first line therapies are based on the results of national surveillance of emerging antimicrobial resistance patterns.

For treatment guidance for uncomplicated gonorrhoea in adults, see Table 7.5.

Table 7.5 Treatment guidance for uncomplicated gonorrhoea in adults

Treatment	**Injection suitable**	**Injection refused or contraindicated**
First line: all uncomplicated anogenital (e.g. urethral, cervical, pharyngeal and rectal) gonorrhoea in adults.	Ceftriaxone 1 g in 3.5 mL 1% lidocaine, when antimicrobial sensitivity known: ciprofloxacin 500 mg orally.	Cefixime 400 mg orally as a single dose *plus* azithromycin 2 g orally.
Second line: all uncomplicated anogenital gonorrhoea in adults.	• In patients with pencillin allergy, all third-generation cephalosporins, such as ceftriaxone (negligible cross-allergy with penicillins). • In cases of penicillin anaphylaxis: ◆ gentamicin 240 mg IM as a single dose plus azithromycin 2 g orally ◆ or if other options unsuitable: spectinomycin* (unlicensed) 2 g IM as a single dose plus azithromycin 2 g orally (grade 1B) ◆ *or* azithromycin 2 g as a single oral dose ◆ NB: Cefixime cannot be used in penicillin anaphylaxis.	• In patients with pencillin allergy, all third-generation cephalosporins, such as cefixime (negligible cross-allergy with penicillins). • If organism known to be sensitive to penicillins: amoxicillin 2 g orally *plus* probenecid 1 g orally.

* Spectinomycin is not recommended for pharyngeal infection due to poor rates of eradication.

Complications

- Epididymo-orchitis.
- Pelvic inflammatory disease.
- Arthritis-dermatitis syndrome (disseminated gonococcal infection [DGI]).
- Conjunctivitis.

Further reading

1. GRASP: The Gonococcal Resistance to Antimicrobials Surveillance Programme (https://assets.publishing.service.gov.uk/government/uploads/system/uploads/attachment_data/file/651636/GRASP_Report_2017.pdf
2. BASHH guidelines (https://www.bashh.org/guidelines).

Syphilis

Pathogenesis

The causative organism for syphilis is the spirochaete *Treponema pallidum*. Syphilis has an incubation period of between 9 and 90 days (average 21 days). Sexual transmission in adults is most common, with non-sexual transmission (e.g. kissing) rare and transmission by fomite rarer still. Individuals remain infectious for approximately 2 years, up to the end of the early latent stage.

Clinical features

These are conventionally divided into early (within 2 years of infection) and late disease (>2 years since infection) (Table 7.6).

Figure 7.5 shows the rash and papular lesions associated with secondary syphilis.

Table 7.6 Clinical signs and symptoms at different stages of syphilis

Stage	Timing after infection	Signs and symptoms
Primary	6 weeks after infection	Classically a single painless ulcer (chancre). Ulcers may be atypical, multiple, painful, purulent, destructive or extra-genital.
Secondary	Within 2 years of infection	Generalised polymorphic rash usually non-pruritic and affecting the palms and soles (Figures 7.5A–C); mucocutaneous lesions including condylomata lata, mucous patches and snail track ulcers; generalised lymphadenopathy. *Less commonly*: patchy alopecia; anterior uveitis; meningitis; cranial nerve palsies; hepatitis and splenomegaly.
Late latent syphilis	2 years after infection	Asymptomatic.
Symptomatic late syphilis		
Meningovascular	2–7 years	Asymptomatic. Focal arteritis inducing infarction/meningeal inflammation; signs dependent on site of vascular injury.
General paresis	10–20 years	Cortical neuronal loss; gradual decline in memory and cognition, emotional lability, personality change, psychosis and dementia. Seizures and hemiparesis are late complications.
Tabes dorsalis	15–25 years	Inflammation of spinal dorsal column/nerve roots; lightening pains, areflexia, paraesthesia, sensory ataxia, Charcot's joints, mal perforans, optic atrophy, pupillary changes (e.g. Argyll Robertson pupil; ➲ see Chapter 18, Argyll Robertson pupils, p. 651).
Cardiovascular	10–30 years	Aortitis (usually ascending); asymptomatic, substernal pain, aortic regurgitation, heart failure, coronary ostial stenosis, angina, aneurysm.
Gummatous	1–46 years Average 15	Inflammatory granulomatous destructive lesions can occur in any organ, but most commonly affect bone and skin.

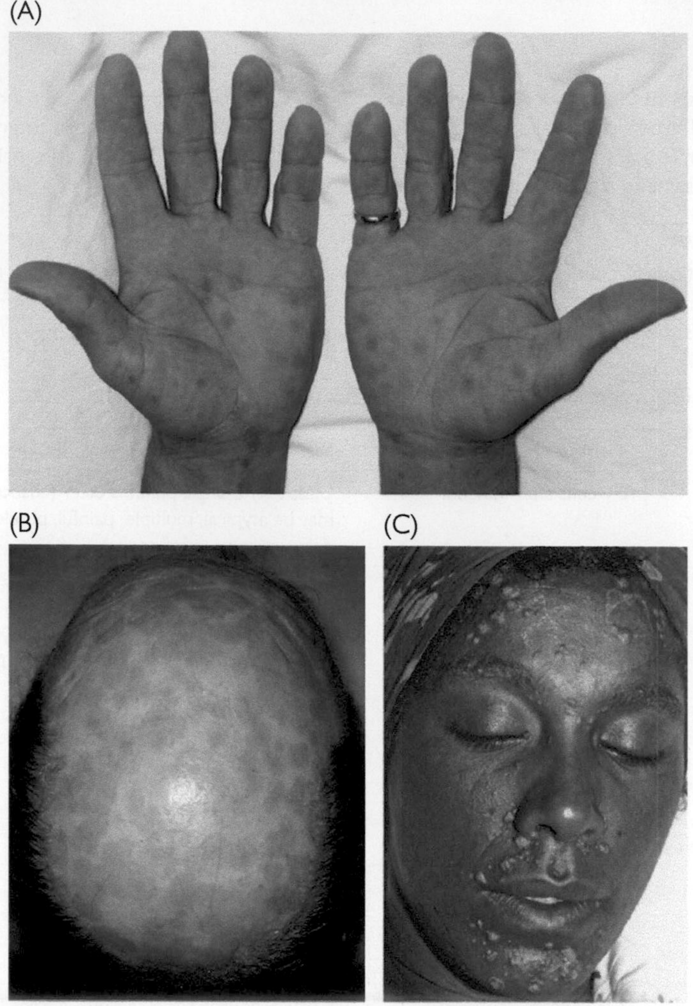

Figure 7.5 (see colour plate section) (A, B) Rash of secondary syphilis on palms and scalp. (C) Papular lesions of secondary syphilis.

Diagnosis

Microscopy

- Demonstration of *Treponema pallidum* from lesions of primary or secondary syphilis by dark ground microscopy (Figure 7.6).

Serological tests for syphilis

- The screening test is a combined specific treponemal IgG/IgA ELISA. If positive, further tests are rapid plasma regain (RPR) and *Treponema pallidum* particle agglutination assay (TPPA).
  - TPPA is a specific treponemal test used to confirm a positive ELISA result.

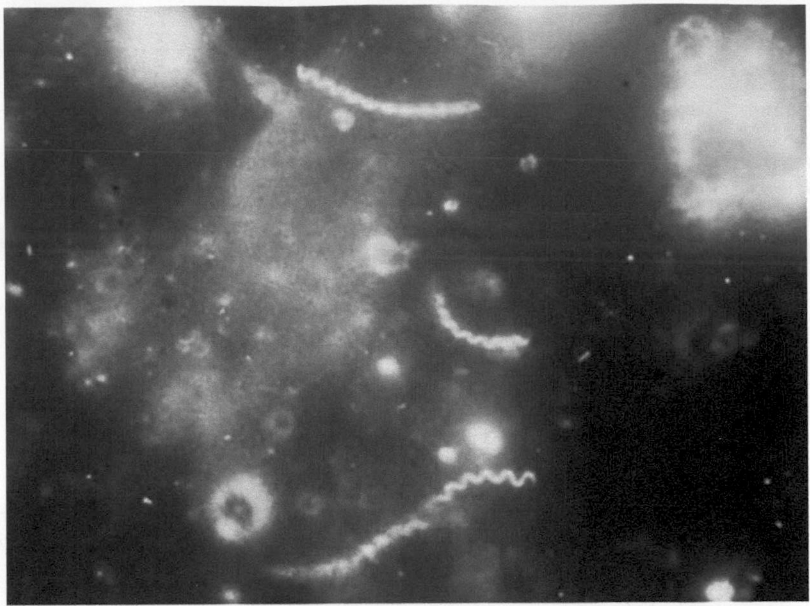

Figure 7.6 *Treponema pallidum* on dark-field examination.

Reproduced with permission from Edson, R.S. Sexually Transmitted Diseases. In *Mayo Clinic Infectious Diseases Board Review*. Temesgen Z (Ed.). Oxford: OUP. Copyright © 2012 Mayo Foundation for Medical Education and Research. DOI: 10.1093/med/9780199827626.001.0001. Reproduced with permission of the Licensor through PLSclear.

  - RPR is a non-specific test, which may be used to stage the infection and to guide treatment response.
- Fluid obtained from genital ulcers can identify primary syphilis using PCR techniques (gold standard test).

For the diagnosis and staging of syphilis, see Table 7.7.

Table 7.7 Diagnosis and staging of syphilis; test interpretation

EIA (enzyme immunoassay)	**TPHA (*Trepnoema pallidum* haemagglutination assay)**	**RPR (rapid plasma reagin)**	**Interpretation**
Negative	Negative	Negative	No serological evidence of syphilis.
Positive	Positive	Positive	Untreated or recently treated syphilis. Follow RPR titre.
Positive	Positive	Negative	Possible syphilis (early or latent) or previously treated syphilis.
Positive	Negative	Negative	Probable false-positive IgG.

Management

A full physical examination is essential to stage the disease at presentation and inform further treatment options. Table 7.8 shows the treatment options.

Table 7.8 Treatment of syphilis

Indication	Treatment
Early syphilis (primary, secondary and early latent): • Patients with neurological or ophthalmic involvement in early syphilis should be managed as per neurosyphilis recommendations.	Benzathine benzylpenicillin 2,400,000 units = 2.4 mega units IM once only (commonly used to encourage compliance) *or* Procaine benzylpenicillin G 600 mg (600,000 units) IM daily for 10 days. If IM injection refused: Doxycycline 100 mg BD PO for 14 days,
Late latent/cardiovascular/gummatous syphilis.	Benzathine benzylpenicillin 2,400,000 units = 2.4 mega units IM weekly for 3 doses (days 1, 8 and 15) *or* Procaine benzylpenicillin 600,000 units IM OD for 14 days *or* If IM injection refused: Doxycycline 100 mg PO BD for 28 days.
Neurosyphilis including neurological/ ophthalmic involvement in early syphilis: • Systemic steroids are used frequently as adjunctive therapy with a lack of consensus amongst guidelines for their use.	Procaine benzylpenicillin 1.2 mega units deep IM in buttock daily *plus* oral probenecid 500 mg PO QDS for 14 days *or* Benzylpenicillin 10.8–14.4 g IV daily given as 1.8–2.4 g every 4 hours for 14 days. If patient declines parenteral treatment: Amoxicillin 2 g TDS PO *plus* probenecid 500 mg QDS PO for 28 days. Alternative oral regime: Doxycycline 200 mg PO BD for 28 days.

Further reading

1. Syphilis and Lymphogranuloma Venereum: Resurgent Sexually Transmitted Infections in the UK: 2009 report. https://assets.publishing.service.gov.uk/government/uploads/system/uploads/attachment_data/file/396987/Syphilis_and_Lymphogranuloma_Venereum_-_Resurgent_Sexually_Transmitted_Infections_in_the_UK.pdf

Epididymo-orchitis

Pathogenesis

- Acute epididymo-orchitis is a clinical syndrome consisting of pain, swelling and inflammation of the epididymis and/or testes.
- The most common route of infection is local extension, arising from direct spread from the urethra (sexually transmitted pathogens) or the bladder (urinary pathogens).
- In older men for whom an STI is not suspected, the most frequent organisms are Gram-negative enteric organisms causing urinary tract infections. Particular risks include recent instrumentation or catheterisation.

For causes of epididymo-orchitis, see Table 7.9.

Table 7.9 Causes of epididymo-orchtits

	Common	Uncommon
Sexually transmitted infection	*Chlamydia trachomatis* *Neisseria gonorrhoeae*	*Mycoplasma genitalium*
Non-sexually transmitted infection	Mumps Gram-negative enteric organisms	*Mycoplasma tuberculosis* *Brucella*
Other causes		Amiodarone Behçet's syndrome

Clinical features

- Unilateral scrotal pain and swelling of relatively acute onset.
- If sexually transmitted, symptoms of urethritis or a urethral discharge. The urethritis is, however, often asymptomatic.
- If uro-pathogen related, symptoms suggestive of urinary infection or a history of bacteriuria.

Important differential diagnoses

- Testicular neoplasm should be considered if a discrete testicular mass is present (i.e. it is not possible to separate the epididymal mass from a testicle). An urgent ultrasound scan and referral is warranted.
- Torsion is more common in men <20 years of age (peak incidence amongst adolescents), but may occur at any age.

Diagnosis

Diagnosis is primarily based on clinical findings. Further investigations may include a urethral smear, urinalysis, MSU, STI screen and imaging studies (ultrasound testes).

Management

- Scrotal support, e.g. jock strap or supportive underwear and avoidance of strenuous exercise/sexual intercourse. Bed rest may be necessary in some instances.
- Simple analgesia (ibuprofen 400 mg BD oral for 14 days).
- Symptoms may take up to a month to resolve. Patients should be advised to abstain from sexual intercourse for the duration of their antibiotic treatment.
- Partner notification should be considered if an STI is suspected. Treatment should include antibiotics known to be effective against gonorrhoea.
- Ofloxacin 200 mg BD oral for 14 days should be reserved for patients likely to have an enteric infective cause.
- If a sexually acquired epididymo-orchitis is suspected, ceftriaxone 1 g IM single dose *plus* doxycycline 100 mg by mouth BD for 14 days is recommended.

Pubic lice and scabies

Pubic lice

Pathogenesis

The crab louse *Phthirus pubis* is transmitted by close body contact. The incubation period is usually between 5 days and 4 weeks, although occasionally individuals appear to have more prolonged, asymptomatic infestation.

Symptoms and signs

Adult lice infest coarse hairs of the pubic area, body hair and, rarely, eyebrows and eyelashes, and lay eggs (nits) which adhere to the hairs (and are commonly visible).

The patient may be asymptomatic or complain of itch due to hypersensitivity to feeding lice and blue macules (maculae caeruleae) may be visible at feeding sites. Eggs attached at the end of hairs (as opposed to close to skin surface) suggest that infection has been present for a longer duration.

Diagnosis

Diagnosis is commonly made on clinical examination by the positive finding of adult lice and/or eggs. Examination under light microscopy can confirm the morphology if necessary.

Management

Patients should be advised to avoid close body contact until they and their partner(s) have completed treatment. Resistance to topical and systemic pediculicide treatment has been reported. If the infestation persists, a different class of pediculicide should be applied

Recommended treatment regimens:

- Malathion 0.5%: apply to dry hair and wash out after at least 2, but preferably, 12 hours (usually left on hair overnight).
- Permethrin 1% cream rinse: apply to damp hair and wash out after 10 minutes.
- Phenothrin 0.2%: apply to dry hair and wash out after 2 hours.

Scabies

Pathogenesis

- This infestation is caused by the mite *Sarcoptes scabiei*. Mites burrow into the skin where they lay eggs; the resulting offspring crawl out onto the skin and make new burrows. They may infest/infect/affect any part of the body. Transmission is by skin-to-skin contact.
- The absorption of mite excrement into skin capillaries generates a hypersensitivity reaction. The predominant symptom is a generalised pruritus, which may take 4–6 weeks to develop and is often worse/more intense at night.

Clinical presentation

- Characteristic silvery lines may be seen in the skin where mites have burrowed. Common sites include the interdigital folds, the wrists and elbows, and around the nipples in women.
- Papules or nodules may result from itching/scratching and often affect the genital area.
- Nodular scabies is a well-known clinical presentation of scabies. The nodules occur in approximately 1:10 patients with scabies, especially in young children, and can persist for many months after treatment. They are thought to be due to hypersensitivity reactions to dead mites.
- Crusted scabies (Norwegian scabies) is a severe form of scabies in which the lesions are often extensive and hyperkeratotic. Nail dystrophy and scalp lesions may be prominent. Crusted lesions teem with mites and pose a significant risk of onward transmission. This type of scabies is well recognised in immunosuppressed individuals.

Diagnosis

The clinical appearance is usually typical, but may pose diagnostic confusion with other pruritic conditions such as eczema. Light microscopy of scrapings from burrows may reveal mites.

Recommended treatment regimens

- Permethrin 5% cream.
- Malathion 0.5% aqueous lotion.

The lotion or cream is applied to every area of the body from the chin and ears downwards. It should be left on for between 8–24 hours depending on which preparation is used. Two applications (1 week apart) are recommended. Resistance to topical treatment has been reported. If the infestation persists, a different agent should be tried. Oral ivermectin has been used with success at a dose of 200 μg/kg, repeated after 1 week. Antihistamines can be used to treat pruritus.

Complications

Secondary infection of the skin lesions can occur following repeated scratching and should be treated appropriately.

Further reading

1. IUSTI guidelines for treatment of pediculosis pubis and scabies. https://www.iusti.org/regions/europe/euroguidelines.htm

Human papilloma virus

Pathogenesis

- There are over 100 genotypes of HPV. HPV types 6 and 11 cause 95% of anogenital warts. HPV types 16 and 18 cause 75% of cervical cancers, 80% of anal cancers, 60% of vaginal cancers and 40% of vulval cancers.
- Oncogenic HPV types are also associated with the development of head and neck cancers.
- The mode of transmission is most often by sexual contact but HPV may be transmitted perinatally. Genital lesions resulting from transfer of infection from hand warts have been reported in children.
- Latent period may be months to years and the condition may recur.

Clinical features

Warts may be single or multiple. Those on the warm, moist, non-hair-bearing skin tend to be soft and non-keratinised; those on dry, hairy areas of skin firm and keratinised. Lesions may be broad based or pedunculated; some are pigmented.

Diagnosis

Diagnosis is made by the recognition of typical warty lesions. In rare cases, where the lesion is atypical or pigmented, a biopsy may be required.

Treatment

Treatment choice depends on morphology, number and distribution of warts, as well as patient preference and cost of therapy. Treatment may be complicated by discomfort and local skin reactions:

- Soft keratinized warts respond well to podophyllotoxin. Podophyllotoxin is a purified form of podophyllin, which is suitable for self-application and is available in a 0.5% solution and 0.15% cream (Warticon® and Condyline®).
- Keratinised lesions are better treated with physical ablative methods, such as cryotherapy, excision or electrocautery. Cryotherapy uses liquid nitrogen spray to cause disruption of the cell membrane at the dermal/epidermal junction resulting in cell injury and death.
- Imiquimod may be suitable for both keratinised and non-keratinised warts. It acts as a toll like receptor-7 agonist that stimulates local tissue macrophages to release interferon alpha and other cytokines as part of a local cell mediated response. Imiquimod is available as a 5% cream (Aldara®).
- Surgical excision: large or pedunculated warts can be removed under local anaesthetic.

Complications

Oncogenic HPV can predispose to intra-epithelial neoplasia and cancer. Physicians must be vigilant about atypical/hyperpigmented lesions and refer for biopsy, especially on a background of immunosuppression (e.g. diabetes, post-transplant, HIV infection).

Vaccination

There are currently three commercially available vaccines: Gardasil® 4; Gardasil® 9 and Cervarix™:

- Gardasil® 4 is a quadrivalent vaccine able to protect against HPV types 6, 11, 16 and 18. Gardasil® 9 is a 9-valent vaccine with additional protection against types 31, 33, 45, 52 and 58. They both reduce the prevalence of anogenital warts and development of pre-malignant/HPV associated malignancies.
- Cervarix™ is a bivalent vaccine providing immunity against HPV types 16 and 18.

Gardasil® and Cervarix™ are designed to elicit virus-neutralizing antibody responses that prevent initial infection with the HPV types represented in the vaccine. The vaccines have been shown to offer 100% protection against the development of cervical precancers and genital warts caused by the HPV types in the vaccine, with few or no side effects. The protective effects of the vaccine are expected to last a minimum of 4.5 years after the initial vaccination. From 2019, all boys and girls in England aged between 12 and 13 are being given a vaccine to protect them against HPV-related disease.

Further reading

1. Vaccinations. https://www.nhs.uk/conditions/vaccinations/hpv-human-papillomavirus-vaccine/
2. Statement on HPV vaccination. https://assets.publishing.service.gov.uk/government/uploads/system/uploads/attachment_data/file/726319/JCVI_Statement_on_HPV_vaccination_2018.pdf

Herpes simplex virus

Pathogenesis

- Herpes simplex virus type 1 (HSV-1) and type 2 (HSV-2) are double-stranded DNA viruses of the herpes virus family, Herpesviridae.
- HSV-1 is the usual cause of oro-labial herpes and is currently the commonest cause of genital infection. HSV-2 was historically associated with sexual transmission, but is now a less common cause.
- Infection may be primary or non-primary, initial or recurrent, symptomatic or asymptomatic.
- HSV-1 and -2 are transmitted by contact with an infectious area of the skin during re-activations of the virus. Approximately 80% and 12% of adults will have been exposed and developed antibodies to HSV 1 and 2, respectively.

Latency and recurrence

Following primary infection, the virus becomes latent in local sensory ganglia, periodically reactivating to cause symptomatic lesions, or infectious asymptomatic viral shedding.

Clinical features of genital herpes

Symptoms

- Local: painful ulcerations (external genitalia ± cervix, rectum); urethral discharge; dysuria; anal discharge; rectal pain/tenesmus; saddle pain.
- Systemic (commoner in primary infection): fevers; myalgia.

Signs

- Vesicles/blisters/ulcers; tender inguinal lymphadenitis; proctitis.
- Atypical presentations: non-specific erythema; erosions; fissures.

Complications

- Auto-inoculation: infected people can transmit the virus and infect other parts of their own bodies, most often the hands, thighs or buttocks.
- Autonomic neuropathy, resulting in urinary retention.
- Aseptic meningitis.

For variant HSV infections, see Box 7.2.

Diagnosis

- PCR for type-specific HSV DNA: swab taken from the base of the lesion (de-roof blister if necessary).
- HSV serology: although not recommended in routine practice for the diagnosis of genital lesions, the detection of HSV-1 IgG, HSV-2 IgG or both, in a single serum sample represents

Box 7.2 Variant HSV infections

- *Localised or disseminated eczema herpeticum*: caused by HSV-1. Commonly develops in patients with atopic dermatitis, burns, or other inflammatory skin conditions. Children are most commonly affected.
- *Herpes whitlow*: vesicular outbreaks on the hand, most commonly due to infection with HSV-1. It usually occurs in children who suck their thumbs, and occurred in health-care workers prior to the widespread use of gloves. The occurrence of herpes whitlow due to HSV-2 is increasingly recognized, probably due to digital–genital contact.
- *Herpes gladiatorum*: caused by HSV-1. It is seen as papular or vesicular eruptions on the torsos of athletes in sports involving close physical contact (classically wrestling).
- *Disseminated HSV infection*: occurs in females who are pregnant and in individuals who are immunocompromised. These patients may present with atypical signs and symptoms of HSV; therefore, the condition may be difficult to diagnose.
- *HSV encephalitis*: presents with fever, encephalopathy and focal neurological signs.
- *Neonatal HSV*: primary HSV infection in late pregnancy can have devastating effects on the fetus. Neonatal HSV usually manifests within the first 2 weeks of life and clinically ranges from localised skin, mucosal or eye infections to encephalitis, pneumonitis, disseminated infection and death.

HSV infection at some time. It can be difficult to establish whether the infection is recent as IgM detection is unreliable and avidity studies are not commonly available. Collection of serum samples a few weeks apart can be used to show seroconversion and this, in turn, can demonstrate/be assumed to represent recent primary infection. HSV-2 antibodies are indicative of genital herpes; HSV-1 antibodies do not differentiate between genital and oropharyngeal infection.

Management of genital herpes

First episode

- General advice: saline baths and simple analgesia.
- Topical anaesthetic agents (e.g. 5% lidocaine [lignocaine] ointment): especially prior to micturition, but should be used with caution because of the risk of potential sensitization.
- Recommended treatment regimens (all for 5 days duration):
  - Aciclovir 200 mg five times daily or aciclovir 400 mg TDS.
  - Valaciclovir 500 mg BD.
  - Famciclovir 250 mg TDS.

Management of complications

- Hospitalisation may be required if complicated by urinary retention, meningism and severe constitutional symptoms.
- Catheterisation: if indicated, suprapubic catheterisation is preferred to prevent the theoretical risk of ascending infection. This may also reduce the pain associated with the catheterisation and allow restoration of normal micturition without the need for multiple recurrent procedures.

Recurrent genital herpes

- Recurrences are self-limiting and generally cause minor symptoms.
- Preventative therapy may be considered in patients with frequent recurrences. If recurrences are identifiable with a prodrome then episodic treatment can be considered to abort an attack, otherwise long-term suppressive therapy may offer an alternative.
- Episodic treatment: aciclovir 800 mg TDS for 2 days or famciclovir 1 g BD for one day or valaciclovir 500 mg BD for 3 days.
- Suppressive treatment: aciclovir 400 mg BD/famciclovir 250 mg BD/valaciclovir 500 mg OD for 6 months to 1 year.

Further reading

1. British Association of Sexual health and HIV Guidelines.(https://www.bashh.org/guidelines.

Trichomonas vaginalis

Pathogenesis

Trichomonas vaginalis is a flagellated protozoon, which affects the squamous epithelium of the genital tract. It is found mainly in the vagina, urethra and para-urethral glands. It is one of the most commonly encountered STIs globally with an estimated 170 million cases occurring each year. In the UK over 90% cases are identified in women and is more commonly isolated in non-white ethnic groups. The mechanisms of pathogenesis are not well understood, although adhesion of TV to vaginal epithelial cells is a critical step.

Clinical presentation

Symptoms and signs in women

- 10–50% are asymptomatic.
- Vaginal discharge, vulval itching, dysuria or offensive odour.
- Occasionally, low abdominal discomfort or vulval ulceration.
- Up to 70% have vaginal discharge, from thin and scanty to profuse and thick.
- Classical frothy yellow discharge occurs in 10–30%.
- Signs of vulvitis, vaginitis and 2% of patients have strawberry cervix.

Symptoms and signs in men

- 15–50% are asymptomatic and usually present as sexual partners of infected women.
- Urethral discharge and/or dysuria.
- Urethral irritation, urinary frequency and rarely purulent urethral discharge or prostatitis.
- Rarely balanoposthitis.

Complications

- Preterm delivery and/or low birthweight infant.
- Predisposition to maternal post-partum sepsis.
- Facilitation of HIV transmission.
- PID.
- Alterations to the normal vaginal flora, increasing susceptibility to bacterial vaginosis.
- Infertility in women and men.
- Acute and chronic prostatitis in men.

Diagnosis

Light field microscopy on the discharge mixed with a drop of normal saline is performed to detect motile trichomonads for men and women presenting with discharge or inflammatory symptoms. NAATs offer the highest sensitivity for the detection of TV and should be the 'gold standard' test of choice where resources allow.

Treatment

First-line

- Metronidazole 2 g orally in a single dose or metronidazole 400–500 mg BD for 5–7 days.

Alternative regimens

- Tinidazole 2 g orally in a single dose.

HIV epidemiology and virology

Globally, 37.0 million people are estimated to be living with HIV and over 35 million are estimated to have died from HIV since the epidemic started. In sub-Saharan Africa nearly 1 in every 20 adults are affected, accounting for 69% of all people living with HIV. Worldwide, HIV is spread mainly through heterosexual sex. While new infection rates have fallen by 50% or more in 25 countries (including 13 in sub-Saharan Africa), they have increased in five countries in Eastern Europe and Central Asia (1,2). Intravenous drug use (IVDU) continues to drive the epidemic in Eastern Europe. Effective control of HIV infection during pregnancy, combined with avoidance of breastfeeding, can almost eliminate mother to child transmission.

The significant advances in HIV therapy (referred to as combination antiretroviral therapy; ART) has resulted in HIV becoming a manageable illness with a near normal life expectancy. Worldwide, however, there remains vast inequity in provision of treatment and care.

UK epidemiology of HIV

100,000 people are estimated to be living with HIV infection in the UK, of whom a quarter are undiagnosed. New diagnoses have declined over the last decade. Overall, HIV prevalence in the UK is approximately 2 per 1000 people, rising to >5 per 1000 in specific areas (e.g. London and Manchester). MSM and persons from black African communities are disproportionately affected in the UK (47 and 37 per 1000 people, respectively).

HIV treatment coverage is high. Of people on ART in 2017, 97% were virally supressed with a viral load ≤200 copies per mL and, therefore, very unlikely to pass on HIV, even if having sex without protection.

HIV virology

HIV is a retrovirus that stores its genetic information as single-stranded RNA (Figure 7.7). An enzyme called reverse transcriptase converts the RNA to DNA, which is subsequently incorporated into the host cell DNA. Thus, the host cell is 'hijacked' to produce further HIV copies.

For modes of transmission of HIV, see Table 7.10.

Immunological effect

- HIV preferentially infects CD4 T cells, macrophages and dendritic cells, primarily through an interaction between the HIV-1 envelope glycoprotein, gp120, with two host cell receptors, CD4 and a chemokine receptor (CCR5 or CXCR4).
- The virus is transferred to CD4 T cells within lymph nodes where most of viral replication occurs.
- During primary HIV infection and seroconversion, there is CD4 proliferation and a concurrent transient peak of HIV replication.
- Without treatment, progressive immunodeficiency occurs, leading to susceptibility to certain opportunistic infections (OIs) and eventually death (Figure 7.8).
- The best surrogate measure of immune function and risk of OIs is measurement of CD4 T cell count.

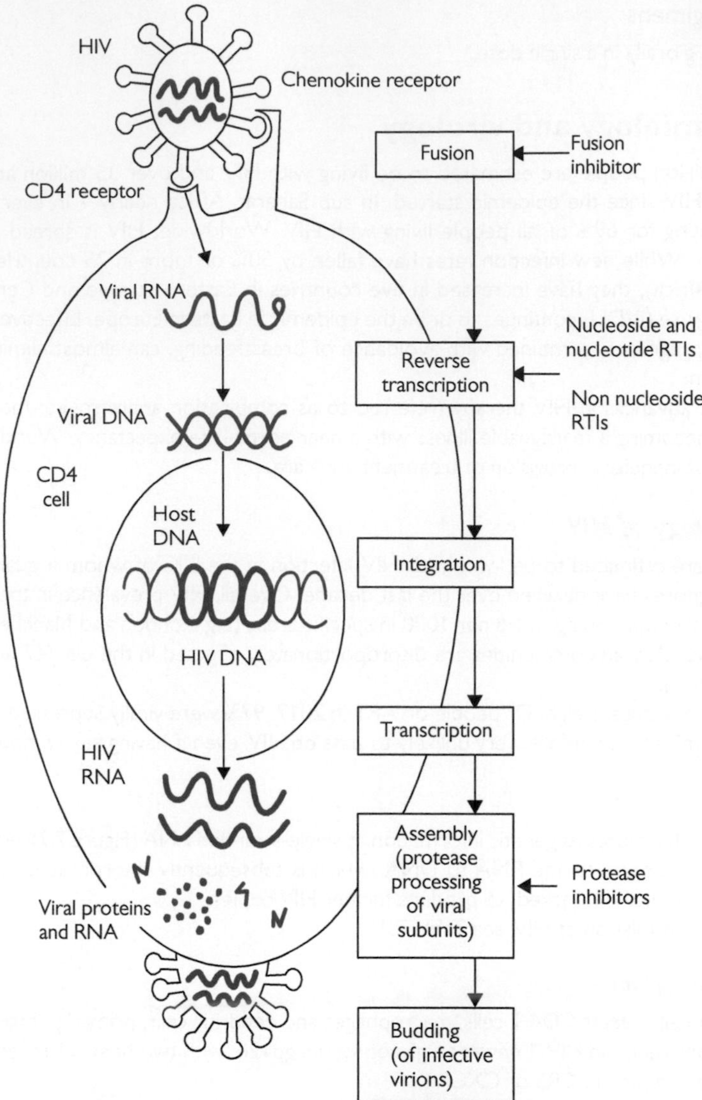

Figure 7.7 HIV life cycle and stages of action of ART.

Reproduced with permission from Handy P. MBE. The standard clinic process and sexual health in primary care. In *Oxford Handbook of Genitourinary Medicine, HIV, and Sexual Health*, 2nd edn, Pattman R. et al. (eds). Oxford: OUP. Copyright © 2010 Oxford University Press. DOI: 10.1093/med/9780199571666.001.1. Reproduced with permission of the Licensor through PLSclear.

Seroconversion, immunosuppression and the natural history of HIV/AIDS

For stages of HIV infection without treatment after transmission, see Figure 7.9.

Primary HIV infection/seroconversion illness

The majority of patients experience some symptoms, which are commonly similar to acute viral illness – general malaise, non-suppurative pharyngitis, lymphadenopathy, mild fever and maculopapular rash.

Table 7.10 Modes of transmission of HIV

Transmission route	Interventions that have been shown to reduce transmission
Sexual intercourse (anal, vaginal and oral)	Condoms. Treatment as prevention (providing HIV treatment to an HIV positive person in order to prevent transmission of HIV). HIV pre- and post-exposure prophylaxis (prevention of HIV in an uninfected person by taking antiretroviral therapy before and around the time of exposure). Male circumcision. Behavioural change.
Contaminated needles	Needle exchange schemes. Post-exposure prophylaxis.
Mother-to-child	HIV treatment to mother during pregnancy and childbirth. HIV treatment to infant post-natally. Avoidance of breastfeeding.
Tissue donation (blood transfusion and organ donation)	HIV screening of samples for donation.

Latent clinical period (± primary generalised lymphadenopathy)

- This stage varies in duration and is asymptomatic apart from possible presence of primary generalised lymphadenopathy (PGL), the main HIV reservoir being lymphoid tissue.

Early symptomatic HIV infection

- The immunosuppressive consequence of HIV predisposes to conditions including oral candida, oral hairy leukoplakia, seborrhoeic dermatitis, herpes zoster, cervical dysplasia or carcinoma in situ, and idiopathic (or thrombotic) thrombocytopenic purpura. These are not acquired immune deficiency syndrome (AIDS)-defining illnesses and classically occur prior to AIDS.

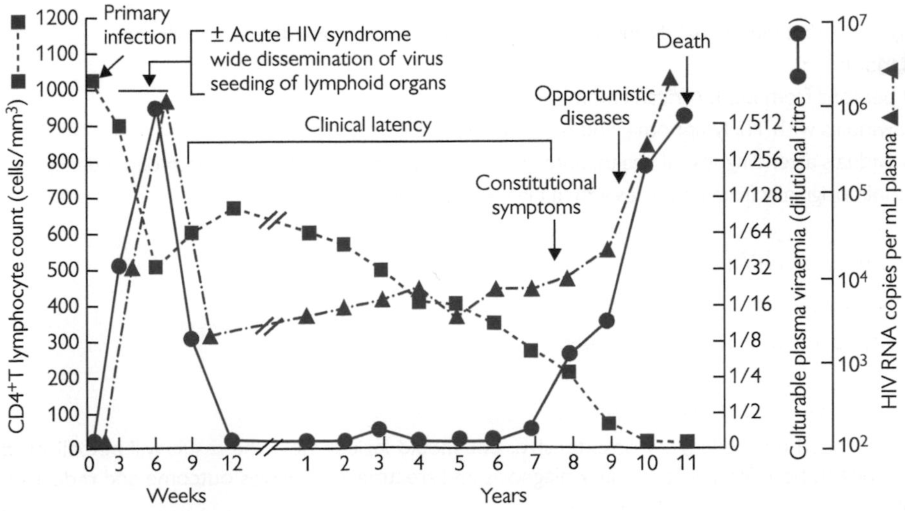

Figure 7.8 Changes in CD4 count and HIV viral load over time and disease susceptibility.

From *The New England Journal of Medicine*, G. Pantaleo et al. The Immunopathogenesis of Human Immunodeficiency Virus Infection. 328:327-335. Copyright © 1993, Massachusetts Medical Society. Reprinted with permission from Massachusetts Medical Society. DOI: 10.1056/NEJM199302043280508.

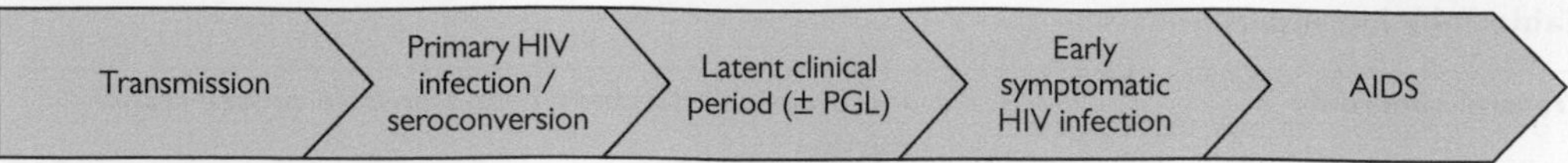

Figure 7.9 Stages of HIV infection without treatment after transmission. PGL = Primary generalised lymphadenopathy.

Acquired immune deficiency syndrome

As CD4 T cells are depleted, a collection of defined illnesses may develop that make up acquired immune deficiency syndrome (see Box 7.3). These OIs usually occur many years after HIV acquisition.

Box 7.3 Common AIDS-defining illnesses

- Pneumocystis *jirovecii* pneumonia (previously known as pneumocystis *carinii* pneumonia; PCP).
- Oesophageal candidiasis.
- Wasting syndrome (unintentional loss of >10% body weight).
- TB.
- *Mycobacterium avium* complex (MAC): disseminated.
- CMV disease (other than liver, spleen or nodes).
- Toxoplasmosis of the brain.
- Recurrent bacterial pneumonia.
- Kaposi sarcoma.
- Cryptococcosis: extrapulmonary.
- Lymphoma (non-Hodgkin's lymphoma, Burkitt's lymphoma, primary CNS lymphoma).

HIV testing

Guidelines from the British HIV Association (BHIVA) state that early recognition, testing and treatment of HIV saves lives and reduces potential onward transmission. BHIVA and NICE suggest universal HIV testing if HIV prevalence is >2 per 1000. In these areas, HIV testing should be offered to all people registered with primary care (GP) or presenting to secondary (hospital) care. In addition, universal HIV testing is also recommended for:

- anyone with a differential diagnosis of HIV seroconversion or an HIV-related illness;
- all MSM;
- all persons from Black African communities;
- individuals with TB, lymphoma, and hepatitis B and/or C;
- individuals attending sexual health, antenatal, termination of pregnancy or drug-dependency services;
- people originally from countries with a high HIV prevalence.

Practicalities of HIV testing

Who can counsel and take the test?

Any nurse, doctor or health-care provider.

What does pre-test counselling consist of?

Counselling need not be lengthy or extensive, but should include how the result will be delivered, the intended health benefits, and that early diagnosis and treatment improves outcome and reduces transmission.

Giving HIV test results

Arrangements for when and how the result will be given should be discussed at the time of testing. Face-to-face provision of HIV test results is encouraged in the following settings:

- ward-based patients;
- patients suspected of having a positive result;
- those with mental health problems/suicide risk;
- highly anxious or vulnerable individuals;
- those for whom English is a second language;
- young people under 16 years.

Which test?

- The preferred HIV test is one that tests for HIV antibody and p24 antigen simultaneously.
- The first detection of p24 occurs approximately 17 days after exposure (range 13–28 days), whereas first detection of HIV antibody is approximately 22 days after exposure (range 18–34 days). The 'window period' is the time in which an HIV serological test may be falsely negative.

Pneumocystis *jirovecii* pneumonia

Pneumocystis *jirovecii* pneumonia (PCP) is a fungus that causes disease in immunosuppressed individuals.

Clinical presentation

- Insidious onset of dyspnoea, cough (mostly non-productive), weight loss and low-grade fever.
- Pneumothorax may cause an acute deterioration and is a poor prognostic indicator.
- Chest auscultation is commonly clear. Extra-pulmonary PCP is rare.
- PCP is usually diagnosed in individuals unaware of their HIV status, or those who decline ART or PCP prophylaxis when CD4 falls <200.

Investigations

- Chest radiograph (Figure 7.10) shows diffuse, bilateral, midzone, interstitial or alveolar infiltrates, and may show pneumothorax.
- Oxygen desaturation on ambulation or exercise.

Diagnosis

- Visualisation of organism using immunofluorescent or Grocott stain from samples, e.g. induced sputum or bronchoalveolar lavage. PCR assays may be available in high-income settings but are not widely available globally.

Treatment

- First line:
  - Supplementary oxygen, ventilatory support.
  - Co-trimoxazole or clindamycin and primaquine for 21 days. Alternatives – pentamidine/atovaquone/trimethoprim + dapsone, although atovaquone and dapsone are only used in milder disease.
- Steroids should be given if pO_2 is <9.3 kPa.

Cytomegalovirus

Cytomegalovirus is a human herpes DNA virus found worldwide, and transmitted through blood, semen and vaginal secretions. In severely immunocompromised patients (CD4<50) end-organ damage results from uncontrolled viral replication.

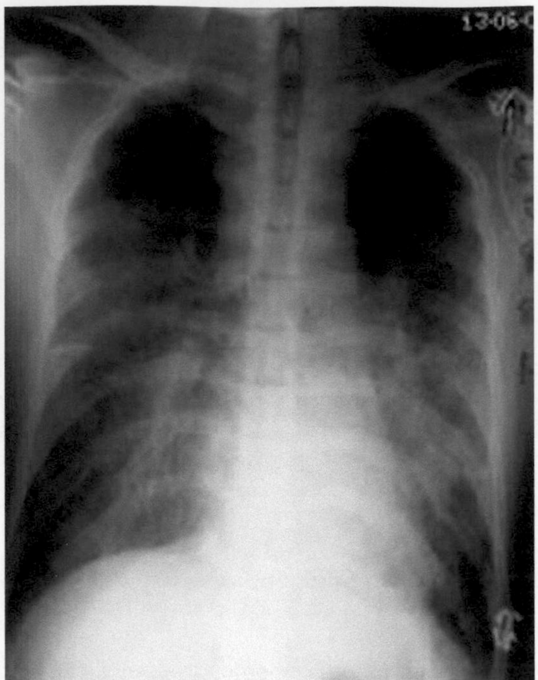

Figure 7.10 Typical Chest X-ray PCP.

Clinical presentation

Common sites include:

1. GI tract (colitis with bloody diarrhoea, oesophageal ulceration with pain and reflux).
2. Retinal (visual disturbance with distinctive fundoscopy; see Figure 7.11).
3. Nervous system: encephalitis or less frequently polyradiculitis.

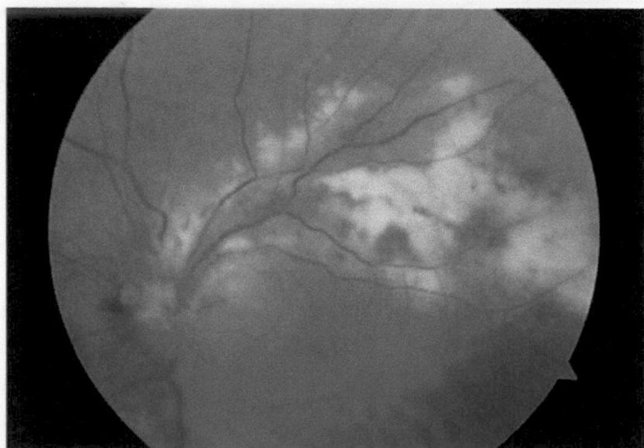

Figure 7.11 (see colour plate section) CMV retinitis, commonly termed 'cheese pizza' or 'pizza pie' retina.
Reproduced with permission from Frith P. The eye in general medicine. In *Oxford Textbook of Medicine*, 5th edn, Warrell D. A. et al. (eds). Oxford: OUP. Copyright © 2013 Oxford University Press. DOI: 10.1093/med/9780199204854.001.1. Reproduced with permission of the Licensor through PLSclear.

Investigations

These depend on clinical presentation. CMV can be identified by immunoglobulins (CMV IgM in acute infection), CMV PCR, biopsy (e.g. GI tract with distinctive 'owl's eyes' appearance on microscopic observation), and culture.

Diagnosis

- Histopathological confirmation provides definitive proof, though often diagnosis is clinical (e.g. retinitis).
- CMV encephalitis: confirmed by a positive CMV PCR on cerebrospinal fluid.
- Serum CMV viraemia in an immunocompromised patient does not in itself indicate end-organ damage.

Treatment

- First line: IV ganciclovir or PO valganciclovir; intraocular ganciclovir device can be used in CMV retinitis. Second line: foscarnet.
- Duration of treatment 2–4 weeks depending on site and severity.
- Secondary prophylaxis (treatment to prevent recurrence/relapse of disease) is indicated for retinitis and can be continued until CD4>100 cells/mm^2 for 3 to 6 months.

Candidiasis, Kaposi's sarcoma and other skin manifestations

Candidiasis

Organism

Candida species, most commonly *Candida albicans*.

Clinical presentation

Occurs in patients with CD4<200, and commonly presents with painless oropharyngeal white lesions (see Figure 7.12). Oesophageal involvement may lead to odynophagia and reflux-type symptoms.

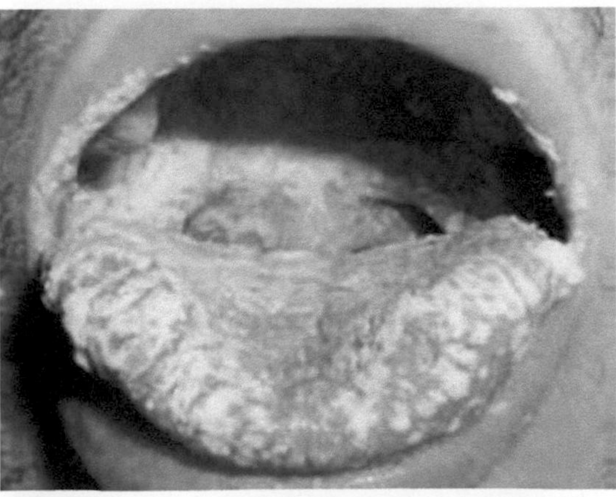

Figure 7.12 (see colour plate section) Oropharyngeal candida.

Republished with permission of MA Healthcare Ltd from Wingfield T., Wilkins E. Opportunistic infections in HIV disease. *Br J Nurs*. 19(10):621–7. Copyright © 2013 MA Healthcare Ltd, a Mark Allen Group company. https://doi.org/10.12968/bjon.2010.19.10.93543. Permission conveyed through Copyright Clearance Center, Inc.

Investigations

- Gastroscopy is limited to individuals with oesophageal symptoms who do not improve with empiric antifungal therapy.
- Swabs, scrapings and biopsies of affected areas for species identification and resistance profiling. This is important for non-albicans infection and for increasingly prevalent '–azole' resistance.

Diagnosis

- Characteristic clinical presentation coupled with known degree of immunosuppression is often sufficient.

Treatment

- First line: topical or oral fluconazole depending on extent of disease. Alternatives include itraconazole and echinocandins.

Kaposi sarcoma (KS) and other skin lesions

Organism

Tumour caused by Human herpes virus-8 (HHV-8).

Clinical presentation

- Most commonly occurs in patients with CD4<200, and presents with multiple skin lesions which are non-tender, raised, dark purple and indurated (Figure 7.13).
- Other sites involved:
  - Intraoral lesions are common.
  - Visceral KS can involve the GI tract (diarrhoea sometimes with protein-losing enteropathy) or pulmonary system (cough, dyspnoea ± haemoptysis).
  - Lymph glands: may lead to lymphoedema.

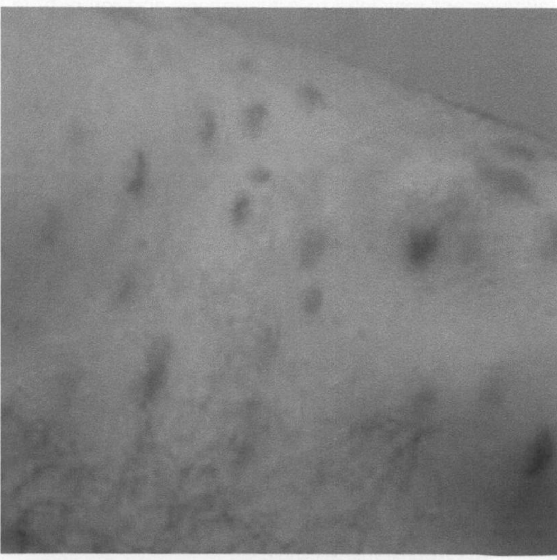

Figure 7.13 (see colour plate section) Kaposi sarcoma lesions.

Investigations

- Bronchoscopy may allow visualisation of endobronchial lesions.
- Radiological findings include interstitial or nodular lesions ± effusions in lung; lymphadenopathy ± hepatosplenomegaly in disseminated disease.

Diagnosis

Cutaneous and oral disease often provide a clinical diagnosis. Histopathological confirmation is required for visceral disease and when chemotherapy is being considered.

Treatment

ART is the mainstay of treatment. Chemotherapy is advocated for advanced cutaneous and visceral disease (e.g. liposomal anthracyclines – doxorubicin).

Other skin lesions

There are a plethora of skin and mucocutaneous manifestations associated with HIV infection, some AIDS defining, and others non-specific but important indicators aiding diagnosis (see Table 7.11).

Table 7.11 Skin infections associated with HIV induced immunosuppression

Organism group	Infection
Virus	*Varicella zoster* virus (multidermatomal), *Herpes simplex* virus, pox viruses (cause molluscum contagiosum), human papilloma virus, HHV-8.
Bacteria	Staphylococcal skin infections, bacillary angiomatosis (caused by *Bartonella henselae* and *quintana*).
Fungal	*Candida* sp. (rarely without mucosal involvement), dermatophytosis ('tinea'), cryptococcosis, histoplasmosis, penicilliosis.
Other	Seborrhoeic dermatitis, Malassezia furfur, severe ('Norwegian') scabies.

Toxoplasma

Organism

Toxoplasma are protozoa found worldwide, transmitted via cat faeces. It is the commonest cause of mass lesions in immunodeficient persons.

Clinical presentation

- Headache0 with rapidly evolving focal neurological deficits (over 1–2 weeks), confusion, seizures.

Investigations

- MRI is preferred over CT with greater sensitivity in picking up the characteristic findings of multiple ring-enhancing lesions in the cortical gray–white matter border and the basal ganglia; often accompanied by significant oedema and potentially midline shift.
- Consider brain biopsy only in suspected cases not responding to treatment.

Diagnosis

- Diagnosis is presumed by a clinical and radiological response to treatment. 85% of people with toxoplasma encephalitis will be serum toxoplasma IgG antibody positive.
- PCR of CSF for toxoplasma is highly specific to exclude the diagnosis, but has poor sensitivity.

For differential diagnosis of space-occupying lesions in immunodeficient persons, see Box 7.4.

Box 7.4 Differential diagnosis of space-occupying lesion in immunodeficient persons

- Cerebral toxoplasmosis.
- Primary CNS lymphoma.
- Progressive multifocal leukoencephalopathy.
- Cerebral tuberculosis.
- Cryptococcosis.
- Metastatic non-Hodgkin's lymphoma.
- Non-HIV related coexistant diagnosis.

Treatment

- First-line: sulfadiazine or clindamycin, plus pyrimethamine and folinic acid.
- Adjunctive steroids: indicated if seizures or signs of raised intracranial pressure.

Cryptococcus

Organism

Encapsulated yeast, *Cryptococcus neoformans*. Spread by inhalation of yeast found in pigeon droppings.

Clinical presentation

- Subacute meningitis or meningoencephalitis is the most common presentation; may be disseminated.
- Severe unremitting headache.
- Other features include confusion, seizures or personality change.

See Figure 7.14 for an MRI showing multiple ring-enhancing cryptococcal lesions.

Investigation

- Serum and CSF cryptococal antigen are highly sensitive and specific. India ink stain and fungal culture should be performed on serum and CSF.
- Interpretation of CSF in cryptococcal meningitis and other infections (➲ see Chapter 8, CSF studies, p. 244 and Table 8.16).

Treatment

- First-line: liposomal amphotericin B and flucytosine (induction phase – 2 weeks), followed by high-dose fluconazole (maintenance phase – 6 weeks).
- Therapeutic LPs may be required repeatedly to relieve symptoms associated with raised ICP.

Mycobacterial disease

Tuberculosis

➲ See Chapter 8, Tuberculosis, p. 260, and Tables 8.8, 8.25, 8.26 and 8.27 and Figure 8.2.

Non-tuberculous mycobacteria

A variety of non-tuberculous mycobacteria (NTM) exist, also known as environmental mycobacteria, atypical mycobacteria, or mycobacteria other than TB. *Mycobacterium avium* complex (MAC) infection is the most common NTM disease requiring treatment. Since the roll out of ART, and earlier diagnosis and initiation of therapy, MAC is not commonly encountered in HIV-positive patients in high-resource settings.

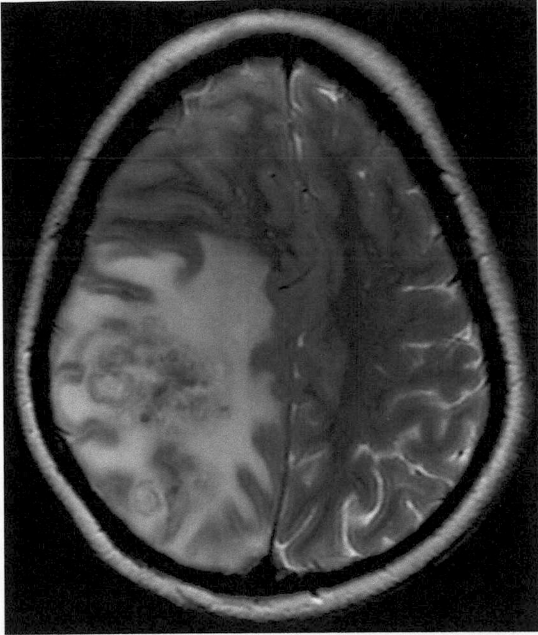

Figure 7.14 T2-weighted MRI showing multiple ring-enhancing cryptococcal lesions with cerebral oedema and mid-line shift in patient with immune reconstitution syndrome.

Reproduced with permission from Wingfield T. et al. Persistent cryptococcal brain infection despite prolonged immunorecovery in an HIV-positive patient. *Case Rep Neurol Med.* 2014(164826). Copyright © 2014 Tom Wingfield et al. doi: 10.1155/2014/164826. This is an open access article distributed under the Creative Commons Attribution License, which permits unrestricted use, distribution, and reproduction in any medium, provided the original work is properly cited.

MAC typically occurs in patients with a CD4 <50 cells/mm^3. Signs are often non-specific, including weight loss, fever, night sweats, fatigue and GI disturbances. Multiple organs may be affected, although local manifestations include lymphadenitis, pericarditis, pneumonitis, osteomyelitis and abscesses. Clinical examination may reveal lymphadenopathy and/or hepatosplenomegaly.

Investigations for MAC include appropriate and repeated mycobacterial culture of body fluids or biopsy. Common laboratory abnormalities include anaemia, pancytopenia, raised alkaline phosphatase (ALP). MAC is diagnosed by positive culture.

Clinical symptoms alongside histopathologic features of granulomas and acid-fast bacilli should prompt initiation of antimycobacterial therapy. Treatment consists of a macrolide plus ethambutol. Third or fourth agents (e.g. rifabutin, aminoglycoside) are reserved for more severe disease or in the absence of ART. Aside from macrolides, clinicians cannot rely on resistance profiles of the agents used to treat MAC as they do not reflect the activity of the drug in the body (i.e. a laboratory report might read 'sensitive', but actually the drug is ineffective in vivo).

Management of HIV in the outpatient setting

- Due to the effectiveness of ART the majority of HIV patient care is delivered in an outpatient setting.
- In the UK approximately 95% of outpatients are taking HIV therapy and 97% have an undetectable viral load.
- OIs are extremely uncommon in individuals on ART with good HIV control.
- The emphasis is now on reducing drug toxicities and co-morbidities which are increased despite virological control. They include:

- Cardiovascular disease and lipid disturbance with increased myocardial infarction risk (secondary to uncontrolled HIV viraemia but also certain HIV treatments including abacavir).
- Renal disease: proximal renal tubulopathy/Fanconi syndrome (treatment related including tenofovir; ➲ see Chapter 16, Fanconi syndrome, p. 562, Table 16.5 and Box 16.4) and renal stones (with atazanavir) (➲ see Chapter 1, Renal calculi, p. 34).
- Bone disease: osteoporosis, osteonecrosis and osteomalacia.
- Viral mediated tumours – include cervical and anal cancer, lymphomas and hepatocellular carcinoma secondary to HPV, EBV, HHV-8 and hepatitis viruses.
- Smoking-related lung disease – COPD and lung cancer.
- Drug interactions – protease inhibitors are liver enzyme inhibitors and may interact with other drugs; acid suppressing agents may reduce absorption of some protease inhibitors and non-nucleoside reverse transciptase inhibitors (NNRTIs).
- CNS problems – neurocognitive impairment (prolonged HIV infection) and depression or psychoses (some HIV treatments, e.g. efavirenz).

Common outpatient management issues include:

- Supporting initiation and continued adherence to ART.
- Monitoring of patients on ART to ensure treatment is effective with minimal toxicity:
  - provision of adherence support and monitoring of HIV viral load;
  - screening for drug toxicity and drug interactions;
  - screening for co-morbidities.
- Providing support on living with a chronic infectious disease. This includes ensuring awareness of effectiveness of treatment as prevention.
- Psychological support for:
  - sexual health screening and partner notification;
  - HIV disclosure;
  - increasing HIV knowledge and promoting self-management skills.
  - use of educational websites (e.g. www.aidsmap.org; www.tht.org.uk).

Antiretroviral therapy

Antiretroviral therapy: principles of treatment

- Different groups of antiretroviral medications target different stages of the HIV lifecycle (see Figure 7.7).
- Antiretroviral medications are given in combination to increase potency and reduce likelihood of acquiring resistance.
- Current standard of care includes three agents, which consists of a backbone of two nucleoside analogues (usually emtricitabine/tenofovir or abacavir/lamivudine) and a third agent (either a NNRTI/protease inhibitor [PI]/integrase inhibitor, see Table 7.12).
- Alternative regimens may be used if there is HIV drug resistance, intolerance or a need to avoid specific toxicities in patients with co-morbidities.
- There can be major interactions between ART and other medications including, e.g. anti-TB therapy. The University of Liverpool's HIV Drug Interactions site gives comprehensive and up-to-date interactive advice for clinicians and healthcare professionals related to these interactions and can be found at https://www.hiv-druginteractions.org/.

The four main ART groups in clinical practice include:

1. Reverse transcriptase inhibitors: inhibit the conversion of HIV RNA to DNA by the enzyme reverse transcriptase. There are two types:
   (a) Nucleoside reverse transcriptase inhibitors (NRTIs) that are analogues of HIV DNA nucleotide that incorporates into the forming HIV DNA blocking its function. Examples include tenofovir, lamivudine, abacavir and emtricitabine.
   (b) NNRTIs that bind to and directly block the reverse transcriptase enzyme. Examples include efavirenz, rilpivirine, etravirine and nevirapine.

2. PIs that inhibit the formation of viral particles by blocking the protease enzyme. Examples include darunavir, atazanavir and lopinavir. They are co-administered with either ritonavir or cobicistat, which boosts the plasma drug level by reducing the breakdown of the PIs in the gut wall and the liver through potent inhibition of cytochrome p450 3A4. This enzyme inhibition is responsible for most of the serious drug interactions associated with this class of medication.
3. Integrase inhibitors that block the integrase enzyme that is responsible for integrating viral DNA into the host cell DNA after reverse transcription. Examples include dolutegravir, raltegravir and bictegravir (see Table 3.4).
4. Chemokine receptor antagonists:
   - Chemokine receptors CCR5 and CXCR4 act as co-receptors to facilitate viral entry into cell.
   - The majority of HIV strains utilise CCR5.
   - CXCR4-using strains can emerge through drug exposure or without drug exposure in individuals who have longstanding HIV or a low CD4 count. Resistance testing using tropism assays identify if CCR5 antagonists, such as maraviroc will have therapeutic benefit (see Table 3.4).

When to start treatment

- Current guidance is that all patients should be offered treatment. The decision to start HIV treatment should be made in close collaboration with the patient as close monitoring and support will be initially required.
- While clinical parameters, CD4 T cell counts and assessment of a patient's readiness to start and comply with ART are all important considerations, the bottom line in HIV guidance is that HIV treatment should be offered to all people with HIV, irrespective of CD4 count as studies show that, with treatment, patients with CD4 counts >500 are less likely to develop AIDS or die, compared with patients who wait to start treatment until they have lower CD4 counts.

Table 7.12 'What ART to start with'

	Preferred	**Alternative**
NRTI backbone	Tenofovir and emtricitabine	Abacavir* and lamivudine
Third agent	Atazanavir/r	Efavirenz
	Darunavir/r	
	Elvitegravir/c Dolutegravir	
	Raltegravir	
	Rilpivirine**	

*Abacavir contraindicated if HLAB5701 positive.
**Only if baseline viral load is <100,000 copies/mL.
Abbreviations: r = ritonavir and c = cobicistat both of which are boosting agents.
Adapted with permission from British HIV Association. British HIV Association guidelines for the treatment of HIV-1-positive adults with antiretroviral therapy 2015 (2016 interim update). Available at: https://www.bhiva.org/file/RVYKzFwyxpgil/treatment-guidelines-2016-interim-update.pdf

Antiretroviral therapy: treatment aims and monitoring

- The average HIV pre-treatment viral load (VL) is 30,000–50,000 copies/mL. The goal of HIV therapy is to suppress viral replication; success is defined as achieving an HIV VL <50 copies/mL within 6 months (most patients have VL <50 by 3 months).
- The risk of OIs is dramatically reduced when virological suppression is achieved irrespective of CD4 recovery.
- High levels of adherence (approximately 90%) are needed to maintain virological suppression.
- HIV patients should undergo monitoring 2–4 times per year, including assessment of adherence, monitoring for drug toxicity and measurement of viral loads to ensure continued treatment success.

- An HIV viral load between 50 and 400 copies/mL (known clinically as a 'blip') does not usually signify treatment failure with 90% individuals re-suppressing on repeat testing. A VL >400 copies/mL is of concern as failure to suppress below this level puts the patient at increased risk of drug resistance.
- The main causes of a detectable viral load whilst on treatment include:
  - suboptimal adherence to ART (including stopping therapy);
  - drug interaction resulting in sub-therapeutic levels of HIV drug;
  - malabsorption;
  - development of drug resistance.

Legal aspects of HIV infection

HIV transmission

Patients on treatment with an undetectable viral load are now considered non-infectious based on long-term follow-up of patients and their partners who have had sex without condoms. There is a multinational campaign to let patients and providers aware of this called U = U ('Undetectable equals Untransmissible'). All persons with HIV should be made aware that untreated HIV is an infectious disease and of the available methods to reduce risk of onward transmission. Partner notification should be discussed if there are contacts who may have been at risk of acquiring HIV infection. Partner notification is usually undertaken by experienced persons who are equipped with the requisite up-to-date knowledge of the legal aspects of diagnosis, along with access to the necessary psychological support services, especially for patients who may be reluctant to disclose for fear of stigma, rejection and domestic violence. Medical practitioners should be aware of the ethical and legal responsibilities related to HIV transmission, particularly around disclosure of information on HIV status (➔ see Chapter 27, Provisions for sexually transmitted disease, p. 888).

Prosecutions for reckless transmission of HIV have been brought in the UK since 2001 (Scotland) and 2003 (England & Wales). Consistent condom use and/or having an undetectable VL may be considered a defence against recklessness. Someone with HIV in England and Wales is only likely to be successfully prosecuted if they:

- knew they were HIV positive at the time of the alleged transmission;
- understood how HIV is transmitted;
- had unprotected sex with someone negative who subsequently tests positive;
- did not disclose their HIV diagnosis before sex;
- can be proven to be the only likely source of transmission.

The GMC offers the following guidance:[1]

> You may disclose information to a known sexual contact of a patient with a sexually transmitted serious communicable disease if you have reason to think that they are at risk of infection and that the patient has not informed them and cannot be persuaded to do so. In such circumstances, you should tell the patient before you make the disclosure, if it is practicable and safe to do so. You must be prepared to justify a decision to disclose personal information without consent.

Health-care workers

A health-care worker who may have been exposed to infection with HIV, in whatever circumstances, must promptly seek and follow confidential professional advice from the Occupational Health Department on whether they should be tested for HIV and with regard to workplace activities. Failure to do so may breach

[1]Reproduced from General Medical Council, Disclosing information about serious communicable diseases. [online] Available at: https://www.gmc-uk.org/ethical-guidance/ethical-guidance-for-doctors/confidentiality–disclosing-information-about-serious-communicable-diseases/disclosing-information-about-serious-communicable-diseases [Accessed 26 Feb. 2019].

the GMC guidance on duty of care to patients. HIV-infected health-care workers have few limitations on their practice, but must not perform exposure prone procedures (EPP), e.g. open surgery or other invasive procedures.

Post-exposure prophylaxis and pre-exposure prophylaxis

Post-exposure prophylaxis (PEP) has two main indications for use: needlestick injury to a health-care worker and following sexual exposure. Prompt treatment post-exposure (within 72 hours) has been shown to reduce risk of HIV acquisition. Animal studies have demonstrated efficacy of PEP following sexual inoculation of HIV with benefit increased if given within 72 hours and continued for 1 month.

Needlestick injury

- *Guidance:* most health-care services have a protocol for needlestick injury and PEP that involves immediate referral to occupational health services. Nevertheless, outside of normal working hours these services may not be directly available.
- *Risk:* a needlestick injury from an HIV positive individual has approximately a 0.3% risk that the recipient will seroconvert with no PEP.
- *Initial advice:*
  - Full history and examination of wound (if dermis not breached then PEP may not be indicated).
  - Wash and irrigate wound with water and soap or alcohol liquid soap.
  - Consent both source case and recipient of injury to take blood for HIV and hepatitis B/C screening. Both the consent and blood samples must be taken by an appropriate health-care professional not involved in the incident.
- *Further advice and treatment:* counsel recipient regarding risk of exposure and risk/side effects of PEP. If PEP is commenced, it should be initiated without delay, the regimen (as dictated by local guidance) should be continued for at least 4 weeks or sooner if the source case tests negative for blood-borne viruses.

Sexual exposure

- *Risk:* a thorough history is essential in estimating risk. This would include the exact type of exposure (oral, anal or vaginal intercourse, associated sexual assault or rape) and any relevant information concerning the source (i.e. known sexually transmitted infections, genital ulceration or HIV). However, it remains difficult to accurately quantify risk given that estimates are based on observational studies.
- PEP for sexual exposure is often initiated in the Emergency department with onward referral to sexual health services for further management.

Pre-exposure prophylaxis and HIV treatment as prevention

- The risk of transmitting HIV sexually to others has been shown to be significantly reduced by taking HIV therapy with an undetectable HIV VL.
- Pre-exposure prophylaxis (PrEP) involves an HIV-negative person taking an OD tablet (e.g. containing the two anti-retroviral drugs, usually tenofovir and emtricitabine) to prevent acquisition of HIV. The tablet can be taken regularly or around the time of having sex. Both MSM and heterosexual study cohorts have shown efficacy with good adherence of oral PrEP in preventing new HIV cases.

Further reading

1. UK National Guidelines for HIV Testing 2008 prepared jointly by British HIV Association British Association of Sexual Health and HIV British Infection Society. http://www.hpa.org.uk/web/HPAweb&HPAwebStandard/HPAweb_C/1245581513121
2. British HIV Association and British Infection Association Guidelines for the Treatment of Opportunistic Infection in HIV-seropositive Individuals 2011. HIV Med. 2011; 12(Suppl. 2):1–5. https://onlinelibrary.wiley.com/doi/epdf/10.1111/j.1468-1293.2011.00944_1.x

3. UK National Guideline for the Use of HIV Post-Exposure Prophylaxis Following Sexual Exposure (PEPSE) 2015. BHIVA and BASSH. https://www.bashh.org/documents/PEPSE%202015%20guideline%20final_NICE.pdf
4. British HIV Association guidelines for the treatment of HIV-1-positive adults with antiretroviral therapy 2015 (2016 interim update). https://www.bhiva.org/file/RVYKzFwyxpgil/treatment-guidelines-2016-interim-update.pdf

Multiple choice questions

Questions

1. In an asymptomatic patient with a diagnosis of HIV without comorbidities or other relevant illnesses, the British HIV Association guidelines recommend commencing antiretroviral therapy if the CD4 count is:
   A. above 500 cells/μL;
   B. below 500 cells/μL;
   C. below 350 cells/μL;
   D. below 200 cells/μL;
   E. At any level.
2. A 35-year-old man presents to the emergency department with a 4-week history of breathlessness and dry cough. His symptoms have not improved despite antibiotic therapy for a presumed community-acquired pneumonia. In addition, he reports 10 kg weight loss in the previous 6 months. He has a history of shingles 3 years ago.

   On examination, he is cachectic with multiple violaceous raised purple lesions on his chest, arms and lower limbs. Auscultation of his chest reveals fine crepitations throughout both lung fields.

   Relevant clinical bedside tests and an arterial blood gas are displayed below:

   - Heart rate: 102 beats/minute.
   - Respiratory rate: 28 breaths/minute.
   - Oxygen saturation: 85% (room air).
   - Investigations:
     - Arterial blood gases breathing air:
       - PO_2 6.8 kPa (11.3–12.6);
       - PCO_2 3.9 kPa (4.7–6.0).

   What is the preferred treatment?
   A. Atovaquone.
   B. Pentamidine.
   C. Clindamycin and pyrimethamine.
   D. Co-trimoxazole.
   E. Trimethoprim and dapsone.
3. A 65-year-old man is diagnosed with HIV infection following investigation for profound weight loss. He reports floaters in both eyes. His fundoscopy image is shown in Figure 7.15.

   What is the most appropriate treatment?
   A. Ganciclovir.
   B. Famciclovir.
   C. Valaciclovir.
   D. Foscarnet.
   E. Cidofovir.

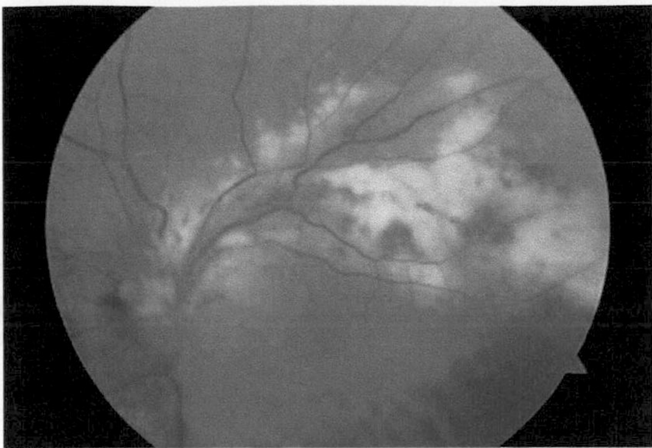

Figure 7.15 (see colour plate section, Fig. 7.11) CMV retinitis, commonly termed 'cheese pizza' or 'pizza pie' retina.
Reproduced with permission from Frith P. The eye in general medicine. In *Oxford Textbook of Medicine*, 5th edn, Warrell D. A. et al. (eds). Oxford: OUP. Copyright © 2013 Oxford University Press. DOI: 10.1093/med/9780199204854.001.1. Reproduced with permission of the Licensor through PLSclear.

4. A 25-year-old man attends GUM clinic reporting a 5-day history of urethral discharge. He last had sexual intercourse with a casual female partner 2 weeks ago. A full sexual health screen is carried out. Gram-negative intracellular diplococci are found on microscopy. What is the most likely diagnosis?
   A. *Neisseria gonorrhoeae*.
   B. *Neisseria menigitidis*.
   C. *Chlamydia trachomatis*.
   D. *Lymphogranuloma venereum*.
   E. *Escherichia coli*.

5. A 50-year-old man presents with a maculopapular rash, fever and oral ulceration with onset over a 7 day period.
   He reports engaging in oral sex with a male partner 6 weeks previously.
   Relevant investigations include:
   - EBV IgG positive, IgM negative.
   - HIV 1/2 antibody and p24 negative.
   - ESR 10 mm/hr (normal values 0–22 mm/hr for men and 0–29 mm/hr for women).
   - ALT 75 iu/L (normal values 0–40 iu/L).

   What is most appropriate next step in management?
   A. Arrange for a repeat HIV test.
   B. Request hepatitis screen and liver ultrasound scan.
   C. Perform syphilis serology.
   D. Request a skin biopsy.
   E. Treat with antihistamines and topical steroids.

Answers

1. E. All patients should commence ART where appropriate, regardless of CD4 count (➲ see Management of HIV in the outpatient setting, Antiretroviral Therapy, When to start treatment, p. 221).

2. D. The history of previous shingles (reactivation of *Varicella zoster* virus) and violaceous raised purple lesions (Kaposi's sarcoma) suggest an underlying HIV infection with significant immunocompromise. The likely diagnosis is PCP, based on dyspnoea and desaturation on mobilisation. The most appropriate first line treatment for severe PCP is co-trimoxazole. Adjunctive steroids would also be of benefit in this patient given pO_2 <9.3 kPa on arterial blood gas. A, B and E may be used as alternative treatments. Clindamycin when prescribed should be given with primaquine not pyrimethamine (➲ see Pneumocystis *jirovecii* pneumonia, Treatment, p. 213).

3. A. Ganciclovir is the preferred treatment for CMV retinitis. D and E are used less commonly used due to higher rate of toxicity (➲ see Cytomegalovirus, Treatment, p. 215).

4. A. A and B are both gram negative diplococci; the clinical scenario indicates a recently acquired sexually transmitted infection. *Neisseria meningitides* is associated with meningitis and not urethral discharge (➲ see Gonorrhoea, p. 196, Figure 7.4 and Table 7.5).

5. C. This is a classical presentation of secondary syphilis and syphilis serology would be diagnostic. The initial HIV test (which checks for antigen and antibody) would have been positive if the rash was due to an HIV seroconversion illness. (➲ see Serological tests for syphilis, p. 200 and Table 7.7).

Chapter 8 **Infectious Diseases and Tropical Medicine**

Douglas Fink and Penelope Smith

Basic microbiology

Nomenclature and taxonomy

The principles of taxonomy date back to the eighteenth century. Traditional identification arranges organisms into groups (or taxa). The most commonly used taxa in clinical medicine refer to the genus and species of bacteria; for example, *pylori* is a species of the genus *Helicobacter*. Molecular techniques allow more precise phylogenetic analysis, describing groups of pathogens according to common genetic descent. Nonetheless, classification does not always inform the clinician about pathogenicity of microorganisms in patients.

Pathogens can be organised into five main groups – viruses, bacteria, protozoa, fungi and metazoa (usually helminths). The structural organisation of these organisms, including that of their genetic material, help define them (see Table 8.1). Eukaryotes are organisms that contain many complex structures enclosed within membranes, including the nucleus. Prokaryotes such as bacteria have no membrane-bound organelles.

Bacteria

Bacteria are described by a number of traditional characteristics:

- Gram stain.
- Appearance under microscope.
- Atmospheric requirements.
- Spore formation.

Table 8.1 Key characteristics of major pathogens

Pathogen	Structure	Basic unit	Example
Virus	Acellular	Virion	*Varicella zoster*
Bacteria	Prokaryote	Unicellular	*Helicobacter pylori*
Protozoa	Eukaryote	Unicellular	*Plasmodium falciparum*
Fungi	Eukaryote	Uni- and multicellular	*Candida albicans*
Helminths	Eukaryote	Multicellular	*Ascaris lumbricoides*

Gram stain

There are five stages to the technique:

1. Heat-fixing the specimen onto a glass slide.
2. Primary stain ('purple' crystal violet [CV] or methylene blue dye).
3. Trapping agent (Gram's iodine).
4. Decolorisation with alcohol or acetone.
5. Counterstain ('red' safranin or basic fuchsin).

Gram-positive bacteria

Peptidoglycan wall retains CV and organisms appear purple.

Gram-negative bacteria

Do not retain CV upon decolorization, but take up safranin counterstain, and appear red or pink.
For common Gram-positive and Gram-negative organisms, see Tables 8.2 and 8.3, respectively.
There are two significant limitations:

1. Low sensitivity: sensitive to populations of approximately 10,000 organisms/mL.
2. Some bacterial species cannot be visualised:
   - No cell wall (such as *Mycoplasma* spp.).
   - Cell wall structure does not retain Gram stain reagents (such as *Chlamydia* spp., *Mycobacterium* spp.).

Appearance under microscope

Bacterial cell walls determine shape that is consistent for each individual genus:

- spherical cocci;
- rod-shaped bacilli;
- spiral bacteria (e.g. *Borrelia* spp. of Lyme disease);
- spirochaetes – tightly coiled bacteria (e.g. leptospirosis).

Atmospheric requirements

There are five main groups of bacteria depending on the relative needs of different genera: obligate anaerobes, obligate aerobes, microaerophiles, capnophiles and facultative anaerobes.

Spore formation

Both *Clostridium* and *Bacillus* produce endospores, which help them survive inhospitable environments (including postage in transcontinental envelopes in the case of *Bacillus anthracis* or anthrax spores).

Table 8.2 Common gram-positive organisms

Microscopic appearance	Atmospheric requirements	Shape	Genus	Further testing	Species
Cocci	Aerobic	Cluster	*Staphylococcus*	Coagulase +	S. *aureus*
				Coagulase -	Coagulase-negative Staph. (CNS)
		Chains	*Streptococcus*; *Enterococcus*	Alpha haemolysis	*Viridans* group
				Beta haemolysis	S. *pyogenes* (Group A); S. *agalacticae*
				Gamma haemolysis	*Enteroccus faecalis*
		Diplococci			*Streptococcus pneumoniae*
	Anaerobic organisms less clinically significant				
Bacilli/rods	Aerobic	Large	*Bacillus*	Spore +	
		Small	*Corynebacterium*		
		Cocco-bacilli	*Listeria*		
		Branching	*Nocardia*		
	Anaerobic	Large	*Clostridium*	Spore +	

Table 8.3 Common gram-negative organisms

Microscopic appearance	Atmospheric requirements	Shape	Further testing	Genus/ species
Cocci	Aerobic	Diplococci		*Neisseria meningitidis, N. gonorrhoeae; Moraxella catarrhalis*
		Cocco-bacilli		*Haemophilus influenzae; Brucella* spp.
		Branching		*Actinomycoses*
	Anaerobic organisms less clinically significant			
Bacilli/rods	Aerobic		Lactose-fermenting	*Enterobacter* spp.; *Escherichia coli; Klebsiella* spp.
			Non lactose-fermenting	*Proteus* spp.; *Shigella* spp.; *Salmonella* spp.; *Pseudomonas* spp. (oxidase +)
	Anaerobic			*Bacteroides* spp.
		'fusiform' or filamentous		*Fusobacterium* spp.

Special cases

1. Obligate intracellular organisms:
   - These can only reproduce within host cells (similarly to viruses).
   - Examples include Rickettsia, *Coxiella* spp., *Chlamydia* spp.
2. *Mycoplasma* spp.:
   - No cell wall at all.
   - Are the smallest form of life capable of independent extracellular existence.

Accurate diagnosis and treatment guidance depends on bacterial culture, which involves five key steps:

- Inoculation of the specimen.
- Incubation.
- 'Reading the plates'.
- Identification.
- Susceptibility testing.

The modern laboratory has automated much of this pathway.

Culture

Many bacterial pathogens grow on non-selective solid media (e.g. blood or chocolate agar).

Selective media (such as MacConkey agar to detect Gram-negative bacteria) are used to inhibit the growth of commensal bacteria that are often present on non-sterile microbiology samples such as sputum. Enrichment media help more delicate fastidious organisms multiply, for example, charcoal enrichment for *Bordetella pertussis* or 'whooping cough'.

Streptococcal species can be classified by their ability to break down red blood cells (RBCs) of red-coloured blood agar:

- *Alpha haemolysis*:
  - Incomplete RBC haemolysis by bacterial hydrogen peroxide (green).
- *Beta haemolysis*:
  - Complete haemolysis by streptolysin (transparent).
- *Gamma haemolysis*:
  - No haemolysis (red).

Protozoa

Protozoa demonstrate limited animal cell-like behaviour. They often have reproductive cycles that involve multiple different hosts, vectors and milieus. Common protozoa are given in Table 8.4.

Fungi

Fungi are mostly yeasts and moulds. Yeasts are usually unicellular, larger than bacteria and form buds. Moulds or filamentous fungi grow multicellular filaments called hyphae. Dimorphic fungi share yeast and filamentous appearances. For common fungi, see Table 8.5.

Helminths

Helminths are parasitic worms. They are multicellular eukaryotes classified by morphology. Cestodes or tapeworms have segmented structures; trematodes or flukes are unsegmented (Table 8.6); nematodes or roundworms have cylindrical structures (Table 8.7).

Additional key terms and definitions

Ziehl–Nielsen stain and mycobacteria

- Staining with carbol-fuchsin or auramine-rhodamine 'Acid fast' species do not decolorise with acidified alcohol and appear vivid pink.
- Positive test for *Mycobacterium* spp. (tuberculous and non-tuberculous), *Nocardia* spp., some protozoa (e.g. *Cryptosporidium* spp.).

Table 8.4 Common protozoa

Locomotion	Location	Species	Transmission	Disease
Flagellate *'whip-like'*	GI	*Giardia*	Ingestion	Giardiasis
	GU	*Trichomonas*	Sexual	Trichomoniasis
	Blood	*Leishmania*	Sand fly	Cutaneous and visceral leishmaniasis
		Trypanosoma		Trypanosomiasis
		T. *gambiense*, T. *rhodesiense*	Tsetse fly	*Sleeping sickness*
		T. *cruzi*	Triatomid bug	*Chagas disease*
Sporozoa *'spore-forming'*	GI	*Cryptosporidium*	Ingestion	Cryptosporidiosis
	Blood	*Toxoplasma*	Ingestion; skin contact	Toxoplasmosis
		Plasmodium	Anopheles mosquito	Malaria
Amoeboid *'cytoplasm extensions'*	GI	*Entamoeba*	Ingestion	Amoebiasis

Table 8.5 Common fungi

Clinical	Species	Microscopy	Transmission	Disease
Superficial = cutaneous	Dermatophytes (*Microsporum*, *Trichophyton*)	Filamentous; spores	Cutaneous	Tinea
Systemic	*Histoplasma*	Dimorphic	Inhalation	Pulmonary; disseminated
	Coccidioides	Dimorphic	Inhalation	'Valley fever'; pulmonary; disseminated
Immunocompromised	*Candida*	Yeast	Cutaneous GI	Oropharyngeal; vulvovaginitis; balanitis; invasive
	Aspergillus	Filamentous	Inhalation	ABPA; pulmonary; chronic pulmonary (± aspergilloma); disseminated

Table 8.6 Common cestode and trematode helminths

Group	Stage	Species	Transmission	Disease
Cestodes = tapeworms	Adult	*Taenia*	Meat consumption	GI symptoms
		T. saginata	Beef	
		T. solium	Pork	
	Larval	*T. solium*	Eggs in human faeces	Cysticercosis (brain, eyes)
		Echinococcus granulosus	Eggs in dog faeces	Hydatid disease (liver, lung, brain)
Trematodes = flukes	Larval	*Schistosoma*	Skin penetration	Schistosomiasis
		S. haematobium		Bladder
		S. japonicum, *S. mansoni*		GI
		Fasciola hepatica	Ingestion (cress)	Liver cysts

Table 8.7 Common nematode helminths

Transmission	Species	Transmission	Disease
Person to person	*Ascaris lumbricoides* 'giant roundworm'	Egg ingestion	Small intestine
	Enterobius vermicularis	Egg ingestion	Large intestine
	Hookworms e.g. *Ancylostoma duodenale*	Larval skin penetration	Small intestine; cutaneous larva migrans
	Strongyloides stercoralis	Larval skin penetration Autoinfection	Larva currens; small intestine; strongyloidiasis
Vector-borne	*Brugia malayi*	Bite of mosquito	'blood filiariasis'
	Wucheria bancrofti	Bite of mosquito	'lymphatic filiariasis'
	Loa loa	Bite of deer fly	Loiasis (calabar swellings, ocular disease)
	Onchocerca volvulus	Bite of *Simulium* fly	Onchocerciasis ('river blindness')
Zoonoses	*Toxicara canis*	Eggs in dog faeces	Visceral *larva migrans*, ocular disease
	Trichinella spiralis	Larvae in pork meat	Muscle cysts

Table 8.8 Antibacterial treatments

Class	Examples	Mechanism of action	Clinical use	Limitations
Beta-lactams				
Penicillins	Natural penicillins (benzylpenicillin); aminopenicillins (amoxicillin); extended-spectrum penicillins (piperacillin)	Inhibit cell wall synthesis	Gram-positive infections. Some Gram-negative infections.	• Resistance. • Spectrum of activity: poor intracellular cover (*Chlamydia* spp., *Legionella* spp.), no cover if no cell wall (*Mycoplasma* spp.). • Adverse effects: 25% mild rashes, 0.5–4% hypersensitivity reactions, 0.05% anaphylaxis, neurotoxicity (if not dose adjusted).
Carboxypenems	Ertapenem, meropenem		Systemic Gram-positive and negative (including *Pseudomonas* spp.) infections.	• Parenteral administration.
Cephalosporins	Second generation (cefuroxime); third generation (cefotaxime, ceftriaxone)		Systemic Gram-positive (and some Gram-negative) infections.	• 10% cross-reactivity with penicillin hypersensitivity.
Glycopeptides	Vancomycin; teicoplanin	Inhibit cell wall synthesis	Systemic Gram-positive infections (including MRSA); pseudomembranous colitis.	• Resistance (>*E. faecium*): 'transferability' to Gram-positive organisms. • Pharmacokinetics: poor GI absorption. • Adverse effects: 15% 'red man' syndrome (histamine release with boluses); renal toxicity (if persistently elevated trough levels); otoxicity (elderly, rare). • Monitoring of levels required.
Aminoglycosides	Gentamicin; amikacin	Inhibit protein synthesis = bactericidal	Systemic Gram-negative infections.	• Pharmacokinetics: no GI absorption; poor tissue, bone, blood–brain barrier (BBB) distribution. • Adverse effects: renal toxicity 10–20% (acute tubular necrosis [ATN] due to accumulation in proximal tubule cells); ototoxicity (if persistently elevated peak levels); neuromuscular paralysis (rare, contraindicated in myasthenia gravis).
Macrolides	Erythromycin; clarithromycin; azithormycin	Inhibit protein synthesis = bacteriostatic	Streptococcal infections in penicillin allergy; atypical pneumonia and URTIs; chlamydial infections; mycobacterial infections.	• Resistance: 'MLS' (inducible 'Macrolide-Lincosamide-Streptogrammin' resistance). • Adverse effects: nausea, vomiting; QT prolongation. • Drug interactions: (macrolides) increased by CYP3A4 inhibitors; (macrolides) inhibit P450 enzymes: statins (myopathy), warfarin (unpredictable INR due to GI flora and P450 interaction).

continued

Table 8.8 *continued*

Class	Examples	Mechanism of action	Clinical use	Limitations
Lincosamides	Clindamycin		Gram-positive infections. Staphylococcal toxic shock syndrome (inhibits staphylococcal toxin); anaerobes (except *C. difficile*).	• Adverse effects: risk of pseudomembranous colitis.
Tetracyclines	Doxycycline; minocycline; tigecycline	Inhibit protein synthesis = bacteriostatic	Rickettsial infections; chlamydial infections.	• Resistance. • Adverse effects: photosensitivity; concentrates in developing bone and teeth (contraindicated in pregnant women and children <8 years).
Quinolones	Ciprofloxacin; levofloxacin; moxifloxacin	Inhibit nucleic acid synthesis (inhibit bacterial DNA gyrase and topoisomerase)	Systemic Gram-negative infections; intracellular infections (Legionella, Salmonella); chlamydial infections; resistant mycobacterial infections.	• Adverse effects: GI upset; tendon rupture <0.5% (associated with steroid use, >60 years); prolonged QT syndrome; lower seizure threshold in epilepsy. • Drug interactions: quinolones inhibit P450 enzymes: aminophylline.
Anti-tuberculosis drugs				
Rifamycins	Rifampicin; rifabutin	Inhibit RNA polymerase and mRNA synthesis	Mycobacterial infections in combination; mengingococcal prophylaxis; prostheses infections in combination.	• Resistance. • Pharmacokinetics: extensive first pass metabolism (older preparations require frequent dosing). • Adverse effects: secretion discoloration (orange urine/sweat/saliva); rash; hepatotoxicity (10%, in combination with other hepatotoxic drugs). • Drug interactions: P450 enzyme inducer (HAART regimen implications).
Isoniazid		Inhibits mycolic acid synthesis	Mycobacterial infections in combination; latent tuberculosis infection as monotherapy.	• Resistance. • Adverse effects: hepatotoxicity (up to 50% in first 2 months); peripheral neuropathy (avoided by co-administration of pyridoxine/B6; risk factors: age, renal and liver disease, HIV, diabetes).
Ethambutol		Inhibits cell wall synthesis (inhibits polymerisation of arabinoglycan)	Mycobacterial infections in combination.	• Resistance. • Adverse effects: optic neuropathy: reduced visual acuity, dose-dependent red-green colour blindness.
Pyrazinamide		Inhibits mycolic acid synthesis	Mycobacterial infections in combination.	• Resistance. • Adverse effects: hepatoxicitiy (in combination with other hepatotoxic drugs); arthralgia.

Lancefield grouping

- Specific carbohydrates in the bacterial cell wall allow agglutination with particular antibodies.
- Used predominantly to classify the species of beta haemolytic streptococci;
  - Group A *Strep*. (GAS), e.g. *S. pyogenes*:
    - Toxin-producing.
    - Specific pathology: necrotising fasciitis; toxic shock syndrome.
  - Group B *Strep*. (GBS), e.g. *S. agalactiae*:
    - Commonly encountered in neonatal and elderly populations.
  - Group D reclassified as *Enterococci*.

Coagulase

- Surface-bound enzyme converts fibrinogen to fibrin, resulting in the clotting of blood ('clumping factor').
- Diagnostic of *S. aureus*, which produces the coagulase enzyme.

Antimicrobial treatments

For antibacterial treatments, see Table 8.8; for antiviral treatments, see Table 8.9; for antifungal treatments, see Table 8.10; and for common antiprotozoan treatments, see Table 8.11.

Table 8.9 Antiviral treatments

Anti-viral	Target virus	Mechanism of action	Clinical use	Limitations
Aciclovir (PO and IV)	HSV > VZV	Inhibits herpes virus DNA polymerase (after phosphorylation by herpes thymidine kinase).	HSV 1 and 2: 1. Encephalitis. 2. Mucocutaneous/ oropharyngeal. 3. Bell's/VII CN palsy (not supported by meta-analysis). VZV: 1. *Varicella pneumonia*. 2. Zoster infection/ 'shingles' (<72 hours symptoms or severe pain). Both viruses: 1. Disseminated disease. 2. Prophylaxis in solid organ transplantation.	Adverse effects: AKI (precipitation of acyclovir crystals in tubules); agitation/ tremor/delirium (rare).
Ganciclovir (IV); Valganciclovir (PO)	CMV >>> other herpes viruses	Inhibits herpes virus DNA polymerase (broader activity than acyclovir).	Prophylaxis in certain transplant recipients; treatment of CMV viraemia or end-organ disease.	• Adverse effects: myelosuppression; AKI. • Drug interactions: co-trimoxazole (overlapping bone marrow and renal toxicity).
Oseltamivir ('Tamiflu®'; PO)	Influenza A and B	Inhibits influenza neuraminidase (sialic acid analogue: prevents viral binding host receptor, reduces release of new virus from host cells).	Post-exposure prophylaxis and treatment (<48 hours fever onset; if either hospitalised, or high risk: >65 years, pregnant, chronic medical conditions).	• Limited evidence: likely only reduces duration of symptoms by 24 hours. • Adverse effects: nausea and vomiting.

Table 8.10 Antifungal treatments

Class and mechanism of action	Agent	Clinical use	Limitations
Triazoles			• Adverse effects: hepatoxicitiy (10% transaminitis). • Drug interactions: *all* inhibit P450 enzyme system (e.g. warfarin control); all metabolised by P450 system to some extent (e.g. rifampicin induction can render undetectable in serum).
Inhibit fungal cell membrane synthesis	Fluconazole	Only yeasts. PO: superficial and invasive candidiasis; endemic fungi (e.g. histoplasmosis). IV: disseminated cryptococcal infection.	Adverse effects: alopecia.
	Itraconazole	PO: endemic fungi; ABPA.	Adverse effects: triad: hypertension, hypokalaemia, peripheral oedema.
	Voriconazole	IV: invasive aspergillosis; invasive candidiasis (resistant to fluconazole).	Adverse effects: visual disturbances (up to 20%), photosensitivity.
Polyenes			
Damages fungal cell membrane directly	Nystatin	Topical: mild oropharyngeal candidiasis.	
	Amphotericin B	Severe invasive fungal infections (all species; typically reserved for life-threatening disease or failed alternative therapy).	Adverse effects: nephrotoxicity (up to 80% incidence of AKI; pre-existing CKD is a risk factor; liposomal preparations have lower incidence of AKI); electrolyte disturbances (distal type 1 RTA; nephrogenic diabetes insipidus); infusion-related reactions (fevers, rigors, nausea).

Infection control

Isolation strategies for infection control are shown in Table 8.12.

Notifiable disease

Registered medical practitioners have a statutory duty to notify a 'Proper Officer' at the local council or health protection team of suspected cases of certain infectious diseases. These include such infections as meningitis, acute infectious hepatitis, food poisoning and tuberculosis (TB) (➲ See Chapter 27, Scenario 4 and Notification in the case of infectious diseases, pp. 886–7).

All Proper Officers are required to pass on the entire notification to Public Health England within 3 days of a case being notified, or within 24 hours for cases deemed urgent. A full list of notifiable diseases can be found on the Public Health England website: https://www.gov.uk/notifiable-diseases-and-causative-organisms-how-to-report.

Table 8.11 Common antiprotozoa treatments

Organism	Disease	Agent	Mechanism of action	Limitations
Flagellates				
Giardia	Giardiasis	PO: Tinidazole single-dose or metronidazole 5 days	Intracellular cytotoxicity	Adverse effects: metallic taste, nausea.
Leishmania	Cutaneous leishmaniasis	Topical: paromomycin	Inhibits protein synthesis	Limited use (predominantly in ulcerating lesions).
		Intralesional injection with cryotherapy or IV: sodium stibogluconate	Inhibits ATP synthesis	Adverse effects: flu-like symptoms, pancreatitis, prolonged QT (and other ECG changes).
	Visceral leishmaniasis	IV: sodium stibogluconate or amphotericin		
		IV: pentamidine	Damages cell membrane	Adverse effects: pancreatitis, dysglycaemia (including diabetes), nephrotoxicity, hepatotoxicity, prolonged QT.
Trypanosoma	West African trypanosomiasis *T. b. gambiense*			
	Early (i.e. no CNS involvement)	IV: pentamidine		
		IV: suramin	Unknown	Adverse effects: rash 90%, nephrotoxicity, hepatotoxicity, myelosuppression, adrenocortical insufficiency. Pharmacokinetics: does not cross BBB.
	Late	IV: eflornithine (± nifurtimox)	Inhibits parasite growth	Adverse effects: vomiting 40%, abdominal pain, myelosuppression. Pharmacokinetics: only IV preparation.
		IV: melarsoprol (± steroids)	Trivalent arsenical compound	Adverse effects: 'arsenic in antifreeze': arsenic encephalopathy 10% (up to 50% mortality), severe extravasation injury, hepatotoxicity, cardiac toxicity.
	East African trypanosomiasi *T. b. rhodesiense*	IV: suramin (plus melarsoprol if CNS involvement)		

continued

Table 8.11 *continued*

Organism	Disease	Agent	Mechanism of action	Limitations
Sporozoa				
Toxoplasma	Toxoplasmosis (typically encephalitis or chorioretinitis)	PO: pyrimethamine plus sulfadiazine (or clindamycin) PO: trimethoprim-sulfmethoxazole (TMP-SMX)	Inhibit folic acid synthesis	Adverse effects: megaloblastic anaemia (folic acid supplementation required). Relapse risk if CD4<200 (chronic suppressive therapy may be indicated).
Entamoeba	Amoebiasis (asymptomatic and invasive)	PO: metronidazole or tinidazole, (plus paromomycin if intraluminal cysts)		

Table 8.12 Isolation strategies for infection control

Type of isolation	Specific precautions	Organisms (suspected or proven)
Contact (enteric)	Glove and gown, handwashing, safe disposal	Bacterial: *C. difficile, E. coli* O157. Viral: RSV, HSV, enterovirus.
Droplet particles >5 microns (travel <1 m)	Plus mask	Bacterial: *N. meningitidis, H. influenzae, Mycoplasma pneumoniae, Bordetella pertussis*. Viral: influenza, rubella, mumps, adenovirus, parvovirus B19, RSV.
Airborne particles <5 microns (prolonged travel in air)	Negative pressure room (air exchanges 6–12/hour)	Bacterial: *Mycobacterium tuberculosis* (TB). Viral: varicella, measles.
Protective	Positive pressure room	—
Category 4	Enhanced precautions (double gloves, fluid-repellent gown, visor); transfer to local high security infectious disease unit (HSIDU)	Viral haemorrhagic fevers excluding dengue (e.g. Lassa, Ebola), rabies.

Healthcare-associated infections

Healthcare-associated infections (HCAIs) encompass both 'hospital acquired infection' and 'nosocomial infections', acquired as a hospital inpatient, outpatient, or nursing home resident. Organisms often have high rates of antibiotic resistance (see Table 8.13).

Chain of infection

HCAIs depend upon a 'chain of infection' (see Figure 8.1). This explains how organisms can be transferred and describes potential prevention strategies.

Table 8.13 Prevalence of healthcare-associated infections organised by body system

Site	% of all HCAIs	Organisms	% isolated organisms
Respiratory	22.8%	Aerobic Gram-negative: *P. aeruginosa, K. pneumoniae, E. coli, Actinetobacter* spp.	>50%
		Aerobic Gram-positive: MRSA>MSSA> *Strep.* spp.>CNS*	20–30%
		Viral: influenza, RSV	<5%
		Fungal	<1%
Urinary	17.2%	*E. coli*	>40%
		ESBL	15%
		Proteus mirabilis	>10%
		P. aeruginosa	>10%
Skin and soft tissue infections	15.7%		
Surgical site	13.8%		
Gastrointestinal	8.8%		
Blood stream infections	7.3%	*Escherichia* spp.	>30%
		Coagulase-negative staphylococcus	14%
		S. aureus	10%
		MRSA	>13%
		Strep. spp.	8%
		Gram-negative: *Klebsiella* spp., *Pseudomonas* spp., *Enterococcus* spp.	0–3%
		Candida	2%

Healthcare-associated **Staphylococcus aureus** *infections*

Key definitions and pathogenesis

- Healthcare-associated *S. aureus* infection encompasses infections acquired:
  - >48 hours after hospital admission (nosocomial);
  - <12 months after exposure to healthcare (non-nosocomial).
- Meticillin-resistant *S. aureus* (MRSA) is distinct from meticillin-sensitive *S. aureus* (MSSA) in its antibiotic sensitivities.
- Healthcare-associated MRSA and MSSA (HA-MRSA and HA-MSSA) remain similar organisms.

Epidemiology

- MRSA represents 13–40% of reported cases of HA-*S. aureus* bacteraemia.
- HA-MRSA carries up to 9× increased risk of inpatient mortality compared with HA-MSSA.

Colonisation

- Represents harmless carriage of the organism (<3% patients during admission screening in the UK are colonised with MRSA; probably >30% colonised with MSSA on admission).

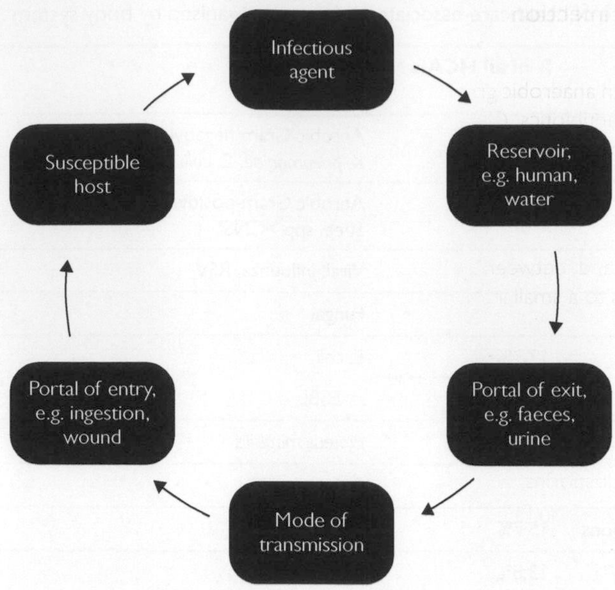

Figure 8.1 Chain of infection.

- >95% of people with nasal colonisation will carry *S. aureus* organisms at other sites.
- Colonisation is associated with increased rates of infection (approximately × 2–3).

Transmission

- Health-care worker contact.
- Fomite contact (including surfaces).
- Direct contact with other patients.
- Aerosolised nasal droplets.

Clinical manifestations

- Both organisms are associated with a wide range of nosocomial infections across body sites (see Table 8.13). HA-MSSA and HA-MRSA bacteraemia have a mortality rate of 20–40%.
- Up to 47% of HA-*S. aureus* infections develop bacteraemia. Up to 30% of patients with bacteraemia will develop metastatic infection (e.g. vertebral osteomyelitis, prosthetic device infection, pulmonary abscess).

Management

- Prevention:
  - Antibiotic stewardship and infection control.
  - Active surveillance: all emergency and elective admissions since 2011.
- Suppression (or 'decolonisation'):
  - Regimen: 5 days topical mupirocin (nasal) and chlorhexidine (shampoo and bodywash).
  - Indications: recurrent MRSA infections, pre-procedure (surgery, invasive non-surgical procedure), outbreaks.
  - Three repeat screens at 1-week intervals should determine success of decolonisation.

Treatment

- Flucloxacillin, vancomycin, teicoplanin, daptomycin, rifampicin, linezolid, depending on a range of bacterial and host factors.

Clostridium difficile infection

Pathogenesis

Clostridium difficile is an anaerobic gram-positive, spore-forming, toxin-producing bacillus. Spores are resistant to heat, acid and antibiotics. *Clostridium difficile* is the causative organism of antibiotic-associated colitis. It colonises the gastrointestinal tract after the normal gut flora have been altered by antibiotic therapy. The organism is capable of elaborating exotoxins that lead to inflammation and diarrhoea.

Epidemiology

In NHS Trusts in England, between 2017 and 2018 there were 13,286 cases of *Clostridium difficile* infection (CDI). This translates to a small increase of 3.4% from 2016/17, and a decrease of 76.1% from 2007/08.

Risk factors

- Age >65 years.
- Colonisation: 30–50% of nursing home residents and 3% healthy adults are colonised.
- Antibiotic exposure; any antibiotic, most frequently, fluoroquinolones, clindamycin, broad-spectrum penicillins, cephalosporins.
- Gastric acid suppression PPI>>H2 blockers.

Clinical manifestations

*C. difficile-**associated diarrhoea***

- Non-severe (mild or moderate).
- Severe:
  - T >38.5°C.
  - Peak leucocytosis > 15 × 10^9/L.
  - Serum creatinine (>50% above baseline).
  - Evidence of severe colitis (at endoscopy or on imaging).
  - *Not* stool frequency.

Pseudomembranous colitis

- 80–90% *C. difficile*-associated diarrhoea (CDAD). Histological diagnosis based on endoscopic findings.
- Life-threatening complications: fulminant colitis, ileus, toxic megacolon (>10 cm caecal dilatation), colonic perforation.

Diagnosis

Testing is indicated in any patient with a *single* episode of diarrhoea that cannot be clearly attributable to an underlying condition or medication.

Stool tests

1. Glutamate dehydrogenase (GDH) enzyme immunoassay (EIA), GDH nucleic acid amplification test (NAAT) or GDH PCR to identify the organism, followed by toxin EIA to identify active *CD* toxin production.
2. Interpretation of stool results:
   - If GDH EIA is positive, and toxin EIA is positive (positive predictive value [PPV] = 91.4%), then *CD* is most likely to be present
   - If GDH EIA is negative, and toxin EIA is negative (negative predictive value [NPV] = 98.9%) then *CD* is very unlikely to be present.
   - If GDH EIA (or NAAT) is positive, and toxin EIA is negative, then *CD* could be present (potential *CD* excretors).
3. Culture testing is not routinely performed.
4. Only re-test to confirm recurrent *CD* infection if the symptoms resolve and then recur.

CT imaging

Endoscopy indicated if:

- High suspicion of CDAD, but stool tests are negative.
- Failure to respond to therapy.
- Atypical presentation with minimal diarrhoea ('silent CDI').

Management

Infection control

- Antibiotic therapy:
  - If non-severe – oral metronidazole 10–14 days.
  - If severe – oral vancomycin 10–14 days.
  - High risk of recurrence: oral fidaxomicin 10–14 days.
  - Poor response to first line: increase oral vancomycin dose, fidaxomicin, add in IV metronidazole.
- Salvage therapy:
  - Stat dose IVIG.
  - Faecal transplantation (infuse 50 g of healthy donor faeces via enema or NG tube to restore microbiota).
  - Surgery (typically if caecal dilatation >10 cm, rising lactate).

Recurrence

Approximately defined as CDAD within 30 days of previous episode:

- 20% risk of recurrence after first episode.
- 50% risk of recurrence after second episode.

Associated with advancing age and ongoing antibiotic therapy.

Upper respiratory tract infections

Rhinitis and the 'common cold'

The 'common cold' is a clinical syndrome caused by numerous viral pathogens. Rhinovirus and Coronaviruses account for >50% of identified cases annually. The syndrome is characterised by mild self-limiting symptoms that typically include rhinorrhoea, low grade fever, sore throat and malaise. In high-risk groups, serious morbidity and mortality can complicate infections with many of these viruses (most notably: influenza, respiratory syncytial virus [RSV] and certain Coronavirus strains).

Pharyngitis and tonsillitis

A range of viral and bacterial organisms commonly causes pharyngitis (see Table 8.14). Of these infections >50% are viral, most of which complicate rhinitis. Streptococcal pharyngitis is the most common bacterial proponent and is associated with significant complications.

Streptococcus pyogenes *throat infection*

Pathogenesis

- Lancefield GAS, also known as *Streptococcus pyogenes*, is responsible for a wide array of conditions. Most commonly worldwide, it causes pharyngitis in all age groups.
- Up to 20% of asymptomatic people carry GAS in their nasopharynx. Transmission is typically by direct contact with respiratory secretions.

Complications

Suppurative

- Local spread: otitis media, sinusitis, mastoiditis.
- Peritonsillar abscess ('quinsy'): infection of fauces and soft palate with risk of airway obstruction.

Table 8.14 Common infectious causes of pharyngitis

Organism	Example	Comment
Viruses	Epstein–Barr virus (EBV)	>80% Pharyngitis in infectious mononucleosis (glandular fever).
	Herpes simplex virus (HSV) type 1	May be severe with ulceration.
	Cytomegalovirus (CMV)	Milder mononucleosis syndrome.
	Primary HIV	Seroconversion illness.
Common bacteria	*Streptococcus pyogenes* (Group A *Streptococcus* [GAS])	10–20% acute pharyngitis; multiple complications.
	Non-Group A *Streptococcus* (Groups C or G)	Not associated with rheumatic fever.
Less common bacteria	*Mycoplasma pneumoniae*	With bronchitis in young healthy adults.
	Neisseria gonorrhoeae	Via orogenital contact.
	Corynebacterium diphtheria	Serious disease in non-immunised countries; 30% develop severe diphtheria caused by exotoxin (formation of grey tough pseudomembrane over pharynx which bleeds on scraping); toxic 'bull neck' swelling of URT may cause stridor. Treatment: antitoxin and penicillin.
	Haemophilus influenzae type B	Acute epiglottitis in non-immunised (>children).
	Fusobacterium necrophorum	Lemierre syndrome (associated septic thrombophlebitis of internal jugular vein and metastatic pulmonary infection).

Non-suppurative

- *Scarlet fever*:
  - Punctate erythematous rash spreading from face to body, sparing the hands and soles, and bright red tongue with prominent papillae; rash desquamates at 1 week.
  - Can be associated with life-threatening cellulitis and sepsis.
- *Acute rheumatic fever (ARF)*:
  - Antibodies against antigens in the GAS cell wall cross-react with heart tissue and other structures (such as neurones).
  - Onset: 2–4 weeks post-acute GAS infection.
  - Peak prevalence between 5–15 years in children; rare, but possible in adults.
  - Long-term sequelae: rheumatic heart disease. 10–20 years post-ARF. Affects up to 50% with carditis as part of ARF.
- *Acute glomerulonephritis*:
  - Streptococcal immune complexes trigger glomerular inflammation and promote antibodies that cross-react with glomerular components.
  - Greatest risk of severe disease in patients >60 years (and children between 5 and 12 years) associated with AKI.
- Streptococcal toxic shock syndrome.

Management

- Antibiotics:
  - Oral phenoxymethylpenicillin or macrolide.
  - Clindamycin may be useful for tissue penetration if significant oedema.
  - Amoxicillin is associated with a maculopapular rash in >50% cases acute EBV.

- Surgical drainage of abscesses may be indicated.
- No vaccination is available.

Meningitis

Pathogenesis

Meningitis is defined by raised white blood cells in the cerebrospinal fluid (CSF). The vast majority of community-acquired meningitis cases in the UK result from invasion of the meninges by organisms that colonise the nasopharynx (see Table 8.15).

Table 8.15 Common causes of acute bacterial meningitis

Organism	Site of entry	Ages affected	Associations
Streptococcus pneumoniae 'pneumococcal'	Nasopharynx; local or distant foci	All	Basal skull or cribriform plate fractures, sinusitis, pneumonia.
Neisseria meningitides 'meningococcal'	Nasopharynx	All	University students.
Listeria monocytogenes	GI tract; placenta	Elderly; neonates	Steroids, pregnancy, alcohol dependence.
Haemophilus influenza	Nasopharynx	All	Local infection.
Staphylococcus aureus	Bacteraemia; skin	All	Foreign bodies, e.g. shunts.
Gram-negative bacilli	Various	Elderly; neonates	Neurosurgery; nosocomial.

Clinical features

Symptoms

- <50% present with the classical triad of fever, neck stiffness and altered mental state.

Signs

- The absence of 'meningism' (nuchal rigidity) on clinical examination is not sufficient to exclude bacterial meningitis and poorly predicts CSF pleocytosis.
- Kernig's sign (with hips flexed at 90°, a patient is unable or unwilling to extend their knee) and Brudzinski's sign (spontaneous flexion of the hips during attempted passive flexion of a patient's neck) have low sensitivity for diagnosis.
- Neurological:
  - seizures: 30%
  - focal neurological deficits: 35%
  - papilloedema: <5% at presentation.
- Skin: *Neisseria meningitides* (meningococcal) meningitis: petechiae or purpura represent subcutaneous (SC) haemorrhage and disseminated intravascular coagulation (DIC).

Diagnosis

CSF studies

- Brain imaging prior to lumbar puncture (LP) is indicated only in patients whose history or examination is suggestive of brain herniation risk during LP. This should include all immunocompromised patients.
- Prior to antibiotic administration, Gram staining is approximately 90% sensitive and approaching 100% specific for the diagnosis of bacterial meningitis (see Table 8.16):
- CSF biochemistry and cytology of bacterial meningitis:

Table 8.16 Expected CSF microscopy findings for common causes of acute bacterial meningitis

Gram stain	Organism
Gram-positive diplococci	*Streptococcus pneumoniae*
Gram-negative diplococci	*Neisseria meningitides*
Gram-positive rods and coccobacilli	*Listeria monocytogenes*
Gram-negative small pleomorphic coccobacilli	*Haemophilus influenza*

- High protein: 100–500 mg/dL.
- Low glucose: ratio of CSF to serum glucose <0.4 (normal CSF ratio >1.4).
- White cell count (WCC):
  - >90% cases have total WCC > 100 cells per μL (LP, seizures and haemorrhage may yield false positive elevated CSF WCCs, but usually <100 cells per μL).
  - >80% of WCC are polymorphonuclear (PMN) cells (acute phase of viral and mycobacterial meningitis may have high PMN count, but usually <80%).

- CSF culture:
  - Before antibiotics: CSF culture 90% sensitivity; <4 hours 75% sensitivity; >4 hours <10% sensitivity.
- Additional investigations:
  - Blood culture.
  - Nasopharyngeal (NP) swabs.

Complications

Mortality

- Delay in antibiotic administration by as little as 3 hours has been shown to significantly increase 3-month mortality.
- Despite antibiotic therapy 25% and 35% mortality rates for community-acquired and nosocomial bacterial meningitis.

Hearing loss

- Permanent sensorineural hearing loss affects approximately 12% of patients.

Management

Any confirmed or probable case of acute bacterial meningitis should be referred to the local public health authority.

Antibiotic therapy

Empiric therapy

Increasing rates of pneumococcal resistance to penicillins (up to 50%) and cephalosporins are common, particularly in infections acquired outside of the UK. If resistance is suspected, adjunctive vancomycin should be considered empirically (see Table 8.17). Where the differential diagnosis includes tuberculosis, specialist advice should be sought for initiation of antituberculous therapy. If herpes simplex meningo-encephalitis is suspected, high dose aciclovir should be given empirically.

Optimising therapy

- Gram staining should narrow therapy within the first 24 hours awaiting culture results.

Table 8.17 Antimicrobial therapy for acute microbial meningitis

Treatment group	Empirical antibiotics
Children and babies >3months	Ceftriaxone.
Babies <3 months	Cefotaxime *and* amoxicillin or ampicillin.
Suspected meningococcal disease other age groups	Ceftriaxone.
Recent travel outside UK or prolonged or recent antibiotic exposure (within 3 months)	Vancomycin in addition to ceftriaxone.
Immunocompromised	Vancomycin *and* ampicillin in addition to ceftriaxone.
Nosocomial	Vancomycin *and* broad spectrum antibiotic with anti-pseudomonal cover (e.g. ceftazidime, meropenem).

Duration of therapy

- 14 days Rx for pneumococcal meningitis.
- 7 days Rx for meningococcal meningitis or other organisms.

Adjunctive steroid therapy

- 10 mg IV dexamethasone 6-hourly for 4 days should be initiated with or before the first antibiotic dose: reduces neurological complication rate if *S. pneumoniae or H. influenzae*.

Prevention

1. Vaccination
2. Chemoprophylaxis:
   - Prolonged close contacts (and transient close contacts if exposed to large respiratory droplets) in 7 days before onset of confirmed or probable meningococcal meningitis infection: 500 mg ciprofloxacin STAT or 600 mg rifampicin BD for 2 days, and full meningococcal vaccination.

Encephalitis

Pathogenesis

Encephalitis is defined as presence of an inflammatory process of the brain parenchyma in association with clinical evidence of neurological dysfunction. The aetiology of the disease is identified in less than 30% of cases. Enteroviruses are the most commonly PCR-isolated virus. Epidemiological factors (in particular geography and animal exposure) and past medical history inform diagnosis (see Table 8.18).

Clinical features

- Encephalitis is characterised by abnormal brain function:
  - Non-specific: seizures, confusion, personality change.
  - Specific: focal neurological deficits.
- Fever may or may not be present.

Diagnosis

Imaging

- Unilateral or bilateral temporal lobe involvement on MRI is strongly suggestive of HSV encephalitis (90% of PCR-proven HSV encephalitis will have MRI changes).

Table 8.18 Common infectious causes of acute encephalitis

Risk factor	Pathogen
Age	
Elderly	*Listeria monocytogenes.*
Immunocompromised	Viral: *Varicella zoster* virus (VZV), cytomegalovirus (CMV), JC virus.
	Non-viral: TB, *Cryptococcus neoformans, Histoplasma capsulatum, Toxoplasma gondii.*
Animal contact	
Birds	West Nile virus.
Cats/dogs	Viral: rabies.
	Non-viral: *Coxiella burnetii, Bartonella henselae, T. gondii.*
Insect contact	
Mosquitoes	St Louis virus, Equine viruses, West Nile virus, Japanese encephalitis virus.
Tick	Viral: tickborne encephalitis virus.
	Non-viral: *Borrelia burgdorferi*, Rocky Mountain Spotted fever (*Rickettsia rickettsii*).
Human contact	*Herpes simplex* virus (HSV), VZV, measles, mumps, Epstein–Barr virus (EBV), HHV-6, enteroviruses.
Vaccination or recent infection in last 1–14 days	Acute disseminated encephalomyelitis (ADEM).

CSF studies

- Often *not* diagnostic.
- Typical CSF findings in viral encephalitis:
  - High WCC, but typically total WCC <250/mm^3 (mostly lymphocytes; early infection may show PMNs).
  - High protein, but total protein typically <150 mg/dL.
  - Normal glucose (>50% serum glucose).

CSF microbiology and virology polymerase chain reaction

- Negative results cannot be used as definitive evidence against the diagnosis.
- Sensitivity and specificity >95% for HSV-1 encephalitis PCR; remains sensitive for up to 7 days after treatment initiation.

Blood tests

- Acute and convalescent (paired) serology.

Electroencephalography (EEG)

- Useful for excluding non-convulsive seizure states.

Complications

- HSV-1 encephalitis: despite treatment, 18-month mortality is approximately 25% (age >30 years, delay in treatment >4 days after symptomatic illness, and low Glasgow Coma Score [GCS] predict poor outcomes).
- Neurological sequelae of all cause viral encephalitis:
  - 60% no sequelae.
  - 25% will not return to work; 1% vegetative state.

Management

Empirical therapy

- Antibiotics: clinical suspicion of bacterial meningitis should prompt empirical antibiotic therapy pending the results of CSF studies.
- Aciclovir: empirical treatment for HSV encephalitis should also be initiated if there is clinical suspicion.

Vaccination

Vaccination is available for: rabies, measles, Japanese encephalitis virus, *Varicella zoster* virus (VZV).

Cerebral abscess

Pathogenesis

Cerebral abscess represents focal collection within the brain parenchyma (see Table 8.19).

Table 8.19 Risk factors for common causes of cerebral abscess

Predisposition	Organisms
Direct spread	
Oral	Strep. spp., *Bacteroides*/ anaerobes
Otogenic	Strep. spp., *Pseudomonas aeruginosa*
Sinus	Strep. spp. (*S. mileri*), *Haemophilus, Fusobacterium*
Neurosurgery	Staph. spp., *Strep.* spp., *Pseudomonas* spp.
Trauma	*Clostridia*
Haematogenous spread	
Chronic pulmonary infections (empyema, bronchiectasis)	Strep. spp., *actinomyces*
Pulmonary AV malformations (10%)	Strep. spp.
Endocarditis (2–4%)	*Viridans strep., S. aureus*
Intra-abdominal	Gram-negative organisms
Immunocompromised	
	Bacteria: *L. monocytogenes, Nocardia*
	Fungal: *Aspergillus, Cryptococcus,*
	Other: *T. gondii, Taenia solium* (cysticercosis)

Direct spread usually results in single abscesses. Haematogenous spread leads to multiple abscess formation in the distribution of the middle cerebral artery and gray–white matter junctions.

Clinical features

Headache is the most common presenting symptom. Signs commonly found are fever (50%), focal neurological deficit (50%) and seizures (25%).

Diagnosis

- Imaging:
  - MRI is preferred to CT.

  - 'Ring enhancing' lesions represent breakdown of the blood–brain barrier and development of an inflammatory capsule.
- Lumbar puncture is typically contraindicated due to risk of transtentorial herniation.
- Stereotactic CT-guided or surgical aspiration.

Management

- Medical:
  - Empirical therapy (see Table 8.20): duration of antibiotics: 4–8 weeks depending on clinical circumstances and radiology.
  - Steroids: if mass effect or low GCS.
- Surgery.

Intra-abdominal infections

Acute viral hepatitis

Table 8.20 Overview of hepatitis viruses A, B, C, D and E

Virus	Transmission	Clinical	Diagnosis	Management
A	Faeco-oral	Incubation: 2-4 weeks. Features: malaise with jaundice by day 7; 0.3% acute liver failure (ALF). No chronic carriage.	Anti-HAV IgM with jaundice.	Contact isolation until 1–2 days. No specific Rx. PEP: HAV vaccine ± IVIG.
B	Blood-borne; sexual	Incubation: 6 weeks–6 months. <30% acute hepatitis (<0.5% ALF; >5% chronic carriage).	HBsAg 2–8 weeks pre-symptoms; HBV DNA, HBeAg and anti-HBc IgM with symptoms.	No specific Rx if not ALF. PEP: HBV vaccine ± IVIG.
C	Blood-borne; sexual	Incubation: 14–60 days. <20% acute hepatitis (rare ALF; >85% chronic carriage).	Anti-HCV IgG in 50% symptomatic patients (8 weeks to 6 months post-exposure); HCV RNA 4 weeks post-exposure often with symptoms.	Consider Rx after 12 weeks. PEP: nil available.
D	Co-infection with HBV	Acute co-infection with HBV, or 'super-infection' of chronic HBsAg carrier.	HDV RNA, HDV IgM and IgG.	No specific Rx or PEP.
E	Faeco-oral	Incubation: 4–8 weeks. 3% ALF (up to 40% mortality in 3rd trimester pregnancy). No chronic carriage unless immunosuppressed.	Anti-HEV IgM.	No specific Rx or PEP.

Other viral causes

Herpes viruses (EBV, CMV, VZV, HSV), adenovirus, Coxsackie, measles, rubella, yellow fever.

Other non-virus causes

Leptospirosis, *Coxiella burnetii*, brucellosis, legionellosis, *Yersinia pestis* (plague).

Infectious diarrhoea

Viral diarrhoea

Norovirus ('winter vomiting bug' or Norwalk virus) is the most common cause of gastroenteritis in the UK. It is transmitted by aerosolised vomitus and fomites. It has a short incubation of 6–36 hours, and causes symptoms for up to 1 week, with up to 2 weeks of subsequent virus shedding. Rotavirus, astroviruses and enteric adenoviruses are the other common causes of viral gastroenteritis. Diagnosis of viral gastroenteritis is by electron microscopy, antigen testing and PCR analysis of stool or vomitus. In practice, viruses are rarely isolated.

Bacterial diarrhoea

Salmonella spp. (non-typhoidal) are the most commonly isolated organisms associated with foreign travel. For common causes of acute bacterial gastroenteritis, see Table 8.21.

Table 8.21 Common causes of acute bacterial gastroenteritis

Organism	Pathogenesis	Associations	History
Escherichia coli (6 pathogenic strains)			Incubation: 1–5 days. Common features: vomiting and diarrhoea for first 6–24 hours followed by watery diarrhoea.
EHEC (enterhaemorrhagic *E. coli*) or VTEC (verocytotoxic *E. coli*): serogroup O157:H7 is most common	Shiga toxin	Outbreaks; food-borne (>beef; very contagious: 10 organisms required).	Features: bloody diarrhoea. Complications: shiga toxin causes haemorrhagic colitis and haemolytic uraemic syndrome (HUS: AKI, microangiopathic haemolytic anaemia, thrombocytopenia) up to 10% mortality.
Non-typhoidal *Salmonella* spp. (>*S. enteritidis* and *S. tymphimurium*)	Epithelial invasion	Food-borne (>poultry, eggs). Summer pattern.	Incubation: 12–36 hours. Features: malaise, vomiting then watery diarrhoea by 24 hours; usually self-limiting by 10 days. Complications: colitis 10%, bacteraemia <5%, metastatic infection (>bone/joints, classically in patients with sickle cell disease).
Campylobacter spp. (*Campylobacter jejuni* is the most common)	Enterotoxin >ileum	Food-borne (>poultry). Summer pattern.	Incubation: 1–7 days. Features: febrile prodrome then vomiting, abdominal pain and watery (bloody <25%) diarrhoea (small volume diarrhoea may be mistaken for surgical abdomen); usually self-limiting by 10 days. Complications: reactive arthritis (onset 1–several weeks after diarrhoea); Guillain–Barré syndrome (GBS; 0.1% after acute *Campylobacter* within 2 months).
Shigella spp. (>75% *S. sonnei* in UK; also known as shigellosis, and 'bacillary dysentery')	Epithelial invasion (>colon) followed by ulceration, abscesses and enterotoxins (including Shiga toxin)	Contaminated food and water. Faeco-oral. Developing >> developed world.	Incubation: 1–7 days. Features: fever, colicky abdominal pain, and mucoid, bloody diarrhoea. Complications: up to 3% toxic megacolon (HUS with *S. dysenteriae* elaborated Shiga toxin).
Cholera (*Vibrio cholerae*)	Cholera toxin	Contaminated food and water (>shellfish). Very rare in developed world.	Incubation: 3–4 days. Features: variable severity: voluminous diarrhoea then pale 'rice-water' stool; usually resolves by 3–6 days; mortality >50% untreated.

Treatment

- Rehydration.
- Antimotility agent if afebrile, non-bloody diarrhoea.
- Empiric antibiotics:
  - Indications – fever, bloody diarrhoea, symptoms >1 week.
  - Antibiotics – fluoroquinolones, macrolides, cephalosporins.

Enteric fever

Pathogenesis

The term 'enteric fever' is used to distinguish both typhoid and paratyphoid fever syndromes from rickettsial typhus infection. *Salmonella enterica* serotype *Typhi*, other serotypes, including *Paratyphi*, produce very similar symptoms. Salmonellae penetrate the gut mucosa through Peyer's patches in the small intestine. Necrosis of submucosal tissues may cause ileal perforation. Organisms may disseminate to the bloodstream and lymphatic system. Organisms persist within macrophages in the liver, spleen and bone marrow.

Epidemiology

Endemic in areas of poor sanitation. Transmitted via contaminated food or water.

Clinical features

- Incubation: 5 to 21 days after ingestion.
- Classical presentation:
  - *First week:* fever, malaise, relative bradycardia, diarrhoea or constipation.
  - *Second week:* abdominal pain, 'rose spots' (salmon-coloured macules on abdomen; transient for hours to days), neurological symptoms (Greek word *typhos* means hazy): headache, delirium, meningitis).
  - *Third week (without treatment):* GI bleeding or perforation (3–10%, risk increases with age).

Diagnosis

- Blood test: early neutrophilia; later neutropenia; abnormal LFTs.
- Culture:
  - Blood 50–70% sensitivity
  - Bone marrow >90% sensitivity (>50% sensitivity after 5 days antibiotic therapy).
  - Stool, urine, rose spot biopsy <40% sensitivity.
- Serology (e.g. Widal test) is generally not used.

Complications

- Relapse: 1–6% of patients will have recurrent bacteraemia within 2–3 weeks after treatment.
- Chronic carriage: 1–5% excrete organisms in stool or urine >12 months. Persistent excretion is associated with contaminated gallstones. Typically, patients do not develop symptomatic disease.

Management

- Fluoroquinolone resistance is common (> Indian subcontinent).
- Empirical antibiotic therapy pending culture results:
  - Uncomplicated: outpatient oral ciprofloxacin or azithromycin.
  - Complicated: inpatient parenteral ciprofloxacin or ceftriaxone.
  - Chronic carriage: ciprofloxacin for 1 month. Consider cholecystectomy.

Prevention

- Immunisation: Not 100% protective against *S. typhi*, and provides no protection against *S. paratyphi*.
- Public health measures: food handlers may return to work once asymptomatic; two negative stool samples post-therapy for food handlers who prepare raw foods.

Liver abscess

Pyogenic and amoebic abscesses are typically symptomatic with fever and abdominal pain. Hydatid liver cysts are often discovered incidentally. For common infectious causes of cystic liver lesions, see Table 8.22.

Table 8.22 Common infectious causes of cystic liver lesions

Organism	Pathogenesis	Complications	Diagnosis
Pyogenic			
Polymicrobial or mono-microbial (*Streptococcus milleri* or *S. anginosus; Staphylococcus aureus; Klebsiella pneumoniae*; TB)	Portal vein pyaemia (biliary, enteric or pelvic infection); haematogenous metastatic infection (>mono-microbial).	Metastatic infection; pylephlebitis (suppurative thrombosis).	CT or US; blood culture; aspirate.
Amoebic			
Entamoeba histolytica	Ingested cysts excyst in the colon and ascend the portal system; <30% associated with intercurrent diarrhoea.	Amoeboma (granulation tissue causing obstruction); rupture (peritonitis, pericarditis, empyemas).	CT: enhancing rim; serology (high false positive rate in endemic areas); aspirate (brown odourless 'anchovy paste').
Hydatid			
Canine tapeworms *Echinococcus granulosus* or *Echinococcus vogeli*	Ingested eggs hatch in the GI tract and ascend the portal system.	Rupture into biliary tree (colic, cholangitis, pancreatitis), peritonitis, pulmonary or pleural hydatidosis; hypersensitivity.	US (95% sensitive), CT or MRI (infoldings of the inner cyst wall, separation of the hydatid membrane from the wall of the cyst); serology; rarely aspirate.

Treatment

Pyogenic

- Medical: Parenteral co-amoxiclav, tazobactam/ piperacillin, ceftriaxone with metronidazole pending culture for 4–6 weeks.
- Drainage: Aspiration: <5 cm abscess; drain insertion: >5 cm abscess; surgical drainage if multiloculated, viscous aspirate, poor response to drain.

Amoebic

- Medical: Invasive amoebiasis requires combined therapies: tissue agent oral metronidazole for 10 days, and intraluminal agent: oral paromomycin for 7 days.
- Drainage: for very large cysts, or uncertain diagnosis.

Hydatid

- Medical: smaller simple cysts: albendazole (up to 6 months therapy); larger simple cysts: PAIR (puncture, aspiration, injection of a scolicidal agent, and re-aspiration) procedure with adjunctive albendazole (1 month pre- and post-procedure).
- Drainage for complex multi-compartment cysts.

Urinary tract infections

Lower urinary tract infections

Asymptomatic bacteriuria

Urine should be sterile. Asymptomatic bacteriuria is defined as isolation of a single organism of ≥ 10^4 colony forming units/mL. The presence of pyuria is inadequate for the diagnosis of bacteriuria. Asymptomatic bacteriuria is not associated with increased morbidity or mortality unless detected in pregnant patients or those undergoing invasive urological procedures. It is present in up to 20% elderly women.

Acute cystitis

Pathogenesis

Bacteria enter the bladder by either ascending the urethra or haematogenously. 20% of women experience a symptomatic urinary tract infections (UTI) during their lifetime. Risk factors include: frequent sexual intercourse, diaphragm use, spermicide use, lack of urination after intercourse. Complicated UTI may be structural (congenital or acquired) or functional (e.g. vesicoureteric reflux). All UTIs in men, pregnant women and children should be considered complicated.

Uncomplicated infections are mostly Gram negative: *E. coli* (75–95%).

Complicated infections:

- Gram negative: *Pseudomonas* spp., *Serratia* spp.
- Gram positive: *Enterococci* (including vancomycin-resistant *Enterococci* [VRE]), *Staphylococci* (*S. aureus* may be suggestive of metastatic infection).
- Fungi (mostly *Candida* spp. in patients receiving antimicrobial therapy).
- Polymicrobial.

Clinical features

Features may be subtle in the elderly.

Symptoms: urinary frequency, dysuria, urgency, suprapubic pain, haematuria.

Diagnosis

- Urinalysis: *if symptomatic*, positive urinalysis has a 92% positive predictive value for UTI. This includes leucocytes (white cells secrete leucocyte esterase, which is detected on dipstick), nitrites (*enterobacteriaceae* convert nitrate to nitrite) and blood.
- Culture of urine and blood.
- Other causes of sterile pyuria: urethritis (*Chlamydia trachomatis, Neisseria gonorrhoeae*, trichomoniasis, *Candida* spp., *Herpes simplex* virus), non-infectious irritants, pelvic inflammatory disease, renal TB.

Complications

Recurrent infection, acute pyelonephritis, prostatitis (50% of men with recurrent UTI).

Management

Empirical antibiotic therapy pending culture results:

- Uncomplicated: 3 days trimethoprim or nitrofurantoin (only if eGFR >60 mL/min).
- Complicated: 7– 14 days fluoroquinolones (better prostatic penetration in men).

Recurrence (infection >2 weeks after initial treatment):

- Longer course of antibiotics ideally based on culture.
- Consider urological assessment.
- Prevention: post-coital voiding, avoid spermicides, cranberry juice.
- Prophylaxis: if ≥3/12 months: continuous or post-coital.

Upper urinary tract infection

Acute pyelonephritis

Pathogenesis

Pyelonephritis implies infection of the upper renal tract with involvement of the kidney. It most commonly occurs after ascending infection secondary to acute cystitis.

Clinical features

Fever and flank pain associated with renal angle tenderness. Symptoms of acute cystitis may or may not be present. Onset is usually over hours, but in cases of complicated infection symptoms may be more insidious over days or weeks.

Diagnosis

- Imaging (US or CT):
  - Uncomplicated: consider if symptoms persist for 48 hours despite treatment.
  - Complicated: early CT imaging is preferred if there is history suggestive of complicated UTI (such as nephrolithiasis or obstruction).

Complications

- Abscess formation: nephric and perinephric.
- Papillary necrosis (and secondary obstruction).
- Emphysematous pyelonephritis:
  - Necrotising multifocal bacterial nephritis.
  - Pathogenesis: >80% associated with diabetes mellitus and typical organisms.
  - Clinical features: flank mass in up to 50% ± crepitation over thigh or flank if advanced infection.
  - Up to 80% mortality if gas extending into perinephric space.

Acute renal failure is rare unless in pregnancy, or renal tract obstruction. However, irreversible renal scarring occurs after even a single episode of pyelonephritis.

Management

- Empirical antibiotic therapy pending culture results:
  - Uncomplicated: 14 days fluoroquinolone PO.
  - Complicated: IV broad spectrum antibiotics (cephalosporin or carbapenem) ± aminoglycoside.

Surgery is indicated for pyonephrosis, abscesses and emphysematous pyelonephritis, if failing to respond to parenteral antibiotic therapy.

Skin and soft tissue infections

Cellulitis

Pathogenesis

- Impetigo: superficial *S. aureus* or GAS infection characterised by small vesicular lesions that develop flaccid bullae, which release yellow discharge that crusts.
- Erysipelas: acute spreading infection of upper dermis and lymphatics.
- Cellulitis: infection that involves deeper dermis and SC fat.
- Risk factors: disruption of skin barrier (bites, trauma, IV drug use, toe web intertrigo, ulcers (venous or arterial); skin inflammation (eczema); pre-existing skin infection (tinea pedis, varicella, impetigo); limb oedema (venous insufficiency, lymphoedema); limb ischaemia; immunosuppression.
- Microbiology: beta-haemolytic streptococci (*S. pyogenes*) and *S. aureus* are the most common pathogens. Up to 96% cases respond to beta-lactam antibiotic therapy, despite no organism being identified in >80%.

Clinical features

Erysipelas classically has a more abrupt onset over hours with clearly demarcated lesions. Cellulitis may have a more indolent course over days with less demarcated spreading erythema. Chills and fever are common at onset.

Diagnosis

- Typically a clinical diagnosis.
- Culture:
  - Skin swabs have no role if skin is intact; culture of pus or bullae fluid.
  - Fungal scrapings of toe webs.
  - Blood cultures if systemic features (<5% yield in patients admitted to hospital with provisional diagnosis of cellulitis).
  - Consider imaging if deeper infection suspected.

Differential diagnosis

- Non-infectious: varicose eczema/stasis dermatitis (early venous insufficiency), lipodermatosclerosis (heavily pigmented areas of firm induration); fibrosing panniculitis in chronic venous insufficiency, deep vein thrombosis, acute gout, drug reactions.

Complications

- Systemic illness (toxic shock syndrome, sepsis)
- Local spread:
  - Soft tissue: SC abscess, pyomyositis, necrotising fasciitis.
  - Bone: osteomyelitis; chronic ulceration.
- Distant spread.
- Recurrent cellulitis.

Management

- Conservative: elevation, emollients.
- Antibiotic therapy:
  - Empirical antibiotics: 5–14 days flucloxacillin, clindamycin or macrolides as monotherapy according to local guidelines.
  - Additional benzylpenicillin is not necessary.
  - Systemic features or significant co-morbidity predisposing to cellulitis: parenteral therapy with switch to oral therapy according to clinical circumstances (average of 3.5 days).
  - MRSA risk: add teicoplanin, vancomycin, linezolid, doxycycline.
- Outpatient parenteral antibiotic therapy (OPAT):
  - Exact role is usually defined locally.
  - May be appropriate for systemically well patients without significant co-morbidities.

Specific forms of cellulitis

Periorbital cellulitis

- Associated with trauma, or contiguous sinus, ear and dental infections.
- Complications: keratopathy, visual loss and ophthalmoplegia, cavernous sinus thrombosis, meningitis.
- Ophthalmic emergency: consider MRI imaging, surgical review, urgent IV ceftriaxone and metronidazole.

Animal bites

- Often polymicrobial:
  - Gram negative: *Pasteurella* spp., *Capnocytophaga canimorsus*, Bacteroides, Fusobacteria.
  - Gram positive: Staphylococci, Streptococci.
- Prophylaxis: if presenting >8 hours after full-thickness bite: 5 days PO co-amoxiclav.
- Vaccination:
  - If completed tetanus primary immunisation: tetanus toxoid only.
  - If incomplete tetanus primary immunisation: tetanus immune globulin and tetanus vaccination.
  - Consider rabies therapy.

Water exposure

- Organisms: five bacteria associated with both fresh and saltwater exposure and subsequent cellulitis: *Aeromonas spp., Edwardsiella tarda, Erysipelothrix rhusiopathiae, Vibrio vulnificus* (typically saltwater), *Mycobacterium marinum* (AEEVM).
- *Aeromonas* and *V. vulnificus* infection may progress rapidly to severe necrotising infection.
- *V. vulnificus* may present as 'primary' sepsis without clear infective focus (30% presentations) and also bullous cellulitis; cirrhosis and hereditary haemochromatosis predispose patients to severe *V. vulnificus* infection.
- Empirical antibiotic therapy: cephalosporin or clindamycin + levofloxacin; consider adding doxycycline if seawater exposure and possible *V. vulnificus* infection.

Necrotising fasciitis

Pathogenesis

Severe acute infection of superficial and deep fascia. Skeletal muscle is often spared.

- Type I (polymicrobial): at least one anaerobic organism (e.g. *Clostridium, Bacteroides, Fusobacterium*) *and* at least one facultative anaerobic streptococcal organism (other than group A) or Enterobacteriaceae (e.g. *E. coli, Proteus, Klebsiella*).
- Type II: GAS (*S. pyogenes*) or other beta haemolytic streptococci isolated alone or in combination, most typically with *S. aureus*. Often in healthy individuals and via haematogenous spread (e.g. secondary to pharyngitis; up to 50% no portal of organisms entry identified). Approximately 5% of GAS skin and soft tissue infections (SSTIs) are necrotising.

Both type I and II infections may have preceding history of skin injury: laceration, trauma, intravenous drug use (IVDU), surgery, burns.

Clinical features

- Systemic toxicity is often present.
- Signs:
  - Most commonly affects lower limbs, but any anatomical site can be affected, e.g. Fournier's gangrene (male genitalia).
  - Exquisitely tender swollen skin (pain out of proportion to appearance).
  - Progression over 24–72 hours to skin necrosis.
  - SC gas possible in type I infection.

Diagnosis

Typically a clinical diagnosis.

Complications

It carries a 34% mortality and risk of compartment syndrome. Worse if complicated by toxic shock syndrome.

Management

- Emergency surgical exploration and debridement should not be delayed.
- Empirical antibiotic therapy: carabapenem or beta-lactamase inhibitor plus clindamycin, and consider agent for MRSA if patient at risk (e.g. vancomycin). If penicillin allergic, try clindamycin, gentamicin and metronidazole.
- Consider intravenous immunoglobulin (IVIG) in toxic shock syndrome.

Pyomyositis

Pathogenesis

- Purulent infection of skeletal muscle associated with haematogenous spread.
- Risk factors: immunosuppression, trauma, IVDU.
- Microbiology: *S. aureus* >> GAS > Gram-negative organisms. However, mycobacterial and fungal pathogens are also recognised.

Clinical features

- Stage 1: fever, crampy pain localised to single muscle group.
- Stage 2 'suppurative' (by 2–3 weeks): fever, muscle swelling, oedema.
- Stage 3: systemic toxicity; fluctuant muscle.

Diagnosis

- Imaging: CT or MRI to localise intramuscular abscesses.

Complications

- Local: compartment syndrome; distant: metastatic infection.

Management

- Empirical antibiotic therapy: IV flucloxacillin for 4 weeks depending on clinical and radiographical circumstances.
- Drainage (percutaneous or open) of abscess is fundamental. Further debridement and fasciotomies may be indicated.
- Formal assessment for additional sequelae of bacteraemia is indicated (e.g. endocarditis).

'Gas gangrene' (Clostridial myonecrosis)

Pathogenesis

Spore-forming *Clostridium* are widespread in soil, and both human and animal GITs. Most (>70%) of clostridial myonecrosis originates from direct 'traumatic' infection.

1. Traumatic 'gas gangrene'
- Direct inoculation of clostridia spores.
    - Associated with vascular compromise to support anaerobic clostridia spores.
    - Other causes: GI surgery, 'skin popping'.
    - Organism: >>*C. perfringens* (bacterial toxins mediate local tissue ischaemia).
2. Spontaneous 'gas gangrene'
- Haematogenous spread from GI source.
    - Organism: >*C. septicum.*

Clinical features

1. Traumatic 'gas gangrene':
- Rapid onset within 24 hours.
    - Severe pain at site of trauma or surgery; crepitus possible.

2. Spontaneous 'gas gangrene':
- Rapid onset.
  - Severe muscle pain without trauma; crepitus possible.

Diagnosis
- Imaging: CT or MRI to delineate deep infection.
- Tissue and blood microscopy and culture: large Gram-variable rods.

Management
Emergency surgical exploration and debridement.

Antibiotic therapy
- Empirical therapy: to cover for necrotising fasciitis.
- Directed Clostridia therapy: IV clindamycin.

Bone and joint infections

Septic arthritis
➲ See Chapter 20, Monoarthropathy, p. 746.

Osteomyelitis

Pathogenesis
For common causes of osteomyelitis and associated risk factors, see Table 8.23.

Table 8.23 Common causes of osteomyelitis and associated risk factors

Mechanism	Clinical scenario	Organisms
Direct or contiguous > polymicrobial	Penetrating trauma, SSTIs, septic arthritis, prosthesis infections, IVDU.	*S. aureus*.
	Ulcers; diabetes; vascular insufficiency.	Anaerobes (e.g. *Bacteroides fragilis*).
	Puncture wounds (through sports shoes).	*Pseudomonas aeruginosa*.
	Bites.	*Eikenella corrodens, Pasteurella multocida*.
Haematogenous > monomicrobial	Bacteraemia.	*S. aureus*.
	UTIs; vascular devices, IVDU.	Gram-negative rods.
	Sickle cell disease.	*Salmonella* spp.
	Endemic area exposure.	*M. tuberculosis; Brucella* spp.; *Coxiella burnetii*.

Site
- Direct/contiguous infection sites vary according to underlying pathology especially pressure areas/bony prominences.
- Haematogenous:
  - Children: long bones, commonly metaphysis.
  - Adult: vertebral, particularly lumbar via bladder to spine through venous plexus.

Duration

- Defined by Lew and Waldvogel.
- Acute: days to weeks.
- Chronic: months to years – implies development of necrotic bone.

Diabetic foot infections

- Typically associated with vascular insufficiency.
- Almost always follows soft tissue infection.
- Acute:
  - Monomicrobial: *S. aureus*, beta-haemolytic *streptococci*.
- Chronic:
  - Polymicrobial (3–5 isolates in samples is common): anaerobes, *P. aeruginosa, Corynebacterium* ('diphtheroids'), *enterococci*.
  - Resistant organisms if multiple hospitalisations and prolonged broad spectrum antibiotics: MRSA, VRE.

Clinical features

- Symptoms: mild dull local pain; constitutional symptoms (fever, malaise).
- Signs:
  - Acute: local swelling and tenderness.
  - Chronic: persistent ulceration over bony prominences, exposed bone, discharging sinus.
  - 'Probing to bone' through diabetic pedal ulcers is highly suggestive (66% sensitivity; 85% specificity).

Diagnosis

Imaging

- Radiography:
  - Common appearances: soft tissue swelling, periosteal reaction, bone destruction (not apparent until 10–21 days of infection).
  - Sensitivity as low as 14%.
- MRI:
  - Useful in early diagnosis (after 1 week), but of less value in monitoring therapy response (bone oedema persists for months).
- Nuclear imaging, e.g. technetium-labelled white cell scans, gallium scans:
  - potential false positive results: fracture, surgery, inflammatory conditions.
- PET FDG (positron emission tomography with fluorine-18-fluoro-D-deoxyglucose).

Blood tests

- Calcium, phosphate and ALP typically normal.
- CRP is more reliable than WCC for monitoring infection.

Microbiology

- Bone biopsy (open, percutaneous, during surgical debridement, CT-guided [vertebral]) is fundamental to direct prolonged antibiotic therapy.
- Blood culture.
- Superficial wound swabs and sinus tract samples have high false positive rates.

Histology

- >5 neutrophils per high-power field suggests infection.
- Granulomatous tissue may suggest TB or fungal infection.

Vascular assessment

- Doppler ultrasonagraphy as first line.
- Angiography may be indicated.

Management

Medical

- Number of agents: Single agent antimicrobial therapy is usually adequate (except in prosthesis-related infection: combination therapy with rifampicin is often used, see Table 8.24).
- Route: ideally IV therapy (often by OPAT); oral acceptable if susceptible organism and good bone penetration.
- Duration: 4–6 weeks (but may be extended until vascularised tissue covers debrided bone); potentially shorter courses post-amputation, rather than debridement as all necrotic tissue can be removed.

Table 8.24 Antibiotic treatment osteomyelitis

Organism	Antibiotic options
S.aureus	Flucloxacillin; OD ceftriaxone; clindamycin; ciprofloxacin with rifampicin, co-trimoxazole with rifampicin.
MRSA	Teicoplanin; vancomycin.
Gram-negative bacilli	Ciprofloxacin; OD ceftriaxone.
P. aeruginosa	Piperacillin-tazobactam; ceftazadime, ciprofloxacin and gentamicin.
Anaerobes	Clindamyin; co-amoxiclav; metronidazole.
Mixed aerobic and anaerobic	Co-amoxiclav; meropenem.
Empiric therapy	Vancomycin and ciprofloxacin (Gram-negative cover).

Surgical

Debridement of necrotic material; revascularisation; prosthesis removal (prosthetic joint infections require different antibiotic protocols in close liaison with surgical teams).

Complications

- Contiguous spread to soft tissue, joints and other structures.
- Malignancy: consider if persistent bone destruction, bleeding, enlarging mass or recalcitrant infection; squamous cell carcinoma is most common.

Tuberculosis

➲ See also Tuberculosis, p. 374; Management of pulmonary tuberculosis, p. 375; and Table 8.8.

Pathogenesis

Mycobacterium tuberculosis complex is part of the *Mycobacterium* genus of more than 50 species of aerobic bacteria. The complex compromises five species: *M. tuberculosis, M. bovis, M. africanum, M. microti*, and *M. ulcerans*. TB describes a range of clinical diseases caused by *M. tuberculosis* and much less commonly *M. bovis*. Mycolic acid cell envelope components confer the ability to resist destaining by acid alcohol after the application of certain dyes. Infection is acquired by inhalation of droplet nuclei (<5 μm diameter).

Epidemiology

- More than 2 billion people (>1/3 world's population) were living with *Mycobacterium tuberculosis* infection in 2010, resulting in 1.4 million deaths in that year.
- 95% prevalence in developing countries. UK incidence is 13.9 per 100,000 population.

Risk factors for TB infection

Host factors

- Infectiousness of person with TB: smear-positive status ('open TB'), culture-positive status, laryngeal or pulmonary (respiratory) TB, lung cavities, presence of cough.
- Susceptibility of respiratory tract: silicosis, smoke exposure (tobacco, cooking fires, occupational).

Environmental factors

- Birth in TB-endemic country (>70% UK TB cases born outside UK).
- Exposure history:
  - Duration of exposure.
  - Concentration of infectious droplet nuclei in air: enclosed space, inadequate ventilation.
  - 'Close contact': nosocomial/household/transport/school/workplace/prison.

Infectiousness

- Infectious TB: all cases of respiratory (pulmonary or laryngeal) TB, which are sputum smear-positive and culture-positive.
- Potentially infectious TB: sputum smear-negative and culture-positive respiratory TB accounts for 10–20% of new TB infections in low incidence countries.
- Non-infectious TB: isolated extra-pulmonary TB, or all cases of respiratory TB, which have two consecutive smear-negative sputum samples and negative culture. Most patients with drug-sensitive TB become non-infectious after 2 weeks of treatment.

Natural history

The natural history of *Mycobacterium tuberculosis* infection is shown in Figure 8.2.

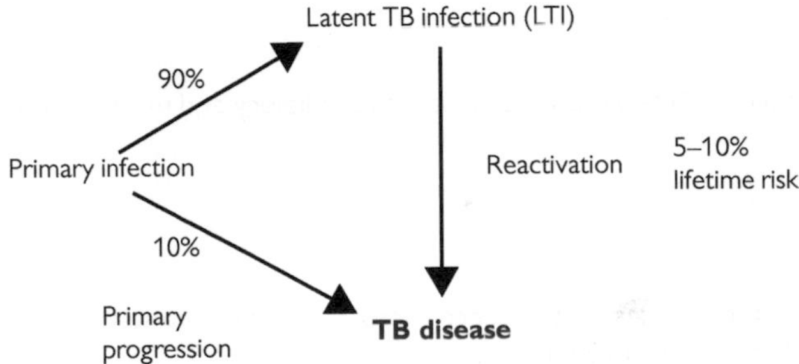

Figure 8.2 Natural history of *Mycobacterium tuberculosis* infection.

Primary infection is caused by inhaled organisms, which multiply within alveolar macrophages leading to an inflammatory response. Multiplying bacilli may enter draining lymph nodes yielding a Ghon complex. By the second week of infection cell-mediated mechanisms control bacilli growth in 90% of primary infections. This leads to persistence of dormant, but viable bacilli within an asymptomatic host and is termed latent TB infection (LTBI). In the lifetime of an immunocompetent individual there is a 5–10% risk of reactivation of these bacilli, which multiply and cause symptomatic disease. Reactivated TB accounts for >70% of TB cases treated in the UK. 'Active TB' is often used clinically to describe symptomatic disease, whether primary or reactivated.

Risk factors for active TB disease

- Impaired immunity (HIV [annual risk of reactivation is 10%], poor nutrition, vitamin D deficiency, substance abuse, smoking, diabetes mellitus, chronic kidney disease, medication: steroids [>15 mg OD >1 month], TNF inhibitors).
- Age (children <5 years, elderly).
- Recent infection.

Multiplying bacilli may spread directly by eroding into lung airways. Haematogenous spread leads to infection of extrapulmonary sites, known as disseminated TB. Miliary TB refers to the specific radiographic appearance of disseminated TB in lung parenchyma, which resembles millet seeds, and can be used to denote all forms of clinical disease resulting from haematogenous dissemination of TB.

Clinical manifestations

- Up to 50% constitutional symptoms in isolation: fever, night sweats, weight loss, malaise.
- Pulmonary disease accounts for 60% of UK presentations (of which up to 30% is pleural disease) and largely affects posterior apical lung segments. Extrapulmonary disease is common in those with advanced HIV infection.

Complications

- Acute pulmonary: haemoptysis, pneumothorax, pleural effusion fistulae, empyema.
- Chronic pulmonary: bronchiectasis, malignancy, chronic pulmonary aspergillosis.
- Extra-pulmonary:
  - Lymphadenitis: 75% cervical lymph nodes; complications – abscess, ulceration, fistula.
  - GI: hepatitis, enteritis, peritoneal.
  - GU: haematuria, proteinuria, 'sterile' pyuria.
  - Bone: especially involving lower thoracic and lumbar vertebrae (often multiple vertebral levels – Pott's disease).
  - CNS: meningitis (2–8-week indolent presentation in immunocompetent), intracranial tuberculoma, spinal arachnoiditis, ocular.
  - CVS: particularly pericardial; mycotic aneurysm.
  - Adrenal (clinical insufficiency in 1% disseminated TB).
  - Scrofuloderma: contiguous extension of deep-seated infection from any structure into overlying skin.

Diagnosis

Combination of compatible clinical syndrome, supportive radiology and testing of clinical specimens.

Active TB infection

Specimen testing

- Acid fast stains:
  - Auramine-staining techniques (fluorescence microscopy) are more sensitive than older carbolfuchsin methods, e.g. Ziehl–Nielsen (ZN).
- Culture:
  - Any clinical specimens including blood in disseminated TB.
- Molecular testing:
  - May identify: (i) *M. tuberculosis* complex, and (ii) common rifampicin (and isoniazid) resistance mutations (as surrogate markers for multidrug resistant [MDR] TB).
  - Advantages: rapid (some <2 hours), sensitivity and specificity similar to culture, minimal training required, increasingly cheap.
- Histology:
  - Caseating granulomas: epithelioid macrophages, Langhans giant cells, and encircling lymphocytes; characteristic caseation ('cheese-like') necrosis is often, but not universally present; organisms may or may not be seen.
  - Differential diagnosis for caseating granulomas:
    - Infectious: leprosy, leishmaniasis, syphilis, fungal (histoplasmosis, cryptococcosis).
    - Non-infectious: sarcoidosis (less likely to caseate, fewer peripheral inflammatory cells), rheumatoid nodules, granulomatosis with polyangiitis (GPA)/Wegener's, Crohn's disease.

Specimens

Sputum

- Spontaneous, induced (ideally three early morning samples 8–24 hours apart), or bronchoscopy and bronchoalveolar lavage.

For sensitivity and specificity of sputum analysis for *M. tuberculosis* , see Table 8.25.

Table 8.25 Sensitivity and specificity of sputum analysis for *M. tuberculosis*

	Smear	Culture	Molecular
Sensitivity	50–80%	80%	Smear positive: 98%; Smear negative: 72–88%
Specificity	98%	98%	95%

Pleural fluid

Typical findings of pleural samples in *M. tuberculosis* infection are shown in Table 8.26.

Table 8.26 Typical findings of pleural samples in *M. tuberculosis* infection

Appearance	pH	Cell count	Glucose	Protein
Straw-coloured; turbid; serosanguinous	<7.40	<2 weeks: neutrophils >2 weeks: lymphocytes (1000–6000 cells/mm^3)	3.3–5.6 mM	>50 g/L (>exudate)

Cerebrospinal fluid

For typical findings of CSF samples in *M. tuberculosis* infections, see Table 8.27 and for associated sensitivity and specificity of CSF analysis, see Table 8.28.

Table 8.27 Typical findings of CSF samples in *M. tuberculosis* infection

Appearance	Cell count	Glucose	Protein
Turbid in late disease	<2 weeks: neutrophils >2 weeks: lymphocytes (100–500 cells/μL)	<2.2 mM (<50% serum glucose)	High, but variable (0.1–6.0 g/dL) depending on subarachnoid blockage

Table 8.28 Sensitivity and specificity of CSF analysis

	Smear	Culture	Molecular
Sensitivity	10–50%	70%	56%
Specificity	-	98%	98%

Latent TB infection

- Tuberculin skin test (TST): Mantoux test in UK measures skin induration 48–72 hours after intradermal injection of TB antigen: >15 mm strongly positive; 6–15 mm hypersensitive; <6 mm negative. False positives occur in previous BCG and non-TB mycobacterial infections; false negatives in immunocompromised and observer error.

- Interferon gamma release assays (IGRA): in UK QuantiFERON-TB Gold In-Tube (QFT-GIT), or T–spot TB test quantifies cell-mediated response after inoculation of patient's blood with *M. tuberculosis* antigens *in vitro*.
  - *Advantages*: not affected by BCG vaccination, no false positive results.
  - *Disadvantages*: does not distinguish between active or latent TB infection; false negatives occur with immunocompromised and anergy of acute active TB infection (negative IGRA does *not* exclude active TB).

Fever in the returning traveller

Approach

Where?

Consider which infections are commonly imported from the region (see Table 8.29).

Table 8.29 Common diagnoses in febrile returning travellers organised by region of travel

Region	Disease	Percentage of imported systemic febrile illness	Local variation
Africa	Malaria	42%	*P. falciparum*
	Diarrhoeal illness	10%	35% parasitic, 25% bacterial
	Respiratory illness	10%	
	No diagnosis	19%	
Asia	Dengue fever	18%	
	Diarrhoeal illness	17%	35% bacterial, 25% parasitic
	Respiratory illness	17%	
	Malaria	7%	
	No diagnosis	22%	
Americas	Diarrhoeal illness	15%	35% parasitic
	Respiratory illness	13%	
	Dengue	9%	
	Malaria	8%	64% *P. vivax*

Common 'cosmopolitan' infections (such as pneumonia) account for approximately 50% of febrile illness in the returning traveller. Defining the setting of travel also helps narrow the differential diagnosis – rural or urban, and the type of accommodation in particular.

When?

Timing of travel and onset of symptoms.

Around 78% of febrile returning travellers had onset of fever during travel or within 1 month of return. If more than 1 month has elapsed since returning from travels, then a significant number of organisms can be excluded (see Table 8.30). GeoSentinel reports that 66% of patients with dengue present within 1 week, and 65% of patients with *falciparum* malaria present within 2 weeks of return.

Table 8.30 Common infections in febrile returning travellers organised by incubation period

Disease	Median incubation	Location
Incubation <14 days		
Viral		
Chikungunya	2–4 days	Tropics; subtropics
Dengue fever	4–8 days	Tropics; subtropics
Arboviral encephalitides	3–14 days	Varies by pathogen
HIV seroconversion	10–28 days	Worldwide
Viral haemorrhagic fevers	3–21 days	Varies by pathogen
Bacterial		
Enteric fever	7–18 days	>Indian subcontinent
Leptospirosis	7–12 days	Worldwide
Bacterial gastroenteritis	1–5 days	Worldwide
Other		
Falciparum malaria	6–30 days; mean 12 days	Tropics; subtropics
Rickettsial infections	Days–weeks	Varies by pathogen
14 days–6 weeks		
Hepatitis A virus	28–30 days	Developing countries
Hepatitis E virus	26–42 days	Developing countries
Acute Q fever (*Coxiella burnetii*)	14–40 days	Livestock exposure
Acute brucellosis	1 week–6 months	Livestock exposure; unpasteurised milk
Acute schistosomiasis	4–8 weeks; mean 40 days	>Africa
Acute African trypanosomiasis (*Trypanosoma brucei rhodesiense*)	6–8 weeks	>East Africa
Early Lyme disease	Weeks–months	USA, Europe, Asia
Amoebic liver abscess	Weeks–months	Developing countries
>6 weeks		
Hepatitis B virus	1–4 months	Worldwide
Tuberculosis	Weeks–years	Worldwide
Visceral leishmaniasis (>*Leishmania donovani* and *infantum*)	2–6 months	>South Asia, East Africa, Middle East, South America, Central Asia

What?

Risk exposures during travel

- Game parks, farms, caves, bites.
- Fresh or saltwater exposure.
- Heath-care facilities.
- Sexual activity.
- Foods.

How?

Prominent associated symptoms or signs

Febrile tropical illness often presents with non-specific features, but it can also be useful to organise the differential diagnosis by systems involved:

- Undifferentiated fever.
- Fever with rash.
- Fever with jaundice:
  - Viral: viral hepatitis, viral haemorrhagic fevers (VHFs), yellow fever.
  - Non-viral: leptospirosis.
- Fever with hepato-/splenomegaly:
  - Bacterial: leptospirosis, brucellosis.
  - Non-bacterial: trypanosomiasis, visceral leishmaniasis, amoebic liver abscess.
- Systemic features: GI, respiratory, CNS.

Pre-exposure history

- Country of birth and residence.
- Malaria: acquired immunity in high transmission areas requires ongoing exposure; 6 months living in non-endemic areas removes this protection (up to 50% of patients with malaria are foreign born nationals visiting friends and relatives [VFRs]).
- Dengue fever: secondary infection with a new dengue virus (four serotypes in total) increases the risk of life-threatening disease, it can be observed in VFRs.
- Age and co-morbidities.
- Vaccinations: fully protective in yellow fever and typhoid.
- Chemoprophylaxis.

First line investigations

For febrile patients returning from the tropics and subtropics within the last 6 months:

- Blood films and rapid diagnostic tests (RDTs) for malaria.
- Blood cultures.
- EDTA for PCR.
- Serum save for serology.
- Relevant microbiology samples.
- CXR.

Viral haemorrhagic fevers

For key viral haemorrhagic fever syndromes, see Table 8.31.

Management of suspected VHF

- Risk assessment available online via https://www.gov.uk/government/collections/ebola-virus-disease-clinical-management-and-guidance.
- Transfer to high security infectious disease unit (HSIDU) if confirmed viral haemorrhagic fevers (VHF).

UK VHF experience since 1970

- 12 imported cases of Lassa fever.
- Two imported cases of Crimean–Congo haemorrhagic fever (CCHF).
- One imported case of Ebola (two evacuated cases of Ebola).

Table 8.31 Key viral haemorrhagic fever syndromes

Disease	Location	Transmission	Features	Specific treatment
Lassa fever	West Africa; sporadic (occasional epidemics)	Reservoir: rodents. Transmission: aerosol, percutaneous, mucosal exposure to: rodent faeces and urine, human body fluids (blood, urine, vomitus). Incubation: 6–21 days.	Fever, protean non-specific manifestations. 20% mortality if hospitalised (80% uncomplicated disease course).	Ribavirin
Ebola virus disease and Marburg haemorrhagic fever (*Filoviridae* virus family)	Sub Saharan Africa; outbreaks	Reservoir: unknown (possibly bats; not primates). Transmission: aerosol, ingestion, percutaneous, mucosal exposure to: bat secretions, human body fluids (blood, urine, vomitus, faeces, sweat). Incubation: 5–14 days.	Fever with prominent diarrhoea, fulminant sepsis possible. Up to 90% mortality in outbreaks (<20% in high-resource setting).	Ongoing trials: monoclonal Abs, vaccination
Crimean–Congo haemorrhagic fever (CCHF)	Africa, Asia, Eastern Europe, Middle East; sporadic (with outbreaks)	Reservoir: small mammals. Transmission: tick bite (> *Hyalomma* tick); percutaneous, mucosal exposure to: livestock tissue and blood, human blood-contaminated body fluids (blood, faeces, vomitus). Incubation: 3–7 days.	Febrile pre-haemorrhagic phase progresses to haemorrhagic manifestations ± multi-organ failure. 10–40% mortality.	Ribavirin
Rift Valley Fever	East Africa (with periods of heavy rainfall); Outbreaks	Reservoir: mammals. Transmission: percutaneous, mucosal exposure to: animal blood, tissue, raw milk; mosquito bites (less common in humans). Incubation: 5–21 days.	Mostly mild febrile illness progresses in minority (<5%) to: ocular disease, meningoencephalitis, haemorrhagic disease. Up to 30% mortality in outbreaks; but often mild disease.	None

Table 8.32 Key characteristics of malaria parasites

Species	Characteristics	Time from bite to parasitaemia	Distribution	Appearance of thin films
P. falciparum	Highest mortality, non-relapsing	Average 10 days	Tropical and subtropical areas: Central & South America, Africa & SE Asia.	Ring forms delicate cytoplasm with 1-2 chromatin dots, multiple infection of single RBC common, Maurer's clefts.
P. vivax	Most common form relapsing	Weeks to months	Central and South America, India and SE Asia.	Ring forms large cytoplasm, fine Schuffner's dots, round RBC.
P. ovale	Rarely fatal, relapsing	Weeks to months	Primarily sub-Saharan Africa.	Ring forms sturdy cytoplasm, round to oval RBC.
P. malariae	Less common, milder	Weeks to months	Tropical and subtropical areas: Central & South America, Africa and SE Asia.	Sturdy cytoplasm, large chromatin.
P. knowlesii	Rarely causes disease in humans		SE Asia.	Delicate cytoplasm, 1-2 chromatin dots.

Malaria

Malaria is arguably the most important of all tropical infections causing high morbidity and mortality in developing countries. It is caused by a protozoal infection transmitted most commonly by the bite of an infected female *Anopheles* mosquito.

Symptoms usually begin 8–15 days after being bitten, and include fever, chills, fatigue, myalgias, vomiting and headaches. There are now known to be five species, which cause disease in humans (see Table 8.32).

Major features of *P. falciparum* severe or complicated malaria include:

- Altered mental status and coma.
- Convulsions.
- Elevated liver enzymes.
- Hypoglycaemia.
- Respiratory distress.
- Renal failure.
- Parasitaemia >2%.
- Shock.
- Severe anaemia.

Treatment

Treatment should be initiated as soon as possible after the diagnosis is confirmed.

Patients with *P. falciparum* should be admitted to hospital for initiation of treatment regardless of parasite count. Patients with severe or complicated malaria, or those who cannot take oral treatment should be given IV infusion.

- Most drugs are active against parasites in the blood including chloroquine, atovaquine-proguanil (Malarone ®), artemether-lumefantrine (Coartem ®), mefloquine, quinine, quinidine, doxycycline (combination with quinine), artesunate.

- Primaquine is active against hypnozoites (dormant liver stage) and should be used to prevent relapse of *P. vivax* and *P. ovale*, once glucose-6-phosphate dehydrogenase (G6PD) deficiency has been excluded.
- Specialist advice should be sought in treatment of the pregnant woman.

Malaria protection – ABCD

A. Be *aware* of the risk, incubation period, possibility of delayed onset, and main symptoms.
B. Avoid being *bitten* by mosquitos: especially between dusk and dawn.
C. *Chemoprophylaxis* when appropriate to prevent infection developing into clinical disease.
D. Seek immediate *diagnosis* and treatment if fever develops 1 week or more after entering endemic area of malaria risk.

Multiple choice questions

Questions

1. A 36-year-old woman is 34 weeks pregnant. She did not contract chickenpox in childhood. She presents to hospital as her sister's 2-year-old son has developed chickenpox. She is asymptomatic. 5 days ago she had protracted exposure to the child who developed the chickenpox exanthem 24 hours later. What is the next step in managing this patient?
   A. Advise the patient to attend if she develops a rash.
   B. Admit to hospital for observation.
   C. Assess index case and swab for VZV PCR.
   D. Test VZV IgG and administer IV aciclovir.
   E. Test VZV IgG and administer *Varicella zoster* immunoglobulin (VZIG).
2. In a UK tuberculosis clinic, which of the following patients should commence tuberculosis chemoprophylaxis of rifamipicin and isoniazid for 3 months?
   A. 76-year-old asymptomatic man with a positive tuberculin skin test whose wife has pulmonary TB. His CXR is normal.
   B. 24-year-old white British lady with severe inflammatory bowel disease, which is poorly controlled with non-immunological therapy whose IGRA is positive.
   C. 24-year-old Somali gentleman whose brother has smear positive TB. He is complaining of a cough for 3 weeks.
   D. 28-year-old asymptomatic Latvian woman with a positive tuberculin skin test who reports that her husband who has recently arrived in the UK has been taking treatment for TB for nearly 2 years.
   E. 21-year-old student nurse who had prolonged exposure without a mask to a patient subsequently diagnosed with smear positive TB. She has no BCG scar. She is asymptomatic and has a normal CXR. She has antiphospholipid syndrome with previous recurrent pulmonary emboli for which she takes warfarin.
3. Which of the following features is not diagnostic for severe malaria?
   A. Thrombocytopenia.
   B. Hypoglycaemia.
   C. Pulmonary oedema.
   D. Seizures.
   E. Parasite load > 2%.

4. A pregnant woman is at 38 weeks gestation. A urine specimen has grown *E. coli*. The antibiogram reports resistance to amoxicillin; it reports susceptibility to ciprofloxacin, trimethoprim and nitrofurantoin. The patient is entirely asymptomatic. What is the best management of this patient?
   A. Repeat urine specimen.
   B. Nitrofurantoin.
   C. Ciprofloxacin.
   D. Co-amoxiclav.
   E. Trimethoprim.

5. An 84-year-old nursing home resident is admitted after 1 week of antibiotic therapy for a recurrent cellulitis. She is mildly tachycardic with otherwise normal observations. On examination, she has mild unilateral leg swelling and erythema. Her white cell count is $16 \times 10^3/\mu L$. She is initiated on combination empirical IV antibiotic therapy on the advice of the microbiology department. At the start of the infusion she begins to complain of pruritus and chest pain. Her blood pressure falls. She is flushed. What is the most likely cause for her deterioration?
   A. Severe sepsis.
   B. Piperacillin/tazobactam.
   C. Co-amoxiclav.
   D. Vancomycin.
   E. Toxic shock syndrome.

Answers

1. E. Without a reliable history of previous chickenpox (VZV), guidelines mandate testing for VZV serology to exclude prior infection. If VZV IgG is negative, implying no immunity to chickenpox, then VZIG is indicated within 10 days of first contact. An individual with chickenpox is infectious 2 days prior to exanthem and until the lesions have crusted over. In the setting of VZV infection during pregnancy, antiviral therapy only has a role in treating symptomatic established infection. (➲ See Table 8.9.)
2. B. Rifampicin and isoniazid for 3 months (or isoniazid monotherapy for 6 months) is recommended treatment for LTBI. Owing to hepatoxicity of the agents, LTBI treatment is only recommended for patients up to 65 years of age. After 65 years of age, the risk of hepatoxicity is greater than the perceived benefit of reducing risk of future TB reactivation. Case D is at risk of MDR TB. Further detail regarding her contact would be required, but there is no role for LTBI treatment in MDR TB contacts. Case E should be screened as a close contact, but should not start treatment empirically. (➲ See Latent TB infection, p. 263 and Tuberculosis, p. 374.)
3. A. All other options are criteria for severe malaria. (➲ See Malaria, p. 268 and Table 8.32.)
4. E. Treatment of asymptomatic bacteriuria in pregnant women is associated with better obstetric outcomes. Nitrofurantoin is associated with haemolytic anaemia in the neonate if used in the third trimester of pregnancy. Trimethoprim is only contraindicated for pregnant women in the first trimester. Ciprofloxacin is recommended against, unless absolutely indicated, given its association with arthropathy in fetal animal studies. Amoxicillin resistance is very common in all urinary isolates. Co-amoxiclav is recommended against in the third trimester owing to the risk of necrotising enterocolitis in the neonate. (➲ See Lower urinary tract infections, p. 253.)
5. D. Red man syndrome is a histamine-mediated response specifically to glycopeptide antibiotics, in particular vancomycin. It does not require prior exposure to the agent and is not thought to be IgE-mediated. It occurs early in infusion of the antibiotic. Although the clinical syndrome may resemble IgE-mediated anaphylaxis it is too early in the therapy to be typical even with a history consistent with antibiotic sensitisation. The microbiologist may have recommended vancomycin given the patient's increased demographic risk of MRSA and healthcare-associated infection. (➲ See Table 8.8.)

Chapter 9 **Haematology**

Nita Prasannan, Christine O. Ademokun and Deepti H. Radia

General haematology

Normal haematopoiesis

The main site for haematopoiesis is the bone marrow; in childhood, all the marrow is haematopoetic, but with increasing age, this becomes restricted to the central skeleton and proximal ends of the long bones (the rest of the bone marrow being made of fat, which is capable of reverting to normal haematopoiesis if required). Stem cells within the bone marrow are crucial for haematopoeisis and function by:

1. Stem cell renewal – production of new stem cells to maintain the stem cell pool.
2. Differentiation to progenitor cells of the different blood cell lineages (Figure 9.1).

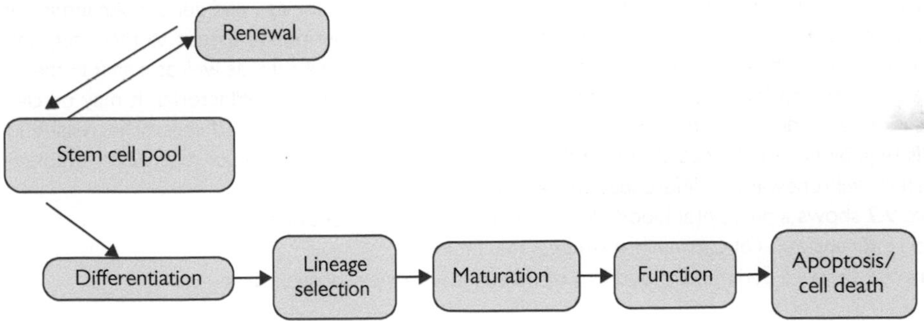

Figure 9.1 Stem cell renewal and differentiation.

A single stem cell is capable of producing 10^6 mature blood cells after 20 divisions and can preferentially produce a particular cell line in response to growth factors (e.g. granulocyte-colony stimulating factor [GCSF]; granulocyte-macrophage colony stimulating factor; erythropoietin; thrombopoietin) when required.

Interpretation of the blood count

Details of the full blood count are shown in Table 9.1.

Table 9.1 Full blood count

Blood cell indices	Purpose and derivation
Hb (haemoglobin)	Iron-containing oxygen-transport metalloprotein in red blood cells.
RBC (red blood cell count)	Number of erythrocytes measured multiplied by a calibration constant.
Hct (haematocrit)	Relative volume of packed erythrocytes to whole blood.
PCV (packed cell volume)	Packed cell volume.
MCV (mean corpuscular volume)	Average volume of individual erythrocytes derived from the histogram of RBC particle size distribution.
MCH (mean corpuscular haemoglobin)	Average amount of Hb per RBC.
MCHC (mean corpuscular haemoglobin concentration)	Average concentration of Hb in RBCs.
RDW (red cell distribution width)	Variation in cellular volume of the RBC population.
Platelets	Number of platelets measured multiplied by a calibration constant.
MPV (mean platelet volume)	Average volume of individual platelets.
WCC (white cell count)	Number of leucocytes measured multiplied by a calibration constant with normal values being: • Total leukocytes: 4.00–11.0 × 10^9/L • Neutrophils: 2.5 × 7.5 × 10^9/L • Lymphocytes: 1.5–3.5 × 10^9/L • Monocytes: 0.2–0.8 × 10^9/L • Eosinophils: 0.04–0.4 × 10^9/L • Basophils: 0.01–0.1 × 10^9/L.

Adapted with permission from Bain, B. (2015) *Blood Cells: A practical guide*. 5th ed. Copyright Wiley Blackwell 2015.

Anaemia

Anaemia is defined as a Hb level that is less than the normal range for age and gender. Anaemic patients have an inadequate red cell mass to deliver sufficient oxygen to peripheral tissues to meet physiological needs. In response, there is increased cardiac stroke volume and heart rate, as well as a shift in the oxygen dissociation curve to favour oxygenating vital organs. Anaemia is often multifactorial. It may be classified by causation: as reduced production of red cells, increased destruction of red cells or increased loss of red cells (e.g. bleeding); or according to red cell size – microcytic, normocytic or macrocytic (Table 9.2).

For stem cell renewal and differentiation, see Figure 9.1.

Figure 9.2 shows a peripheral blood film of a patient with iron deficiency anaemia.

For an interpretation of plasma iron studies, see Table 9.3.

Figure 9.3 shows a peripheral blood film of a patient with megaloblastic anaemia.

Haemolytic anaemia

- Due to increased destruction of red cells.
- May be:
  - Intravascular:
    - Red cells broken down in the blood vessels.
    - Free Hb accumulates in the blood stream (haemoglobinaemia) and is filtered by the glomeruli causing haemoglobinuria and haemosiderinuria.
  - Extravascular:
    - Red cells broken down in the reticuloendothelial system.
- Key features in the clinical history:
  - Family history and previous episodes (suggestive of inherited aetiology).
  - Diet (relevant in G6PD deficiency).

Table 9.2 Causes of anaemia

Type of anaemia	Causes	Key points for assessment
Microcytic anaemia MCV <80 fl MCH <27 pg	Iron deficiency	Very common, many causes. Clinical history invaluable, to include: dietary habits, blood loss from GI, genitourinary and/or respiratory tracts, blood donation, drugs (e.g. antithrombotics), previous peptic ulcer disease and/or gastric surgery, and symptoms of coeliac disease. Management: identify and treat the underlying cause. Ix: Peripheral blood film (PBF) (Figure 9.2), iron studies (Table 9.3), coeliac screen. Iron replacement and the iron stores of most patients can be restored via the oral route. Side effects of oral iron include nausea, epigastric pain, constipation and diarrhoea, which are improved if it is taken with food or by dose reduction (ideally 200–300 mg of elemental iron per day is required). Parenteral iron therapy is available and is helpful in late pregnancy, oral iron intolerance, ongoing haemorrhage and chronic renal failure.
	Anaemia of chronic disease	Characterised by reduced availability of iron, erythropoietin levels and red cell lifespan (~70–80 days instead of 120). Pathogenesis: chronic infection, chronic immune activation and/or malignancy lead to increased levels of interleukin-6 (IL-6). IL-6 stimulates hepcidin production and release from the liver, which increases the internalisation of ferroportin molecules on cell membranes reducing access of iron to the circulation. Increases in pro-inflammatory cytokines also hasten destruction of red cell precursors and reduction of erythropoietin receptors. Ix: ESR, CRP, autoimmune screen.
	Lead poisoning	Ix: lead levels.
	Thalassemia	➲ See Thalassemia, p. 277 and Table 9.5.
	Sideroblastic anaemia	May be congenital or acquired (clonal in myelodysplasia or reversible due to alcohol excess, pyridoxine deficiency, lead poisoning, copper deficiency, excess zinc, and drugs e.g. isoniazid, chloramphenicol, cycloserine and linezolid). Ix: bone marrow biopsy, iron studies, copper levels, caeruloplasmin, lead levels, zinc levels.
Normocytic anaemia	Early microcytosis/macrocytosis	
	Myeloma	➲ See Myeloma, p. 303.
	Mixed deficiencies	Dietary history. Ix: haematinics (Vitamin B_{12}, folate, ferritin), autoantibodies.
	Bone marrow failure	➲ See Bone marrow failure syndromes, p. 307 and Table 9.15.
	Anaemia of chronic disease (may also be microcytic)	See above.
	Aplastic anaemia	➲ See Aplastic anaemia, p. 307.

continued

Table 9.2 *continued*

Type of anaemia	Causes	Key points for assessment
Macrocytic anaemia MCV>95 fl	Vitamin B_{12} deficiency (megaloblastic*)	Previous gastric surgery, dietary habits. Ix: Vitamin B_{12}, folate, PBF (Figure 9.3.)
	Folate deficiency (megaloblastic*)	Dietary habits, use of medication, e.g. methotrexate. Ix: Vitamin B_{12}, folate, PBF.
	Haemolysis	➲ See Haemolytic anaemia, p. 272.
	Myelodysplasia	➲ See Myelodysplasia, p. 293 and Box 9.1.
	Alcohol excess	Clinical history and examination (➲ see Chapter 15, Blood tests, p. 523, Investigation of liver disease, p. 523 and Presentations associated with liver disease, p. 523, and Tables 15.2 and 15.3).
	Liver disease	Clinical history and examination for stigmata of liver disease (➲ see Chapter 15, Blood tests, p. 523, Investigation of liver disease, p. 523 and Presentations associated with liver disease, p. 523, and Tables 15.2 and 15.3). Ix: Hepatitis virology, autoimmune screen, caeruloplasmin.

fl, femtolitres; pg, picograms; Ix, investigations; LDH, lactate dehydrogenase.
*Megaloblastic anaemia results from inhibition of DNA synthesis during RBC production, leading to continuing cell growth without division. It is characterised by many large immature and dysfunctional red blood cells (megaloblasts) in the bone marrow and hypersegmented neutrophils (exhibiting five or more nuclear lobes ['segments'; normal ≤4]) in the peripheral blood.

Table 9.3 Interpretation of plasma iron studies

	Iron	Total iron binding capacity	Ferritin
Iron deficiency	Decreased	Increased	Decreased
Anaemia of chronic disease	Decreased	Decreased	Increased
Chronic haemolysis	Increased	Decreased	Increased

Data from Provan D et al., *Oxford Handbook of Clinical Haematology*, Third Edition, Oxford, UK: Oxford University Press, 2009.

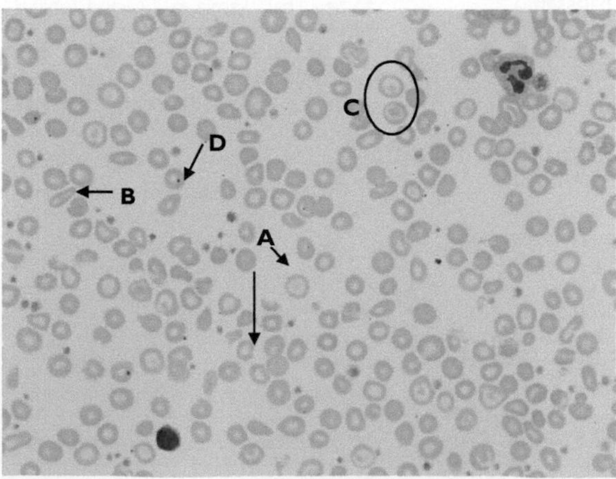

Figure 9.2 (see colour plate section) Peripheral blood film of a patient with iron deficiency anaemia, post splenectomy (Oil immersion ×100 magnification). (A) Hypochromic, microcytic red cells typical of iron deficiency. (B) Pencil cells typical of iron deficiency. (C) Target cells with haemoglobinised dark areas, both centrally and peripherally (as a band), with a white ring of relative pallor in between, are due either to increased red cell surface area or to decreased intracellular haemoglobin content; commonly seen post-splenectomy. (D) Howell–Jolly bodies (histopathological findings of basophilic nuclear remnants in circulating erythrocytes, usually signifying a damaged or absent spleen).

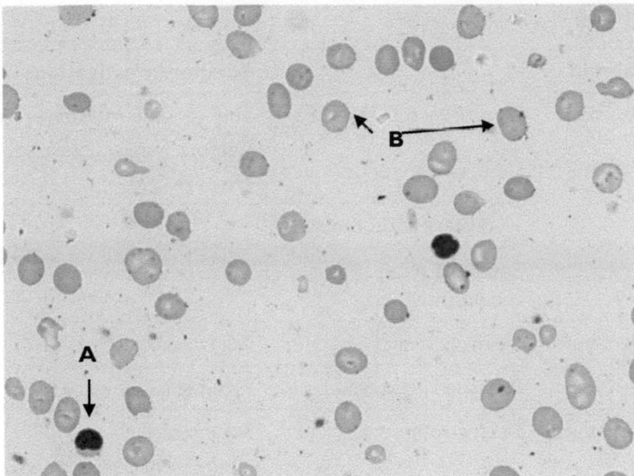

Figure 9.3 Peripheral blood film of patient with megaloblastic anaemia due to vitamin B_{12} deficiency (Oil immersion ×100 magnification). (A) Normal lymphocyte. (B) Ovalocyte/macro-ovalocyte (enlarged oval-shaped erythrocyte).

  - Drug history (e.g. cephalosporins, levofloxacin, nitrofurantoin, dapsone, levodopa, methyldopa).
  - Infective symptoms (relevant to mycoplasma, malaria).
  - Constitutional symptoms (relevant to inflammatory or malignant causes).
- Clinical examination may reveal jaundice, splenomegaly and lymphadenopathy.
- Baseline investigations:
  - FBC – showing macrocytosis and raised reticulocyte count.
  - Peripheral blood film (PBF) (Figure 9.4).
  - Direct antiglobulin test (DAT):
    - This test detects IgG or C3d bound-red cells. In warm autoimmune haemolytic anaemia (AIHA), the red cells are often coated with IgG autoantibodies. In cold AIHA, the antibody involved is IgM, which causes complement activation. The IgM autoantibody then dissociates at higher temperatures, leaving complement behind, which is picked up by the DAT. In mixed AIHA, both IgG and C3d may be present.

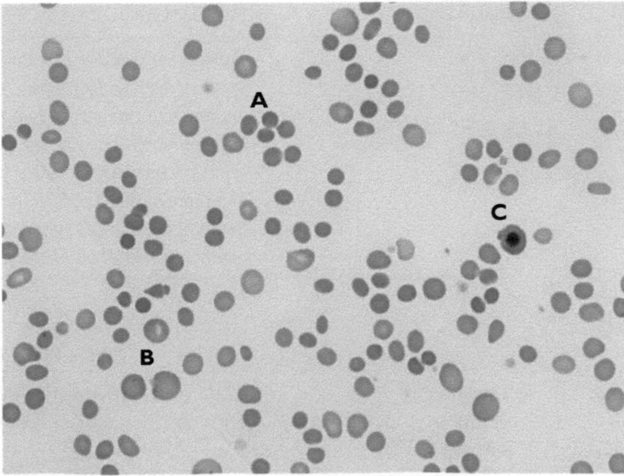

Figure 9.4 (see colour plate section) Peripheral blood film of patient with warm autoimmune haemolytic anaemia (Oil immersion ×100 magnification). (A) Spherocyte (sphere-shaped erythrocyte). (B) Polychromasia (erythrocytes of different shades of colour, typically greyish blue, due to premature release of immature erythrocytes [reticulocytes] from the bone marrow). (C) Nucleated red blood cell.

Table 9.4 Types of haemolytic anaemia

Type of haemolytic anaemia			Further investigations
Inherited	Membrane disorders	Hereditary spherocytosis	EMA (eosin-5-maleimide) binding or cryohaemolysis. Osmotic fragility (less used). Negative DAT.
		Hereditary elliptocytosis	
		Southeast Asian ovalocytosis	
	Metabolic disorders	G6PD deficiency	G6PD assay.
		Pyruvate kinase deficiency	Pyruvate kinase assay.
	Haemoglobinopathies	Sickling syndromes	Sickle screen. Haemoglobin electrophoresis.
		Unstable haemoglobins	Mass spectrometry.
Acquired	Immune	AIHA: Warm	DAT.
		AIHA: Cold	DAT. Mycoplasma serology, EBV serology.
		Haemolytic disease of the newborn	DAT. Maternal and fetal blood group.
		Haemolytic transfusion reactions	DAT.
		Cold haemagglutin disease	
	Mechanical	Cardiac prosthetic valve-associated	
		March haemolysis	
	Drugs	Methyldopa Rifampicin Penicillin	
	Infections	Malaria	Malaria testing.
	Paroxysmal cold haemoglobinuria		Donath Landsteiner test that involves mixing a patient's serum with P antigen positive, group O red blood cells and fresh donor serum (which serves as a source of complement). The patient and donor serum mixture is incubated in a melting ice bath (0°C) for 30 minutes and then warmed to 37°C for 1 hour. The tube is centrifuged, and the supernatant is examined for haemolysis, which, if present, constitutes a positive test.
	Paroxysmal nocturnal haemoglobinuria		Flow cytometry. Ham test that involves demonstration of lysis of red blood cells when the pH of plasma is reduced to 6.5.
	Microangiopathic syndromes (➲ see Chapter 16, Thrombotic microangiopathies, p. 578)	Thrombotic thrombocytopenic purpura (TTP)	ADAMTS (A Disintegrin And Metalloprotease with ThromboSpondin 1 repeats) 13 assay.
		Haemolytic uraemic syndrome (HUS)	
		Malignant hypertension	

- LDH as a marker of cell turnover.
- Haematinics (folate, vitamin B_{12}, iron studies):
  - Stores depleted in the context of haemolysis, particularly folate.
- LFTs – raised bilirubin levels.
- Urinalysis for haemoglobinuria/haemosiderinuria.
- Red cell alloantibodies if recently transfused.
- Viral serology.

For types of haemolytic anaemia, see Table 9.4.

Management of haemolysis depends on the underlying cause. Immune cases are often treated with immunosuppressive agents such as steroids, IVIG, rituximab, cyclophosphamide, and eculizumab (a humanized monoclonal antibody against complement C5; see Table 3.4). In chronic haemolytic states, splenectomy is an option with careful consideration of the immediate and long-term complications (➲ see Chapter 6, Vaccines, p. 175).

Haemoglobinopathies

Haemoglobin (Hb) normally consists of a single haem unit attached to 4 globin chains (2 α chains and 2 β chains). Other globin chains produced at different periods of development (e.g. in utero) include δ, ζ, γ. Hb's main function is oxygen transport between the lungs and the tissues/organs to allow aerobic respiration.

Sickling disorders

This occurs due to an abnormal Hb 'S' inherited from one parent combined with an S, C, D, O or beta thalassaemia from the other parent. The genotype abnormalities resulting from a single amino acid change in the beta globin gene include HbSS ($\beta^S\beta^S$), SC ($\beta^S\beta^C$), S-beta thal ($\beta^S\beta$-thalassaemia), S-D Punjab ($\beta^S\beta^D$) and S-O Arab ($\beta^S\beta^O$). There is a wide geographical distribution, particularly of the compound sickling disorders. Hb AS (the 'sickle trait') is the carrier state. It does not have the clinical manifestations associated with the other sickling disorders except in situations of extremely low oxygen tension when sickling can occur.

Diagnosis can be made prenatally through screening of at-risk parents (amniocentesis, chorionic villus sampling) or newborns. Confirmatory tests can be performed using high performance liquid chromatography, isoelectric focusing and cellulose acetate electrophoresis. The classic 'sickle cells', and features of haemolysis and hyposplenism are seen on the PBF.

Sickle cells have an elongated structure and adhere to vascular endothelium particularly under conditions of low oxygen tension (Figure 9.5). This predisposes them to occlude small blood vessels, impairing blood flow. Their relatively short life span causes anaemia.

The clinical manifestation varies widely from asymptomatic to frequent acute symptomatic attacks (called vaso-occlusive crises) or marked chronic haemolysis. There is a steady state anaemia (Hb usually between 60–90 g/L). Types of crises include hand-foot syndrome (in children), hepatic or splenic sequestration, acute chest and aplastic (temporary red cell aplasia due to parvovirus B19 infection) crises. Management is mainly preventative and symptomatic, with warmth, hydration and analgesia. Any evidence of sepsis should be promptly managed according to local protocols with particular note to cover for Streptococcus pneumonia, mycoplasma, haemophilus influenza and *Legionella*.

Patients are monitored for the chronic vaso-occlusive effects of the disease such as avascular necrosis (➲ See Chapter 5, Case 16, p. 140), splenic infarction and hyposplenism with consequent immune compromise (➲ for vaccination recommendations against encapsulated organisms see Chapter 6, Vaccines, p. 175), chronic renal disease, pulmonary hypertension, proliferative retinopathy, cerebrovascular disease, pigment gallstones, priapism and leg ulcers. Folic acid supplements are prescribed for the chronic haemolysis. Patients with severe disease can be treated with hydroxycarbamide (to increase the level of HbF (fetal haemoglobin [$\alpha_2\gamma_2$]), regular red cell exchange transfusions or a bone marrow transplant (BMT) (in the most severe cases).

Thalassemia

This set of disorders occurs due to a reduction or complete lack of one or more of the chains that make up the globin portion of Hb. The type of thalassemia depends on which of the globin chains is affected

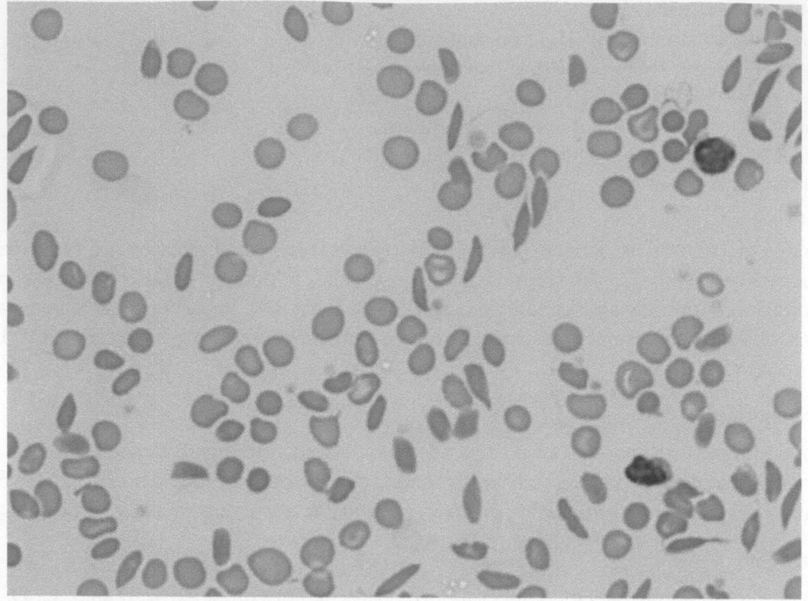

Figure 9.5 Peripheral blood film of patient with HbSS sickle cell disease showing many sickle shaped red cells (Oil immersion ×100 magnification).

and the number affected (Table 9.5). There are 2 α globin genes on chromosome 16 (normal = αα/αα) and, as such, α thalassaemia is a very heterogeneous disorder with a wide spectrum of clinical manifestations. Patients need prenatal counselling, ideally pre-conception, to evaluate their risk of having a severely affected child.

Erythrocytosis

- Hb >185 g/L in men; >165 g/L in women.
- Hct >0.55.
- Red cell mass >25% of mean predicted value.
- Neutrophil and platelet counts are often raised (in primary erythrocytosis).

A raised Hct with a normal red cell mass is termed apparent erythrocytosis (e.g. resulting from dehydration).

Causes

For causes of absolute erythrocytosis, see Table 9.6.

Presenting symptoms of primary erythrocytosis

Presenting symptoms of primary erythrocytosis include: pruritus; painful splenomegaly; gout; thrombosis; haemorrhage.

Management of primary erythrocytosis

The aim of management is to reduce the complications:

- Aspirin 75 mg/day.
- Screen and treat vascular risk factors (smoking, hypertension, hypercholesterolaemia).
- Venesect to Hct <0.45.
- Cytoreductive therapy (with hydroxycarbamide) if venesection not tolerated.

Table 9.5 Types of thalassemia

Thalassemia type	Globin chain abnormality	Clinical symptoms	Laboratory results	Treatment
α thalassemia trait	(αα/α-) deletion of a single gene.	Usually asymptomatic.	Slight reduction in MCV/MCH.	Nil specific.
α^+ thalassemia and α^0 thalassemia	(αα/-- or α-/α-).	Usually asymptomatic but patients may be anaemic.	Low MCV/MCH.	Folic acid supplementation may be beneficial in patients with elevated reticulocyte counts.
Haemoglobin H disease	(α-/--) 3 genes deleted.	Marked anaemia, hepatosplenomegaly and haemolysis.	Characteristic PBF with target cells, reticulocytosis, microcytosis, nucleated red blood cells (NRBCs) and HbH inclusions (tetramers of β globin seen on cresyl blue stain that have polymerised due to lack of α chains).	Folic acid supplementation may be beneficial in patients with elevated reticulocyte counts, red cell transfusions for severe anaemia, iron chelation for those requiring chronic transfusions.
Hb Barts	(--/--) all 4 α chains deleted.	Incompatible with life; affected fetuses are born hydropic.	No functional adult haemoglobin.	
β-thalassemia trait	Abnormality in one β globin gene.	Carrier state mild microcytic anaemia.	Basophilic stippling on blood film, raised Hb A2 ($\alpha_2\delta_2$) fraction on Hb electrophoresis.	Nil specific.
β thalassemia intermedia	Absence or reduction in production of both β globin allelic products.	Anaemia (Hb 60–110 g/L) with hepatosplenomegaly.		Patients require intermittent blood transfusions particularly at times of physiological stress, e.g. pregnancy.
β thalassemia major	Absence or reduction in production of both β globin allelic products.	Chronic anaemia, skeletal deformities, hepatosplenomegaly.	Red cell anisopoikilocytois and NRBCs on blood film.	Regular blood transfusions (taking care to manage transfusional iron overload in the liver, heart, pancreas and skin with iron chelation therapy) and hydroxycarbamide to increase HbF, and/or BMT.

Table 9.6 Causes of absolute erythrocytosis

Primary	**Secondary**
PRV (polycythaemia rubra vera) • *JAK 2 positive requires both.* A1 High haematocrit (>0.52 in men, >0.48 in women) OR raised red cell mass (>25% above predicted). A2 Mutation in JAK 2. • *JAK 2 negative requires A1-4, plus A5 or A6 or 2 B criteria.* A1 Raised red cell mass (>25% above predicted) OR haematocrit≥0.60 in men, ≥0.56 in women. A2 Absence of mutation in JAK2. A3 No cause of secondary erythrocytosis. A4 Bone marrow histology consistent with polycythaemia vera (hypercellular with trilineage hyperplasia). A5 Palpable splenomegaly. A6 Presence of an acquired genetic abnormality (excluding BCR-ABL1) in the haematopoietic cells. B1 Thrombocytosis (platelet count >450 310^9/L). B2 Neutrophil leucocytosis (neutrophil count >10 310^9/L in non-smokers, ≥12.5$310^9$/L in smokers). B3 Radiological evidence of splenomegaly. B4 Low serum erythropoietin.	*Congenital causes* • High oxygen affinity states (2,3 bisphosphonate deficiency, erythropoietin receptor mutation, Von-Hippel Lindau disease). *Acquired conditions* (erythropoietin-mediated) • Hypoxia (chronic lung disease, right to left cardiopulmonary shunts, CO poisoning, hypoventilation). • Renal hypoxia (renal artery stenosis, renal failure, polycystic kidney disease). • Erythropoietin generating tumours (renal cell carcinoma, hepatocellular carcinoma, pheochromocytoma, cerebellar haemiangioblastoma). • Exogenous erythropoietin administration (androgen-based drugs). • Post-renal transplant erythrocytosis. • Idiopathic erythrocytosis.

Leukocytosis and leucopenia

Causes

For causes of leukocytosis and leucopenia, see Table 9.7.

Thrombocytosis (raised platelet count)

Causes

- Iron deficiency and other causes of anaemia.
- Systemic infection.
- Inflammation and other acute phase responses.
- Hyposplenism.
- Myeloproliferative disorders.

Often, no treatment is required for reactive/secondary thrombocytosis. In patients with reactive thrombocytosis >1000 × 10^9/L, daily low dose aspirin to minimise the risk of thrombosis may be considered.

Thrombocytopenia (reduced platelet count)

Causes

- Viral infections (including hepatitis and HIV).
- Autoimmune conditions, e.g. SLE.
- Helicobacter pylori infection.
- Drugs, e.g. sodium valproate, methotrexate, carboplatin, quinine, vancomycin.
- Chronic liver disease.
- Acute leukaemia.
- Immune thrombocytopenic purpura (ITP).

Table 9.7 Causes of leukocytosis and leucopenia

	Infectious causes	Other causes
Neutrophilia	Acute bacterial infections – may progress to leukemoid reaction (WCC>50 × 10^9/L) in severe infection. Rickettsial infections.	Haematological malignancy. Can be associated with DIC.
Neutropenia	Viral infections, e.g. rubella, CMV.	Ethnic variant. Drugs, e.g. propylthiouracil, penicillamine, clozapine, sodium valproate. Primary autoimmune neutropenia. Cyclic neutropaenia – neutropenia tends to occur every 3 weeks and lasts 3–6 days at a time due to changing rates of cell production by the bone marrow; result of autosomal dominantly inherited mutations in ELA2 gene encoding neutrophil elastase; estimated to occur in 1 in 1 million individuals worldwide; treatment includes GCSF and usually improves after puberty.
Eosinophilia	Parasitic infections.	Allergy syndromes, e.g. asthma, hay fever, pemphigus, dermatitis herpetiformis, allergic reactions to drugs including DRESS (drug reaction with eosinophilia and systemic symptoms) with anticonvulsants, sulfonamides, allopurinol, non-steroidal anti-inflammatory drugs and risperidone.
Monocytosis	Chronic bacterial infections. Malaria. Trypanosomiasis. Tuberculosis.	
Monocytopenia		SLE. Hairy cell leukaemia.
Lymphocytosis	Brucella. Toxoplasma. Pertussis. Viral infections e.g. EBV, CMV, coxsackie, adenovirus. Chronic infection with TB, syphilis.	Haematological malignancy, e.g. CLL, ALL, lymphoproliferative disorders.
Lymphopenia	Viral infections e.g. HIV. Legionella.	Malignancy e.g. Hodgkin's lymphoma (HL). Inflammatory conditions e.g. SLE, rheumatoid arthritis, sarcoidosis. Pancreatitis. Uraemia.
Basophilia	Viral infections, e.g. influenza, VZV.	Myeloproliferative disorders, e.g. CML, myelofibrosis. Hypothyroidism. Inflammatory disorders, e.g. ulcerative colitis.
Basopenia	As part of leucocytosis in response to infection.	Thyrotoxicosis. Hypersensitivity reactions (urticaria, anaphylaxis). Cushing's syndrome.

DIC, disseminated intravascular coagulation; CMV, cytomegalovirus; ALL, acute lymphoblastic leukaemia; CML, chronic myeloid leukaemia; VZV, varicella zoster virus.

As a general rule, a platelet count >20 × 10^9/L is considered safe and <10 × 10^9/L is considered high risk of spontaneous bleeding. Counts >50 × 10^9/L can be safe for basic surgery; a count >100 × 10^9/L is desirable for CNS surgery or intra-ocular bleeding. Treatment is mainly of the underlying cause and, in most cases, platelet transfusions achieve a safe platelet count.

Immune thrombocytopenic purpura

- Acquired, immune-mediated, isolated thrombocytopenia (platelet count <100 × 10^9/L).
- Equal gender incidence.
- Short-lived disorder, usually requiring no treatment in children, but may be a chronic disorder in adults.
- No gold standard test; relies on excluding other causes of thrombocytopenia.
- Treatment rarely indicated in patients with platelets >50 × 10^9/L unless there is a clear reason, such as surgery or ongoing bleeding.
- Platelet transfusions are only used in emergencies as they are rapidly destroyed by the antibodies. Concurrent treatment with steroids enable the platelets to last longer.
- Therapies of proven benefit include corticosteroids, IVIG, rituximab and the new thrombopoetin agonists, eltrombopag and romiplostim.
- In chronic cases, immunosuppressive medication such as vincristine, ciclosporin and mycophenylate mofetil are valid options.
- Splenectomy has been used successfully but, due to post-splenectomy complications, is reserved as a third- or fourth-line treatment option.
- Bleeding is uncommon, but when it occurs standard measures, such as haemostatic pressure, tranexamic acid (which is an antifibrinolytic agent) or desmopressin (which promotes release of von Willebrand factor [vWF] and subsequent increase in factor VIII survival secondary to vWF complexing), may be helpful.
- Pregnancy is a particularly challenging time for diagnosis and treatment as many of the therapies are contraindicated in pregnancy. Around the time of delivery, it is critical to have a platelet count sufficient to prevent bleeding; steroids and IVIG (sometimes with platelets) are the drugs of choice in this situation.

Blood transfusion

Blood components

The main blood components, red cells, platelets and plasma are separated by centrifuging:

- Red cells:
  - Can be stored for 35 days at 4–6°C.
  - Should be transfused within 4 hours of removal from a refrigerated environment.
- Platelets:
  - May be from a single donor or pooled from several donors.
  - Stored at room temperature.
  - Bacterial contamination commonly implicated.
- Plasma:
  - Fresh frozen plasma (FFP) is formed when plasma is rapidly frozen at –30°C to prevent loss of coagulation factors. When required, FFP should be thawed and transfused within 24 hours. During this period it should be stored at 4°C. Cryoprecipitate is formed when FFP is thawed from a single donor at 4°C. The important clotting factors within cryoprecipitate are factor VIII, vWF, factor XIII and fibrinogen.

Blood groups

A blood type/group is based on the presence/absence of antibodies and/or presence/absence of inherited antigenic substances on the surface of red blood cells. More than 30 blood group systems are recognized by the International Society of Blood Transfusion; the 2 most important ones being the ABO (Table 9.8) and Rhesus (Rh) systems. Patients should receive their own type-specific blood products to minimise the risk of a transfusion reaction (➲ see Complications of blood transfusion, p. 284 and Tables 9.10 and 9.11). To determine the patient's ABO and Rh group and screen the plasma for the presence of red cell alloantibodies, which may potentially result in a transfusion reaction, a group and screen sample is required. Cross-matching involves mixing a sample of the recipient's serum with a sample of the donor's red blood cells and checking if the mixture agglutinates, showing that that particular donor's blood cannot be transfused to that particular recipient. Blood group AB individuals have both A and B antigens on the surface of their RBC and do not have antibodies against either A or B antigen. Therefore, an individual with type AB blood can receive blood from individuals of any ABO group, but cannot donate blood to any group other than AB. Blood group O individuals do not have either A or B antigens on the surface of their RBCs and their blood serum contains anti-A and anti-B antibodies. Therefore, a group O individual can receive blood only from a group O individual, but can donate blood to individuals of any ABO blood group (Table 9.9).

Table 9.8 ABO blood group system

	Group A	**Group B**	**Group AB**	**Group O**
Antigens in red blood cell	A antigen	B antigen	A and B antigens	None
Antibodies in plasma	Anti-B	Anti-A	None	Anti-A and anti-B

Adapted from Norfolk, D. (2013). *Handbook of Transfusion Medicine*, Fifth Edition, The Stationery Office. Crown copyright information is reproduced with the permission of the Controller of HMSO and the Queen's Printer for Scotland.

Table 9.9 ABO red blood cell compatibility table

Recipient	**Donor**			
	O	**A**	**B**	**AB**
O	✓	✗	✗	✗
A	✓	✓	✗	✗
B	✓	✗	✓	✗
AB	✓	✓	✓	✓

Adapted from Norfolk, D. (2013). *Handbook of Transfusion Medicine*, Fifth Edition, The Stationery Office. Crown copyright information is reproduced with the permission of the Controller of HMSO and the Queen's Printer for Scotland.

The Rh system consists of five antigens: C/c, E/e and D, the latter being the most relevant clinically. Unlike the ABO system, RhD negative individuals do not have naturally occurring anti-D antibodies. Instead, anti-D antibodies are found in RhD negative individuals who have been previously 'sensitised' by being exposed to RhD positive red cells through either a transfusion or via pregnancy with a RhD positive fetus. If a RhD negative patient has developed anti-D antibodies, a subsequent exposure to RhD positive blood leads to a potentially dangerous transfusion reaction. Since anti-D antibodies are IgG antibodies which can cross the placenta, they can bind to RhD positive fetal cells resulting in haemolytic disease of the fetus/newborn. This may be prevented by administration of anti-D immunoglobulin to RhD negative mothers during pregnancy to bind any RhD positive fetal red blood cells before the mother is able to produce an immune response and form anti-D IgG antibodies. RhD positive patients, however, do not react to RhD negative blood.

Indications for transfusion of red cells and platelets

- Massive haemorrhage:
    - Defined as loss of one blood volume (7% of the ideal body weight in an adult) in 24 hours or as 50% loss of blood volume in 3 hours.

    - Hb should be maintained >80g/L.
    - Platelets should be maintained $>75 \times 10^9$/L (and $>100 \times 10^9$/L in major trauma or CNS haemorrhage).
- Bone marrow failure.
- Chemotherapy:
    - Hb should be maintained >80 g/L.
    - Platelets should be maintained $>10 \times 10^9$/L, unless there is sepsis in which case platelets should be maintained $>20 \times 10^9$/L or bleeding in which case platelets should be maintained $>50 \times 10^9$/L.
- Haemoglobinopathies:
    - Patients with sickle cell anaemia may be on a long term transfusion programme (top up or exchange) to prevent complications of the disease.
    - Patients with thalassemia major require regular transfusion to prevent extramedullary haematopoiesis.

Indications for FFP

- Massive transfusion: to replace coagulation factors and aid haemostasis.
- Liver failure.
- DIC if a patient is actively bleeding.
- Thrombotic thrombocytopenic purpura (TTP).
- Haemorrhagic disease of the newborn.
- Single clotting factor deficiency in cases when no specific factor concentrate is available.

Indications for cryoprecipitate

- Massive haemorrhage: to replace fibrinogen.
- Liver failure.
- DIC if a patient is actively bleeding.
- Clotting factor disorders when no specific factor concentrate is available.

Unlike FFP, compatibility testing is not strictly necessary for cryoprecipitate administration but it is given as ABO compatible when possible.

Complications of blood transfusion

For different types of transfusion reaction, see Table 9.10. For transfusion reaction symptom severity and management, see Table 9.11.

All patients with suspected transfusion reactions should have the following investigations:

- FBC, U&Es, LFTs.
- Blood cultures if pyrexia.
- Haemolysis screen:
    - Lactate dehydrogenase (LDH).
    - DAT.
    - Repeat compatibility and antibody testing.
    - Haptoglobin.
    - Urinalysis for haemoglobinuria.

All moderate and severe transfusion reactions should be reported to Serious Hazards of Transfusion (SHOT).

Safety and consent

The commonest cause of acute haemolytic transfusion reaction is clerical error. To ensure that the correct patient receives the correct blood, each of the following steps need to be instated and performed by trained staff:

- *Patient identification*: name, date of birth, NHS and hospital number.
- *Sample labelling*: pre-transfusion sampling at the bedside.

Table 9.10 Different types of transfusion reaction

Type of transfusion reaction	Pathogenesis	Timing of reaction	Specific features	Prevention
Acute haemolytic transfusion reactions, e.g. ABO blood group incompatibility	IgM mediated; intravascular haemolysis secondary to activation of complement.	Immediate.		Safe administration of blood as per the National Patient Safety Agency.
Delayed haemolytic transfusion reactions	IgG mediated; extravascular haemolysis; due to the development of clinically significant alloantibodies which may not have been detected during pre-transfusion testing.	Between 1 and 14 days after transfusion.		Use of antibody card; previous transfusion history including liaising with other hospitals where the patient has been transfused previously.
Non-haemolytic allergic reactions	Occur due to reactions to plasma protein.			Leucodepletion of blood products.
Febrile non-haemolytic reactions	Due to antibodies against human leucocyte antigens (HLA).			Pre-medication with paracetamol.
Transfusion associated circulatory overload (TACO)	Fluid overload.		Increased risk with patients over the age of 60 and patients with cardiac or pulmonary failure.	Use of diuretics; slowing the rate of transfusion; reassessing clinical need for each subsequent unit of transfusion.
Transfusion associated graft versus host disease (GvHD)	Due to discrepancy between the histocompatibility antigens when lymphocytes are transfused from a donor (➲ See Chapter 6, Mechanisms of rejection, p.172 and Prevention of graft rejection and complications of transplantation, p. 173).			Leucodepletion; irradiation of blood products.
Post-transfusion purpura	Alloantibodies against human platelet antigen (HPA)-1a most commonly and HPA-1b occasionally resulting in a fall in platelet count.	7 days after transfusion.	Usually in multiparous women or previously transfused patients.	Use of HPA-1a negative blood products.

Adapted from Norfolk, D. (2013). *Handbook of Transfusion Medicine*, Fifth Edition, The Stationery Office. Crown copyright information is reproduced with the permission of the Controller of HMSO and the Queen's Printer for Scotland.

Table 9.11 Transfusion reaction symptom severity and management

Severity of symptoms	Symptoms	Management
Mild	Urticaria, flushing, temperature rise* <2°C.	Paracetamol, antihistamines.
Moderate	Wheezing, angioedema, hypotension, temperature rise* >2°C.	Stop transfusion immediately. Assess whether pyrexia is in keeping with the patient's clinical history; if not, send unit of blood for culture and take blood cultures from the patient. If severe/incompatible transfusion reaction, acute management of airway, breathing and circulation is needed. Specific measures such as adrenaline IM 1:1000 are needed if there is evidence of anaphylaxis.
Severe	Hypotension with evidence of shock or respiratory compromise such as stridor or anaphylaxis, temperature rise* >2°C.	As for moderate symptoms.

*Compared with pre-transfusion temperature.
Adapted from Norfolk, D. (2013). *Handbook of Transfusion Medicine*, Fifth Edition, The Stationery Office. Crown copyright information is reproduced with the permission of the Controller of HMSO and the Queen's Printer for Scotland.

- *Laboratory*: robust IT systems with warning flags for patients with special requirements.
- *Blood product collection*: robust IT system that only trained staff can access.
- *Administration of blood*: observations taken regularly throughout transfusion.

Informed consent for transfusion of blood products is important. Jehovah's witnesses, who believe that they should not receive blood transfusions, should be identified early and given appropriate counselling of the risks associated with not having a blood transfusion. In elective situations, Hb should be optimised early, through alternative measures such as iron replacement, erythropoietin therapy, and antifibrinolytic agents such as tranexamic acid, and appropriate surgical techniques undertaken to reduce bleeding during surgery. It should also be clearly documented what blood products the patient will have and in what circumstances.

Haemostasis

Overview of haemostasis

Coagulation begins after an injury has damaged the endothelial lining of a blood vessel. Exposure of blood to the subendothelium initiates two processes: changes in platelets and the exposure of subendothelial tissue factor to plasma factor VII. Platelets immediately form a plug at the site of injury; this is called primary haemostasis. Secondary haemostasis occurs simultaneously with additional coagulation factors responding in a complex cascade (Figure 9.6) to form fibrin strands, which strengthen the platelet plug.

Components of haemostatic pathway

Platelets

- Derived from cytoplasm of megakaryocytes in bone marrow.
- Number regulated by thrombopoetin.
- Function in haemostasis mediated by glycoproteins (Gp) on the cell surface and granules in the cytoplasm (α granules contain haemostatic proteins and δ granules contain pro-aggregation factors).
- Form a platelet plug at sites of vascular breach:
  - Plug initially unstable with platelets adhering to the vessel wall (adhesion via GpIa and Ib receptors) and to each other (aggregation via GpIIb/IIIa receptors and vWF).
  - Granule release consolidates the initial plug to make it stronger.

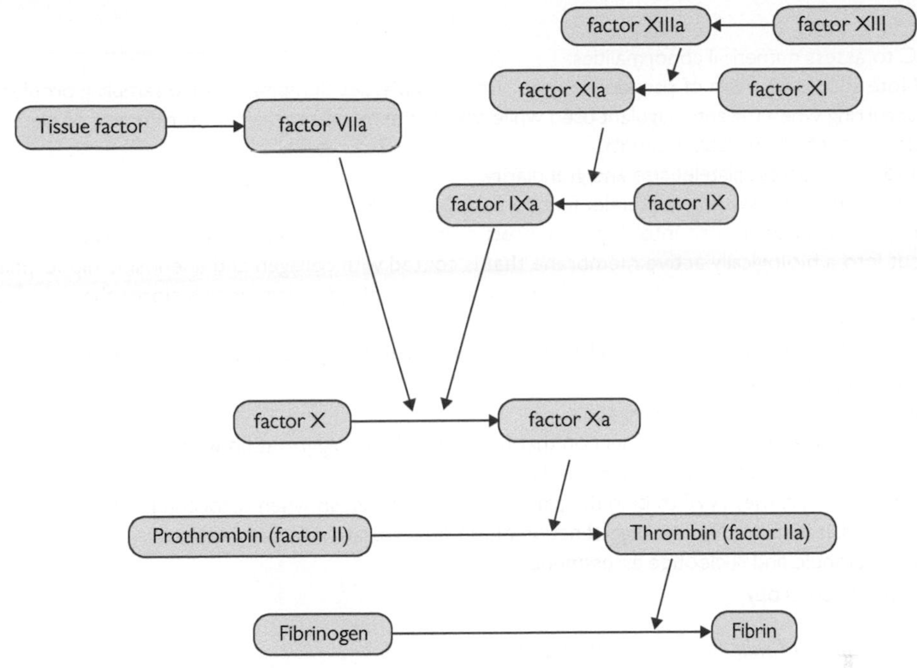

Figure 9.6 The coagulation cascade.

Coagulation factors

Coagulation factors are generally serine protease enzymes which act by cleaving downstream proteins (Figure 9.6). There are some exceptions, e.g. factors V and VIII are glycoproteins and factor XIII is a transglutaminase.

Coagulation factor inhibitors are proteins that inhibit specific coagulation factors, serving to limit unchecked progression of the coagulation cascade that would otherwise occur. They include tissue factor pathway inhibitor (TFPI), antithrombin, and Protein C and Protein S that both inhibit factors V and VIII.

Fibrinolytic system

Fibrin clot is broken down by plasmin into fibrin degradation products (FDPs) that are subsequently cleared by proteases in order to prevent uncontrolled clot formation and/or persistence. Plasmin is the active form of plasminogen, this activation being catalysed by urokinase and tissue plasminogen activator (tPA). Urokinase circulates in the blood stream and tPA is released from damaged endothelium. Urokinase and tPA are in turn inhibited by PAI (plasminogen activator inhibitor) 1 and PAI 2. Plasmin is inhibited by α-1-antiplasmin, α-2-macroglobulin and tissue activator plasmin inhibitor.

Vessel wall

Tissue factor, without which the coagulation cascade cannot be triggered, is bound to the vessel walls. In addition, vasoconstriction reduces blood flow to an injured area and gives more opportunity for platelet activation and coagulation factor interaction with the injured area.

Disorders of coagulation

Platelet disorders

Platelet disorders are either quantitative (thrombocytosis and thrombocytopenia) or qualitative. Qualitative platelet disorders are rare and can broadly be described as inherited and acquired.

Platelet tests

- FBC to assess numerical abnormalities:
  - Note should be made of pseudothrombocytopenia/platelet clumping (in vitro sampling problem occurring when the anticoagulant used while testing the blood sample causes clumping of platelets that mimics a low platelet count).
- Blood film to assess platelet size and granularity.
- Platelet function assay (PFA)/platelet function analyser –100:
  - Aspirates blood in vitro into disposable test cartridges through a microscopic aperture cut into a biologically active membrane that is coated with collagen and adenosine diphosphate (ADP) or collagen and epinephrine inducing a platelet plug to form, which closes the aperture.
  - Dependent on platelet function, plasma vWF level, platelet number and (to some extent) the Hct.
- Platelet aggregometry.
- Ristocetin-induced platelet aggregation:
  - Ex vivo assay for live platelet function that measures platelet aggregation with the help of vWF and exogenous ristocetin added in a graded fashion.
    - Ristocetin causes vWF to bind the platelet receptor GpIb, so when ristocetin is added to normal blood, it initiates the initial agglutination phase of aggregation of live platelets.
- Platelet granule and nucleotide assessment.
- Electron microscopy.

General principles of management of platelet disorders

- Conservative measures: e.g. pressure, avoidance of antiplatelet drugs, tranexamic acid.
- Platelet transfusion with prolonged bleeding or prior to an invasive procedure:
  - If possible it is useful to have HLA platelet typing to minimise the development of platelet antibodies that can occur in multiply transfused patients.
- Recombinant activated factor VII with severe bleeding, although the evidence base is lacking.

Inherited platelet disorders

- Glanzmann's thromboaesthenia:
  - Autosomal recessive.
  - Due to mutations in genes encoding GpIIb/IIIa (integrin $\alpha_{IIb}\beta_3$).
  - Results in a lack of platelet aggregation.
  - Platelet aggregation normal with ristocetin, but impaired with other agonists, such as ADP, thrombin, collagen or epinephrine.
- Bernard Soulier syndrome:
  - Autosomal recessive.
  - Due to mutations in the gene that encodes GpIb.
  - Causes defective platelet binding.
  - May be associated with thrombocytopenia.
  - Platelet function tests demonstrate a lack of aggregation to ristocetin that is not corrected by addition of normal plasma, distinguishing it from von Willebrand disease.
- Platelet granule abnormalities including:
  - Grey platelet disorder of α granules.
  - Hermansky Pudlak syndrome and May Hegglin abnormality of δ granules.

Acquired platelet disorders

- Drugs include:
  - Antiplatelet drugs, e.g. aspirin, dipyridamole, clopidogrel, ticagrelor.
  - Drugs that inhibit platelet function including nitrates, calcium channel blockers, beta-lactam antibiotics and selective serotonin reuptake inhibitors.
- Some foods and herbal remedies, which can affect platelets both qualitatively and quantitatively, including ginseng, turmeric, ginger and garlic.

- A variety of medical conditions including liver failure, uraemia, hypergammaglobulinaemia, myeloproliferative disorders and cardiopulmonary bypass.

Coagulation factor disorders

Inherited coagulation disorders

Haemophilia A

- Most common inherited coagulation factor disorder.
- X-linked deficiency of factor VIII.
- Presents in childhood with joint bleeding and bruising.
- Severity increases with decreasing baseline levels of factor VIII.
- Without treatment, patients suffer spontaneous bleeding into joints, causing arthropathy, muscle bleeds and haematuria; bleeds in the CNS or retroperitoneum can be fatal.
- Diagnosed with prolonged activated partial thromboplastin time (APTT) that corrects with the addition of normal plasma followed by measuring plasma levels of factor VIII:
  - Mild disorder cannot be excluded when APTT is normal.
  - Diagnosis aided by a strong history of bleeding and family history.
- Treated ideally in specialized haemophilia centres by a multidisciplinary team with focus being to replace factor VIII prophylactically with a recombinant product (or purified plasma derived products) to a level of ~30–50%:
  - Higher thresholds of factor VIII are required for operative interventions with a known bleeding risk.
  - Desmopressin may be used for minor procedures.
  - Treatment may be complicated by the development of inhibitors that are antibodies to factor VIII causing patients to be refractory to therapy:
    - This can sometimes be managed with agents such as factor eight inhibitor bypass activity and/or with immunosuppression.

Haemophilia B

- Deficiency of factor IX.
- Similar disease in many ways to haemophilia A in terms of mode of inheritance and treatment principles.
- Desmopressin of no value in haemophilia B.

Von Willebrand disease

- Characterised by a reduction in amount or function of vWF whose main function is as a ligand for platelet adhesion and as a carrier molecule for factor VIII.
- Usually inherited in an autosomal dominant form.
- Grouped into three subtypes:
  - type 1 – qualitative partial deficiency;
  - type 2 – functional abnormality; further subdivided into types 2A, 2B, 2M and 2N;
  - type 3 – total deficiency.
- Symptoms are mainly bleeding from mucosal surfaces and after invasive procedures except type 3, where severe bleeding including haemarthrosis occurs.
- Management via:
  - Avoidance of antiplatelet agents.
  - Use of tranexamic acid, desmopressin and vWF rich clotting factor concentrates.
- Advisable to ensure patients are vaccinated against transmissible viruses such as hepatitis.

Other inherited coagulation factor deficiencies include factor VII deficiency, factor X deficiency, factor XI deficiency and dysfibrinogenaemia/afibrinogenaemia, all of which cause a coagulopathy of varying severity. There are recombinant products for replacement in factor VII deficiency and purified concentrates available in factor XI and XII deficiency.

Acquired coagulation disorders

The most common acquired coagulation disorders include drugs (Table 9.13), DIC, acquired clotting factor inhibitors, massive transfusion and liver disease.

Disseminated intravascular coagulopathy

- Systemic reaction to inflammatory conditions including severe sepsis, trauma, malignancy, organ necrosis, toxins and obstetric complications including placental abruption, pre-eclampsia/eclampsia and amniotic fluid embolism.
- Causes widespread activation of the coagulation and fibrinolytic pathways with a resultant consumption coagulopathy.
- No specific diagnostic test but in conjunction with the clinical state of the patient there is thrombocytopenia, a fall in fibrinogen levels, and a rise in FDP, prothrombin time (PT) and APTT; results should be monitored sequentially as they can worsen alongside the clinical condition.
- Treatment is mainly of the underlying condition but it is useful to keep the platelet count > 20×10^9/l (or higher if there is significant bleeding), and clotting factors should be transfused if a patient is bleeding or about to undergo an invasive procedure.

Acquired clotting factor inhibitors

- Commonly caused by autoantibodies to coagulation factors that result in a reduction in circulating levels of factors and a coagulopathy with bleeding at unusual sites.
- Patients tend to be over the age of 60 years.
- Patients with haemophilia who have been heavily treated with replacement clotting factors may also develop inhibitors.
- Commonly treated with immunosuppression as replacing the deficient clotting factor may aggravate the underlying process; bypassing agents may also be used with variable effect.

Thrombosis

Arterial and venous thrombosis

Virchow's triad can be used to understand the 3 important factors contributing to thrombus formation:

1. Stasis of blood
2. Endothelial injury
3. Hypercoagulability

Traditionally it was understood that endothelial injury as a result of rupture of an atherosclerotic plaque was the dominant component in the formation of an arterial thrombus, whereas stasis and hypercoagulability were the most important factors in venous thrombosis. More recent epidemiology studies suggest an overlap between arterial and venous thrombosis pathogenesis. For risk factors for thrombosis, see Table 9.12.

Therapeutic anticoagulation

Indications for anticoagulation include:

- Treatment and prevention of venous thromboembolic events (VTEs).
- Patients with atrial fibrillation (AF) with a moderate to high risk of thromboembolic events (➲ see Chapter 13, Supraventricular tachycardias, p. 467 and Table 13.48).
- Patients with mechanical heart valves.

For anticoagulant drugs, see Table 9.13. For cytochrome P450 drug and food interactions with warfarin, see Table 9.14.

Heparins are the drug of choice for VTE in patients with cancer. Warfarin is the drug of choice for patients with mechanical heart valves. Warfarin is contraindicated in pregnancy as is it teratogenic

Table 9.12 Risk factors for thrombosis

Risk factors for arterial thrombosis	Risk factors for venous thrombosis
Hypertension	Endothelial injury, e.g. surgery.
Hypercholesterolaemia Diabetes Cigarette smoking Abdominal obesity	Hypercoagulable states, e.g. malignancy, pregnancy and post-partum state, thrombophilias.

1) Adapted with permission from Lowe, G. Common Risk factors for both arterial and venous thrombosis. *British Journal* of Haematology, 140(5):488-95. https://doi.org/10.1111/j.1365-2141.2007.06973.x. © 2008 John Wiley & Sons Ltd. 2) Adapted with permission from Hoffbrand, A.V. & Moss, P. *Essential Haematology*, Sixth Edition (2011). Copyright © 2011, John Wiley and Sons.

(➲ see Chapter 23, Management, p. 815). Anticoagulation is contraindicated in conditions where the risk of bleeding outweighs the benefit associated with anticoagulation. Examples include:

- Intracerebral haemorrhage.
- Inherited and acquired bleeding disorders, e.g. haemophilia, von Willebrand disease, liver/renal failure.
- Lesions, which may bleed, e.g. active peptic ulcer disease, oesophageal varices, aortic aneurysm.
- Recent stroke.
- Major surgery within the last 72 hours.
- Severe hypertension with a systolic BP >200 mmHg or diastolic BP >120 mmHg.

Newer oral anticoagulants (e.g. dabigatran, rivaroxaban, apixaban, edoxaban) have a rapid onset and offset, broad therapeutic window and predictable pharmacokinetics. As such, they do not need regular monitoring. Unfractionated heparin infusions require regular monitoring of APTT.

Complications of anticoagulation include:

- Haemorrhage, particularly CNS haemorrhage and GI haemorrhage.
- Heparin-induced thrombocytopenia (HIT):
  - Occurs when IgG antibodies bind to heparin bound to platelet factor 4 and further activate platelets resulting in new thrombosis that results in a consumptive thrombocytopenia.
- Heparin-induced osteoporosis.

Thrombophilia

Thrombophilia is a tendency to form clots. Patients with a heritable thrombophilia may present at a young age with an unprovoked VTE at an unusual site. Patients should be counselled appropriately; a positive diagnosis may not change the duration or intensity of anticoagulation. Inherited thrombophilias have variable penetrance and are diagnosed in <30% of cases of VTE, reinforcing it to be only one risk factor. Thrombophilia testing should not be carried out in an acute setting when coagulation factors are consumed, and ideally should wait until after anticoagulation therapy has been completed.

Factor V Leiden mutation

- Factor V Leiden mutation (FVL) is the most prevalent genetic risk factor for VTE.
- Penetrance is low with only 10% of heterozygotes and 44% of homozygotes developing thrombosis in their lifetime. The combination of FVL with other inherited thrombophilias or acquired high risk situations, such as pregnancy or surgery particularly predisposes patients to a significant risk of VTE.

Prothrombin allele G20210A variant

Prothrombin allele G20210A is a variant that is associated with increased prothrombin levels and with a relative risk of VTE of 3.

Table 9.13 Anticoagulant drugs

Drug (oral administration unless otherwise stated)	**Method of action**	**Effect on coagulation tests**	**Reversal agent**
Warfarin (and other Vitamin K antagonists)*	Antagonises factors II, VII, IX and X (vitamin K dependent clotting factors).	Raised PT and INR.	Omit dose. Vitamin K. PCC. FFP not indicated.
Low molecular weight heparin (subcutaneous)	Anti-thrombin (factor II) and factor Xa.	May increase APTT in overdose. Raised anti- factor Xa.	Protamine sulfate (less predictable than for unfractionated heparin).
Unfractionated heparin (subcutaneous or IV)	Anti-thrombin (factor II) and factor Xa.	Raised APTT and anti-factor Xa and thrombin time.	Discontinue the drug. Protamine sulphate (1 mg/80–100 units unfractionated heparin, maximum 50 mg); usually not required if normal renal function and >4 hours have elapsed.
Danaparoid (subcutaneous or IV)	Heparinoid (anti-factor II and X activity).	Raised anti-factor Xa.	Plasmapheresis in emergency.
Fondaparinux (subcutaneous or IV)	Indirect factor Xa inhibitor.	Raised anti- factor Xa.	Recombinant factor VIIa in critical bleeding.
Argatroban (IV)	Direct thrombin inhibitor.	Raised APTT ratio. Also prolongs thrombin time and PT.	Discontinue the drug. General haemostatic measures.
Apixaban, Rivaroxaban, Edoxaban	Direct factor Xa inhibitor.	Raised anti- factor Xa. PT prolonged.	PCC. Recombinant factor VIIa in critical bleeding.
Dabigatran	Direct thrombin inhibitor.	Raised anti-factor IIa and thrombin time and ecarin clotting time. Prolongs APTT sometimes.	Discontinue drug. General haemostatic measures. Activated charcoal <2 hours after administration. Idarucizumab. Haemodialysis. PCC/recombinant factor VIIa in extreme bleeding.

PCC, prothrombin complex concentrate; INR, international normalised ratio.

*Warfarin has variable pharmocodynamic and pharmacokinetic properties. It is metabolised by the cytochrome P450 enzyme system and has a narrow therapeutic window with a number of cytochrome P450 drug and food interactions which affect the INR to varying degrees (Table 9.14). The effect of warfarin is monitored using the PT, from which the INR is derived by comparing the patient's PT to a normal (control) sample. The target INR depends on the reason for anticoagulation e.g. target INR of 2.5 for treatment of VTE; target INR of 3.5 for patients with antiphospholipid syndrome and arterial thrombosis. The duration of anticoagulation also depends on the reason for anticoagulation e.g. 3 months for provoked VTE with temporary risk factors; long-term for AF and mechanical prosthetic valves.

Data from Makris, M. et al. Guideline on the management of bleeding in patients on antithrombotic agents. *British Journal of Haematology*, 2012, 160(1), 35-46. https://doi.org/10.1111/bjh.12107; and data from NICE (2016) KTT16 Anticoagulants, including non-vitamin K antagonist oral anticoagulants (NOACs). Available from https://www.nice.org.uk/guidance/ktt16.

Table 9.14 Cytochrome P450 drug and food interactions with warfarin

Cytochrome P450 inhibitors (increase effect of warfarin)	**Cytochrome P450 inducers (decrease effect of warfarin)**
Grapefruit juice	Carbamazapine
Ritonavir	Phenytoin
Sodium valproate	Rifampicin
Isoniazid	Alcohol (chronic ingestion)
Alcohol (acute intake)	
Ciprofloxacin	

Adapted with permission from Hoffbrand, A.V. & Moss, P. *Essential Haematology*, Sixth Edition (2011). Copyright © 2011, John Wiley and Sons.

Deficiencies in natural anticoagulants (antithrombin, protein C and protein S)

Antithrombin deficiency

- Autosomal dominant inheritance.
- Two types: type 1 is quantitative; type 2 is qualitative.
- Associated with a relative risk of VTE >25-50.

Protein C deficiency

- Autosomal dominant inheritance.
- Associated with a relative risk of VTE of 6.5.
- Heterogenous condition with variable penetrance; hence, risk of recurrence of VTE may vary.

N.B. Protein C levels can also be affected by other factors such as vitamin K deficiency and liver disease.

Protein S deficiency

- Autosomal dominant inheritance.
- Associated with a relative risk of VTE of 2–3.

N.B. Acquired protein S deficiency can occur with vitamin K deficiency, liver disease and pregnancy.

Haematological malignancy

Myeloid malignancy

Myelodysplasia (MDS)

- Heterogeneous group of clonal disorders.
- Characterised by ineffective haematopoiesis and, as a consequence, cytopaenia:
  - Anaemia (Hb<100 g/L): fatigue; dyspnoea; heart failure.
  - Neutropenia (<1.8×10^9/L): asymptomatic and incidental finding on a blood test; infection.
  - Thrombocytopenia (platelets <100×10^9/L).
- Affects 5 in 100,000 people.
- Incidence increases with age.
- May be primary or secondary to previous exposure to alkylating agents.

Box 9.1 WHO classification of myelodysplasia

- Refractory cytopenia with unilineage dysplasia (RCUD):
  - FBC: single cytopenia.
  - PBF: blasts <1%.
  - Bone marrow: blasts <5%, dysplasia >10% in one cell lineage.
- Refractory cytopenias of multilineage dysplasia (RCMD):
  - FBC: ≥2 cytopenias.
  - PBF: blasts <1%.
  - Bone marrow: blasts <5%, dysplasia >10% in ≥2 lineages.
- Refractory anaemia with ringed sideroblasts (RARS):
  - FBC: anaemia.
  - PBF: blasts <1%.
  - Bone marrow: ring sideroblasts >15%, blasts <5%.
- Refractory anaemia with excess blasts-1 (RAEB-1):
  - FBC: cytopenia.
  - PBF: 2–4% blasts, monocytes $<1 \times 10^9$/L.
  - Bone marrow: unilineage or multilineage dysplasia, 5–9% blasts, no auer rods (cytoplasmic clumps of azurophilic [stainable with a Romanowsky stain] granular material composed of fused lysosomes/primary neutrophilic granules containing peroxidase, lysosomal enzymes and large crystalline inclusions).
- Refractory anaemia with excess blasts-2 (RAEB-2):
  - FBC: cytopaenia.
  - PBF: 5–19% blasts.
  - Bone marrow: unilineage or multilineage dysplasia, 10–19% blasts, auer rods present.
- MDS – unclassified:
  - Bone marrow: blasts <5%, unilineage or no dysplasia, but typical cytogenetics associated with MDS.
- MDS associated with 5q deletion:
  - FBC: anaemia and thrombocytosis.
  - Bone marrow: unilineage erythroid dysplasia.

Data from BSH Guidelines for Diagnosis and Management of Adult MDS/WHO Classification of MDS. Swerdlow 2008.

Classification

The previous French-American-British (FAB) classification system has been replaced by the WHO criteria (Box 9.1) that relies on the results of:

1. FBC: number of cytopaenias.
2. PBF: percentage of blasts seen.
3. Bone marrow: number of lineages with dysplasia and percentage of blasts seen.

Complications

- Progression to an acute leukaemia.
- Complications of treatment:
  - Recurrent blood transfusions are associated with risk of transfusion reactions, development of alloantibodies and iron overload that can result in multiple organ failure.
  - Side effects of chemotherapy agents: e.g. azacitidine can affect liver function; ciclopsorin has been associated with renal dysfunction.

Prognosis

- Prognosis depends on the percentage of blasts in the bone marrow; a higher percentage conferring a poorer prognosis.

- International Prognostic Scoring System (IPSS) is calculated from the percentage of blasts in the bone marrow, the number of cytopenias and the presence or absence of prognostically relevant cytogenetic abnormalities (including 5q and 20q deletions):
  - IPSS low risk (score 0) and intermediate-1 risk (score 0.5–1.0) have a prognosis of 3–5 years.
  - IPSS intermediate-2 risk (score 1.5–2) and high risk (score >2.5) have a prognosis of 4 months.

Investigations

- FBC.
- PBF.
- Haematinics (iron studies, vitamin B_{12}, folate).
- Erythropoietin levels.
- Bone marrow aspirate and trephine and cytogenetics and iron studies.
- Special tests, e.g. HLA typing if the patient is a candidate for BMT.

Treatment

Supportive management

- Red cell and platelet transfusions.
- GCSF if recurrent bacterial infections with neutropenia.
- Tranexamic acid for bleeding.
- Iron chelation if more than 20–30 red cell transfusions.
- Erythopoietin replacement if low erythropoietin level. An adequate iron store is necessary for erythropoietin replacement to be effective.
- Psychosocial support.

Disease-specific treatments

- For low/intermediate risk patients:
  - Erythropoietin if levels are low.
  - Immunosuppression with ciclosporin and anti-thymocyte globulin (ATG) if erythropoietin levels are adequate.
  - Hypomethylating agents such as azacitidine or decitabine if there is inadequate response to immunosuppression or patients are unlikely to respond.
  - Lenalidomide is effective in reducing red blood cell transfusion requirements in patients with a 5q deletion cytogenetic abnormality.
- For intermediate/high risk patients:
  - Allogenic BMT if a suitable donor is available in a patient fit for intensive treatment.
  - Azacitidine or decitabine if there is no suitable donor for BMT or the patient is not fit for intensive treatment.

Myeloproliferative neoplasms

Myeloproliferative neoplasms incorporate polycythaemia rubra vera (PRV), essential thrombocythaemia (ET), myelofibrosis and chronic myeloid leukaemia (CML) that are clonal haematopoietic stem cell neoplasms that often involve constitutive activation of tyrosine kinase.

Essential thrombocythaemia

ET is defined as a platelet count >450 × 10^9/L in the presence of a known mutation such as JAK 2 V617F (substitution of phenylalanine for valine at position 617 on the *JAK 2* tyrosine kinase gene increasing JAK 2 kinase activity with cytokine-independent growth of cell lines), or CALR (calreticulin) gene mutation (generating a novel terminal peptide of the resulting protein that causes a loss of endoplasmic reticulum KDEL [lysine, aspartic acid, glutamic acid, leucine] retention signal). ET may also be considered with thrombocytosis (platelet count >450 × 10^9/L) with no secondary causes (such as iron-deficiency) or reactive causes and typical bone marrow findings of staghorn (large hyperlobulated) megakaryocytes and no increase in reticulin.

Patients may present in a variety of ways including:

- Incidental finding on a routine blood test.
- Thrombosis.
- Haemorrhage: bleeding normally associated with very high platelet counts (>1500 × 10^9/L).

Complications

- Transformation to an acute leukaemia: occurs when blasts are >20%.
- Thrombosis.
- Haemorrhage.
- Microvascular symptoms:
  - Erythromelalgia (syndrome characterised by redness, heat and pain, usually affecting one or more extremities).
  - Migraine.

Risk classification

- High risk: includes any one of the following: aged >60 years, previous ET-related thrombosis/haemorrhage, platelet count >1500 × 10^9/L.
- Intermediate risk: aged 40–60 years with no high risk features.
- Low risk: aged <40 years with no high risk features.

Investigations

- FBC: platelet count >450 × 10^9/L.
- JAK 2 V617F mutation (55% of patients), *CALR* gene mutation.
- Iron studies and CRP to exclude secondary causes.
- Bone marrow biopsy: staghorn megakaryocytes with no increase in reticulin.

Treatment

Supportive management

- Aspirin:
  - Antiplatelet agent that can reduce the risk of thrombosis.
  - Contraindicated if platelet counts >1000 × 10^9/L, as such high platelet counts may be associated with bleeding, and in patients with asthma or previous history of peptic ulcer disease.
- Screen and treat risk factors for thrombosis, i.e. hypertension, hypercholesterolaemia, diabetes mellitus, cigarette smoking.
- Long-term warfarin only if recurrent VTE/life-threatening thrombosis.

Cytoreductive treatment

- High risk patients:
  - First line treatment: hydroxycarbamide:
    - Known side effects: GI symptoms, rashes, leg ulcers, teratogenicity.
  - Second line treatment: anagrelide:
    - Known side effects: GI symptoms, headache, heart failure, bone marrow and pulmonary fibrosis.
- Low risk patients:
  - Only consider cytoreductive therapy if patients are symptomatic or as part of a clinical trial.

Myelofibrosis

- Patients usually aged 50–60 years.
- Presenting symptoms include:
  - Anaemia.
  - Constitutional symptoms (weight loss, lethargy, night sweats).
  - Gout.

    - Painful splenomegaly.
- FBC shows anaemia and a leucoerythroblastic blood film (left shift in myeloid series, presence of nucleated red cells).
- Diagnosis confirmed by bone marrow aspiration and trephine that shows increased marrow cellularity and megakaryocyte proliferation, with evidence of bone marrow fibrosis.
- JAK 2 V617F mutation present in approximately 50% of patients.
- Myeloproliferative leukaemia (MPL) virus W515 mutation present in approximately 10–15% of patients, leading to the production of an abnormal thrombopoietin receptor protein resulting in the overproduction of abnormal megakaryocytes that stimulate fibroblasts to produce collagen in the bone marrow.
- Complications include:
    - Acute myeloid leukaemia (AML): 15–20% progress to AML.
    - Infection.
    - Haemorrhage.
    - Portal hypertension secondary to splenomegaly.
- Poorer prognosis with:
    - Age >65 years.
    - White cell count >25 × 10^9/L.
    - Hb <100 g/L.
    - Blasts in PBF.
- Patients may be classified as:
    - Low risk: no poor prognosis factors.
    - Intermediate risk-1: 1 poor prognosis factor.
    - Intermediate risk-2: 2 poor prognosis factors.
    - High risk: ≥3 poor prognosis factors.
- Treatment options:
    - Low risk patients may be observed.
    - Erythropoietin for anaemia if there is no splenomegaly.
    - Red cell transfusion.
    - Allopurinol for hyperuricaemia.
    - Hydroxycarbamide; prednisolone; danazol; thalidomide; lenalidomide if splenomegaly.
    - Splenectomy for splenomegaly in patients refractory to drug treatment.
    - Ruxolitinib (JAK inhibitor) in intermediate/high-risk patients:
        - Side effects include: opportunistic infections, *Herpes zoster*, weight gain, hypercholesterolaemia, liver dysfunction, anaemia, thrombocytopenia.
        - Allogenic BMT for high risk patients.

Chronic myeloid leukaemia

CML is a neoplasm of the haematopoietic stem cells characterized by an increase in the granulocyte series and the presence of the Philadelphia chromosome t(9,22) that involves a reciprocal translocation between chromosomes 9 and 22, resulting in a fusion gene BCR-ABL. This in turns results in the production of an abnormal 210 kDa protein resulting in constitutive tyrosine kinase activity and increased cell proliferation and survival.

Patients usually present in their 50s. CML is more common in females. There may be a history of exposure to irradiation. Patients may present with constitutional symptoms, gout or painful splenomegaly, or as an incidental finding following an abnormal FBC. Occasionally, when the white cell count is significantly raised, patients may present with symptoms of leucostasis (blurred vision, headaches, dizziness), which is a medical emergency.

Most patients present in the chronic phase when the PBF shows <10% blasts. In the accelerated phase, there are 10–19% blasts in the PBF and in blast crisis there are >20% blasts in the PBF. In the accelerated phase, patients can also have a basophilia, thrombocytopenia and splenomegaly despite treatment. Complications include infection and progression to an acute leukaemia. A number of risk stratification scores exist, based upon age, spleen size, platelet count, basophil and eosinophil counts, and blast %.

For a peripheral blood film of a patient with CML, see Figure 9.7.

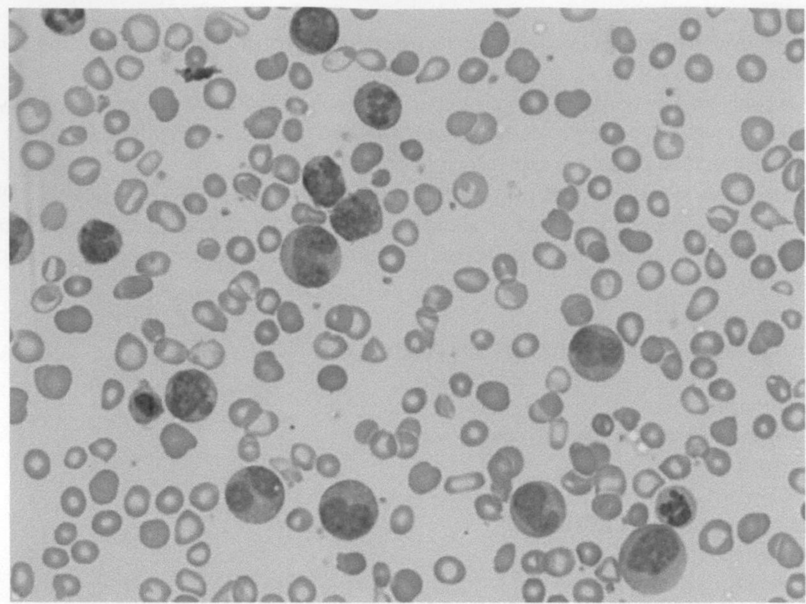

Figure 9.7 (see colour plate section) Peripheral blood film of patient with chronic myeloid leukaemia showing many immature myeloid precursors (Oil immersion x100 magnification).

FBC shows raised WCC with neutrophilia and basophilia, anaemia and thrombocytosis/thrombocytopenia. Serum LDH and urate levels (secondary to high cell turnover) are often raised. Neutrophil alkaline phosphatase (NAP) is low in contrast to a leukemoid reaction due to infection or inflammation when it is raised. Bone marrow biopsy shows hypercellularity with myeloid hyperplasia. Cytogenetics and molecular tests show the presence of t(9,22) and BCR-ABL.

The only curative treatment for CML is a BMT or an allogenic stem cell transplant. There are four other major mainstays of treatment:

- Tyrosine kinase inhibitors: imatinib, dasatinib, nilotinib, radotinib.
- Myelosuppressive or leukopheresis therapy (to counteract the leucocytosis during early treatment).
- Splenectomy.
- Interferon α in pregnancy.

Chronic myelomonocytic leukaemia

- Classified as an MDS/myeloproliferative overlap disorder.
- Blood monocyte count >1 × 10^9/L.
- No Philadelphia chromosome.
- No mutation in platelet-derived growth factor receptor alpha polypeptide or beta-type platelet-derived growth factor receptor.
- Blast count <20%.
- Dysplasia of at least one lineage of myeloid blood cell.
- Azacitidine and stem cell transplantation are approved treatments.

Acute myeloid leukaemia

AML is a neoplasm of the haematopoietic myeloid precursor cells characterised by >20% blasts in a bone marrow sample. It is the commonest acute leukaemia in adults, with the majority of patients being over 60 years of age. Risk factors include:

- Previous history of MDS.
- Cytotoxic therapy, e.g. alkylating agents, ionising radiation, benzene.

Box 9.2 WHO classification system of acute myeloid leukaemia

- AML associated with genetic abnormalities:
  - translocation between: chromosomes 8 and 21, chromosomes 9 and 11, chromosomes 15 and 17, chromosomes 6 and 9, chromosomes 1 and 22.
  - translocation or inversion in: chromosome 16, chromosome 3.
- AML associated with MDS.
- Therapy-related AML.
- AML not otherwise specified
  - M0-M7:
    - M0 – undifferentiated acute myeloblastic leukaemia.
    - M1 – acute myeloblastic leukaemia with minimal maturation.
    - M2 – acute myeloblastic leukaemia with maturation (commonest form).
    - M3 – acute promyelocytic leukaemia (APML):
      - associated with the reciprocal translocation t(15,17) which results in an abnormal fusion protein called PML-RARA;
      - haematological emergency.
    - M4 – acute myelomonocytic leukaemia and acute myelomonocytic leukaemia with eosinophilia (M4 eos).
    - M5 – acute monoblastic leukaemia.
    - M6 – acute erythroid leukaemia.
    - M7 – acute megakaryocytic leukaemia.
  - Acute basophilic leukaemia.
  - Acute panmyelosis with fibrosis.
- Myeloid sarcoma (also known as granulocytic sarcoma or chloroma).
- Myeloid proliferations related to Down syndrome.
- Undifferentiated and biphenotypic acute leukaemia with both lymphocytic and myeloid features; sometimes called acute lymphoblastic leukaemia (ALL) with myeloid markers, AML with lymphoid markers, or mixed phenotype acute leukaemia.

- Chromosomal defects, e.g. Down syndrome, Fanconi anaemia.
- Cigarette smoking.

Box 9.2 shows the WHO classification of AML.

Clinical features

- Symptomatic anaemia (especially in the elderly): lethargy, shortness of breath, chest pain.
- Infection–neutropenic sepsis, atypical infection, e.g. HSV, VZV.
- Constitutional symptoms: fevers, weight loss, night sweats.
- Specific features of different types of AML:
  - M3 can be associated with DIC and present with haemorrhage (gum bleeding, epistaxis).
  - M4 and M5 is associated with gum hypertrophy.
- Symptoms and signs of leucostasis: hypoxia, confusion, retinal haemorrhage.
- Hepatosplenomegaly if previous CML.

Complications

- Neutropenic sepsis.
- DIC and haemorrhage.

Investigations

- FBC and PBF demonstrate pancytopaenia (anaemia, neutropenia and thrombocytopenia).
- Bone marrow aspirate and trephine cytogenetics and molecular analysis: >20% blasts.

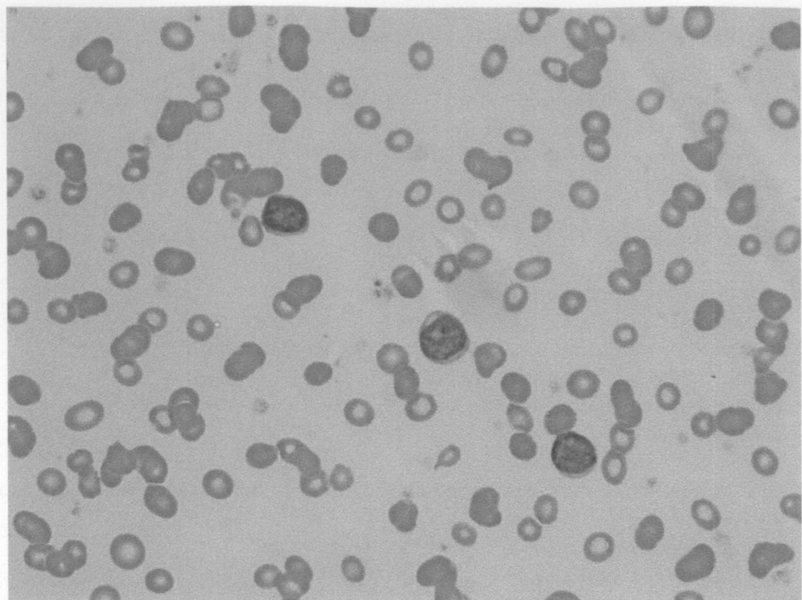

Figure 9.8 (see colour plate section) Peripheral blood film of patient with acute myeloid leukaemia showing three large immature blasts with nucleoli (Oil immersion ×100 magnification).

- Bone marrow immunophenotyping confirms acute leukaemia based on the presence of markers on cells.
- LDH: usually raised.
- Urate: may be raised by rapid cell turnover.
- Renal and liver function to determine dosing and adverse effects of chemotherapy agents.
- Coagulation: DIC in M3.

For a peripheral blood film of a patient with AML, see Figure 9.8.

Treatment

- Explanation of diagnosis and counselling.
- Monitoring for and use of allopurinol and hydration to prevent tumour lysis syndrome/acute renal failure (➲ see Chapter 10, Tumour lysis syndrome, p. 334).
- Treatment of neutropenic sepsis with broad spectrum antibiotics.
- Leucopheresis if symptoms or signs of leucostasis.
- Red cell and platelet transfusion support:
  - Aim for platelets >20 × 10^9/L if septic, or >50 × 10^9/L if bleeding or acute promyelocytic leukaemia (APML; due to the associated increased risk of bleeding).
- Chemotherapy:
  - Usually involves a cardiotoxic anthracycline, e.g. daunorubicin, idarubicin; patients require echocardiography prior to treatment.
  - Intrathecal chemotherapy needed if evidence of CNS involvement e.g. methotrexate, cytarabine.
  - All-trans-retinoic acid (ATRA) or arsenic trioxide should be started as soon as APML is suspected:
    - ATRA dissociates the nuclear receptor co-repressor-histone deacetylase complex (whose interaction is enhanced by the PML-RARA fusion protein) from the retinoic acid receptor and allows DNA transcription and differentiation of immature leukaemic promyelocytes into mature granulocytes, reducing the risk of DIC.

    - ATRA therapy is associated with the potentially fatal 'differentiation syndrome' involving cytokine release, fever, peripheral and pulmonary oedema, pleural effusions and renal impairment.
  - Post-chemotherapy bone marrow sampling to assess response to chemotherapy.
- Allogenic BMT if the AML is associated with high risk cytogenetics and the patient is less than 60 years of age and otherwise medically fit.

Lymphoid malignancy

Acute lymphoblastic leukaemia

- Commonest leukaemia in children (with a good prognosis).
- Associated with:
  - Down syndrome;
  - Fanconi anaemia;
  - Klinefelter syndrome;
  - exposure to chemicals;
  - paternal exposure to radiation.
- FAB classification[1]:
  - L1: small cells with homogenous nuclear chromatin, small or absent nucleoli and small amounts of cytoplasm (most common form in children).
  - L2: large cells with variable nuclear chromatin and ≥1 nucleoli (most common form in adults).
  - L3: large homogenous cells with large nucleoli and significant basophilic cytoplasm and vacuolation (very aggressive form).

Like AML, patients with acute lymphoblastic leukaemia (ALL) also present with symptoms of bone marrow failure involving symptomatic anaemia, recurrent infections (fungal and bacterial), symptoms of leucostasis, and bleeding secondary to low platelets. CNS involvement, occurs more commonly than in AML, and patients may present with symptoms of meningism (headache, neck stiffness, vomiting). Lymphadenopathy and hepatosplenomegaly may be present on examination. The main complications are immunosuppression, associated with risk of life threatening infections, and risk of relapse.

Investigations

- FBC demonstrates anaemia and thrombocytopenia and may show a significantly raised white cell count with a lymphocytosis.
- PBF: lymphoblasts >20%.
- Bone marrow biopsy: immunophenotyping will confirm whether ALL is T or B cell-mediated.
  - Some cytogenetics will be favourable, while others such as BCR-ABL are associated with a poorer prognosis.
- CT neck, chest, abdomen, pelvis (CT-NCAP) to investigate for evidence of lymphadenopathy and organomegaly.
- Lumbar puncture: need a platelet count of $>80 \times 10^9/L$.
- Echocardiography to assess baseline cardiac function (as chemotherapy agents may be cardiotoxic).

Treatment

Supportive management

- Prompt treatment of neutropenic sepsis with antibiotics.
- Antifungal and anti-viral treatment.
- Red cell and platelet transfusions.
- Hydration and allopurinol to prevent tumour lysis syndrome (➔ see Chapter 10, Tumour lysis syndrome, p. 334).

[1] Reproduced from *Journal of Clinical Pathology*, Bennett JM, Catovsky D, Daniel MT, et al., Proposals for the classification of chronic (mature) B and T lymphoid leukaemias. French-American-British (FAB) Cooperative Group, 42, pp. 567–584. Copyright © 1989, with permission from BMJ Publishing Group Ltd and the Association of Clinical Pathologists. http://dx.doi.org/10.1136/jcp.42.6.567.

Definitive management

The aim is to achieve a complete remission that is defined as recovery of the FBC and blasts <5% in the bone marrow.

- Involves four stages:
  - Induction chemotherapy to bring about bone marrow remission, e.g. prednisolone, vincristine and an anthracycline drug.
  - Consolidation therapy to eliminate any remaining leukaemia cells, e.g. methotrexate and 6-mercaptopurine.
  - CNS prophylaxis involving intrathecal chemotherapy ± craniospinal radiotherapy.
  - Maintenance chemotherapy.
- Allogenic BMT may be appropriate for high-risk or relapsed patients.

Chronic lymphocytic leukaemia

Chronic lymphocytic leukaemia (CLL) is the commonest leukaemia in the western world, accounting for 25–30% of all leukaemias, with patients usually presenting in their 70s. A lymphocytosis is defined as a lymphocyte count $>5 \times 10^9$/L and in CLL this lymphocytosis persists for greater than 3 months. The lymphocytes are mature, but not functional, and are found in the blood, bone marrow, lymph nodes, spleen and liver. Often there is no associated cause. Genetics may play a part as CLL is much more common in the relatives of those with lymphoid malignancies; also CLL has a low incidence in Japan.

Presentation is usually asymptomatic, with lymphocytosis being found incidentally on a FBC. Other patients may present at later stages with lymphadenopathy, hepatosplenomegaly or symptoms of bone marrow failure (night sweats, bruising/bleeding, recurrent infections). CLL may be complicated by AIHA, immune thrombocytopenia and/or transformation to a lymphoma.

Investigations

- FBC demonstrating lymphocytosis.
- PBF demonstrating smear cells and mature lymphocytes (Figure 9.9).
- Haemolysis screen as CLL may be associated with AIHA.

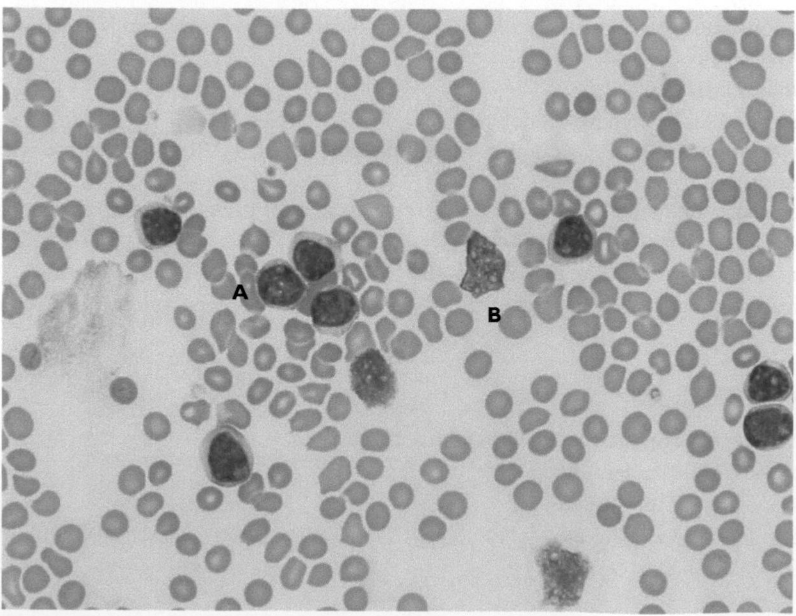

Figure 9.9 (see colour plate section) Peripheral blood film of patient with chronic lymphocytic leukaemia (Oil immersion ×100 magnification). (A) Mature lymphocytes – some with nucleoli. (B) Smear cell.

- Peripheral immunophenotyping (detection of markers on cells to identify the cell type using monoclonal antibodies); lymphocytes in CLL have a characteristic immunophenotype.
- Lymph node biopsy.

For a peripheral blood film of a patient with CLL, see Figure 9.9.

Treatment

Asymptomatic patients may be observed over time. Chemotherapy should be considered in those who are symptomatic, have autoimmune haemolysis, immune thrombocytopenia, which is not responding to steroids, or a rapidly increasing lymphocyte count. The choice of treatment depends on performance status (➲ see Chapter 10, Performance status assessment, p. 327 and Table 10.6) and the presence/absence of the p53 deletion:

- Patients with poor performance status are given chlorambucil.
- Patients with good performance status and the p53 deletion are given alemtuzumab (a monoclonal antibody that binds to the CD52 protein on the surface of lymphocytes).
- Patients with good performance status but not the p53 deletion are given a combination of fludarabine, cyclophosphamide and rituximab (FCR).

Patients who receive alemtuzumab or fludarabine need lifelong irradiated blood products to prevent transfusion-associated graft versus host disease. These agents are also associated with prolonged lymphopenia and, therefore, patients should be given *Pneumocystis jirovecii* prophylaxis with cotrimoxazole or pentamidine nebulisers for 3–6 months following treatment.

Myeloma

Myeloma is a haematological malignancy of plasma cells with an incidence of 60 per million people. The majority of patients are aged ≥70 years and it is more common in Afro-Caribbean individuals.

Patients can present with complications of myeloma:

1. Hyper**C**alcaemia: abdominal pain, constipation, kidney stones, depression.
2. **R**enal impairment (➲ see Chapter 16, Myeloma cast nephropathy, p. 576).
3. **A**naemia: dyspnoea, lethargy, cardiac failure.
4. **B**ony disease: lytic lesions, spinal cord compression (medical emergency) (➲ see Chapter 10, Metastatic spinal cord compression, p. 335).

Presentation of myeloma can also be with symptoms of hyperviscosity (headache, retinal haemorrhages, shortness of breath) that is a medical emergency.

Myeloma is diagnosed if the following are present:

1. Paraprotein (M protein) >30 g/L*.
2. Bone marrow plasma cell population >10%.
3. Presence of end-organ damage due to myeloma (if present, the paraprotein and plasma cell population in the bone marrow do not have to meet the above criteria).

*The UK Myeloma Forum and Nordic Myeloma Study Group define an M-protein/paraprotein as 'a monoclonal immunoglobulin secreted by an abnormally expanded clone of plasma cells in an amount that can be visualised by immunofixation of serum and/or urine'. The M-protein may involve the whole immunoglobulin or the free light chain portion only, in which case it is referred to as a serum-free light chain.

Myeloma is often preceded by a monoclonal gammopathy of unknown significance (MGUS) with M-protein <30 g/L and no evidence of end organ damage.

Investigations

- FBC.
- U&E.
- Serum protein electrophoresis: to identify if a paraprotein is present.
- Urine protein electrophoresis: for presence of Bence Jones protein (monoclonal globulin protein or immunoglobulin light chain).
- Skeletal survey for presence of lytic lesions.

- Fundoscopy: for possible retinal haemorrhages.
- Plasma viscosity if there are symptoms of hyperviscosity.

Treatment

Patients with MGUS are monitored in an outpatient setting for development of myeloma, and similarly asymptomatic patients with myeloma are monitored for evidence of end-organ damage. Management of symptomatic myeloma includes supportive treatment and chemotherapy:

- Supportive treatment/management of medical emergencies:
  - Hyperviscosity: plasma exchange.
  - Hypercalcaemia: IV hydration and bisphosphonates; dose of bisphosphonates may need to be reduced if the patient has renal impairment.
  - Spinal cord compression (➲ see Chapter 10, Metastatic spinal cord compression, p. 335).
  - Infection: broad spectrum antibiotics.
  - Bone disease: analgesia and local radiotherapy.
- Chemotherapy:
  - The majority of patients are not candidates for intensive chemotherapy due to their age and multiple comorbidities.
  - Main chemotherapy drugs are bortezomib, thalidomide and lenalidomide:
    - Thalidomide and lenalidomide are associated with an increased risk of VTE and so patients are started on venous thromboprophylaxis pre-emptively.

Amyloidosis

Amyloidosis occurs when insoluble amyloid fibrils are deposited in soft tissues. There are many different types of amyloid, which can be clinically subdivided into localised and systemic forms. Localised amyloidosis usually affects the skin (➲ see Chapter 21, Amyloidosis, p. 771), whereas systemic amyloidosis (such as AL and aplastic anaemia [AA] amyloidosis) can affect any visceral organ. AL amyloidosis is a clonal plasma cell disorder with deposition of the fibrous protein, resulting in organ dysfunction, particularly of the kidneys, heart, liver and peripheral nervous system. AL amyloidosis is associated with myeloma, Waldenstrom's macroglobinaemia and lymphoma. AL amyloidosis is 20 times more common than AA amyloidosis that occurs with increased production of amyloid protein, often as a complication of chronic inflammatory diseases (e.g. rheumatoid arthritis, inflammatory bowel disease) and infections (e.g. osteomyelitis, tuberculosis).

Clinical features

- Localised amyloidosis:
  - Skin plaques/nodules.
- Systemic amyloidosis:
  - Organ dysfunction/involvement associated with amyloid deposition including:
    - Renal failure (most common) including nephrotic syndrome (➲ see Chapter 16, Amyloidosis, p. 577).
    - Cardiac failure leading to shortness of breath, peripheral oedema, hepatosplenomegaly.
    - Liver dysfunction.
    - Sensory and autonomic neuropathies.
    - Hypothyroidism.
    - Susceptibility to bleeding with bruising around the eyes, termed 'racoon-eyes' (due to amyloid deposition in blood vessels and reduced activity of thrombin and factor V as a result of amyloid binding).
    - Macroglossia that may lead to dysphagia and obstructive sleep apnoea.
    - Carpal tunnel syndrome.

Investigations

- FBC.
- U&E.
- LFT.
- 24-hour urine collection for proteinuria.
- Myeloma screen:

- serum and urine electrophoresis;
- skeletal survey.
- Bone marrow biopsy with Congo red stain for presence of amyloid fibrils.
- Echocardiogram.
- SAP (serum amyloid P component) scanning:
  - Involves injecting radiolabelled SAP into the patient to detect amyloid deposits in the body without the need for an invasive biopsy.

Treatment

- Excision or laser removal of localised amyloidosis lesions.
- Treating underlying inflammatory disorder or infection in AA amyloidosis to reduce serum amyloid A protein production.
- Treating underlying myeloma in AL amyloidosis, usually with bortezomib-based chemotherapy.
- Management of secondary organ dysfunction, e.g. nephrotic syndrome, cardiac failure.

Lymphoma

Lymphomas are essentially 'cancers of the lymph nodes' and are best subdivided into Non-Hodgkin's lymphomas (NHL) and HL.

Non-Hodgkin's lymphoma

85% of NHL is of B cell origin and the remaining 15% is of T cell origin. B cell NHLs include:

- Follicular lymphoma.
- Diffuse large cell B-cell lymphoma (DLBCL): commonest variant (30% of all NHLs).
- Burkitt's lymphoma: an aggressive form of lymphoma which tends to affect young adults.
- Mantle cell lymphoma: tends to affect the elderly, presenting in advanced stages with a poor prognosis.

Present symptoms

- B symptoms (drenching night sweats, 'lumps and bumps', weight loss, recurrent infections).
- Local mass effects of lymph node enlargement.
- Bone marrow failure: bruising/bleeding secondary to thrombocytopenia; lethargy, shortness of breath and/or heart failure secondary to anaemia; and recurrent infections secondary to leucopaenia.
- Hepatosplenomegaly.

Investigations

- FBC and PBF: to investigate for cytopaenias secondary to bone marrow failure and abnormal lymphocytes on the blood film such as Burkitt cells.
- LDH: raised with high cell turnover.
- Serum biochemistry:
  - Renal impairment may result from the mass effect of lymph node enlargement or secondary to tumour lysis associated with high tumour bulk.
  - Hyperkalaemia, hyperphosphataemia, hyperuricaemia and hypocalcaemia may occur with tumour lysis.
- Hepatitis B surface antigen, hepatitis B core antibody, hepatitis C and HIV are routinely tested prior to starting chemotherapy since:
  - Chemotherapy is immunosuppressive and, therefore, patients are prone to viral reactivation that is associated with increased mortality and morbidity, e.g. rituximab has been associated with hepatitis B reactivation.
  - There are drug interactions between certain antiretroviral medications and chemotherapy agents, which can increase risk of chemotherapy toxicity.
  - Burkitt's lymphoma is associated with EBV and HIV.

- Human T-cell lymphotropic virus (HTLV) type 1 serology: may be positive in adult T cell leukaemia (ATLL).
- Echocardiogram to assess baseline cardiac function as chemotherapy regimens often incorporate cardiotoxic agents such as doxorubicin.
- Excision lymph node biopsy: required for definitive diagnosis.
- Bone marrow biopsy for staging purposes:
  - Immunophenotyping in combination with immunochemistry can aid diagnosis.
  - Cytogenetics may be useful as some lymphomas such as Burkitt's lymphoma are associated with the translocation t(8,14).
- CT-NCAP for staging.
- PET scan pre- and post-treatment to assess response.

The Ann Arbor classification used to stage NHL[2]

- Stage I: involvement of a single lymph node group or lymphoid structure.
- Stage II: involvement of two or more lymph node groups or one lymph node group and one extranodal site, all on the same side of the diaphragm.
- Stage III: involvement of multiple lymph node groups or lymphoid structures on both sides of the diaphragm.
- Stage IV: disseminated involvement of one or more extralymphatic organs including liver, bone marrow or lungs.

New diagnoses are discussed at a multidisciplinary meeting with lymphoma specialists and histopathologists. The diagnosis and type of lymphoma is confirmed to form an individualised management plan incorporating:

- Supportive management:
  - Hydration and allopurinol with electrolyte monitoring to reduce the risk of tumour lysis syndrome.
  - Blood product support.
- Chemotherapy: e.g. DLBCL is treated with R-CHOP (rituximab, cyclophosphamide, daunorubicin, vincristine and prednisolone); for patients with significant concerns regarding cardiotoxicity, chemotherapy regimens such as mini-RCHOP (where the dose of doxorubicin is reduced) or RCVP (rituximab, cyclophosphamide, vincristine and prednisolone) may be used.

Hodgkin's lymphoma

HL is relatively uncommon and, due to advances in treatment, has a high cure rate. It can be classified into two types:

- Classical HL: hallmark is the bi/multinucleated Reed Sternberg B cell.
- Nodular lymphocyte pre-HL.

Patients affected are usually between the ages of 15 and 30 years. As with NHL, patients may present with B symptoms and/or a cervical mass or symptoms from local effect from a mediastinal mass. Diagnosis is confirmed via biopsy of the lymph node/mass. Investigations including CT-NCAP and PET scanning, and bone marrow aspirate and trephine with immunophenotyping facilitate staging in a similar fashion to NHL. Disease staging is particularly important as it has implications for treatment selection:

- Early stage: non-bulky disease; absence of B symptoms; Ann Arbor stage I/II.
- Advanced stage: bulky disease; presence of B symptoms; Ann Arbor stage III/IV.

HL used to be treated with a chemotherapy regimen called MOPP (mustargen, Oncovin® [also known as vincristine], procarbazine and prednisolone), but this was associated with a significant risk of a second malignancy (e.g. AML) within 20 years and infertility. Early stage HL is now treated with 2–4 cycles of ABVD (Adriamycin®, bleomycin, vinblastine and dacarbazine) chemotherapy and involved field radiation therapy (IFRT). In comparison, advanced stage HL is treated with six cycles of chemotherapy. Patients who relapse and are fit for intensive chemotherapy will undergo this treatment followed by an autologous BMT.

[2] Adapted by permission from the American Association for Cancer Research: Carbone PP, Kaplan HS, Mushoff K, et al: Report of the committee on Hodgkin's disease staging classification, *Cancer Research*, 31:1860, 1971. Copyright © 1971, American Association for Cancer Research.

The main complications of HL are related to the side-effects and long-term complications of chemotherapy, and include pulmonary fibrosis (e.g. bleomycin) and cardiotoxicity (e.g. anthracyclines such as doxorubicin). Intensive chemotherapy carries a risk of myelodysplasia and AML. Post-BMT complications include immunosuppression, fatigue, psychosocial effects, secondary malignancies (e.g. AML) and infertility. Long-term follow up is of particular importance due to risks of secondary malignancies and hypothyroidism from radiation.

T cell lymphomas

T cell lymphomas are rare. ATLL is an aggressive form associated with HTLV. It has a high incidence in Japan and the Caribbean and is transmitted sexually, vertically or parenterally. It has a very poor prognosis and requires intensive chemotherapy (e.g. bi-weekly CHOP [cyclophosphamide, vincristine, doxorubicin and prednisolone]).

Biological therapeutic agents in haemato-oncology

Rituximab, an anti-CD20 monoclonal antibody, has revolutionised the management of many haematological conditions in which B cells play an important role including ITP, NHLs as well as autoimmune conditions. It is administered as an infusion. The main side effects of rituximab are:

- Allergic reactions (nausea, flu-like symptoms, anaphylaxis).
- Immunosuppression:
  - increased risk of reactivation of hepatitis B;
  - patients should avoid live vaccines, such as yellow fever and tuberculosis until 6 months post-treatment.
- Bruising/bleeding due to low platelets.
- Anaemia.
- Unknown effects on a fetus, such that pregnancy should be avoided until 12 months post-treatment.

Bone marrow failure syndromes

Bone marrow failure occurs when haematopoiesis is unable to meet physiological demand for the production of healthy blood cells. Bone marrow failure can be acquired (e.g. AA) or inherited (including Fanconi anaemia, Diamond Blackfan anaemia [DBA], dyskeratosis congenita [DC] and congenital dyserythropoietic anaemia [CDA]; Table 9.15).

Aplastic anaemia

AA is defined as a pancytopaenia with a hypocellular marrow in the absence of an abnormal infiltrate. It has an incidence of 4 per million people and is more common in East Asia. It has a bimodal prevalence, presenting between 10 and 25 years of age or in those aged >60 years. Most cases are idiopathic, but other causes include:

- Drugs: chloramphenicol, chloroquine, penicillamine.
- Occupational exposure: benzene, pesticides.
- Infections: EBV, hepatitis, HIV, Parvovirus B19.
- ALL.
- Pregnancy.

Patients present with bone marrow failure symptoms of anaemia, thrombocytopenia and/or neutropenia. The British Committee for Standards in Haematology states the diagnosis of AA requires two out of three of the following criteria[3]:

1. Hb <100 g/L.

[3] Reproduced with permission from Killick, S. B. et al. Guidelines for the diagnosis and management of adult aplastic anaemia. *British Journal of Haematology*, 172(2):187-207. © 2015 British Society for Haematology and John Wiley & Sons Ltd. https://doi.org/10.1111/bjh.13853.

2. Platelets $<50 \times 10^9$/L.
3. Neutrophils $<1.5 \times 10^9$/L.

AA is classified further according to severity:

- Severe AA: two out of three of:
  - platelets $<20 \times 10^9$/L;
  - neutrophil count $0.2–0.5 \times 10^9$/L;
  - reticulocyte count $<20 \times 10^9$/L.
- Very severe AA: neutrophil count $<0.2 \times 10^9$/L.
- Non-severe AA: neutrophil $>0.5 \times 10^9$/L.

Complications of AA include iron overload due to repeated blood transfusions, AML, MDS and paroxysmal nocturnal haemogloburia that is an acquired disease characterised by a triad of thrombosis, haemolysis and bone marrow failure.

Investigations include:

- FBC and reticulocyte count.
- PBF to exclude other causes of bone marrow failure such as AML.
- Haematinics: vitamin B12/folate/iron studies.
- Virology (hepatitis, HIV and EBV).
- Haemolysis screen: LDH, bilirubin, DAT.

Treatment involves:

- Supportive treatment to prevent infections and manage complications of anaemia and bleeding:
  - Antifungal and neutropenic sepsis prophylaxis.
  - PCP prophylaxis.
  - Iron chelation therapy once ferritin is >1000 μg/L.
  - Platelet and blood transfusions if platelet count $<10 \times 10^9$/L and Hb <80 g/L; exceptions to this are in sepsis in which case the platelet count is maintained $>20 \times 10^9$/L and bleeding when it is maintained $>50 \times 10^9$/L.
- Immunosuppressive therapy and BMT for patients with severe/very severe AA:
  - In patients aged <40 years with a matched sibling, BMT is first line treatment.
  - Patients aged <40 years with no matched sibling are given immunosuppressive therapy with ATG and ciclosporin as first-line treatment.

Pure red cell aplasia

Pure red cell aplasia (PRCA) is a rare condition characterised by an isolated marked reduction or absence of erythroid activity in the bone marrow. The other cell lineages remain unaffected. PRCA can be congenital (DBA) (Table 9.15) or acquired due to:

- Viral illness such as parvovirus B19 or EBV:
  - More common in patients with an existing red cell disorder, such as sickle cell anaemia.
- Drugs including azathioprine and co-trimoxazole.
- Autoimmune conditions such as rheumatoid arthritis and SLE.
- Thymomas.
- CLL.
- Anti-erythropoietin antibodies secondary to erythropoietin injections in chronic renal failure patients.

Patients usually present with symptoms of anaemia or of the underlying condition.

Investigations include:

- FBC and PBF:
  - If the PRCA is associated with an AIHA, the reticulocyte count may be elevated.
  - Changes in keeping with an underlying red cell disorder such as sickle and target cells in sickle cell anaemia may be present.
  - Lymphocytosis may be present if the underlying cause is CLL.

Table 9.15 Inherited bone marrow failure syndromes

Bone marrow failure syndrome	Pathogenesis	Genetic defect	Clinical features	Diagnosis	Treatment	Complications
Fanconi anaemia (commonest of inherited bone marrow failure syndromes)	Cells hypersensitive to DNA damaging agents, e.g. DEB (diepoxybutane), MMC (mitomycin C), ionising radiation.	17 genes identified; most commonly Fanconi A and C; primarily autosomal recessive genetic disorder but may be X-linked; carrier frequency in Ashkenazi Jewish population about 1/90.	Bone marrow failure symptoms; short stature; microcephaly; hyperpigmentation; gonadal abnormalities; malformations of kidney; majority present aged <20 years.	DEB /MMC test (a positive result confirms chromosomal breakage in peripheral blood lymphocytes' DNA in the presence of DEB or MMC).	Transfusions; GCSF; allogenic BMT (curative); androgens (oxymetholone).	Malignancies (liver especially if androgen treatment).
Diamond Blackfan anaemia (DBA)	Defect in ribogenesis.	Mutation in *RPS19* gene; autosomal dominant disorder.	Anaemia; radial anomalies; renal abnormalities; cleft palate; cardiac and urogenital abnormalities; presents in first year of life.	Macrocytic anaemia; decrease in erythoid precursors on bone marrow biopsy; genetic analysis.	Steroids; blood transfusions; BMT (curative); Some patients display spontaneous recovery.	AML (risk lower than Fanconi anaemia).
Dyskeratosis congenita (DC)	Defect in telomere maintenance.	Mutations that directly or indirectly affect the vertebrate telomerase RNA component, e.g. DKC1, TERC, TERT or TINF2 genes; may be autosomal dominant, autosomal recessive or X-linked disorder.	Abnormal nails; reticulated skin rash; oral leukoplakia; scleroderma skin; osteopenia.	Genetic analysis.	Androgens; GCSF; BMT (curative).	Restrictive lung disease; immunodeficiencies; AML; MDS.
Congenital dyserythropoietic anaemia (CDA)	Ineffective erythropoiesis.	Type 1: *CDAN* gene. Type 2: *SEC23B* gene. Type 3: *KIF 23* gene. Type 4: *KLF1* gene.	Type 1: moderate to severe macrocytic anaemia; syndactyly; absent radial phalanges, skin pigmentation, sensorineural deafness, hypoplastic right 3rd rib. Type 2: moderate anaemia, hepatosplenomegaly. Type 3: mild anaemia and retinal degeneration. Type 4: severe anaemia; splenomegaly.	Multinucleated erythroblasts on bone marrow biopsy.	Blood transfusions and chelation therapy.	

Adapted with permission from Hoffbrand, A.V. & Moss, P. *Essential Haematology*, Sixth Edition (2011). Copyright © 2011, John Wiley and Sons.

- DAT.
- Virology (parvovirus, EBV, CMV).
- Bone marrow aspirate and trephine that will reveal almost absence of erythroid precursors.
- Peripheral immunophenotyping if the underlying cause is CLL.

In children, PRCA is usually transient and self-limiting, and management is often expectant, unless a red cell transfusion is clinically indicated. Specific treatments are avoided if possible to minimise complications. Various immunosuppressive agents have been used in PRCA such as corticosteroids, ciclosporin, azathioprine and rituximab. Approximately one-third of patients with thymoma respond to a thymectomy, and treatment of other underlying causes have also led to beneficial outcome of PRCA. For refractory cases, autologous and allogenic stem cell transplant is considered. Patients on regular transfusions may need iron chelation in the long-term.

Haematological aspects of pregnancy

Pregnancy is a time of significant changes in the haematological system (many of which are physiological and do not need medical intervention):

- Anaemia due to:
  - Increased plasma volume causing a dilutional anaemia.
  - Increased red cell mass.
  - Increased iron requirements to support increased red cell mass, fetal and placental requirements.
  - Increased folate use.
- Rise in MCV in association with the aforementioned causes of anaemia.
- Thrombocytopenia:
  - Platelet count of 100–150 × 10^9/L is common in pregnancy and is not associated with an increased risk to mother or baby, or to childbirth.
  - ITP is sometimes diagnosed in pregnancy and often treated with a combination of intravenous immunoglobulin and/or steroids.
  - Specific obstetric causes (that all need aggressive management to ensure safe delivery) including (➔ see Chapter 23, Pre-eclampsia and eclampsia, HELLP syndrome, Thrombocytopenia, p. 811.):
    - pre-eclampsia;
    - eclampsia;
    - HELLP (haemolysis, elevated liver enzymes, low platelet count) syndrome;
    - obstetric complications, such as placental abruption, amniotic fluid embolism and retention of a dead fetus that are associated with DIC commonly cause thrombocytopenia.

Platelet levels are particularly important in the third trimester when adequate plans for safe delivery must be made in conjunction with the obstetric, anaesthetic and neonatal teams. Safe levels of platelets for delivery can be a contentious issue, but the thresholds listed in Table 9.16 are considered safe. It is important to be aware of coagulation test results as these can affect bleeding, particularly in the context of altered liver function. Sequential changes in platelet count and the time interval between readings should also be noted.

Table 9.16 Platelet thresholds for obstetric interventions

Intervention/procedure	Platelet threshold (×10^9/L)
Normal vaginal delivery	50
Caesarean section	50
Epidural insertion	80
Epidural removal	100

Pregnancy is regarded as a hypercoagulable state in which there is an increased risk of thrombosis throughout pregnancy and continuing until 6 weeks post-partum. This is due to an increase in the prothrombotic clotting factors (fibrinogen, factor VIII and vWF) with no corresponding increase in anti-thrombotic clotting factor levels. As pregnancy progresses, increased venous stasis due to abdominal pressure on the large veins and reduced mobility add to the risk. Women are anticoagulated in pregnancy and the post-partum period according to the number of risk factors:

- ≥ 4 risk factors are anticoagulated from 12 weeks gestation;
- ≤ 3 risk factors are anticoagulated from 28 weeks;
- 2 risk factors are anticoagulated postnatally.

Risk factors that are taken into account include:

- Pre-existing risk factors: previous VTE, the existence of a heritable thrombophilia, the presence or detection of an acquired thrombophilia, a previous VTE (except if provoked by surgery), medical comorbidities, age >35 years, obesity (BMI >30 kg/m^2), smoking, parity >3, gross varicosities and paraplegia.
- Obstetric risk factors: multiple pregnancies and the presence of pre-eclampsia.
- Birth-related factors: a Caesarean section.
- Other risk factors include: surgical procedures, hyperemesis/dehydration, immobility/hospital admission, systemic infections, ovarian hyperstimulation syndrome (1st trimester only) and bone fracture.

The ideal anticoagulant treatment modality is low molecular weight heparin as this does not cross the placenta. Warfarin is teratogenic in the first trimester and associated with an increased risk of CNS abnormalities if taken in any trimester; therefore, it is rarely given in pregnancy except in specific cases with appropriate counselling (➲ see Chapter 23, Management, p. 815). There is currently no data on the novel oral anticoagulants in pregnancy so these are not advised. Low dose aspirin has no role in prophylaxis or treatment of VTE in pregnancy. Other agents such as fondaparinux and danaparoid should only be given in conjunction with a haematologist with expertise in thrombosis.

Many drugs used in the treatment of haematological and oncological disorders, including chemotherapy, are teratogenic. As such, pregnancy tests are required for female patients of childbearing age to determine dosing and adverse effects of treatments. Options of sperm and oocyte saving may be considered (➲ see Chapter 10, Oocyte and sperm saving, p. 328).

Further reading

1. BloodRef: the online reference for hematology professionals. http://bloodref.com/
2. British Committee for Standards in Haematology Guidelines. https://b-s-h.org.uk/guidelines/.
3. Hoffbrand VA, Higgs DR, Keeling DM, Mehta AB. *Postgraduate Haematology,* 7th edition. Oxford: Wiley-Blackwell, 2016.
4. Provan D, Baglin T, Dokl I, de Vos J. *Oxford Handbook of Clinical Haematology*. Oxford: Oxford University Press, 2015.

Multiple choice questions

Questions

1. Which of the following drugs is a direct thrombin inhibitor?

   A. Rivaroxaban.
   B. Warfarin.
   C. Edoxaban.
   D. Dabigatran.
   E. Apixaban.

2. A patient with AML on chemotherapy is admitted with neutropenic sepsis. His platelet count is 5×10^9/L. Which of the following statements is correct?
   A. He does not need a platelet transfusion as he is not bleeding.
   B. He should have a platelet transfusion to keep his platelet count above 20×10^9/L as he is septic.
   C. He should have a target platelet count of 50×10^9/L.
   D. He should have a target platelet count of 10×10^9/L.
   E. He should have a target platelet count of 100×10^9/L.
3. A 30-year-old lady with post-partum haemorrhage complicating her third pregnancy was transfused a pool of platelets. 8 days later a repeat FBC revealed her platelet count had decreased from 80×10^9/L to 7×10^9/L. What is the likely diagnosis?
   A. Acute haemolytic reaction.
   B. TRALI.
   C. Post-transfusion purpura.
   D. Transfusion transmitted infection.
   E. AML.
4. An 18-year-old lady presents with increasing breathlessness over 1 month and has a large mediastinal mass on CXR. What is the most likely underlying haematological pathology?
   A. Myeloma.
   B. Acute myeloid leukaemia.
   C. Hodgkin's lymphoma.
   D. Sickle cell disease.
   E. Acute lymphoblastic leukaemia.
5. Which of the following viruses are not routinely tested for as part of a lymphoma diagnostic work up?
   A. Hepatitis B.
   B. Hepatitis C.
   C. HIV.
   D. Hepatitis E.
   E. EBV.
6. Which one of the following is not associated with aplastic anaemia?
   A. Parvovirus B19.
   B. CLL.
   C. EBV.
   D. Chloramphenicol.
   E. Penicillamine.
7. Which one of the following options is a curative management option for Fanconi anaemia?
   A. Transfusion.
   B. GCSF.
   C. Corticosteroids.
   D. Stem cell transplant.
   E. Androgen

Answers

1. D. Dabigatran is a direct thrombin inhibitor whilst rivaroxaban, edoxaban and apixaban are direct factor Xa inhibitors. Warfarin inhibits the vitamin K epoxide reductase enzyme, and thus prevents vitamin K epoxide being recycled back to vitamin K. The resultant depletion of vitamin K in its hydroquinone form limits the γ-carboxylation of coagulation factors II, VII, IX and X, restricting the biological activity of these factors and producing an anticoagulant effect. (➲ See Table 9.13.)
2. B. As a general rule, a platelet count $>20 \times 10^9$/L is considered safe and $<10 \times 10^9$/L is considered high risk of spontaneous bleeding. Counts $>50 \times 10^9$/L can be safe for basic surgery and a count $>100 \times 10^9$/L is desirable for central nervous system surgery or intraocular bleeding. When treating patients with AML, platelet counts $>20 \times 10^9$/L are advised if the patient is septic, or $>50 \times 10^9$/l if the patient is bleeding or has acute promyelocytic leukaemia (due to the associated increased risk of bleeding). (➲ See Thrombocytopenia, p. 280, and Acute myeloid leukaemia, p. 298.)
3. C. A number of complications of transfusion of blood products exist (see Table 9.10). In post-transfusion purpura, alloantibodies against human platelet antigens result in a fall in platelet count approximately 7 days after transfusion. This usually occurs in multiparous women or previously transfused patients.
4. C. Myeloma is a haematological malignancy of plasma cells with the majority of patients being aged ≥70 years. Patients can present with hypercalcaemia, renal impairment, anaemia, bony disease and/or symptoms of hyperviscosity (headache, retinal haemorrhages, shortness of breath). AML is the commonest acute leukaemia in adults, with the majority of patients being aged >60 years. Patients may present with symptomatic anaemia, infection, constitutional symptoms of fevers, weight loss and night sweats, and/or specific features of different types of AML (e.g. M3 can be associated with DIC and present with haemorrhage; M4 and M5 are associated with gum hypertrophy). Patients with Hodgkin's lymphoma are usually between the ages of 15–30 years and may present with B symptoms (including drenching night sweats and weight loss), symptoms of bone marrow failure (including bruising/bleeding secondary to thrombocytopenia, lethargy and shortness of breath secondary to anaemia, and recurrent infections secondary to leucopaenia), and/or a cervical mass or symptoms from local effect from a mediastinal mass. Sickle cell disease is a haemoglobinopathy with symptomatic vaso-occlusive crises and chronic haemolysis. Like AML, patients with ALL also present with symptoms of bone marrow failure involving symptomatic anaemia, recurrent infections and bleeding secondary to low platelets. (➲ See Myeloma, p. 303, Acute myeloid leukaemia, p. 298 and Box 9.2, Hodgkin's lymphoma, p. 306, Sickling disorders, p. 277, and Acute lymphoblastic leukaemia, p. 301.)
5. D. Hepatitis B surface antigen, hepatitis B core antibody, hepatitis C, EBV and HIV are routinely tested prior to starting chemotherapy for lymphoma (➲ see Investigations, p. 305.)
6. B. Aplastic anaemia is not associated with CLL. (➲ See Aplastic anaemia, p. 307.)
7. D. Treatments for Fanconi anaemia include transfusions, granulocyte colony stimulating factor, androgenic steroid therapy and allogenic bone marrow transplantation. Only the latter is curative. (➲ See Table 9.15.)

Chapter 10 **Principles of Oncology and Palliative Care**

Elizabeth Smyth, Elisa Fontana and David Cunningham

Biology of cancer

Hallmarks of cancer

1. Cancer cells demonstrate sustained proliferation via:
   - Increased expression of growth factor receptor proteins on the cell surface thus increasing sensitivity to ligand stimulation.
   - Changes in intracellular signalling pathways leading to constitutive signalling activation:
     - e.g. B-rapidly accelerated fibrosarcoma (BRAF) mutation in 40% of melanomas leading to sustained mitogen-activated protein kinase (MAPK) pathway activation – known as a 'driver mutation' that transforms a normal gene into an 'oncogene'; in many cases, these tumours are 'oncogene addicted' for growth and this may present a target for drug treatment.
   - Production of growth factors resulting in autocrine (self) stimulation of proliferation, or stimulation of local non-cancerous cells, which in turn produce growth factors (paracrine stimulation).
2. Cancer cells evade growth suppressors:
   - For example, evasion of retinoblastoma (RB) associated tumour suppressor gene pathway:
     - RB protein interacts with cyclins and cyclin-dependent kinases (CDKs) and is responsible for the important G1 checkpoint, which blocks the entry of a cell into the DNA replication S-phase and cellular growth.
     - RB1 mutation is associated with childhood retinoblastoma; in inherited cases the *RB1* gene mutation is inherited from a parent (germline) and a second mutation occurs during childhood

(somatic) – this is an example of Knudson's two-hit hypothesis where both alleles of a tumour suppressor gene must be inactivated in order to facilitate cancer growth.

- For example, evasion of tumour protein (TP) 53 tumour suppressor gene pathway:
  - The function of TP53 is to sense intracellular stressors and be the 'guardian of the genome':
    - TP53 does not allow a cell to enter the replicative cycle if there is excessive DNA damage or if oxygen and glucose levels are insufficient.
    - TP53 induces apoptosis if there is irreparable intracellular damage.
- TP53 is the most commonly mutated gene in cancer (>50%); in cancers without TP53 mutations the *TP53* gene may be inactivated by other mechanisms.
- Inherited mutations in TP53 are associated with Li-Fraumeni syndrome in which patients have an increased risk of breast cancer, sarcoma, leukaemia and glioblastoma.

3. Cancer cells resist cell death:
   - Loss of TP53 function, increased expression of anti-apoptotic proteins such as B cell lymphoma (Bcl)-2, and decreased expression of pro-apoptotic regulators such as Bcl-2-associated X protein (Bax) and Bcl-2-like protein 11 (Bim) are examples of mechanisms by which cancer cells avoid apoptosis (programmed cell death – a control mechanism by which the growth of abnormally proliferating cells is curtailed).
4. Cancer cells can replicate indefinitely:
   - The capacity of normal cells to undergo cell division cycles is finite. In contrast, most cancer cells have unlimited replicative capacity or are 'immortalised'. Telomeres (repetitive nucleotide repeat segments located at the end of chromosomes) play a key role in this process by shortening with each cell division (and therefore with age). When telomeres are completely eroded, chromosomal instability, cellular senescence or apoptosis may occur. The DNA polymerase telomerase enzyme that adds telomeric DNA to the end of shortening telomeres is rarely expressed in non-cancer cells but is upregulated in most (85–90%) cancer cells facilitating endless replication and 'immortalisation'.
5. Cancers initiate and sustain angiogenesis:
   - Angiogenesis is the process by which tumour growth is sustained beyond microscopic size (when glucose, oxygen and other nutrients are provided through tissue diffusion).
   - The 'angiogenic switch' is governed by pro-angiogenic factors, such as vascular endothelial growth factor (VEGF)-A and anti-angiogenic factors such as thrombospondin (TSP)-1.
   - Tumour-associated neo-vasculature is characteristically distorted and 'leaky'.
   - Neo-angiogenesis is variable across tumour subtypes, e.g. pancreatic cancer is poorly vascularised.
   - Angiogenesis has been successfully targeted in cancer treatment, e.g. the anti-VEGF-A monoclonal antibody bevacizumab (active in metastatic colorectal and non-small cell lung cancer [NSCLC]) and the tyrosine kinase inhibitors sunitinib and pazopanib (active in renal cancer) (Table 10.8).
6. Cancer is associated with invasion and metastasis:
   - Cancer cells may spread via the lymphatic system to lymph nodes, via the haematogenous route to lung, liver and bone, or directly to body cavities such as the peritoneum or pleura. Cancer cells intravasate into local lymphatic or blood vessels, and extravasate into distant tissues where they may develop into micrometastases followed by macrometastases. Colonisation of distant tissues and the growth of macrometastases require collaboration between tumour cells and those of the microenvironment such as mesenchymal stem cells and tissue-associated macrophages, which produce chemokines and metalloproteinases that facilitate metastatic growth; this process is known as the 'seed and soil hypothesis'. A key enabling process in the 'invasion-metastasis cascade' is epithelial-mesenchymal transition (EMT). Characteristics of cells that have undergone EMT include change in morphology (epithelial/polygonal to fibroblast/spindle cell shape), loss of adherens junctions and increased cellular motility; decreased expression of the cell adhesion molecule E-cadherin facilitates many of these changes.
7. Cancer cells have dysregulated cellular metabolism:
   - Cancer cells display high levels of glucose uptake and less efficient glucose metabolism by glycolysis pathways in preference to oxidative phosphorylation. Although the glycolytic pathway produces less ATP (with less energy efficiency) than oxidative metabolism, the products of the pathway are helpful in generating nucleosides and amino acids required to generate new cells.

This 'aerobic glycolysis' is facilitated by upregulating GLUT1 glucose transporters on cells which enhance glucose importation; this characteristic of cancer cells is demonstrated by the uptake of the radioactive sugar fluorodeoxyglucose on PET scans.

8. Cancer cells must evade immune surveillance/destruction (➲ see also Chapter 6, The immune system and malignancy: principles of immune surveillance and malignancy of the immune system, p. 166).
   - Supported by evidence of increased rates of cancer in immunocompromised patients and in experimental models of mice deficient in selected lymphocyte subsets.
   - The process of 'immunoediting' is suggested in non-immunocompromised hosts, whereby immunogenic clones are destroyed by the host immune system, leaving behind less immunogenic tumours, which escape immune destruction.
   - The anti-tumoral immune response is suggested by the improved survival of resected colon cancer patients whose tumours are heavily infiltrated with cytotoxic T lymphocytes.
   - Developments in immunotherapies such as anti-cytotoxic T-lymphocyte-associated protein (CTLA) 4 (ipilimumab) and anti-programmed death (PD) 1 antibodies (nivolumab, pembrolizumab), which stimulate the immune system to detect and destroy tumours have significantly extended survival for patients with melanoma, renal cell and NSCLCs.

Factors enabling development of cancer

Genetic instability

Mutations in genes relating to cellular proliferation, signalling, apoptosis and the other hallmarks of cancer facilitate acquisition of the hallmark capacities described above. It is notable that tumours vary significantly in mutational burden and genomic instability. Melanoma, which may occur following extensive exposure to ultraviolet radiation, or lung cancer, which occurs following chronic tobacco exposure, are associated with a high mutation load, but many paediatric cancers have low mutational burdens. Determination of which mutations are 'driver' mutations, on which the tumour is functionally dependent, versus 'passenger' mutations is an important goal for effective pharmaceutical development. However, the activity of any given driver mutation is context dependent; for example, melanoma tumours with BRAF mutations are exquisitely sensitive to BRAF inhibitor drugs such as vemurafenib or dabrafenib, but BRAF-mutated colorectal tumours are insensitive to BRAF inhibitors.

DNA damage and repair

DNA may be damaged by exogenous factors (e.g. ultraviolet light, ionising radiation) or errors may be made during DNA replication. In order to preserve genomic stability a number of DNA repair pathways exist. Among the most important of these are the mismatch repair (MMR) and nucleotide excision repair (NER) systems:

- The MMR system corrects DNA replication errors such as base-base mismatches and is composed of several subunits. These include MLH1, MSH2, MSH6 and PMS2. A heterodimer of MSH2 and MSH6 recognises insertion deletion loops and base pair mismatches; this complex then interacts with the MLH1-PMS2 heterodimer to initiate the DNA repair process. Germline mutations in these mismatch repair proteins lead to hereditary non-polyposis colon cancer (HNPCC)/Lynch syndrome. Patients with Lynch syndrome have a high lifetime risk of colorectal cancer (up to 80%) and an increased risk of gastric, endometrial, small bowel and other tumours, with MSH2 or MLH1 being the genes most commonly affected (70% patients). Loss of MMR function also occurs in sporadic tumours, frequently through promoter methylation of MHL1. Tumours that are mismatch repair deficient accumulate mutations in short (mono, di, tri and tetra) nucleotide repeats – this is known as microsatellite instability (MSI). Up to 15% of sporadic (non-familial) colorectal cancers demonstrate MSI; these tumours are associated with proximal colon location, lymphocytic infiltrate and improved prognosis.
- The NER system repairs more complex (up to 30 bases) DNA strand damage caused by ultraviolet light and chemicals. Patients with xeroderma pigmentosum (XP), who are extremely sensitive to ultraviolet light-induced DNA damage and develop frequent skin cancers, have high pyrimidine dimer mutation rates and NER activity reduced by up to 95%.

The DNA damage response pathway is responsible for repair of single and double-strand DNA breaks and interstrand cross-links. Germline mutations of genes involved in the DNA repair process predisposing to cancer include *BRCA1*, *BRCA2*, *PALB2* and Fanconi anaemia genes. *BRCA1* and *BRCA2* work together to maintain genomic integrity by repairing double-stranded DNA during DNA replication. *BRCA1* and *BRCA2* germline mutations act in an autosomally dominant fashion and increase the risk of breast (*BRCA1*>*BRCA2*), ovarian (*BRCA1*>*BRCA2*), pancreatic and prostate cancer. Recent research has shown that if *BRCA* is impaired in a tumour cell, then the role of poly-ADP ribose polymerase (PARP) becomes increasingly important in repairing single- and double-stranded DNA breaks. If the function of PARP is then blocked, this leads to 'synthetic lethality' due to almost complete inhibition of double-strand break repair and cell death. Use of PARP inhibitors such as olaparib in patients with BRCA mutations has been effective in several cancers including ovarian and breast cancer.

Inflammation and the microenvironment

Although cytotoxic T lymphocytes may have a role in immune destruction of tumours by the adaptive immune system, other cells of the innate immune system, which invade early neoplastic lesions may promote tumourigenesis by inducing inflammation (by substances such as growth and pro-angiogenic factors), and extra-cellular matrix modifiers that induce EMT and promote invasion and metastasis. Infiltrating immune inflammatory cells consist of certain macrophage subtypes, mast cells and neutrophils in addition to several types of T and B lymphocyte. Known inflammatory and tumour-promoting mediators, which are secreted by these cells include epidermal growth factor (EGF), VEGF, fibroblast growth factor (FGF) 2 and matrix degrading enzymes such as matrix metallopeptidase (MMP)-9.

Cancer stem cells

A small proportion of cells in tumours have an increased ability to seed new tumours in immunodeficient mice. These cells have similar RNA patterns to non-cancer stem cell populations and are called 'stem-like' or 'cancer stem cells (CSCs)'. It is possible that some derive from normal tissue, which has been transformed and others may derive from less differentiated progenitor cells, which have also undergone malignant transformation. Stem-like cells are thought to be more resistant to chemotherapy than other cell types, and may explain tumour recurrence following successful eradication with chemo/radiotherapy.

Growth factors: biology and target manipulation

Growth factor receptors and their intracellular downstream signalling pathways play a crucial role in cancer development and have been a key target for modern oncology drug development. Pathways common to activation of many growth factor pathways include:

1. Binding of ligand to receptor.
2. Receptor dimerisation:
   - homodimerisation (binding to the same receptor), e.g. VEGF;
   - heterodimerisation (binding to a non-identical receptor), e.g. EGF.
3. Receptor activation with autophosphorylation.
4. Downstream signalling activated by phosphorylated receptors.

In this way, extracellular signals are transmitted via the receptor and the cytoplasm to the nucleus. Pharmacologically directed blockade of this pathway may target either the ligand or the receptor. One of the most commonly altered growth factor pathways is that of the EGF receptor, which incorporates four structurally similar receptor tyrosine kinases (ERBB1 (EGFR), ERBB2 (human epidermal growth factor receptor [HER]2), ERBB3 (HER3) and ERBB4 (HER4)). The EGF receptor pathway provides an excellent example of the many ways in which genes and their protein receptors may be dysregulated in cancer. In lung adenocarcinoma, frequent mutation of the kinase domain of EGFR occurs, which leads to constitutive receptor activation and sustained intracellular signalling. This pathway has been successfully exploited therapeutically using oral anti-EGFR tyrosine kinase inhibitors such as erlotinib or gefitinib. In contrast, amplification of HER2 is commonly demonstrated in breast and oesophagogastric cancer, and oncogene addiction in these tumours has been treated effectively with the anti-HER2 monoclonal antibody trastuzumab (Table 10.8).

Intracellular signalling pathways

The rat sarcoma (RAS)/RAF/MAPK pathway is one of the most important signalling transduction pathways in cancer. Mutations in the RAS family (h-Ras, k-Ras and n-Ras) are found in up to 30% of all cancers. Guanosine triphosphate (GTP)-bound RAS binds with high affinity to c-RAF and, subsequently, RAF signals downstream to the MAPK pathway, which is a key mediator of transmembrane to nuclear signalling. This pathway is constitutively active in cancers which have mutations of components such as RAS or RAF leading to uncontrolled cell growth.

Other key signalling pathways that are frequently dysregulated in cancer include phosphoinositide 3-kinase/protein kinase B (AKT)/mechanistic target of rapamycin (mTOR) and CDK pathways. The mTOR pathway regulates nutrient metabolism and cellular energy, while the CDK pathway and co-factor cyclins controls cell cycle regulation through entry into phases of DNA replication (S phase) and division (M phase). Both pathways have been successfully pharmacologically blocked by mTOR inhibitors (everolimus) and CDK inhibitors (palbociclib), respectively.

Clonality and heterogeneity

All tumours evolve as an evolutionary process, implying that tumours may dynamically adapt. The somatic alterations (mutations, chromosomal changes or epigenetic changes), which lead to cancer are initially acquired in a single cell, and any of these which increase the chances of a cell surviving (increased evolutionary fitness) will increase the proportion of this cell's progeny in any future population. This process is known as clonal selection. The process is repeated over time leading to acquisition of further genetic changes in a stepwise manner. However, the instrinsic genomic instability of tumours may lead to development of new mutations or changes, which only affect one spatial component of the tumour. This leads to intratumoural heterogeneity and is a major determinant of resistance to targeted therapies. Subclones with a specific alteration may respond to targeted therapy leading to tumour shrinkage; however, subclones without the alteration may then expand to fill this niche. Heterogeneity also poses a challenge when performing tumour biopsies as only a single area of the tumour is sampled; plasma circulating tumour DNA may overcome this issue in the future.

Epidemiology of cancer

- Globally, in 2012, there were 14.1 million cases of cancer and 8.2 million deaths due to cancer.
- Lung cancer is the most common cancer (1.8 million cases diagnosed annually), and is the most common cause of cancer death in men worldwide.
- Breast cancer is the second most common cancer (1.6 million cases diagnosed annually), and is the most common cause of cancer death in women worldwide.
- Other important cancers worldwide include:
  - colorectal cancer (1.4 million cases annually);
  - stomach cancer (951,600 cases annually);
  - liver cancer (782,500 cases annually).
- 57% of cancer diagnoses and 65% of deaths due to cancer occur in developing countries.
- Cancers display regional variation in prevalence due to differences in underlying risk factors:
  - prostate, colorectal and female breast cancers are more common in developed countries;
  - stomach and liver cancers are more frequently diagnosed in developing countries.

Tobacco and cancer

- Approximately 2.1 million premature deaths per year occur as a result of tobacco use and, in developed countries, approximately half of cancer cases relate to smoking.
- The carcinogenic properties of tobacco include ingredients, such as polycyclic aromatic hydrocarbons (e.g. benzo[a]pyrine), nitrosamines, formaldehyde and polonium; carcinogens cause

the formation of DNA adducts leading to mutations in oncogenes and tumour suppressor genes, and epigenetic inactivation of tumour suppressors through promoter methylation.

- The International Agency for Research on Cancer has determined that tobacco is causal for the following cancers: bladder, cervical, colorectal, laryngeal, liver, lung, oesophageal, oral, pancreatic, renal, sinonasal and stomach; use of cigars and pipes is strongly associated with cancers of the oral cavity, larynx and oesophagus, and causally with lung cancer.
- Tobacco acts synergistically with alcohol to produce cancers of the oral cavity and oesophagus, and with radon and asbestos to cause lung cancer.
- The effect of tobacco on DNA is variable due to the effect of germline polymorphisms in genes relating to the cytochrome P450 (CYP450) system, which is responsible for tobacco metabolism.

Oncogenic viruses

Approximately 15% of cancers are due to chronic viral infection. However, most individuals infected with oncogenic viruses do not go on to develop cancer because of the protective role of the host immune system. Virally induced cancers are therefore more common in immunosuppressed or immunocompromised individuals.

- EBV causes Burkitt's lymphoma (a translocation brings the *c-myc* oncogene under persistent stimulation by an immunoglobulin enhancer, which promotes persistent, rapid proliferation) and is also implicated in endemic nasopharyngeal carcinoma, Hodgkin's lymphoma, gastric carcinoma (EBV subtype) and AIDS-related lymphoma.
- HPV subtypes 16 and 18 are implicated in cervical cancer, anal cancer, penile cancer and specific head and neck cancers:
  - HPV genes *E6* and *E7* become integrated into the human genome and interrupt the function of the tumour suppressors p53 and RB.
  - Vaccination against high risk subtypes of HPV decreases the risk of cervical neoplasia and is recommended for all girls and boys aged 12–14 years (➲ see Chapter 7, Vaccination, p. 205).
- Hepatitis B virus (HBV) and hepatitis C virus (HCV) infections increase the risk of hepatocellular carcinoma (HCC), with co-infection increasing the risk further and HBV vaccination reducing the risk.

Lifestyle

Migrants from developing countries to developed countries begin to demonstrate cancers associated with developed countries within a short time frame; this supports the hypothesis that lifestyle factors such as diet are associated with cancer risk. Up to one-third of cancers in developed countries could be avoided by changes in diet and physical activity, while maintaining a normal weight.

- Obesity is associated with increases in post-menopausal breast cancer, colorectal cancer, endometrial cancer, oesophageal adenocarcinoma, pancreatic cancer and renal cancer.
- Red meat ingestion (beef, pork, lamb, processed meat) is associated with colon and rectal cancer; up to 10% of UK colorectal cancers may be associated with dietary processed meat consumption.
- Alcohol consumption is associated with cancers of the oral cavity, larynx, oesophagus, colon and breast.
- Dietary fibre protects against colorectal cancer; consumption of green leafy vegetables, brassicas and fruit protect against oral cavity, larynx, oesophageal and gastric cancers.

Investigation of cancer

Imaging

Chest X-ray

- Inexpensive, widely available.
- Small (<1-cm) lesions difficult to detect.

- Blind to retrocardiac and retrodiagphragmatic spaces.
- Only bulky mediastinal lymph nodes will be detected.

Computerised tomography

- Most frequently used cross-sectional imaging modality for staging.
- IV contrast used to enhance images and differentiate tumour from normal tissue:
  - hypervascular tumours more prominent in the arterial phase of contrast injection (e.g. colorectal, HCC);
  - most other tumours best seen during later venous phase.
- Lymph nodes must be >10 mm in short axis to be classified as abnormal, but size alone cannot determine if a lymph node is malignant.

Magnetic resonance imaging

- Useful for determining local cancer invasion through walls of viscera, in particular in rectal, cervical, bladder and prostate cancer.
- More sensitive for detection of small liver metastases than CT.
- Imaging modality of choice for CNS malignancies.

Ultrasound

- Inexpensive.
- No ionising radiation.
- Useful for distinguishing solid from cystic masses.
- Helpful for taking ultrasound-guided tissue biopsies.
- Operator-dependent (subjective) and dependent on patient body habitus.

Positron emission tomography

- ^{18}F-FDG-PET uses the fluorescent sugar ^{18}F-FDG, which is taken up by glucose transporters in cancer cells to identify locations of cancer spread not seen on conventional imaging.
- Frequently used as an addition to other cross-sectional imaging tools.
- May be falsely positive in inflammation (including granulomatous disease and following radiotherapy) and infection.
- Physiological increased uptake is frequently seen in the brain, ureter, brown fat and thymus.
- Falsely negative in tumours with low glucose uptake, such as mucinous tumours or tumours that are well differentiated with a low growth rate (e.g. low grade neuroendocrine tumour).
- Specific situations exist where PET-CT may help to avoid futile surgery including:
  - Non-small cell lung cancer: PET-CT is more sensitive than CT alone for staging, and will upstage or lead to a change in treatment for up to 30% of patients.
  - Oesophageal cancer: PET-CT will detect CT-occult metastatic disease in up to 15% of patients.
  - Metastatic colorectal cancer with apparently operable liver limited disease: PET-CT will detect non-resectable disease or metastatic disease in up to 25% of patients.

Radiographic scintigraphy

➲ See Chapter 5, Nuclear medicine, p. 115.

- Involves administration of radioisotopes to patients and subsequent measurement of emitted radiation by gamma cameras to form two-dimensional images:
  - Octreotide scan – octreotide, a drug similar to somatostatin, is radiolabelled with indium-111 and injected IV; the radioactive octreotide attaches to tumour cells that have receptors for somato-

statin (neuroendocrine tumours, phaeochromocytoma and medullary thyroid cancer; ➲ see Chapter 19, Neuroendocrine tumours, p. 700).
- Iodine-131 scan – radiolabelled iodine-131 is administered orally with uptake assessed for differentiated papillary and follicular thyroid cancer (➲ see Chapter 19, Scintigraphy, p. 679 and Thyroid nodules, p. 682).
- Technetium-99m scan – technetium-99m is a metastable nuclear isomer of technetium-99 and administration is used for identification of lymphatic drainage pathways for sentinel node resection.

Circulating tumour markers

➲ See Chapter 6, Tumour antigens, p. 166.

Helpful in surveillance for relapse in resected patients and for monitoring response to treatment in patients on systemic therapy:

- Cancer antigen (CA)-125 in women who have undergone treatment for ovarian cancer.
- Carcinoembryonic antigen (CEA) following resection of colorectal cancer to monitor for early relapse.
- LDH, alpha fetoprotein (αFP) and βHCG to monitor for relapse in testicular cancer.
- Prostate specific antigen (PSA):
  - May be elevated due to benign prostatic hyperplasia, prostatic inflammation or infection, sexual activity or digital rectal examination, in addition to prostate cancer.
  - Useful to detect recurrence and monitor response to treatment in men who have undergone radical prostatectomy for prostate cancer:
    - American Urological Association definition of biochemical relapse is serum PSA ≥0.2 ng/mL followed by a second confirmation of the same level;
    - following radiotherapy an increase in PSA level by 2 ng/mL above the nadir or three successive rises confirms relapse.

Histology

The International Classification of Diseases for Oncology (ICD-O) system classifies cancer by:

- Topography (anatomic site of disease, e.g. oesophagus).
- Morphology (histological type of tumour [e.g. adenocarcinoma] together with behaviour [e.g. malignant]).

For categories of cancer, see Table 10.1.

Table 10.1 Categories of cancer

Descriptor	Site of origin
Carcinoma	>80% of cancer cases. Arise from the epithelial lining of the inside or the outside of the body: - adenocarcinoma arises from glands/organs. - squamous cell carcinoma arises from squamous epithelium.
Sarcoma	Arise from connective tissue (bone, muscle, cartilage) or fat. Frequently a cancer of young adults (e.g. osteosarcoma – bone; rhabdomyosarcoma – skeletal muscle; angiosarcoma – blood vessels).
Lymphoma	Derived from lymphoid cells in lymph glands or extra-nodal locations (➲ see Chapter 9, Lymphoma, p. 305).
Myeloma	Derived from bone marrow plasma cells (➲ see Chapter 9, Myeloma, p. 303).
Leukaemia	Overproduction of bone marrow-derived white cells (myeloid, granulocytic, lymphocytic or erythroid) (➲ see Chapter 9, Chronic myeloid leukaemia to Chronic lymphocytic leukaemia, pp. 297–303).
Mixed	

Histological grade is a measure of how similar the tumour is to the original tissue from which it is derived:

- Grade 1 – well differentiated.
- Grade 2 – moderately differentiated.
- Grade 3 – poorly differentiated.
- Grade 4 – undifferentiated.

Many cancers have histological subclassifications which impact on tumour behaviour and response to specific treatments (as they may be associated with an underlying different genotype).

For histological subtypes of cancer, see Table 10.2.

Table 10.2 Histological subtypes of cancer

Lung cancer histological subtypes	**Features**
Squamous NSCLC	Central; cavitating; hypercalcaemia.
Adenocarcinoma NSCLC	Peripheral; more common in non-smokers; *EGFR* mutation; *ALK*, *ROS* and *RET* translocations.
SCLC	Rapidly proliferating; frequent brain metastases.
Breast cancer histological subtypes	**Features**
Infiltrating ductal carcinoma	Most common (>70%); fibrous tissue response leads to palpable mass.
Infiltrating lobular carcinoma	5–10% of breast cancer; infiltrates as single cells; may have no mass lesion; more often multicentric/bilateral; spreads to peritoneum/meninges.
Medullary carcinoma	High-grade syncytial growth with lymphoplasmacytic infiltrate; increased in BRCA1 mutation carriers; improved survival.
Tubular carcinoma	More common in screened population; low grade; metastases infrequent; favourable prognosis.
Renal cancer histological subtypes	**Features**
Clear cell (proximal tubule)	75–80% of renal cancer; frequent loss of chromosome 3p; associated with von Hippel–Lindau gene alterations.
Papillary (proximal tubule)	15% of renal cancer; exists as type I (good prognosis, MET mutation) and Type II (poor prognosis).
Chromophobe (collecting ducts)	3–7% of renal cancer; high TERT expression.
Oncocytoma (collecting ducts)	Multiple/bilateral in tuberous sclerosis and Birt–Hogg–Dube/ Hornstein–Knickenberg syndrome (autosomal dominant genetic disorder with susceptibility to renal cancer, renal and pulmonary cysts, and noncancerous fibrofolliculomas).
Testicular cancer histological subtypes	**Features**
Seminoma	50% of all testicular cancers; median age 40 years; tumour markers usually normal although βHCG may be mildly elevated.
Non-seminomatous germ cell tumours including:	Median age 30 years.
• Embryonal carcinoma	Does not produce αFP.

continued

Table 10.2 *continued*

Testicular cancer histological subtypes	Features
• Choriocarcinoma	Most aggressive; widespread metastases via blood; very high βHCG; does not produce αFP.
• Yolk sac tumour	Produces αFP.
• Teratoma	Tumour with tissue or organ components resembling normal derivatives of more than one germ layer.
Sex cord stromal tumours including:	Median age 40–50 years.
• Leydig cell tumour	Virilising or feminising; precocious puberty.
• Sertoli cell tumour	Feminising more common; associated with Peutz–Jeger syndrome.
Ovarian cancer histological subtypes	**Features**
High grade serous	Up to 80% of ovarian cancer; advanced presentation at diagnosis; poor prognosis; BRCA1 or 2 mutations in up to 10% of patients.
Endometrioid	10% of ovarian cancer; diagnosed at early stage with good prognosis; associated with MSI, Lynch syndrome and endometrial cancer.
Clear cell	5–10% of ovarian cancer; more common in East Asia; associated with MSI and Lynch syndrome; less sensitive to platinum chemotherapy.

ALK, anaplastic lymphoma kinase; MET, MET proto-oncogene receptor tyrosine kinase; RET, rearranged during transfection; ROS, proto-oncogene tyrosine-protein kinase enzyme encoded by the *ROS1* gene; SCLC, small cell lung cancer; TERT, telomerase reverse transcriptase.

Immunohistochemistry

Immunohistochemistry tests identify antigens (typically proteins) in a cell using complementary antibody binding (Table 10.3). The tumour is then viewed under a light or fluorescent microscope.

Table 10.3 Immunohistochemistry tests used in cancer diagnosis

Immunohistochemistry test	Diagnosis
Cytokeratins	Carcinoma
TTF1	Lung or thyroid cancer
S-100	Melanoma
Vimentin	Mesenchymal origin cancer
CD20	B-cell lymphoma
CD3	T-cell lymphoma
CD30	Hodgkin's lymphoma
αFP	Hepatocellular carcinoma, yolk sac tumour

CD, cluster of differentiation; TTF1, thyroid transcription factor 1.

Fluorescence in-situ hybridisation

- Uses fluorescent probes, which bind to complementary DNA sequences to identify changes (amplification, deletions, translocations) at the DNA level in cells.

For commonly used fluorescence in-situ hybridisation (FISH) assays in oncology, see Table 10.4.

Table 10.4 Commonly used FISH assays in oncology

FISH assay	Diagnosis ± clinical application
HER2 amplification	Breast cancer and gastroesophageal cancer; predicts response to anti-HER2 therapy (e.g. trastuzumab).
ALK translocation	NSCLC; predicts response to crizotinib therapy.
MYC t(8:14)	Burkitt's lymphoma.
Bcl2 t(14:18)	Follicular lymphoma.
CCND1 t(11:14)	Mantle cell lymphoma.

CCND1, gene encoding cyclin-D1; MYC, myc oncoprotein transcription factor.

Assessment of mutations in cancer

Several sequencing modalities are available including:

- Sanger (direct sequencing):
  - useful if the mutation is not known;
  - expensive, slow and not highly sensitive.
- Allele specific testing with PCR:
  - faster;
  - cheaper and more sensitive;
  - mutation must be known to design a primer.
- Next generation sequencing:
  - can perform parallel analysis of many genes at once;
  - requires expensive hardware and bioinformatics expertise;
  - currently mostly limited to research.

For cancer genotypes predictive of response to targeted therapies, see Table 10.5.

Table 10.5 Cancer genotypes predictive of response to targeted therapies

Cancer	Mutation	Predicts positive response to:	Predicts negative response to:
Melanoma	BRAF mutation	Vemurafenib, dabrafenib	
Lung adenocarcinoma	EGFR mutation	Erlotinib, gefitinib, afatinib	
Ovarian cancer	BRCA1 mutation	Olaparib (PARP inhibition)	
CML	BCR-ABL translocation	Imatinib, dasatinib, nilotinib	
Colorectal cancer	KRAS or NRAS mutation		Cetuximab, panitumumab

BCR-ABL, breakpoint cluster region-Abelson; CML, chronic myeloid leukaemia.

Gene expression profiling

Gene expression profiling is used to measure the expression (at the messenger [m] RNA level) of hundreds or thousands of genes simultaneously. Gene expression patterns in cancers with the same histological classification (e.g. breast adenocarcinoma or gastric adenocarcinoma) reveal new molecularly divided groups of tumours, which may differ in prognosis. In breast cancer, common subtypes include:

- Luminal A tumours:
  - more common;
  - high expression of oestrogen receptors;
  - good prognosis.
- Luminal B tumours:
  - less strongly expressed oestrogen receptor-related genes;
  - more expression of proliferation-related genes;
  - worse prognosis.
- Basal type cancers:
  - low expression of luminal type genes and *HER2*-related genes.
- HER2 enriched cancers:
  - high expression of *HER2*-related genes and proliferative genes;
  - low expression of luminal type genes.

One of the most useful applications of gene expression profiling in oncology has been the development of the 21-gene recurrence score that stratifies women with node negative oestrogen receptor positive breast cancer into high- and low-risk categories. Women in high-risk categories are candidates for adjuvant chemotherapy, whereas those in low-risk categories are spared the toxicity of adjuvant chemotherapy from which they are unlikely to benefit.

Staging of cancer

The aim of staging is to establish the extent of cancer spread in the body with accurate staging being essential to avoid under- or over-treatment.

The American Joint Committee on Cancer (AJCC)/Union for International Cancer Control (UICC) TNM (tumour, node, metastases) Cancer Staging System is shown in Box 10.1.

Box 10.1 The American Joint Committee on Cancer (AJCC)/Union for International Cancer Control (UICC) TNM (tumour, node, metastases) Cancer Staging System

T category reflects assessment of the primary tumour

- TX: the primary tumour is not evaluable.
- T0: no evidence of a primary tumour.
- Tis: carcinoma in situ.
- T1–T4: description of size and/or extent of a primary tumour which is evaluable.

N category reflects involvement of nearby lymph nodes

- NX: regional lymph nodes are not evaluable.
- N0: no regional lymph node involvement with cancer.
- N1–N3: involvement of regional lymph nodes (number dependent on cancer subtype).

M category is descriptive of the presence or absence of distant metastases:

- M0: no distant metastasis.
- M1: presence of distant metastases.

Adapted with permission from Brierley, J. et al. (2016). *TNM Classification of Malignant Tumours*, Eighth Edition, Wiley-Blackwell.

Each cancer has different criteria for T, N and M stages that provide prognostic information. Some cancers also include other histological factors, such as grade, ulceration or tumour markers as a component of their staging systems.

Cancer staging may be clinical, radiological or pathological. Pathological staging following neoadjuvant therapy uses the prefix yp, e.g. ypT3N1. Radiological and other investigative modalities are useful for staging, including:

- CT.
- MRI.
- FDG PET: helpful in excluding the presence of CT occult metastases.
- Endoscopic ultrasound (EUS): helpful for T-staging in endoluminal cancers (e.g. oesophageal, gastric) and for confirming the presence of malignant lymph nodes.
- Laparoscopy: helpful for pre-operative staging of intra-abdominal malignancies as peritoneal spread of cancer is poorly visualised on CT; 15–20% of gastric cancers may have occult peritoneal metastases.

Staging systems outside of AJCC/UICC of relevance include:

- International Federation of Gynaecology and Obstetrics (FIGO) staging system for gynaecological cancers.
- Ann Arbor staging system for lymphoma (➔ see Chapter 9, The Ann Arbor classification used to stage NHL, p. 306).
- Testicular cancer staging algorithms incorporating serum tumour markers (LDH, αFP, βHCG).

Principles of oncological treatment

The aim of treatment should be defined prior to initiating therapy; this may be curative or palliative. The risks and benefits of treatment must be considered alongside the patient's symptoms, co-morbidities and desire for treatment.

Performance status assessment

Performance status is used to assess the capacity of patients to participate in daily activities. Patients with a lower performance status are more likely to experience treatment-related toxicity. The Eastern Cooperative Oncology Group (ECOG) Performance Status Scale is shown in Table 10.6.

Table 10.6 Eastern Cooperative Oncology Group (ECOG) Performance Status Scale

ECOG PS Category	Description
0	Fully active, able to carry on all pre-disease performance without restriction.
1	Restricted in physically strenuous activity, but ambulatory and able to carry out work of a light or sedentary nature, e.g. light housework, office work.
2	Ambulatory and capable of all self-care, but unable to carry out any work activities; up and about more than 50% of waking hours.
3	Capable of only limited self-care; confined to bed or chair more than 50% of waking hours.
4	Completely disabled; cannot carry on any self-care; totally confined to bed or chair.
5	Dead.

Co-morbidity assessment

- Co-morbidities may significantly impact on oncology treatment; these may be formally assessed using the Charleston co-morbidity index.
- Renal and hepatic impairment may limit the use of drugs metabolised or eliminated via these organs.
- Concomitant medications may interact with treatment, e.g. imatinib activity being increased by cytochrome P450 3A4 inhibitors, such as ketoconazole, itraconazole and clarithromycin (➲ see Chapter 3, Metabolism, p. 69, and Table 3.12).
- Diabetes is associated with poorer survival outcomes in resected colorectal cancer.
- Increased body mass index is associated with worse survival in ovarian cancer.
- Depression is associated with worse cancer specific survival; up to 24% of patients with cancer may meet criteria for major depressive disorder.

Multidisciplinary cancer care

Cancer care in the UK is focused on the concept of the multidisciplinary team (MDT). This includes surgeons, medical oncologists, radiation (clinical) oncologists, pathologists, radiologists, nurses and support staff with expertise in a specific cancer area. The MDT meets to discuss a patient's cancer case (history, examination, imaging, pathology) and a personalised recommendation is made for care in line with evidence-based treatment guidelines.

Oocyte and sperm saving

Many cancer treatments carry risks of infertility or gonadal failure, and oocyte and sperm saving strategies are available for patients. Girls who have entered puberty with signs of sexual maturity are eligible for oocyte or embryo cryopreservation. Single women may cryopreserve oocytes in the presence of normal ovarian reserve. Women in a relationship may have embryo cryopreservation. Boys who have entered puberty and show signs of sexual maturity are eligible for sperm cryopreservation. All patients must:

- Be stable and well enough to defer chemotherapy for time allocation for fertility treatment.
- Undergo screening for hepatitis B and C and HIV so that positive and negative samples are stored separately.
- Not have started chemotherapy prior to fertility preservation treatment.

Following chemotherapy, which may lead to gonadal failure, women should be assessed by oncofertility services to assess ovarian function and fertility status, and men should have assessment of fertility 1–2 years post-treatment to see if fertility has returned so that preserved sperm may be discarded.

Principles of radiation oncology

Radiotherapy uses ionising radiation to cause cellular DNA damage, which predisposes to cell death. It exploits the differential ability of normal and malignant cells to undergo DNA repair in response to radiation. The underlying genetic changes that have led to malignant transformation render cancer cells less able to repair and, therefore, more susceptible to cell death. However, normal tissue may also be damaged by radiotherapy, causing potentially permanent toxicity. Each tissue has a defined susceptilibity or tolerance to radiation. Careful treatment planning is therefore essential to maximise dose to the tumour, while maintaining the radiation exposure to normal tissues below the tolerance dose and minimising the volume of normal tissue exposed to radiation.

The anatomic boundaries of the tumour must be located and mapped (usually with a CT scan), while the patient is immobilised (to maintain a constant position during treatment). The 'target volume' is delineated using imaging. To this, a margin of normal tissue will often be added, to account for any microscopic disease spread that cannot be visualised and/or to take into account any movement of the tumour during the radiation treatment. Patients may be tattooed or have fiducial markers (metal seeds) placed internally to allow accurate localisation of the tumour.

Toxicity of radiotherapy

The toxicity of radiotherapy depends on the target area, and the volume and type of normal tissue, which will be exposed to radiation. Oral mucositis occurs as a result of head and neck radiotherapy, and nausea, vomiting and diarrhoea may occur as a result of abdominal radiotherapy. Late side effects include fibrosis, infertility and secondary cancers.

Types of radiotherapy

Radiation is most commonly delivered with a machine known as a linear accelerator that 'accelerates' electrons to a high energy state and produces either photon or electron beams. External beam radiotherapy is most commonly delivered with photons that penetrate more deeply into the body than electrons. Electrons are used for superficial areas, such as the skin or breast where depth of penetration is not desired.

Proton therapy is a form of 'particle therapy' in which heavy particles are produced by specialised equipment. Proton therapy may be useful when crucial normal anatomic structures are close to the area of interest as proton therapy is associated with a rapid dose fall-off. This has been useful in some paediatric tumours, and also in uveal melanoma.

Targeting radiotherapy

- In conformal radiotherapy, the target volume and normal tissues are delineated on a CT scan. The position of the radiotherapy beams is then chosen to optimise the radiation dose to the tumour and limit radiation to normal tissue thus reducing toxicity. Lead shielding may be used to help reduce the dose to normal tissues.
- Intensity modulated radiotherapy (IMRT) is a type of radiotherapy that uses advanced computer programmes to modulate the intensity of the radiation beam at different sites concurrently. This helps to shape the radiation beam more accurately, particularly around concave structures.
- Stereotactic radiotherapy involves combining highly conformal radiotherapy, usually with multiple radiation beams, with very precise treatment delivery. This type of radiotherapy gives a high dose of radiation in a small number of treatments (≤ 5). In tumours that are small and well-defined, stereotactic radiotherapy may result in long-term efficacy (e.g. small brain metastases, liver metastases).
- Brachytherapy involves placing a radioactive source adjacent to or within the target area delivering a high dose of radiation to the tumour, but limiting the dose to healthy tissue (e.g. in cervical cancer). In prostate cancer, radioactive seeds may be placed into the prostate gland.

Infusional radionucleotide treatments

- Radium 223, an alpha particle emitter, which accumulates in bone, has efficacy in prostate cancer bone metastases.
- Radioactive iodine (I-131) that accumulates in thyroid cancer cells may be used to treat local or metastatic disease.
- 177-lutetium-dotatate is accumulated by octreotide-avid neuroendocrine tumours and may be used to treat metastatic neuroendocrine disease.
- Yttrium radioactive microspheres may be directed into the liver for the treatment of liver metastases, e.g. in colorectal cancer.

Chemotherapy

Chemotherapy involves the administration of cytotoxic agents either IV, orally, or, more rarely, locoregionally. The efficacy of chemotherapy is determined by factors such as the proportion of tumour cells, which are actively dividing (growth fraction) and the number of tumour cells in the population. Most human tumours do not become clinically apparent until they are at least 1 cm^3 in volume (at least 10^9 cells). Larger tumours typically have fewer cells, which are actively dividing due to limitations in tumour blood flow and nutrient distribution. Therefore, tumours grow more rapidly when they are smaller, and have a lower growth rate at larger sizes; this is known as Gompertzian kinetics. Cells that are not actively dividing are less sensitive to chemotherapy, and therefore the fractional cell kill using chemotherapy may be less for larger cancers. The Norton–Simon hypothesis, based on Gompertzian kinetics, proposed that tumours that are given less opportunity to re-grow between chemotherapy sessions will have higher proportions of the tumour destroyed by chemotherapy; this led to the development of dose-dense chemotherapy, in particular for the adjuvant treatment of breast cancer.

Chemotherapy may be administered before curative surgery (neo-adjuvant), or after (adjuvant), or before and after (peri-operative). The purpose of neo-adjuvant chemotherapy is to reduce tumour bulk prior to surgery potentially to allow a less extensive resection and to eliminate radiologically occult micrometastases prior to surgery. The purpose of adjuvant chemotherapy is to reduce the risk of cancer recurrence in patients who have undergone a potentially curative resection by eliminating radiologically occult micrometastases. Adjuvant chemotherapy is a standard of care for resected breast, colon and ovarian cancers, which have a moderate to high risk of recurrence. As tumours that are micrometastatic are small, it is proposed that their growth fraction is higher and that they may be more susceptible to chemotherapy than larger tumours. However, many patients who do not have micrometastatic disease and are already cured by surgery receive unnecessary chemotherapy.

Chemotherapy delivered locoregionally increases concentrations in the area of tumour, while decreasing exposure to healthy tissue. Examples include intraperitoneal chemotherapy for ovarian cancer, isolated limb perfusion for melanoma, intra-hepatic arterial infusion for liver metastases and intra-thecal infusion for leptomeningeal metastases.

For specific chemotherapy drugs, see Table 10.7.

Table 10.7 Specific chemotherapy drugs

Drug type (examples)	Mechanism of action	Toxicities
Anthracyclines (doxorubicin, epirubicin)	Intercalate between base pairs in RNA/DNA, thereby preventing synthesis. Inhibit topoisomerase II.	Myelosuppression. Cardiotoxicity. Leukaemia (doxorubicin).
Alkylating agents (cyclophosphamide, ifosfamide)	Cross-link DNA strands.	Haemorrhagic cystitis.
Taxanes (paclitaxel, docetaxel)	Disrupt microtubule function.	Neuropathy.
Platinums (cisplatin, carboplatin, oxaliplatin)	Cross-link DNA strands.	Neurotoxicity. Nephrotoxicity. Thrombogenicity.
Anti-metabolites • Purine (fludarabine) • Pyrimidine (5-fluorouracil, gemcitabine) • Folate (methotrexate, pemetrexed)	Mimic naturally occurring metabolites to inhibit DNA, RNA or protein synthesis.	Cytopenia (fludarabine). Diarrhoea and mucositis (5-fluorouracil). Gastrointestinal upset. Hepatotoxicity, ulcerative stomatitis, leucopenia, pneumonitis, pulmonary fibrosis (methotrexate). Cytopenia (permetrexed, gemcitabine, fludarabine).
Topoisomerase inhibitors • topoisomerase I (irinotecan) • topoisomerase II (etoposide)	Regulate DNA unwinding (uncoiling).	Diarrhoea (irinotecan). Second cancers (etoposide).
Vinca alkaloids (vincristine, vinblastine)	Disrupt microtubule function.	Neuropathy.

Hormone therapy

Steroid hormones such as oestrogen and testosterone are powerful drivers of endocrine sensitive tumours such as breast cancer or prostate cancer. Inhibition of the action of such hormones has been effective in treating many hormonally driven cancers, both in the adjuvant setting and for patients with metastatic disease.

Hormone therapy for women

- Selective oestrogen receptor modulators (SERMs) may act as oestrogen receptor agonists in selected tissues, and antagonists in others:
    - Tamoxifen acts as an agonist in the endometrium, but an antagonist in breast tissue. Tamoxifen is the hormone therapy of choice for premenopausal women with breast cancer who require endocrine therapy, but women taking it must be monitored for the risk of developing endometrial cancer (4% increased risk). Side effects of tamoxifen also include increased risk of thromboembolic disease, hot flushes and sexual dysfunction.
    - Fulvestrant is also a SERM, but only has oestrogen receptor antagonist and no agonist activity. It is used for the treatment of hormone receptor-positive metastatic breast cancer in post-menopausal women with disease progression following anti-oestrogen therapy.
- Aromatase inhibitors that inhibit the aromatase enzyme converting androgens into oestrogens (aromatisation) are approved for and have been shown to be superior to tamoxifen in the treatment of breast cancer in post-menopausal women. Two types exist:
    - Irreversible steroidal inhibitors (e.g. exemestane) that form a permanent and deactivating bond with the aromatase enzyme.
    - Non-steroidal inhibitors (e.g. anastrozole and letrozole) that inhibit the synthesis of oestrogen via reversible competition for the aromatase enzyme.

Side effects of aromatase inhibitors include osteoporosis, cardiovascular disease, hypercholesterolemia and aromatase inhibitor-associated musculoskeletal syndrome (AIMSS) (consisting of arthalgia, stiffness and bone pain), which may be responsible for treatment discontinuation in 10–20% of patients.

- Endocrine therapies may be combined with targeted therapies in patients with metastatic breast cancer who are resistant to hormonal therapy alone, e.g. palbociclib plus fulvestrant; everolimus plus exemestane.
- Immunohistochemistry for oestrogen receptors predicts response to hormone therapy; patients with tumours with <1% staining are not recommended for anti-oestrogen therapy.
- Ovarian ablation in younger women may be achieved through oophorectomy or use of a gonadotropin-releasing hormone (GnRH) analogue such as goserelin, leuprolide or triptorelin.

Hormone therapy for men

- For men with prostate cancer, androgen-deprivation therapy (ADT) is an important component of treatment for high-risk localised disease and for metastatic disease. The aim of ADT is to decrease testosterone to 'castrate' levels. This can be achieved by bilateral orchidectomy (rarely performed) or medically using a GnRH agonist, such as goserelin, leuprolide, triptorelin or buserelin. Importantly, the initial effect of such medical therapy is to stimulate testosterone production, which may result in a clinical 'tumour flare' leading to increased symptoms of bony pain in the patient with bone metastases. This can be prevented by concurrent use of an anti-androgen therapy. Side effects of ADT include sexual dysfunction, osteoporosis, hot flushes and possible increased risk of cardiovascular disease.
- Anti-androgen therapies, such as bicalutamide, block the binding of dihydrotestosterone to the androgen receptor. They are usually given in conjunction with ADT. Side effects include gynaecomastia and breast tenderness, hot flushes and sexual dysfunction.
- A novel anti-androgen drug, which has improved survival for patients with metastatic castrate-resistant prostate cancer is abiraterone. This is an inhibitor of the cytochrome P450 17A1 (CYP17A1) enzyme that blocks biosynthesis of testosterone. Toxicities include hypokalaemia and

hypertension, and patients must be treated concurrently with steroids due to the risk of adrenal insufficiency.

Targeted therapies

Personalised oncology

Tumour subtyping by genetics has led to the understanding that even in cancers with the same histology, underlying molecular drivers may differ; so-called 'inter-tumour heterogeneity'. Furthermore, even within the same tumour, subclones may evolve which have distinct molecular drivers and respond differentially to targeted therapy; so-called 'intratumour heterogeneity'.

When targeted drugs are assessed in unselected patient groups, the treatment benefit is frequently marginal, but when a group of patients with an underlying targetable oncogene addiction is targeted the results are more successful:

- EGFR inhibitors such as erlotinib or gefitinib provide a very small benefit in an unselected NSCLC population but a very large benefit when used only in patients with specific EGFR mutations (➲ see Chapter 11, Targeted therapy, p. 364).
- Cetuximab or panitumumab lack efficacy if a RAS mutation is present in colorectal cancer (➲ see Table 3.4).

Many mutations have disease-specific effects (they are context specific), e.g. BRAF V600E mutations in melanoma predict for response to BRAF inhibition with vemurafenib, but the same mutation does not predict for response to single agent BRAF inhibition in colorectal cancer because of differences in EGFR activation between these two cancer types.

Molecularly targeted drugs

Molecularly targeted therapy may be classified as drugs that inhibit cancer growth or kill cancer cells by targeting specific molecules upon which the cancer cells rely for growth or survival. This is distinct from traditional cytotoxic chemotherapy, which kills all rapidly dividing cells, and is therefore associated with a different spectrum of side effects. The most commonly targeted pathways in cancer cells are growth factor receptors, intracellular signalling molecules, regulators of angiogenesis, and immune checkpoint modulators (Table 10.8).

Oncological emergencies

Neutropenic sepsis

The definition of neutropenic sepsis is any patient receiving chemotherapy and presenting with neutrophil count $\leq 0.5 \times 10^9$/L and a temperature ≥ 38°C ± signs or symptoms of clinically significant sepsis.

Pathogenesis/risk factors

Both the chemotherapy regimen and patient-related factors must to be taken into account when evaluating the risk of developing neutropenic sepsis:

- Chemotherapy regimens are classified as:
  - High risk (>20%) – prophylactic GCSF therapy recommended.
  - Intermediate risk (10–20%).
  - Low risk.
- Patient-related risk factors include:
  - Previous chemotherapy/radiotherapy.
  - Bone marrow involvement.
  - Recent surgery or presence of open wounds.
  - Liver or kidney dysfunction.
  - Age >65 years.

Table 10.8 Molecularly targeted drugs

Drug	Target	Measurable bio-marker	Disease in which therapy is employed
Monoclonal antibodies			
Trastuzumab[1]	HER2	HER2	Breast and gastro-oesophageal cancer.
Cetuximab[1] Panitumumab[1]	EGFR	KRAS and NRAS	Colorectal cancer.
Rituximab[2]	CD20	CD20	B-cell lymphoma.
Bevacizumab[3]	VEGF		Colorectal cancer, NSCLC, renal cell cancer, glioblastoma.
Ramucirumab[3]	VEGFR2		Gastro-oesophageal cancer, NSCLC, colorectal cancer.
Aflibercept[4]	VEGF		Colorectal cancer.
Antibody drug conjugates (containing a cytotoxic agent delivered directly to the cancer cell using a monoclonal antibody to an expressed protein)			
TDM1	HER2	HER2	Breast cancer.
Brentuximab	CD30	CD30	Hodgkin's lymphoma, anaplastic T cell lymphoma.
Tyrosine kinase inhibitors			
Imatinib	BCR-ABL, PDGFR, c-KIT	BCR-ABL	CML, GIST.
Erlotinib, gefitinib	EGFR	EGFR mutation	NSCLC.
Sunitinib	Multiple tyrosine kinases		Renal cell cancer.
Pazopanib, axitinib	VEGFRs, PDGFRs, c-KIT		Renal cell cancer.
Everolimus	mTOR		Breast cancer, renal cell cancer, pancreatic neuroendocrine tumours.
Crizotinib	ALK, c-MET, ROS1	EML4-ALK fusion	NSCLC.
Vemurafenib	BRAF	BRAF mutation	Melanoma.
Cabozantanib	RET, VEGFR2, c-MET		Medullary thyroid cancer.
Ibrutinib	Bruton's tyrosine kinase		CLL, follicular NHL, mantle cell NHL.

c-KIT, mast/stem cell growth factor receptor; CLL, chronic lymphocytic leukaemia; EML4-ALK, echinoderm microtubule-associated protein-like 4-anaplastic lymphoma kinase; GIST, gastrointestinal stromal tumour; NHL, non-Hodgkin's lymphoma; PDGFR, platelet-derived growth factor receptor; RET, RET proto-oncogene receptor tyrosine kinase; TDM1, ado-trastuzumab emtansine.

[1]Directly blocks target; [2]Immune system affected by antibody dependent cytotoxicity; [3]Inhibits tumour angiogenesis; [4]Binds to circulating VEGF thus acting as 'VEGF trap' inhibiting angiogenesis.

Assessment and investigations

- History and full physical examination including assessment of vital signs and level of consciousness, and presence of central access devices or any other type of catheter.
- Urgent blood tests including FBC with differential, clotting profile, kidney and LFTs, glucose, CRP, lactate and a minimum of two blood cultures (from peripheral sites and indwelling devices if present).
- Urinalysis, skin swabs, sputum and stool samples, CXR.
- If persistent pyrexia occurs despite appropriate treatment, second-level investigations may be considered, for example, HRCT scan of the chest ± broncho-alveolar lavage.

Management

All patients with suspected neutropenic sepsis should be treated as an acute medical emergency and offered empiric antibiotic therapy with no need to confirm a neutrophil count before commencing treatment:

- Prompt IV fluid resuscitation and oxygen therapy are recommended in the presence of unstable vital signs.
- Broad-spectrum IV antibiotic treatment should be commenced without waiting for blood results, ideally within the first hour from presentation:
  - A beta-lactam antibacterial agent, such as piperacillin and tazobactam is usually the preferred monotherapy, unless otherwise specified in local antibiotic policies or penicillin-allergic patients.
  - A second agent is frequently added, most frequently an aminoglycoside (gentamicin or amikacin), although there is no definitive consensus.
  - An agent with broad Gram-positive cover (e.g. vancomycin or teicoplanin) should be considered for a potentially infected venous access device.
  - Metronidazole should be considered with intra-abdominal sepsis.
- Patients with prolonged neutropenia (e.g. haematopoietic transplant patients) who are at risk of fungal infections, and who do not respond to broad spectrum antibiotics, but who remain febrile after 3–5 days should receive empiric anti-fungal therapy; cultures for fungal infection should be obtained prior to initiating treatment.
- Patients with vesicular lesions or suspicion of viral infection should be treated with anti-viral therapy (e.g. aciclovir, ganciclovir).
- There is no evidence that use of GCSF improves survival, but it may reduce the duration of neutropenia and length of hospital stay.
- Oral antibiotics and outpatient management may be considered in a limited number of patients with low risk febrile neutropenia with no signs of sepsis.

Tumour lysis syndrome

Tumour lysis syndrome (TLS) occurs when a large number of rapidly proliferating cells die leading to release of high volumes of intracellular components such as nucleic acids and other intracellular metabolites. TLS usually occurs during the first cycle of chemotherapy, but may arise spontaneously. The malignancies that are most commonly affected are high-grade haematological malignancies, such as aggressive NHL, Burkitt's lymphoma and acute leukaemias (lymphoblastic and myeloid). Other risk factors include high LDH, bulky disease, high white cell count, high uric acid and pre-existing renal impairment.

The Cairo–Bishop criteria[1] for diagnosis of biochemical TLS require the presence of ≥2 of the following abnormalities in a patient with cancer, or undergoing treatment for cancer, within 3 days prior to and up to 7 days after initiation of treatment:

- Uric acid ≥ 476 μmol/L or 25% increase from baseline.
- Potassium ≥6.0 mmol/L or 25% increase from baseline.

[1] Reproduced with permission from Cairo, M. S., and Bishop, M. Tumour lysis syndrome: new therapeutic strategies and classification. *British Journal of Haematology*, 127(1):3–11. © 2004 British Society for Haematology and John Wiley & Sons Ltd. https://doi.org/10.1111/j.1365-2141.2004.05094.x.

- Phosphate ≥1.45 mmol/L or 25% increase from baseline.
- Calcium ≤1.75 mmol/L or 25% decrease from baseline.

Patients at high risk of TLS should be identified prior to commencing chemotherapy. In the presence of risk factors, prophylactic measurements should include:

- IV hydration in order to maintain a high urinary output (3 L/24 hours).
- Allopurinol (xanthine oxidase inhibitor that blocks the conversion of purine metabolites to uric acid) prior to commencement of chemotherapy and continuation for at least 1 week following chemotherapy.
- Consideration of rasburicase (recombinant version of urate oxidase that converts uric acid to allantoin which is more easily excreted in urine) in place of, but never with allopurinol:
  - Rasburicase may cause anaphylaxis and is contra-indicated in patients with G6PD deficiency (due to production of hydrogen peroxide in the urate oxidase reaction).
  - Rasburicase causes falsely low urate levels unless the sample is sent on ice to the laboratory.

Management of established tumour lysis syndrome

Admission to a critical care unit with cardiac monitoring should be considered in clinically symptomatic patients. Treatment should include:

- IV hydration with an isotonic solution without potassium to maintain urinary output ≥100 mL/hour.
- IV rasburicase, unless contraindicated in which case allopurinol should be considered.
- Calcium gluconate infusion in cases of symptomatic hypocalcaemia; asymptomatic hypocalcaemia should not be treated as this increases the risk of calcium phosphate deposition in the kidneys.
- Renal dialysis in cases of significant and intractable fluid overload, hyperkalaemia, hyperuricaemia, hyperphosphataemia or hypocalcaemia.

Metastatic spinal cord compression

Metastatic spinal cord compression (MSCC) is defined as spinal cord or cauda equina compression by direct pressure ± induction of vertebral collapse, or instability by metastatic spread, or direct extension of malignancy that threatens or causes neurological disability. MSCC occurs in up to 5% of patients with cancer, and is the presenting feature in up to 20% of patients with an underlying malignancy. The risk of MSCC is higher in cancers with a known propensity for bone metastases (breast cancer, prostate cancer, lung cancer, multiple myeloma and lymphoma). Although most cases of MSCC are due to bone metastases, up to 15% are related to epidural/leptomeningeal disease.

Assessment and investigations

- As early diagnosis of MSCC is fundamental to prevention of permanent neurological disability, patients with bony metastases and their caregivers should be informed of potential symptoms including:
  - Spinal pain exacerbated by coughing or sneezing.
  - Radicular pain.
  - Nocturnal pain preventing sleep.
  - Localised spinal tenderness.
  - Limb weakness, sensory alteration, ataxia.
  - Bladder or bowel dysfunction.
- If MSCC is suspected, MRI should be performed within 24 hours (➲ see Chapter 5, Case 14, p. 137).

Management

- MSCC should be managed in a timely and multidisciplinary manner.
- High-dose corticosteroids should be commenced (usually dexamethasone 16 mg/day), with proton pump inhibitor cover, and continued while the management plan of MSCC is taking place, and may be weaned after surgery or the start of radiotherapy.

- Surgical referral should be considered in all patients with a life expectancy of >3 months; improved neurological outcomes have been shown in patients undergoing surgery and post-operative radiotherapy compared with radiotherapy alone.
- External beam radiotherapy represents the treatment of choice when surgical decompression is not possible and should be commenced as soon as possible.
- Analgesia should be offered according to the WHO 3-step ladder (➲ see Management of pain, p. 338).
- Bisphosphonates may reduce bone pain and the risk of fracture in patients with breast cancer and myeloma, and reduce bone pain in prostate cancer which has failed to respond to other analgesia.
- Patients with possible spinal instability should be nursed flat and immobilised with spinal alignment.
- Prophylactic anticoagulation should be considered in immobilised patients.
- A urinary catheter should be placed in case of bladder dysfunction.
- Prevention of constipation related to autonomic dysfunction or opioids is necessary with a low threshold for laxative use.
- After definitive treatment, rehabilitation and local supportive care should be organised to facilitate discharge.

Superior vena cava obstruction

Superior vena cava obstruction (SVCO) occurs when there is obstruction of blood flow though the superior vena cava (SVC) due to internal thrombosis, tumoural invasion or external compression. The consequent increase in venous pressure in the upper body results in tissue oedema with airway obstruction and cerebral swelling. If gradual compression of the SVC occurs then development of collateral vessels draining into the inferior vena cava system may compensate for the obstruction; hence, an acute onset of compression is more likely to cause SVCO.

The most common cause of SVCO is NSCLC; other causes include highly proliferative tumours (e.g. lymphomas), germ cell tumours and small cell lung cancer (SCLCs). Central venous access devices are also a risk factor; thrombotic occlusions are more frequently related to peripherally inserted central catheters (PICCs) due to inadequate catheter tip placement than portacath/Mediport devices.

Assessment and investigations

- In the presence of risk factors, new onset of facial oedema, upper limb swelling, distension of neck and chest wall veins, laryngeal oedema or shortness of breath should trigger investigations to rule out SVCO.
- Symptoms also include cough, stridor, hoarseness and headache (characteristically worse on leaning forward or lying down).
- Symptoms may be made worse by holding the hands above the head (Pemberton's sign).
- JVP is usually raised and typically non-pulsatile.
- CXR will be abnormal in most patients.
- Doppler ultrasound may demonstrate thrombus in axillary or subclavian veins.
- Contrast-enhanced CT is the imaging modality of choice, and delineates the site, cause, level and extension of the obstruction, and the presence of collateral vessels.
- FBC and clotting profile should be monitored in case an extensive thrombosis is associated with platelet sequestration.

Management

- If SVCO is related to central access device thrombosis the treatment is anticoagulation.
- In other cases, treatment should target the underlying disease in order to shrink the mass and reduce compression.

- If histology is unknown, the underlying lesion should be biopsied prior to initiating treatment, if feasible and safe.
- Symptomatic measures include raising the head to reduce orthostatic pressure, diuretics and glucocorticoids (although glucocorticoids should not be initiated prior to diagnosis if lymphoma is suspected as they are cytotoxic to many lymphomas).
- Patients with high risk of sudden respiratory failure or presenting with symptomatic cerebral oedema require immediate emergency treatment; endovascular stent placement will provide more immediate relief of pressure than radiotherapy or chemotherapy.

Metabolic complications of cancer

Malignant hypercalcemia

➲ See Chapter 1, Hypercalcaemia, p. 3.

Syndrome of inappropriate antidiuretic hormone production (SIADH)

➲ See Chapter 19, Syndrome of inappropriate antidiuretic hormone, p. 692.

Prevention and screening

Prevention

- Lifestyle modification:
  - smoking cessation;
  - reduction of alcohol intake;
  - physical activity;
  - sun protection;
  - balanced diet with low intake of animal fat;
  - safe sexual activity.
- Chemoprevention, e.g. tamoxifen in women with high risk of breast cancer.
- Surgical prevention in patients with specific genetic alterations:
  - Oophorectomy and bilateral mastectomy in BRCA mutation carriers.
  - Colectomy in the presence of hereditary colorectal cancer syndromes such as familial adenomatous polyposis (➲ see Table 2.5).
- Vaccination:
  - HPV and HBV vaccination.

Screening

Cancer screening involves early identification of cancer for which an acceptable curative treatment is still possible. The ideal screening test must:

- Have high sensitivity and specificity.
- Be valid and reproducible.
- Be safe, easy to perform and widely available.
- Have a low cost.
- Result in survival prolongation.

Approved screening tests include:

- Mammography for breast cancer every 2 years for women aged 50–69 years.
- Cervical screening smear tests every 3 years for women aged 25–49 years and every 5 years for women aged 50–64 years, and additional testing for high risk HPV genotypes.
- Faecal occult blood test for bowel cancer every 2 years between the ages of 60 and 74.

NB: Serum PSA screening for early detection of prostate cancer is not associated with significant survival benefits, but is associated with increased risks of over-diagnosis and overtreatment with potential detrimental effects on quality of life. Instead of routine PSA screening in the UK, there exists an informed choice programme (prostate cancer risk management) for healthy men aged 50 and over such that if, following discussion of the risks and benefits of PSA testing, a patient wishes to proceed, testing will be performed by the NHS.

Principles of palliative care

Palliative care is: 'an approach that improves the quality of life of patients and their families facing the problem associated with life-threatening illness, through the prevention and relief of suffering by means of early identification and impeccable assessment and treatment of pain and other problems, physical, psychosocial and spiritual'.

A palliative care approach:

- Offers relief from pain and other symptoms.
- Neither hastens nor postpones death.
- Addresses psychological and spiritual aspects of care.
- Supports the patient to live as actively as possible until death.
- Supports the family through the patient's illness and bereavement.

Palliative care should start as soon as possible for patients with terminal illnesses, and not necessarily when no active treatment options are available; multiple aspects of palliation of care are beyond physical symptoms and related to the distress caused at any stage of the disease, from diagnosis to end of life.

Physiology of pain

- Nociceptors in the skin, joints, bones, muscles and soft tissues transduce somatic pain, while visceral nociceptors transduce visceral pain.
- Large, myelinated, fast-conducting (5–30 m/s) A-delta fibres transmit pain that is well-localised and sharp.
- Small, unmyelinated, slow-conducting (0.5–2 m/s) C fibres transmit pain that is diffuse and dull.
- A-delta and C fibres synapse on second order neurons in the substantia gelatinosa of the spinal cord; the second order fibres then cross the cord via the anterior white commissure and ascend in the spinothalamic tract.
- Before reaching the brain, the spinothalamic tract splits into the lateral neospinothalamic tract and the medial paleospinothalamic tract:
  - Second order neospinothalamic tract neurons carry information from A-delta fibres and terminate at the ventral posterolateral nucleus of the thalamus, where they synapse on third order neurons (dendrites of the somatosensory cortex).
  - Paleospinothalamic neurons carry information from C fibres and terminate throughout the brain stem.
- Neuropathic pain is triggered by abnormal activation of the nocioceptive system which can persist in the absence of a noxious stimulus, e.g. trigeminal neuralgia, post-herpetic neuralgia, phantom limb pain.

Management of pain

Up to 74% of patients with advanced cancer have pain. Pain should be fully described in terms of site, nature, radiation, severity (using a scale if possible), and effect on quality of life and mood. Nerve pain is characteristically burning or shooting, liver pain may cause right upper quadrant symptoms, bone pain is worse on movement, headache due to raised intracranial pressure is worse on lying down, and pain due to bowel obstruction is intermittent and colicky. Identification of the source of the pain should also be sought, i.e. direct invasion by cancer; treatment toxicity; non-cancer pain.

The pharmacological approach to pain consists of a WHO 3-step 'analgesic ladder' consisting of:

- First step: non-opioids with or without co-analgesics.
- Second step: 'weak opioids' plus non-opioids.

- Third step: 'strong opioids' with or without non-opioids.

Key features of treatment include:

- Starting at the most appropriate step of the ladder based on the severity.
- If pain is not controlled, the next step should be considered.
- A rescue drug in appropriate dosage between fixed administrations should always be available.
- The oral route should be preferred when possible.
- Analgesia should be administered around the clock (every 3–6 hours), rather than as required.
- Co-analgesia or adjunctive treatments (e.g. non-steroidal anti-inflammatory drugs [NSAIDs], paracetamol, transcutaneous electrical nerve stimulation [TENS]) should be considered for all patients.
- The 'correct' dose is individual and a clear written prescription must be provided to the patient and family.

Non-opioid analgesics

Non-opioid analgesics include paracetamol, aspirin and NSAIDs (e.g. ibuprofen, ketorolac, indometacin), and the cyclo-oxygensase (COX)-2 inhibitors celecoxib and meloxicam. In view of their different toxicity profile and mechanisms of action, non-opioid analgesics are frequently used with opioid analgesics to provide synergistic activity and reduction in opioid demand.

COX enzymes convert arachidonic acid to prostaglandins, prostacyclin and thromboxane A2. Prostaglandins may directly activate nociceptors, but more commonly act as sensitisers, for example, by reducing the activation threshold for selected nociceptor sodium channels or by sensitising afferent sensory neurons to bradykinin. There are two major isoforms of the COX enzyme:

- COX-1: present in most tissues, playing a role in normal physiology, in particular gastric cytoprotection, renal function and platelet aggregation.
- COX-2: only expressed in the inflammatory state, except in brain, kidney and bone, where it is constitutively expressed.

Paracetamol acts predominantly in the CNS by reduction of the active form of COX, which leads to a decrease in COX catalytic ability. The reductive capacity of paracetamol is dependent on low levels of brain peroxidase, which also accounts for the lack of peripheral anti-inflammatory activity of paracetamol (as peroxidase levels are high in areas of inflammation). The centrally acting analgesic effects of paracetamol is mediated via the endogenous cannabinoid system; this may be responsible for the feeling of well-being which is described by some paracetamol users. Paracetamol is associated with a low rate of side effects with prolonged administration, although overdose can cause liver toxicity (➲ see Chapter 3, Paracetamol, p. 83 and Figure 3.3).

Most traditional NSAIDs (e.g. ibuprofen, diclofenac) inhibit both COX-1 and COX-2. The putative benefit associated with selective COX-2 inhibition is a reduction in gastrointestinal toxicity compared with unselective inhibitors with comparable analgesic effects. It is also proposed that selective COX-2 inhibition leads to reduced vascular endothelial prostacyclin production, but not reduced levels of prothrombotic platelet thromboxane A2 predisposing to endothelial activation and cardiovascular events. Non-selective NSAIDs are associated with an increased risk of cardiovascular events (including ischaemic heart disease, congestive cardiac failure and hypertension). Careful patient selection is advised when prescibing both traditional NSAIDs and COX-2 inhibitors.

NSAIDs are effective in controlling the pain related to bone metastases, and muscular and soft tissue inflammation. Non-prostaglandin-mediated mechanism of NSAID action may also play a role in pain reduction; these include inhibition of granulocyte migration to areas of inflammation, by reducing neutrophil-endothelial cell adherence, and reduction in nitric oxide synthetase production by decreased NF-κB-dependent transcription.

Opioids

Opioids bind to specific opioid receptors in the nervous system and other tissues. There are three principal classes of opioid receptors, μ, κ, δ, although up to 17 have been reported, and include the ε, ι, λ and ζ receptors. There are three subtypes of μ-receptor: μ_1, μ_2 and μ_3. These are all G-protein coupled receptors acting on gamma-aminobutyric acid (GABA)-ergic neurotransmission. The pharmacodynamic response to an opioid depends upon its unique binding affinity to the various classes of opioid receptors, and whether the opioid is an agonist or an antagonist, which allows for a range of opioid effects to exist. For example, the supraspinal analgesic properties of the opioid agonist morphine are mediated by activation of the μ_1 receptor; respiratory depression and physical dependence by the μ_2 receptor; and sedation and spinal analgesia by the κ receptor. Opioids' individual molecular structures are also responsible for their different duration of action.

Classical 'weak' opioids, such as codeine and tramadol represent the second step on the WHO analgesic ladder and are indicated for mild to moderate pain. Codeine may be administered as a single drug or in combination with paracetamol in pre-prepared formulations. When the maximum dose of step 2 drugs is insufficient to control pain, switching to a 'strong' opioid, such as morphine, on step 3 is recommended. Morphine is the first-line recommended opioid for moderate to severe pain and oral, subcutaneous (SC) or IV formulations are available. Immediate-release formulations should be started and when pain is controlled at a stable dose, the opioid may be changed to a modified release version. Fentanyl and buprenorphine may be administered as transcutaneous patches and are indicated in the presence of poor compliance to oral medication, but are not suitable for acute, uncontrolled pain.

- Nausea may occur initially with opioids that may be treated with anti-emetics.
- All patients treated with opioids require laxatives.
- Signs of opioid toxicity include drowsiness, vivid dreams, twitching and pinpoint pupils.
- The opioid antagonist naloxone should only be considered if there is significant respiratory depression, as pain control will be significantly reduced.

Management of bone pain

- NSAIDs are useful for bone pain, but consideration of side effects is essential.
- Bisphosphonates should be considered as an adjunct to analgesia:
  - They directly inhibit osteoclast activity leading to a decrease in bone reabsorption and an increase in bone mineralisation.
  - Examples include zoledronic acid or pamidronate.
  - Patients should be advised of a possible flare of bone pain, transient arthralgia and temperature following the first infusion of bisphosphonate therapy, and warned of the rare side effect of jaw osteonecrosis.
- Palliative radiotherapy may be useful.
- Vertebroplasty may be helpful for isolated vertebral collapse.
- Surgical referral for prophylactic fixation of long bone metastases may be considered based on patient prognosis and Mirels score (tool based on bone tumour site, pain, lesion and size).

Management of neuropathic pain

Neuropathic pain may be caused by invasion of cancer into the spinal cord, nerve roots, plexuses or peripheral nerves, or by chemotherapy drugs, such as oxaliplatin or taxanes. First-line therapeutic agents include the calcium channel alpha 2-delta ligands gabapentin and pregabalin, or tricyclic anti-depressants such as amitriptyline. The serotonin norepinephrine reuptake inhibitor duloxetine may be effective for pain, which has not responded to first-line therapy. Standard analgesics may be used as adjuncts to neuropathic agents.

If neuropathic pain is caused by compression of a nerve and decompression is possible, this should be performed. Radiotherapy may be helpful for compression which cannot be surgically relieved. Locoregional treatment using local anaesthetic and steroid may also be helpful.

Key symptom management

- Breathlessness:
  - Highly distressing symptom.
  - Underlying cause should be sought:

- ▪ Reversible causes include:
  - Pleural effusions – may be drained.
  - Upper airway compression – may be treated with stent placement.
  - Pulmonary embolism or pneumonia – may be treated medically.
- ▪ Non-reversible causes (for which pharmacological palliation is recommended with oxygen, bronchodilators, steroids, opiates ± benzodiazepines) include:
  - Disease infiltrating the lung parenchyma or the chest wall.
  - Lymphangitic carcinomatosis.
  - Phrenic nerve palsy.
- Liver capsular stretch pain:
  - May be treated with dexamethasone or NSAIDS.
- Nausea/vomiting (Table 10.9):
  - Resistant nausea may be treated with levomepromazine.

Table 10.9 Causes and treatments for nausea and vomiting in palliative care settings

Cause	Treatment
Chemotherapy	5 hydroxytryptamine (HT)$_3$ receptor antagonists (e.g. ondansetron, granisetron); neurokinin-1 receptor antagonists (aprepitant); dexamethasone; metoclopramide; domperidone; cyclizine.
Radiotherapy	5HT$_3$ receptor antagonists ± dexamethasone, metoclopramide, domperidone, cyclizine.
Gastritis	Proton pump inhibitors or H$_2$ histamine receptor antagonists.
Brain metastases/raised intracranial pressure	Dexamethasone.
Metabolic complications, e.g. hypercalcaemia, renal failure, liver failure	Correction/medical treatment of metabolic abnormalities.
Intestinal obstruction	MDT management to include: • nil by mouth • IV rehydration • SC cyclizine, haloperidol or levomepromazine • parenteral opiates and hyoscine butylbromide to control pain • parenteral dexamethasone to reduce peritumoural oedema • SC infusion of octreotide to reduce secretions.
Constipation	Laxatives; suppositories; enemas.
Anxiety	Benzodiazepines.

End of life care

The care of dying patients aims to relieve the physical, emotional, spiritual and social distress of patients and their families. Before the active dying phase occurs, a discussion related to the preference for the place of end of life care and the 'do not attempt resuscitation' (DNAR) status is imperative (➲ see Chapter 27, Breaking bad news/do not attempt cardiopulmonary resuscitation, p. 889). A rational review of interventions and medications is recommended with cessation of what is not expected to be beneficial. This should include decisions regarding clinically assisted hydration (via IV or SC fluids), focusing on potential relief from distressing symptoms associated with dehydration, but a lack of a significant prolonging of life. If clinically assisted hydration is commenced, this should be reviewed regularly for signs of benefit (relief of symptoms) or harm (e.g. fluid overload). The patients' wishes and preferences should be respected at all times:

- SC infusions via syringe drivers are preferential routes of drug administration.
- Pharmacological intervention aims to control symptoms such as pain, agitation and respiratory secretions:
  - Opioids can address pain and dyspnoea.
  - Haloperidol is the preferred choice in the presence of delirium.
  - Midazolam is usually recommended for sedation of distressed patients.
  - Benzodiazepines are employed in the presence of seizures.
  - Anticholinergic agents, such as hyoscine hydrobromide, may reduce secretions.
- Frequent mouth care should be offered to dying persons, who should also be offered the opportunity to drink if they wish to and are able.
- After-death care includes timely death certificate completion, acknowledgement of family bereavement, and communication of the death to the GP and other clinicians involved in the patient's care.

Further reading

1. Hanahan D, Weinberg RA. Hallmarks of cancer: the next generation. *Cell*. 2011; 144:646–74.
2. Amin MB, Greene FL, Edge SB, et al. The Eighth Edition AJCC Cancer Staging Manual: Continuing to build a bridge from a population-based to a more "personalized" approach to cancer staging. *Cancer*. 2017; 67(2):93–9.
3. ESMO Factsheets on Biomarkers. http://oncologypro.esmo.org/Science-Education/Factsheets-on-Biomarkers.
4. ESMO Clinical Practice Guidelines: Supportive and Palliative Care. http://www.esmo.org/Guidelines/Supportive-Care.

Multiple choice questions

Questions

1. Based on investigations performed due to a positive family history, a young man is diagnosed with Lynch syndrome. The cancer he is most likely to be diagnosed with is:
   A. Gastric cancer.
   B. Pancreatic cancer.
   C. Melanoma.
   D. Colon cancer.
   E. Testicular cancer.
2. The ERBB2 (HER2) receptor is commonly over expressed in:
   A. Lung cancer.
   B. Breast cancer.
   C. Oesophagogastric cancer.
   D. Lung cancer and breast cancer.
   E. Breast cancer and oesophagogastric cancer.
3. The Epstein–Barr virus is associated with all of the following except:
   A. Burkitt's lymphoma.
   B. Hodgkin lymphoma.
   C. Merkel cell carcinoma.
   D. Nasopharyngeal carcinoma.
   E. AIDS related lymphoma.
4. A 62-year-old female presents with an ulcerating mass on the posterior calf. The nodule is asymmetric and pigmented with an irregular border. Staging investigations reveal lung and liver metastases. Molecular diagnostics performed on the resection specimen are most likely to reveal:

A. EGFR mutation.
B. NRAS mutation.
C. KRAS mutation.
D. BRAF mutation.
E. BRCA1 mutation.

5. A pre-menopausal female is diagnosed with early breast cancer, which is oestrogen receptor-positive. She is treated with surgery followed by adjuvant chemotherapy and is then commenced on tamoxifen. Her treating oncologist warns her that tamoxifen is associated with an increased risk of:
   A. Thromboembolic disease.
   B. Oestrogen receptor-positive renal cell carcinoma.
   C. Endometrial cancer.
   D. Thromboembolic disease and oestrogen receptor positive renal cell carcinoma.
   E. Thromboembolic disease and endometrial cancer.

6. A 72-year-old male currently undergoing chemotherapy treatment for metastatic colorectal cancer presents to A&E complaining of dysuria for 2 days and rigors for the past 4 hours. His temperature is 38.5°. BP is 110/70 mm Hg, pulse rate is 95 beats/minute and oxygen saturations are 97% on room air. What is the next best course of action?
   A. Dipstick urine and if positive send mid-stream urine to the laboratory and prescribe oral amoxicillin empirically.
   B. Septic screen, urgent labs and commence broad spectrum antibiotics if neutrophil count is <1.0.
   C. Septic screen, urgent labs and empirically start broad spectrum IV antibiotics before FBC result is known.
   D. Discharge with paracetamol.
   E. Start GCSF.

7. A 40-year-old male is diagnosed with Burkitt's lymphoma and is scheduled to commence intensive chemotherapy. Which of the following statements regarding prevention and treatment of tumour lysis syndrome (TLS) is true?
   A. A low lactate dehydrogenase is a risk factor for TLS.
   B. Established TLS is associated with hypokalaemia, hypercalcaemia and hyperphosphataemia.
   C. Established TLS is associated with hyperkalaemia, hypocalcaemia and hyperphosphataemia.
   D. IV hydration and immediate initiation of allopurinol and rasburicase is recommended to treat established TLS.
   E. IV calcium gluconate should be used routinely to treat hypocalcaemia.

Answers

1. D. Lynch syndrome is an autosomally dominant inherited disorder associated with an increased risk of mismatch repair deficient tumours. Lynch syndrome is most commonly associated with colon cancer, although cancers may also occur in other organs, such as the gastric, endometrium and small bowel (➲ see Factors enabling development of cancer, Genetic instability, DNA damage and repair, p. 317).
2. E. The ERBB2 receptor is commonly over-expressed in breast cancer and oesophagogastric cancer. It may be therapeutically targeted using anti-HER2 therapies, such as trastuzumab (➲ see Growth factors: biology and target manipulation, p. 318).
3. C. EBV is associated with Burkitt's lymphoma, Hodgkin lymphoma, nasopharyngeal carcinoma and AIDS related lymphoma (➲ see Oncogenic viruses, p. 320).
4. D. The patient's signs are consistent with a malignant melanoma. Malignant melanoma is most frequently associated with the presence of a BRAF mutation (➲ see Table 10.5).

5. E. Tamoxifen treatment is associated with an increased risk of thromboembolic disease and endometrial cancer (➲ see Hormone therapy for women, p. 331).
6. C. Empiric treatment of suspected febrile neutropenia with broad spectrum antibiotics does not require confirmation of neutropenia. Treatment should commence immediately once the diagnosis is suspected (➲ see Oncological emergencies, Neutropenic sepsis, p. 332).
7. C. The risk of TLS is increased in patients with a high lactate dehydrogenase. Rasburicase and allopurinol are not administered concurrently. Symptomatic hypocalcaemia may be treated with IV calcium gluconate, asymptomatic hypocalcaemia should not be treated with IV calcium gluconate as this may increase the risk of calcium phosphate deposition in the kidneys (➲ see Oncological emergencies, Tumour lysis syndrome, p. 334).

Chapter 11 **Respiratory Medicine**

Richard Lee, Brintha Selvarajah* and William L. G. Oldfield*

Asthma and specific variants

Asthma

Asthma is a chronic inflammatory disease that is characterised by reversible airflow obstruction, and presents clinically as wheeze, cough and dyspnoea. It is the commonest chronic respiratory disease in the UK with an estimated 5.4 million sufferers. The pathogenesis of asthma is shown in Figure 11.1.

Aetiology

The aetiology of asthma is multifactorial and thought to involve a combination of genetic and environmental factors including:

- Susceptibility loci in the genes *ADAM33, GPRA* and *ORMDL3*, and polymorphisms of tumour necrosis factor.
- Infection (rhinovirus, influenza, mycoplasma), allergens (pollen), occupational exposures and stress.

'Atopic' asthmatics produce IgE-antigen complexes when exposed to a relevant antigen that bind to mast cells, basophils and macrophages, leading to histamine release, causing airway constriction and oedema.

* Joint first authors.

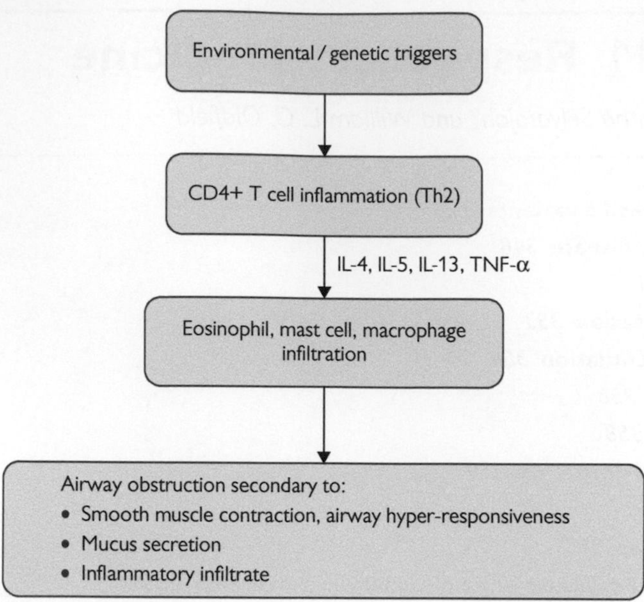

Figure 11.1 The pathogenesis of asthma.

Clinical features

A detailed history identifies diurnal variability in symptoms and risk factors, such as allergy, family history, nasal polyposis, obesity, aspirin use and reflux oesophagitis.

Typical symptoms include:

- Wheeze.
- Shortness of breath.
- Cough.
- Chest tightness.
- All classically worse at night or in the early morning.

Examination is often normal although, in chronic asthmatics and in acute exacerbations, expiratory wheeze may be heard. Atopic features, such as eczema and nasal polyposis may be present.

Diagnosis

Investigations

- Blood tests: FBC, eosinophilia (e.g. ABPA or Churg Strauss), IgE and aspergillus precipitins.
- Imaging: CXR may show hyperinflation.
- Spirometry: peak expiratory flow rate (PEFR) or 'Peak flow':
  - Airways obstruction leads to a decreased PEFR and forced expiratory volume in one second (FEV_1).
  - Airways obstruction is confirmed by a FEV_1 < 70% and FEV_1/ forced vital capacity (FVC) <70%.
  - May be normal between episodes due to variability.

A confident diagnosis of asthma can be made if there is:

- 15% diurnal PEFR variation on >3 days a week.
- FEV_1 >15% decrease after 6 minutes of exercise.
- Reversibility with bronchodilator – FEV_1 increase >12% or 200 mL increase.

- Allergy testing: If there is suspicion of an allergic trigger, a specific IgE test (formerly known as a Radioallergosorbant test) or skin prick test can be performed.
- Bronchial challenge test: used in diagnostic uncertainty, this test uses inhaled histamine or metacholine to measure bronchial hyperresponsiveness (BHR).

Risk stratification in acute asthma

It is important to categorise the patient with acute asthma according to their severity:

- Moderate exacerbation:
  - Increasing symptoms.
  - PEFR 50–75% predicted.
  - Current guidelines suggest patient may be discharged from hospital if PEFR >75% 1 hour post-bronchodilator treatment.
- Acute severe asthma:
  - PEFR 33–50% best or predicted.
  - Respiratory rate (RR) >25 breaths/minute.
  - HR ≥110 bpm.
  - Inability to complete sentences.
- Life-threatening asthma:
  - PEFR <33% best or predicted.
  - SaO_2 <92%, PaO_2 < 8kPa, normal $PaCO_2$.
  - Poor respiratory effort and silent chest on auscultation.
  - Cyanosis.
  - Arrhythmia/hypotension.
  - Confusion/exhaustion.
  - Coma.
- Near-fatal asthma:
  - Raised $PaCO_2$.
  - Requiring mechanical ventilation.
  - Risk factors: previous near-fatal asthma, patient taking ≥3 asthma medications, psychosocial features, frequent A&E attendances.

Acute management

- Oxygen therapy if oxygen saturations are <92% in which case arterial blood gas (ABG) analysis is required.
- Nebulised β2 agonist (e.g. salbutamol, terbutaline), repeated if no clinical improvement.
- Nebulised anticholinergic drug (e.g. ipratropium) if no improvement despite initial therapy.
- Steroids should be given early (IV if the patient is unable to take orally or concerns exist regarding absorption).
- A severe presentation may warrant a single dose of IV magnesium sulfate. Magnesium sulfate has bronchodilator activity, possibly due to inhibition of calcium influx into airway smooth muscle cells.
- Methylxanthines, such as aminophylline are no longer routinely used in the acute setting as there is limited evidence for their benefit above intense β2 agonist therapy. Furthermore, they are associated with an increased risk of adverse effects.

Long-term management

- A multifaceted approach is required to achieve symptom and exacerbation control.
- Focus on patient education, e.g. inhaler technique, patient self-management with asthma action plans and identifying and avoiding possible triggers.

The British Thoracic Society (BTS) advocates the step up/step down management plan depending on symptom control (1):

- Step 1: Mild intermittent asthma:
  - Short-acting β2 agonist.
  - Check compliance, consider spacer device.
  - Use of more than one inhaler per month is a marker of poorly controlled disease; move to Step 2.
- Step 2: Regular preventer therapy (200–800 μg equivalent of betamethasone):
  - Start at 400 μg/day of inhaled steroid and titrate up to 800 μg if needed.
- Step 3: Add on therapy:
  - Add a long-acting inhaled β2 agonist (LABA) and consider increasing the inhaled steroid dose to 800 μg.
  - If no response to LABA, stop this treatment, and increase the inhaled steroid to a dose of 800 μg/day (if not done already), and consider a leukotriene antagonist (e.g. montelukast).
- Step 4: Addition of fourth drug:
  - Monitor for toxic effects of methylxanthines; symptomatically and with drug level monitoring initially. Side effects may include arrhythmias and nausea.
  - If no improvement, then a trial of a leukotriene antagonist (if not already trialled) or methylxanthine is warranted.
  - Increase steroid to 2000 μg/day.
- Step 5: Refer to specialist care.

Further treatment for chronic asthma

Specialist centres may recommend:

- Daily oral steroid may be commenced at the lowest dose that gains control.
- Steroid sparing agents if poor control persists. Methotrexate and ciclosporin are recommended, but there is limited evidence to support their use.
- Continuous terbutaline (β2 agonist) infusions via a portable syringe driver.
- Omalizumab (an IgE recombinant monoclonal antibody) has been approved by NICE as an add-on therapy to step 5 treatment in patients with severe atopic asthma. It has been shown to reduce exacerbation rates and asthma symptoms with a reduction in steroid usage (2).
- Mepolizumab (an anti-IL-5 monoclonal antibody) may also be considered in severe eosinophilic asthma.

All patients require an asthma action plan, a self-management plan, which monitors PEFR, highlights warning signs of severe attacks and facilitates exacerbation self-management.

Smoking cessation advice and support should be offered to all smokers. Patient education may include trigger avoidance as well as nutrition and weight control.

References

1. British Thoracic Society. British guideline on the management of asthma (revised 2019) https://www.brit-thoracic.org.uk/standards-of-care/guidelines/btssign-british-guideline-on-the-management-of-asthma/.
2. Holgate S, Chuchalin AG, Hébert J, et al. Efficacy and safety of a recombinant anti-immunoglobulin E antibody (omalizumab) in severe allergic asthma. *Clin Exp Allergy*. 2004;34(4):632–8.

Further reading

1. Asthma UK. Stop asthma attacks. Cure asthma. http://www.asthma.org.uk.
2. NICE. Asthma. NICE quality standard QS25. https://www.nice.org.uk/guidance/qs25.
3. Royal College of Physicians. National review of asthma deaths. https://www.rcplondon.ac.uk/projects/national-review-asthma-deaths.

Interstitial lung disease

Interstitial lung disease (ILD) describes any process that results in diffuse inflammatory change or fibrosis within the interstitium (1). It can be classified by the aetiology, the most common of which are as follows:

- Inorganic dusts:
  - Coal, silica, beryllium and asbestos cause disease through inhalation, often termed pneumoconiosis.
- Organic materials:
  - Cause a Type 4 hypersensitivity pneumonitis (HP) with subsequent granuloma formation, resulting from inhalation of an organic antigen in a previously sensitised individual:
    - NB: this is not an allergic response mediated by a Type 1 reaction.
  - Antigens include thermophilic actinomycetes (farmer's lung), *Aspergillus clavatus* (malt worker's lung) and bird proteins (bird fancier's lung).
- Drug-induced:
  - Common culprits include amiodarone, chemotherapy agents (e.g. bleomycin, methotrexate), sulfasalazine, gold, nitrofurantoin and radiation (see Table 3.8).
- Connective tissues disease (CTD):
  - Conditions commonly associated with lung fibrosis include rheumatoid arthritis, SLE, polymyositis, dermatomyositis, systemic sclerosis (SSc), Sjogren's syndrome and ankylosing spondylitis.
  - An evolving subgroup of patients possess 'interstitial pneumonia with autoimmune features' (IPAF), but do not meet established criteria for a CTD (2).
- Sarcoidosis.

Idiopathic interstitial pneumonias

- These comprise of a heterogenous group of disorders, classified according to their radiological and histopathological findings. The most common is idiopathic pulmonary fibrosis (IPF), which conveys a very poor prognosis with limited treatment options currently available. Table 11.1 describes the clinical features and management of each idiopathic interstitial pneumonias (IIP) subtype.

Malignancy

- Rarely malignancies can cause ILD, e.g. lymphangitic carcinomatosis. Patients with ILD have an increased risk of lung cancer.

Symptoms and clinical findings

- Progressive shortness of breath and a chronic non-productive cough. In acute presentation, such as hypersensitivity pneumonitis, there may also be symptoms of fever, myalgia and arthralgia.
- There may be peripheral manifestations of CTD e.g. rheumatoid arthritis (➲ see Chapter 20, Clinical features, p. 706 and Box 20.1).
- Clubbing is seen in IPF, but is rare in sarcoidosis or hypersensitivity pneumonitis.
- Pulmonary findings may be non-specific, but classic descriptions include fine basal-end inspiratory crackles. Hypersensitivity pneumonitis usually presents with crackles in the upper and mid zones. Patients with advanced pulmonary fibrosis may have signs of pulmonary hypertension.

Investigations

Imaging

- *CXR and HRCT*: are key investigations since radiological abnormalities and their distribution can point to a specific causation (➲ see Chapter 5, Case 4, p. 122, for the typical radiological changes seen on CXR and HRCT).
- *Blood tests*: erythrocyte sedimentation rate (ESR), CRP, FBC, U&Es, LFT, calcium, autoimmune screen, serum IgG precipitins for a particular antigen and serum angiotensin-converting enzyme (ACE).
- *Lung function tests*: typically demonstrates a restrictive picture (➲ see Obstructive vs restrictive lung disease, p. 377) with reduced forced vital capacity and transfer factor for carbon monoxide (TLCO).

Table 11.1 Classification of idiopathic interstitial pneumonias

Subtype	Nomenclature	Clinical features	Radiological findings	Treatment and prognosis
UIP (IPF)	Usual interstitial pneumonia (idiopathic pulmonary fibrosis)	Dry cough and progressive breathlessness. Clubbing, fine-end interstitial crackles.	Peripheral, subpleural, basal reticulation with honeycombing.	Treatment with immunosuppression has fallen out of favour since the PANTHER trial showed increased mortality (3). Pirfendione and nintedanib, two anti-fibrotics are currently licenced for patients with FVC 50–80% predicted. Poor median survival of 3–5 years. Holistic care, O_2 therapy and palliation of symptoms is important.
DIP	Desquamative interstitial pneumonia	Dry cough, SOB. Common in smokers.	Lower zone ground glass opacities.	Most patients improve with steroids.
RBILD	Respiratory bronchiolitis ILD	Cough, SOB. Common in smokers.	Ground glass opacities with nodular changes in no particular distribution.	Resolution with smoking cessation, but some patients may need steroids.
AIP	Acute interstitial pneumonia	Similar to ARDS. Hypoxia and respiratory failure.	Patchy infiltrates throughout the lung.	Rapid progression, needs prompt supportive treatment with ICU monitoring.
COP	Cryptogenic organising pneumonia	SOB, dry cough, fever.	Bilateral diffuse opacities with lower and peripheral preference.	Once other underlying infective or inflammatory causes are ruled out, treatment is with systemic steroids with good prognosis.
LIP	Lymphoid interstitial pneumonia	Associated with autoimmune, lymphoproliferative disorders and HIV.	Linear nodular opacities and honey combing.	1/3 of patients progress to extensive fibrosis. Steroids are often used.
NSIP	Non-specific interstitial pneumonia	SOB, cough and weight loss.	Diffuse symmetrical ground glass ± reticulation.	Corticosteroids; patients usually remain stable on treatment.

Data from *American Journal of Respiratory Critical Care Medicine*, 188, 6, William D. Travis, Ulrich Costabel, David M. Hansell, et al, An Official American Thoracic Society/European Respiratory Society Statement: Update of the International Multidisciplinary Classification of the Idiopathic Interstitial Pneumonias, pp. 733–748, 2013; and British Thoracic Society, 'Interstitial lung disease guideline', *Thorax* 2008;63;v1-v58

- *Video assisted thoracoscopic surgery (VATS) assisted lung biopsy* may be indicated if there is a diagnostic uncertainty. This is rarely undertaken, given the risk of complications, with the majority of diagnoses made on clinical and radiological findings.

Management

- If present, any underlying cause should be identified to guide treatment.
- Idiopathic pulmonary fibrosis may meet criteria for nintedanib/pirfenidone.
- Hypersensitivity pneumonitis is managed mainly by antigen avoidance. If no clinical improvement, a tapered course of corticosteroids may dampen the immune response.
- Drug-induced pneumonitis is treated by drug cessation, but steroids maybe used in severe cases.
- CTD-related ILD is managed by treatment and maintenance of stability of the underlying CTD activity. Damage sustained prior to treatment may not be reversible.

References

1. Raghu G, Remy-Jardin M, Myers JL, et al. Diagnosis of idiopathic pulmonary fibrosis. An official ATS/ERS/JRS/ALAT clinical practice guideline. *Am Journal Resp Crit Care Med* 2018;198(5): e44-e68. https://www.thoracic.org/statements/resources/interstitial-lung-disease/diagnosis-IPF-full-length.pdf
2. Fischer A, Antoniou KM, Brown KK, et al. An official European Respiratory Society/American Thoracic Society research statement: interstitial pneumonia with autoimmune features. *Eur Resp J*. 2015; 46:976–87.

Sarcoidosis

Sarcoidosis is a multisystem granulomatous disorder of unknown aetiology. It usually presents between 20 and 49 years of age. In the UK, the incidence of sarcoidosis is 5–10:100,000. It is more common in people of Afro-Caribbean and Scandinavian descent and slightly more common in females.

Immunopathogenesis

Sarcoidosis is thought to occur in a genetically susceptible person who is exposed to a specific, but unknown environmental agent (Figure 11.2):

- Geographical cluster studies have not identified a specific infective or occupational trigger.
- An association has been noted between sarcoidosis and Class 2 MHC region chromosome 6p and 3p.
- The underlying pathology is a CD4+ T cell alveolitis leading to non-caseating granulomas and fibrosis.

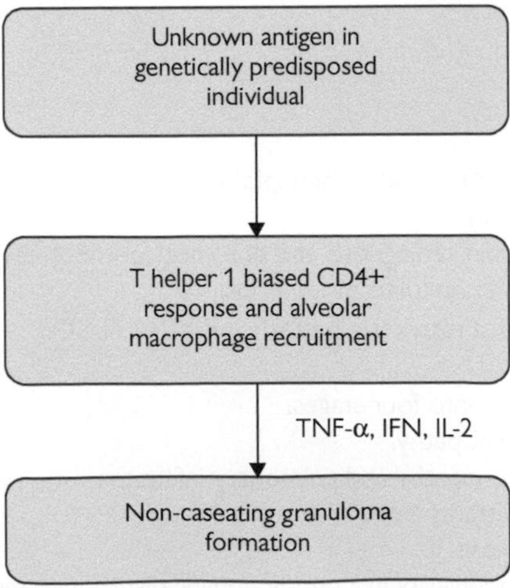

Figure 11.2 The immunopathogenesis of sarcoidosis.

Clinical presentation

Sarcoidosis is a multisystem condition and as such may present in a variety of ways.

- Pulmonary involvement:
  - 90% of patients;
  - dry cough;
  - breathlessness.
- Cutaneous involvement (➲ see Chapter 21, Clinical presentations, p. 771):
  - lupus pernio – chronic indurated purplish lesions of the face;
  - erythema nodosum.
- Ocular involvement:
  - anterior uveitis (➲ see Chapter 18, Uveitis, p. 665).
- Cardiac sarcoidosis:
  - may result in heart block or cardiomyopathy and is therefore potentially life-threatening.
- Renal vasculitis.
- Hypercalcaemia.
- Non-specific symptoms:
  - low-grade fever;
  - fatigue;
  - weight loss;
  - night sweats;
  - arthralgia.
- Löfgren's syndrome:
  - mild acute form of sarcoidosis;
  - bilateral hilar lymphadenopathy;
  - fever;
  - ankle arthritis;
  - erythema nodosum;
  - good prognosis, resolves completely in 80% of patients within 1–2 years.

Examination

- Peripheral lymphadenopathy ± skin manifestations.
- There may be few positive findings on respiratory examination even in the context of an abnormal CXR. Patients who have developed fibrosis may have fine-end inspiratory crackles in the upper lobes.

Investigations

- *Blood tests*:
  - FBC, LFTs, U&Es, serum calcium and immunoglobulins (to exclude common variable immunodeficiency disease, see Table 6.2).
  - Serum ACE has a limited role in diagnosis and does not contribute as a marker of disease activity.
- *Urine microscopy*: red cell casts: vasculitis or nephritis.
- *Spirometry*: may manifest with a restrictive pattern and a low TLCO.
- *Radiology*:
  - CXR findings can be divided into four stages:
    - Stage 1 – Hilar lymphadenopathy.
    - Stage 2 – Hilar lymphadenopathy and pulmonary infiltrates.
    - Stage 3 – Pulmonary infiltrates alone.
    - Stage 4 – Pulmonary fibrosis.
  - HRCT may demonstrate nodularity in a peri-lymphatic distribution with upper and middle zone predominance.

- *Histological diagnosis*:
  - Lymph node biopsy, transbronchial biopsy or endobronchial ultrasound (EBUS) guided mediastinal lymph node sampling may be required to obtain histological confirmation of the diagnosis.
  - A biopsy may also be required to exclude possible differential diagnoses, including lymphoma or tuberculosis.

Management

- The majority of patients remain asymptomatic and require no treatment.
- Steroids form the mainstay of medical treatment for sarcoidosis. Indications for treatment include:
  - Respiratory: increasing symptoms with deteriorating lung function and worsening changes on CXR.
  - Absolute indications for steroids include cardiac or neurological involvement, and hypercalcaemia.
- The BTS recommends starting prednisolone at 0.5 mg/kg/day for 4 weeks and to slowly taper down over 6 months. There may be a need to maintain a low dose of 5–7.5 mg of prednisolone a day.
- If steroid treatment fails or there is a life-threatening indication, pulsed IV methylprednisolone may be required.
- Steroid-sparing agents such as azathioprine and cyclophosphamide may be required if there is need for long-term steroid use. TNF inhibitors such as infliximab may also be considered.

Prognosis

As many patients are asymptomatic and many regress spontaneously, prognosis is good with 60% achieving clinical remission. Patients with a chronic clinical picture have a worse prognosis with a mortality of between 1 and 6%.

Further reading

1. Spagnolo P, Rossi G, Trisolini R, et al. Pulmonary sarcoidosis. *The Lancet Respiratory Medicine*, 2018; 6(5): 389–402.

Lung transplantation

The first successful lung transplant in the UK was done in the early 1980s. Since then, the number of patients requiring lung transplants have increased, but with an ongoing shortfall of donor organs. Currently approximately 150 lung transplants and 5 heart–lung transplants are carried out in the UK annually with an average waiting time of 12 months.

Indications for lung transplantation

- Chronic end-stage lung disease, despite maximal medical therapy with a life expectancy of ≤ 2–3 years.
- WHO performance status ≤ 3.
- No significant cardiac, renal or hepatic impairment. Age <55 years for heart–lung transplant, <60 years for bilateral lung and <65 years for single lung transplant.

Common conditions requiring lung (heart–lung) transplantation

- Chronic obstructive pulmonary disease (COPD): BODE (body mass index, airflow obstruction, dyspnoea and exercise capacity) index of 5, FEV1 <20%.
- Cystic fibrosis (CF): FEV1 <30% with rapid deterioration (if associated with severe RV dysfunction).
- IPF.
- Idiopathic pulmonary arterial hypertension (if associated with severe RV dysfunction).
- Pulmonary hypertension secondary to congenital cardiac disease.

Transplant assessment and procedure

- Prior to referral for lung transplantation, it is important to optimise nutritional status, baseline physical abilities and other comorbidities.

- Essential investigations required prior to referral for lung transplant include:
  - Full pulmonary function test.
  - 6-minute walk test.
  - Sputum analysis.
  - ECG, echocardiogram (ECHO).
  - Chest HRCT.
  - Viral serology.
- The majority of lung transplants are single, but they can be bilateral, or as part of a heart and lung transplant. Following surgery, there will usually be a prolonged inpatient stay followed by close outpatient review.
- Immunosuppresive drugs such as tacrolimus, mycophenolate mofetil, azathioprine and prednisolone must be taken lifelong post-transplant. Levels of these drugs should be closely monitored to avoid toxicity or under treatment.

Complications

- Acute rejection: presents within 3 months of transplantation and is treated with enhanced immunosuppression. Early graft rejection has a high mortality, and is demonstrated by pulmonary infiltrates and hypoxia with a fall in spirometry >10%. Transbronchial biopsy shows perivascular and interstitial mononuclear cell infiltration.
- Chronic graft rejection: affects 50–60% of patients within 5 years of transplant. Histologically, it is characterised by bronchiolitis obliterans, which conveys a poor prognosis, marking failure of the organ.
- Malignancy: post-transplant lymphoproliferative disorders.
- Infection: commonly Gram-negative organisms especially *Pseudomonas*, but also CMV and aspergillus.
- Drug-related complications include renal impairment and osteoporosis.

Prognosis

- Survival rates are 85% at 1 year and 50% at 5 years.
- Grafts typically perform well for 3–5 years before showing signs of failure.

Further reading

1. Orens JB, Estenne M, Arcasoy S, et al. International guidelines for the selection of lung transplant candidates: 2006 update. *J Heart Lung Transplant*. 2006;25:745–55.

Non-invasive ventilation

Non-invasive ventilation (NIV) delivers ventilatory support to improve respiratory failure via an interface that does not cross the larynx. Continuous positive airway pressure (CPAP) is often included in this description, although technically it does not provide ventilatory support as there is no assistance with inspiration.

Continuous positive airway pressure

CPAP applies a constant pressure throughout the respiratory cycle and works by splinting open and recruiting collapsed alveoli, thus reducing pulmonary circulatory shunting and improving lung compliance. This improves oxygenation and reduces the work of breathing. Sometimes the term positive-end-expiratory pressure (PEEP) is used interchangeably to describe the pressures set on the ventilator.

Indications for continuous positive airway pressure

- Worsening Type 1 respiratory failure by either bridging to or avoiding intubation.

- Acute cardiogenic pulmonary oedema by improving lung compliance and oxygenation when drug treatment has been optimised. CPAP also assists in the translocation of interstitial fluid to the alveolar capillaries surrounding the alveoli, further improving gas exchange.
- In the domiciliary setting, CPAP can be used as a treatment of obstructive sleep apnoea/ hypoapnoea syndrome (OSAHS) by splinting open the airways and improving oxygenation.

Settings

- The usual pressure applied is between +5 cmH_2O to +10 cmH_2O via a mask. Oxygen can be entrained to maintain saturations >94% if there is no evidence of hypercapnia.

Non-invasive ventilation

NIV delivers alternating higher inspiratory pressures, which increase tidal volume and lower expiratory pressures that allows recruitment of alveoli at the end of expiration.

Indications for non-invasive ventilation

NIV is used in the treatment of type 2 respiratory failure in both acute and chronic settings.

Acute exacerbation of COPD

- Respiratory acidosis ($PaCO_2$ >6 kPa and pH <7.35), no improvement despite optimal medical management and appropriate controlled oxygen therapy (usually aiming for peripheral capillary oxygen saturation [SpO_2] 88–92%).
- Reduces mortality and the need for intubation.
- Patients with pH <7.25 or H^+ >56 nmol/L respond less well and should be managed in a high dependency unit (HDU)/intensive care unit (ICU) for consideration of intubation.

Decompensated obstructive sleep apnoea/obesity hypoventilation syndrome

- NIV can be used if there is evidence of type 2 respiratory failure or CPAP fails to correct obstructive sleep apnoea (OSA)/obesity hypoventilation syndrome (OHS).

Respiratory failure secondary to neuromuscular weakness or chest wall deformity

- These include kyphoscoliosis, post-polio, motor neurone disease, spinal cord injury and myopathies, which can cause type 2 respiratory failure.
- NIV is administered overnight to reduce daytime hypercapnia and reduce nocturnal hypoxaemia.

Non-invasive ventilation settings (example regime)

- Set the initial inspiratory positive airway pressure (IPAP) at 12 cmH_2O and the expiratory positive airway pressure (EPAP) at 4 cmH_2O.
- Increase IPAP by 2–4 cmH_2O every 15 minutes until an adequate tidal volume is achieved, or more slowly according to comfort and ABG analysis.
- Increase EPAP ± oxygen entrained to achieve saturations between 88 and 92%.

Patient monitoring on non-invasive ventilation/continuous positive airway pressure

- For both CPAP and NIV, there should be continuous pulse oximetry and ECG monitoring for the first 12 hours, and regular RR, pulse, BP measurements and assessments of consciousness.
- ABG should be taken as a minimum at 1, 4 and 12 hours after the initiation of NIV. This will guide changes in settings, escalation plans to intubation and ceilings of treatment.

Contraindications for non-invasive ventilation

It is important to assess the need for NIV in a patient who has severe respiratory failure but *not to delay* intubation if success is unlikely.

Relative contraindications to its use

1. Impaired consciousness or confusion – the patient will not be able to trigger sufficient breaths and should be assessed for intubation immediately.
2. Life-threatening hypoxaemia.
3. Haemodynamic instability or arrest. NIV reduces preload so can lower blood pressure further, so patients should be considered for admission to ICU.
4. Facial surgery or burns.
5. Undrained pneumothorax: the positive pressure ventilation may convert a simple pneumothorax to a tension pneumothorax.
6. Vomiting.
7. Inability to protect airway, e.g. GCS < 8.

Further reading

1. BTS guideline – BTS/ICS guidelines for the ventilatory management of acute hypercapnic respiratory failure in adults. *Thorax* 2016;71:ii1-ii35.

Bronchiectasis

- Bronchiectasis is characterised by irreversible abnormal luminal airway dilatation and bronchial wall-thickening, secondary to a repeating cycle of infection and chronic inflammation.
- Worldwide prevalence varies due to differences in vaccination programmes and antibiotic therapies. In the UK, incidence is estimated at 1.06–1.3 per 100,000 population.

Pathogenesis

- An initial insult, usually infective in nature, is thought to damage the airways and lead to an inflammatory response and further damage to the mucociliary apparatus.
- This renders the airways susceptible to bacterial colonisation and an ongoing vicious cycle of chronic inflammation and lung damage.
- Neutrophils are the most prominent cell type in the bronchial lumen and release mediators, particularly proteases and elastases, which cause bronchial dilation.
- The inflammatory infiltrate within the airway is predominantly composed of macrophages and lymphocytes.

Aetiology

The possible causes fall into the following categories:

- Causes of generalised bronchiectasis include:
  - Post-infectious: include TB, whooping cough, severe pneumonia, non-tuberculous mycobacterium and ABPA.
  - Genetic: most common in childhood is CF (➲ see Cystic fibrosis, p. 358), alpha-1-antitrypsin deficiency, primary ciliary dyskinesia including Kartagener's syndrome (dextrocardia, chronic sinusitis and bronchiectasis), Marfan's syndrome, Ehlers–Danlos syndrome and Young's syndrome (bronchiectasis, sinusitis and azoospermia).
  - Immunodeficiency: primary hypogammaglobinaemia, HIV, CLL and nephrotic syndrome.
  - Aspiration and inhalation injury.
  - Systemic conditions: associated with rheumatoid arthritis, CTD, inflammatory bowel disease and yellow nail syndrome (lymphoedema, yellow discolouration of nails, pleural effusion).
  - Mounier–Kuhn syndrome (tracheobronchial dilation associated with recurrent lower respiratory tract infections).
  - Williams–Campbell syndrome (a congenital syndrome characterised by absence of cartilage in subsegmental bronchi leading to bronchiectasis distal to the collapsed airways).

 - Swyer–James syndrome (MacLeod's syndrome) caused by a childhood bronchiolitis obliterans infection, which may lead to bronchial wall damage with localised or generalised bronchiectasis, air-trapping and stunted pulmonary arterial development.
 - Idiopathic.
- Causes of localised bronchiectasis include:
 - Bronchial atresia.
 - Post-infection (typically the upper lobes or apical segment of lower lobes in patients with old TB).
 - Bronchial airway obstruction: foreign body or a mass, e.g. bronchogenic cancer.
 - Swyer–James syndrome (localised or generalised bronchiectasis).
- Traction bronchiectasis is seen in the context of pulmonary fibrosis.

Clinical features

- Productive purulent cough ± haemoptysis.
- Dyspnoea.
- Wheeze.
- Intermittent pleuritic pain.
- Exacerbations are characterised by increased sputum production, sputum colour and consistency change with fever and lethargy.

Examination

- Clubbing may be present.
- Coarse inspiratory and expiratory crackles may be heard, as well as expiratory wheeze.
- Full systemic examination to establish a possible underlying cause.

Investigations

The aim of the investigations should be to confirm the diagnosis, identify and treat any underlying causes, and optimise management to prevent exacerbations:

- *Blood tests*: CRP, white blood cells (WBCs), immunoglobulins, aspergillus serology, including IgE, and further specialised tests such as CF genotyping, alpha-1-antitrypsin levels and an autoimmune screen may be indicated.
- *Sputum microscopy and culture* can guide tailored antimicrobial therapy.
- *Spirometry* commonly shows an obstructive picture and possible reversibility (ABPA).
- *Chest radiography* classically demonstrates linear markings ('tram lines'). ➲ See also Chapter 5, Case 1, p. 118.
- *HRCT*: lack of bronchial tapering, airway dilatation to the periphery, bronchial wall-thickening and the signet sign, where the airway is larger than the corresponding vessel due to dilatation.

Management

- Antibiotic therapy to treat infections promptly and prevent recurrent exacerbations to stop the inflammatory cycle. Tailoring treatment to sputum microbiology is important.
- Empirical treatment should be started while waiting for sputum culture. First-line treatment includes amoxicillin for 14 days (or clarithromycin if penicillin allergic) unless previous cultures have shown this to be inappropriate.
- IV antibiotics should be considered if the patient is very unwell, hospitalised or has a resistant organism that has failed to respond to oral therapy in the past (especially *Pseudomonas aeruginosa*). Prolonged use of antibiotics should be considered in patients who have >3 exacerbations per year or progressive lung function decline.
- Micro-organisms commonly responsible for colonisation are *Staphylococcus aureus, Haemophilus influenza, Moraxella catarrhalis* and *Pseudomonas* species.
- Long-term nebulised antibiotics or combination antibiotics, especially if chronically colonised with *Pseudomonas*, may be required.

Additional medical treatments

- Physiotherapy and postural drainage, optimised with nebulised normal/hypertonic saline can help. There is no evidence for the routine use of inhaled or oral steroid or bronchodilators unless there is evidence of airways obstruction.
- Mucolytics such as carbocisteine may help, but lack robust evidence for use.

Interventional therapy and surgery

- Bronchial embolisation: indicated for massive haemoptysis.
- Surgical resection may be indicated for localised bronchiectasis once all medical measures have been exhausted.
- Lung transplantation is a common outcome in patients with CF, but is otherwise only routinely offered if there is rapid progressive respiratory deterioration despite optimum medical management.

Further reading

1. Barker AF. Bronchiectasis. *New Engl J Med*. 2002;346:1383–93.
2. Pasteur MC, Bilton D, Hill AT, et al. British Thoracic Society guideline for non-CF bronchiectasis. *Thorax*. 2010;65(Suppl. 1):i1–i58.

Cystic fibrosis

Pathogenesis

Cystic fibrosis is an autosomal recessive disease caused by mutations in the CF transmembrane conductance regulator (*CFTR*) gene on chromosome 7. The gene encodes an ion channel protein regulating chloride transport across the epithelial cells lining the lungs, liver, pancreatic ducts, intestines, sweat glands and reproductive organs. In the lungs, this leads to a viscous mucus, which cannot be removed by the cilia, resulting in recurrent infections. Common pathogens include *Haemophilus influenzae, Staphylococcus aureus, Pseudomonas aeruginosa, Burkholderia cepacia* and *Klebsiella* species.

Clinical features

- Repeated episodes of cough and chest infections.
- Nasal polyposis, sinusitis.
- Pancreatic dysfunction: steatorrhoea, chronic diarrhoea with malabsorption and failure to thrive in children.
- Cholelithiasis and liver disease.
- Meconium ileus in neonates.
- Rectal prolapse.

Investigations

- Sodium sweat test: positive if sweat chloride content > 60 mmol/L.
- Genetic testing.

Management

- Mucolytics.
- Airway clearance measures.
- Antibiotics.
- Supplemental pancreatic enzymes, calories, and fat-soluble vitamins to support growth and nutrition.

Prognosis

Although life expectancy is considerably shorter, in the past 50 years, the average survival has increased dramatically to almost 38 years of age.

Pneumonia and empyema

'Pneumonia' usually referring to community acquired pneumonia (CAP) has an incidence of 500–1000 per 100,000 adults in the UK. Between 20 and 40% of cases are admitted to hospital with a median length of stay of 5 days. Inpatient 30-day mortality for CAP is up to 18% and, of patients admitted, 1–10% require intensive care where mortality is even higher (~30%).

Pathogenesis

- An inflammatory response of the lung to infection with one of several common, usually bacterial micro-organisms.
- Inflammatory cell infiltration of the lung parenchyma results in accumulation of fluid and micro-organisms, and production of purulent sputum.
- Development of consolidation impairs gas exchange and is usually associated with a fever, rise in inflammatory markers and the evolution of a systemic inflammatory response, which if untreated, leads to sepsis, cardiovascular compromise and multi-organ failure.

A number of risk factors are associated with atypical presentations or more severe disease:

- COPD.
- Diabetes mellitus.
- Old age.
- In those with high alcohol consumption there is an increased risk of aspiration pneumonia. Alcohol intake may also influence responsible organisms and disease course by relative immunosuppression.

For common organisms causing pneumonia, see Table 11.2.

Table 11.2 Pneumonia: common organisms

Organism	Frequency (hospital diagnoses)	Classical features
Streptococcus pneumonia	39%	Commoner in winter.
Chlamydophila pneumoniae	13%	Longer incubation period, may be associated with headaches.
Viral pneumonia	13%	Inflammatory markers maybe normal. 'Flu-like' illness, e.g. muscle aches and coryzal symptoms.
Mycoplasma pneumonia	11%	Epidemics ~4–5 yearly.
Haemophilus influenza	5%	
Legionella pneumophila (and related species)	4%	Related to travel, e.g. in relation to water containing systems. May have diarrhoea/neurological symptoms, e.g. encephalopathy. Haematuria/deranged LFTs.
Chlamydophila psittaci	3%	Usually transmitted from birds/animals.
Staphylococcus aureus	2%	Cavitatory organisms. Often severe respiratory distress.
Moraxella catarrhalis	2%	
Coxiella burnetii	1%	Relation to animal sources (usually sheep) and epidemics. Dry cough, high fever.

Data from Maskell N, Millar A. (2009) *Oxford Desk Reference: Respiratory Medicine*. Oxford, UK: Oxford University Press.

Terminology

- *Atypical pneumonia* is an outdated term referring to pneumonia caused by atypical organisms that do not respond to 'typical' antibiotics (*M. pneumoniae, C. pneumoniae, C. psittaci* and *C. burnetii; Legionella* spp.). These organisms often use intracellular replication and therefore are usually not beta lactam sensitive.
- *Hospital-acquired pneumonia (HAP)* (developing 48 hours after admission to a health-care institution) or *ventilator-associated pneumonia* (intubated patients) are associated with unusual and often resistant organisms, e.g. *Pseudomonas aeruginosa*, MRSA or Gram-negative bacteria, which can be difficult to treat and is associated with high mortality.
- *Aspiration pneumonia* describes soiling of the lungs with gastric contents providing a double insult of anaerobic organisms and a chemical pneumonitis secondary to the acidic stomach contents.

Clinical features

Common symptoms

- Cough (which can be dry or productive/purulent).
- Fever, sweating and malaise.
- Haemoptysis.
- Chest pain (suggests pleurisy, pleural effusion or empyema).
- Respiratory compromise; tachypnoea or dyspnoea.

On examination

- Focal crepitations.
- Dullness and increased vocal resonance may be identified.
- Signs of a pleural effusion indicating possible empyema.
- Pleural thickening post-empyema may result in persisting dullness.

Diagnosis

Blood tests

- WBC and CRP.
- U&Es to assess severity (CURB65; ➲ see Pneumonia prognostic indices, p. 361 and Box 11.1).
- Blood film: 'rouleux' formation or stacking of RBC can be suggestive of mycoplasma pneumonia due to the production of cold agglutinins.

Microbiology

- Sputum/blood cultures.
- Pneumococcal and legionella antigen/serology tests.

Pulse oximetry and arterial blood gas analysis

Imaging

- CXR is indicated in all cases admitted to hospital.
- Opacification of airspaces occupying one or more lobes, classically highlighted with 'air bronchograms'.
- Cavitation: associated with *Staphylococcus, Klebsiella* (upper lobe predilection) and TB.
- Radiographic features should resolve within 6 weeks, thereafter underlying pathology should be considered.
- Note that radiological resolution frequently lags behind clinical improvement.

Interventional procedures

- Parapneumonic effusions should be assessed at an early stage by diagnostic (± therapeutic) pleural aspiration, ideally under ultrasound guidance.

- Pleural fluid is sent for Gram stain, culture and assessment of Light's criteria.
- Pleural ultrasound can identify turbidity and loculations, suggestive of an empyema.

Pneumonia prognostic indices

Poor prognostic features of CAP include:

- Age (e.g. >50 years).
- Comorbidity.
- Hypoxaemia.
- Multilobar involvement.

CURB65 score (Box 11.1) is commonly utilised as a prognostic indicator of CAP outcomes such as survival. The 'pneumonia severity score' is another less widely used severity score.

Treatment failure is predicted by cavitation, pleural effusion, acidaemia, hyponatraemia, legionella/ Gram-negative infection and multilobar involvement.

Box 11.1 CURB65 score

1 point for each of the following:

- Confusion.
- Urea > 7 mmol/L.
- Respiratory rate >30/min.
- sBP $\leq$90 ± dBP<60 mmHg.
- Age >65 years.

Adapted by permission from BMJ Publishing Group Limited. Lim WS, et al. Defining community-acquired pneumonia severity on presentation to hospital: an international derivation and validation study. *Thorax* 58:377–82. Copyright © 2003, BMJ Publishing Group Ltd and the British Thoracic Society. http://dx.doi.org/10.1136/thorax.58.5.377.

Complications

Failure of pneumonia to improve

- Early (within 72 hours) versus late failure (after 72 hours).
- Ineffective (e.g. suboptimal or allergic response to) anti-microbial therapy.
- Unusual or resistant pathogens.
- Impaired mechanical or immune defence.

Pleural effusion

- Complicates over 50% of CAP.
- Loculations and progression to empyema.

Lung abscess

- Rare, although alcohol use and specific organisms increase the risk, e.g. anaerobes, *S. aureus*, *Klebsiella* spp., Gram-negative organisms or *Streptococcus milleri* (poor dental hygiene).
- Septic emboli may result in meningitis, endocarditis and septic arthritis.

Management

- Oxygen therapy: aim: $PaO_2 \geqslant 8$ kPa, $SpO_2 \geqslant 94\%$). Patients with COPD or known risk of CO_2 retention require careful titration of oxygen (aiming SaO_2 88–92%) and consideration of ventilatory support.
- Circulatory support.
- Nutrition and smoking cessation should also be encouraged.

Lung cancer staging

- Accurate staging is critical for prognostication and treatment selection.
- The IASLC (International Association for the Study of Lung Cancer) TNM classification uses anatomical involvement and size by imaging and biopsy. TNM correlates closely with survival and is used to select the most appropriate treatment.
- Small cell lung cancer is also described in terms of limited and extensive stages.
- Performance status (PS) e.g. the ECOG score is the next most significant factor in defining a patient's potential therapy. Late presentation and poor performance status is a major factor in limiting treatment options.

Management

- A lung cancer MDT discussion ensures chest physicians liaise closely with oncologists and thoracic surgeons.
- Resection, radical radiotherapy or interventional procedural treatment e.g radiofrequency ablation (RFA) of early stage lung tumours can result in cure. This requires detailed preoperative imaging and lung function testing (including diffusion capacity [DLCO]), and assessment of surgical fitness.
- Surgical options include lobectomy, pneumonectomy and wedge resection. Video-assisted thoracoscopic surgery ('VATS') allows a less invasive approach.

Management of small cell lung cancer

- Chemotherapy can be extremely effective initially, although is usually of palliative intent.
- Prophylactic cranial irradiation against brain metastases or more focused approaches (stereotactic radiotherapy or surgery) for limited volume disease is sometimes offered.

Management of non-small cell lung cancer

- Surgery is the preferred intervention, where appropriate, in early stage disease, e.g. stage I or II.
- 'Radical radiotherapy' or techniques, such as stereotactic body radiation therapy (SBRT) or radiofrequency ablation is considered in patients who may not tolerate surgery or the associated complications.
- In more advanced disease (e.g. stage 3 N2 disease), multimodality therapy, that may include chemotherapy in addition to surgery and/or radiotherapy is considered.
- Stage IV is associated with particularly poor prognosis and is usually limited to palliative approaches with chemotherapy or radiotherapy, or best supportive care.
- The focus of lung cancer awareness drives and screening campaigns is often prompt recognition of symptoms to encourage an early medical opinion.

Targeted therapy

- Genetics:
  - ◆ Oncogenic mutations in 'epidermal growth factor receptor' (EGFR; ➲ see Chapter 10, Personalised oncology, p. 332) predict:
    - ▪ Response to novel EGFR 'tyrosine kinase inhibitors' (TKI [e.g. gefitinib and erlotinib]); mutations include *L858R* 'deletion in exon 19'.
      - EGFR TKI are more effective than standard chemotherapy in patients with activating EGFR mutations.
    - ▪ Poor response to treatment with first line EGFR TKI, e.g. *T790M* mutation (where the EGFR TKI Osimertinib would be more appropriate).
  - ◆ Other genes of interest in targeted therapy include KRAS, the ALK-Ros translocation and c-Met.
- Immunotherapy, e.g. nivolumab: blockade of PDL1 action blocks the tumour cells' defence against the host immune response.

Lung cancer emergencies

- *Upper airway obstruction* may develop rapidly. Urgent transfer to a surgical unit for rigid bronchoscopy/debulking is required if clinically appropriate, taking into consideration fitness for further treatment and risk of transfer to a surgical centre.
- *SVCO obstruction* (➲ see Chapter 10, Superior vena cava obstruction, p. 336). Treat cancer, e.g. chemotherapy/radiotherapy and consider stenting.
- *Massive haemoptysis* requires rapid anaesthetic review and tilting the patient to decubitus position to point the bleeding point downwards to prevent soiling of the other lung.

Holistic care

- Smoking cessation should be offered to all patients as it can influence treatment outcomes.
- Symptom palliation, also described as 'best supportive care' can be as effective as active approaches in advanced stage lung cancer in influencing quality of life and survival.
- Opiates are given for pain and breathlessness and benzodiazepines for anxiety/restlessness.
- Other aspects may include physiotherapy, nutrition and optimising the patient's home environment.

Lung cancer screening

Large randomised trials have confirmed that lung cancer screening can reduce mortality by finding curable, early stage disease. Also known as 'Targeted Lung Health Checks', a nationwide implementation pilot commissioned by NHS England will invite 600,000 patients between 2019 and 2023.

Further reading

1. Lung cancer: diagnosis and management.NICE guideline [NG122]. Published date: March 2019. https://www.nice.org.uk/guidance/ng122

Rare lung disease

A rare lung disease is one that affects less than 1 in 2000 people and, although this comprises a small number of patients compared with other lung diseases, the burden on individual patients can be worse.

For key features of rare lung disease, see Table 11.3.

Thromboembolic disease and pulmonary hypertension

Pulmonary embolism and pulmonary hypertension (PH) both compromise right heart function. PE is usually an acute presentation, and is the leading cause of preventable hospital death. In contrast, PH is more commonly assessed in a subspecialist respiratory clinic.

The annual incidence of thromboembolic disease (TED) is 70–110 cases per 100,000. It encompasses deep vein thrombosis (DVT) and PE with a ratio of DVT:PE, 2.3:1.3. 50% are related to immobility, 30% idiopathic and remaining 20% secondary to cancer, surgery and trauma. 25–50% test +ve for a thrombophilia screen (➲ see Diagnosis, p. 367 and Table 11.4).

Pulmonary embolism

Pathogenesis

Pulmonary embolism results in sudden, partial or complete occlusion of the pulmonary circulation with impaired perfusion of lung segments and consequent hypoxia. Lung infarction, right heart strain and failure may ensue.

Risk factors

Virchow's triad is a useful aide memoire of risk factors:

- Venous stasis (e.g. immobility [hospitalisation, long haul flights], heart failure, malignancy).
- Hypercoagulable state (e.g. thrombophilia, dehydration, pregnancy).
- Vessel wall damage (e.g. surgery, trauma, inflammatory conditions).

Table 11.3 Key features of rare (orphan) lung diseases

	Pathogenesis	Clinical features	Associations	Diagnosis	Treatment
Amyloidosis	Due to abnormal protein folding there is accumulation of proteinaceous insoluble fibrils in the extracellular space. Can affect the lung parenchyma, larynx, lymph nodes, trachea and bronchi.	• Dyspnoea. • Cough. • Can be asymptomatic.	Bronchiectasis. Sjogren's syndrome. Plasmocytoma. Castleman tumours. Depends on subtype of amyloidosis (AA/AL).	• CXR/HRCT: solitary or multiple nodules or diffuse alveolar pattern. • Lung/lymph node biopsy: Congo red stain shows typical apple green birefringence. • ^{123}I-labelled scintigraphy localises radiolabelled serum amyloid P.	There are limited clinical trials so limited effective treatment. • Generalised AA/AL may benefit from chemotherapy/steroid therapy. • Localised AA/AL: may benefit from resection or laser therapy.
Pulmonary alveolar proteinosis	Abnormal surfactant clearance by macrophages leading to alveoli filling with proteinaceous material. There is failure of GMCSF (granulocyte-macrophage: CSF) signalling secondary to anti-GMCSF antibodies leading to macrophage dysfunction.	• Dyspnoea. • Cough. • Increased risk of infection due to macrophage dysfunction.		• CXR: bilateral consolidation. • HRCT: 'crazy paving' pattern. • Lung biopsy: periodic acid Schiff (PAS) positive. • 90% associated with anti-GMCSF antibodies in bronchoalveolar lavage (BAL). • Milky BAL fluid.	• Prognosis is variable with 1/3 going in to spontaneous remission and 1/3 progressing. • Symptomatic patients can be treated with whole lung lavage with 95% positive response.
Adult pulmonary Langerhans' cell histiocytosis (previously called histiocytosis X)	Infiltration of the lung with granulomatous organisation of Langerhans cells. Can affect lungs, bone, skin and the pituitary gland. Higher prevalence in smokers.	• 20–40 years old. • Exertional SOB. • Cough. • Pneumothorax. • Systemic symptoms. • 25% asymptomatic.	• Pulmonary hypertension. • Diabetes insipidus. • Lymphoma. • Lung cancer: smoking link.	• CXR: micronodular and reticular opacities with lower lobe sparing. • HRCT: disseminated nodules ± cavitation that can form cysts. • Lung biopsy: cytoplasmic Birkbeck granules on electron microscopy.	• Variable prognosis: median survival 12–13 years. • 50% improve spontaneously. • Steroids can be used, but its use is not validated. • Smoking cessation. • Lung transplant: but may reoccur.
Lymphangioleiomyomatosis	Proliferation of immature smooth muscle cells (lymphangioleiomyomatosis [LAM] cells) throughout the lungs, which leads to cyst formation.	• Women of childbearing age. • SOB. • Cough. • Haemoptysis. • Chylothorax. • Secondary pneumothorax.	• Angiomyolipoma of the kidney. • Tuberous sclerosis complex. • Pulmonary hypertension.	• CXR: hyperinflated, reticular shadowing. • HRCT: multiple round cysts. • Lung biopsy: cysts.	• Prognosis variable. • 70% are alive at 10 years. • No effective treatment. • Avoid oestrogens (HRT): seems to be hormone dependent. • Lung transplant.

Data from S Chapman et al. (2009) *Oxford Handbook of Respiratory Medicine*, Third Edition. Oxford, UK: Oxford University Press

Table 11.4 Assessment of clinical pretest probability

Modified Well's score	Pulmonary embolus rule out criteria (PERC) score
• Signs and Symptoms of DVT: Localised tenderness/leg > 3cm larger than other/asymmetrical pitting oedema/ superficial veins (3) • PE most/equally likely diagnosis (3) • Tachycardia (>100/min) (1.5) • 3 days immobility/surgery ≤ 4 weeks (1.5) • Previous DVT/PE (1.5) • Haemoptysis (1) • Malignancy (1) Wells > 4 suggests PE (28% incidence vs 3%) (1)	• Age >50 • Tachycardia (>100/min) • Hypoxia on room air (<95%) • Previous DVT/PE • Recent surgery/trauma • Haemoptysis • Unilateral swollen leg • Oestrogen therapy • ALL criteria absent gives PE probability <2% if pre-test probability low (<15%) (2)

(1) Reproduced with permission from: Wells P, Anderson D, Rodger M et al. Derivation of a simple clinical model to categorize patients probability of pulmonary embolism: increasing the models utility with the SimpliRED D-dimer. *Thrombosis and Haemostasis*, 2000; 83 (3): 416–420. Copyright © 2000, Rights Managed by Georg Thieme Verlag KG Stuttgart • New York. DOI: 10.1055/s-0037-1613830
(2) Reproduced with permission from Kline J. A. et al., Clinical criteria to prevent unnecessary diagnostic testing in emergency department patients with suspected pulmonary embolism. *Journal of Thrombosis and Haemostasis*, 2(8):1247–55. © 2004 International Society of Thrombosis and Haemostasis and John Wiley & Sons Ltd. https://doi.org/10.1111/j.1538-7836.2004.00790.x

Sepsis, oral contraceptive use (oestrogen exposure) and previous TED are additional risk factors. 25% of patients with a PE have no identifiable risk factor (termed 'unprovoked PEs').

Clinical features

- DVT: asymmetrical leg discomfort, swelling, oedema, discolouration and heat.
- PE: pleuritic chest pain, tachycardia, dyspnoea, syncope, sudden haemodynamic instability.

Diagnosis

Evidence-based literature supports the practice of determining the clinical pretest probability of pulmonary embolism before proceeding with diagnostic testing (Table 11.4). There are three validated systems: Modified Wells Scoring System, Revised Geneva Scoring System, and Pulmonary Embolism Rule Out Criteria (PERC).

- PE – NICE guidance also suggests using Wells score.
  - Geneva score includes age, heart rate > 100 bpm, PaO_2 and $PaCO_2$.
- Highest risk factors for PE:
  - Surgery: general or orthopaedic surgery.
  - Major trauma.
  - Thrombophilia: severe anti-thrombin or protein C or S deficiency, anti-phospholipid syndrome, factor V Leiden mutation homozygous.
- ECG changes (in a patient who has suffered a PE) include:
  - Non-specific: sinus tachycardia, anterior T wave inversion.
  - Evidence of right heart strain (massive PE) – classical S wave in lead 1, Q and T waves in lead 3 'S1Q3T3' pattern, tall R waves V1, right axis deviation, right bundle branch block (RBBB).
- D-dimers: degradation products of cross-linked fibrin. Raised levels are linked with thrombotic activity. High sensitivity (and so a useful rule-out test) in patients with a low pretest probability, but specificity can be < 50% with false positives in infection, inflammation, cancer, surgery and pregnancy.
- Doppler US: sensitivity higher for proximal DVT (versus distal), whole-leg USS is performed in high pretest probability or following positive d-dimer. If distal veins are difficult to visualise, repeat USS in 1/52 or perform *venography*.
- ECHO: may show a dilated, pressure-overloaded right ventricle with inappropriate bowing of the interventricular septum. A thrombus in the RV may also be seen.
- Radiological investigations include CTPA and VQ scan (➲ see Chapter 5, Case 12, p. 134).
  - CXR shows few specific signs: pulmonary oedema, cardiomegaly or 'prominent' pulmonary vessels.
  - CTPA remains the gold standard test.

- V:Q scanning – indications include:
  - certain stages of pregnancy;
  - low risk young patients with normal lungs;
  - contraindication to CTPA (e.g. high risk of contrast induced nephropathy).

Pregnancy and PE

➲ See Chapter 23, Venous thromboembolism and pulmonary embolism, p. 814.

Disease classification and prognosis

- DVT: there are three types – ascending (> 60% of cases), transfascial and descending (more common in pregnancy).
- PE: risk stratified according to haemodynamic status, presence of RV dysfunction (RVD) or myocardial injury.
  - High risk (or massive) PE: acute PE with sustained hypotension (SBP < 90 mmHg or drop ≥40 mmHg >15minutes).
  - Intermediate risk (or sub-massive) PE: presence of RVD or injury (e.g. troponin) in absence of hypotension.
  - Low risk PE: absence of hypotension, and absence of RVD or injury.
- High sensitivity troponin T has negative predictive value of 98% for adverse outcome.
- Without PE, DVT alone does not cause mortality, but 10–20% of patients will die secondary to related disease.

Complications

- Specific to PE:
  - Acute: haemodynamic instability, death.
  - Chronic: pulmonary arterial hypertension (if progresses to NYHA III to IV consider pulmonary thromboendarterectomy).
- Specific to DVT:
  - Acute: PE.
  - Chronic: post-thrombotic syndrome (50% of patients with DVT; treat with compression therapy), superficial thrombophlebitis, and venous hypertension ± secondary varices or ulcers.

Management

- Key treatment goals to control:
  - Thrombus progression and thereby risk of massive PE.
  - Risk of acute and chronic pulmonary and peripheral venous hypertension.
  - Relapsing disease.

Management of PE

- Heparin:
  - In cases with high suspicion of PE, it is usual to instigate anticoagulation with a low molecular weight heparin (LMWH), while awaiting the outcome of diagnostic tests.
  - Use LMWH or fondaparinux unless severe kidney disease, high risk of bleeding, >80 years or underweight, in which case unfractionated heparin (UFH) is preferable since it is readily reversible.
  - No routine measurement of anti-factor Xa levels (unless pregnant).
  - Continue heparin for at least 5 days and until INR > 2 for 2 consecutive days.
  - Long-term heparin is sometimes preferable, e.g. in cancer patients (rapid reversibility if require procedures or if bleeding events).
  - Heparin-induced thrombocytopenia: rapid drop in platelets to <50% of baseline value). Perform HIT antibody tests, stop heparin, replace with alternative anticoagulation. Avoid future exposure.

- Oral anticoagulants:
  - Commence on same day as heparin in haemodynamically stable patients.
  - Novel anticoagulants (NOVACs) such as rivaroxaban and dabigatran are alternatives that do not require monitoring. They are associated with a lower risk of intracranial bleed, but higher GI bleed risk.

For duration of anticoagulation in patients diagnosed with PE, see Table 11.5.

- Thrombolysis:
  - In a confirmed, life-threatening PE with the following findings the use of thrombolysis (e.g. IV alteplase 50 mg) may be justified (➲ see also Chapter 12, Shock [especially section Pulmonary embolus], p. 394 and Table 12.2):
    - Collapse.
    - Evidence of shock (increased lactate, hypotension).
    - Evidence of right heart strain (on ECG/ECHO/CTPA).
    - Evidence of myocardial injury (increased troponin).
- Cardiac arrest with suspected PE. Intra-vessel thrombolysis/clot retrieval or surgical embolectomy are used in some centres.
- Inferior vena cava (IVC) filters used for primary or secondary prevention (usually where anticoagulation is contraindicated).
- Patients should be monitored for chronic thromboembolic pulmonary hypertension, with an echocardiogram 1 year after PE (looking for RVD); may result in lifelong anticoagulation.
- *Contraindications for thrombolysis*: ➲ see Chapter 13, Acute medical management, p. 428.

Table 11.5 Duration of anticoagulation in patients diagnosed with PE

Scenario	Anticoagulation treatment
Provoked PE with temporary cause, e.g. fracture, long flight	3 months of warfarin (INR 2–3) or rivaroxaban.
Unprovoked PE	Usually longer duration (e.g. 6–12 months +) of anticoagulation (warfarin or rivaroxaban) after risk–benefit assessment.
Secondary to cancer	Low molecular weight heparin continued until cancer considered cured or at least 6 months.
Two or more episodes of PE regardless of underlying risk factors	Extended anticoagulation (no scheduled stop date).
Pregnant women with acute VTE	Low molecular weight heparin is continued until the end of pregnancy.

Data from NICE Clinical Knowledge Set: Pulmonary Embolism last revised in January 2015. https://cks.nice.org.uk/pulmonary-embolism; and C Kearon et al., 'Antithrombotic Therapy for VTE Disease: CHEST Guideline and Expert Panel Report', *Chest*, 149, 2, 2016, pp. 315–52.

Management of deep vein thrombosis

- 80–90% can be treated at home if low acute bleeding risk and full compliance.
- Oral anticoagulants:
  - Commence on same day as heparin in haemodynamically stable patients.
  - Continue heparin for at least 5 days or until INR > 2 for 2 consecutive days.
- Compression stockings advised, elevate leg when sitting, undergo regular exercise.
- Duration of anticoagulants:
  - 6 weeks if isolated calf vein DVT;
  - 3 months for femoro-popliteal DVT;
  - 6 months for massive DVT involving iliac vein or IVC.

Emerging prognostic markers and therapies

- Other biomarkers evolving as adverse prognostic markers, including H-FABP and GDF-15.
- The Pulmonary Embolism Thrombolysis Study (PEITHO): randomised patients to heparin ± tenecteplase based on positive troponin and evidence of RVD in patients with acute PE. There was a significant reduction in primary endpoint (all-cause mortality or haemodynamic collapse < 7days), but with a significant increase in number of strokes (2.4% versus 0.2%).
- The novel oral anticoagulants will likely supersede warfarin in the future.

Further reading

1. European Society of Cardiology (ESC) Guidelines on the management and diagnosis of acute pulmonary embolism. *Eur Heart J*. 2014;35(43):3033–73.
2. NICE. Venous thromboembolic diseases: diagnosis, management and thrombophilia testing. Clinical guideline CG144, 2013. https://www.nice.org.uk/guidance/cg144.
3. Konstantinides S, Goldhaber SZ. Pulmonary embolism: risk assessment and management. *Eur Heart J*. 2012;22:3014–22.
4. British Thoracic Society guidelines for the management of suspected acute pulmonary embolism. *Thorax* 2003;58(6):470.

Pulmonary hypertension

Pulmonary hypertension refers to increased pressure in the pulmonary arteries due to elevation in the pulmonary arteries, or secondary to rises in pressure in the pulmonary venous and pulmonary capillary system. It is defined by a mean pulmonary arterial pressure (mPAP)> 25 mmHg at rest, (normal mPAP is <20 mmHg).

PH is divided into the following subtypes:

- Group 1: Pulmonary arterial hypertension (PAH): idiopathic or related to another underlying condition, e.g. systemic sclerosis.
- Group 2: PH relating to left-sided heart disease.
- Group 3: PH relating to lung disease or hypoxia, e.g. pulmonary fibrosis.
- Group 4: Chronic thromboembolic PH.
- Group 5: Unknown or multifactorial.
- Unresolved thrombus occurs in 0.5–4% of cases of PE resulting in chronic thromboembolic pulmonary hypertension (CTEPH).
- Most other causes are due to increased *resistance* in the pulmonary vascular bed and an imbalance of vasoactive mediators including endothelin 1, prostacyclins and nitric oxide.
- The 'obstructed' right ventricular outflow tract leads to increased 'afterload' and right heart failure.
- PH in cardiac disease arises from raised left atrial pressure.
- In lung disease, PH commonly results from hypoxic vasoconstriction or damage to lung vasculature.
- PH associated with CTD can arise from damaged lung architecture, chronic hypoxaemia and small vessel obstructive vasculopathy.
- Up to 40% of patients with idiopathic PAH (IPAH) have a mutation in BMPR2 (~20% of carriers develop PH).

Clinical features

Dyspnoea may be acute in onset, with subsequent progression, and is usually accompanied by pleuritic pain. Other cardiac symptoms include exertional dizziness, syncope, angina and palpitations.

Examination findings include:

- Right-sided cardiac failure or functional tricuspid regurgitation, e.g. elevated jugular venous pulse (JVP), ankle oedema and ascites.

- Loud, palpable P2 and right ventricular heave.
- Cyanosis.
- Fine end inspiratory crackles of pulmonary fibrosis.
- Underlying aetiology:
  - Systemic sclerosis (e.g. tightening of skin of face and hands [sclerodactyly], Raynaud's phenomena ± digital amputation or gangrenous infarction), or other rheumatological joint involvement.

Diagnosis of pulmonary hypertension

A detailed history and examination is required to reveal possible underlying aetiology and guide appropriate testing.

- Blood tests:
  - clotting studies;
  - auto-antibodies (e.g. anti-nuclear antibodies [ANA], anti-dsDNA);
  - iron studies;
  - thyroid function tests (TFT);
  - sickle screen;
  - HIV testing;
  - brain natriuretic peptide (BNP)/N-terminal brain natriuretic peptide (nt-BNP).
- Chest radiography:
  - pulmonary oedema;
  - cardiomegaly or 'prominent' pulmonary vessels;
  - 'pruning' (rapidly tapering diameter) of the pulmonary vessels.
- ECG:
  - 'right heart strain' pattern with right axis deviation and prominent R waves.
- Lung function testing:
  - decreased 'transfer factor' (± restrictive picture if underlying fibrosis) suggests PH, rather than a parenchymal/airways pathology.
- Transthoracic echo (TTE):
  - 'right ventricular systolic pressure' estimates 'peak' pulmonary pressures.
- Right heart catheterization:
  - Gold standard investigation (mPAP ≥ 25 mmHg is diagnostic).
  - Pulmonary pressures, cardiac output/index, right atrial pressure, pulmonary vascular resistance/ pulmonary artery saturations and pulmonary artery wedge pressure are assessed.
- Further investigations:
  - 6-minute walk distance (6MWD) has a prognostic role.
  - Overnight sleep oximetry is a screening test for a sleep-related cause (e.g. OSA).

Management of pulmonary hypertension

Patients with PH should be managed at a dedicated National Pulmonary Hypertension Centre.

Medical therapies

- Vasodilator therapy: calcium channel blockers; infused or nebulised prostanoids (e.g. iloprost or treprostinil); endothelin receptor antagonists (e.g. bosentan); phosphodiesterase-5 (PDE-5) inhibitors (sildenafil). These therapies have significantly improved mortality and symptoms.
- Warfarin is used in CTEPH and IPAH, but its benefit in other forms of PH is less clear.
- Diuretics, digoxin and long-term oxygen therapy (LTOT).
- Annual influenza vaccination.

Surgical options

- Pulmonary endarterectomy: improves symptoms, haemodynamics and survival.
- Lung transplant for severe PAH (5-year survival 50%).

Complications of pulmonary hypertension

- Right heart failure is a major complication and may manifest as worsening dyspnoea or deterioration in exercise tolerance.
- PH carries an increased risk of thromboembolic events.
- Pregnancy is associated with a high mortality in PH (17–33%) and contraceptive advice should be given.

Prognosis

- Prognosis varies with underlying diagnosis:
  - IPAH: median survival of 5 years achievable with treatment; or if untreated median survival is 2.8 years.
  - Systemic sclerosis: carries a particularly poor prognosis.

Further reading

1. ESC/ERS Guidelines for the diagnosis and treatment of pulmonary hypertension *Eur Heart J*. 2016;37:67–119.

Pulmonary vasculitis and pulmonary eosinophilias

Pulmonary vasculitis and eosinophilia are rare, but command high morbidity and mortality. Diagnosis can be challenging, but should be considered with unusual or non-resolving presentations, particularly when systemic features suggest an associated CTD.

Pathogenesis

- Inflammatory cells, blood and exudate infiltrate the alveolar spaces to cause a diffuse alveolar haemorrhage (DAH).
- Pathological features described include true pulmonary capillaritis, but also diffuse alveolar damage and DAH (without other damage).
- 40% of anti-neutrophil cytoplasmic antibodies (ANCA)-associated vasculitis (AAV) present with DAH.
- Systemic vasculitis can be classified by vessel size affected (➲ see Chapter 20, Vasculitis, p. 735).

ANCA-associated vasculitis

ANCA-associated vasculitis is a collective term for ANCA-associated vasculitides, which are historically known as Wegener's granulomatosis (granulomatosis with polyangiitis [GPA]; ➲ see Chapter 20, Granulomatosis with polyangiitis (previously Wegner's granulomatosis), p. 736) and Churg–Strauss syndromes (eosinophilic granulomatosis with polyangiitis (EGPA; ➲ see Chapter 20, Eosinophilic granulomatosis with polyangiitis (previously Churg– Strauss syndrome), p. 735).

GPA is caused by C-ANCA (against proteinase 3 [PR3]), which predominantly affects the upper airways. EGPA is caused by P-ANCA (against neutrophil myeloperoxidase [MPO]), which commonly presents with an evolving asthma that later develops eosinophilia and subsequently vasculitis. Granulomata-forming, ANCA can cause a pulmonary renal vasculitis syndrome (➲ see Chapter 16, Systemic vasculitis and the kidney, p. 575).

Goodpasture's syndrome

Causes alveolar haemorrhage resulting from anti-glomerular basement membrane (GBM) antibodies that can also cause crescentic glomerulonephritis (➲ see Chapter 16, Systemic vasculitis and the kidney, p. 575).

Other diseases associated with pulmonary vasculitis/diffuse alveolar haemorrhage

Other diseases associated with pulmonary vasculitis/DAH include SLE, SSc, mixed CTD (MCTD), rheumatoid arthritis, Henoch Schonlein purpura, cryoglobuliaemia and HIV.

Pulmonary eosinophilia

Pulmonary eosinophilia are a heterogenous group of diseases (see Box 11.2) associated with eosinophilic alveolar infiltrates and peripheral eosinophilias. Pulmonary infiltrates in peripheral eosinophilia can be

Box 11.2 Causes of a pulmonary eosinophilia

- Parasitaemia, e.g. helminthic infections.
- Resolving pneumonia.
- Hydatid disease.
- Sarcoidosis.
- Polyarteritis nodosa.
- ABPA.
- EGPA.
- Acute and chronic eosinophilic pneumonia.

transient, chronic and even migratory (Loffler's syndrome) as seen in response to organisms such as *Wuchereria bancrofti* and *Ascaris lumbricoides*.

Eosinophilia localisation varies with the parasite/disease process. Some are associated with an 'asthmatic picture' as in EGPA.

Clinical features

- Severe haemoptysis is recognized, but is often absent.
- More subtle symptoms may include cough, dyspnoea, pleuritic pain.
- Clinical examination may reveal evidence of underlying extra thoracic and thoracic disease, e.g. purpuric rash, joint pain/inflammation.
- Pulmonary vasculitis should be considered in any persistent, aggressive or unusual presentation of pneumonia.

Diagnosis

Blood tests

- FBC.
- Inflammatory markers suggestive of co-existent or superadded infection.
- U&E.
- Coagulation studies (for alternative causes of pulmonary haemorrhage).
- A blood film (blood dyscrasias).
- Auto-antibodies:
  - ANCA and if positive anti-MPO or anti-PR3 (AAV).
  - ANA ± anti-dsDNA/centromere/Scl-7070/C1q/Jo1/Ro and La/antiphospholipid antibodies (APLA).
  - RF.
  - IgE and aspergillus precipitins (aspergillosis).

Urine

- Red cell casts.

Radiology

- *CXR*: alveolar infiltrates, which can be migratory or transient.
- *CT thorax*: diffuse ground glass shadowing of alveolar inflammation that may be accompanied by airspace opacification secondary to haemorrhage.

Prognosis

Mortality in systemic vasculitis is high and reflects an often aggressive, inflammatory infiltration of the lungs, which may also include the kidneys and other organs. Dialysis at presentation for such diseases is a poor prognostic sign.

Management

The immediate priority is to stabilise the patient and ensure early assessment by the appropriate specialist teams including Rheumatology and Critical Care.

Asphyxia/respiratory compromise commonly presents a more immediate threat to life than blood loss, and for this reason patients may require early respiratory support.

- *AAV*: severe disease is usually treated with pulsed IV cyclophosphamide and high-dose methylprednisolone. Plasma exchange is used for renal disease but its role in pulmonary disease is less clear.
- Remission can be sustained with less aggressive agents, such as azathioprine. Methotrexate can be used as an alternative in less severe renal disease.
- *Goodpasture's syndrome*: corticosteroids and pulsed cyclophosphamide alongside plasmapheresis/albumin. Treatment may be continued until anti-GBM is undetectable, followed by tapering corticosteroids then cyclophosphamide or similar agent.
- *Drug induced vasculitis*: stop offending drug, some centres recommend corticosteroids.
- *Pulmonary eosinophilia*: identify and treat underlying condition and consider immunosuppressive treatment (corticosteroid). Advise smoking cessation. Parasitic infections require appropriate anti-microbial agent.

References

1. Rhee CK, Min KH, Yim NY, et al. Clinical characteristics and corticosteroid treatment of acute eosinophilic pneumonia. *Eur Resp J*. 2013; 41(2):402–9.
2. Lee RW, D'Cruz DP. Pulmonary renal vasculitis syndromes. *Autoimmunity Rev*. 2010; 9(10):657–60.

Tuberculosis

Pathogenesis and Epidemiology; ➲ see Chapter 8, Tuberculosis, p. 260.

Clinical features of pulmonary tuberculosis

- Chronic productive cough.
- Haemoptysis.
- Fever.
- Weight loss.
- Night sweats.
- Respiratory examination:
  - Crackles and reduced breath sounds, usually in the upper lobes.
  - Lower zone dullness and decreased percussion note related to pleural effusion.
- Presence of a BCG scar should be sought.

Investigations

Blood tests

- Inflammatory markers (FBC and CRP).
- LFTs, U&Es (baseline required before treatment).
- Calcium and vitamin D levels: vitamin D plays an important role in the host response against TB.
- HIV test: latent TB is more likely to be activated and more severe in presentation.

Sputum culture

- Sputum culture is the gold standard investigation (➲ see Chapter 8, Specimen testing, p. 262 and Specimens, p. 263). Acid-fast bacilli (AFB) are available within hours and confirms need for isolation. Cultures take up to 6–8 weeks and to determine full anti-mycobacterial sensitivities. If AFB are smear negative, treatment based on a clinical diagnosis may be necessary while awaiting culture results. A history of close contacts with active TB is helpful, as is identification of necrotising granulomas from lymph node or extra-pulmonary biopsy specimens.

Radiology

- *CXR* is indicated in all cases; upper zone abnormalities.
- Cavitation or the characteristic 'tree-in-bud' sign.
- Pleural effusions.
- Apical fibrosis indicative of old TB.

Further investigations

- *Bronchoscopy* is employed in cases where TB culture cannot be confirmed by sputum, but clinical suspicion is high, particularly where immunocompromise raises the possibility of other co-infections. Necrotising granulomas from EBUS are strongly suggestive of TB.
- *Induced sputum* can be an effective and less invasive means of obtaining sputum where experience is available.
- *Pleural fluid sampling*:
  - Often an exudate.
  - Organisms rarely cultured.
  - Usually lymphocytic.
  - Pleural adenosine deaminase (ADA), a lymphocytic enzyme, is often increased.
- *Pleural biopsy*:
  - High diagnostic yield.
  - Biopsy using Abrams needle, thoracoscopic approach or radiologically guided techniques (e.g. tru-cut biopsy).
- *Rapid diagnostic tools:*
  - 'Xpert' is a rapid (2 hours), point-of-care mycobacterium tuberculosis (MTB)/resistance to rifampicin (RIF) assay, offering diagnosis from sputum in 2 hours, as well as information on rifampicin resistance. This is of particular value for predicting multidrug resistance in high prevalence areas and heralds a new way of diagnosing TB.

Management of pulmonary tuberculosis

- Hospital admission is not necessary for the majority of patients unless they are at risk of deterioration, MDR-TB or loss to follow-up.
- A side room with negative pressure facilities is preferable to minimise the risk of spread to the open ward (essential for MDR-TB).
- Masks should be worn if suspected to be smear positive, particularly if MDR-TB is suspected or aerosol generating procedures are being performed (e.g. chest physiotherapy, induced sputum or bronchoscopy).

Unless resistant organisms are suspected, active TB is treated according to WHO guidance with quadruple therapy:

- *R*ifampicin (6 months).
- *I*soniazid (6 months).
- *P*yrazinamide (2 months).
- *E*thambutol (2 months).

Drugs used in the treatment of TB; ➲ see Table 8.8.

Multi-drug resistant tuberculosis

- In 2013, 7% of UK cases of TB were resistant to first-line drugs.
- Resistance arises through selection of resistant strains through inappropriate or incomplete treatment.
- *MDR-TB:* resistant to at least the two most effective anti-TB drugs isoniazid and rifampicin.
- *Extensively drug resistant (XDR) TB*: resistance to isoniazid and rifampicin and additionally a fluoroquinolone and any second line injectable agent (e.g. amikacin or capreomycin).

Surgical approaches

Older patients may have clinical evidence of historical treatments:

- Thoracoplasty: marked volume loss on the affected side.
- Phrenic nerve crush: short supraclavicular fossa scar.
- Plombage: an inert substance (e.g. plastic balls) inserted into the pleural space, thus compressing the adjacent lung.

Latent tuberculosis

Screening is routinely performed in:

- New entrants from areas of high endemicity.
- Close contacts (e.g. >12 hours/day) of newly diagnosed cases.
- Health care workers.
- Those with a significant risk of reactivation (e.g. receiving immunomodulatory therapy such as infliximab).

Tuberculosis screening tests for latent TB

➲ See Chapter 8, Latent TB infection, p. 263.

Management

Standard regime includes:

- Isoniazid for 6 months.
- Combination of rifampicin and isoniazid (given as Rifinah®) for 3 months.
- Appropriate treatment group: 16–35-year-olds who are TST or IGRA positive without a positive sputum smear or other feature of active TB.

References

1. NICE. Tuberculosis: updated 2016. https://www.nice.org.uk/guidance/ng33.
2. World Health Organisation – Global TB Report 2018. http://www.who.int/tb/publications/global_report/en/.

Pulmonary function tests

Pulmonary function testing is a widely available diagnostic tool. Pulmonary function tests (PFTs) are cheap, easy to perform and non-invasive with good inter-operator reproducibility.

Indications

- Investigation of respiratory symptoms (e.g. cough, dyspnoea).
- Monitoring respiratory disease (progression or treatment response).
- Screening for respiratory complications, e.g. in CTD or neuromuscular disease or in 'at-risk' populations, e.g. pneumotoxic chemotherapy or occupational toxin exposure.
- Pre-operative assessment.
- Post-lung transplant surveillance.

Contraindications

- Recent MI (4–6 weeks).
- Unstable angina.
- Recent thoracic/abdominal/ophthalmic surgery.
- Aortic aneurysm.
- Current pneumothorax.
- Active tuberculosis; wait until risk of contagion has subsided or take measures to avoid cross-contamination.

Spirometry

- Forced vital capacity (FVC): from full inspiration patient exhales as long and as forcefully as possible.
- Forced expiratory volume in 1 second (FEV1): amount of air forcibly exhaled in 1 second.
- Total lung capacity (TLC): Measured using helium dilution or body plethysmography.
- Functional residual capacity (FRC): derived by displacement of air from a closed box (change in pressure by Boyle's Law), within which the patient sits. FRC is the remaining volume at the end of a normal expiratory effort.
- Residual volume is the remaining volume after a maximal forced expiratory effort (~500 mL). This increases when there is gas trapping. Also expressed as percentage of predicted TLC.
- Diffusion capacity (DLCO): calculated by uptake of carbon monoxide (CO) by haemoglobin and describes the diffusion of alveolar gases into the pulmonary capillary vasculature as determined by the area.
- Transfer factor (KCO): the rate constant (K) for alveolar-capillary carbon monoxide (CO) transfer (= permeability factor, kCO) corrects for alveolar volume.

For lung volumes and capacities, see Figure 11.3.

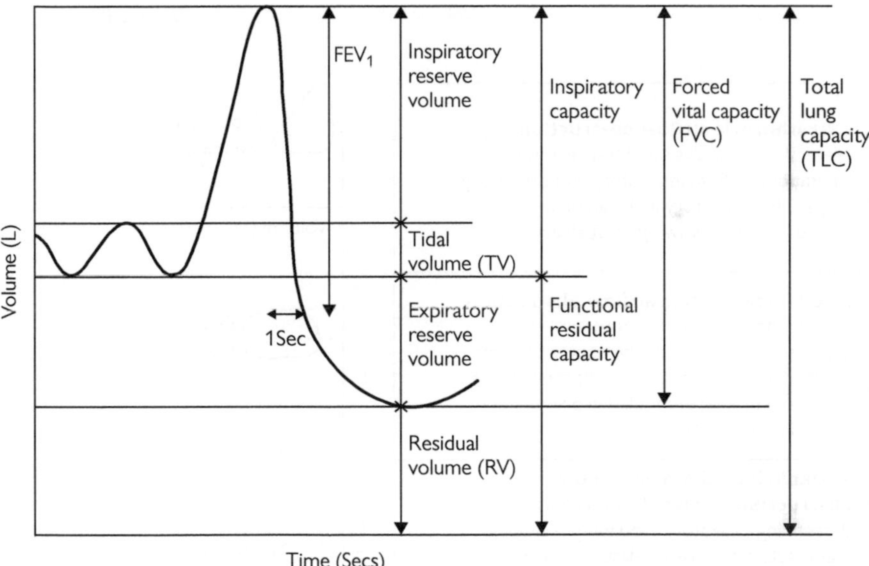

Figure 11.3 Lung volumes and capacities.

Reproduced with permission from Bessant R. *The Pocketbook for PACES*. Oxford: OUP. Copyright © 2012 Oxford University Press. Reproduced with permission of the Licensor through PLSclear.

Obstructive vs restrictive lung disease (FEV1/FVC)

- *Obstructive patterns* (e.g. asthma/COPD) compromise airway flow greater than elastic recoil and, hence, disproportionately reduce FEV1 compared with FVC (FEV1/FVC <0.7).
- *Restrictive lung diseases* show reduction in spirometry values with (FEV1/FVC >0.7), e.g. pulmonary fibrosis, kyphosis.
- *Emphysema:* Alveolar volume (VA) is low and leads to incomplete gas mixing (inspired/residual volume). KCO is also low (loss of alveolar-capillary surface) with reduced transfer factor for carbon monoxide (TLCO).

Flow volume loops

Allows visual assessment of inspiratory and expiratory effort – the inspiratory or expiratory limbs reflect particular presentations:

- In restrictive defects the loops tend to be smaller in a linear pattern.
- Obstructive problems tend to be more concave (with sagging of the expiratory loop) and influenced by the location of the obstruction.

For flow volume loops, see Figure 11.4.

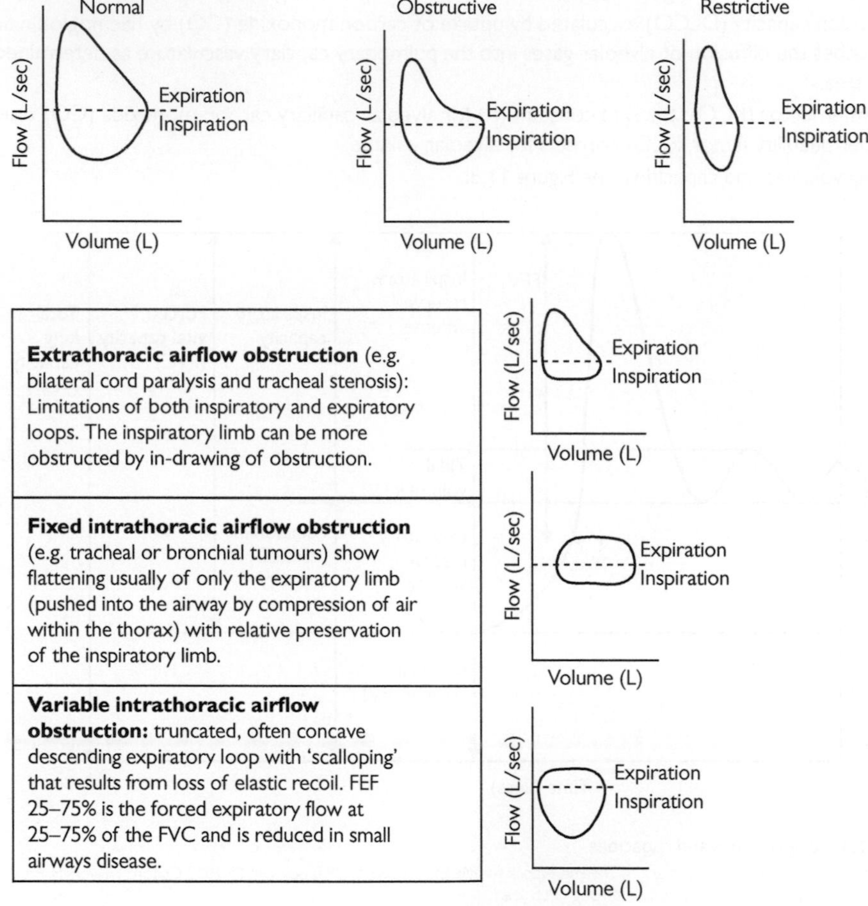

Figure 11.4 Flow volume loops.

Respiratory muscle testing

FVC is also reduced in neuromuscular diseases (e.g. Guillain–Barré syndrome, MND). Reduced FVC can indicate diaphragm weakness when measured supine.

Maximal inspiratory and expiratory pressures (MIP and MEP) are a more accurate test of respiratory muscle function.

For characteristic findings of lung function testing in disease states, see Table 11.6.

Table 11.6 Characteristic findings of lung function testing in disease states

Picture	Description	PFT values	Diseases
Mechanical/chest wall	E.g. incomplete expansion.	Low FVC, low alveolar volume (VA) associated with elevated KCO (TLCO falls by only 3% per 10% fall in VA).	Neuromuscular disease. Kyphoscoliosis. Obesity. Pleural effusion or a poorly performed test.
Diffuse loss of alveolar units	E.g. those affected by disease process (remaining lung also affected).	Low VA, low to normal KCO and a markedly reduce TLCO.	Diffuse fibrosis (IPF, CTD, pneumoconiosis). Alveolar infiltrates (inflammatory). Non-specific interstitial pneumonia (NSIP) PCP. Cardiovascular disease (pulmonary oedema, cardiac failure)
Discrete loss of alveolar units	Loss of a whole or part lung/lobe with preservation of remaining normal lung.	Low VA, but KCO slightly increased as blood flow diverted: TLCO falls relatively less than VA (but much more than in incomplete expansion – cf. above).	Surgical resection (lobectomy/ pneumonectomy). Local destruction (TB/ bronchiectasis). Localised infiltrate (sarcoidosis).
Pulmonary vascular disorders		Decreased KCO (with proportionally reduced TLCO) with normal or near normal VA.	PAH. CTEPH. Vasculitis. Sickle cell disease. Hepatopulmonary syndrome.
Increased pulmonary blood volume		Increases KCO and TLCO.	High cardiac output or left to right shunt.
Alveolar haemorrhage		VA mildly reduced by alveolar filling of blood. Gives markedly increased KCO (150% or 30% above baseline) as CO reacts with extravascular Hb. KCO returns to baseline 24 hours after haemorrhage has ceased – take care to correct to Hb.	Anti-GBM. Vasculitis. SLE. Idiopathic haemosiderosis.

Data from Fitting W. 'Transfer factor for carbon monoxide: a glance behind the scenes'. *Swiss Medical Weekly*, (2004) Jul 24;134(29–30):413–8.

Further reading

1. Moore V. Spirometry: Step by Step ERS. *Breathe J*. 2012;8:232–40.
2. Hancox, R, Whyte K. *McGraw-Hill's Pocket Guide to Lung Function Tests*, 2nd edn. Lance Medical, 2006.
3. Fitting W. Transfer factor for carbon monoxide: a glance behind the scenes *Swiss Med Wkly*. 2004;134(29–30):413–18.
4. Ranu H. *et al*. Pulmonary function tests. *Ulster Med J*. 2011;80(2):84–90.
5. Stanojevic. The Global Lung Function Initiative: dispelling some myths of lung function test interpretation. https://breathe.ersjournals.com/content/9/6/462.

Pneumothorax and pleural effusions

Diseases of the pleura affect over 3000 people per 1 million population each year. Pneumothorax and pleural effusions are the most common manifestations of pleural disease and may have specific disease associations.

Pathogenesis of pleural effusions

- Normal pleural fluid production is ~0.15 mL/kg/day allowing close apposition and frictionless interaction between the visceral and parietal pleura.
- Diseases of either pleural membrane or underlying structures can compromise production or drainage of pleural fluid leading to an effusion.
- Infection, inflammation and cancer result in loss of protein into the pleural space (an exudate), while in cardiac or renal failure, a transudate is more common.

Pathogenesis of pneumothoraces

- These arise most commonly from sub-pleural bullae of unknown aetiology, which may relate to an inflammatory response leading to a protease to anti-protease imbalance, which can be exacerbated by smoking.
- Bullae result in communication between airways and pleural space leading to escape of air during inspiration into the pleural space with lung collapse.
- Pneumothoraces typically occur in tall, young males with a low BMI.
- Primary pneumothoraces occur where no underlying pulmonary pathology is apparent.
- Secondary pneumothorax infers underlying pulmonary pathology, e.g. emphysema.
- Tension pneumothorax is a respiratory emergency and occurs where air escapes into the pleura, but cannot return leading to escalating pleural pressures, displacement of the lungs and heart, and eventually cardiac compromise.
- The risk in smokers is increased by up to 20-fold in a dosage-dependent manner.
- COPD and *Pneumocystis carinii* are also recognised risk factors for 'secondary pneumothorax'.

Clinical features

Pneumothoraces present acutely with pleuritic chest pain and breathlessness. In contrast, pleural effusions usually present chronically with accompanying symptoms reflecting fluid overload or indicative of underlying pathology of the pleura itself, such as infection or malignancy.

A comparison of the clinical features of pleural effusion and pneumothorax are given in Table 11.7.

Table 11.7 Comparison of the clinical features of pleural effusion and pneumothorax

Signs	Pleural effusion	Pneumothorax
Chest expansion	Reduced	Reduced
Percussion	Stony dullness	Hyper-resonance
Bronchial breathing	Above level of pleural effusion	Not present
Mediastinal shift	Away from the effusion if large	Away from the pneumothorax if large or tension pneumothorax
Cardiac compromise	Not present	Assess for tension pneumothorax

Diagnosis

Chest radiograph

- Pleural effusion:
  - Blunted costophrenic angles with a meniscus (note, in contrast, a flat fluid–air transition suggests hydropneumothorax).
  - Additional signs may suggest underlying pathology (e.g. tumours, consolidation or upper lobe disease).

- Pneumothorax:
  - Often a thin line can be seen with lung markings visible only on one side of this.
  - Look for unexpectedly lucent areas of thorax, particularly under the first rib/clavicle where easily concealed.
  - A supine chest radiograph may show a 'deep sulcus sign' (where the costophrenic recess is accentuated).
  - The size of a pneumothorax is assessed by measuring the distance between the pleura and chest wall at the level of the hilum.

Pleural ultrasound

- Gold-standard investigation for pleural disease, both for diagnostic imaging and safe pleural sampling and drainage.
- Vital organs can be imaged to avoid damage to viscera.
- Used for pleural effusions but can also identify pleural thickening and pneumothorax.

Pleural aspirate/'tap' (thoracocentesis)

- Under US guidance. Diagnostic pleural fluid samples should be sent for biochemistry (protein/LDH), cytology and culture in addition to serum LDH (see Table 11.8).

Light's criteria are useful to help distinguish between transudates and exudates. The presence of ≥1 of the following is suggestive of an exudate:

- Pleural:serum protein ratio > 0.5;
- Pleural:serum LDH > 0.6; or
- Pleural:serum LDH > 0.66 ULN.

Table 11.8 Typical characteristics of pleural effusions

Type	Protein	Pleural:serum protein ratio	Pleural:serum LDH ratio	Glucose	pH	Appearance
Transudates, e.g. CCF, renal failure, fluid overload	<30	<0.5	<0.6 *or* <0.66 ULN	Normal/ low	7.3–7.45	Straw colour, clear
Exudates, e.g. pleurisy/para-pneumonic	>30	>0.5	>0.6 *or* >0.66 ULN	Low	If low, as for Empyema	Straw colour/ turbulent
Empyema	>30	>0.5	>0.6 *or* >0.66 ULN	Low	Low. Drain if <7.2	Purulent ± odorous.
Rheumatoid effusion	>30	>0.5	>0.6 *or* >0.66 ULN	V. low	7.3–7.45	Yellow/green
Tuberculosis	>30: often higher	>0.5	>0.6 *or* >0.66 ULN	Low	7.3–7.45	Straw colour ± cloudy/ bloody
Malignancy	>30	>0.5	>0.6 *or* >0.66 ULN Very high (suggestive of lymphoma)	Low	7.3–7.45	Blood-stained

ULN, upper limit of normal. Data from Light RW, Macgregor MI, Luchsinger PC, Ball WC (1972). 'Pleural effusions: the diagnostic separation of transudates and exudates'. *Annals of Internal Medicine*, 77 (4): 507–13. doi:10.7326/0003-4819-77-4-507.

Thoracoscopy

Video assisted thoracoscopic surgery (VATS) or 'medical' thoracoscopy allow visualisation of the pleura for procedures such as biopsy, drainage and pleurodesis.

Pleural biopsy

Pleural biopsy may be performed at time of thoracoscopy or under US or CT guidance. If high suspicion of TB a blind pleural biopsy with an Abrams needle may be considered, although image-guided techniques are now favoured.

Management of pneumothorax

- Size will influence decision to aspirate or drain.
- Small pneumothoraces with <2 cm rim at the level of the hilum may resolve spontaneously in comparison with larger pneumothoraces.
- Secondary pneumothoraces are less likely to resolve with simple aspiration.
- The BTS guidelines clearly defines how pneumothoraces should be managed (see Figure 11.5) (1).
- Pneumothoraces commonly result in hospitalisation for several days
- In-patient surgical referral maybe required if no resolution or recurrence; open thoracotomy and pleurectomy remains the procedure with the lowest recurrence rate. VATS with pleurectomy and pleural abrasion is better tolerated, but has a higher recurrence rate.
- Uncomplicated cases can respond well to simple aspiration.

Management of pleural effusion

- These are often managed in outpatient clinics after a diagnostic aspirate.
- Transudates are most often managed conservatively, with correction of fluid overload and treatment of cardiac/renal failure.
- Exudates require careful diagnosis of underlying infection or cancer, and either definitive treatment of the cause or palliation (e.g. ~1.5 L therapeutic needle aspirate) as appropriate. Therapeutic aspiration may also be useful while awaiting a more definitive thoracoscopy.
- Pleurodesis uses talc insufflation (thoracoscopic) or talc slurry (via a chest drain) to cause an inflammatory reaction that fuses the pleura to limit further fluid accumulation. This causes considerable discomfort and requires analgesia. An in-dwelling semi-permanent drain may be a preferable option.

Complications

- Para-pneumonic effusions may progress to empyema ± permanent pleural scarring and adhesions, loculations or trapped lung.
- Pneumothorax reoccurs in approximately one-third of cases, most within 6 months to 2 years.
- Pleural procedures have a significant risk of injury to underlying lung/vital organs. In 2008 the National Patient Safety Agency (NPSA) recognised a high rate of severe and fatal complications arising from chest drain insertion which has led to widespread implementation of US-guided drain insertion (2).

References

1. Maskell N, on behalf of the British Thoracic Society Pleural Disease Guideline Group. British Thoracic Society Pleural Disease Guidelines – 2010 update. *Thorax*. 2010;65(8):667–9.
2. National Patient Safety Agency Rapid Response Report 1065 – Chest drain insertion. 2008. http://www.nrls.npsa.nhs.uk/resources/entryid45=59887.

Further reading

1. Miserocchi G. Physiology and pathophysiology of pleural fluid turnover. *Eur Resp J*. 1997;10(1):219–25.
2. Sahn SA, Heffner JE. Spontaneous pneumothorax. *N Engl J Med*. 2000;342:868–74.

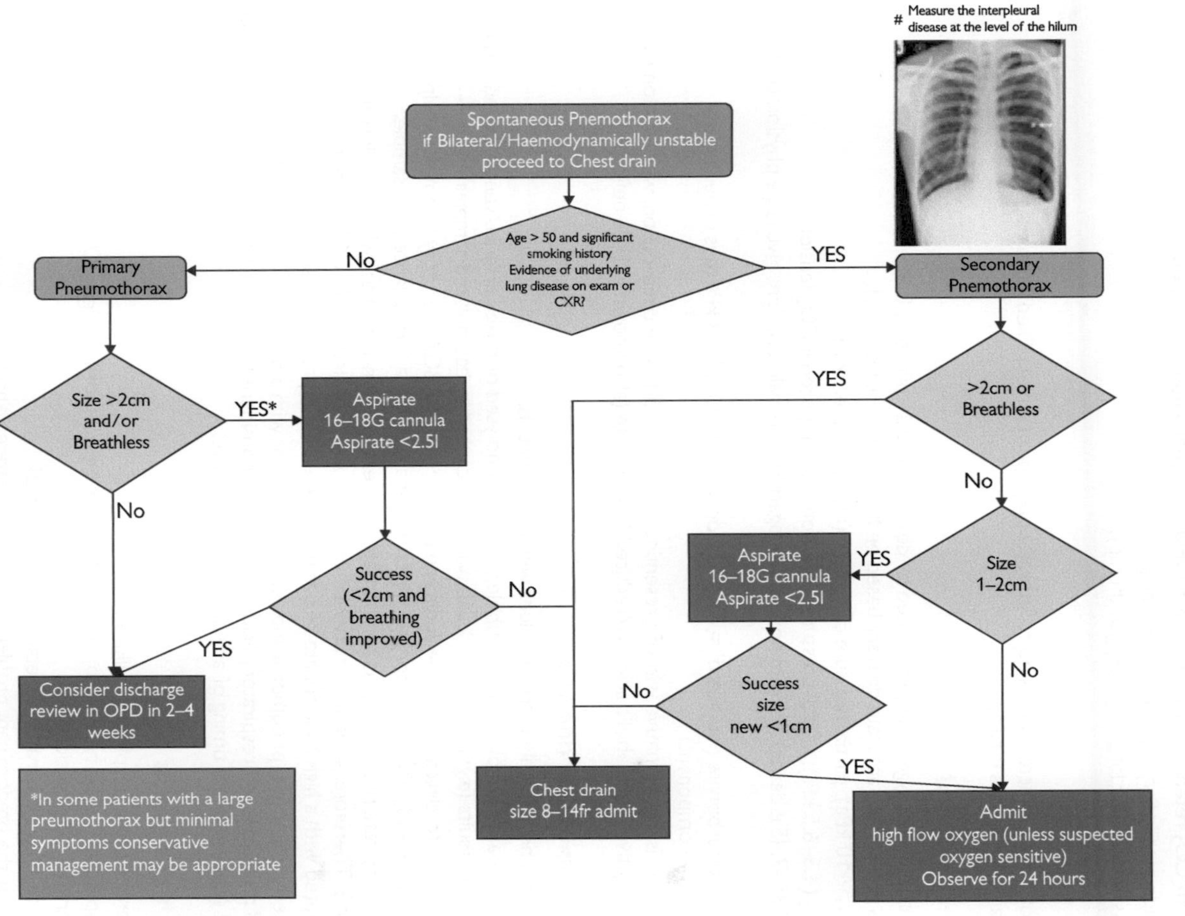

Figure 11.5 Management of spontaneous pneumothorax.

Reproduced from *Thorax*, Hooper C. et al. on behalf of the BTS Pleural Guideline Group. Investigation of a unilateral pleural effusion in adults: British Thoracic Society pleural disease guideline 2010. 65(Suppl. 2):ii4–ii17. Copyright © 2010, Published by the BMJ Publishing Group Limited. http://dx.dci.org/10.1136/thx.2010.136978. With permission from BMJ Publishing Group Ltd.

Arterial blood gas analysis

Indications

- Severe or unexplained hypoxia, e.g. in pneumonia or pulmonary embolus.
- Differentiate type 1 or 2 respiratory failure.
- Confirm CO_2 retention/narcosis (e.g. COPD, hypoventilation, exhaustion).
- To guide respiratory support and weaning.
- Assessing need for long-term oxygen therapy.

Contraindications

- Do not sample where there is no collateral supply (perform modified Allen's test) or if there is a local arterio-venous fistula.

Key definitions and terms

- FiO_2: delivered oxygen – approximated by device, e.g. 0.21 (air) to 0.8 (non-rebreathe). 'Venturi' masks allow more accurate delivery based on flow (Bernoulli principle).
- PaO_2 (>~10 kPa): partial pressure of oxygen (arterial O_2 tension).
- $PaCO_2$ (4.5–6.5 kPa): partial pressure of carbon dioxide (arterial CO_2 tension).
- pH (7.35–7.45): deviations from normal are logarithmic (small variations give large physiological changes).
- Standard bicarbonate ('standard' = adjusted for normal CO_2 of 5.3 kPa thus excluding any respiratory component).
- *Base excess* is an alternative way of presenting metabolic acid/base contribution, which becomes more negative in metabolic acidosis/reduced bicarbonate (also known as base deficit).

Important points for analysis

- Compare unexpectedly extreme values with clinical details.
- Poorly prepared samples, e.g. air bubbles, clots, haemolysed or mixed arterial/venous blood can give unreliable results (e.g. hypo/hyperkalaemia can be caused by haemolysed samples).
- Comparison to clinical features including an ECG or recent ABG/laboratory sample can help to avoid errors and, where appropriate, repeat the analysis with a formal laboratory sample.
- Respiratory rate rises quickly to compensate for metabolic abnormalities (which are slower to correct). Therefore, a metabolic acidosis should be accompanied by a low CO_2; high CO_2 should be associated with a high bicarbonate or positive base excess if present for some time.
- A mixed picture (e.g. pneumonia and sepsis in a patient with a background of COPD) producing a mixed metabolic and respiratory acidosis should be considered in light of current pathology, previous blood gas results and timing of any biochemical change.

Approach to analysis

1. Is there hypoxia (respiratory failure)?
2. Is respiratory failure type 1 (normal/low CO_2) or type 2 (normal/high CO_2)?
3. Is there acidosis/alkalosis?
4. Does this have respiratory/metabolic components?
5. Which is the predominant problem and is there compensation?

For common presentations of ABG analysis, see Box 11.3.

Box 11.3 Arterial blood gas analysis: common presentations

- Respiratory failure/respiratory acidosis: rise in CO_2 (type 2 respiratory failure) results in low blood pH.
- Respiratory acidosis with metabolic compensation: with time bicarbonate production is increased (giving positive base excess) to compensate for excess CO_2 ($H_2O + CO_2 \rightarrow HCO_3^- + H^+$).
- Metabolic acidosis (low bicarbonate/negative base excess).
- Low anion gap (calculated from 'standard' cations/anions – $Na^+ + K^+) - (Cl^- + HCO_3^-)$: (normal is 10 [6–14] mmol/L), e.g. excess normal saline, diarrhoea or renal tubular acidosis. Chloride usually high from H^+/Cl^- exchange in renal tubules.
- High anion gap (exogenous/unmeasured anions)
  - Aide memoire 'KUSMALE': *K*etoacidosis, *U*rea, *S*ugar (glucose), *M*ethanol, *A*lcohol, *L*actic acidosis (poor organ perfusion, e.g. sepsis or ischaemic bowel), *E*thylene glycol (anti-freeze).
- Metabolic acidosis with respiratory compensation (low $PaCO_2$): in such circumstances, respiratory rate quickly increases to drive down CO_2 (more dependent on ventilation/tidal volume) and, hence, neutralise blood PH.

Less common pictures

Pulse oximetry saturation discrepancy with PO_2/SaO_2 on ABG

Carboxyhaemoglobin (CO poisoning) is more red and methaemoglobin (e.g. toxicity from nitrate fertiliser, sulfonamides and some local anaesthetics) is more blue; result in unreliable oximetry calculations. ABG analysers use a different mechanism that does not rely on the same spectral properties.

Additional analysis

- Alveolar:arterial (A:a) gradient: quantifies alveolar gas exchange.
- A:a = ($[FiO_2]$ × [atmospheric pressure - H_2O pressure] - $[PaCO_2/0.8]$) – PaO_2.
  - Normal gradient estimate = (Age/4) + 4.
  - High values seen in V:Q mismatch, shunt and alveolar hypoventilation.
  - P/F ratio (PaO_2/FiO_2) is similar, but easier to calculate (normal >~50).

Useful tips

- Partial pressure values (e.g. $PaCO_2$) can be approximately converted from KPa to mmHg (older units) by multiplying by 7.
- A number of medical calculators exist online or via smartphones to assist with ABG calculations and conversions.

Further reading

1. Cowley NJ, Owen A, Bion JF. Interpreting arterial blood gas results. *Br Med J*. 2013; 346:f16.

Multiple choice questions

Questions

1. A 25-year-old woman with known asthma presents to A&E with severe shortness of breath and wheeze. She receives nebulised salbutamol. On admission, her PEFR was 88 L/min (Normal PEFR 550 L/min) with a respiratory rate of 33/min. Auscultation reveals a silent chest.

Arterial blood gas results reveal:

- pH 7.37 (7.35-7.45).
- $PaCO_2$ 5.3 (4.7–6.0 kPa).
- PaO_2 8.1 (10–14 kPa).
- Standardised bicarbonate 30 (22–26 mmol/L).

What would be the next most appropriate step?

A. Organise an urgent CXR.
B. Increase inhaled steroid.
C. Contact the intensive care registrar to consider intubation and ventilation.
D. Prescribe IV aminophylline.
E. Commence an IV salbutamol infusion.

2. A 40-year-old Nigerian man presents with a facial rash and dry cough. Chest radiograph shows bilateral reticular shadowing in the upper zones.

   Which one of the below statement is true concerning sarcoidosis?

   A. Serum ACE is the gold standard diagnostic test.
   B. Histology characteristically reveals necrotising granulomas.
   C. First line treatment for hypercalcaemia in sarcoidosis is IV bisphosphonates.
   D. Hilar lymphadenopathy is the most common abnormality seen on chest radiography.
   E. The majority of patients require long-term steroid treatment.

3. A 75-year-old man with a history of COPD is brought into the Emergency Department complaining of increasing shortness of breath, fever and a productive cough. On examination, coarse crackles are heard in the left base.

   Bedside observations:

   - Respiratory rate 28 breaths/minute.
   - Pulse 90 bpm.
   - BP 145/60 mmHg.
   - SpO_2 82% (room air).
   - Chest radiograph: consolidation in the left lower zone.
   - Arterial blood gas on room air demonstrates:
     - pH 7.39.
     - $PaCO_2$ 8.8 kPa.
     - PaO_2 6.3 kPa.
     - Bicarbonate 36 mmol/L.

   He receives bronchodilators and antibiotics. What should be the next step in his management?

   A. Start on NIV.
   B. Start on CPAP.
   C. Increase FiO_2 until oxygen saturations are between 88 and 92%.
   D. Intubate.
   E. Start doxapram.

4. A 35-year-old woman presents with a history of shortness of breath and wheeze. A chest radiograph reveals left upper zone bronchiectasis and she is noted to have a peripheral eosinophilia and elevated Total IgE on blood tests.

   What is the most likely diagnosis?

   A. Eosinophilic granulomatosis with polyangiitis (Churg–Strauss syndrome).
   B. Allergic bronchopulmonary aspergillosis (ABPA).
   C. Schistosomiasis infection.
   D. Rheumatoid arthritis.
   E. Peanut allergy.

5. A 56-year-old woman attends the Respiratory clinic for assessment. She has a 35-pack/year smoking history and has been referred with a persistent cough, without breathlessness, which has failed to

improve despite three courses of antibiotics. She reports a single episode of haemoptysis. She remains active and is able to undertake gardening. On examination, finger clubbing and percussion dullness at the right lung base are noted. CT thorax demonstrates a 2-cm mass at the right hilum with no lymphadenopathy.

Which of the following statements are true?

A. This patient should be referred directly to the medical oncologists for immediate chemotherapy.
B. This patient should be discussed with thoracic surgeons at a lung cancer MDT.
C. Small cell lung cancer is the most likely diagnosis.
D. Urgent radical therapy is indicated irrespective of lung function.
E. Pre-operative assessment would not include a CT-PET scan.

6. A 40-year-old man with an 18-month history of breathlessness presents to the Emergency Department with worsening dyspnoea over a 2-week period. He has a history of a pulmonary embolism 10 years ago and is a lifelong non-smoker.

Bedside observations:

- Oxygen saturations: 94% (room air).

On examination:

- Bipedal ankle oedema, a loud P2 and right ventricular heave.
- Chest radiograph: normal.
- Transthoracic echocardiogram:
    - Right ventricular systolic pressure: 35 mmHg above right atrial pressure (normal range 15–25 mmHg).

Which one of the following statements is true?

A. Right heart catheterisation would be an appropriate next management step.
B. A CTPA would offer conclusive evidence of elevated pulmonary pressures.
C. Oral prostaglandins are likely to be the initial therapeutic choice.
D. Pulmonary endarterectomy is unlikely to offer substantial improvement.
E. He should be assessed and managed at his local hospital.

7. A 32-year-old woman presents with a 1-month history of haemoptysis, myalgia and flu-like symptoms. Her past medical history includes persistent nasal crusting. Bronchoscopy following an episode of haemoptysis 10 years ago was reported as normal. The chest radiograph shows an infiltrate at the left lower zone and there is evidence of renal impairment. Her haemoglobin is 9.4 g/dL.

Which one of the following statements is true?

A. Initial approach should include blood tests for haemoglobin, antinuclear antibodies and antineutrophil cytoplasmic antibodies and a specialist Rheumatology opinion.
B. The FVC is likely to be increased.
C. Red cell casts in the urine would suggest nephrolithiasis.
D. 4 units of blood should be cross-matched urgently.
E. She should receive anticoagulation and undergo an urgent CT-pulmonary angiogram (CTPA).

8. A 24-year-old medical student attends clinic accompanied by his partner, having recently returned from a medical elective in South Africa. He reports a productive cough, weight loss and night sweats. Despite this, since returning to the UK he has been able to continue his medical studies. Examination reveals a single large painless right cervical lymph node. Chest radiograph demonstrates apical shadowing with a prominent right hilum.

Which of the following statements is true?

A. One sputum specimen sent for acid-fast bacilli (AFB) will be sufficient.
B. He should be admitted for a 14-day course of ciprofloxacin.
C. He can continue examining patients as part of his medical studies.
D. Fine needle aspiration (FNA) of a lymph node may yield the diagnosis.
E. Tuberculin skin test (TST) and interferon gamma immunoglobulin release assay (IGRA) should be performed urgently.

9. A 56-year-old patient presents with a 6-month history of dyspnoea and ankle swelling. He is currently under investigation for arthropathy and a skin rash. Chest radiograph shows basal opacification, but no other focal opacity.

   Pulmonary function tests and arterial blood gas are displayed in Figure 11.6.

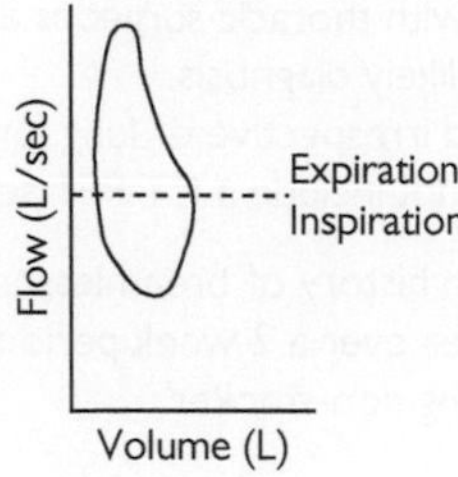

Figure 11.6 Pulmonary function tests and arterial blood gas.

Lung function test results:

- FEV_1 2.3L.
- FVC 2.7L.
- VA 4.2L.
- DLCO 9L.

Arterial blood gas results:

- pH 7.35 (7.35–7.45).
- $PaCO_2$ 5.3kPa (4.7–6.0 kPa).
- PaO_2 7.8kPa (resting).
- Standardised bicarbonate 19 mmol/L.

Which of the following statements is true?

A. The flow loop is typical of emphysema.
B. There is proportionate reduction in the DLCO relative to the FVC.
C. Serum autoantibodies would not be a useful test.
D. Right heart studies on echocardiography should be considered.
E. An obstructing tumour might be present and account for the severity of hypoxia.

10. A 55-year-old smoker of 15 cigarettes/day presents with cough and left-sided pleuritic chest pain.

    Bedside observations:

- HR 78/min.
- BP 145/98 mmHg.
- SpO_2 94% on room air.
- Temp 37.3°C.

Chest radiograph: consolidation at the right lung base, blunting of the right costophrenic angle and prominent mediastinal lymphadenopathy. Which if the following statements is true?

A. A pleural aspiration should be performed removing 50 mL of pleural fluid for pH, protein, culture and cytology.
B. A chest drain should be inserted into the second intercostal space.
C. He requires immediate pleural drainage.

D. If the pleural aspirate demonstrates a pH 7.8 there would be an increased urgency to insert a chest drain.
E. Talc should be inserted into the pleural space via the drain following resolution of the effusion to prevent its recurrence.

Answers

1. C. The clinical presentation is of life-threatening asthma and there should be early contact with the ITU team for closer monitoring (➲ See Risk stratification in acute asthma, p. 347).
2. D. Histologically, non-caseating granulomas are found in sarcoidosis, as well as in patients with malignancy or common variable immunodeficiency; necrotising granulomas occur in TB. First-line treatment of hypercalcemia secondary to sarcoidosis includes IV hydration and steroids (➲ see Sarcoidosis, p. 351 and Figure 11.2).
3. C. The initial priority is to increase the FiO_2 with the aim of improving oxygenation. Titrating and improving oxygenation initially may reduce the respiratory effort required by the patient, resulting in less fatigue and leading to better ventilation.
   This blood gas shows evidence of chronic Type 2 respiratory failure, which may worsen with increased oxygenation. If increasing the FiO_2 results in worsening hypercapnia then NIV should be considered. CPAP would be considered in the context of Type 1 respiratory failure. Pneumonia in the context of severe Type 2 respiratory failure should prompt consideration of intubation. Doxapram is a respiratory stimulant, which has been shown to be inferior to NIV in improving Type 2 respiratory failure and can cause agitation. It may be considered as a bridge to NIV (➲ see Arterial blood gas analysis, p. 384, and Non-invasive ventilation, p. 355).
4. B. Patients with ABPA become colonised with aspergillus, with subsequent bronchial obstruction and a cycle of inflammation that leads to bronchiectasis (particularly of the upper lobes). A peripheral eosinophilia is common (➲ see Bronchiectasis, p. 356).
5. B. The probable diagnosis is an early stage NSCLC. It is likely to be visible at bronchoscopy, allowing for tissue biopsy and histological assessment. If resection is considered likely, a CT-PET at an early stage may help to avoid delay prior to surgery. Lung function studies are an important part of pre-operative assessment and should also be organised early in appropriate patients (➲ see Lung cancer, p. 362).
6. A. The TTE is abnormal and right heart catheterisation would be indicated. The symptoms described could be the result of a pulmonary embolus (or recurring emboli) or chronic thromboembolic pulmonary hypertension. A CTPA will help to establish any acute or resolving emboli, but while signs such as an enlarged right atrium, right ventricle or pulmonary artery suggest pulmonary hypertension, they give no definitive evidence of pulmonary artery pressure.
   Vasodilators are a mainstay of pulmonary hypertension therapy and include prostaglandins, but oral preparations have poor biostability so infusions or nebulisers are used. Thromboarterectomy offers significant improvements in symptoms and survival in patients with chronic thromboembolic pulmonary hypertension (CTEPH) (➲ see Thromboembolic disease and pulmonary hypertension, p. 365).
7. A. This scenario is suggestive of pulmonary haemorrhage (haemoptysis in the context of acute kidney injury and systemic illness), rather than infection or pulmonary embolism. The history of nasal crusting and renal disease (red cell casts are pathognomonic of glomerulonephritis) suggest ANCA-associated vasculitis. Fresh haemoptysis can cause an elevated KCO not FVC; KCO is less likely to be increased if there has been a few days without bleeding. Priorities in the acute setting are to stabilise the patient and treat the inflammatory disease. Respiratory compromise is one of the greatest immediate concerns, often more so than the risk of blood loss (➲ see Pulmonary vasculitis and pulmonary eosinophilias, p. 372).

8. D. The clinical history is suggestive of active TB with a high risk of transmission. Standard assessment includes three sputum samples for AFB, preferable on early-morning specimens. Community-acquired pneumonia is unlikely and prescribing other antibiotics may complicate treatment. The risk of TB transmission in this clinical context poses a significant public health concern. Occupational health can assess the risk of prior exposure to patients and provide advice on the period of absence from his clinical duties, while undergoing assessment. FNA of the lymphadenopathy may be sufficient to identify an AFB-positive smear/culture. TST and IGRA are unlikely to be helpful here as he has signs of active TB disease; TST can ulcerate in such cases (➔ see Chapter 8, Tuberculosis, p. 260).
9. D. There is a reduced FVC with preserved FEV1/FVC ratio and a flow loop pattern typical of a restrictive defect. An arthropathy and skin rash suggests there may be an undiagnosed CTD. The disproportionate reduction in DLCO and marked Type 1 respiratory failure are suggestive of associated pulmonary hypertension. Further diagnostic tests would include autoantibodies, HRCT scan thorax and ECHO to screen for pulmonary hypertension. (➔ see Pulmonary function tests, p. 377).
10. A. This patient has a pleural effusion with possible underlying empyema or malignancy. Diagnostic aspiration of fluid can differentiate a transudate and exudate and may point to infection or malignancy.

    Pleural procedures, where possible, are performed via the safe triangle under the axilla, alternatively the posterior aspect of the thorax may be suitable. In most cases, pleural ultrasound will help identify a safe location.

    Since the patient here is not unstable, chest drain insertion (which is not without risk) should be performed during routine working hours by appropriately trained staff. The presence of a low pH <7.2 suggests an empyema, for which there would be an increased urgency to drain the fluid. Pleurodesis is not indicated as this is a first and a causative diagnosis has not been established (➔ see Pneumothorax and pleural effusions, p. 380 and Table 11.8).

Chapter 12 **Critical Care**

Matthew C. Frise and Ingeborg Welters

Essential concepts in critical care

Introduction

Critical care is unique as a specialty in defining its patient population not according to the nature of illness, but rather its severity. Patients in modern-day intensive care units (ICUs) include those with multi-organ failure requiring specialised support, and those at high risk of deterioration who may require urgent intervention. Box 12.1 gives a classification of levels of care according to the UK Intensive Care Society (ICS). ICUs often consist of a mixture of level 2 and level 3 beds, although there is considerable variation in the organisation of individual units. In many hospitals separate high dependency units (HDUs) exist, which closely interact with the ICU. ICUs and HDUs require a high ratio of nursing and medical staff to patients and, although such care is expensive, it is cost-effective.

Box 12.1 Levels of care as defined by the ICS

- *Level 0*: hospitalized, but needs can be met through normal ward care.
- *Level 1*:
  Recently discharged from a higher level of care.
  - Requires additional monitoring, clinical interventions, clinical advice or input.
  - Receiving critical care outreach service support.
- *Level 2*:
  Requires pre-operative optimization.
  - Needs extended post-operative care.
  - Receiving single organ support (except advanced respiratory support – level 3).
  - Receiving basic respiratory and/or basic cardiovascular support.
- *Level 3*:
  Receiving advanced respiratory support alone.
  - Receiving support of two or more organ systems (except basic respiratory with basic cardiovascular support – level 2).

Basic respiratory support includes NIV; intubation for airway protection without ventilatory support; CPAP via a tracheostomy and use of more than 50% oxygen delivered by face mask. Basic cardiovascular support includes use of a CVP line or an arterial line; provision of a single intravenous vasoactive drug and use of IV antiarrhythmic agents.

Haemodynamic monitoring

The scope for continuous and invasive monitoring sets the ICU apart from other ward areas. The circulation is a particular focus, and an understanding of basic physiology is essential to interpret the data obtained.

Cardiac physiology and anatomy, as well as arterial and central venous waveforms are covered in ➲ Chapter 13, Cardiac physiology and anatomy, p. 409. Arterial blood pressure may be continuously measured using an arterial line, which also permits frequent blood gas analysis to guide ventilation and other therapies. Typical sites include the radial, femoral and brachial arteries. Central venous catheters (CVCs) allow central venous pressure (CVP) monitoring, and permit continuous and bolus infusion of multiple medications into the central circulation concomitantly.

Highly invasive haemodynamic monitoring may be performed with a pulmonary artery catheter (PAC, also known as a Swan–Ganz catheter). This device consists of a pressure transducer, thermistor and balloon, and is inserted via a central vein and floated across the tricuspid valve into a distal pulmonary artery. Inflating the balloon allows occlusion of the vessel and the pulmonary capillary 'wedge pressure' to be measured. Cardiac output (CO) may be measured by using indicator dilution principles, with temperature serving as indicator. Injection of cold saline into the right atrium followed by downstream temperature measurement generates a thermodilution curve, which is inversely proportional to the stroke volume. Multiplication of stroke volume (SV) and heart rate serves to calculate CO.

While the PAC is the gold standard, other techniques such as PiCCO (Pulse Contour Cardiac Output) have replaced its use, because evidence for therapeutic benefit from routine insertion of PACs is lacking. PiCCO uses a CVC and arterial line to estimate CO based on thermodilution and waveform analysis. Oesophageal Doppler probes, an additional approach to record blood flow continuously in the descending aorta, and serial transthoracic echocardiography, may also be used to assess SV, CO and the response to fluid challenges and vasoactive drugs. Data obtained from invasive monitoring are valuable in distinguishing different causes of circulatory embarrassment. An explanation of common variables measured is given in Box 12.2.

Box 12.2 Common invasively measured haemodynamic variables

Cardiac output

Total volume of blood pumped by the heart in one minute; the product of stroke volume (SV) and heart rate (HR). Normal range of 4–8 L/min.

Cardiac index

CO divided by body surface area (BSA) with a normal range at rest of 2.6–4.2 L/min/m^2.

Pulmonary artery occlusion pressure (PAOP) or pulmonary capillary wedge pressure (PCWP)

Back pressure measured by wedging an inflated balloon into a distal pulmonary artery; provides an indirect assessment of left atrial pressure (LAP), but may be unrepresentative in some settings. Normal range 6–15 mmHg.

Right atrial pressure

Normal range 0–7 mmHg. The JVP waveform is the corresponding physical sign. CVP can be measured using a CVC.

Pulmonary artery pressure

Systolic (15–28 mmHg), diastolic (6–15 mmHg) and mean pulmonary artery pressure (PAP) can be measured.

Systemic vascular resistance (SVR)

The resistance offered to blood flow by the peripheral circulation. Has a variety of units. Normal range 9–20 mmHg/min/L (Woods units).

Vasoactive drugs

Situations in which an adequate circulation cannot be maintained despite optimisation of volume status are common in critically ill patients. Agents that act directly on the cardiovascular system are then required to support the circulation, including adrenoreceptor agonists, phosphodiesterase inhibitors and calcium sensitisers. These agents fall into two groups – inotropes and vasopressors – but many have characteristics of both. Vasoactive drugs have potentially serious side effects, so continuous invasive blood pressure monitoring and frequent clinical reassessment are required.

Inotropes

- Act on the heart increasing force and rate of myocardial contraction.
- Tend to increase CO and blood pressure.
- Increase cardiac work and myocardial oxygen demand.
- Increase risk of tachyarrhythmias, which would be undesirable in a heart with already compromised contractility.

Vasopressors

- Act on the circulation causing vasoconstriction.
- Main function is to increase mean arterial pressure (MAP).
- Have the potential to compromise blood flow to limbs and vital organs – the opposite of their desired effect.

Catecholamines

For adrenoreceptor agonists commonly used in critical care, see Table 12.1.

Table 12.1 Adrenoreceptor agonists commonly used in critical care

<table>
<tr><th></th><th>β_1 receptor</th><th>β_2 receptor</th><th>α_1 receptor</th><th>α_2 receptor</th></tr>
<tr><td rowspan="2"></td><td colspan="4">Inotropy</td></tr>
<tr><td>Chronotropy</td><td>Broncho- and vaso-dilatation</td><td colspan="2">Vasoconstriction</td></tr>
<tr><td>Adrenaline</td><td colspan="2" rowspan="2">Predominant effect at low doses</td><td colspan="2" rowspan="2">Predominant effect at high doses</td></tr>
<tr><td>Noradrenaline</td></tr>
<tr><td>Dobutamine</td><td colspan="2">Potent action</td><td>Weak action</td><td></td></tr>
<tr><td>Metaraminol</td><td colspan="3"></td><td>Potent action</td></tr>
</table>

Adapted from Bersten, A. and Soni, N. (2013). *Oh's Intensive Care Manual*, Seventh Edition, Butterworth-Heinemann Elsevier.

Phosphodiesterase inhibitors

These drugs inhibit phosphodiesterase and thereby prevent the inactivation of intracellular cAMP, a molecule downstream to β-adrenergic receptor activation that increases activation of protein kinase A, which in turn phosphorylates many components within cardiomyocytes, such as calcium and potassium channels and components of the myofilaments. Phosphorylation of calcium channels permits an increase in calcium influx into the cell permitting increased contractility; phosphorylation of potassium channels promotes their action in repolarisation of cardiomyocytes therefore increasing the rate at which cells can depolarise and generate contraction; phosphorylation of components on myofilaments allows actin and myosin to interact more easily, thus increasing contractility and the inotropic state of the heart. Amrinone, enoximone and milrinone are occasionally used in cardiogenic shock, but evidence of efficacy is lacking.

Levosimendan

This agent is a calcium-sensitiser and acts as a lusitrope, improving myocardial relaxation. There is some evidence to suggest it may be superior to dobutamine in myocardial infarction complicated by cardiogenic shock.

Vasopressin

This naturally occurring posterior pituitary hormone is used in hypotensive vasoplegic shock if there is insufficient response to noradrenaline alone. There is also considerable interest in whether it may have a role in cardiopulmonary resuscitation.

Shock

Shock describes the state of imbalance between tissue oxygen supply and demand. Hypotension is often wrongly assumed to be a universal feature; patients may be normo- or even hypertensive, but still shocked. Indeed, one of the first changes during significant haemorrhage in previously healthy individuals is a rise in diastolic blood pressure due to reflex sympathetic vasoconstriction.

In physiological terms, tissue hypoxia may be viewed as a consequence of:

- Low partial pressure of oxygen (hypoxaemic hypoxia).
- Low haemoglobin (anaemic hypoxia): due to an absolute haemoglobin reduction or functional deficit as in carboyxhaemoglobinaemia or methaemoglobinaemia.
- Low cardiac output (stagnant hypoxia).
- Histotoxicity of poisons such as cyanide (oxygen available, but cannot be used).

The different types of shock are shown in Table 12.2 and outlined below. ➲ Cardiogenic shock is considered in Acute heart failure, p. 401.

Table 12.2 Subtypes and haemodynamic profiles of shock.

	Type of shock			
	Distributive	**Hypovolaemic**	**Obstructive**	**Cardiogenic**
Aetiology	Loss of vascular tone	Loss of circulating volume	Blood flow obstructed	Pump failure
Examples	Sepsis Anaphylaxis Spinal cord injury	Major haemorrhage Volume depletion	Massive PE Tamponade	Anterior MI Mitral valve rupture CCB overdose
CO	High	Low	Low	Low
CVP/JVP	Low or normal	Low	High	High or normal
SVR	Low	High	High	High
PAOP	Normal or low	Low	Normal or high	High

PE, pulmonary embolism; MI, myocardial infarction; CCB, calcium channel blocker; other abbreviations, see Box 12.2.

Anaphylactic shock

Definition

Anaphylaxis results from a type 1 hypersensitivity reaction to a triggering allergen causing histamine release (➲ see Chapter 6, Type I hypersensitivity, p. 160). In its severest form, anaphylactic shock involves massive vasodilatation and capillary leak leading to hypotension, and respiratory distress; either one alone or a combination of both may contribute rapidly to death despite immediate treatment. The speed of onset of anaphylactic shock and short interval between onset and cardiopulmonary arrest is often underestimated. (Table 12.3).

The mortality rate remains high even if resuscitation is successful, mainly due to hypoxic brain injury. Treatment must therefore be rapidly instituted according to the standard ABCDE approach; specific interventions include the following (although not based on randomised controlled trials):

- Adrenaline: this is the cornerstone of therapy and should be given without delay if anaphylaxis is suspected. It is often wrongly held in reserve while other measures are implemented by which time its effectiveness may be reduced and the patient seriously ill. The aim is to prevent the development of anaphylactic shock, since this is much harder to treat than to prevent. The initial dose in adults

Table 12.3 Intervals between exposure and cardiac or respiratory arrest in anaphylaxis

Type of precipitant	Median (range) time before cardiopulmonary arrest
Iatrogenic	5 (1–80) minutes
Foodstuffs	30 (6–360) minutes
Venom	15 (4–120) minutes

Data from Pumphrey RS. Lessons for management of anaphylaxis from a study of fatal reactions. *Clinical and Experimental Allergy: Journal of the British Society for Allergy and Clinical Immunology*, 2000;30:1144-50.

is 0.5 mL of 1:1000 adrenaline (0.5 mg) IM. In the setting of severe shock, which may compromise muscle perfusion, and in cardiac arrest, adrenaline should be given IV by an appropriately experienced individual. The long-term management of individuals at risk of anaphylaxis involves provision of an adrenaline auto-injector.

- Fluids: if the patient is shocked, large volume fluid resuscitation should be given. If it is possible that anaphylaxis has been triggered by a colloid, such as gelofusin, this should be discontinued and resuscitation continued with crystalloid.
- Oxygen: since respiratory distress and impending airway compromise are highly likely, high-flow oxygen therapy should be the default until the patient's condition is clearly stabilised.
- Intubation: if there are any signs of airway compromise an intensivist or anaesthetist should be called; the incidence of difficult intubation is very high in this group and instrumentation of the airway by an inexperienced individual may exacerbate the problem.
- Inhaled β-agonists: nebulised salbutamol may be given for bronchospasm; nebulised adrenaline may also be given for laryngeal oedema.
- Hydrocortisone: is usually given at a dose of 100–200 mg IV.
- Antihistamines: chlorphenamine can be given at a dose of 10 mg IV.

Obstructive shock

Obstructive shock results from physical impairment of the outflow of blood from the left or right ventricular cavity. The commonest causes are massive pulmonary embolus and cardiac tamponade.

Pulmonary embolus

Thrombolysis is controversial due to a lack of large properly controlled clinical trials. It is clearly indicated in the setting of cardiac arrest, and is also recommended in the presence of haemodynamic compromise. Surgical embolectomy can be considered in patients not responding to thrombolysis or in whom this is contraindicated. Optimising preload with fluid resuscitation has theoretical advantages, but may lead to worsening right ventricular dysfunction.

Tamponade

A fluid collection within the relatively non-expansile pericardial sac compromises LV and RV filling, thus impairing CO. Bedside echocardiography can rapidly confirm or refute this diagnosis, and allows immediate percutaneous drainage of the pericardial effusion under ultrasound guidance (➲ see Chapter 5, Case 7, p. 127). Fluid resuscitation and vasoactive drugs may be beneficial as temporising measures, while drainage is being organised.

Hypovolaemic shock

Hypovolaemic shock is due to a significant reduction in circulating volume. The cause may be obvious, although a massive haemorrhage may be concealed in the retroperitoneum or GI tract. Haemodilution takes time to occur and the haemoglobin concentration will therefore not fall acutely in this setting. GI or renal losses from profuse diarrhoea or polyuria severe enough to cause hypovolaemic shock are typically accompanied by significant electrolyte disturbances. Acute management is volume resuscitation with crystalloid or blood, while the underlying cause is sought and addressed. Failure to recognise hypovolaemia as a cause of escalating vasopressor requirements can lead to worsening tissue ischaemia as a consequence of profound vasoconstriction, and death, if an adequate circulating volume is not restored.

Spinal shock

Spinal shock results from disordered autonomic activity following spinal cord injury. In high cord injuries sympathetic supply to the heart and peripheral circulation is lost in the presence of preserved vagal tone, leading to profound veno- and vasodilatation without an ability to mount a tachycardia and preserve CO. In the setting of acute cord injury, volume resuscitation and vasoactive drugs may be required.

Sepsis and septic shock

Pathophysiology

Bacteraemia is the presence of viable bacteria in the blood. This may give rise to the systemic inflammatory response syndrome (SIRS), defined as any two of:

- Temperature > 38°C or < 36°C.
- Heart rate > 90 bpm.
- Respiratory rate > 20.
- WBC count > 12 or < 4 × 10^9/mL.

Emphasis was previously placed on SIRS as a possible indicator of bacterial infection, but SIRS can be caused by a variety of infectious agents, such as bacteria and fungi, as well as non-infectious conditions, such as trauma, pancreatitis and burns.

The contemporary view places less emphasis on these criteria, and instead defines sepsis as life-threatening organ dysfunction caused by a dysregulated host response to infection, driven either by microbial molecules such as lipopolysaccharide or by substances arising from tissue injury. Local inflammation activates the innate immune system, coagulation pathways, and a cascade of pro-inflammatory cytokines such as TNF-α, IL-6, IL-8 and IL-1β. Up-regulation of inducible nitric oxide (NO) synthase leads to high levels of NO production, loss of vascular tone and hypotension. Endothelial dysfunction is evident with up-regulation of cell adhesion molecules and increased permeability leading to capillary leak. The microcirculation is disrupted by microthrombi from intravascular coagulation. Tissue perfusion is thus compromised and mitochondrial dysfunction leads to defective oxygen utilisation, even if an adequate circulation can be restored. Patients with septic shock have a mortality greater than 40%, and are identified by persisting hypotension requiring vasopressors to maintain MAP ≥65 mmHg, or a serum lactate level >2 mmol/L despite adequate volume resuscitation.

Management

Early goal-directed therapy (EGDT) describes an approach to managing sepsis and septic shock, whereby patients are resuscitated according to physiological targets with the aim of correcting tissue hypoxia. The concept of 'bundles' of interventions that when provided together improve outcome has also gained acceptance (Box 12.3). One key component of management is source control, with timely administration of antibiotics and drainage of infected fluid. A thorough search for the source of infection (e.g. an intra-abdominal collection or empyema) is mandatory, and if found requires radiological or surgical drainage. The septic process may otherwise fail to resolve or recrudesce after apparently successful therapy.

Fluids

The three key questions for critically ill patients are:

1. How much fluid should be given?
2. How rapidly?
3. Which fluid is best?

The answers to these questions vary between clinical scenarios, but a few guiding principles are:

Box 12.3 Surviving Sepsis care bundles

To be completed within 3 hours

- Measure lactate level.
- Obtain blood cultures prior to administration of antibiotics.
- Administer broad spectrum antibiotics.
- Administer 30 mL/kg crystalloid for hypotension or lactate ≥ 4mmol/L.

To be completed within 6 hours

Apply vasopressors for hypotension that does not respond to initial fluid resuscitation to maintain a mean arterial pressure (MAP) ≥ 65 mmHg with noradrenaline being the drug of choice (adding or switching to adrenaline if noradrenaline fails).

In the event of persistent arterial hypotension despite volume resuscitation (septic shock) or initial lactate ≥ 4 mmol/L:

- Measure CVP: target: ≥ 8 mmHg.
- Measure central venous oxygen saturation ($ScvO_2$) – target: ≥ 70%.
- Re-measure lactate if initial lactate was elevated; target: normalisation.

Adapted with permission from Dellinger R.P. et al., Surviving sepsis campaign: international guidelines for management of severe sepsis and septic shock: 2012, *Critical Care Medicine*, 2013 Feb;41(2):580-637. doi: 10.1097/CCM.0b013e31827e83af.

- Give enough fluid, but not too much: fluid overload from excessive resuscitation is associated with increased mortality in sepsis.
- Decide on a target value for MAP, CVP or urine output before administration.
- Administer a small fluid challenge rapidly enough that a change in physiological parameters will be evident if effective (e.g. 250 mL of crystalloid over 5–10 minutes) and reassess the patient afterwards. A smaller volume (100 mL) may be used in patients with anuria or cardiac disease.
- Crystalloids are the fluid of choice for resuscitation. Albumin can be added in individuals requiring very large volume resuscitation.
- There is no evidence from randomised controlled trials that resuscitation with colloids reduces the risk of death compared with crystalloids and may actually be harmful. Hydroxyethylstarch is contraindicated in sepsis due to an increased incidence of acute kidney injury (AKI) and worse outcome.
- Large volume infusion of sodium chloride may cause a hyperchloraemic metabolic acidosis and increase the risk of acute kidney injury; the use of balanced fluids such as Hartmann's may be preferable.
- A modest amount of fluid and a modest amount of noradrenaline are better than very large quantities of either in isolation – the two should be used in conjunction.

Adjunctive therapies

Noradrenaline is the most widely used vasoactive drug in sepsis, but further therapies exist that are of use depending on the clinical situation:

- Corticosteroids: can be considered as a continuous infusion of 200–300 mg hydrocortisone over 24 hours in septic shock with ongoing haemodynamic instability despite fluid resuscitation and vasopressors.
- Vasopressin: should not be used in isolation, but may reduce noradrenaline requirements.
- Dobutamine: if there is evidence of impaired contractility and/or a low CO despite adequate MAP, myocardial dysfunction may be improved by addition of an inotropic agent.
- Blood transfusion: in the acute setting EGDT suggests using packed red cells to achieve a haematocrit of >30% in patient with SvO_2 <70%; subsequently, however, evidence supports adopting a transfusion threshold of 70 g/L haemoglobin in the absence of acute bleeding, cardiac ischaemia or profound hypoxaemia.

Sedation, analgesia and neuromuscular blockade

Historically, mechanically ventilated patients on ICUs were routinely heavily sedated and paralysed to facilitate invasive ventilation, and to treat pain and discomfort. However, reduced sedation and neuromuscular blockade to allow patients to be conscious and orientated for prolonged periods, and to permit early rehabilitation, are associated with improved outcomes. Table 12.4 lists examples of commonly used agents.

Table 12.4 Anaesthetic drugs commonly used in critical care

Sedatives	**Description**	**Advantages**	**Disadvantages**
Propofol	IV anaesthetic agent for intubation and continuous sedation.	Short distribution half-life. Smooth and rapid induction.	Hypotension. Relatively expensive.
Midazolam	IV benzodiazepine for continuous sedation.	Cardiovascular stability.	Slow to wear off.
Ketamine	IV dissociative anaesthetic agent for intubation, sedation and analgesia.	Bronchodilator. Potent analgesic at low doses.	Increases HR and BP due to sympathomimetic activity.
Etomidate	IV anaesthetic agent for intubation.	Cardiovascular stability.	Adrenal suppression; no longer given as an infusion or during emergency intubation.
Analgesics			
Morphine	IV opioid analgesics for continuous or short-term analgesia.	Cheap.	Slow to wear off. Histamine release. Accumulates in renal failure. Respiratory depression.
Fentanyl		Minimal histamine release. Cardiovascular stability.	Respiratory depression.
Alfentanil		Rapid onset.	Potent respiratory depression.
Remifentanil		Very short half-life so wears off quickly.	Expensive. Potent respiratory depression. May cause respiratory muscle rigidity.
Neuromuscular blockers			
Suxamethonium	Depolarising blocker for intubation.	Excellent intubating conditions. Short-acting.	Numerous side effects and contraindications in critical illness.
Rocuronium	Non-depolarising blocker for intubation.	Paralytic effects reversed by sugammadex.	Inferior intubating conditions to suxamethonium.
Atracurium	Non-depolarising blocker for intubation or continuous paralysis.	Continuous infusion when paralysis required. Spontaneous degradation.	Histamine release.

Critical illness polyneuropathy and myopathy

An acute sensorimotor axonal polyneuropathy and myopathy is associated with critical illness, especially in the setting of sepsis. Prolonged use of neuromuscular blocking drugs is a major risk factor. Accordingly, guidelines now recommend keeping paralysis to a minimum. In some settings, especially status asthmaticus, paralysis is unavoidable in order to ventilate patients adequately.

Delirium

Delirium is very common in critically ill patients and can present as a hyperactive or hypoactive form, the latter being difficult to detect. Reducing the use of sedatives, especially benzodiazepines, along with environmental approaches and a pro-active approach to screening for delirium are now accepted as the standard of care. Haloperidol is commonly used to treat delirium in ICU patients though evidence is lacking to support this approach.

Severity scoring and outcome prediction

A variety of systems exists for quantifying illness severity, most of which correlate with outcome. No scoring system can reliably predict outcome in an individual patient; two patients with apparently similar illness severity and organ dysfunction may have very different subsequent clinical courses. The APACHE scoring system has been used for decades and has been refined a number of times. It includes a number of parameters measured within the first 24 hours of admission to ICU, including age, pulse rate, mean blood pressure, temperature, respiratory rate, partial pressure of oxygen in the arterial blood (PaO_2)/fractional inspired oxygen (FiO_2) ratio, haematocrit, white cell count (WCC), creatinine, urine output, urea, sodium, albumin, bilirubin, glucose, acid base status, and neurological abnormalities based on Glasgow Coma Score. Also taken into consideration are chronic health variables such the presence of AIDS, cirrhosis, hepatic failure, immunosuppression and haematological or metastatic malignancy. ICU admission diagnosis, location from which the patient was admitted, and length of stay before ICU admission, are also included.

Another system, the Sequential Organ Failure Assessment (SOFA), assigns a value to the levels of dysfunction in six different systems: respiratory, cardiovascular, hepatic, coagulation, renal and neurological. An acute change in total SOFA score ≥2 points in the context of suspected or proven infection identifies the organ dysfunction that constitutes sepsis. An abbreviated version, the quick-SOFA (qSOFA) score is a bedside tool that can rapidly identify patients with suspected infection outside an ICU setting. It uses three criteria, assigning one point for each of the following: low blood pressure (SBP ≤100 mmHg), high respiratory rate (≥22 breaths per min), and altered mentation (Glasgow coma scale <15). A score of >2 is associated with poorer outcome and prolonged stay in an ICU.

Organ support

The aetiology, pathogenesis and management of individual organ failures are addressed in their relevant chapters. This section considers the situations in which patients with different organ failures come to the attention of the critical care physician and how they are then managed.

Acute respiratory failure and ARDS

The consequences of respiratory insufficiency may be considered as hypoxia and hypercapnia, with either predominating initially. However, they are not independent and as a patient tires, both become inevitable. Acute respiratory failure may occur in the setting of essentially normal lungs (e.g. as a consequence of neurological disease such as Guillan–Barré syndrome or botulism) or from acute pathological processes affecting the lungs (e.g. pneumonia, aspiration). In the case of the latter there is often pre-existing lung disease, or another chronic illness that does not directly affect the lung, but predisposes to respiratory failure with further insult (e.g. immunosuppression, motor neurone disease or severe kyphoscoliosis). The commonest medical indication for admission to an ICU in the UK is pneumonia.

Acute respiratory failure in chronic obstructive pulmonary disease

Though acute deteriorations of any chronic lung disease may lead to severe illness, chronic obstructive pulmonary disease (COPD) is one of the most common existing lung pathologies in patients needing respiratory support. Appropriate medical therapy, type I and type II respiratory failure, and the use of non-invasive ventilation (NIV) are discussed in ➲ Chapter 11, Non-invasive ventilation, p. 354. Specific indications for invasive mechanical ventilation are:

- Reduced consciousness level and thus failure to protect the airway.
- Inability to manage secretions.

- Refractory hypoxaemia.
- Fatigue and impending collapse despite NIV.
- Respiratory arrest.

Status asthmaticus

A minority of asthmatics will deteriorate despite maximal therapy. Oxygenation can usually be maintained relatively easily in acute asthma with little or no supplementary oxygen; varying degrees of hypocapnia are common. Progressive hypoxaemia, normo- or hypercapnia, haemodynamic instability and confusion are ominous, and suggest that the patient is tiring and mechanical ventilation will be necessary. Additional treatments available in the ICU setting include:

- The inhalational anaesthetic agent isofluorane, which has a bronchodilator action.
- Ketamine or adrenaline infusions, both of which cause bronchodilatation.
- Extracorporeal CO_2 removal and/or membrane oxygenation (ECMO) when adequate oxygenation and/or carbon dioxide clearance cannot be achieved despite maximal therapy and an appropriate mode of mechanical ventilation.

NIV may avoid intubation in acute severe asthma, but its role has yet to be clearly defined. If used it should be in an environment where intubation can be undertaken quickly and safely.

Acute respiratory distress syndrome

Acute respiratory distress syndrome (ARDS) is a condition characterised by the rapid onset of diffuse bilateral alveolar damage, classified according to the severity of hypoxaemia relative to the FiO_2:

- Mild: $PaO_2/FiO_2 \leq 300$ mmHg.
- Moderate: $PaO_2/FiO_2 \leq 200$ mmHg.
- Severe: $PaO_2/FiO_2 \leq 100$ mmHg.

The condition has a wide range of precipitants (Table 12.5). The pathophysiology is complex and probably varies according to the underlying diagnosis. The key features are disruption of the alveolo-capillary barrier, recruitment of inflammatory cells (especially neutrophils) and surfactant dysfunction. Recovery may be characterised by the development of fibrosing alveolitis. Management involves aggressive treatment of the underlying cause, avoidance of fluid overload and lung-protective ventilation. These same principles can be applied to prevent ARDS in those at risk of its development.

Table 12.5 Conditions leading to ARDS.

Lung pathology	Non-lung pathology
Pneumonia	Extrapulmonary sepsis
Gastric aspiration	Pancreatitis
Lung trauma	Transfusion-related acute lung injury
Submersion injury	Polytrauma
Smoke inhalation	
Marrow embolism	

Lung protective ventilation

Aggressive mechanical ventilation with high tidal volumes in an effort to maintain a normal $PaCO_2$ is harmful. Critically ill patients with, or at risk of, ARDS, should be ventilated with a low tidal volume and optimal positive end-expiratory pressure to improve outcome. Permissive hypercapnia is a term that denotes acceptance of a moderately raised $PaCO_2$, which is not usually associated with significant deleterious effects in this setting.

Acute heart failure

Acute heart failure most commonly takes the form of a significant decompensation of chronic heart failure (➲ see Chapter 13, Heart failure, p. 451). Acute heart failure requiring critical care input may also occur in patients with a previously normal heart, most commonly following an acute myocardial infarction. There are two reasons why patients with acute heart failure require organ support; first, pump failure that leads to an inadequate cardiac output to meet the body's requirements, necessitating circulatory support; and second, pulmonary oedema of such severity that ventilatory support is required. Cardiogenic shock carries an extremely high mortality even in the presence of a reversible cause. Complications include acute oliguric renal failure, ischaemic hepatitis (shock liver) and gut ischaemia. Supportive measures should be instituted prior to definitive treatment to correct the underlying cause, e.g. severe pulmonary oedema may require intubation before angiography can be performed safely.

Specific therapies that may be employed include:

- Intra-aortic balloon counterpulsation (balloon-pump): a bridging therapy involving the percutaneous insertion of an arterial balloon catheter via a femoral artery until just distal to the left subclavian artery. The balloon is inflated with helium during diastole with the aim of improving coronary blood flow and myocardial perfusion, and actively deflated during systole to reduce afterload. A common setting in which it is used is following emergency revascularisation in anterior myocardial infarction. Complications include gut, renal, cerebral and limb ischaemia, vascular injury and balloon rupture. Evidence for a mortality benefit is lacking, so the decision on its use should be jointly made by senior members of the cardiology/cardiothoracic and critical-care teams.
- Vasoactive drugs: inotropes such as adrenaline or milrinone, or the lusitrope levosimendan.
- Ventricular assist devices (VAD): usually while awaiting transplantation, although have been successfully used in patients with reversible underlying pathologies such as viral myocarditis. These are mechanical pumps that take over the work of driving blood through the systemic circulation (left [L]VAD), pulmonary circulation (right [R]VAD) or both.
- Temporary pacing wire: may be necessary in complete heart block.

Acute kidney injury

Acute kidney injury (➲ see Chapter 16, Acute kidney injury, p. 583, Table 16.10 and Figure 16.4), is a common reason for admission to ICU, but patients admitted to ICU with other organ failures frequently develop AKI as a complication. Those admitted with AKI as a primary diagnosis often have features such as oligo- or anuria with worsening metabolic acidosis and hyperkalaemia, meaning that acute renal-replacement therapy (RRT) cannot safely be undertaken elsewhere. Factors that commonly contribute to AKI in critically ill patients include:

- Pre-renal:
  - hypovolaemic shock.
- Renal:
  - sepsis;
  - contrast media;
  - antimicrobials, e.g. gentamicin, amphotericin, penicillins, aciclovir.
- Post-renal:
  - renal tract obstruction – must be excluded radiologically with bedside US being a convenient option.

Indications for RRT in the ICU (Box 12.4) are different from the criteria typically used in a more stable patient with single organ failure, or acute-on-chronic renal failure in a renal unit. RRT in critical care can be given in the form of continuous venovenous haemofiltration (CVVH), continuous venovenous haemodiafiltration (CVVHDF) or continuous venovenous haemodialysis (CVVHD). Intermittent haemodialysis can also be used, but there is theoretically a greater risk of haemodynamic instability, fluctuation in urea clearance and acidaemia and, thus, risk of disequilibrium in a vulnerable patient population.

Furosemide, sometimes as a continuous infusion, may be used in an attempt to avoid RRT when the primary problem is volume overload, rather than metabolic derangement. It has been suggested that furosemide may be renoprotective in some way but evidence is lacking. Similarly, the use of 'renal dose dopamine'

Box 12.4 Suggested indications for renal replacement therapy in the ICU

Blood chemistry abnormalities

- Hyperkalaemia: $K^+ > 6.5$ mmol/L, or lower but rapidly rising, e.g rhabdomyolysis.
- Urea > 35 mmol/L, or lower with evidence of uraemic encephalopathy or pericarditis.
- Creatinine > 400 μmol/L.
- Severe hypo- or hypernatremia: $Na^+ < 110$ mmol/L or > 160 mmol/L.
- Uncompensated metabolic acidosis.

Volume overload

Pulmonary oedema refractory to diuretics, or diuretics not appropriate.

Low urine output

Oliguria (urine output 0.25–0.5 mL/kg body weight/hour).

Anuria (urine output <0.25 mL/kg body weight/hour).

Removal of dialysable toxins

Note haemodialysis and haemofiltration have different efficacies.

Adapted from Bersten, A. and Soni, N. (2013). *Oh's Intensive Care Manual*, Seventh Edition, Butterworth-Heinemann Elsevier.

is obsolete; though dopamine has a diuretic action and may increase urine output, there is no evidence for improved outcomes with its use in critically ill patients with AKI.

Acute liver failure

The pathophysiology of acute liver failure (ALF) is discussed in Chapter 15 ➲ Acute liver failure, p. 526. ALF may arise in a previously normal organ, but is common in patients with even mild and sometimes undiagnosed (e.g. alcohol-related) existing liver disease, who fare badly with decompensation in ICU. Patients with ALF may require admission to ICU for the following reasons:

- Airway protection: required due to encephalopathy.
- Variceal bleeding.
- Sepsis: liver patients are immunocompromised and may develop spontaneous bacterial peritonitis.
- Concomitant renal failure: especially in paracetamol overdose or in hepatorenal syndrome.
- Metabolic acidosis: discussed below.

Altered consciousness and airway protection

Any cause of altered consciousness in a patient who is unable to protect their airway may necessitate ICU admission. The primary concern is aspiration of gastric contents, which can cause severe lung injury but may not be immediately clinically evident. A GCS of ≤ 8 is often considered the threshold for intubation. A patient with an identifiable precipitant, such as a single seizure, may be monitored closely in a suitable environment as their consciousness level improves. Some conditions where airway protection may be necessary are given in Box 12.5.

Raised intracranial pressure

Intracranial pressure (ICP) is normally 7–15 mmHg in a supine adult, but may be raised in a variety of medical conditions including:

- Intracranial haemorrhage.
- Hepatic encephalopathy.
- Extensive cerebral infarction.
- Prolonged hypoxia.

ICP monitoring can be performed using pressure transducers inserted intraventricularly or transcranially into the brain parenchyma or subarachnoid space by drilling a hole in the skull. The role of routine ICP

Box 12.5 Examples of situations in which intubation for airway protection may be appropriate

Status epilepticus

Intubation and mechanical ventilation is necessary both because of ongoing reduced consciousness and a requirement for agents, such as propofol, thiopentone or midazolam to control seizures.

CNS infection

E.g. meningitis, encephalitis.

Encephalopathy

Aetiologies include hepatic, uraemic, septic, hypertensive and hypoxic-ischaemic.

Drug intoxication

Especially mixed overdoses with or without alcohol.

Stroke

In patients with malignant stroke, intracerebral haemorrhage or cerebral venous sinus thrombosis, intracranial pressure may rise rapidly causing unconsciousness and decompressive craniotomy may be lifesaving.

monitoring in comatose patients is unclear. The cerebral perfusion pressure (CPP) can be calculated by subtracting the ICP from the MAP. In healthy individuals cerebral blood flow remains relatively constant with a CPP between 50 and 100 mmHg due to autoregulatory mechanisms. In raised ICP, increasing the MAP with vasoactive drugs will increase CPP, thereby increasing cerebral blood flow. Additional therapies are also used to lower ICP:

- Mannitol: osmotic diuretic that will dehydrate the brain parenchyma.
- Hypertonic saline: similar action to mannitol.
- Hyperventilation: acutely lowering $PaCO_2$ causes cerebral vasoconstriction, which reduces ICP by lowering the volume of intracranial blood; this is only effective for short periods and the long-term aim is to maintain eucapnia.
- Barbiturates: reduce brain metabolism and cerebral blood flow.

Nutritional support

All critically ill patients require nutritional support and evidence favours introduction of enteral feeding (usually via nasal or orogastric tube) as soon as possible. Contraindications include diseases associated with ileus, intestinal obstruction, active GI haemorrhage or bowel ischaemia. If the enteral route is not available TPN may be used (➲ see Chapter 1, Principles of enteral and parenteral nutrition, p. 15).

Total parenteral nutrition

TPN in critical illness is associated with a number of complications:

- Line-related sepsis and other complications of central venous cannulation.
- Hepatic dysfunction.
- Electrolyte and acid-base abnormalities: hypokalaemia, hypophosphataemia, hyperchloraemia and associated acidosis.
- Refeeding syndrome.

Tight glycaemic control

Many critically ill patients without a previous diagnosis of diabetes will develop stress hyperglycaemia. Treatment with continuous infusion of human soluble insulin should be adjusted according to blood glucose levels with an aim to maintain levels below 10 mmol/L. Evidence suggests that the morbidity associated with hypoglycaemia offsets the benefits of a narrow target range of 4.5–6 mmol/L.

Stress ulcer prophylaxis

Gastric and duodenal stress ulceration is common in critical illness. It is standard practice for prophylactic H_2-receptor antagonists or proton pump inhibitors to be used, although the evidence for this approach is not strong. It may be unnecessary in patients who have been established on enteral nutrition and acid suppression may increase the risk of nosocomial pneumonia.

Skin failure and burns

Skin failure is a particularly challenging organ failure to address, often necessitating transfer to specialised centres to optimise outcome. Causes include:

- Extensive burns.
- Toxic epidermal necrolysis.
- Stevens–Johnson syndrome.
- Autoimmune blistering syndromes.

Irrespective of the cause, the key challenges result mainly from loss of the barrier and homeostatic functions of the skin, and are as follows:

- Fluid balance: huge volumes of fluid can be lost leading to hypovolaemia and electrolyte disturbances.
- Sepsis.
- Thermoregulatory failure.
- ARDS: massive cytokine release can precipitate lung injury.

Specific situations

Lactic acidosis

Lactic acidosis is a commonly encountered problem in critical care. Lactate is metabolised by several organs including the brain, skeletal muscle, liver and kidneys, such that levels in health are usually <2 mmol/L. Strenuous exercise in healthy individuals produces a marked lactic acidosis which resolves with rest. A similar phenomenon is seen following a generalised tonic-clonic seizure. A marked lactic acidosis in an obtunded patient, which resolves with little or no intervention often points retrospectively to an unwitnessed seizure.

In critical illness a lactic acidosis is usually due to shock and a consequence of a combination of three processes:

- Tissue hypoxia increasing anaerobic respiration (e.g. cardiogenic shock and ischaemic bowel).
- Hepatic hypoperfusion impairing lactate clearance.
- Impaired mitochondrial function in septic shock.

A classification for lactic acidosis is given in Box 12.6. In practice, critically ill patients often have several contributing factors. Treatment is withdrawal of likely culprit agents, coupled with appropriate resuscitation. In the peri-arrest setting sodium bicarbonate may have a role as a temporising measure, but correction of the underlying problem is paramount.

Cardiac arrest and therapeutic hypothermia

In individuals remaining comatose following successful resuscitation from out-of-hospital cardiac arrest, therapeutic cooling to a temperature of 32–34°C for a period of 24 hours was thought to improve neurological outcome and mortality. The effectiveness of this approach has been called into question more recently and avoiding hyperthermia, rather than inducing hypothermia, may be of most benefit. If undertaken, cooling can be achieved with the following procedures:

- Delivering a bolus of cold crystalloid.
- Use of cooling blankets.
- Application of ice packs near major vessels in axillae and groins.
- Insertion of IV cooling catheters.
- Prevention of shivering using neuromuscular blockade and/or magnesium infusion.

Box 12.6 Classification of lactic acidosis

Type A: tissue hypoxia present (shock states)

- Severe hypoxaemia, hypovolaemia or anaemia.
- Carbon monoxide poisoning.
- Ischaemic bowel.
- Low cardiac output.

Type B: tissue hypoxia absent

Underlying disorders

- Sepsis.
- Malignancy: especially hepatic or haematological.
- Liver or renal failure.
- Thiamine deficiency.

Drugs

- β-agonists, e.g. adrenaline, salbutamol.
- Propofol.
- Methanol.
- Ethylene glycol.
- Biguanides, e.g. metformin.
- Isoniazid.
- Sorbitol: constituent of TPN.
- Salicylate.
- Iron.
- Cyanide.

Inborn errors of metabolism (rare)

➲ See Chapter 1, Inherited metabolic disorders, p. 29

Data from Woods, Hubert Frank; Cohen, Robert (1976). *Clinical and Biochemical Aspects of Lactic Acidosis*. Oxford: Blackwell Scientific.

Brainstem death

In the UK brain death is defined as the absence of clinical function of the brainstem involving:

- Loss of consciousness.
- Unresponsiveness.
- Inability to breathe.
- Loss of brainstem reflexes.

The diagnosis of brainstem death must be confirmed by two independent doctors. If both are in agreement, then the time of death is taken as that at which the first set of tests was performed. The following are prerequisites:

- The patient is apnoeic and comatose, and therefore ventilator dependent.
- There must be underlying structural brain injury in keeping with brainstem death.
- The causal disorder must have been determined.
- Reversible causes of coma must have been excluded:
  - alcohol or drug intoxication;
  - sedatives or neuromuscular blocking agents;
  - disturbance in blood glucose or electrolytes;
  - hypothermia.

The diagnosis is established by clinical examination:

- Fixed, unreactive pupils (usually but not always dilated).
- Absent corneal reflexes.

- No response to pain in trigeminal nerve distribution.
- No gag or cough reflex.
- Absent caloric responses: no eye movements upon slow irrigation of each ear canal in turn with at least 50 mL of ice-cold water.
- Failure of respiratory effort despite $PaCO_2$ > 6.5 kPa and pH < 7.35 (apnoea test); following pre-oxygenation, mechanical ventilation is ceased for a time to assess the response to hypercapnia.

Further reading

1. Myburgh JA, Mythen MG. Resuscitation fluids. *N Engl J Med*. 2013;369:1243–51.
2. Gotts JE, Matthay MA. Sepsis: pathophysiology and clinical management. *Br Med J*. 2016;353:i1585.
3. Sweeney RM, McAuley DF. Acute respiratory distress syndrome. *Lancet*. 2016;388:2416–30.
4. Kraut JA, Madias NE. Lactic acidosis. *N Engl J Med*. 2014;371:2309–19.
5. Resuscitation Council (UK). Information for professionals. https://www.resus.org.uk/information-for-professionals/.

Multiple choice questions

Questions

1. A 64-year-old man suffers an extensive anterior myocardial infarction and develops florid pulmonary oedema. He is intubated and taken for primary percutaneous coronary intervention to his proximal left anterior descending coronary artery. He is stable in the ICU for 6 hours following the procedure, but then develops a metabolic acidosis and oliguria. His mean arterial pressure falls to 55 mmHg. A pulmonary artery catheter reveals a PCWP of 5 mmHg and cardiac index (CI) of 2.3 L/min/m^2.
   Which of the following is most likely to account for the change in his condition?
   A. Acute left ventricular failure.
   B. Bacterial sepsis.
   C. Cardiac tamponade.
   D. Occult bleeding.
   E. Mitral valve rupture.

2. An obese 54-year-old woman is brought to the Emergency Department having been found unconscious on the floor at home. Her GCS on arrival is 6 and she is normotensive. An arterial blood gas on 15 L/min oxygen via a non-rebreathe mask reveals the following:
   - pH: 7.15.
   - pCO_2: 5.2 kPa.
   - pO_2: 14.5 kPa.
   - Lactate: 8.6 mmol/L.

   Of the following, which is most in keeping with the presentation?
   A. Use of high flow oxygen in a patient with unrecognised obesity-hypoventilation syndrome.
   B. Mixed drug overdose complicated by aspiration of gastric contents.
   C. Severe infective exacerbation of COPD.
   D. Unwitnessed generalised tonic-clonic seizure.
   E. Overdose of metformin prescribed for type 2 diabetes mellitus.

3. What is the correct dose of adrenaline for the initial treatment of anaphylaxis in an adult?
   A. 0.5 mg 1:10,000 IM.
   B. 0.5 mg 1:1,000 IM.
   C. 0.5 mg 1:10,000 IV.
   D. 0.5 mg 1:1,000 IV.
   E. 0.5 mg 1:1,000 SC.

Answers

1. D. A large retroperitoneal haemorrhage from a femoral access site for PCI may have occurred. The haemodynamic variables indicate hypovolaemic shock. The CI would not be expected to be this low in septic shock. Though cardiogenic shock and tamponade may complicate an extensive anterior MI the PCWP of only 5 mmHg argues against these diagnoses. In acute MR the PCWP is generally grossly elevated. ➲ See Box 12.2, Table 12.2 and Hypovolaemic shock, p. 395 for further information.
2. B. The ABG is consistent with a severe lactic acidosis with a lack of appropriate respiratory compensation in the setting of reduced consciousness. The PaO_2 is far too low for the high fraction of inspired oxygen. The patient is not hypercapnic, so this cannot explain the coma. A single seizure in isolation would normally be followed by hyperventilation to compensate for the metabolic acidosis. An overdose of metformin is possible, but the best answer is B since this would explain the metabolic acidosis, respiratory depression, raised alveolar-arterial gradient and coma. Agents might include opioids, benzodiazepines, tricyclic antidepressants and alcohols, including ethylene glycol. Sepsis also commonly gives this presentation but this is not offered as an option (➲ see Lactic acidosis, p. 404 and Box 12.6, for further discussion of the causes of a lactic acidosis).
3. B. The initial treatment should be 0.5 ml of 1:1,000 adrenaline IM, a dose of 0.5 mg. IV administration should only be undertaken by clinicians experienced in its use (➲ see Anaphylactic shock, p. 394, for further discussion of the management of anaphylactic shock).

Chapter 13 **Cardiology**

David Holdsworth, Rupert P. Williams* and Nicholas Gall*

Cardiac physiology and anatomy

Physiology

- The cardiovascular system maintains blood flow (cardiac output) through all body tissues. CO from the left ventricle must, over several beats, equal total venous return (VRet) to the right atrium (RA).
- Mean arterial pressure (Box 13.1) is maintained by CO and total peripheral resistance (TPR):

$$\text{MAP} = \text{CO} \times \text{TPR}$$
$$\text{CO} = \text{SV} \times \text{HR}$$

where HR is heart rate; SV is stroke volume.

* Joint first authors.

Box 13.1

The relationship of systemic arterial blood pressure to cardiac output and peripheral resistance is akin to Ohm's law relating potential difference to electrical current and resistance.

- At a given MAP, tissue flow is autoregulated by regional vasodilation proportional to local metabolic activity.
- The small muscular arteries and arterioles are at branch points in the vascular tree. Vasomotor tone is controlled by:
  - Shear-induced, NO-mediated vasodilatation matching flow to the downstream metabolic requirements.
  - Central control to maintain whole-body blood pressure through
    - sympathetic stimulation of VSM;
    - the effect of circulating catecholamines on VSM.
- The simplified Poisuille–Hagen equation describes flow as proportional to the 4th power of the radius. Hence, blood flow is exquisitely sensitive to vasomotor changes.
- The total cardiac output is equal to the stroke volume multiplied by the heart rate.

MAP, mean arterial pressure; NO, nitric oxide; VSM, vascular smooth muscle.

Stroke volume

Stroke volume is determined by five factors:

1. *Preload* (venous return), is maintained by:
   - The intravascular filling status (most blood volume resides in the venous compartment).
   - Venomotor tone.
   - RA pressure (increased RA pressure will decrease the gradient for venous return and so reduce VRet).
2. *Afterload*: MAP against which the LV volume is ejected:
   - As afterload increases, the degree of end diastolic stretch of the LV increases, enhancing contractility. Pathologically high afterload (e.g. severe hypertension or aortic stenosis) significantly reduces SV. It may lead to hypertrophy of a non-dilated LV with a small volume, or LV dilatation beyond the physiological parameters of the Starling relationship.

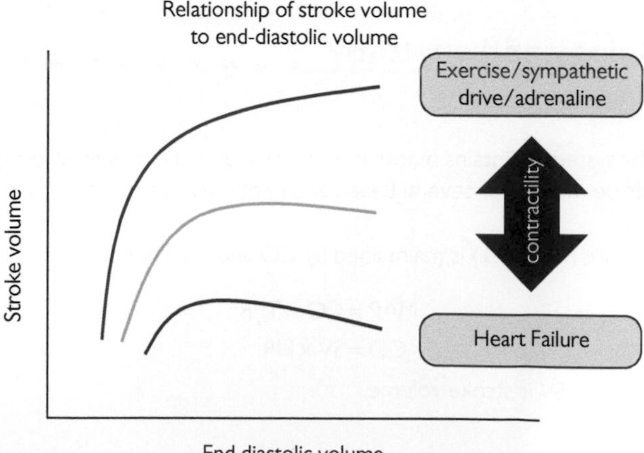

Figure 13.1 The influence of ventricular filling on stroke volume, as described by Otto Frank and Ernest Starling. Within the physiological range, an increase in the resting fibre length increases the tension developed during myocardial contraction.

3. *Contractility*: the sensitivity (or *gradient*) of the Starling relationship between end diastolic volume (EDV) and force of contraction is described as contractility (Figure 13.1):
   - Factors intrinsic to the myocardium (e.g. ageing or heart failure) reduce force of contraction at any given EDV.
   - Extrinsic factors (e.g. sympathetic nervous stimulation, circulating catecholamines and positive inotropes) increase contractility.
4. *HR*: the volume of filling is proportional to the duration of diastole. As HR increases, cardiac filling time reduces, limiting SV.
5. *Coordinated cardiac contraction*:
   - Sinus rhythm – allows consistent diastolic filling time.
   - Coordinated atrial contraction – to 'prime' ventricles.
   - Atrioventricular (AV) node delay – allows for complete ventricular filling.
   - Coordinated ventricular contraction – simultaneous biventricular depolarisation from apex to base (i.e. narrow QRS on surface ECG).
   - Absence of coordinated contraction (e.g. atrial fibrillation [AF] or bundle branch block [BBB]) may cause a marked reduction in CO. This underscores the benefits of cardioversion or cardiac resynchronsiation therapy in selected patients.

Heart rate

HR is determined by three factors:

1. *Neural stimulation of the sinoatrial node* (pacemaker potential):
   - Parasympathetic/sympathetic stimulation slows/increases HR.
2. *Humoral factors*:
   - Circulating positive chronotropes (endogenous, e.g. adrenaline, and exogenous, e.g. isoprenaline) increase HR.
   - Circulating negative chronotropes (exogenous, e.g. β-blockers, verapamil) reduce HR.
3. *Atrial filling*:
   - Increasing RA stretch increases HR via a mechanically-coupled ion channel influence on pacemaker potential (the 'Bainbridge reflex').

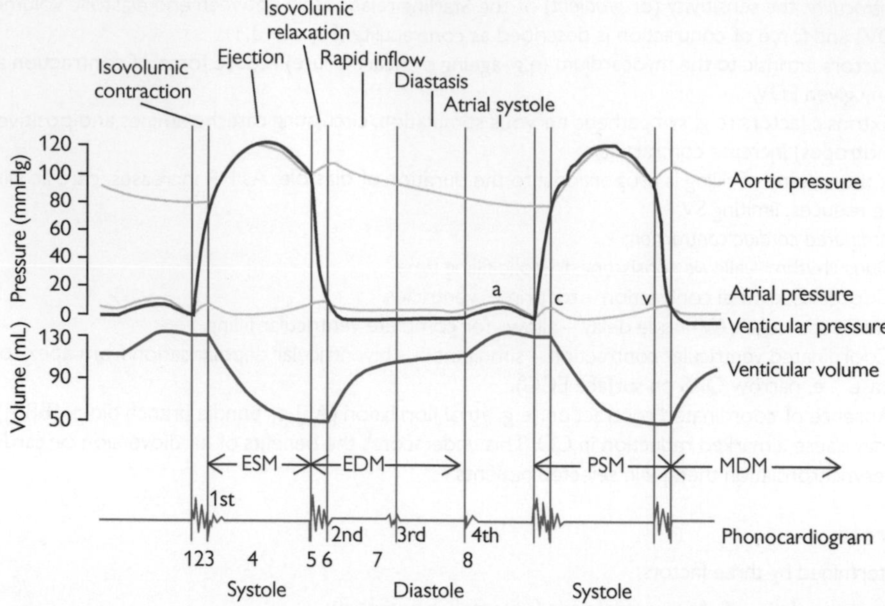

Figure 13.2 The 'Wiggers' diagram displays the simultaneous variation in key cardiovascular parameters with time, across the cardiac cycle. Aortic, ventricular and atrial pressure and ventricular volume are shown. The heart sounds (phonocardiogram) are also displayed. ESM (ejection systolic murmur), EDM (end diastolic murmur), PSM (pan systolic murmur), MDM (mid-diastolic murmur).

Cardiac cycle

This is the haemodynamic, electrical and mechanical events which occur during one iteration of systole and diastole (Figure 13.2). Pathological changes to this cycle explain certain cardiovascular examination findings.

For a diagram of arterial waveform, see Figure 13.3.

Jugular venous pulse

The internal JVP reflects the atrial pressure waveform (see Figure 13.4 and Table 13.1). The JVP is measured with a patient reclined at 45°.

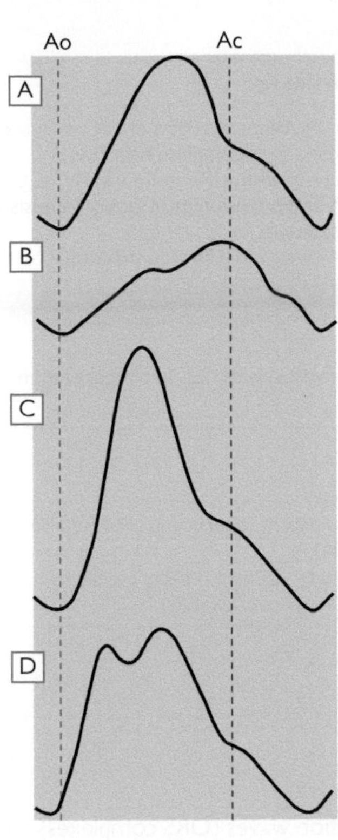

Ao–aortic valve opens (immediately follows S1)
Ac–aortic valve closes (coincides with S2)

A. Normal arterial pulse, dicrotic notch in the descending limb represents the closure of the aortic valve and subsequent elastic recoil of the elastic aorta

B. Aortic stenosis (AS)–slow rising, late peaking pulse

C. Aortic regurgitation (AR)–brisk, high volume upstroke and rapid, early pressure drop. The extremely rapid fall in blood pressure acounts for the low diastolic pressure. The area under the curve reflects the forward stroke volume. Note that in AR stroke volume is both increased and ejected more rapidly and transiently. This accounts for the palpation of a 'collapsing pulse'

D. Bisferiens pulse–most commonly associated with coincident pathology of aortic stenosis and aortic regurgitation, there is a biphasic ejection with a palpable mid systolic 'dip' in pressure wave

Figure 13.3 Diagram of arterial waveform.

Reproduced with permission from Hall, R. and Simpson, I. The Cardiovascular History and Physical Examination. In *The ESC Textbook of Cardiovascular Medicine*, 2nd edn, Camm AJ et al. (Eds). Oxford: OUP. Copyright © 2009 European Society of Cardiology. DOI: 10.1093/med/9780199566990.001.0001. Reproduced with permission of the Licensor through PLSclear.

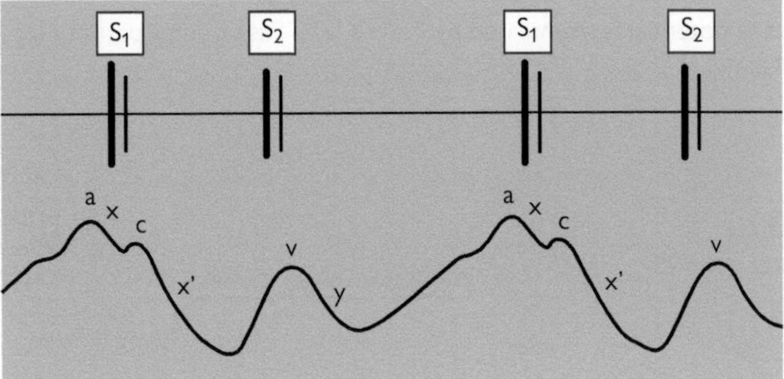

Figure 13.4 The pressure waveform of the jugular venous pulsation, which reflects the changing pressure in the right atrium is shown alongside the heart sounds S1 (representing closure of the atrioventricular valves) and S2 (closure of the semilunar valves through which blood flows into the aorta and pulmonary artery). The a-wave represents the effect of atrial contraction; the x-descent that follows represents atrial relaxation. The c-wave represents the conducted pressure of the bulging of the tricuspid valve back into the right atrium during isovolumic contraction of the right ventricle. The x'-descent occurs during systole, as the tricuspid annulus moves down towards the cardiac apex, as blood is ejected from the pulmonary artery, this 'sucks' blood into the right atrium. The v-wave represents the pressure rising in the right atrium as the atrium fills passively from venous blood returning to the heart, the y-descent follows the opening of the tricuspid valve and emptying of the right atrium into the right ventricle.

Reproduced with permission from Hall, R. and Simpson, I. The Cardiovascular History and Physical Examination. In *The ESC Textbook of Cardiovascular Medicine*, 2nd edn, Camm AJ, et al. (Eds). Oxford: OUP. Copyright © 2009 European Society of Cardiology. DOI: 10.1093/med/9780199566990.001.0001. Reproduced with permission of the Licensor through PLSclear.

Table 13.1 Jugular venous pulse

JVP feature	Physiology	Pathophysiology
a-wave	Retrograde venous pressure of atrial contraction.	Cannon a-waves: contraction of RA when tricusid valve is closed (e.g. complete heart block). Giant a-waves: *obstruction* to flow in RV (e.g. pulmonary hypertension, pulmonary stenosis or tricuspid stenosis). Loss of a-waves: atrial fibrillation/flutter.
c-wave	Bulging of the closing tricuspid valve in early ventricular systole.	
v-wave	Pressure rising in the atrium due to filling from the venous return.	Giant v-waves: severe tricuspid regurgitation.
x-descent	'Suction' effect of the relaxing right atrium.	
y-descent	'Suction' effect of relaxing right ventricle.	Blunted y-descent reflects impaired RV filling (e.g. tamponade). Accentuated y-descent reflects accelerated filling (e.g. constrictive pericarditis).

Electrocardiography

Morphology of the electrocardiogram

- Records electrical activity over time.
- Atrial depolarisation waves (P waves), ventricular depolarisation waves (QRS complexes) and ventricular repolarisation waves (T waves) are recorded for each cardiac cycle.
- *Positive* deflections in the ECG result from electrical activity *towards* a surface electrode (e.g. V5).
- Depolarisation occurs from subendocardium towards subepicardium, their sum producing the surface ECG.
- Cardiac action potential (see Figure 13.5).
- Resting membrane potential is maintained by Na^+/K^+/ATPase pump (partitioning Na^+ extracellularly and K^+ intracellularly).

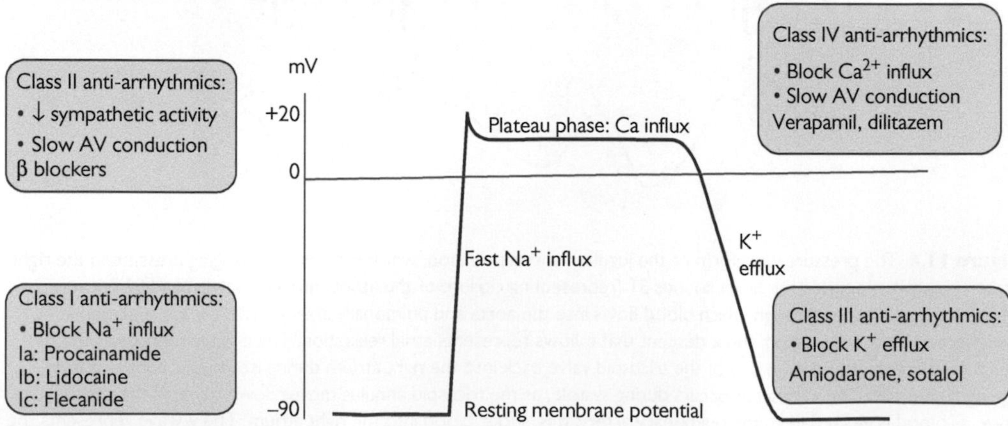

Figure 13.5 The action potential and Vaughan Williams classification of anti-arrhythmic drugs.

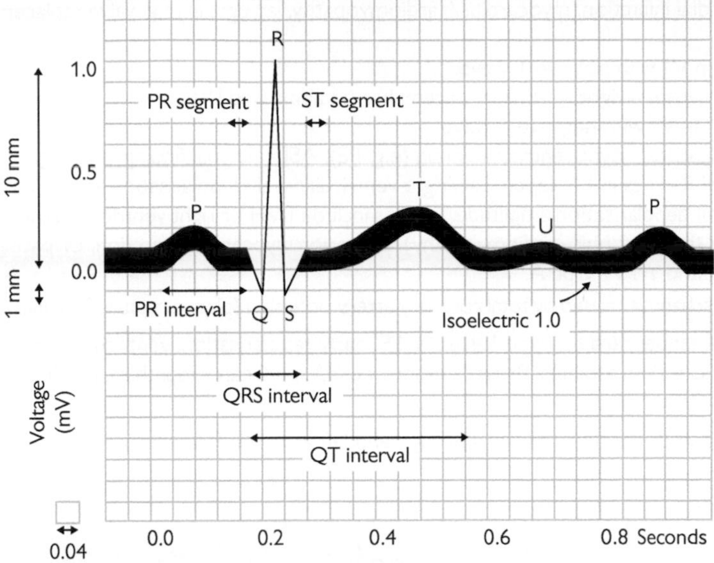

Figure 13.6 ECG morphology in a lead facing left ventricular free wall (e.g. V5).

Reproduced with permission from Cardiovascular medicine. In *Oxford Handbook of Clinical Medicine*, 10th edn, Wilkinson IB, et al. (Eds). Oxford: OUP. Copyright © 2017, Oxford University Press. DOI: 10.1093/med/9780199689903.001.0001. Reproduced with permission of the Licensor through PLSclear.

Normal electrocardiogram characteristics

- Axis: *Normal* = –30° to +90°; *Left* = –30° to –90°; *Right* = +90° to +180°.
- All cardiomyocytes have automaticity (sinus node has highest).
- Sinus rhythm implies a P wave originating from the sinoatrial (SA) node; the P wave is +ve in I, II, aVF, V2-6, and –ve in aVR.
- PR interval: isoelectric and duration 0.12–0.2 seconds.
- QRS duration < 0.12 seconds. R wave height <25 mm in V5+6; <20 mm in lead I; and <16 mm in lead aVL.
- T wave is usually +ve in all leads except in aVR and V1, may be -ve in V2, and also another -ve in the limb leads; any further -ve leads would be abnormal.
- A small U wave can be a normal finding.

ECG morphology in a lead facing a left ventricular free wall is shown in Figure 13.6.

Common electrocardiogram abnormalities

- *Pathological Q waves* are > 0.04 seconds, > 2mm deep and >25% of the following R wave amplitude. Causes: any transmural scar/fibrosis (transmural infarction, amyloidosis, neoplastic infiltration, cardiomyopathy), LBBB, Wolff–Parkinson–White (WPW), dextrocardia.
- *Left axis deviation*: axis –30° to –90°.
  - Causes – cardiomyopathy, primum atrial septal defect (ASD), left ventricular hypertrophy (LVH), LBBB, left anterior hemi-block, tricuspid atresia.
- *Right axis deviation*: axis +90° to +180°.
  - Causes – right ventricular hypertrophy (RVH) (e.g. secondary to PE, lung disease, large secundum ASD), infancy, RBBB.
- *Bundle branch block*: (QRS >0.12 seconds) myocardial scarring affecting the conduction tissue may cause RBBB or LBBB, delaying depolarisation to the corresponding myocardium. Causes include

post myocardial infarction, myocarditis/cardiomyopathy, iatrogenic (e.g. valve replacement) and idiopathic.

- *LBBB* – *rS* in V1 with positive T wave.
  - Specific causes – right ventricular pacemaker (at apex) and LVH.
- *RBBB* – *rsR* in V1 with negative T wave.
  - Specific causes – right ventricular strain (e.g. PE), ASD; normal finding in young.

- *Dominant/tall R waves in V1*: septal wall/right ventricular wall depolarisation amplitude > left posterior wall depolarisation amplitude. Causes include RVH or right ventricular strain, septal hypertrophy (hypertrophic cardiomyopathy), posterior myocardial infarction, LV pacing, dextrocardia and WPW type A.
- *ST elevation*: Ischaemia caused by total coronary artery occlusion (plaque rupture/coronary artery spasm).
  - Other causes: pericarditis, hyperkalaemia, PE, early repolarisation, ventricular aneurysm, cardioversion, LVH, athletes, Brugada syndrome (➲ see Channelopathies, p. 476 and Figure 13.27).

For a normal ECG and intentional reversal of right and left arm, see Figure 13.7.

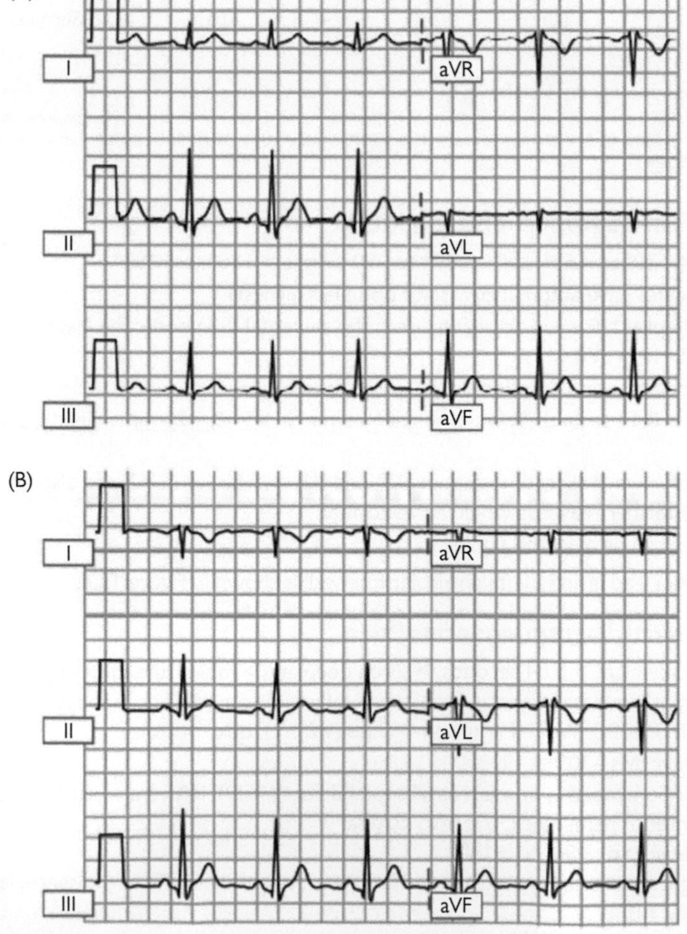

Figure 13.7 Normal ECG (A) and intentional reversal of right and left arm in (B).

Other electrocardiogram abnormalities

- *Left atrial enlargement*: biphasic P wave in V1.
- *Right atrial enlargement*: tall P wave in II.
- *Athletes hearts:* sinus bradycardia, first degree heart block, Wenkebach phenomenon, voltage criteria for LVH, early repolarisation.
- *Transient Q waves:* coronary spasm, hypoxia, hypothermia.

Metabolic electrocardiogram abnormalities

- *Hypothermia:* prolonged PR, QRS and QTc; 'Osborne' J-waves, ventricular ectopy and shivering artefact.
- *Hypokalaemia:* tall P waves, flat/inverted T waves ± ST depression, tall U waves, prolonged PR interval, long QT interval, ± broad QRS.
- *Hyperkalaemia:* absent P waves, tall T waves, broad QRS developing into a sinusoidal pattern (comprising QRS and T waves: pre-arrest).
- *Hypocalcaemia*: long QT interval.
- *Hypercalcaemia*: short QT interval.

Prolonged electrocardiogram monitoring

- *Holter monitor*: continuous monitoring for 24 hours to 7 days, with a patient diary for correlation with symptoms. Ventricular ectopic frequency > 20% of total beats (over a 24-hour period) places patient at risk of developing future cardiomyopathy; consider β-blocker and arrange echocardiogram.
- *External recorders*: intermittent monitoring – patient places monitor on chest at onset of symptoms.
- *Wearable loop recorders*: continuous monitoring (on a self-erasing loop); at onset of symptoms patient activates recorder, which records minutes of continuous ECG traces before and after event.
- *Implantable loop recorders*: records ECG when rhythm activates pre-specified alarm criteria (e.g. irregular R-R interval, HR > 150 bpm), implanted for 3+ years.

Further reading

1. Bayes de Luna A, Batchvarov VN, Malik M. The morphology of the electrocardiogram. *The ESC Textbook of Cardiovascular Medicine*, 2nd edn, 2009. Oxford: Oxford University Press.

Imaging

Indications

Cardiac structure and function

- Chamber sizes, wall thickness and function.
- Tissue characterisation (e.g. cardiomyopathy, intracardiac masses).
- Pericardium.
- Congenital heart disease (morphology, connections and shunts).

Valve anatomy and function

- Valve leaflets, valve apparatus (annulus, chordae, papillary muscles) and pathology (e.g. vegetation).
- Valve haemodynamics (stenosis and regurgitation).

Coronary artery anatomy and coronary ischaemia

Stable chest pain with suspected coronary artery disease (CAD):

- CAD is confirmed by *anatomical imaging*:
  - CT calcium scoring.
  - CT coronary angiography.
- Myocardial ischaemia is confirmed by *functional imaging*:
  - Stress echo (US).
  - Stress myocardial perfusion scan (nuclear).
  - Stress cardiac magnetic resonance (CMR; not widely available).

Known CAD and impaired LV function (ischaemic cardiomyopathy):

- Perfusion defect: a segment of myocardium with reduced perfusion under 'stress' (exercise or drug induced [e.g. dobutamine]).
- Viable myocardium: a segment of reduced contractile function with potential to improve with revascularisation.
- Viablity is indicated by:
  - Wall thickness >6 mm at end-diastole.
  - Improved contractile function with low-dose inotropes.
  - Scar <50% of wall thickness (late gadolinium enhancement on CMR).
  - Intact, functioning cell membrane (PET scanning techniques).

Aorta

- Anatomy (aneurysm, dissection, coarctation).
- Haemodynamics (of coarctation).

The choice of investigation will depend on various factors. Transthoracic echocardiogram is accessible, but insensitive in diagnosis. CMR and transoesophageal echocardiogram (TOE) are both sensitive, but difficult to organise rapidly. In most hospitals CT aortography (with contrast) is the best emergency imaging.

Imaging: modality characteristics and indications for cardiovascular imaging

See Table 13.2 for imaging modality characteristics and Table 13.3 for indications for cardiovascular imaging and appropriate modality.

Invasive cardiology

Indications for left heart catheter catheterisation

- Acute coronary syndrome.
- Stable chest pain: if high or very high pre-test probability of coronary artery disease. If lower probability consider functional imaging test or CT coronary angiography (1).
- Prior to cardiac (e.g. valvular) or high risk non-cardiac surgery.

Table 13.2 Imaging modality characteristics

	Classic roles	Advantages	Disadvantages	Recent developments
ECHO TTE TOE *Most commonly used modalities*	Anatomy and function: myocardium (systolic and diastolic). Valve (and structure). Pericardium. Aorta (moderate sensitivity).	Cheap. Safe. Widely available. Portable. Excellent functional, haemodynamic data from Doppler, e.g. diastolic function, blood flow parameters.	Subject to 'ECHO windows'. Poor in obesity and COPD.	3D ECHO in valve assessment/LV function. Increasing use of IV contrast: Myocardial perfusion Enhance LV endocardial border: LV function. Thrombus detection.
Nuclear SPECT PET	Mainly functional assessment; not used for anatomy. Coronary perfusion (ischaemia). Viability (amount of scar). Accurate ejection fraction.	Accurate functional assessment of both perfusion and viable myocardium. Superior stress test to echo in obese patients and patients with COPD or renal impairment.	Ionising radiation. Limited availability. Limited anatomical information.	PET – quantification of metabolism (aerobic and anaerobic). 'Hybrid' imaging, e.g. coregistration with MSCT data.
Cardiac MSCT	Coronary artery assessment. Total coronary calcium score – risk stratification. Exclusion of significant coronary stenoses. Good aortic imaging.	Very good anatomical imaging. Reasonable availability.	Ionising radiation. Quite expensive. Contrast induced nephropathy.	Use of contrast to exclude non-calcified plaque, reducing doses of radiation.
Cardiac magnetic resonance	Anatomy and function. Accurate volumes and EF. Perfusion and viability.[1] Good tissue characterisation with gadolinium contrast. Non-invasive angiography is available, but inferior to CTCA.	Excellent anatomical imaging. Very high spatial resolution; temporal resolution is inferior to echo. Answers most questions posed of cardiovascular imaging.	Expensive. Restricted availability. Contraindications: some ferromagnetic implants (e.g. some pacemakers and ICDs, and most CRT[D]s). Claustrophobia. Nephrogenic systemic fibrosis.	Phase-contrast (velocity-coded) CMR can now give flow information, including volumes, mean and peak velocities.

Abbreviations: TTE, transthoracic echo; TOE, transoesophageal ECHO; SPECT, single positron emission computed tomography; PET, positron emission tomography; MSCT, multi-slice computed tomography; COPD, chronic pulmonary obstructive disease; CTCA, computed tomography coronary angiogram; CMR, cardiac magnetic resonance; EF, ejection fraction; ICD, implantable cardiac defibrillator; CRT(D), cardiac resynchronisation therapy defibrillator.

[1]Perfusion is possible with 'first pass' gadolinium contrast; late gadolinium enhancement represents scar (volume of scar estimated) giving viability assessment.

Table 13.3 Indications for cardiovascular imaging and appropriate modality

Indication	Echocardiography (US)	Nuclear imaging	Cardiac computed tomography (CCT)	Cardiac magnetic resonance (CMR)
LV assessment	++	++	++	+++
Size /volume				
Systolic function and EF	++	++	++	+++
Diastolic function	+++ a major advantage	–	–	+
Coronary artery anatomy for coronary artery disease	–	–	+++ 'Gold standard' is invasive coronary angiography	–
Functional testing for ischaemia (Δ rest:stress) *imaging during rest and stress*	+++ Using wall motion changes (IV contrast makes perfusion assessment possible)	+++ Using perfusion changes (adenosine and exercise stress)	–	+++ Using perfusion (adenosine) *or* wall motion changes (dobutamine)
Myocardial viability	++ Wall thinning[1] and contractile reserve[2]	+++	–	++ wall thinning[1], contractile reserve[2] and scar assessment[3]
RV size and function	++	–	++	+++
Valve disease	+++	–	+ For stenosis	++ For regurgitation. + For stenosis
Cardiac masses	++	–	++	+++
Aortic disease	+ TTE ++ TOE	–	+++ accurate image whole aorta	+++ accurate image whole aorta
Pericardial disease	+++ Diagnosis *and* haemodynamics (not sensitive for pericardial thickness)	–	++ For pericardial thickness. + For haemodynamics	++ For pericardial thickness. + For good haemodynamics
Congenital cardiac disease	++	–	+ Ionising radiation inappropriate in young cohort	+++

[1]Wall thinning: segments with an end-diastolic wall thickness <5.5 mm are unlikely to improve with revascularisation.
[2]Contractile reserve: if resting regional wall motion abnormality responds to low-dose dobutamine this suggests malperfusion that will improve with revascularisation.
[3]Scar assessment: based on thickness of CMR late gadolinium enhancement (LGE) across the wall from none (0%) to transmural (100%). LGE prediction of myocardial viability: <50% are probably viable and will respond to revascularisation; >75% probably non-viable.

Concepts of left and right heart catheterisation

- Left heart catheterisation (LHC) requires arterial access and is used to visualise ± treat significant coronary artery stenoses with percutaneous coronary intervention (PCI). Multiple views of the same artery are required to avoid missing an 'eccentric' stenosis.
- LHC visualises the left and right coronary arteries (Figure 13.8).
- Fractional flow reserve (FFR) is a physiological test used to assess whether a coronary artery stenosis is flow limiting. FFR represents the maximum possible flow achievable (in the presence of a stenosis, compared with the absence of a stenosis), assuming minimal microvascular resistance during hyperaemia. Distal coronary artery pressure is measured with an intra-coronary pressure wire during pharmacological hyperaemia (e.g. adenosine).
  - FFR = distal coronary pressure divided by aortic pressure. FFR < 0.8 indicates significant flow limitation.
- LHC also enables aortography and therefore diagnosis of aortic regurgitation; coarctation of aorta; identification of bypass grafts; aortic root dilatation and patent ductus arteriosus.
- Right heart catheterisation (RHC) requires central *venous* access. It is used to:
  - Measure pressure and oxygen parameters in the RA, RV, PA and pulmonary capillaries.
  - Provide access for the treatment of arrhythmias and to obtain cardiac biopsies.
  - Insert closure devices to repair ASD.

Complications from left heart catheterisation

- Uncommon (< 1% risk of major complications): coronary/aortic dissection, air embolism (coronary ischaemia or stroke, depending on location), ventricular arrhythmias, tamponade (more common after RHC). Mortality < 0.1%.
- 5% chance of contrast allergy (e.g. rash), contrast-induced nephropathy, arterial access complications (haemorrhage, false aneurysm).

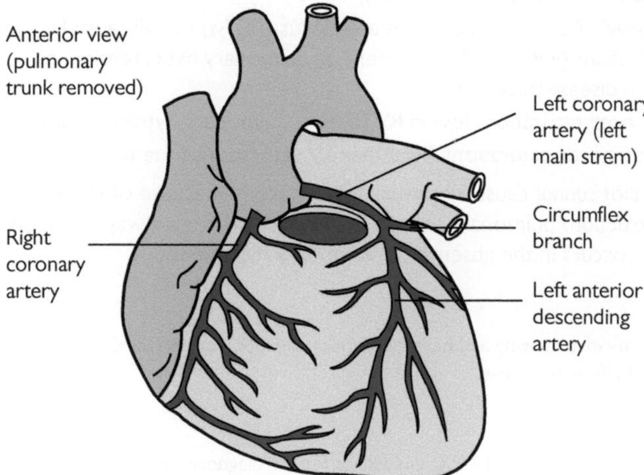

Figure 13.8 Coronary anatomy of LCA and RCA.

Haemodynamic measurements

Pressure

- Systolic LV pressure = systolic aortic pressure. When >10 mmHg drop across valve consider aortic stenosis.
- Normally pulmonary capillary wedge pressure (PCWP) = left ventricular end-diastolic pressure (LVEDP).
- Mean pulmonary artery pressures > 25 mmHg suggest pulmonary arterial hypertension.

Blood oxygen and shunt calculations

- Right heart saturations should be < 75%. If > 75% suggests L to R shunt.
- Left heart saturations should be > 96%. If < 95% suggests R to L shunt or severe lung disease.
  - If R to L shunt increasing inspired oxygen content will not increase oxygen saturations.
- Cardiac output is calculated with the *Fick principle* (oxygen consumption divided by arteriovenous oxygen difference).

Cases

- Primum ASD: step up in *saturations* in *low* RA (+ elevated RV and PA pressures).
- Secundum ASD: step up in *saturations* in *mid* ± *high* RA (+ elevated RV and PA pressures).
- Pericardial constriction: elevated and equal RA and LA pressures, and elevated and equal right ventricular end-diastolic pressure (RVEDP) and LVEDP.
- Mitral stenosis: PCWP > LVEDP by > 5 mmHg.
- Patent ductus arteriosus (PDA) with L to R shunt: step up in *pressure and saturations* in *PA* (e.g. RV 22/5 mmHg and 74% saturations, PA 35/14 mmHg and 94% saturations).
- Ventricular septal defect (VSD) with *L to R shunt*: step up in *pressure and saturations* in *RV* (vs RA), although LV pressure >> RV pressure initially.
- VSDs (small or large), ASDs, patent ductus arteriosus (PDAs) can all cause Eisenmenger's syndrome: L to R shunt (initially), development of pulmonary hypertension, polycythaemia, then R to L shunt (later in disease process).
- VSD with *R to L shunt*: saturations low in RV (due to pulmonary hypertension), LV and aorta.
- Tetralogy of Fallot: aortic saturations *lower* than LV saturations (due to overriding aorta).
  - Tetralogy of Fallot *cannot* cause Eisenmenger's syndrome because of severe right ventricular outflow tract obstruction/pulmonary atresia; thereby RV pressure always > LV pressure, with R to L shunt (cyanosis occurs in the absence of pulmonary hypertension).

Further reading

1. Seiler C, Di Mario C. Invasive imaging and haemodynamics. *The ESC Textbook of Cardiovascular Medicine*, 2nd edn, 2009. Oxford: Oxford University Press.

Reference

1. Knuuti J, Wijns W, Saraste A, *et al*. 2019 ESC Guidelines for the diagnosis and management of chronic coronary syndromes: The Task Force for the diagnosis and management of chronic coronary syndromes of the European Society of Cardiology (ESC). *European Heart Journal*, 425.

Ischaemic heart disease

Chronic ischaemic heart disease

Ischaemic heart disease (IHD) affects 4–7% of people aged 45–64 years, increasing to 12% in those aged 65–84 years. IHD is more prevalent in men, except in middle age, during which more women are affected.

Pathophysiology

- Stable atherosclerotic plaque: thick fibrous cap, small necrotic core.
- Vasospastic angina: vasoconstriction of hyper-reactive vascular smooth muscle ± endothelial dysfunction.
- Microvascular dysfunction: primarily due to endothelial dysfunction (e.g. secondary to diabetes, LVH).

Risk factors

- Primary: hypercholesterolaemia (high LDL), hypertension, smoking.
- Secondary: diabetes, reduced HDL, obesity, family history, stress, gout, race (South Asians), male, age, chronic renal failure, low social class, increased homocysteine levels, low weight at 1 year of age.
- Protective: exercise, low cholesterol diet, high HDL:LDL ratio.

The risk assessment and management of dyslipidaemia is discussed in Chapter 1 (➲ Lipids and atherosclerosis, p. 20, including Cardiovascular risk assessment, p. 22, Figure 1.5, and Table 1.3).

Clinical features

- Constricting anterior chest discomfort radiating to neck, shoulders, jaw or arms (left > right), precipitated by exertion.
- Relieved by rest or GTN within about 5 minutes.
- *Unstable* angina occurs at rest or lasts > 20 minutes.

Diagnosis

- *Bloods:* FBC (including to exclude anaemia), HbA1c, renal function, fasting lipid profile, ± BNP.
- *ECG:* identify signs of ischaemia at rest (if present consider acute coronary syndrome).
- *ECHO:* identify regional wall motion abnormalities and evaluate LV ejection fraction.
- *Determine likelihood of CAD* to determine first line investigation (Table 13.4):
  - If CAD risk 10–29%: perform CT calcium scoring (if score 0: look for alternative diagnosis, if 1–400: perform CT coronary angiography, if > 400 perform invasive angiography).
  - If CAD risk 30–60%: perform functional imaging (myocardial perfusion scintigraphy [MPS], SPECT, stress MRI, stress ECHO).
  - If CAD risk 61–90%: perform invasive coronary angiography (gold standard).

Table 13.4 Table to determine likelihood of coronary artery disease. Percentage of people estimated to have CAD according to typicality of symptoms, age, sex and risk factors

	Non-anginal chest pain				Atypical angina				Typical angina			
	Men		Women		Men		Women		Men		Women	
Age (years)	Lo	Hi	Lo	Hi	Lo	Hi	Lo	Hi	Lo	Hi	Lo	Hi
35	3	35	1	19	8	59	2	39	30	88	10	78
45	9	47	2	22	21	70	5	43	51	92	20	79
55	23	59	4	25	45	79	10	47	80	95	38	82
65	49	69	9	29	71	86	20	51	93	97	56	84

Lo, no risk factors; Hi, diabetes, smoking, high cholesterol.

Prognosis

- Annual mortality 1.2–2.4% in stable angina. No difference in clinical outcome with percutaneous coronary intervention (PCI) versus optimal medical therapy (OMT) (COURAGE study). However, if FFR ≤0.8 then PCI reduces composite end-point of death, MI and urgent revascularisation versus OMT (FAME-2 study).
- Adverse prognosis given by any risk factor for CAD, and also elevated resting HR.

Management

Optimal medical therapy

- Aspirin (or clopidogrel), statin, and angiotensin-converting enzyme inhibitors (ACE-i) if heart failure, hypertension or diabetes.
- ≥1 anti-anginal medication. First-line medications are nitrates, β-blockers and/or calcium-channel blockers, with trimetazidine as last line of therapy (see Table 13.5).

Table 13.5 Side effects and contraindications of drugs used in chronic stable angina

	Side effects	**Contraindications**
Nitrates	Headache, hypotension, syncope, methaemaglobinaemia.	Hypertrophic cardiomyopathy (HCM).
β-blockers	Fatigue, depression, bronchospasm, heart block, impotence, hypoglycaemia.	2nd-degree heart block, asthma/severe COPD, severe PVD.
Ca-channel blockers (heart rate slowing)	Constipation, gingival hyperplasia, heart block.	Congestive heart failure.
Ca-channel blockers (dihydropyridine)	Ankle swelling, headache.	Severe aortic stenosis, HCM.
Ivabradine (I_f/'funny' channel inhibitor)	Visual disturbances, atrial fibrillation, heart block.	Severe liver disease.
Nicorandil	Oral/anal/GI ulceration, headache, hypotension.	Congestive heart failure.
Trimetazidine (inhibits fatty acid metabolism)	Movement disorders.	Parkinson's disease, tremors and movement disorders, renal disease.
Ranolazine (prevents calcium overload)	CU prolongation, constipation.	Severe liver disease.
Allopurinol	Gastric discomfort.	Hypersensitivity.

Coronary angiography ± fractional flow reserve ± PCI

- Revascularisation indicated *to improve prognosis* when left main stem (LMS) or proximal left anterior descending (LAD) stenosis, 2–3 vessel disease, diabetes, > 10% ischaemia, FFR ≤0.8.
- Revascularisation indicated with the aim *to improve symptoms despite OMT* (3 anti-anginal medications) when any stenosis proven to be significant (defined by FFR or functional stress imaging).
- Revascularisation strategy (coronary artery bypass grafting [CABG] versus PCI): CABG shown to have better prognosis in complex CAD (SYNTAX SCORE: anatomical risk score based on location,

complexity and number of coronary artery stenoses) and diabetic patients (FREEDOM study; [1]). Patients with proximal LAD or LMS stenoses require multi-disciplinary discussion.

- After PCI: aspirin lifelong, second anti-platelet for ≥1 month if bare metal stent, and ≥3–12 months if drug-eluting stent. Tailor duration of dual anti-platelets depending on ischaemic versus bleeding risk.

Acute coronary syndromes

One in six men and one in seven women will die from myocardial infarction (MI).

- *STEMI (ST-segment elevation myocardial infarction)*: incidence is 77/100,000 population (slight trend decrease).
- *NSTEMI (non-ST-segment elevation myocardial infarction) and unstable angina*: incidence is 132/100,000 population (slight trend increase).

Pathophysiology

- Rupture of thin fibrous cap with exposed necrotic core, which is highly inflammatory and prothrombotic, and triggers occlusive or sub-occlusive thrombosis.
- *STEMI*: fibrin-rich thrombus, which is completely occlusive.
- *NSTEMI*: platelet-rich thrombus, which is partially or intermittently occlusive. Platelet-rich thrombus may embolise.

Clinical features

- Severe central crushing chest pain, nausea ± sweating, signs of left/right heart failure.
- There may be evidence of AV block (especially inferior MI). AV block seen with anterior MI is a poor prognostic sign.

Diagnosis

- *Definition of myocardial infarction:* rise and fall of cardiac biomarker > 99th percentile of the upper reference limit (Table 13.6), *with ≥ 1 of*: symptoms of ischaemia, ST-T changes or new LBBB, development of Q waves, new regional wall motion abnormality (echo), intracoronary thrombus seen on coronary angiogram or on autopsy.
- *NB:* Troponin is a regulatory cardiac protein involved in actin-myosin interaction. *Troponin I is more specific than T* for cardiac muscle. Troponin T can be found in low levels in some skeletal muscle.
- *Echocardiogram:* all patients should have an ECHO performed to assess LV function and identify regional wall motion abnormalities

Table 13.6 Cardiac biomarkers in acute myocardial infarction

Cardiac Biomarkers	Initial rise	Peak	Return to normal	Notes
Myoglobin	1–4 h	6–7 h	24 h	Low specificity.
Creatinine phosphokinase	4–8 h	18 h	2–3 days	CPK-MB is principle enzyme.
Troponin	3–12 h	24 h	3–10 days	Troponin I more specific than T.
Lactate dehydrogenase	10 h	24–48 h	14 days	Not as specific as troponin.

Table 13.7 Causes of a raised troponin, ST-segment elevation and myocardial infarction with normal coronary arteries.

Causes of raised troponin	Causes of ST elevation	Causes of myocardial infarction with normal coronary arteries
Myocardial infarction	Myocardial infarction	Coronary artery spasm (e.g. secondary to amphetamines).
Coronary spasm	Pericarditis (saddle-shaped and diffuse)	
Tachyarrhythmias		Coronary artery embolus (e.g. from LV thrombus/vegetation).
Myocarditis and cardiomyopathy	Hyperkalaemia	
DC cardioversion	DC cardioversion	Coronary arteritis (e.g. polyarteritis nodosa).
Pulmonary embolus	Pulmonary embolus	
Pneumonia	Left ventricular hypertrophy	Hypertrophic cardiomyopathy.
Exacerbation of COPD	Left bundle branch block	Aortic stenosis.
Rhabdomyolysis	Brugada syndrome	Hypertension.
Renal failure	Normal variant	Severe anaemia.
Septicaemia		Thyrotoxicosis.
Subarachnoid haemorrhage		Phaeochromocytoma.

Causes of a raised troponin are shown in Table 13.7.

- *ECG:*
  - *STEMI.*
    - (a) ST-segment elevation (≥1 mm in ≥2 consecutive limb leads, or ≥2 mm in ≥2 consecutive chest leads).
    - (b) new-onset LBBB. Consider Sgarbossa criteria.
    - (c) *ISOLATED V1–V3 prominent R waves with ST-segment depression* (>0.05mV – indicative of *posterior STEMI*).

For progression of infarction following STEMI, see Figure 13.9, and for posterolateral STEMI, see Figure 13.10.

  - *NSTEMI*: distinguished from unstable angina with biomarkers, e.g. troponin:
    - (a) ST-segment depression or T-wave inversion.
    - (b) Lead aVR ST-segment elevation + 0.1 mV ST segment depression in ≥8 surface leads indicates left main stem occlusion or multi-vessel disease.

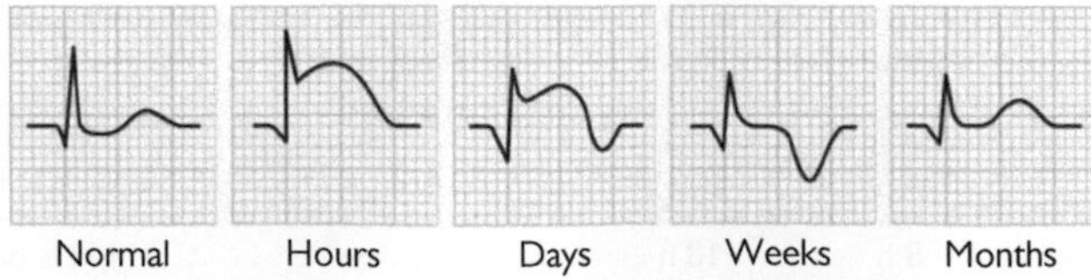

Figure 13.9 Progression of infarction following STEMI.

Reproduced with permission from Cardiovascular medicine. In *Oxford Handbook of Clinical Medicine*, 10th edn, Wilkinson IB, et al. (Eds). Oxford: OUP. Copyright © 2017, Oxford University Press. DOI: 10.1093/med/9780199689903.001.0001. Reproduced with permission of the Licensor through PLSclear.

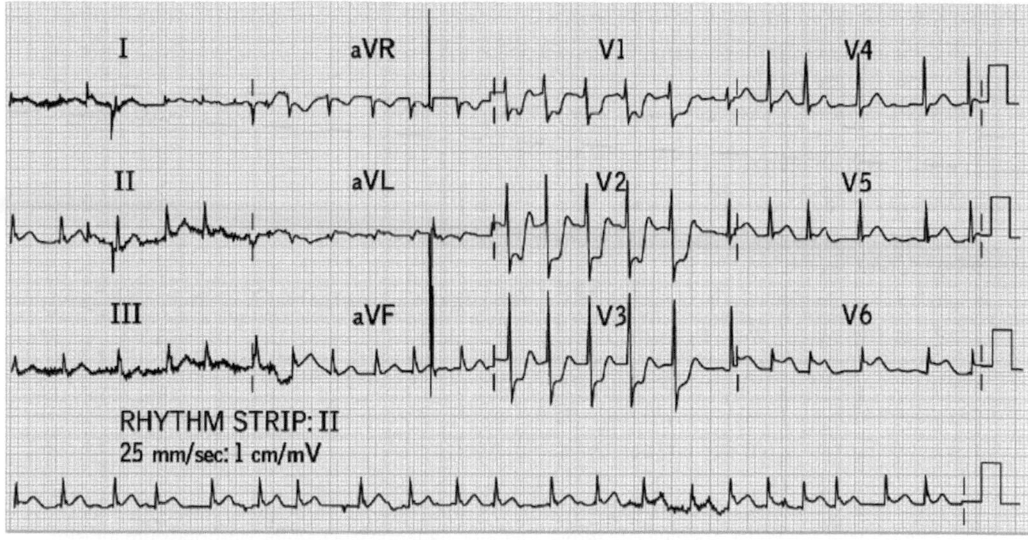

Figure 13.10 Posterolateral STEMI.

Reproduced with permission from Cardiovascular medicine. In *Oxford Handbook of Clinical Medicine*, 10th edn, Wilkinson IB, et al. (Eds). Oxford: OUP. Copyright © 2017, Oxford University Press. DOI: 10.1093/med/9780199689903.001.0001. Reproduced with permission of the Licensor through PLSclear.

Prognosis

- In-hospital mortality: STEMI (4.6%) > NSTEMI (4.3%).
- 12-month mortality: NSTEMI (12%) > STEMI (9%).
- Cardiogenic shock: very high mortality (50–80% within 48 hours).
- Predictors of poor prognosis:
  - LV dysfunction.
  - 'GRACE score' predictors of poor prognosis: age, HR, BP, ST segment deviation, cardiac arrest, raised creatinine or raised cardiac enzymes, Killip class (degree of heart failure).

Complications following myocardial infarction

- Heart failure, pericarditis (Dressler's syndrome), LV aneurysm and/or thrombus.
- Cardiogenic shock: defined as cardiac index <2.2 L/min/m^2, urine output <20 mL/hour or systolic BP only < 90 mmHg despite inotropes or intra-aortic balloon pump.
- LV wall rupture.
- Arrhythmias: AF (most common), non-sustained ventricular tachycardias (NSVT) and high-degree AV block (NB. The RCA supplies the AV-node in 80% of patients).
- Life-threatening arrhythmias: ventricular tachycardia (VT)/ventricular fibrillation (VF).
- Mitral regurgitation (e.g. restriction of posterior leaflet, papillary muscle rupture).

Invasive management (revascularisation)

- *STEMI*: Primary percutaneous coronary intervention (PPCI):
  - Immediate reperfusion with PPCI, unless it will take >2 hours from first medical contact to performing PPCI (in this case give thrombolysis).
  - *Always* performed immediately with symptoms <12 hours duration, and performed if symptoms >12 hours *and evidence of ongoing ischaemia*.
  - Reperfusion of a totally occluded artery is not indicated in stable patients with symptoms >48 hours duration.

- *NSTEMI: PCI*
  - PCI should be performed urgently if there is ongoing ischaemia (pain, ST depression/T wave inversion) despite OMT.
  - Early PCI (within 72 hours) has additional prognostic benefit.

Acute medical management

➲ See Disease prevention, p. 429.

- These apply to both STEMI and NSTEMI except where otherwise indicated. Treatment must not delay transfer for PPCI:
  - Inhalational: oxygen – SpO_2 target 94–98% unless risk of CO_2 retention (88–92% until ABG confirms normal or low pCO_2).
  - Oral: aspirin + ADP-receptor blocker (clopidogrel/prasugrel/ticagrelor). (See Figure 13.11.) β-blocker (contraindicated in acute heart failure).
  - SC (NSTEMI only): LMW heparin (for ~72 hours or until PCI is performed: fondaparinux is a selective factor Xa inhibitor and most efficacious) (Figure 13.11).
  - Intra-arterial: (during PCI): unfractionated heparin or bivalirudin (Figure 13.11).
  - IV: consider Gp IIb/IIIa inhibitors (e.g. abciximab) if thrombus or 'slow reflow' post-PPCI, or during transfer for PCI if ongoing ischaemia. Diabetic patients: glucose-insulin-potassium infusion (DIGAMI study).
- RV infarction (e.g post-inferior/posterior STEMI): may need significant filling with fluids to maintain LV filling pressure.
- Avoid β-blockers in STEMI precipitated by cocaine overdose (due to theoretical risk of alpha driven hypertensive crisis).
- Thrombolysis (STEMI only): recombinant tPA (e.g. tenecteplase) is preferred to streptokinase (which carries risk of hypotension and anaphylaxis [*can only be given once*]). Consider streptokinase in patients > 75 years as lower incidence of intracranial bleeding.

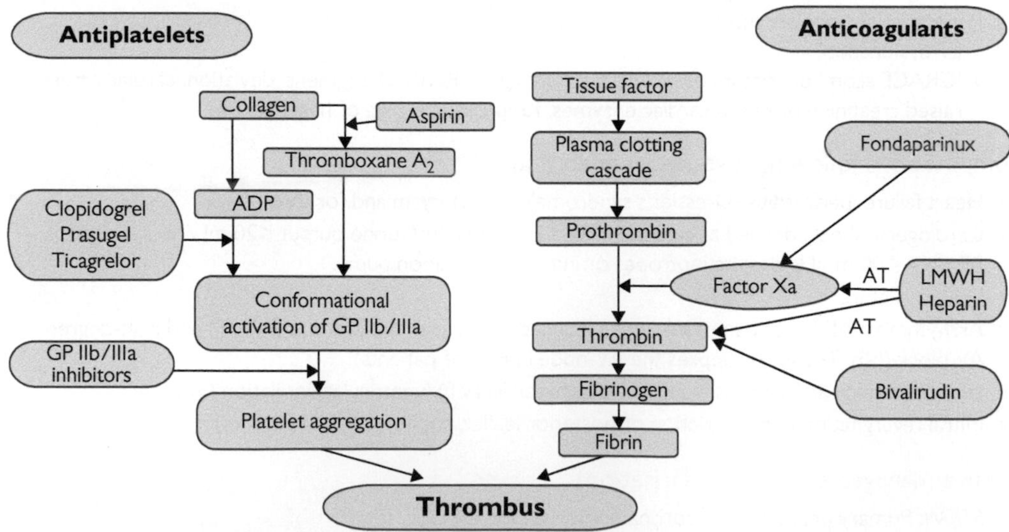

Figure 13.11 Targets for anti-thrombotic drugs (antiplatelets and anticoagulants). Aspirin irreversibly inhibits platelet isoenzyme cyclo-oxygenase 1 (COX-1) suppressing thromboxane production. ADP-receptor blockers cause irreversible changes in platelet receptor $P2Y_{12}$ (inhibiting platelet aggregation).

Key: AT, antithrombin; GP, glycoprotein; LMWH, low molecular weight heparin. Adapted from Roffi, M. and Patrono, C., 2015 ESC Guidelines for the management of acute coronary syndromes in patients presenting without persistent ST-segment elevation: Task Force for the Management of Acute Coronary Syndromes in Patients Presenting without Persistent ST-Segment Elevation of the European Society of Cardiology (ESC), *European Heart Journal*, 2016, 37, 3, by permission of Oxford University Press and the European Society of Cardiology.

- Absolute contraindication to thrombolysis:
  - *Any history of*: previous intracranial haemorrhage, cerebrovascular accident (CVA) of unknown cause, CNS neoplasm or arterio-venous (AV) malformation, known bleeding disorder, or aortic dissection.
  - Previous proven ischaemic CVA in last 6 months, GI bleeding in last month, head injury/major trauma in last 3 weeks.
- Relative contraindication to thrombolysis:
  - Refractory hypertension (systolic >180 mmHg, diastolic >110 mmHg).
  - Transient ischaemic attack (TIA) in last 6 months.
  - Surgery within the last 10 days.
  - Pregnancy or within 1 week post-partum.
  - Active peptic ulcer.
  - Oral anticoagulant therapy.
  - Non-compressible puncture (e.g. lumbar puncture, liver biopsy).

Disease prevention

- Risk scores such as 'SCORE chart' and 'Framingham cardiovascular disease risk' include cholesterol, age, BP and smoking to evaluate the 10-year CVD risk.
- 'Highest risk' patients: previous MI, previous diagnosis of CVD, ischaemic stroke, diabetes with target organ damage (e.g. microalbuminuria), eGFR < 30 mL/min, risk SCORE ≥ 10%.

Lifestyle changes: primary prevention

(a) *Smoking cessation:* nicotine replacement, buproprione and antidepressants.
(b) *Diet and weight reduction:* aim for a BMI < 25, weight reduction if waist >102 cm (man), >88 cm (woman).
(c) *Physical activity and avoidance of physical inactivity:* 30 minutes moderate intensity exercise > 5 times per week to reduce the rate of progression of coronary plaques and improve collaterals, improve endothelial function, reduce thrombotic risk.
(d) *Blood pressure:* office ≤140/90 mmHg, home ≤135/85 mmHg, night ≤120/70 mmHg.
(e) *Stress management:* possible benefit of cognitive behavioural therapy to reduce stress.

Lifestyle changes: secondary prevention (i.e. following MI)

(a) *Blood pressure:* Systolic <140 mmHg, *but not <110 mmHg.*
(b) *Exercise-based rehabilitation programme:* reduces all-cause mortality and risk of recurrent MI and improves quality of life (QOL).
(c) *Driving*: cannot drive for 4 weeks unless successful PCI/PPCI *and* LVEF > 40% (then 1 week).

OMT: primary prevention

(a) *Lipid-lowering therapy*: (➲ see Chapter 1, Lipids and atherosclerosis, p. 20 and Table 1.3). Start treatment in patients with 'high' or 'highest' risk of CVD: target LDL <1.8 mmol/L (general population <3 mmol/L)
(b) *Anti-hypertensives:* ➲ see Hypertension, p. 430, Tables 13.8–13.17 and Figure 13.12).
(c) *Anti-diabetic medication*: to fulfill target HbA_{1c} < 7%.

OMT: secondary prevention (i.e. following MI)

(a) *Anti-thrombotic therapy:* aspirin lifelong, clopidogrel (CURE study) or other ADP-receptor blocker for 12 months.
(b) *Lipid-lowering therapy:* high dose statins to lower LDL-cholesterol concentration to <1.8 mmol/L.

(c) *Minimise adverse LV remodelling*: ACE-i and β-blockers in all patients (unless contraindicated, e.g. renal failure, acute LV failure, hypotension, high-grade AV block), aldosterone antagonists if left ventricular ejection fraction (LVEF) < 40% and either clinical evidence of heart failure or diabetes. Both β-blockers and ACE-inhibitors require up-titration to licensed dose or maximal tolerated dose to achieve best prognostic benefit. If there is contraindication to β-blockers, verapamil and diltiazem can be considered as long as there is no heart failure (negatively inotropic).

Emerging therapies/investigations

- *Chronic IHD*: stem cell therapy, spinal cord stimulation, referral to refractory angina centre.
- *Acute coronary syndrome (ACS)*: stem cell therapy, reducing reperfusion injury (e.g. anti-oxidants).
- *Disease prevention*: PCSK9 inhibitors, use of biomarkers to gauge CVD risk (e.g. high sensitivity CRP), measurement of lipoprotein A in familial IHD.

Reference

1. Farkouh ME, Domanski M, Sleeper L, et al. Strategies for multivessel revascularisation in patients with diabetes. *N Engl J Med*. 2012;367:2375–84.

Further reading

1. NICE guideline: Chest pain of recent onset (2010). https://www.nice.org.uk/guidance/cg95
2. European Society of Cardiology (ESC) Guidelines for the management of acute myocardial infarction in patients presenting with ST-segment elevation (2012) and in those presenting without persistent ST-segment elevation (2015).
3. European Society of Cardiology (ESC) Guidelines on cardiovascular disease prevention in clinical practice (2012).

Hypertension

Hypertension affects 1 billion humans worldwide. It causes half of all IHD and stroke. Primary ('essential') hypertension accounts for the majority of cases – a secondary cause is found in approximately 10%.

Pathophysiology of hypertension

Primary

- Multi-factorial pathology including renin-angiotensin system (RAS) activation and vascular remodelling with increased total peripheral resistance. RAS activation is less significant in black people.
- Linked to ageing.
- In the developed world, modifiable lifestyle risk factors are common: obesity, physical inactivity, alcohol consumption, high salt intake and smoking.

Secondary

- Often severe or of sudden onset and/or resistant to treatment.
- A secondary cause should be sought carefully if <40 years of age.

All patients should have urine analysis and serum creatinine carried out, with further investigations, as appropriate, to establish the underlying cause.

For causes of secondary hypertension, see Table 13.8.

Clinical features

Hypertension is generally asymptomatic. Malignant hypertension may be associated with visual disturbances (papilloedema and retinal haemorrhage), confusion (cerebral oedema) or heart failure.

For clinical features of end organ damage or secondary aetiology, see Table 13.9.

Table 13.8 Causes of secondary hypertension

Seondary hypertension	Diagnostic investigation
Renal parenchymal disease (5% of all adult hypertension)	➲ See Chapter 16, Assessment of renal function, p. 549; Direct and indirect measurements of renal function, p. 550.
Renovascular disease (2% of all adult hypertension)	➲ See Investigations, p. 572.
Coarctation of the aorta (association with bicuspid aortic valve and Turner's syndrome)	Echocardiogram ± cardiac CT or MRI.
Phaeochromocytoma	➲ See Chapter 19, Phaeochromocytoma and paraganglionoma, p. 696.
Cushing's syndrome	➲ See Cushing's syndrome, p. 687 and Table 19.7.
Conn's syndrome	➲ See Primary hyperaldosteronism, p. 695.
Associated with female sex hormones	Pregnancy test. (➲ Chapter 23, Pre-eclampsia and eclampsia, p. 811 and Table 23.6)

Diagnosis and staging

- Diagnosis by ambulatory measurement or by home BP measurement are better indicators of prognosis and more cost effective, than clinic measurements.
- Cardiovascular risk is continuous with the magnitude of hypertension. Nevertheless, set values can be combined with a total cardiovascular risk score, to guide the initiation and urgency of treatment.

For NICE staging of hypertension, see Table 13.10, and for diagnostic criteria of hypertension, see Table 13.11.

Investigations

See Table 13.12.

Risk stratification and treatment initiation

For treatment of hypertension, see Table 13.13 and for cardiovascular risk calculators, see Table 13.14.

Table 13.9 Clinical features of end organ damage or secondary aetiology

Examination features	
General and associated conditions	Cushingoid appearance, marks of glucometer fingerprick testing.
Fundoscopy	Hypertensive retinopathy.
Neurological	Focal signs of previous stroke.
Cardiovascular examination	BP measurement (➲ see Diagnosing and staging, p. 431 and Tables 13.10 & 13.11).
	Heaving apex beat of LVH.
	Coarctation: mid (and later, pan-) systolic precordial murmur radiating to the back. High BP in upper extremities and low/unrecordable BP in legs (± toenail clubbing).
	Carotid bruits: vascular disease.
	Lateralising abdominal bruit of renovascular disease.
Urine dip and analysis	Microalbuminuria may indicate subclinical renal disease (lab albumin: creatinine ratio is more reliable). Pregnancy testing (βHCG).

Table 13.10 NICE staging of hypertension

Stage (NICE CG127)	Clinic blood pressure (CBP)	Ambulatory blood pressure monitoring (ABP) or home blood pressure monitoring (HBPM)
Stage 1	≥140/90	≥135/85
Stage 2	≥160/100	≥155/95
Stage 3 (severe)	≥180/110	Consider same-day referral if adverse clinical features.

Table 13.11 Diagnostic criteria of hypertension (NICE CG 127)

Blood pressure measurement (NICE CG 127)	Direction
CBP	At least 2 measurements (>1 min apart) if BP >140 SBP or >90 DBP arrange ABPM.
ABP monitoring	At least 2 measures per hour in waking hours, mean of 14 measurements over 24 hours.
HBPM	At least 2 measures per day. For a minimum of 4 days (up to 7). Discard records from Day 1, record the mean.

Table 13.12 Investigations for hypertension

Diagnosis of causes of secondary hypertension	see Table 13.8: Secondary hypertension	
Assessment of sub-clinical end-organ damage	Fundoscopy	Hypertensive retinopathy
	ECG	LVH
	Echo (if LVH on ECG)	
	Urinalysis (albumin: creatinine ratio)	Hypertensive nephropathy
Assessment of cardiovascular risk profile	Fasting lipid profile	Input to risk calculator
	Fasting glucose	>7 mM
	Oral glucose tolerance test (if borderline)	>7.8 mM = IGT >11.1 mM = diabetes

Table 13.13 Treatment of hypertension

Stage	Treatment
Stage 2	Offer treatment regardless of risk factors/comorbidity.
Stage 1	Offer treatment if: • Target organ damage. • Established cardiovascular disease. • Renal disease. • Diabetes. • 10-year cardiovascular risk ≥20%.
All patients	Lifestyle modification.

Table 13.14 Cardiovascular risk calculators

Cardiovascular risk calculators		NICE Recommendation
Framingham Risk Calculator 1991.		Withdrew recommendation for Framingham calculator (2010). No stated preference for available calculators.
Joint British Societies 2 (JBS2) – based on Framingham. BNF risk charts are based on this calculator.		
Joint British Societies 2 (JBS3) – is the first calculator to provide an output on lifetime (as well as 10-year) risk.		
Q-RISK 2 UK primary care population cohort.	Includes a social deprivation index.	
ASSIGN Scottish primary care cohort.		

Calculators available via: http://heartuk.org.uk/health-professionals/resources/risk-calculators

Management

For treatment protocol, see Figure 13.12. For common antihypertensive drug side effects and contraindications, see Table 13.15 and for condition-specific preferences for anti-hypertensives, see Table 13.16.

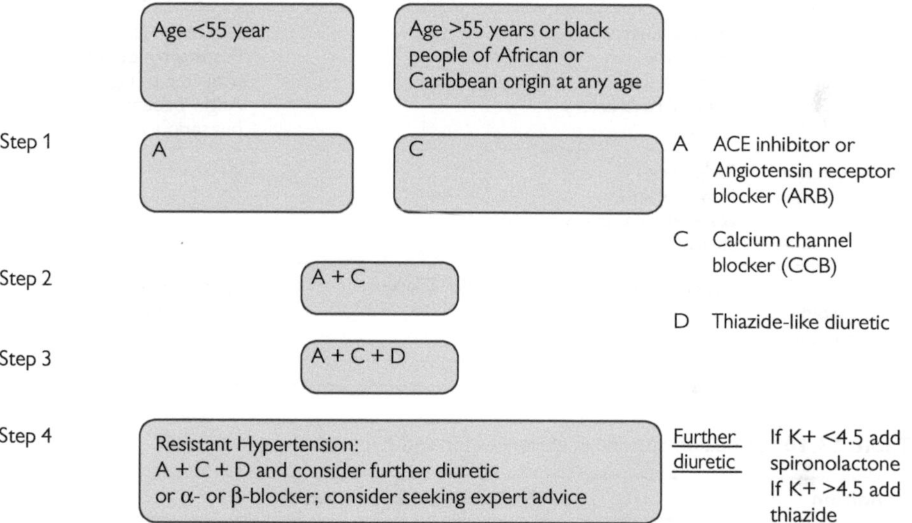

Figure 13.12 Treatment protocol from the British Hypertension Society and NICE (CG127).
Data from NICE. Clinical guideline (CG127). Hypertension in adults: diagnosis and management. London, UK: NICE. Copyright © 2011 NICE. https://www.nice.org.uk/guidance/CG127.

Hypertension clinical guidelines and key trials

All patients between 40 and 74 years old should be screened for hypertension.

For key trials in hypertension, see Table 13.17.

Emerging therapies for resistant hypertension

Renal sympathetic denervation is a recent technique involving radio-frequency ablation of sympathetic nerves to both kidneys, delivered from a catheter passed from femoral access site to each renal artery in turn.

For more information see NICE Interventional Procedure Guideline 418 (January 2012).

Table 13.15 Common antihypertensive drug side effects and contraindications

Anti-hypertensive drug	Absolute contraindication	Relative contraindication	Side effects
Thiazides	Gout.	Metabolic syndrome. Glucose intolerance.	Hyponatraemia, hyperuricaemia, hypokalaemia and may worsen the metabolic syndrome/glucose intolerance.
Calcium channel blockers (dihydropyridines, e.g. amlodipine)		Ankle swelling.	Ankle swelling (common for amlodipine).
Calcium channel blockers (verapamil/diltiazem)	Heart failure. Heart block (2nd/3rd degree).		Ankle swelling (rarely occurs).
β-blockers	Asthma. Heart block (2nd/3rd degree).	PVD. COPD. Metabolic syndrome. Glucose intolerance.	Erectile dysfunction, marked fatigue and may worsen metabolic syndrome/glucose intolerance.
ACE-i	Angio-oedema. Pregnancy. Hyperkalaemia. Bilateral renal artery stenosis.		Dry cough (common). Postural hypotension may be mitigated by night-time dosing. Angio-oedema (uncommon, but serious).
Angiotensin receptor antagonists (ARAs)	Pregnancy. Hyperkalaemia. Bilateral renal artery stenosis.		
Diuretics (mineralocorticoid receptor antagonists, e.g. spironolactone)	Hyperkalaemia.	Renal failure.	Spironolactone can cause gynaecomastia.

Table 13.16 Condition-specific preferences for anti-hypertensives

Condition	Preferred antihypertensive
Angina	β-blockers and calcium channel blockers (dihydropyridines).
Heart failure	ACE-i. Angiotensin receptor antagonists (ARAs). Mineralocorticoid receptor antagonists. β-blockers.
Previous MI	ACE-i. ARAs. β-blockers.
Atrial fibrillation (permanent)	β-blockers. Calcium channel blockers (non-dihydropyridines).
Microalbuminuria & renal dysfunction	ACE-i. ARAs.
Peripheral vascular disease	Calcium channel blockers (dihydropyridines).

Table 13.17 Key trials in hypertension

Trial	Critical findings
International Society of Hypertension. *Global burden of blood pressure related disease.* (2001. Lancet 2008; 371(9623):1513–18).	Hypertension causes 47% of IHD and 54% of stroke.
HOPE study (N Engl J Med 2000; 342:145–53). >9000 patients with known vascular disease randomised to 10 mg ramipril (ACE-i) vs placebo.	ACE-i reduced composite primary endpoint MI/CVA/ vascular death by 22%. The clinical benefit was significantly greater than that justified by the modest reduction in BP.
ALLHAT study (J Am Med Ass 2002; 288:2981–97). >42,000 patients with HTN and ≥ one cv risk factor randomised to chlortalidone (thiazide), amlodipine (CCB), lisinopril (ACEi) or doxazosin (α-blocker). Target BP <140/90.	Primary outcome: composite fatal CHD and non-fatal MI. Doxazosin arm stopped early due to superiority of chlortalidone. No difference in *primary* endpoint between thiazide, CCB and ACE-i. Including *secondary* vascular endpoints shows thiazide superior to ACE-i and CCB.
LIFE study (Lancet 2002; 359(9311):995). >9000 patients with HTN and LVH. Double-blinded losartan versus atenolol.	BP reduction: no difference. ARB reduced primary endpoint. Mortality/MI/CVA by 14%.
ASCOT study (Lancet 2005; 366(9489):895). >19,000 patients with HTN and ≥3 other cv risk factors. Double-blinded atenolol (with bendroflumethiazide as necessary to achieve target BP) versus amlodipine (with perindopril as necessary).	Primary endpoint: composite fatal CHD and non-fatal MI. Trial stopped early due to strong trend towards amlodipine superiority. Fewer patients developed diabetes on amlodipine.
SPRINT study (N Engl J Med 2015; 373:2103–16). >9000 patients with HTN (SBP>130) and increased CV risk (but not T2DM) randomised to tight (SBP<120 mmHg) or standard (SBP<140 mmHg) BP control.	Primary endpoint: composite MI, other ACS, CVA, HF or cv death. Trial stopped early due to decreased primary outcome in intensive treatment group (hazard ratio 0.75). NB. There was a higher incidence of new renal impairment in the intensive treatment group.
PATHWAY-2 study (Lancet 2015; 386:2059–68). 335 patients with HTN (SBP>140) already established on three drugs randomised to all of placebo, bisoprolol, doxazosin and spironolactone in 12 week blocks to test the best 4th line agent.	Primary endpoint: systolic BP. SBP was lowest in the spironolactone as 4th line agent group. Spironolactone reduced SBP by 4–4.5 mmHg (average) vs. doxazosin and bisoprolol, respectively.

ACE-i, angiotensin-converting enzyme inhibitor; MI, myocardial infarction; CVA, cerebrovascular accident; HTN, hypertension; cv, cardiovascular; CCB, calcium channel blocker; CHD, coronary heart disease; LVH, left ventricular hypertrophy; ARB, angiotensin receptor blocker; T2DM, type 2 diabetes mellitus; ACS, acute coronary syndrome; HF, heart failure.

References

1. NICE hypertension: clinical management of primary hypertension in adults. Clinical Guideline CG127, 2011. http://www.nice.org.uk/cg127
2. European Society of Cardiology (ESC) Management of arterial hypertension, (2007) www.escardio.org/gudelines/clinical-practice-guidelines/arterial-hypertension-management-of

Valvular heart disease

Valvular heart disease affects 1.8–2.5% of people in the developed world (13% of those aged above 75 years). The decreasing incidence of rheumatic heart disease and ageing population has changed the pattern of valve disease:

- Aortic stenosis (AS) and mitral regurgitation (MR) are more common.
- Mitral stenosis (MS) and aortic regurgitation (AR) are decreasing in frequency.
- In the developing world rheumatic fever and therefore MS remain common.

Congenital valvular heart disease is rare, with the exception of bicuspid aortic valve (BAV; 0.5–1% of the population).

Causes of valvular heart disease

See Table 13.18.

Table 13.18 Causes of valvular heart disease

AS	Calcific degeneration associated with atherogenic risk factors and renal disease (raised serum calcium). Degeneration occurs faster in bicuspid aortic valve.		
	Rheumatic (now rare in Europe and US).		
	Congenital.		
MR	Organic (leaflet pathology)	Degenerative disease with prolapse. Rheumatic heart disease. Endocarditis. Rare: SLE, radiation, weight loss drugs (e.g. fenfluramine).	
	Ischaemic	Acute: papillary muscle rupture. Chronic: regional wall motion abnormality restricting leaflet closure (e.g. inferior MI).	
	Functional	Dilated LV leading to dilated mitral annulus and central MR.	
AR	Acute	Aortic dissection. Infective endocarditis with virulent pathogen (e.g. *Staph. aureus*). Traumatic leaflet rupture.	
	Chronic	Primary leaflet pathology	Rheumatic. Degenerative. Connective tissue disease.
		Secondary to aortic root dilatation	Seronegative arthropathies (e.g. ankylosing spondylitis). Hypertension.
		Both root and leaflet pathology	Bicuspid aortic valve. Marfan's syndrome.
MS	Rheumatic mitral valve disease is the commonest cause. Degenerative disease, with progression of annular calcification onto the valve leaflets (12.5%). Rare causes: SLE, Fabry's disease, amyloid, Whipple's disease.		
PS	Congenital.		
PR	Pulmonary hypertension is the most common. Connective tissue disease. Right heart endocarditis.		
TR	Pulmonary hypertension. 'Functional' right heart dilatation. Right heart endocarditis.		
TS	Mitral stenosis. Carcinoid.		

Clinical features

Careful history and physical examination, combined with clinical suspicion are essential to diagnostic sensitivity. NB. Patients often under-report symptoms after adjusting their daily living to accommodate their pathology.

- Disease progression: careful objective questions on changing exercise tolerance over time.
- Aetiology (see Table 13.18).
- Prognosis: the following are ominous prognostic signs (may relate to comorbidities, e.g. heart, lung, renal and neurological disease):
  - Heart failure and collapse.
  - Rapid progression of symptoms.

- Valve disease typically presents with:
  - Exertional breathlessness; ankle swelling; abdominal distension.
  - Exertional chest pain – angina (with severe AS).
  - Dizziness/collapse/syncope (with severe AS).

For clinical signs of valvular heart disease, see Table 13.19.

Table 13.19 Clinical signs of valvular heart disease

Characteristics	Signs	
	Aortic stenosis	**Aortic regurgitation**
Pulse	Small volume pulse. Slow rising (= late-peaking) pulse.	Collapsing pulse (pulse pressure > diastolic pressure).
BP	Narrow pulse pressure.	Wide pulse pressure. DBP <50 mmHg is an ominous sign.
JVP		Visible carotid pulsation – Corrigan's pulse.
Apex beat	Heaving (pressure loaded) apex.	Thrusting, displaced (volume-loaded) apex; not in acute AR.
Auscultation	ESM – radiation to carotids (neither amplitude nor radiation is a marker of severity). Quiet or absent second heart sound.	Early diastolic murmur (best heard along left sternal border in end expiration with patient leaning forward – shorter murmur indicates more severe AR [aortic and LV pressures equalise more rapidly]). A long ejection systolic (flow) murmur due to the obligate increase in stroke volume; occurs *very* commonly.
Heart failure	Signs of left heart failure.	Signs of left heart failure.
Other signs	Pallor of associated anaemia.	There are many eponymous signs which all reflect raised stroke volume, wide pulse pressure and arterial collapse in diastole.
	Mitral stenosis	**Mitral regurgitation**
Pulse	Irregular secondary to AF caused by left atrial dilatation.	Irregular secondary to AF caused by left atrial dilatation.
BP	Low BP.	
JVP	Loss of 'a-wave' if in atrial fibrillation.	Loss of 'a-wave' if in atrial fibrillation.
Apex beat	Non-displaced apex.	Thrusting (volume loaded apex).
Auscultation	Mid-late diastolic (low pitch) murmur with pre-systolic accentuation heard at apex with minimal radiation; pre-systolic accentuation does not occur if in AF. Opening snap at beginning of diastolic murmur, early after S2 (indicates high left atrial LA pressure). Wide splitting of S2 due to late P2.	Pansystolic murmur (radiation to axilla) louder on *expiration*. Mid-late systolic murmur in MV prolapse (radn. to axilla, louder on *inspiration*). 3rd heart sound. Wide splitting of S2 due to early A2.
Heart failure		Signs of left heart failure.
Other signs	*Mitral facies* (dilated vessels in cheeks).	

continued

Table 13.19 *continued*

Characteristics	Signs	
	Pulmonary stenosis	**Pulmonary regurgitation**
JVP	Raised JVP.	
Apex beat	Left parasternal heave of RV hypertrophy.	
Auscultation	ESM at the upper left sternal border. Pansystolic murmur of TR if RV dilated.	EDM heard along the left sternal border.
Heart failure	Signs of right heart failure.	Signs of right heart failure.
Other signs	Cyanosis – if a right to left shunt occurs.	
	Tricuspid stenosis	**Tricuspid regurgitation**
JVP	Prominently raised.	Raised, with giant V waves.
Auscultation	Mid-diastolic murmur at the lower left sternal border.	Pan-systolic murmur at the lower left sternal border.
Heart failure	Peripheral oedema and severe venous congestion.	Often severe right heart failure.
Other signs		Pulsatile liver.

Investigations

Echocardiography is the main modality for investigating valve disease. Often TTE is sufficient; TOE is more sensitive and can be used intra-operatively to guide interventions.

Echo provides:

- A 2D, real-time image of the valves and chambers of the heart.
- Doppler-encoded velocity of blood flow data:
  - Colour flow mapping.
  - Peak and mean velocities of forward jets in stenosis allowing estimate of the pressure drop across a valve.
  - Peak velocities of regurgitant jets allowing estimation of regurgitant volume.
- 3D images (advanced echo).

Cardiac catheterisation:

- Valuable in coronary artery assessment.
- Indications (European Society of Cardiology [ESC] guideline) for coronary angiography pre-operatively include all men over 40 years and all post-menopausal women.

CT and CMR may contribute to surgical planning (➲ see Imaging, p. 417 and Table 13.2).

An exercise test (± exercise echo) may elicit under-reported symptoms and demonstrate haemodynamic or echo signs of adverse prognosis, e.g. fall in BP (severe AS) or pulmonary hypertension (severe MR).

Treatment

Patients with valve disease should be reviewed at appropriate intervals in specialist clinics with a dedicated ECHO service. Valve intervention should be timed to minimise risk and maximise benefit.

- The standard intervention for AS, AR and MR is open surgery on cardiopulmonary bypass.
- Surgical risk is assessed with validated scoring systems (Euroscore II).
- Valve repair (where possible) is superior to valve replacement for MR.
- Valve replacement has several options:
  - Bioprosthesis: xenogenic material (e.g. bovine/porcine pericardium): may be within a pre-made cylinder (stent) or on a simple annulus (stentless).
  - Mechanical prosthesis: bileaflet and single tilting disc valves are available ('ball and cage' valves now rarely used). Valve development is focused on improving flow characteristics, durability and reducing thrombogenicity.
  - Autograft/homograft: aortic valve disease can be treated by transposing the native pulmonary valve to the aortic position, the latter replaced with a homograft (Ross procedure). Advantages include no anticoagulation requirement and, in young patients the aortic valve can 'grow with the patient' (homografts do not grow).
  - Bioprosthesis or mechanical valve? Mechanical valves:
    - Last longer (less susceptible to structural valve deterioration [SVD]).
    - Require anticoagulation.
    - Are generally recommended in younger patients.
    - Women of childbearing age may elect for bioprostheses to avoid anticoagulation in pregnancy. Haemodynamic changes of pregnancy may accelerate SVD.
- SVD is a particular problem in young patients who experience accelerated deterioration of bioprosthetic valves.
- A catheter-based technique may be undertaken when the risk of open surgery is considered too high:
  - Transcatheter aortic valve implantation (TAVI) for severe aortic stenosis.
  - Transcatheter balloon valvuloplasty for MS (and to palliate AS).
  - Percutaneous (catheter deployed) mitral valve intervention (i.e. mitral clipping) for severe mitral regurgitation.
- The roles for medication in valve disease are:
  - Treating symptoms/complications of valve disease.
  - Secondary prevention of cardiovascular risk factors.
  - Palliation where intervention is not possible.

Rheumatic heart disease

Up to 3% of infections (often pharyngitis) with Group A (beta haemolytic) *Streptococcus* (GAβ-HS) will cause an episode of acute rheumatic fever (ARF). ARF is the result of molecular mimicry, by several GAβ-HS epitopes of proteins which occur in human tissues (synovium, skin, heart and CNS). The resulting inflammation accounts for the symptoms and signs which define the major and minor criteria for ARF (*Revised Jones criteria*) (Table 13.20).

Table 13.20 Revised Jones Criteria for Acute Rheumatic Fever

Evidence of previous GAβ-HS infection *and* either
2 MAJOR or
1 MAJOR and 2 MINOR criteria

Major criteria	**Tissue involved**	**Notes**
Arthritis	Synovium of joints	Commonest symptom (occurs in 75%). Migratory polyarthritis.
Carditis *pancarditis*	Heart (all layers: pericardium, myocardium, endocadium (hence, an *acute valvulitis*)	The mid-diastolic murmur of LV filling across an acutely inflamed mitral valve is a *Carey-Coombes* murmur. Rheumatic heart disease occurs: • in 40–60% of patients with carditis; • only in those with carditis complicating the ARF; • often after many years. Recurrent episodes ARF increase risk rheumatic heart disease.
Chorea	Central nervous system	Chorea may occur, but only after a delay of several months.
Erythema marginatum	Skin	Pink 'rings' (caused by central clearing) on the *trunk* and *extensor surfaces* of limbs. It migrates and may last several months. Occurs in < 5% of cases of ARF.
Subcutaneous nodules		Typically found around bony prominences on extensor surfaces (elbows, knees).
Minor criteria	**Tissue involved**	**Notes**
Acute fever	Systemic immune response	
Raised ESR and CRP		
Arthralgia	Synovium of joints	Pain without objective evidence of inflammation (arthritis).
Prolonged PR interval	Heart (AV node)	This heart block usually responds to antibiotic treatment of the infection.

Adapted with permission from Gewitz, M. H. et al. Revision of the Jones Criteria for the Diagnosis of Acute Rheumatic Fever in the Era of Doppler Echocardiography. *Circulation*, 2015;131:1806–1818. Copyright © 2015, American Heart Association and Wolters Kluwer Health. https://www.ahajournals.org/doi/10.1161/CIR.0000000000000205.

Treatment of ARF includes:

- Early IV antibiotics benzylpenicillin G or ceftriaxone. Follow on doses of 4-weekly IM benzylpenicillin or oral penicillin V should be continued daily for up to 10 years or into adulthood after an episode of ARF to reduce the risk of late complication with rheumatic heart disease.
- Acute carditis: oral prednisolone treatment (1 mg/kg daily) to a maximum of 80 mg daily.
- Acute arthritis responds to high-dose aspirin.

Mitral valve prolapse

See Table 13.21.

Table 13.21 Mitral valve prolapse (MVP)

Definition	MVP is defined by imaging, when the anterior or posterior mitral valve leaflets cross the valve plane by >2 mm into the left atrium during ventricular systole.		
Symptoms	Caused by MR	SOB from pulmonary congestion. Fatigue from reduced forward flow.	
	Reports of female preponderance and association with atypical chest pain are erroneous.		
Examination	Heart sounds	There may be a 'late'[1] systolic click, followed immediately by the murmur (caused by the 'prolapse' across the valve plane and the start of MR).	
	Murmur	A 'late'[1] crescendo murmur lasts until the end of systole (S2). As severity of MVP increases, the murmur becomes pansystolic.	
		Unlike most[2] left-sided murmurs, which are accentuated by manoeuvres that increase LV volume and therefore LV flow (increased afterload [squatting] and temporary increased left venous return [expiration]) the reverse is true of the murmur of MVP. As the LV volume increases, the subvalvular apparatus is pulled apically, thus reducing the degree of prolapse.	
Investigation	ECHO is the central investigation providing:	Exact site of prolapse. Degree of MR. Size and function of left ventricle. Size (degree of dilatation) of left atrium. Pulmonary pressure and effects on right heart.	All of this information is used to guide the decision of whether surgery/catheter intervention is indicated and feasible.
	Stress ECHO:	The maximum degree of prolapse, MR and pulmonary hypertension.	
Treatment	Surgical treatment	Gold standard treatment for MVP with severe MR is by open surgical repair. Surgical indication (Europe) is when the left ventricle has dilated to an end-systolic diameter of >4 cm.	

[1]'Late' in this sense means 'not beginning immediately after S1'. The click and murmur may, however, occur very shortly after S1.
[2]The murmur of hypertrophic cardiomyopathy with LV outflow tract obstruction ('HCM') is also sometimes *reduced* by increased LV volume because the increase in LV diameter may 'lift' the septal obstruction 'out' of the LV outflow tract.

Infective endocarditis

Infective endocarditis (IE) affects 3–10/100,000 persons annually. 30% of cases have no prior valvular heart disease (VHD).

Pathophysiology and epidemiology

Vegetations mainly consist of inflammatory cells, platelets and fibrin. IE of the valvular endothelium results from:

- *Mechanical damage* exposing extracellular matrix proteins, resulting in tissue factor production and fibrin and platelet deposits: termed non-bacterial thrombotic endocarditis (NBTE). Turbulent blood flow (e.g. VHD) predisposes to damage to valvular endothelium. Bacterial adherence and infection usually form on the low-pressure side of the valve.
- *Local inflammation* promoting expression of transmembrane proteins that bind fibronectin. Fibronectin adheres to these proteins, allowing certain pathogens (e.g. *Staphlyococcus aureus*) which carry fibronectin binding protein to adhere to this inflammatory surface. This often occurs on previously normal valves.
- *Increased risk:* male, elderly, immunocompromised, haemodialysis and transplant patients.

Box 13.2 Diagnostic criteria: the 'Duke criteria'

2 major criteria *or* 1 major + 3 minor criteria *or* 5 minor criteria.

Major criteria

Blood cultures: >1* +ve BC of typical pathogen.

*Only one blood culture required if *Coxiella burnetii*.

Echocardiography: vegetation, abscess or prosthesis dehiscence or new valvular regurgitation.

Minor criteria

Positive BC of atypical pathogen, predisposition to IE (VHD, IVDU), fever > 38°C, septic embolic phenomena, immune complex phenomena, serology positive for pathogen.

Adapted from *The American Journal of Medicine*, 96, Durack D.T. et al. New criteria for diagnosis of infective endocarditis: utilization of specific echocardiographic findings. Duke Endocarditis Service, pp. 200–209. Copyright © 1994 Published by Excerpta Medica Inc. https://doi.org/10.1016/0002-9343(94)90143-0

Clinical features

- Non-specific sub-acute symptoms: fever, chills, malaise and night sweats. Symptoms may resolve following antibiotics, but usually relapse after stopping.
- Cardiac murmur(s) on auscultation.
- Vasculitic phenomena: splinter haemorrhages, petechial rash.
- Immune complex phenomena: Roth spots (retinopathy), Osler nodes (painful), microscopic haematuria, (rheumatoid factor positivity).
- Septic embolic phenomena: dependent on site of IE (e.g. stroke, digital ischaemia and Janeway lesions [painless] for left-sided valvular vegetations).
- Persistent bacteraemia: hepatosplenomegaly, anaemia.

Diagnosis and disease classification

- Serial blood cultures (BC): three sets of BCs, which should be taken >1 hour apart, and all within 24 hours.
- Echocardiography: TOE (gold standard for excluding IE) – higher sensitivity to visualise vegetations compared with TTE.
  - TTE is the first line investigation following blood cultures.
  - TOE is the first line investigation in prosthetic valve infective endocarditis (PVE).

For diagnostic criteria – Duke criteria, see Box 13.2.

There are two principal classifications:

(a) IE according to the localization of infection and presence or absence of intracardiac material:
 (i) left-sided native valve IE; (ii) left-sided PVE, subdivided into early PVE (<1 year after surgery) and late PVE (>1 year after surgery); (iii) right-sided IE; (iv) device-related IE (either permanent pacemaker [PPM] or implantable cardioverter defibrillatory [ICD]).

(b) IE according to the mode of infection:
 (i) Health care-associated (ia) nosocomial; (ib) non nosocomial; (ii) community acquired; (iii) IVDU associated.

For causes of infective endocarditis, see Table 13.22.

NB. When native valve IE and PVE cases are combined together, staphylococci are the most common pathogen.

There has been a significant increase in the incidence of staphylococcal IE over the last 10 years.

Prognosis

- In-hospital mortality 15–22%.
- 30–50% of patients with IE undergo surgery.

Poor prognostic features

- PVE (*early PVE* has 20–40% in-hospital mortality).

Table 13.22 Causes of infective endocarditis

Blood culture positive endocarditis: causative pathogens (starting with most common) ~90% of IE cases		
Native valve IE BCs positive *Streptococcus viridans* *Staphylococcus aureus* *Streptococcus bovis* (associated with carcinoma of the colon) Enterococci	*Early PVE (< 1 year)* *Staphylococcus aureus* Coagulase-negative staphlyococci, enterococci, fungi *similar organisms when IE associated with PPM or ICD	*PVE (> 1 year)* Same as native valve IE

Blood culture negative endocarditis (and tests used to detect them – successful in~60% of cases)~10% of IE cases		
Infective organism	*Test (NB. PCR = Polymerase chain reaction)*	*Non-infective*
Typical organism above but BC taken *after* antibiotics		SLE (Libman-Sacs).
Brucella spp.	Serology, PCR of surgical material	Marantic endocarditis (metastatic related)
Coxiella burnetti	Serology, PCR of surgical material	
Bartonella spp.	Serology, PCR of surgical material	
Chlamydia spp.	Serology, PCR of surgical material	
Mycoplasma spp.	Serology, PCR of surgical material	
Legionella spp.	Serology, PCR of surgical material	
Histoplasmosis	Prolonged culture +1- PCR (not yet clear)	
Tropheryma whipplei	Histology + PCR of surgical material	
Fungi	Lysis-centrifugation & culturing on special fungal media	
HACEK group	Prolonged culture (*Haemophilus* spp, *Actinobacillus*, *Cardiobacterium* spp, *Eikenella*, *Kingella* spp)	

- Comorbidity (insulin-dependent diabetes mellitus [IDDM], old age, previous cardiovascular, renal or pulmonary disease).
- Staphylococcal, fungal or Gram-negative bacilli infection.

Complications of IE and indications for surgery

See Table 13.23.

- Complications of IE are indications for surgery:
  - Septic embolisation in left heart IE can cause:
    - Neurological impairment from transient symptoms; mycotic aneurysms; ischaemic or haemorrhagic stroke.
    - Limb, abdominal (kidney, spleen) or even coronary ischaemia.
  - Septic embolisation in right heart IE can cause pulmonary emboli, presenting with pleuritis/ pneumonia.

Table 13.23 Indications for surgery in IE

Native valve endocarditis	Prosthetic valve endocarditis
Heart failure with acute AR or MR	Heart failure.
Annular or aortic root abscess (prolongation of PR interval on ECG)	Annular or aortic root abscess (prolongation of PR interval on ECG).
Large (>10 mm) mobile vegetation or recurrent embolism	Large (>10 mm) mobile vegetation or recurrent embolism.
Fungal infection on culture	*Staphylococcus aureus* or fungal infection on culture.
Persistent infection >10 days after starting antibiotics (fever, bacteraemia, leucocytosis)	Persistent fever >10 days after starting antibiotics.
	Early PVE ≤2 months after surgery.
	Prosthetic valvular dehiscence or dysfunction.

Management

Bactericidal antimicrobial drugs (see Table 13.24). Bacteriostatic antimicrobials are ineffective. In treatment failure surgery is required to remove infective material (including possible abscesses) ± replace incompetent valves.

- Aminoglycosides (e.g. gentamicin) synergize with cell wall inhibitors (e.g. benzylpenicillin) for bactericidal activity.

Table 13.24 Antibiotic regimens for IE (1)

Pathogen	Native valve IE	Duration (weeks)	Prosthetic valve IE*	Duration (weeks)
Unclear or before culture	Ampicillin 12 g/day IV in 4 doses	4–6	Vancomycin 30 mg/kg/day IV in 2 doses	6
	or co-amoxiclav 12/day IV in 4 doses	4–6	*and* rifampicin 1200 mg/day PO in 2 doses	6
	and gentamicin 3 mg/kg/day IV in 2–3 doses	4–6	*and* gentamicin 3 mg/kg/day IV in 2 doses	2
			*Late PVE treated same as native valve IE	
Streptococci (oral + group D)	Benzylpenicillin G12–18 million U/day[1,2] IV in 6 doses	4	Rare to be secondary to *Streptococcus*, seek specialist microbiology advice	
	or amoxicillin 100 mg/kg/day IV in 4–6 doses	4		
	or Ceftriaxone 2g/day IV or IM in 1 dose	4		
N.B. *2/52 course only if non-complicated IE*	Benzylpenicillin G12–18 million U/day[1,2] IV in 6 doses	2		
	or amoxicillin 100 mg/kg/day IV in 4–6 doses	2		
	or ceftriaxone 2 g/day IV or IM in 1 dose	2		
	and gentamicin 3 mg/kg/day IV in 1 dose	2		
Staphylococci *Meticillin-susceptible*	Oxacillin or flucloxacillin or nafcillin 12 g/day IV in 4–6 doses	4–6	Oxacillin or flucloxacillin or nafcillin 12 g/day IV in 4–6 doses	≥6
	± gentamicin 3 mg/kg/day IV in 2 doses	0.5	*and* rifampicin 1200 mg/day PO in 2 doses	≥6
			and gentamicin 3 mg/kg/day IV in 2 doses	2
Meticillin-resistant or penicillin allergic	Vancomycin 30 mg/kg/day IV in 2 doses	4–6	Vancomycin 30 mg/kg/day IV in 2 doses	≥6
	± gentamicin 3 mg/kg/day IV in 2 doses	0.5	*and* rifampicin 1200 mg/day PO in 2 doses	≥6
			and gentamicin 3 mg/kg/day IV in 2 doses	2
***Enterococcus* spp.**	Amoxicillin *200* mg/kg/day IV[3] in 4–6 doses	4–6	Rare to be secondary to *Streptococcus* seek specialist microbiology advice	
	and gentamicin 3 mg/kg/day IV in two doses	4–6		

[1]If penicillin allergic give vancomycin 30 mg/kg/day IV in 2 doses (4 weeks).
[2]If penicillin strains (MIC0. 125–2 mg/L) give 24 million U/day penicillin (4 weeks) *and* gentamicin (2 weeks).
[3]If pencillin allergic give Vancomycin 30mg/kg/day IV in 2 doses (6 wks).
Data from Hoen, B., and Duval, X. (2013). Infective endocarditis. *The New England Journal of Medicine*, 368:1425–1433; and data from *BNF* https://bnf.nice.org.uk/treatment-summary/cardiovascular-system-infections-antibacterial-therapy.html.

- PVE requires a longer duration of antibiotics (at least 6 weeks, compared with 2–6 weeks for native valve IE).
- Duration of antibiotics should always be calculated from the first day of appropriate antibiotics.
- Anticoagulation: patients with PVE complicated by ischaemic and non-haemorrhagic stroke, and who are taking oral anticoagulants, should stop and replace these with heparin for 2 weeks.
- Drug side effects (generic side effects include rash, allergy, GI symptoms):
  - Gentamicin – nephrotoxicity, ototoxicity, tinnitus.
  - Rifampicin – increases hepatic metabolism of warfarin and other drugs, hepatitis, breathlessness.
  - Vancomycin – nephrotoxicity (accentuated in the presence of gentamicin), thrombocytopenia.

Antibiotic prophylaxis

- European guidance (2): prophylactic antibiotics in patients undergoing an invasive dental procedure with:
  - Prosthetic valve.
  - History of IE.
  - Unrepaired cyanotic congenital heart disease.
- NICE guidance (3): no antibiotic prophylaxis recommended in any circumstances, although permitted in patients who were previously offered antibiotic prophylaxis.
- Good oral, dental and skin hygiene is recommended by all guidelines.

Evidenced-based clinical guidelines and references

1. BNF. https://bnf.nice.org.uk/treatment-summary/cardiovascular-system-infections-antibacterial-therapy.html
2. European society of cardiology (ESC) Guidelines on Prevention, Diagnosis and Treatment of Infective Endocarditis (2015). www. escardio.org/guidelines/clinical-practice-guidelines/infective-endocarditis-guidelines-on-prevention-diagnosis-and-treatment-of.
3. NICE Prophylaxis against infective endocarditis: antimicrobial prophylaxis against infective endocarditis in adults and children undergoing interventional procedures, CG 64. http://www.nice.org.uk/CG064.

Myocardial disease

Primary cardiomyopathies

Hypertrophic cardiomyopathy

Hypertrophic cardiomyopathy is an autosomal dominant condition affecting 1 in 500 (0.2%) of the population. It is the commonest cause of sudden cardiac death in the young. There is incomplete, age-related penetrance.

Seventy per cent of cases of HCM results from mutations in the cardiac sarcomere that cause *increased* energy demand, leading to hypertrophy and *mechanical inefficiency, myofilament disarray* and *fibrosis*. Hypertrophy predominantly affects the LV, usually with asymmetrical severe interventricular septal hypertrophy, which may cause outflow obstruction. Apical HCM is also quite common. Patients with presyncope and syncope must be investigated for both left ventricular outflow tract (LVOT) obstruction and arrhythmic aetiology.

For clinical features of HCM and their cause, see Table 13.25; for an ECG of a patient with HCM see Figure 13.13.

Investigations are undertaken following a careful history, family history and physical examination. Investigations are shown in Table 13.26.

Patients with HCM should have annual surveillance including symptom review, exercise testing (BP not increasing by >25 mmHg is a risk factor for sudden cardiac death [SCD]), Holter ECG monitoring (NSVT is a risk factor for SCD) and AF (common due to left atrial [LA] dilatation).

First degree relatives of patients with HCM, should undergo lifelong surveillance (due to delayed age-related penetrance), beginning in adolescence.

Table 13.25 Clinical features of HCM and their cause

HCM presentation	Pathophysiology
Chest pain	Poor myocardial perfusion during diastole.
SOB or SOBOE	Diastolic heart failure and/or LVOT obstruction.
Palpitations	Ectopics, atrial or ventricular arrhythmia.
Pre-syncope or syncope	Ventricular arrhythmia or LVOT obstruction.
Sudden cardiac death	Ventricular arrhythmia or *severe* LVOT obstruction.

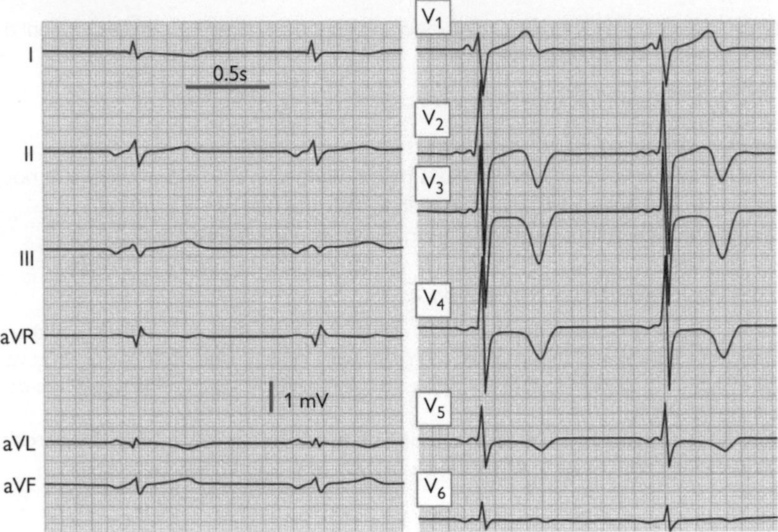

Figure 13.13 ECG of HCM. Note the large amplitude QRS complexes and deep, symmetrical T wave inversion from V2–V5.

Table 13.26 Investigations in HCM

Investigation	Findings
ECG	Left ventricular hypertrophy by voltage criteria. Widespread T-wave inversion of anterolateral leads. *ECG pattern may precede hypertrophy.*
ECHO	Wall thickness/asymmetrical septal hypertrophy (ASH). Septal:posterior LV wall thickness >1.5:1. Systolic anterior movement (SAM) of the mitral leaflet. LVOT pressure gradient (>30 mmHg at rest). LA diameter. Caution: may miss apical changes. Findings may be difficult to distinguish from *athlete's heart.*
CMR	Sensitivity for anatomical diagnosis approaches 100% (➲ see Chapter 5, Case 17, pp. 141–142).
Gene studies	Required for definitive *inherited* HCM diagnosis, access limited. Fabry's disease (X-linked α-galactosidase deficiency), a treatable *phenocopy* of HCM.
Endomyocardial biopsy	Confined to research studies only since the advent of CMR.

Table 13.27 Treatment for HCM

Treatment	Notes
Lifestyle	Avoidance of competitive and high-intensity sport.
Drugs: Verapamil *or* beta blockade	Verapamil – is *lusitropic* (aids ventricular relaxation) and negatively inotropic, which reduces LVOT gradient. β-blockers: increase diastolic filling; decrease LVOT gradient. NB. β-blockers are an *alternative* to verapamil. They are not safe in combination: risk of heart block and –ve inotropic HF.
Antiarrhythmic drugs: Disopyramide (Class Ia) Amiodarone (Class III)	Disopyramide: negatively inotropic and improves Ca^{2+} balance. Amiodarone: useful treatment for arrhythmia in HCM.
Pacing	To deliberately induce dyssynchrony and improve LVOT gradient.
Alcohol septal ablation	For severe LVOT obstruction the septum can be treated with angiographically guided alcohol septal ablation.
Surgical myectomy	For severe LVOT obstruction the septum can be treated with surgical myectomy (on bypass [median sternotomy]).
ICD	Secondary prevention is indicated for VT and aborted SCD. In high risk cases (➲ see Table 13.28) ICD for primary prevention.

Table 13.28 Risk stratification for sudden cardiac death in HCM

Risk stratification for ICD implantation	Notes
Presence of NSVT on Holter monitoring	≥3 ventricular beats at >120 bpm, lasting <30 seconds is non-sustained VT. This is a risk factor for SCD.
Septal thickness >30 mm	Risk is proportional to the thickness of the septum.
Family history	Significant risk if a first degree relative suffered SCD <45 years of age.
Abnormal BP response to exercise	Systolic BP failing to rise by ≥25 mmHg.
Hx of syncope	Unexplained syncope is a poor prognostic sign.
Resting LVOT gradient >30 mmHg	Resting gradients typically worsen with exertion.

For treatment of HCM, see Table 13.27. For risk stratification for sudden cardiac death in HCM, see Table 13.28.

The presence of ≥2 risk factors for SCD is an indication for ICD implantation. Fibrosis, as assessed by late gadolinium enhancement on MRI is also a potential risk factor. Where there is one risk factor decisions should be made by a multidisciplinary team.

Dilated cardiomyopathy

Dilated cardiomyopathy (DCM) is the third commonest cause of heart failure and the commonest cause for cardiac transplant. In DCM, the heart chambers (especially the LV) become dilated and the systolic function is impaired, due to apoptosis and fibrosis of the LV wall. 30–50% of cases are caused by inherited mutations (mostly autosomal dominant). The pathogenesis of DCM is shown in Table 13.29.

Table 13.29 Pathogenesis of DCM

Pathogenesis of DCM phenotype	Notes
Genetic. Mostly AD, but also AR, X-linked and mitochondrial	Structural (nuclear envelope, contractile apparatus, cell adhesion), transcription, splicing and metabolic protein encoding genes.
Pathogenesis of DCM phenocopy	**Notes**
Ischaemia	>50% occlusion of one coronary artery as a minimum finding.
Hypertension	Likely due to the interaction of the hypertensive insult with a genetic predisposition.
Infection (see also myocarditis)	Viral (adenovirus, coxsackie, parvovirus, HIV). PCR has detected viral nucleic acid in up to 35% of DCM patients. Bacterial, fungal, rickettsial, mycobacterial and parasitic.
Tachycardia	Prognosis on restoration of controlled ventricular rate is very good.
Toxins and chemotherapy	Alcohol, cocaine. Chemotherapy (anthracylclines, e.g. doxorubicin, biologic, e.g. trastuzumab, Herceptin®). Trace element (e.g. cobalt, lead, mercury, arsenic) poisoning.
Endocrine/metabolic	Diabetes. Hypothyroid and hyperthyroid (prolonged tachycardia). Phaeochromocytoma (see also Takatsubo [Table 13.36]).
Nutritional disorders	Thiamine (Vit B1), selenium, carnitine deficiencies.
Peripartum	Presenting between 1 month pre- and 5 months post-partum.
Inherited muscular dystrophies	Duchenne and Becker (X-linked dystrophin mutations). Emerry-Dreiffus (X-linked 'Emerin' [nuclear lamin] mutation). Barth syndrome (X-linked, 'Tafazzin' [mitochondrial protein]).
Autoimmune and collagen vascular disorders	e.g. SLE.

The presentation, investigation and management of dilated cardiomyopathy are the same as for heart failure. Specialist referral is indicated.

Arrhythmogenic right ventricular cardiomyopathy

Arrhythmogenic right ventricular cardiomyopathy (ARVC) is an *autosomal dominant* condition. Prevalence is 1 in 1:5000, with a male preponderance of 3:1. Presentation is commonly between adolescence and age 40 years. Fifty per cent of ARVC is caused by mutations in genes encoding structural proteins of cardiac desmosome proteins – desmoplakin, plakoglobin, plakophilin 2, desmoglein 2, and desmocollin 2. Structural deficits in desmosomes cause changes predominantly affecting the RV, but may affect both ventricles or even predominantly the LV.

- Direct cell damage and ultimately apoptosis of cardiac myocytes.
- Remodelling of gap junctions leading to arrhythmias (potentially fatal).
- Disruption of extracellular-nucleus signalling, resulting in fibro-fatty infiltration.

Clinical features of ARVC include palpitations, which may represent VT (LBBB pattern with inferior directed axis); syncope resulting from ventricular arrhythmia; heart failure, if there is significant dysfunction of the ventricular myocardium – especially if this extends to the left ventricle; sudden death.

Investigations are undertaken following a careful history, family history and physical examination. For investigations in ARVC, see Table 13.30. An ECG of the epsilon waves characteristic of abnormal repolarization in ARVC is shown in Figure 13.14.

Table 13.30 Investigations in ARVC

ARVC investigations	Findings
ECG and signal averaged ECG	T wave inversion in V1–3 (and beyond) in the absence of RBBB. Epsilon wave (terminal notch in the QRS complex). Late potentials on signal averaged ECG.
24-hour Holter monitor ECG	For RV origin ectopy and arrhythmia burden.
Exercise tolerance test (ETT)	For exercise-provoked arrhythmias.
ECHO	Regional RV akinesia, dyskinesia or aneurysm and outflow tract dilatation.
CMR	Regional RV akinesia, dyskinesia or dyssynchronous RV contraction, and either raised RV end diastolic volume or RV ejection fraction ≤40%.
RV angiography	Regional RV akinesia, dyskinesia or aneurysm.
Gene studies	Not required in Task Force criteria. May aid research studies/family screening.
Endomyocardial biopsy	Indicated if diagnosis unclear by history, ECG and imaging.

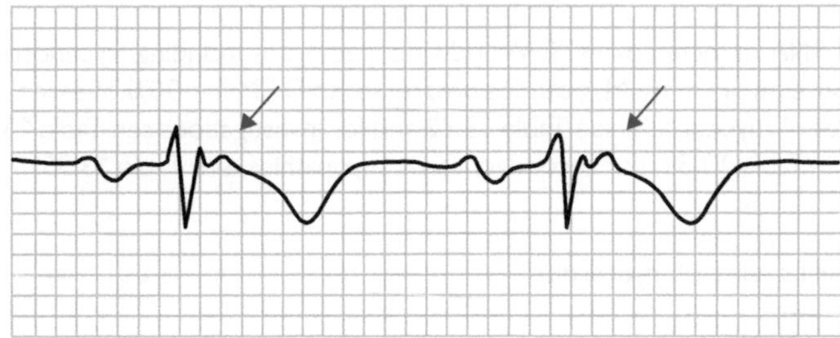

Figure 13.14 ECG showing the 'epsilon waves' (arrows) characteristic of abnormal repolarisation in ARVC, seen here in V1.

Diagnosis is made by 'Modified, Standardised Task Force criteria' (Circulation. 2010; 121:1533–41).

Management

Management of ARVC requires risk stratification and is aimed at preventing SCD. Indicators of high risk include family history, complex ventricular arrhythmia, arrhythmia at a young age, exercise-induced symptoms and any syncope or pre-syncope. For treatment of ARVC, see Table 13.31.

Myocarditis and viral cardiomyopathy

Inflammatory cardiomyopathy can be categorised into:

- Infectious.
- Autoimmune.
- Idiopathic.

In the West, cardiotropic viral infections are responsible for most acute myocarditis. Common agents include parvovirus B19, HHV-6 (a herpes virus), Coxsackie (an enterovirus), EBV, CMV and adenovirus. 35%

Table 13.31 Treatment for ARVC

Treatment		Notes	
Management of heart failure		Isolated severe right ventricular failure or biventricular failure is treated according to standard heart failure guidelines (➲ see Heart failure, p. 451, Table 13.36 and Figures 13.15–13.19).	
		Treatment-resistant heart failure may require transplant.	
Management of arrhythmias	Drugs	Amiodarone and β-blockers with caution.	
	Ablation	Well-localised monomorphic VT may be treated with radiofrequency catheter ablation (multiple procedures may be needed).	
	ICD	Indications	Family history of sudden death.
			History of syncope.
			Documented VT.
			Aborted SCD.
Screen family members		Autosomal dominant condition with variable penetrance.	

of DCMs have viral RNA detected by PCR. Worldwide, pathogens including trypanosomes, spirochaetes and rickettsia can cause myocarditis. Myocarditis progresses to DCM in ~20% of cases.

For clinical features of myocarditis, see Table 13.32 and for investigations see Table 13.33. Treatment of myocarditis is given in Table 13.34. For secondary cardiomyopathies, see Table 13.35.

Table 13.32 Clinical features of myocarditis

Clinical features	Notes
Prodrome	A flu-like prodrome may proceed acute myocarditis (by days to weeks).
Palpitations	These include sinus tachy or bradycardia, atrial and ventricular extrasystoles, VT and VF.
Chest pain	*Myocarditis* may present with pain that mimics angina. *Pericarditis* typically causes a positional, sharp pleuritic pain.
SOB/SOBOE	A very sudden onset of severe heart failure symptoms, with severe LV dysfunction and pulmonary oedema, particularly in acute fulminant myocarditis.
Syncope and sudden death	Both syncope and SCD, often during exertion, may be the first presentation.

Table 13.33 Investigations in myocarditis

Investigation	Findings
ECG	A wide variety of rhythm disturbance and morphology changes are possible: AV block, LBBB, RBBB. Q waves, ST depression and T-wave inversion.
Cardiac enzymes	Often raised: from mild to high (reflecting myocardial damage) High troponin confers poor prognosis.
Coronary angiogram	Normal (or coronary disease disproportionate to the LV dysfunction).
ECHO	LV function ranges from normal to severe LV dysfunction (acute fulminant type). There may be regional wall motion abnormalities and pericardial effusion (if pericardial extension).

Table 13.34 Treatment of myocarditis

Treatment	Notes	
Exclude reversible causes	Angiography to exclude coronary obstruction.	
Inpatient monitoring	During acute phase of inflammation.	
Management of heart failure	According to standard heart failure guidelines (➲ see Heart failure, Table 13.36 and Figures 13.15–13.19).	
Endomyocardial biopsy (if LV function not improving)	Transvenous sampling through RV endocardium Immunohistochemistry of biopsy sample.	
Immunosuppressant drugs (rarely required)	Guided by biopsy findings and include:	Steroids; Azathioprine; interferon-β.

Table 13.35 Secondary cardiomyopathies

Subtype	Aetiology	Treatment (in addition to standard heart failure therapy; ➲ see Heart failure, Table 13.36 and Figures 13.15–13.19)
Hypertensive cardiomyopathy	Secondary to poorly controlled hypertension.	BP control.
Alcohol-related (toxic)	Excess alcohol.	Alcohol abstinence.
Metabolic	Diabetes, thiamine deficiency.	Treatment of cause.
Tachycardia-related	Raised HR over several weeks or months.	Rate control (may include thyrotoxicosis Rx).
Stress-related (Takatsubo)	Uncertain. Physical triggers > emotional triggers. ?Catecholamine surge.	Good prognosis (when no cardiogenic shock present), but high risk of recurrence.
Peripartum cardiomyopathy (➲ see Chapter 23, Peri-partum cardiomyopathy, p. 804)	Specific pregnancy endocrine aetiology.	Strict avoidance of future pregnancies. Rx with dopamine agonists to suppress prolactin.

Heart failure

Epidemiology and pathophysiology

The prevalence of heart failure (HF) is ~1.5% (900,000) of the UK population rising to >10% in those over 70 years. HF accounts for 5% of UK emergency medical admissions.

Heart failure has a heterogenoeous pathophysiology, which results in a *cardiac output insufficient for the body's metabolic requirements*. Progressive, pathological remodelling of the LV is usually driven by a neuro-endocrine axis in which there is increased sympathetic drive and over-activation of the renin-angiotensin system (RAS), with raised levels of angiotensin II and aldosterone. Interruption of sympathetic drive and the RAS are the basis of most effective drug treatment of HF.

The heart failure syndrome is divided into:

- HF with reduced ejection fraction (HFrEF) (commonest in men >65).
- HF with preserved ejection fraction (HFpEF) (commonest in women aged >75). The aetiology of HFpEF is poorly understood. Hypertension and LVH appear to be central to the pathophysiology.

Causes of heart failure are given in Table 13.36.

Table 13.36 Causes of heart failure

Coronary artery disease	Atheromatous coronary disease (~2/3 of systolic HF). Coronary artery spasm (cocaine use). Vasculitis.		
Hypertension	Increased afterload directly on the LV. Renal disease. Arterial disease.		
Valve disease	Aortic stenosis.	↑Afterload (pressure loaded LV).	
	Mitral regurgitation. Aortic regurgitation.	↑Preload (volume loaded LV).	
Idiopathic	<15% of HF is idiopathic.		
Metabolic	Diabetes. Obesity. Thyrotoxicosis/hypothyroidism.		
Toxins	Anthracycline chemotherapy (e.g. doxorubicin). Biologic chemotherapy (trastuzumab [Herceptin ®]). Alcohol.		
Inherited cardiomyopathy (see Table 13.29)	Hypertrophic cardiomyopathy. Arrythmogenic right ventricular dysplasia. Inherited dilated cardiomyopathy.		
Acquired cardiomyopathies	Tachyarrhythmia, e.g. AF with fast ventricular response (AF can be a cause or a result of HF). Peri-partum cardiomyopathy. Catecholamine-induced (Takatsubo).		
	Restrictive and infiltrative cardiomyopathies		Amyloid. Sarcoid. Haemochromatosis. Endomyocardial fibrosis. Anderson–Fabry disease.
Infection (see Table 13.29)	Viral myocarditis, bacterial, fungal, rickettsial, mycobacterial, South American trypanosomiasis (Chagas' disease).		

Clinical features

Heart failure is a clinical syndrome, not a diagnosis. It comprises a collection of signs and symptoms that reflect cardiac pump failure and consequent circulatory congestion (Table 13.37).

Document:

- History of ischaemia (MI, angina, prior revascularisation).
- Vascular risk factors: smoking, hypertension, diabetes, dyslipidaemia, family history or chronic inflammatory conditions (rheumatoid, gout).
- History of structural heart disease or arrhythmia.
- Family history of structural heart disease or sudden death.
- Prescription/non-prescription drugs and alcohol history.
- Symptoms during current/past pregnancies may be relevant.

Signs of heart failure are given in Table 13.38. For the New York Heart Association (NYHA) functional classification of heart failure severity, see Table 13.39.

Diagnosis, investigations and classification

Three investigations are central in confirming the diagnosis: ECG, natriuretic peptides and echocardiography (Table 13.40). For heart failure diagnostic protocol, see Figure 13.15.

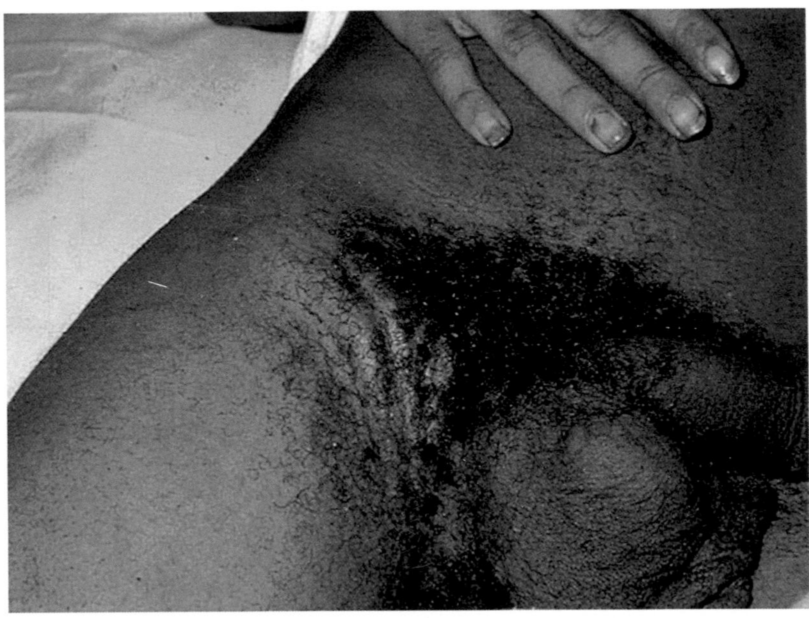

Figure 7.3 Groove sign in lymphogranuloma venereum.

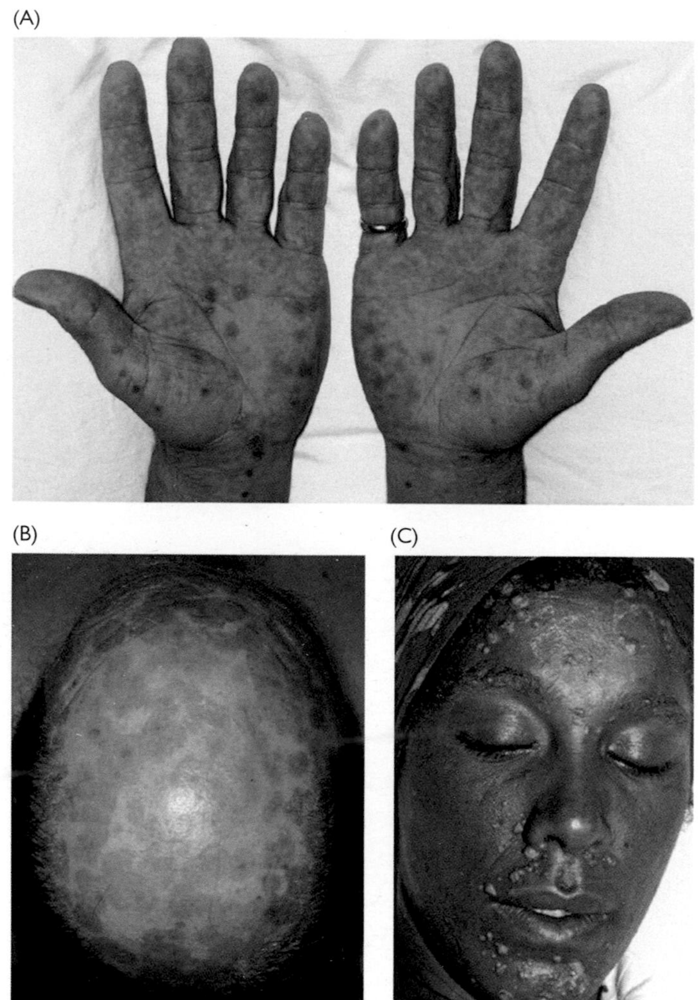

Figure 7.5 (A, B) Rash of secondary syphilis on palms and scalp. (C) Papular lesions of secondary syphilis.

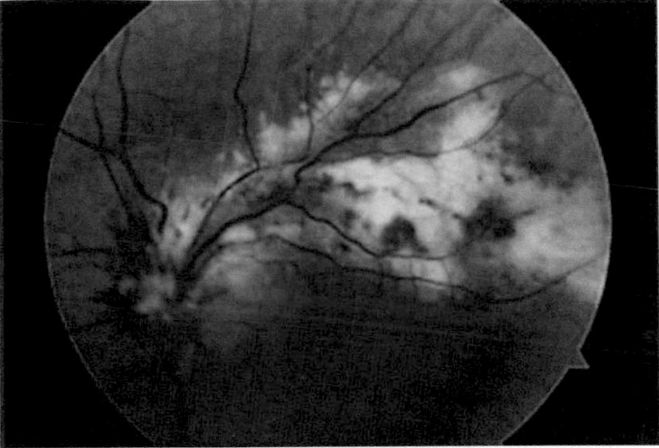

Figure 7.11 CMV retinitis, commonly termed 'cheese pizza' or 'pizza pie' retina.

Reproduced with permission from Frith P. The eye in general medicine. In *Oxford Textbook of Medicine*, 5th edn, Warrell D. A. et al. (eds). Oxford: OUP. Copyright © 2013 Oxford University Press. DOI: 10.1093/med/9780199204854.001.1. Reproduced with permission of the Licensor through PLSclear.

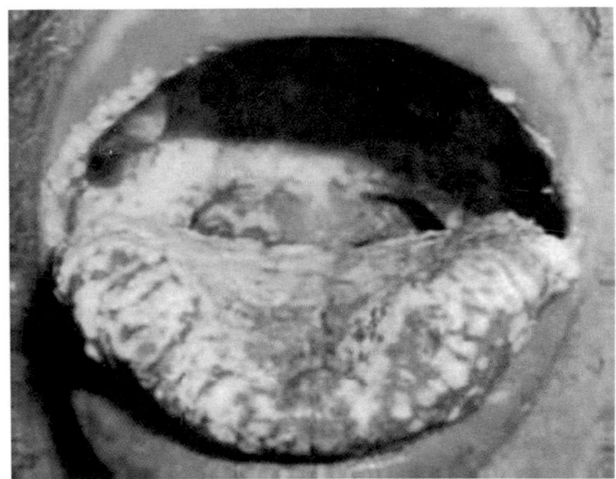

Figure 7.12 Oropharyngeal candida.

Republished with permission of MA Healthcare Ltd from Wingfield T., Wilkins E. Opportunistic infections in HIV disease. *Br J Nurs.* 19(10):621–7. Copyright © 2013 MA Healthcare Ltd, a Mark Allen Group company. https://doi.org/10.12968/bjon.2010.19.10.93543. Permission conveyed through Copyright Clearance Center, Inc.

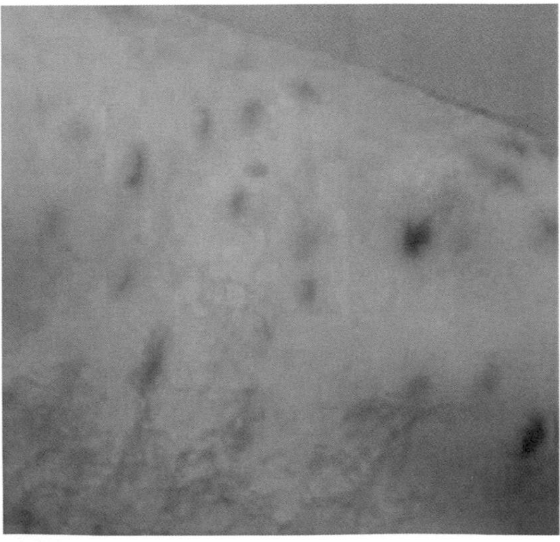

Figure 7.13 Kaposi sarcoma lesions.

Republished with permission of MA Healthcare Ltd from Wingfield T., Wilkins E. Opportunistic infections in HIV disease. *Br J Nurs.* 19(10):621–7. Copyright © 2013 MA Healthcare Ltd, a Mark Allen Group company. https://doi.org/10.12968/bjon.2010.19.10.93543. Permission conveyed through Copyright Clearance Center, Inc.

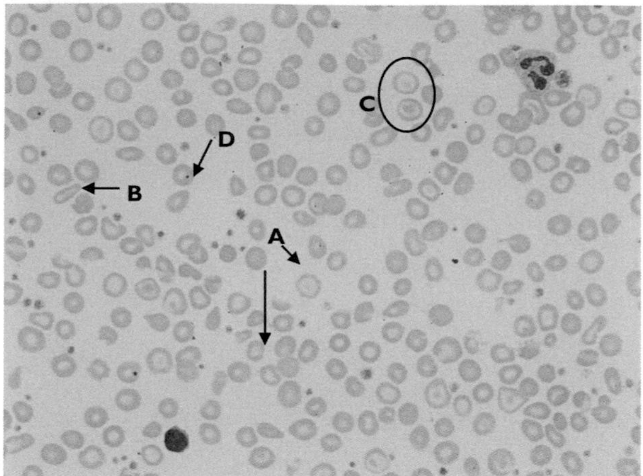

Figure 9.2 Peripheral blood film of a patient with iron deficiency anaemia, post splenectomy (Oil immersion ×100 magnification). (A) Hypochromic, microcytic red cells typical of iron deficiency. (B) Pencil cells typical of iron deficiency. (C) Target cells with haemoglobinised dark areas, both centrally and peripherally (as a band), with a white ring of relative pallor in between, are due either to increased red cell surface area or to decreased intracellular haemoglobin content; commonly seen post-splenectomy. (D) Howell–Jolly bodies (histopathological findings of basophilic nuclear remnants in circulating erythrocytes, usually signifying a damaged or absent spleen).

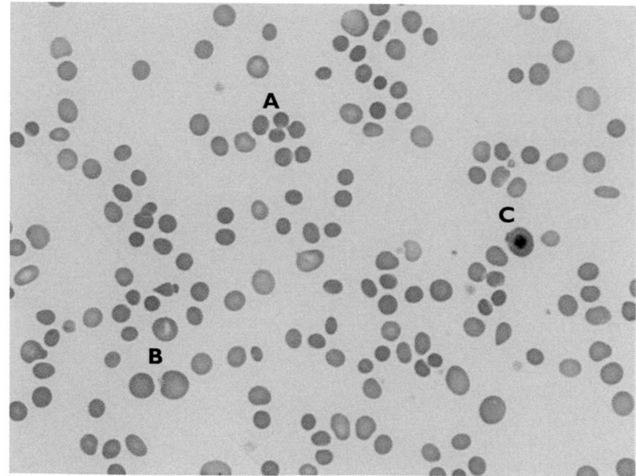

Figure 9.4 Peripheral blood film of patient with warm autoimmune haemolytic anaemia (Oil immersion ×100 magnification). (A) Spherocyte (sphere-shaped erythrocyte). (B) Polychromasia (erythrocytes of different shades of colour, typically greyish blue, due to premature release of immature erythrocytes [reticulocytes] from the bone marrow). (C) Nucleated red blood cell.

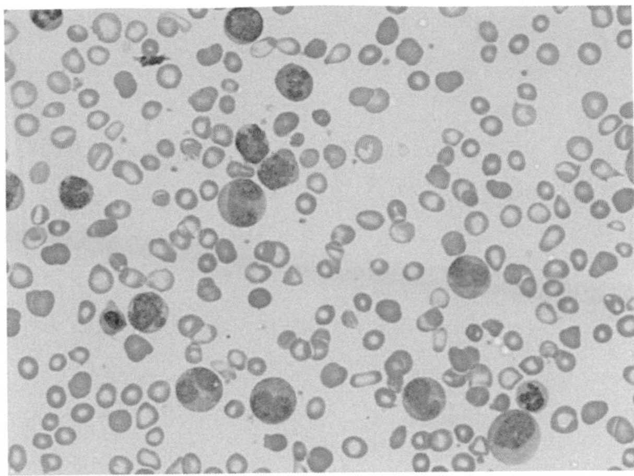

Figure 9.7 Peripheral blood film of patient with chronic myeloid leukaemia showing many immature myeloid precursors (Oil immersion x100 magnification).

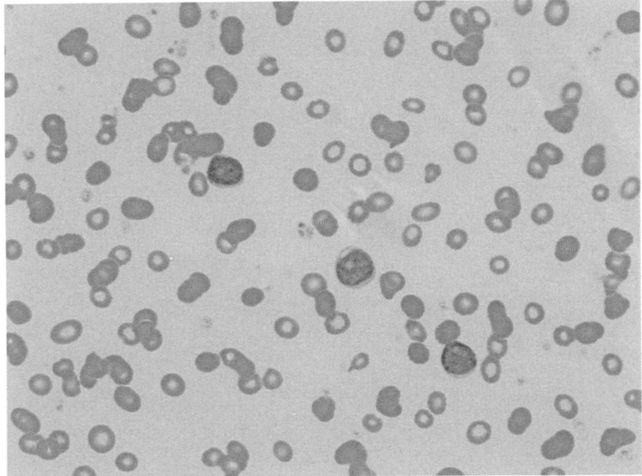

Figure 9.8 Peripheral blood film of patient with acute myeloid leukaemia showing three large immature blasts with nucleoli (Oil immersion ×100 magnification).

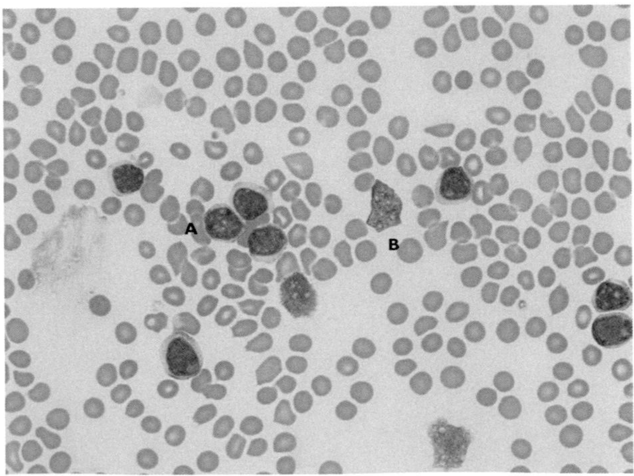

Figure 9.9 Peripheral blood film of patient with chronic lymphocytic leukaemia (Oil immersion ×100 magnification). (A) Mature lymphocytes – some with nucleoli. (B) Smear cell.

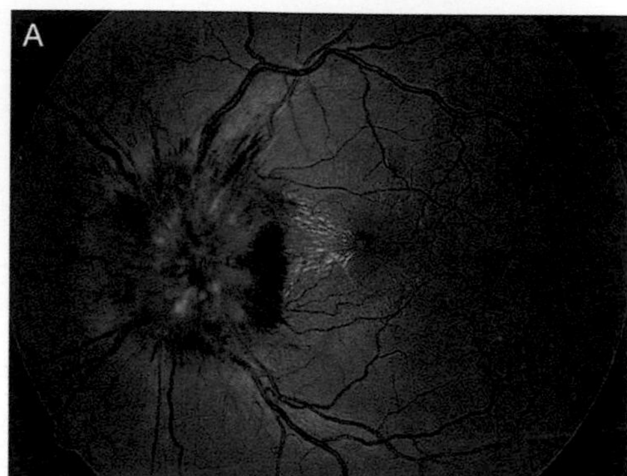

Figure 18.7 Papilloedema. The optic disc appears hyperaemic, with blurred margins, splinter haemorrhages, and engorged, dilated surrounding veins. There is early development of tiny hard exudates tracking along the maculopapular bundle.

Courtesy of Brian R. Younge, MD, Mayo Clinic, Rochester, Minnesota. Used with permission.

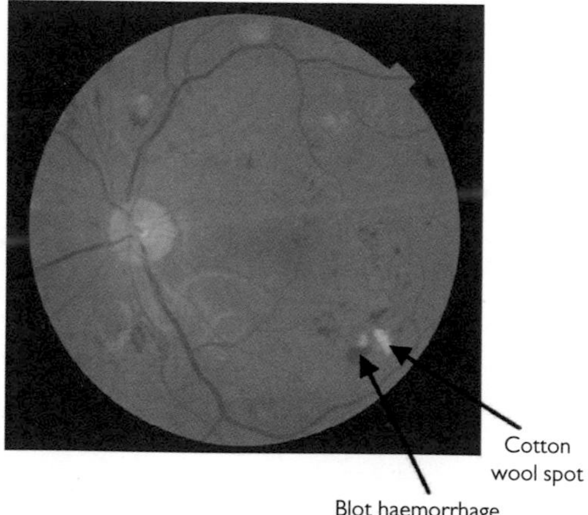

Figure 18.9 Pre-proliferative diabetic retinopathy. Cotton wool spots and blot haemorrhages are indicated.

Reproduced with permission from Leigh R. Pre-proliferative and proliferative retinopathy. In *Diabetic Retinopathy Screening to Treatment*, Dodson, P. (Ed). Oxford, UK: Oxford University Press. Copyright © 2008 Heart of England Retinal Screening Centre. DOI:10.1093/med/9780199544967.003.0007.

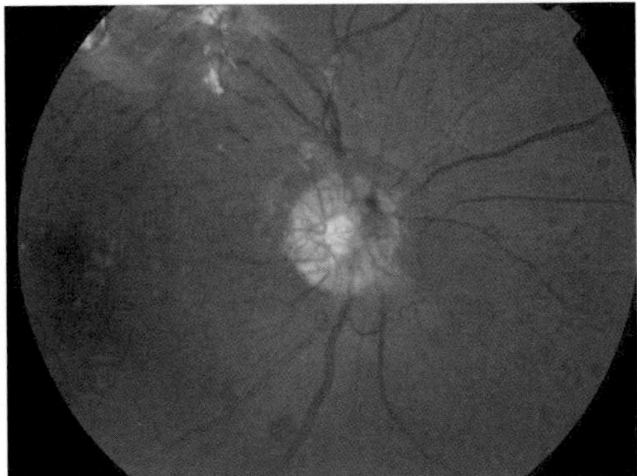

Figure 18.10 Proliferative diabetic retinopathy. New vessels have formed all over the optic disc. They are fine, looping, and aimless.

Reproduced with permission from Imaging Service Moorfields Eye Hospital.

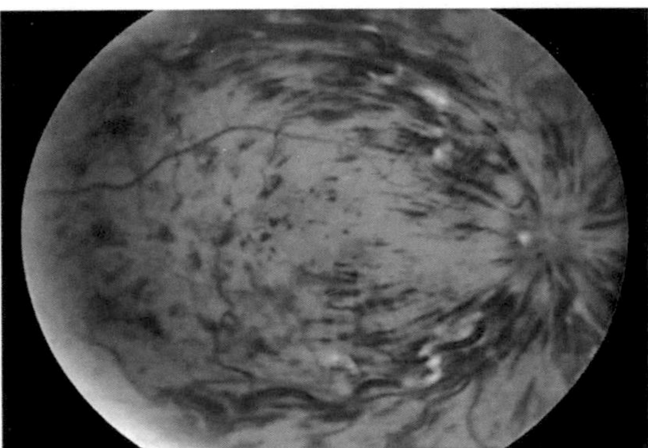

Figure 18.12 Central retinal vein occlusion. Profuse flame haemorrhages have formed between the nerve fibres in all quadrants. Cotton wool spots representing microinfarcts are often also present.

Reproduced with permission from Frith P. The eye in general medicine. In *Oxford Textbook of Medicine*, Fifth Edition, Warrell D. A. et al. (Eds.). Oxford, UK: OUP.

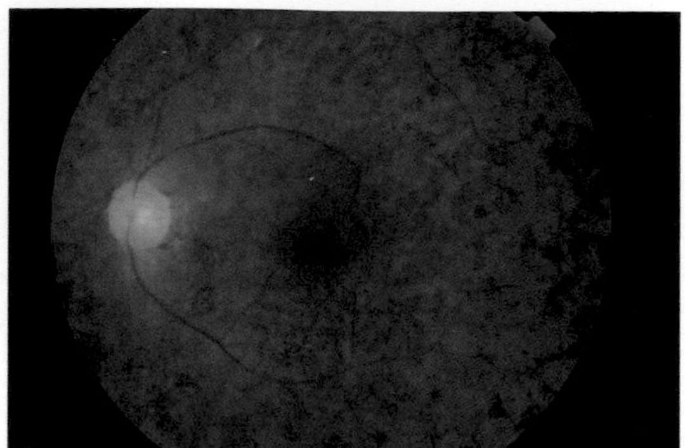

Figure 18.13 Retinitis pigmentosa: Peripheral retinal pigmentation classically occurs in a 'bone-spicule' pattern (like the branches of a tree) although it may also take the form of multiple small black spots.

Reproduced with permission from Imaging Service Moorfields Eye Hospital.

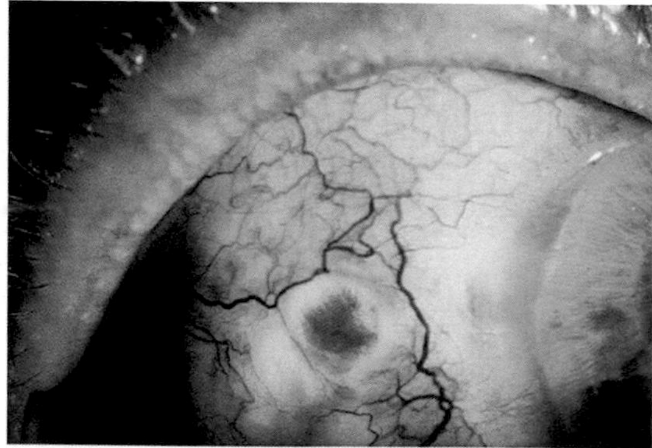

Figure 18.14 Scleritis demonstrating scleromalacia. Vasculitis results in focal ischaemia, with translucency and thinning of the sclera, which may perforate.

Reproduced with permission from Frith P. The eye in general medicine. In *Oxford Textbook of Medicine*, Fifth Edition, Warrell D. A. et al. (Eds.). Oxford, UK: OUP. Copyright © 2013 Oxford University Press. Reproduced with permission of the Licensor through PLSclear.

Table 13.37 Symptoms of heart failure

Symptom	Description	Consider
Shortness of breath (SOB)	Initially occurring on exertion (SOBOE) and then with reducing effort until occurring at rest (SOBAR).	Nature of onset (sudden/recent) and precipitating event (e.g. MI). Exercise tolerance in distance and duration.
Orthopnoea	Breathlessness worse lying flat.	Angle/pillows used.
Paroxysmal nocturnal dyspnoea (PND)	Waking breathless at night with desperate need to be upright.	
Ankle swelling	Bilateral swelling of dependent areas.	Duration/progression. Dihydropyridines can cause ankle swelling (e.g. amlodipine).
Fatigue	A common, non-specific symptom of poor forward flow.	
Angina	Central, exertional chest pain or tightness (often radiating to left arm, neck); may suggest an ischaemic aetiology.	
Palpitations	May suggest aetiology or be a complication of heart failure.	Atrial arrhythmias. VT.

Table 13.38 Signs of heart failure

Abnormalities	Signs	Cause
Left HF	Low BP.	Reduced contractility of LV. Reduced stroke volume.
	Low volume central pulse.	
	Apex: (infero)laterally displaced and palpable over a diffuse area (*thrusting*).	Reflecting LV dilatation.
	3rd heart sound.	Sound of diastolic filling of blood into stiff LV with raised end diastolic pressure.
	Pansystolic murmur.	Dilatation of LV causing 'functional' mitral regurgitation.
	Bilateral end inspiratory crepitations.	Transudation of pulmonary venous fluid into interstices.
Right HF	Elevated JVP; ≥4cm vertical above clavicle with patient at 45° angle.	
	Bilateral pitting oedema of the ankles; progresses proximally.	Note the most proximal extent of oedema.
	Tender hepatomegaly, ascites in severe RV failure.	The liver is pulsatile only where there is severe tricuspid regurgitation.
Associated signs	Cachexia.	Tissue wasting due to poor blood supply.
	Pulse rate and rhythm.	May cause tachycardia and/or AF.
	Needlestick marks on fingertips of non-dominant hand.	Glucose monitoring of a patient with diabetes.
	Peripheral scars of bypass conduit harvest.	Anteromedial course of long saphenous vein in the legs.
	Median sternotomy scar.	CABG (NB: if no scar on leg, internal mammary graft may have been used) and valve surgery (commonest causes); congenital heart disease correction and transplant (both associated with increased risk HF).
	Clinical signs of valve disease (see Table 13.19).	

Table 13.39 New York Heart Association (NYHA) Functional classification of Heart Failure Severity

NYHA I	*No limitation* of physical activity	Subclinical
NYHA II	*Slight limitation* of physical activity	Mild
NYHA III	*Marked limitation* of physical activity	Moderate
NYHA IV	*Inability* to carry out *any* physical activity without discomfort	Severe

Table 13.40 Investigations in heart failure

Investigation		**Finding**	**Significance**
ECG		Normal ECG	Negative predictive value for heart failure: Acute presentation: 98% Chronic presentation: 86%
		Tachyarrhythmia Atrial Ventricular	May reflect the cause or a complication of heart failure.
		LVH by voltage criteria (Sokalow)	LVH. HCM.
		Q waves	Previous transmural infarction.
		Conduction disease Heart block Intraventricular conduction delay esp. LBBB	May indicate benefit for biventricular pacing. (NB. Standard RV pacing may worsen systolic function). Cardiac resynchronisation therapy (biventricular pacing) can improve outcomes.
Natriuretic peptides, e.g. BNP and NT-proBNP		Peptide hormones secreted by cardiac myocytes when the heart is diseased or the cardiac chambers are stretched.	Natriuretic peptides are non-specific but very sensitive and so a normal level virtually excludes heart failure.
Echocardiography		Widely available. Relatively cheap. Portable. Non-ionising.	The mainstay of cardiac imaging in heart failure. Diagnosis and classification: HFrEF. HFpEF. Severity (ejection fraction, etc.). Aetiology (e.g. severe AS or regional wall motion abnormality). Alternative diagnosis (e.g. pulmonary hypertension).
Blood tests	Biochem	U&E. Fasting glucose and lipids.	Renal function and use of diuretics and potassium sparing agents (ACE-i, MRAs, etc.). Diabetes or dyslipidaemia.
	Haem	FBC, Hct and ferritin.	Anaemia, iron overload, prognosis.
	Other	Thyroid hormones.	Thyrotoxicosis can exacerbate and mimic HF.

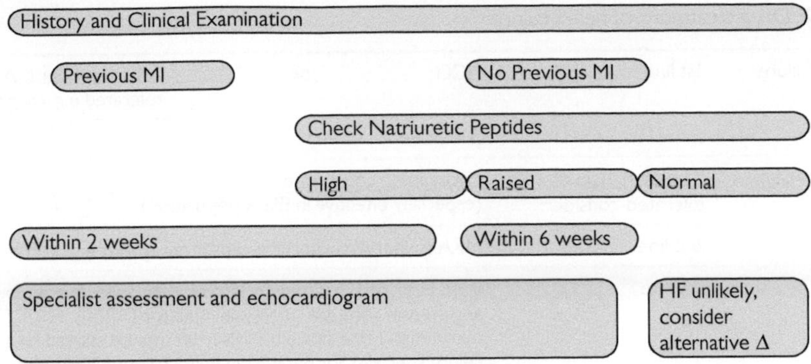

Figure 13.15 Heart failure diagnostic protocol from NICE CG108 (2010 update).

Treatment

See Tables 13.41 and 13.42.

Table 13.41 Heart failure treatment

Lifestyle modification	Graded exercise training. Smoking cessation. Alcohol. Diet and nutrition. Weight loss.	Cardiac rehabilitation: Education for lifestyle modification. Support. Group therapy. Graded exercise.
Pharmacological	Heart failure targeted treatment.	see Table 13.42.
	Treatment for associated conditions.	Hypertension. Diabetes. Dyslipidaemia.
Coronary revascularisation	Coronary angioplasty or coronary bypass surgery may be indicated in cases where imaging demonstrates 'viability' in the context of blocked coronary arteries.	'Viable' or 'hibernating' myocardial segments are those which contract poorly, but remain alive.
Devices	Cardiac resynchronisation therapy.	Cardiac resynchronisation therapy (pacemaker only): CRT (P).
	Defibrillators.	Implanted cardiac defibrillator: ICD.
		Cardiac resynchronisation therapy (with added defibrillator): CRT (D).
Ventricular assist devices	For carefully selected patients as a 'bridge to transplant'. This technology cannot (in the UK, according to NICE) be used as a 'destination therapy' (i.e. not instead of transplant).	
Heart transplant	For carefully selected (usually younger) patients.	

Table 13.42 Drug treatment of heart failure

Systolic heart failure HFrEF	1st line	ACEi	or	ARB (consider if ACEi not tolerated e.g. *cough*)
	and	β-blocker		
Specialist assessment	If neither ACEi or ARB tolerated-consider:	Hydralazine and nitrate (especially effective in Black population)		
	2nd line	MRA (mineralocorticoid receptor antagonist e.g. spironolactone)		
	3rd line	If ACEi or ARB has been tolerated then substitute an angiotensin receptor neprilysin inhibitor (ARNI). NICE [TA388] recommend that sacubitril valsartan may be started by a heart failure specialist for patients in heart failure NYHA class II–IV, with an ejection fraction <35% and already taking a stable dose of ACE-i or ARB. Consider ivabradine if on max tolerated dose of β-blocker and SR >70/75 (ESC/NICE) bpm. Consider digoxin to reduce hospitalisation		
Diastolic heart failure HFpEF	NICE recommend treatment of associated HTN, DM and IHD. ESC recommend treatment of associated HTN and IHD, but also rate control in AF. In HFpEF, unlike HFrEF, rate controlling Ca channel blockers (e.g. verapamil) may be used. No treatment has convincingly been shown to reduce morbidity and mortality.			

Cardiac resynchronisation therapy

Cardiac resynchronisation therapy (CRT) uses a pacemaker that can stimulate the left ventricle. This is a very effective means of improving HF, particularly where there is sinus rhythm and LBBB.

Combining an ICD with a cardiac resynchronisation therapy-pacemaker (CRT-P) results in a cardiac resynchronisation therapy defibrillator (CRT-D). These devices can be distinguished on CXR (Figures 13.16–13.19).

For indications for cardiac resynchronisation therapy, see Table 13.43 and for implantable cardiac defibrillators, see Table 13.44.

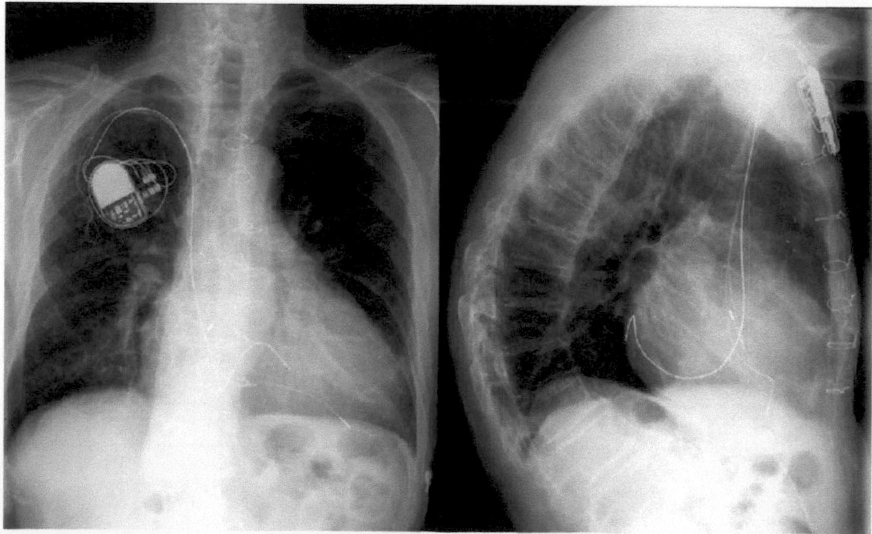

Figure 13.16 PA and lateral CXR films of a CRT(P) – no defibrillating charge coils visible on leads. RA, RV and LV leads seen.

Reproduced with permission from Mc Murray J, et al. Heart failure. In *The ESC Textbook of Cardiovascular Medicine*, 2nd edn. Camm AJ, et al. (Eds). Oxford: OUP. Copyright © 2009 European Society of Cardiology. DOI: 10.1093/med/9780199566990.001.0001. Reproduced with permission of the Licensor through PLSclear.

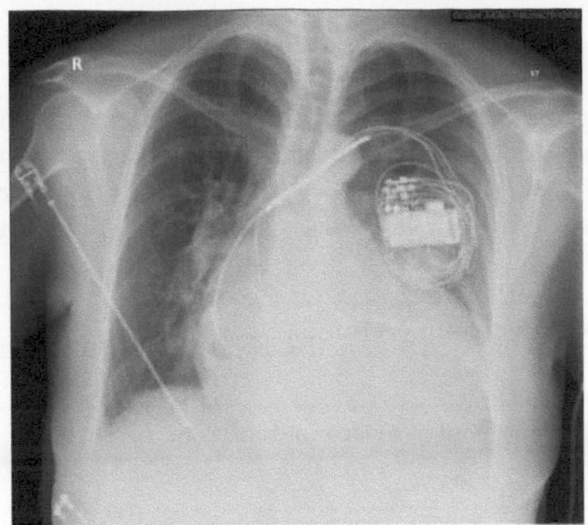

Figure 13.17 PA CXR of a CRT(D) – lead tips visible in RA, RV apex and on LV lateral wall. Defibrillator coils are clearly visible.

Reproduced with permission from Mc Murray J, et al. Heart failure. In *The ESC Textbook of Cardiovascular Medicine*, 2nd edn. Camm AJ, et al. (Eds). Oxford: OUP. Copyright © 2009 European Society of Cardiology. DOI: 10.1093/med/9780199566990.001.0001. Reproduced with permission of the Licensor through PLSclear.

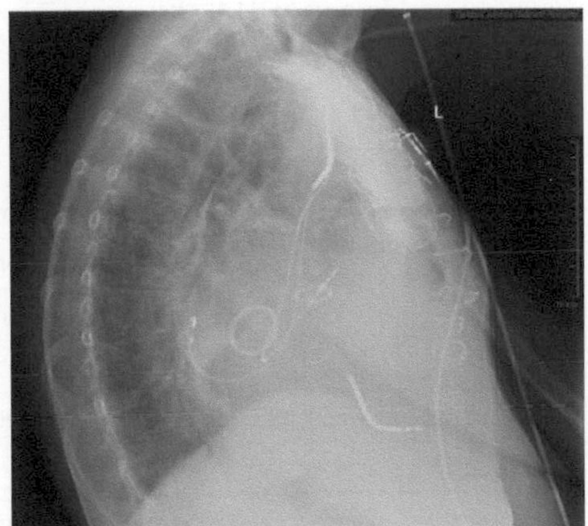

Figure 13.18 Lateral CXR of a CRT(D) – the 'dorsally placed' lead is the LV lead and the supero-anterior is the RA lead.

Reproduced with permission from Mc Murray J, et al. Heart failure. In *The ESC Textbook of Cardiovascular Medicine*, 2nd edn. Camm AJ, et al. (Eds). Oxford: OUP. Copyright © 2009 European Society of Cardiology. DOI: 10.1093/med/9780199566990.001.0001. Reproduced with permission of the Licensor through PLSclear.

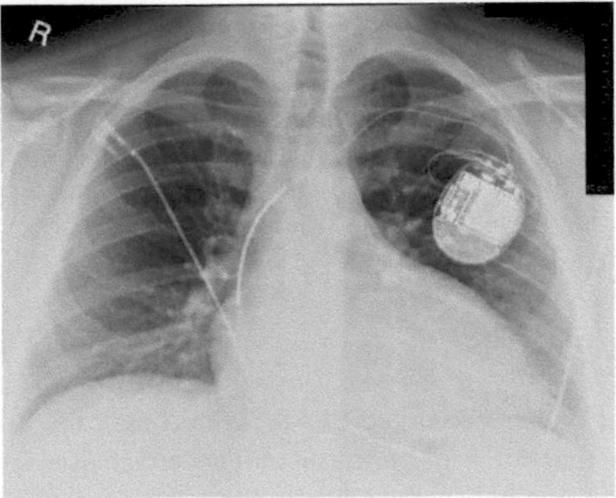

Figure 13.19 A single lead ICD device. The lead is placed in the RV apex and the two defibrillator coils are clearly visible.

Reproduced with permission from Mc Murray J, et al. Heart failure. In *The ESC Textbook of Cardiovascular Medicine*, 2nd edn. Camm AJ, et al. (Eds). Oxford: OUP. Copyright © 2009 European Society of Cardiology. DOI: 10.1093/med/9780199566990.001.0001. Reproduced with permission of the Licensor through PLSclear.

Table 13.43 Indications for cardiac resynchronisation therapy and/or implantable cardiac defibrillator in heart failure. Implantable cardioverter defibrillators (ICDs), cardiac resynchronisation therapy (CRT) with defibrillator (CRT-D) or CRT with pacing (CRT-P) are recommended as treatment options for people with heart failure who have left ventricular dysfunction with a left ventricular ejection fraction (LVEF) of ≤35% as specified

	NYHA class			
QRS duration	**I**	**II**	**III**	**IV**
< 120 ms	ICD if high risk of sudden cardiac death			ICD and CRT not indicated
120–149 ms + no LBBB	ICD	ICD	ICD	CRT-P
120–149 ms + LBBB	ICD	CRT-D	CRT-P or CRT-D	CRT-P
>150 ms	CRT-D	CRT-D	CRT-P or CRT-D	CRT-P

Reproduced from © NICE (2014) TA314 Implantable cardioverter defibrillators and cardiac resynchronisation therapy for arrhythmias and heart failure. Available from https://www.nice.org.uk/guidance/ta314 NICE guidance is prepared for the National Health Service in England. All NICE guidance is subject to regular review and may be updated or withdrawn. NICE accepts no responsibility for the use of its content in this product/publication.

Table 13.44 Indications for implantable cardiac defibrillator (ICD)

Primary arrhythmia prevention	Selected patients with familial cardiac conditions with a high risk of sudden cardiac death.	Brugada syndrome.
		Long QT syndrome.
		Hypertrophic cardiomyopathy.
		Arrhythmogenic cardiomyopathy.
	Selected patients who have undergone surgical repair of congenital heart disease.	
Secondary arrhythmia prevention	Survived VF arrest.	
	Symptomatic sustained VT with haemodynamic compromise.	

Data from Technology appraisal guidance [TA314], Implantable cardioverter defibrillators and cardiac resynchronisation therapy for arrhythmias and heart failure, 2014.

Heart failure clinical guidelines and key trials

See Table 13.45.

Further reading

1. NICE. Chronic heart failure in adults: diagnosis and management. NICE guideline NG106, 2018. https://www.nice.org.uk/guidance/NG106.
2. Ponikowski P, Voors AA, Anker SD, et al. 2016 ESC Guidelines for the diagnosis and treatment of acute and chronic heart failure. *European Heart Journal* 2016; 37:2129–200. http://eurheartj.oxfordjournals.org/content/ehj/early/2016/06/08/eurheartj.ehw128.full.pdf.

Pericardial disease

Pericarditis accounts for 5% of patients admitted to A&E with chest pain. It is caused by inflammation of one or both layers (visceral and parietal) of pericardium. Pericardial disease can be subdivided into pericarditis, constrictive pericarditis, and pericardial effusion and cardiac tamponade (Table 13.46). For typical ECG changes in acute pericarditis, see Figure 13.20. For the semiquantitative assessment of pericardial effusion size, see Figure 13.21. Pressure/volume curve of the pericardium is shown in Figure 13.22.

Table 13.45 Key trials in heart failure

	Trial	Critical findings
ACEi	*CONSENSUS* N Engl J Med. 1987. NYHA IV (severe symptomatic HF), no ECHO. n = 247, RCT Enalapril (target 20 mg BD) versus placebo.	Stopped after 6 months due to 41% relative risk reduction in all-cause mortality.
	SOLVD N Engl J Med. 1991. EF ≤35% *and* asymptomatic prevention (n = 4228) *or* symptomatic (NYHA II-IV) treatment (n = 2569), RCT Enalapril (10 mg BD) versus placebo. 3 years follow-up.	In 'prevention' group: reduced hospitalisation, but no mortality benefit. In 'treatment' group: reduced mortality 16% and hospitalisation 26%.
ARBs	*ValHeFT* N Engl J Med. 2001. EF <40% and symptomatic with HF n = 5010, RCT valsartan (target 160 mg BD) versus placebo. Most patients already on ACE-i. 2 years median follow-up.	Primary endpoint – all-cause mortality: no benefit. Secondary composite endpoint: mortality and HF morbidity: 13% relative risk reduction with valsartan. Subgroup analysis of pts not on ACE-i: all-cause mortality benefit.
	CHARM Lancet 2003. RCT candesartan (up to 32 mg OD) versus placebo. n = 7601 in 3 arms: '*Alternative*' median follow up 34/12 intolerant of ACE-i. '*Added*' 41/12 in addition to ACE-i. '*Preserved*' 37/12 pts with HFpEF. Primary composite endpoint – CV death and hospitalisation for HF.	'*Alternative*': 23% reduction in primary endpoint. '*Added*': 15% reduction in primary endpoint. '*Preserved*': no reduction in primary endpoint, but fewer hospitalisations and 40% less development of Type 2 DM. Overall non-significant (p = 0.055) reduction in mortality.
β-blocker	*CIBIS II* Lancet 1999. At a time when β-blockers were considered *unsafe* in HF and the 1-year mortality for acute HF admission was 50%. EF ≤35% and NYHA III or IV n = 2647, RCT bisoprolol (target 10mg OD) versus placebo.	34% reduction in primary endpoint: all-cause mortality. Also reduced hospitalisations for HF. This study marked a paradigm shift in HF treatment.
	MERIT-HF J Am Med Ass 2000. Recruited before CIBIS II result known. EF ≤40% and NYHA II-IV (less severe cohort). n = 3991, RCT slow release metoprolol (CR/XL) (target 200 mg OD) versus placebo.	34% reduction in primary endpoint: all-cause mortality.
	COPERNICUS N Engl J Med. 2001. After it was established that β-blockers were indicated in stable HF this trial examined an acute, severe HF cohort: EF <25% and NYHA III and IV. n = 2289, RCT carvedilol (target 25 mg BD) versus placebo.	35% reduction in primary endpoint: all-cause mortality.
MRAs	*RALES* N Engl J Med. 1999. EF ≤ 35% and NYHA III and IV *and* on ACE-i, diuretic *and* K^{+}<5.0 mmol/L. n = 1663, RCT spironolactone (12.5–50 mg, most on 25 mg) versus placebo.	Stopped early due to 30% reduction in all-cause mortality. Also 35% reduction in hospital admission and reduced NYHA class. Mean rise in K+ (<0.3 mM) and only 2% > 6.0 mmol/L.

continued

Table 13.45 *continued*

	Trial	Critical findings
	EMPHASIS EF <35% and NYHA class II (mild symptoms) *and* recent hospitalisation or raised natiuretic peptides. n = 2737, RCT eplerenone (target 50 mg OD) versus placebo.	24% reduction in primary endpoint: all-cause mortality. 37% reduction in composite of CV death and hospitalisation for HF.
Digoxin	*DIG* (Digitalis Investigators Group) *Trial* N Engl J Med. 1997. EF ≤45% and NYHA II-IV (any symptoms) in SR. n = 6800, RCT digoxin (target 250 μg) versus placebo.	NB. this trial was pre-β-blocker Rx for HF. 28% reduction in hospitalisation for HF over a mean 3-year follow-up period. No mortality benefit.
Isosorbide dinitrate and hydralazine	*V-HeFT-II* N Engl J Med. 1991. Mild to moderate stable HF (NYHA II-III) on a diuretic and digoxin. n = 804 (men), RCT H-ISDN versus enalapril.	28% trend towards mortality increase with H-ISDN.
	A-HeFT N Engl J Med. 2004. Moderate to severe stable HF (NYHA III-IV) on β-blocker, ACE-i/ARB, diuretic and digoxin. n = 1050 (*African-American* men and women), RCT H-ISDN (target 40 mg ISDN and 75 mg hydralazine TDS) versus placebo.	Trial stopped at 10 months due to: 43% all-cause mortality benefit of H-ISDN. 33% reduction in hospitalisation.
Ivabradine	*SHIFT* Lancet 2010. EF ≤ 35%, symptomatic HF (NYHA II-IV), sinus rhythm >70 bpm and >90% on β-blocker and either ACE-i or ARB. n = 6588 RCT ivabradine (target 7.5 mg BD) versus placebo. Primary composite: CV death or HF hospitalisation.	NB. Only 26% of patients were on a full dose of β-blocker. 18% reduction in composite endpoint (CV death and HF hospitalisation), but *no significant* reduction in CV death. 26% reduction in HF hospitalisation.
Cardiac resynchronisation therapy/ biventricular pacing	*CARE-HF* N Engl J Med. 2005. EF<35%, NYHA III or IV and QRS >150 ms *or* 120–150 ms and ECHO evidence of dyssynchrony. n = 813 RCT of CRT(P) versus standard pacing. Primary endpoint: all-cause mortality.	33% reduction in all-cause mortality.
ICD implantation	*MADIT-II* N Engl J Med. 2002. EF <30%, MI >1/12 prior. n = 1232 RCT (3:2) ICD or OMT. Primary endpoint: all-cause mortality.	Terminated (early) at 20/12 due to reduction in all-cause mortality from 19.8 to 14.2%.
Coronary revascularisation	*STICH* N Engl J Med. 2011 (& 2016). EF ≤35%, NYHA I-III and coronary artery disease (2 [30%] or 3 [60%] vessel disease). n = 2012 RCT medical therapy alone versus + medical therapy + CABG.	No change in primary endpoint: all-cause mortality. 19% reduction in CV death. 26% reduction in all-cause mortality and CV hospitalisation. NB. 10-year data – reduction in mortality with CABG.
Neprilysin inhibition (combined with ARB)	*Paradigm-HF* N Engl J Med. 2015. EF <40% and NYHA II and III. LCZ696 (valsartan-sacubitril). n = 8442 RCT of LCZ696 versus enalapril (10 mg BD [SOLVD dose]).	20% reduction in CV mortality. 16% reduction in all-cause mortality.

HF, heart failure; ACE-i, angiotensin-converting enzyme inhibitor; CV, cardiovascular; ARB, angiotensin receptor blocker; MRA, mineralocorticoid receptor antagonist; H-ISDN, hydralzine and isosorbide dinitrate; OMT, optimal medical therapy.

Table 13.46 Pericardial disease

	Pericarditis	Constrictive pericarditis	Pericardial effusion ± cardiac tamponade
Epidemiology	5% of patients admitted A&E. Aetiology: 90% post-viral/idiopathic, 2% bacterial, 4% tuberculosis (TB), 5–7% neoplastic, 4% autoimmune	Rare. Aetiology: idiopathic 45%, post-surgical 35%, post-radiation 7%. Other causes: TB (usually post-effusion), bacterial/uraemic/recurrent pericarditis, mallignancy, CTD.	Pericardial effusion common (>50 mL of fluid within pericardial sac). Aetiology: viral (echovirus + coxsackie most common), bacterial TB, fungal, autoimmune (e.g. SLE), neoplastic, post-PCI/cardiac surgery, uraemic, drugs.
Pathophysiology	Inflammation of one or both layers of pericardium.	Scarred and inelastic pericardium, resulting in restriction of diastolic filling of both RV and LV.	Effusion –>↑ intracardiac pressure: sudden 100–200 mL ↑ post-op can cause tamponade, slow 2L effusion may not.
Clinical features	Retrosternal, sudden, pleuritic pain. Eased on sitting forwards 85% have audible pericardial rub. Suddenly raising legs can precipitate pain.	Signs of right HF, soft heart sounds, atrial fibrillation, non-pulsatile hepatomegaly, *Kussmaul's sign +ve* (JVP ↑ on inspiration: [RV unable to accommodate normal increased venous return during inspiration]) . *Prominent X & Y descent in JVP* (severely restricted diastolic filling). *Pericardial knock* (halt in rapid LV filling) ± *pulsus paradoxus* (>10 mmHg ↓ inspiration).	Pericardial effusion: may be asymptomatic. Signs of cardiac tamponade: hypotension, signs of right heart failure, soft heart sounds, *Kussmaul's sign -ve. Prominent X (no Y) descent in JVP. No pericardial knock. Pulsus paradoxus present.*
Diagnosis *CXR* (➲ See Chapter 5, Case 7, p. 127)	Exclude pneumothorax, ? TB.	Pericardial calcifications, pleural effusions.	Enlarged silhouette with clear lung fields.
ECG	85% have widespread concave ST-segment elevation and PR depression.	Normal or low voltages, T wave inversion, atrial fibrillation, AV block.	Small complexes, *electrical alternans* (of ORS and rarely T wave).
ECHO	Small pericardial effusion common.	Thickened pericardium, normal size RV and LV, normal function, large atria, restricted filling of RV and LV with >25% respiratory variation.	Diastolic collapse RA -> RV > LA ± LV, ↑ TV flow + ↓ MV flow during inspiration.
		NB. Key features to distinguish *constrictive pericarditis* from *restrictive cardiomyopathy*: (i) *absence of LVH, MR/TR and conduction abnormalities in constrictive pericarditis.* (ii) *absence of calcification in restrictive cardiomyopathy.*	

continued

Table 13.46 *continued*

	Pericarditis	Constrictive pericarditis	Pericardial effusion ± cardiac tamponade
Cardiac catheterisation	Not indicated	'Square root' sign in RV ± LV pressure trace, LVEDP + RVEDP ~ equal. Constrictive pericardium limits effects of inspiration on RV/LV.	RA pressure elevated, RV mid-diastolic pressure = RA pressure. Interventricular dependence (i.e. ↑ RV SV –> ↓ LV SV).
Other	*Bloods:* elevated WCC, CRP, ESR & troponin (40% of patients) ± ANA, RF, complement (if autoimmune), ± urea (if ESRF), ± HIV ±. *Pericardial fluid:* AFB, cytology.	*Cardiac CT and cardiac MRI: to look for* evidence of myocardial atrophy and fibrosis, respectively (both adverse prognostic signs).	*Fluid: protein, LDH, glucose, cell count, PCR (e.g. TB), tumour markers (e.g. CEA, CYFRA 21-1), cultures, acid fast bacilli.*
Disease classification	*Acute:* resolves in <2–3 weeks. *Recurrent:* ≥1 repeated episodes (includes intermittent and incessant). *Chronic:* pain ± fever >3 months.	Multiple pathoanatomical forms of constrictive pericarditis (versus restrictive cardiomyopathy): *annular form (AV grooves), left* or *right* sided, *global* ± pericardial fibrosis.	*Onset:* Acute (<1/52), (subacute (1-12/52). Chronic (>12/52). Size (mm): mild<10, mod 10-20, severe >20. *Distribution:* circumferential versus loculated.
Prognosis	Good, unless poor prognostic indicators: *fever* < 38°C, subacute onset, low *BP*, immunosuppressed, effusion >2 cm, myopericarditis, JVP elevated, history anticoagulants.	Poor, unless indication for surgery noted early (long-term survival similar to general population). Prognosis considerably worse in presence of myocardial fibrosis or atrophy or adhesions.	Small effusions: depends on aetiology; large effusions and tamponade: poorer prognosis. Poor prognositc indicators: aortic dissection, coagulopathy/anticoagulants, platelets < 50.
Complications	Tamponade (in 15% idiopathic, but 40% of bacterical, TB or neoplastic). Constrictive pericarditis.	Acute peri-operative cardiac insufficiency and ventricular wall rupture.	Large effusions: 33% chance of tamponade. Chronic effusions may cause constrictive pericarditis.
Management	Treat cause and hospitalise if poor prognostic signs/ non-idiopathic. High dose: aspirin/ NSAIDs 1–2/52 (use aspirin post-AMI) ± colchicine: recurrent or pain >2/52 0.5 mg BD for 3–6 months (side effects: GI upset, neutropenia) ± steroids if pain despite above 0.5 mg/kg/day for 2–4/52.	Pericardectomy (unless extensive myocardial fibrosis/ atrophy, severe disease + NYHA IV). Mortality 6–12% in patients suitable for surgery. Symptomatic management (diuretics, digoxin, β-blockers) for congestion or arrhythmias, pre-operatively. Cardiac CT used prior to surgery to detect myocardial fibrosis or atrophy pre-op.	Treat specific cause (60% associated with known disease), but when cause unclear: trial aspirin/NSAIDs 1–2 weeks (± colchicine ± steroids [if recurrent/ prolonged]) (until <30 mL/ 24 hours). Consider pericardial window or pericardectomy if recurrent.

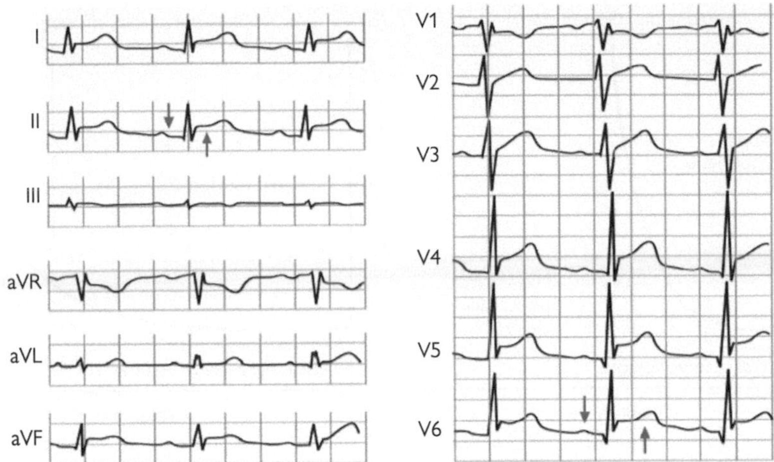

Figure 13.20 Typical ECG changes in acute pericarditis: PR depression, concave ST-segment elevation.

Reproduced with permission from *The ESC Textbook of Cardiovascular Medicine*, 1st edn. Camm AJ (Eds.). Oxford: Wiley. Copyright © 2006 European Society of Cardiology.

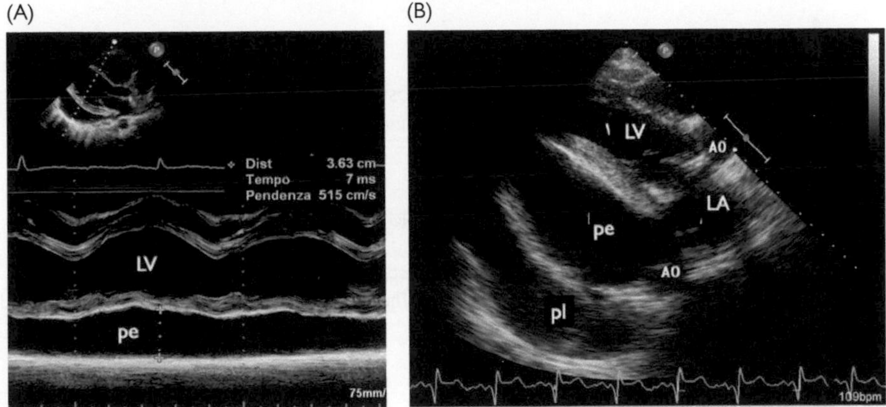

Figure 13.21 Semiquantitative assessment of pericardial effusion size: visualized in M-mode (A) and 2D (B) trans-thoracic echocardiography.

Abbreviations: LV, left ventricle; pe, pericardial effusion; pl, pleural effusion; Ao, aorta; LA, left atrium).

Reproduced with permission from Imazio M, Adler Y. Management of pericardial effusion. *Eur Heart J*. 2012; 34(16):1186–97, by permission of European Society of Cardiology and Oxford University Press. Copyright © 2012, European Society of Cardiology. https://doi.org/10.1093/eurheartj/ehs372.

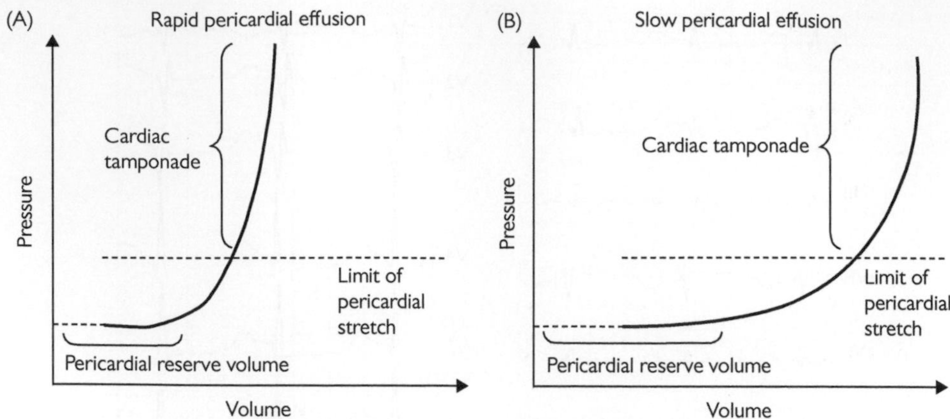

Figure 13.22 Pressure/volume curve of the pericardium with fast-accumulating pericardial fluid leading to cardiac tamponade with a smaller volume (A) compared with the slowly accumulating pericardial fluid reaching cardiac tamponade only after larger volumes (B).

Emerging therapies

1. Pericarditis: IVIG and interleukin-1B antagonists of possible benefit in refractory cases.
2. Pericardial effusion: intrapericardial therapies (triamcinolone) to reduce steroid usage.

Evidence-based clinical guidelines and references

1. Imazio M, Brucato A, Cemin R, et al. A randomized trial on colchicine for acute pericarditis. *N Engl J Med*. 2013;369:1522–8.
2. Imazio M, Adler Y. Management of pericardial effusion. *Eur Hosp J*. 2013;34:1186–97.
3. Maisch, B, Soler-Soler J, Hatle L, Ristic A. Pericardial diseases. *The ESC Textbook of Cardiovascular Medicine*, 2nd edn, 2009. Oxford: Oxford University Press.

Arrhythmias

Relevant anatomy and pathophysiology

- SA node to AV node to bundle of His to bundle branches (right and left, left divides: anterior and posterior fascicles).
- Conduction system innervated by parasympathetic and sympathetic nervous system at all levels: parasympathetic tone slows SA node automaticity and slows AV nodal conduction, sympathetic tone the opposite.
- Damage to the myocardium or autonomic nerves (e.g. local or CNS ischaemia, infarction, infection, infiltration or degeneration) can result in any cardiac arrhythmia.
- The RCA supplies the SA node, and in ~ 90% of cases the AV node.

Definition, clinical features and aetiologies

- Bradycardia: <60 bpm (but resting HR 50–59 often considered normal).
- Sinus arrhythmia is normal and reflects intact vagal tone.
- If stroke volume maintained despite profound bradycardia patients may be asymptomatic.
- Syncope (usually requires pause >6 seconds), presyncope and light headedness can all occur.

For causes of bradycardia, see Table 13.47.

Table 13.47 Causes of bradycardia

Intrinsic (local) causes of bradycardia	Extrinsic causes of bradycardia
Idiopathic degeneration (ageing)	Increased vagal tone (acute): vasovagal syncope, carotid sinus hypersensitivity.
Infiltrative diseases: sarcoidosis, amyloidosis, haemochromatosis	Increased vagal tone (chronic): exercise training.
Infectious diseases: endocarditis, Gram-negative sepsis, typhoid fever, diphtheria	Electrolyte imbalance: hypokalaemia, hyperkalaemia, hyponatraemia.
Collagen vascular disease (auto-immune inflammation): SLE, RA, scleroderma	Metabolic disorders: hypothyroidism, hypothermia, obstructive sleep apnoea.
Inherited diseases: myotonic dystrophy, SA and AV nodal disease	Neurological disorders: raised intracranial pressure, CNS tumours/infection/infiltration.
Trauma: valve replacement	Drugs (negatively chronotropic ± bathmotropic [degree of excitability]): clonidine, lithium, amiodarone, propafenone, cocaine (overdose), β-blockers, calcium channel blockers, digoxin.

Disease classification system of bradycardias

- Sinus node dysfunction (sick sinus syndrome):
  - Includes abnormal SA nodal and atrial conduction, and tachycardia-bradycardia syndrome (Figure 13.23A and B(i)).
  - Associated atrial fibrillation or flutter and thromboemboli.
- AV conduction dysfunction (can cause mortality due to SCD [prolonged ventricular standstill or bradycardia-induced ventricular tachyarrhythmias]):
  - First degree AV block (PR interval > 200 ms).
  - Second degree AV block: mobitz type I and II. Atrial rhythm partially conducted to ventricles (Figure 13.23). Mobitz I rarely leads to syncope. Mobitz II has much higher risk of third degree AV block (complete heart block [CHB]).
  - CHB: complete dissociation of P and QRS complexes. Higher risk of ventricular standstill with infra-nodal disease (broad QRS).
- Interventricular block (i.e. bundle branch block) causes broad QRS:
  - Right bundle branch block (RBBB): rSR' pattern in V1 and qRs pattern in V6.
  - LBBB: rS pattern in V1 and RsR' pattern in V6.
  - RBBB leads to *inter*-ventricular dyssynchrony. LBBB leads to *inter*-ventricular dyssynchrony (with dysfunction of both fascicles) or *intra*-ventricular dyssynchrony (if only left anterior or left posterior hemifascicle affected).
  - Left anterior hemiblock: left axis deviation, rS pattern inferior leads.
  - Left posterior hemiblock: right axis deviation, tall R wave in inferior leads.
- Bifascicular block: RBBB and either left anterior or left posterior hemiblock (therefore two fascicles); LBBB (due to involvement of both fascicles).
- Trifascicular block: first degree heart block and RBBB, and either left anterior or left posterior hemiblock.

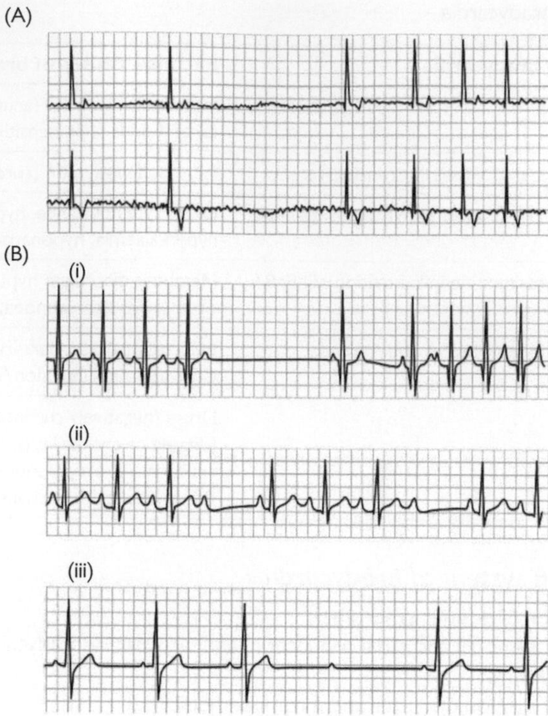

Figure 13.23 (A) Tachycardia-bradycardia syndrome. (B) (i) Sinus arrest; (ii) Mobitz type I: gradually increasing PR until non-conducted P wave; (iii) Mobitz type II: abrupt conduction failure of p waves.

Diagnosis, prognosis and management

- Look for adverse features: chest pain, shortness of breath at rest, systolic BP < 90 mmHg, depressed consciousness.
- Investigate with:
  - *ECG.*
  - *Ambulatory ECG*: intermittent bradycardia.
  - *Echocardiography*: for structural heart disease.
  - *Exercise testing*: for chronotropic response if chronotropic incompetence suspected.
- Annual mortality of acquired, untreated CHB is 15%. Poor prognostic features: increasing age (especially >80 years), structural heart disease, AV block post *anterior* MI.
- Management (if stroke volume maintained treatment may not be necessary):
  - IV atropine ± isoprenaline if symptomatic.
  - Treat reversible causes (e.g. metabolic abnormality or stop offending drug).
  - Consider pacemaker insertion.

For indications for pacing, see Box 13.3.

Pacemakers

- Terminology: four letters in order (e.g. DDDR):
  - 1st – chamber paced (ventricle [V], atria [A], dual [D])
  - 2nd – chamber sensed (V, A, D).
  - 3rd – response to sensing (inhibitory [I], trigger [T], dual: triggering and inhibition [D]).
  - 4th – rate response (enables HR increase with exercise).

Box 13.3 Indications for temporary and permanent pacing

Indications for pacing

- Sinus node disease (e.g. chronotropic incompetence):
  - When symptoms clearly linked to bradycardia.
- Acquired AV block:
  - Mobitz type II second degree AV block and CHB even if asymptomatic.
  - Mobitz type I second degree AV block if symptoms.
  - First degree AV block if PR interval 300 ms and significant symptoms. Post-AV node ablation (e.g. atrial fibrillation with poor rate control).
- Congenital AV block (even if asymptomatic if satisfy following):
  - Second or third degree AV block and wide QRS or rate <50 bpm or pauses.
- Neurocardiogenic syncope:
  - ➲ See Syncope and sudden cardiac death, p. 473.
- Overdrive pacing for artial tachyarrhythmias (e.g atrial fibrillation):
  - No longer a stand-alone indication for pacing.
- Left ventricular outflow tract obstruction (e.g. HCM):
  - If contraindication to alcohol septal ablation and no indication for ICD.
- Acquired long QT syndrome:
  - Temporary pacing only, e.g. secondary to amiodarone overdose.

- Pacemakers selection: DDDR unless:
  - Permanent atrial fibrillation – VVIR.
  - Pure sinus node dysfunction: AAIR or DDDR.
  - EF<35%: CRT-P or CRT-D (➲ see Cardiac resynchronisation therapy, p. 456, Tables 13.41 and 13.43 and Figures 13.16–13.18).

Supraventricular tachycardias

Definition, clinical features and aetiology

- Tachycardia: HR > 100 bpm, and SVT with narrow QRS duration unless BBB (permanent or rate-related) or accessory pathway.
- Paroxsymal (sudden onset) or persistent.
- Asymptomatic, or palpitations, chest pain, dyspnoea, anxiety, dizziness, syncope or polyuria.

For tachyarrhythmia predisposition/precipitation, see Box 13.4.

Box 13.4 Tachyarrhythmia predisposition/precipitation

Predisposing or precipitating factors inducing tachyarrhythmias

- Non-cardiac causes:
  - Stress: exercise stress, mental stress, anxiety, lack of sleep.
  - Stimulants: alcohol, caffeine (e.g. coffee, energy drinks), nicotine.
  - Drugs: antibiotics, anti-arrhythmics, antidepressants.
  - Systemic causes: fever, infection, anaemia, electroyte disturbances (low K^+ or Mg^{2+}), hyperthyroidism, premenstruation, menstruation.
- Cardiac causes:
  - Myocardial fibrosis: previous myocardial infarction, other (e.g. sarcoidosis, HCM).
  - Inherited:
    - ➲ see SCD, p. 475 and Box 13.7
    - Congenital: WPW type A and type B, congenital heart disease.
    - Other: cardiomyopathy, valvular heart disease, accessory pathways.

Disease classification system of supraventricular tachycardias

- *Sinus tachycardia*: either physiological or inappropriate (excess sympathetic/reduced parasympathetic tone). Consider β-blockers, diltiazem/verapamil/ivabradine to rate control if inappropriate.
- *Postural orthostatic tachycardia syndrome (POTS)*: persistent postural sinus tachycardia within 10 minutes of standing, without postural hypotension or autonomic neuropathy. Management:
  - Encourage high salt diet, fluids, compression stockings.
  - Consider β-blockers, fludrocortisone, midodrine.
- *Atrial and AV junctional extrasystoles* (or atrial premature beats [APB]): common, especially > 50 years, due to increased automaticity. Management:
  - Avoid stimulants.
  - Consider β-blockers (± class I anti-arrhythmics).
- *Sinus node re-entry tachycardia*: re-entrant circuits involving SA node, usually triggered and terminated by APB. P wave identical to sinus. Rare. Management: adenosine/vagal maneouvres acutely, β-blockers if recurrent.
- *Atrial tachycardia* (AT: differentiated from atrial flutter by isoelectric baseline between P waves): atrial depolarisation with rates 110–300 bpm. Can be focal (small area responsible, like SA node), multi-focal (rare: usually elderly patients with COPD). Management: as for atrial flutter, except in elderly patients with COPD and multi-focal AT: consider amiodarone ± diltiazem.
- *Atrial flutter/macro re-entrant atrial tachycardia* (atrial rate 240–350 bpm (unless diseased atria or on drugs, e.g. flecainide [190–220 bpm]), absence of isoelectric baseline between P waves): rare < 50 years, increased in COPD, pneumonia, heart failure. Most common form (85%) involves the cavo-tricuspid isthmus (CTI). In mitral valve disease much more likely to be LA related. AV conduction can be 1:1, 2:1 or variable (depending on drugs, rate, AV node). Management:
  - Rate control: if asymptomatic (diltiazem, β-blockers, verapamil).
  - Cardioversion (anticoagulate for ≥3 weeks, unless episode <48 hours): DC-cardioversion or class III antiarrhythmics (ibutilide and amiodarone superior to class Ic).
  - Drug therapy for prevention; Class 1c drugs e.g. flecainide which has no AV nodal slowing, so risk of 1:1 AV conduction which is potentially fatal. Flecainide should, therefore, be prescribed with AV nodal blocking agents in addition.
  - Catheter ablation: treatment of choice if CTI atrial flutter. Anticoagulate as CHA_2DS_2VASC score as persistent AF risk even post-ablation.
- *Atrial fibrillation*: multiple random atrial impulses, driven by pulmonary vein atrial ectopy. Atrial remodelling increases atria instability, reducing the chance of restoring normal sinus rhythm (NSR).
  - Incidence 1–2%.
  - Paroxsymal, persistent (>7 days, but 'cardiovertable') or permanent (>7 days + NSR not possible).
  - All forms associated with a 5-fold increase risk of stroke.

For causes of atrial fibrillation and flutter, see Box 13.5, and for risk scores, see Table 13.48.

Box 13.5 Causes of atrial fibrillation and flutter

Causes of atrial fibrillation/flutter

- Valvular heart disease: Especially mitral stenosis, also mitral regurgitation (both dilate left atrium).
- Non-valvular heart disease: IHD, HTN, myocarditis, pericarditis, cardiomyopathy, WPW, dilated left atrium.
- Lung disease: Pulmonary emboli, lung malignancy, COPD, severe pneumonia.
- Other: Thyrotoxicosis, alcohol abuse, cocaine abuse, caffeine excess.

  - Management:
    - Thromboembolic risk assessment.
    - Reversal of cause.
    - Rate control ± rhythm control.

Table 13.48 Risk scores in atrial fibrillation and flutter

CHA_2DS_2 VASC score (risk of stroke)	HASBLED score (risk of bleeding)
Congestive heart failure	**H**ypertension
Hypertension	**A**bnormal renal/liver function
Age ≥ 75 years	Previous **S**troke
Diabetes	**B**leeding (previous major bleed)
Previous **S**troke/TIA/ systemic emboli	**L**abile INR (time in therapeutic range <60%)
Vascular disease*	**E**lderly (> 65 years)
Age 65–74 years	**D**rugs (e.g. antiplatelets/NSAIDs)/alcohol
Sex **C**ategory (female = 1)	
Explanation Each of above scores 1 or 2	Explanation Each of above scores 1
Implication Higher score = increase risk stroke score ≥ 2 = lifelong anticoagulation	Implication Score > 2 indicates need for caution (but does NOT = contraindication to anticoagulation)

NB. Annual stroke risk: CHA_2DS_2VASC score of *2 = 2.2%, 4 = 4%, 6 = 10%, 9 = 15%*. Female sex only scores 1 when combined with another risk. Score ≥2 indicates requirement for lifelong anticoagulation (warfarin or new oral anticoagulants [NOACs]: dabigatran, rivaroxaban, apixaban). *Aspirin is no longer considered appropriate* as an alternative. NOACs (approved for *non-valvular AF*): as effective as warfarin, no monitoring needed. Lower risk of CNS haemorrhage.

* Vascular disease defined by any of: significant coronary artery disease, peripheral artery disease or aortic plaque.

- Rate control: first line therapy if: elderly, contraindications to cardioversion or asymptomatic. β-blockers, verapamil, diltiazem; digoxin second-line. AV node ablation and pacemaker if rate or rhythm control fails.
- Rhythm control (acute) (in younger, symptomatic patients):
  - If 'adverse features' perform DC cardioversion (DCCV).
  - If onset AF ≥ 48 hours anticoagulate (≥3 weeks)/exclude left atrial thrombus (TOE) pre-cardioversion.
  - Use DCCV as most effective.
  - Medical cardioversion possible: flecainide, propafenone, ibutilide or vernakalant *if no evidence of structural heart disease*, amiodarone if present.
  - Post-cardioversion anticoagulate ≥ 4 weeks or lifelong if CHA_2DS_2VASC score ≥2.
- Rhythm control (chronic):
  - Regular flecainide, propafenone, sotalol, dronedarone, amiodarone or consider catheter ablation.

- *Atrioventricular node re-entry tachycardia (AVNRT):* Most common SVT, more in females, normal heart.
  - AV nodal conduction has two pathways: one fast and one slow with different properties.
  - AVNRT is a circuit rhythm using one pathway anterogradely and the other retrogradely.
  - Management:
    - Acute: vagal manoeuvres, carotid sinus massage, adenosine, β-blockers/verapamil.
    - Chronic: ablation, or any anti-arrhythmic drug.

- *Atrioventricular re-entry tachycardia (AVRT)*: due to extra-nodal accessory pathways (AP):
  - WPW syndrome, congenital, prevalence 0.1–1%.
  - Diagnosis of WPW is *only* when:
    - pre-excitation in NSR (when AV conduction occurs anterogradely through AP *and* AVN) *and*
    - tachyarrhythmias (AVRT/AF) occur.
  - Two types (subclassified by location of AP): type A (left-sided pathway) and type B (right-sided).
  - WPW with AF may degenerate into VF and requires urgent DCCV.
  - WPW associations: Ebstein's anomaly, HCM, mitral valve prolapse.
  - Management for arrhythmias (asymptomatic pre-excitation does not mandate treatment):
    - Slow AVN conduction: *AVN blockers are contraindicated* in WPW because if AF occurs they may increase pathway conduction and VF.
    - Slow AP conduction: class 1a, 1c or class 3 drugs (see Figure 13.5). Consider ablation.

  The mechanism of AVRT versus AVNRT is shown in Figure 13.24.

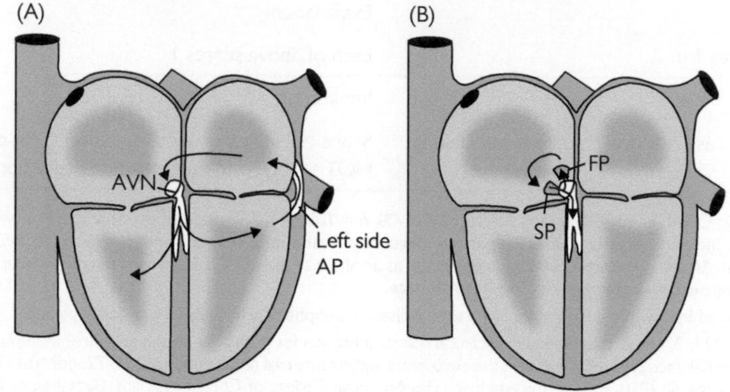

Figure 13.24 Mechanism of AVRT versus AVNRT. (A) Orthodromic AVRT via a left-sided AP. Activation from atria (A) to ventricle (V) is down the AVN, then across V and back from V to A up the AP, completing the circuit. (B) Typical AVNRT activates from A to AVN via the slow pathway (SP) and from the AVN to A via fast pathway (FP), thus completing the circuit.

Diagnosis

- Look for adverse features: chest pain, shortness of breath at rest, systolic BP <90 mmHg, depressed consciousness.
- *ECG*: obtain traces during the episode and at rest (may show pre-excitation):
  - Identification of two consecutive P waves within R-R cycle suggests AT.
  - AVNRT (typical): retrograde P waves hidden at end of QRS, difficult to see.
  - Pre-excitation: short PR interval, wide QRS with slurred upstroke (delta wave).
  - Type A WPW (left-sided pathway): upright/postive delta wave in V1 (negative if type B).
  - Orthodromic AVRT: narrow QRS with retrograde P waves, often seen in the ST segment.
  - Antidromic AVRT: wide QRS with either RBBB (type A) or LBBB (type B).
  - WPW with AF: broad QRS, irregular, varying QRS morphology, ventricular rate up to 250–300 bpm.
- *ECHO:* exclude structural heart disease.
- *Electrophysiology (EP) studies*: To define ± ablate the pathway (with cauterisation or cryotherapy); used to risk stratify WPW patients.

Prognosis and general management

- Normal life expectancy unless:
  - In WPW, if SVT degenerates into AF and subsequently VF.
  - Systemic embolism (e.g. stroke with AF).
  - Persistent SVT results in LV failure.
- Management:
  - Adverse features – immediate DCCV.
  - No adverse features:
    - Regular narrow QRS tachycardia – vagal manoeuvres, carotid sinus massage, adenosine (NB. adenosine has no effect on macro re-entrant AT).
    - Other – ➲ see Acute coronary syndromes, p. 425.
  - Lifestyle measures: avoid tobacco, caffeine, alcohol.
  - Radiofrequency catheter ablation (RFCA) success rates: ~ 95% AVNRT and AVRT, typical atrial flutter, >90% focal AT, 60–80% atypical atrial flutter, 57–87% AF (AF free at 1 year).

Ventricular tachycardias

Definition, clinical features, aetiology and disease classification system

- QRS broad, 100–300 bpm. Aetiology of broad complex tachycardia is VT in 80%.
- Symptoms depend on ventricular rate (e.g. >190 bpm resulting in presyncope or syncope) and duration (e.g. persistent VT can lead to pulmonary congestion).
- VT is:
  - Sustained or non-sustained (NSVT: ≥3 beats, but <30 seconds duration).
  - Polymorphic or monomorphic.
- Polymorphic VT (Figure 13. 25a): beat to beat morphology variation, with progressive cyclical changes. Torsades de pointes is polymorphic VT caused by prolonged QT.
- Monomorphic VT (Figure 13.25b): morphology is constant for a given ECG lead:
  - Majority are re-entrant, originating from border zone of scarred myocardium.
  - Minority are driven by hypoxaemia, electrolyte distrubance or ischaemia/infarction.

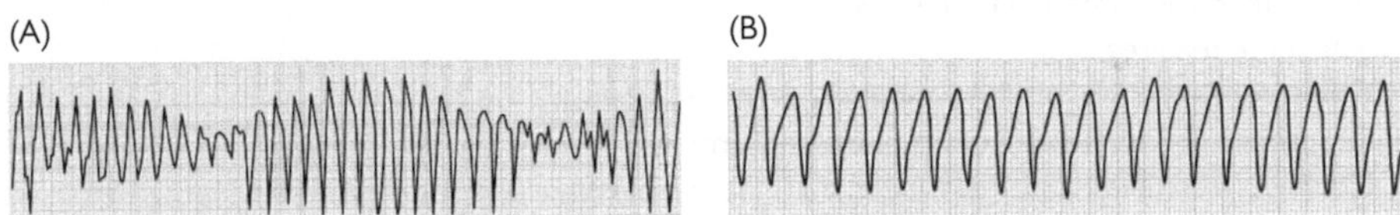

Figure 13.25 (A) Polymorphic VT . (B) Monomorphic VT .

Reproduced with permission from Cardiovascular medicine. In *Oxford Handbook of Clinical Medicine*, 10th edn. Wilkinson IB, et al. (Eds). Oxford: OUP. Copyright © 2017, Oxford University Press. DOI: 10.1093/med/9780199689903.001.0001. Reproduced with permission of the Licensor through PLSclear.

Diagnosis

- Look for adverse features (same as for supraventricular tachycardia [SVT]).
- *ECG*:
  - The following features favour VT over SVT with aberrancy:
    - extreme QRS axis: –90 to ± 180°;
    - QRS >140 ms;
    - altered QRS from NSR;
    - dissociated P waves;
    - concordance of precordial leads (either negative or positive);
    - capture beats (see Figure 13.26A);
    - fusion beats (see Figure 13.26B).

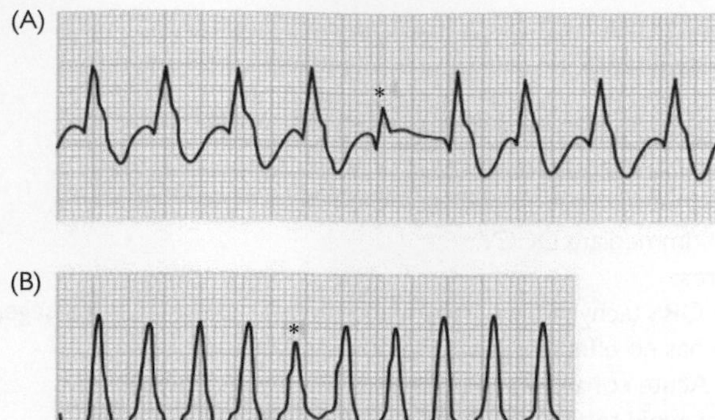

Figure 13.26 (A) Capture beat. (B) Fusion beat.

Reproduced with permission from Cardiovascular medicine. In *Oxford Handbook of Clinical Medicine*, 10th edn. Wilkinson IB, et al. (Eds). Oxford: OUP. Copyright © 2017, Oxford University Press. DOI: 10.1093/med/9780199689903.001.0001. Reproduced with permission of the Licensor through PLSclear.

- ◆ Determine origin of VT:
  - ▪ LBBB-type pattern = LV septum or right ventricular outflow tract;
  - ▪ RBBB-type pattern = LV origin.
- *Ambulatory ECG monitoring*: to correlate with intermittent symptoms.
- *Echocardiography*: to assess cardiac function.
- *Electrophysiology studies*: to prove the daignosis if uncertain or during VT ablation.

Prognosis and management

- Polymorphic VT and V rate >220 bpm have high chance to progress to VF.
- VT is major cause of mortality in patients with structural heart disease.
- Management:
  - ◆ Adverse features – immediate DCCV.
  - ◆ No adverse features:
    - ▪ Chemical cardioversion (e.g. amiodarone or llidocaine).
    - ▪ Suppress VT with β-blockers ± additional anti-arrhythmics.
    - ▪ Correct reversible cause (e.g. electrolyte abnormalities, reperfusion if AMI).
  - ◆ If polymorphic VT: give $MgSO_4$, IV β-blockers ± overdrive pacing/isoprenaline (to increase HR and shorten QT interval). Class I and III anti-arrhythmics are *contraindicated*.
  - ◆ Long-term:
    - ▪ Implantation of an ICD.
    - ▪ Consider ablation if drug resistant.

Drug-induced VT

- Tricyclic antidepressant (TAD) overdose: epileptic seizures and VT, also dilated pupils and urinary retention. Management: IV sodium carbonate (correct hypoxia and acidosis), avoid class 1 anti-arrhythmics.
- Lithium overdose: epileptic seizures and VT, also myoclonic jerks. Management: haemodialysis.
- Digoxin toxicity: nausea, visual disturbances and hyperkalaemia. Management: digoxin-specific Fab antibody and reversal of hyperkalaemia.
- Cocaine: present with:
  - ◆ VT: treat with IV sodium chloride.
  - ◆ Coronary spasm ± rupture: treat with GTN ± reperfusion.

Complications

- Pacemakers:
  - Early: tamponade, pneumothorax, haematoma, infection, lead malposition.
  - Late: infection, lead malposition, lead fracture.
- Anti-arrhythmic drugs:
  - Arrhythmias.
  - QT prolongation (class 1: procainamide, flecainide, llidocaine, quinidine; class III: amiodarone, sotalol, dofetilide, ibutilide).
- Ablation: radiation injury, haematoma, AV fistula, thromboembolism, tamponade, AVN block. AF ablation specific: atrioesophageal fistula, PV stenosis, phrenic nerve injury.

Clinical guidelines and references

1. Kappenberger L, Linde C, Toff WD. Bradycardia. *The ESC Textbook of Cardiovascular Medicine*, 2nd edn, 2009. Oxford: Oxford University Press.
2. Farre J, Wellens HJ, Cabrera JA, Blomstrom-Lundqvist. Supraventricular tachycardia. *The ESC Textbook of Cardiovascular Medicine*, 2nd edn, 2009. Oxford: Oxford University Press.
3. Priori SG, Blomström-Lundqvist C, Mazzanti A *et al*. 2015 ESC Guidelines for the management of patients with ventricular arrhythmias and the prevention of sudden cardiac death: The Task Force for the Management of Patients with Ventricular Arrhythmias and the Prevention of Sudden Cardiac Death of the European Society of Cardiology (ESC), *European Heart Journal*, 2015: 36(41);2793–2867. https://doi.org/10.1093/eurheartj/ehv316

Syncope and sudden cardiac death

Syncope

Transient loss of consciousness (T-LOC) due to global cerebral hypoperfusion, from a drop in cardiac output or total peripheral vascular resistance. (In normals when systolic ≤60 mmHg).

Pathogenesis, clinical features and epidemiology

- Syncope characterised by:
  - rapid onset;
  - short duration (usually <1 minute);
  - spontaneous rapid and complete recovery (retrograde amnesia possible).
- NB. Seizures: shorter aura (3–30 seconds), longer duration/recovery, and skin colour may turn red or blue during LOC.

Syncope and seizures can cause urinary incontinence, tongue biting and limb jerks.

- Bimodal distribution of presentation:
  - Young patients: reflex syncope is most common cause.
  - Patients over 65 years: cardiac and orthostatic causes are most common.
- Incidence of syncope in elderly: 0.5%, 60–69 years; 1–2%, 70–79 years. Epileptic seizures in similar age uncommon: <1%.

Disease classification system of syncope

- Neurogenic syncope ('reflex syncope' – transient, vasodilation ± bradycardia):
  - Vasovagal: mediated by orthostatic/emotional stress, e.g. fear, pain.
  - Situational: cough, sneeze, post-micturition, post-exercise, post-prandial.
  - Carotid sinus syncope (triggered by manipulation of carotid sinuses, e.g. shaving).
  - Atypical (without a clear trigger).
- Orthostatic hypotension (common in elderly: peripheral vasocontriction is either deficient [primary autonomic failure] or insufficient [in response to hypovolaemia]):
  - Primary autonomic failure (e.g. Parkinson's Plus, multiple system atrophy [MSA]).
  - Secondary autonomic failure (e.g. diabetes, uraemia, spinal cord injury).
  - Volume depletion: diarrhoea, vomiting, haemorrhage.
  - Drug-induced: diuretics, vasodilators, alcohol, antidepressants, phenothiazines.

- Cardiac disease:
  - Brady/tachyarrhythmias.
  - Structural heart disease: aortic stenosis, HCM, cardiac masses, cardiac tamponade, pulmonary embolus, acute aortic dissection or MI, congenital anomalies of coronary arteries.

Diagnosis

- History of episode:
  - Details of onset, duration and recovery, witnesses.
  - Ascertain high risk features:
    - Syncope on exertion/whilst supine.
    - Known structural heart disease.
    - Palpitations with syncope.
    - Family history of SCD under 40.
    - Palpitations, breathlessness or chest discomfort on exertion.
- Lying/standing BP (may be negative in delayed orthostatic hypotension: perform tilt test).
- *ECG:* may show unifying diagnosis or high risk features:
  - Features of higher grade AV block:
    - *Mobitz type II AV block.*
    - Bifascicular block (RBBB & left axis deviation or LBBB).
    - Symptomatic sinus bradycardia (<50 bpm).
    - Sinus pauses ≥3 seconds.
  - Previous myocardial infarction.
  - Long (or short) QT syndrome: inherited or secondary to drugs (Box 13.6).
  - Brugada syndrome (➲ see Channelopathies, p. 476 and Figure 13.27).
  - Negative T waves in V1–3: suggestive of arrhythmogenic right ventricular dysplasia.
  - Accessory pathway: pre-excitation (short PR, delta waves).
  - Broad QRS: suggestive of ventricular arrhythmias.
- *ECHO:* for evidence of structural heart disease.
- *Carotid sinus massage* (if over 60 years; pressure applied over common carotid bifurcation for 5 seconds): positive test if symptoms occur with asystole ≥3s, AV block or a fall in systolic BP fall ≥50 mmHg.
- *Ambulatory ECG monitoring* (➲ see Prolonged electrocardiogram monitoring, p. 417): Holter (continuous) monitoring if frequency >1 per week, otherwise loop recorder monitoring (external versus implantable [can remain in situ for 3 years]).
- *Tilt table testing*: to precipitate neurogenic syncope if potential cause.
- *Exercise testing*: if syncope associated with exertion.

Box 13.6 Acquired causes of long QT syndrome

- Electrolyte disturbances:
  - hypokalaemia, hypomagnesaemia, hypocalcaemia.
- Drugs:
  - Class I (flecainide) and III (amiodarone) anti-arrhythmic drugs. Tricyclic anti-depressants and neuroleptic agents.
  - Erythromycin and ketoconazole.
  - Some anti-histamines.
- Cardiovascular diseases:
  - Mitral valve prolapse, myocardial infarction, Sick sinus syndrome, complete heart block.
- Other:
  - Subarachnoid haemorrhage, liquid protein diet.

NB. Normal range 380–440 ms, but varies with age, gender and HR.

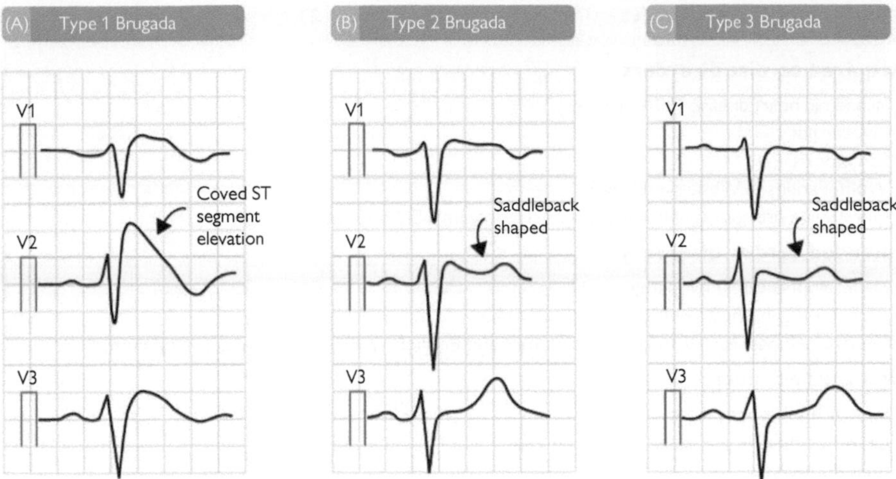

Figure 13.27 Brugada syndrome ECGs. Type 1 is only pattern diagnostic of the disease, with highest risk of SCD. ECG changes may be provoked by an ajmaline challenge.
Reproduced with permission from Clinical ECG Interpretation (2019), Araz Rawshani (www.ecgwaves.com).

Prognosis and management

Key treatment goals: (i) prolong survival; (ii) prevent recurrences; (iii) improve quality of life.

- Good prognosis: neurogenic syncope, young age, normal ECG, reversible orthostatic hypotension.
- Poor prognosis: structural heart disease, arrhythmias, exertional syncope, family history of SCD.

Neurogenic syncope and orthostatic hypotension

- Lifestyle measures: avoid triggers (e.g. hot crowded environment, volume depletion), manoeuvres to abort syncope (e.g. lying supine, leg crossing and handgrip to cause peripheral vasoconstriction).
- Drugs (better evidence for orthostatic hypotension): midodrine (α-agonist), fludrocortisone.
- Permanent pacemaker: generally if > 40 years with syncope, documented bradycardia and all else failed.

Cardiac syncope

Treat specific cause – ➲ see Arrhythmias, p. 464 and Ventricular tachycardias, p. 471): Indication for:

- Permanent pacemaker: for symptomatic bradycardia.
- ICD: for symptomatic VT in structural heart disease (Table 13.44; [2]). Other ICD indications:
    - Primary prevention: prior myocardial infarction (>4 weeks ago) with *either* LVEF < 35% *or* DCM with EF <35% or a cardiac condition with high risk of SCD.
    - Secondary prevention:
        - post-cardiac arrest due to VT/VF;
        - sustained syncopal VT;
        - sustained VT without syncope or cardiac arrest, but LVEF <35%.

Sudden cardiac death

- SCD, likely from fatal cardiac arrhythmias, is the most common cause of sudden adult death syndrome.
- 500 cases per year; ECG may be diagnostic.
- First degree relatives of sudden adult death syndrome victim should be screened in a specialist clnic.
- Most cases, however, relate to ischaemic and other structural heart disease.

For causes of sudden cardiac death, see Box 13.7.

Box 13.7 Causes of sudden cardiac death

Acquired cardiac disorders

- Ischaemic heart disease (80% of cases).
- Myocarditis.
- Sarcoidosis.
- Wolff–Parkinson White syndrome.
- Mitral valve prolapse (controversial: association with SCD on autopsies).

Inherited cardiac disorders

- Hypertrophic cardiomyopathy.
- Arrhythmogenic right ventricular cardiomyopathy.
- Ion channelopathies: e.g. long QT syndromes and Brugada syndrome, coronary artery anomalies.

Non-cardiac causes

- Subarachnoid haemorrhage.
- Drug overdose (e.g. cocaine, amphetamines).
- Rhabdomyolysis.
- Commotio cordis (sudden trauma to chest).
- Heatstroke (e.g. marathon runners).

Channelopathies

- Brugada syndrome:
  - Mutations to sodium ion channel SCN5A in many.
  - Autosomal dominant.
  - Prevalence 0.15%, males >> females, more common in Far East Asia.
  - Fatal cardiac arrhythmias mostly *during sleep* and in males.
  - Diagnostic criteria: ECG pattern (Figure 13.27) and one of:
    - Documented VF.
    - Self-terminating polymorphic VT.
    - Family history of SCD < 45 years.
    - Syncope.
    - Nocturnal agonal respiration.
  - Management: ICD implantation if VT/ VF or unexplained syncope.
- Inherited/idiopathic long QT syndrome:
  - Defect within transmembrane ion channels cause repolarisation abnormalities.
  - Both potassium (KVLQT1: chromosome 11 [*LQT1*] and HERG gene: chromosome 7 [*LQT2*]) and sodium (SCN5A: chromosome 3 [*LQT3*]) transport channel proteins.
  - Autosomal dominant (Romano–Ward syndrome), autosomal recessive (Jarvell–Lange–Neilsen syndrome rarer, with associated congenital nerve deafness) forms.
  - Prevalence approximately 1:2500, long QT diagnosed on ECG/genetics.
  - LQT2 and LQT3 have a higher risk of cardiac arrest than other types.
  - Fatal cardiac arrhythmias in situations with *increased sympathetic activity* (physical exertion, emotion, sudden loud noises).
  - Management: β-blockers ± ICD.
  - Isoprenaline is contra-indicated in *inherited* LQTS, useful in *acquired* LQTS.
- Catecholaminergic polymorphic ventricular tachycardia (CPVT):
  - Mutation with cardiac ryanodine receptor (or rarely calsequestrin).
  - Autosomal dominant in 60%, prevalence 1:10,000.
  - Diagnosed on treadmill testing or catecholamine provocation.
  - Fatal cardiac arrhythmias in situations with *increased sympathetic activity*.
  - Management: β-blockers ± ICD implantation ± cervical sympathectomy.

Cardiomyopathies

➲ See Myocardial disease, p. 445, Tables 13.25–13.35 and Figures 13.13 and 13.14.

- HCM:
  - Management: β-blockers ± ICD implantation if ≥2 risk factors for SCD.
- Arrhythmogenic right ventricular cardiomyopathy/dysplasia (ARVD):
  - Management: β-blockers ± amiodarone ± ICD implantation if (syncope or VT despite Rx).

Clinical guidelines and references

1. Brignole M, Moya A, de Lange FK, et al. 2018 ESC Guidelines for the diagnosis and management of syncope. *European Heart Journal*, 2018: 39(21);1883–1948. https://doi.org/10.1093/eurheartj/ehy037.
2. NICE. Implantable cardioverter defibrillators for arrhythmias, 2006. NICE guideline TA95. https://www.nice.org.uk/Guidance/TA95.
3. Priori SG, Wilde AA, Horie M. HRS/EHRA/APHRS Expert consensus statement on the diagnosis and management of patients with inherited primary arrhythmia syndromes. *Heart Rhythm*. 2013; 10(12):1932–63.

Thromboembolic disease

➲ See Chapter 11, Thromboembolic disease and pulmonary hypertension, p. 365 and Tables 11.4 and 11.5.

Aortic disease

See Table 13.49.

Cardiac tumours

Cardiac tumours are rare. Most are secondary, and are malignant. Most (90%) primary cardiac tumours are benign. The majority of malignant tumours are sarcomas and lymphomas. Secondary, metastatic tumours of the heart mostly arise from carcinomas of the liver, kidney, lung and breast.

For adult cardiac tumours, see Table 13.50.

Presentation

- Constitutional symptoms: non-specific flu-like illness.
- Obstruction: e.g. shortness of breath (SOB)/syncope.
- Embolism: stroke/other organ ischaemia.

Imaging and tissue diagnosis

- Imaging:
  - Echocardiography provides the best combination of spatial and temporal resolution. It is also the cheapest and most accessible imaging modality.
  - CMR and, to a lesser extent, cardiac CT offer superior tissue characterisation.
- Tissue diagnosis: not routinely required prior to surgical excision of a symptomatic tumour. Right-sided masses can be biopsied more easily.

Treatment

- Surgery: optimal if no metastasis.
- Radiotherapy: with primary cardiac sarcomas neo-adjuvant radiotherapy improves the success of resection and adjuvant radiotherapy reduces recurrence.
- Chemotherapy: many effective anthracycline agents (e.g. doxorubicin and epirubicin) are cardiotoxic. Nevertheless, treatment of primary cardiac lymphoma with chemotherapy is unique among the primary cardiac malignancies in carrying a reasonable prognosis.

Table 13.49 Aortic pathology

Aortic disease	Thoracic aortic aneurysm		Acute aortic syndromes		
Definition	Pathological dilation of the aorta between the aortic valve and the diaphragm.		Acute aortic dissection	Intramural haematoma (IMH)	Deep penetrating ulcer (DPU)
			The entry of blood from a 'true' lumen to a 'false' lumen via an intimal tear.	An ectopic collection of blood within the aortic wall in the absence of an intimal tear.	The erosion into, or through, the aortic wall of an atherosclerotic plaque.
Aetiology	Atherosclerotic risk factors.[1]		All risk factors for aortic aneurysm are also risk factors for dissection.	Believed to be secondary to a bleed of the *vasa vasorum*.	Advanced atheromatous disease, likely to represent the 'early phase' of IMH.
	Cystic medial degeneration: *loss of smooth muscle cells, fibrosis and elastic fibre degeneration*		Deceleration trauma, e.g. road traffic collision or fall from height. Iatrogenic e.g. catheter manipulation during angiography (coronary ± aortic dissection possible).		
		Bicuspid aortic valve.[2]			
		Marfan's syndrome.			
		Ehler–Danlos syndrome.			
		Loeys–Dietz.			
		Pseudoxanthoma elasticum.			
	Aortitis – inflammatory pathology	Infectious: syphilis, bacteria, fungal.			
		Non-infectious: atherosclerosis, rheumatoid arthritis, seronegative arthropathy, Wegener's disease, Takayasu arteritis, giant cell arteritis, Kawasaki's disease.			
Frequency and classification	Much less common than AAA. Incidence 10 per 100,000 patient years.		Rare: incidence ~3 per 100,000 patient years.	Very rare, often considered a 'precursor' to acute aortic dissection.	Seen in advanced atheromatous disease, usually in elderly 'vasculopaths'.
	Ascending aorta	60%	Classification (Stanford)[3]		
	Aortic arch	10%	A Involves ascending aorta.		
			B Origin distal to left subclavian artery.		
	Descending thoracic aorta	20%	0.5% of presentations of acute chest or back pain.		
	Thoraco-abdominal (crosses diaphragm)	10%			

Presentation Clinical features	Variable presentation, often asymptomatic (incidental imaging finding). Occasionally pain: ischaemia (of branch vessels, including coronaries) or from compression effect (chest, back or limb). Rarely hoarseness from compression of recurrent laryngeal nerve.		Pain (95% of patients) of which 85% is abrupt in onset, radiating to the central chest or back and ~50% is 'tearing' in nature. Painless in 5% of cases. Symptoms relating to hypoperfusion of aortic branches (MI, stroke, limb ischaemia, renal failure/oliguria) or with aortic regurgitation (20–50%). Loss of pulses (20%) is an indicator of poor progosis	
Diagnosis and investigations	Radiological investigations include CXR, CT and CMR: ➲ See Chapter 5, Case 6, p. 126.		CXR: widened mediastinum. ECG: ST or T wave changes (55% patients).	
Complications	Continued dilatation of aneurysm. Aortic rupture (risk rising abruptly at 6 cm). Aortic regurgitation (secondary to root dilatation).		Aortic rupture. Aortic regurgitation. Cardiac tamponade. 'Malperfusion': MI, stroke, renal failure, acute limb ischaemia, bowel infarction.	Rupture. Dissection. Aneurysmal dilatation.
Management	Management vascular risk factors (including hypertension). Annual serial imaging follow-up with the same modality (CMR or contrast CT).		Immediate diagnostic imaging and monitor in critical care. BP control: opiates and IV β-blockers (Target: <110 mmHg systolic).	Management vascular risk factors (including hypertension).
Medical				
Surgical	Indications for open surgical root replacement[4]		Type A: cardiopulmonary bypass and surgery to surgically reconstruct ascending aorta (with either native valve preserved or aortic valve replacement). Type B: onservative treatment (BP management). Complicated Type B: endovascular stenting is superior to open surgery.	Width >2 cm or depth >1 cm: intervention may be considered (high risk of rupture). Endovascular stenting or open surgical repair.
	Tricuspid (normal) aortic valve	≥ 5.5 cm		
	Bicuspid	≥ 5.0 cm		
	Marfan syndrome	≥ 4.5 cm		

[1]The aorta ages throughout life. Ageing involves both lumen dilatation and increased wall stiffness, with increased pulse wave velocity and impaired perfusion distally, especially during diastole. The rate of ageing is proportional to conventional vascular risk and is faster in men (median age thoracic aortic aneurysm in men 65 years; women 77 years).
[2]Bicuspid aortic valve. Aortic dissection is 10 times more likely in patients with bicuspid, than in normal tricuspid aortic valves. In patients undergoing aortic root replacement for aneurysmal dilatation, cystic medial degeneration was detected in 75% of BAV patients (14% of cases with tricuspid valves).
[3]Classification of aortic dissection is prognostically important as Standford Type A dissection (ascending aorta) carries >50% mortality within 30 days (even with full medical therapy) and therefore mandates early surgical intervention. Type B dissection has a 10% 30-day mortality and can often be managed with medical therapy and possible endovascular repair (EVAR – stenting). See Chapter 5, Case 6, p. 126.
[4]European Society of Cardiology '2014 ESC Guidelines on the diagnosis and treatment of aortic diseases'.

Table 13.50 Adult cardiac tumours

Tumour classification				Frequency	Location	Notes
Non-neoplastic mass	Mural thrombi (clot adherent to the wall)			Common.	Left atrial appendage	In AF and with regional wall motion abnormality.
					LV apex Endocardium overlying region of infarction Within aneurysm	Common post-infarction. Inflamed endocardium. Sluggish atrial flow in the absence of atrial systole. Left atrial appendage clot is common.
	'Vegetation' of fibrin and pathogenic organisms			Quite common.	Valve leaflets	(➔ See Infective endocarditis, p. 441, Tables 13.22–13.24 and Box 13.2.)
	Lipomatous hypertrophy of atrial septum			Quite common.	Inter-atrial septum	The extension into the atrial septum of epicardial fat. Seen in elderly obese patients.
Benign neoplasm	Cardiac myxoma			Rare, <0.05% in autopsy series.	80% LA, 18% RA, 2% RV, <1% LV	Can present at any age, peak in 6th decade. Female:male preponderance 2:1. Most are sporadic, ~7% are part of an autosomal dominant familial syndrome: the Carney complex (recurrent cardiac myxomas, skin hyperpigmentation and multiple endocrine neoplasms).
Malignant neoplasm	Primary	Sarcomas	Angiosarcoma. Leiomyosarcoma. Fibrosarcoma. Osteosarcoma. Rhabdomyosarcoma.	Very rare <0.005% in autopsy series.		May be surgically resected, usually in association with neo-adjuvant and adjuvant radiotherapy. Treatment of lymphoma by chemotherapy has a better prognosis.
		Lymphoma				
	Secondary metastatic	Carcinoma	Lung. Breast. Hepatocellular carcinoma. Renal cell carcinoma.	20 times more common than primary cardiac tumours. ~1% in autopsy series.	Commonly by direct invasion, frequently involving pericardium.	Often complicated by effusion.
		Sarcoma				
		Melanoma				

Congenital heart disease

Epidemiology, aetiology and associations

- The rate of congenital cardiac abnormalities in live births is 0.8%.
- 250,000 adults in the UK have congenital cardiac disease.
- Bicuspid aortic valve constitutes a *further* 0.5–1% of the population (~600,000).
- Over the last 70 years, prognosis has improved dramatically.
- Cardiac intervention has improved:
    - Higher rates of definitive primary corrective surgery and fewer palliative procedures.
    - Shift towards 'structural intervention' catheter-based techniques.
- Imaging (ECHO and CMR) has revolutionised diagnosis and treatment.
- Prior to intervention: mortality in infancy >85%.
- Since intervention: survival to adulthood >85%.
- The number of adults with congenital cardiac disease now exceeds the number of children.

For risk factors for congenital cardiac abnormalities, see Table 13.51, and for chromosomal and other genetic abnormalities associated with cardiac abnormalities, see Table 13.52.

Pathological patterns in congenital cardiac disease: non-cyanotic and cyanotic

Non-cyanotic congenital heart disease

Left to right shunts: usually result from anatomical defects with higher left-sided pressures (the commonest congential lesions):

- VSD (32% of cardiac abnormalities).
- ASD (8%).
- PDA (7%).
- Anomalous pulmonary venous drainage (1%).

Table 13.51 Risk factors for congenital cardiac abnormalities

Risk factor	Associated cardiac abnormality	Notes
Maternal rubella during pregnancy	Patent ductus arteriosus (PDA). Pulmonary stenosis.	Congenital rubella syndrome. (Triad: deafness, cataract and cardiac abnormalities.) Much less frequent since vaccination (MMR).
Alcohol	Ventricular septal defect (VSD). Atrial septal defect (ASD).	
Maternal age	The risk of chromosomal abnormalities increases with age.	
Maternal diabetes	Double outlet right ventricle. Truncus arteriosus (an undivided artery arising from both ventricles). Transposition of the great arteries VSD. Hypoplastic left heart syndrome.	Congenital cardiac abnormality rate is up to 8.5% of live births (>10 times non-diabetic rate). Multifactorial pathophysiology.
Prescription drugs	E.g. NSAIDs have been implicated in risk of septal and arterial defects. (A link between lithium and Ebstein's anomaly has not been borne out in most studies.)	Teratogens should be given to women of childbearing age only with advice on risks and contraception.

Table 13.52 Chromosomal and other genetic abnormalities associated with cardiac abnormalities

Risk Factor	Associated cardiac abnormality		Notes
Trisomy 21 *Down* syndrome	Atrioventricular septal defect (AVSD): ASD. VSD. PDA. Tetralogy of Fallot.		~50% of Down syndrome babies have a significant cardiac abnormality. AVSD is often associated with a single, trileaflet atrioventricular valve, which may be regurgitant.
XO *Turner* syndrome	Bicuspid aortic valve (30%). Coarctation of aorta (10–12%). AS. Hypoplastic left heart syndrome. Partial anomalous pulmonary venous drainage drainage (≥1 pulmonary vein[s] draining from lung to right atrium).		Turner syndrome is consequently frequently associated with some left ventricle outflow obstruction. (➲ See Chapter 5, Case 5, p. 124.)
Trisomy 18 *Edwards* syndrome	VSD, ASD and PDA.		
Trisomy 13 *Patau* syndrome	VSD, ASD and dextrocardia.		
Microdeletion Chromosome 7 *Williams* syndrome	Supravalvular AS.		Elfin facies. 'Cocktail party' disposition (voluble, gregarious manner).
Microdeletion Chromosome 22 *DiGeorge* syndrome	Associated with disorders of the arterial trunk: Tetralogy of Fallot. Truncus arteriosus. Interrupted aortic arch. VSD.		Interrupted aortic arch behaves like a 'completed' form of coarctation. 15% of patients with Tetralogy of Fallot are found to have DiGeorge syndrome.
Noonan syndrome AD mutation in RAS-MAPK genes	Pulmonary stenosis (~55%). HCM (up to 35%). ASD (up to 25%). VSD (up to 20%).		Flat nasal bridge. Webbed neck. Kyphoscoliosis. Short stature. Learning disability (~25%).
Marfan syndrome AD (FBN-1 gene, Chromosome 15)	Aortic root dilatation	Aortic aneurysm and dissection risk. Aortic regurgitation.	Fibrillin mutation leads to cystic medial degeneration of aorta.
	Mitral valve prolapse.		
Holt–Oram syndrome *TBX5* gene mutation	ASD. First degree heart block.		Triphalangeal thumb, polydactyly, absent radius in forearms.

Left to right shunts and Eisenmenger's syndrome

The pathological significance of a left to right shunt is determined by the relative flow rate across the shunt in proportion to the final forward flow rate in the aorta. A high shunt fraction (e.g. pulmonary flow [Qp]/ systemic flow [Qs] >2.0) leads to increased blood flow and shear stress in the lungs and a reactive pulmonary hypertension. Pulmonary hypertension causes secondary right ventricular hypertrophy and raised right-sided pressures. This may result in shunt reversal (right to left flow) termed Eisenmenger's syndrome, causing cyanosis and associated with reduced life-expectancy. Once shunt reversal has occurred then the shunt cannot be closed due to the likelihood of acute right ventricular failure, i.e. the RV is unable to pump its full stroke volume against the excessive pulmonary pressures.

Left-sided obstruction

- Subvalvular stenosis: fibromuscular membrane arising from ventricular septum; surgically resectable, but has a high risk of recurrence.
- Aortic stenosis (4% of cardiac abnormalities).
- Supravalvular stenosis (as seen in Williams syndrome).
- Coarctation of the aorta (5% of cardiac abnormalities).
- Interrupted aortic arch.

Cyanotic congenital heart disease

Cyanosis results when overall oxygenation is so poor that circulating deoxygenated blood >5 g/dL.

- Cyanotic cardiac conditions include:
  - Pulmonary stenosis (with right to left shunting) (7% of cardiac abnormalities).
  - Tetralogy of Fallot (5%):
    - RV outflow tract obstruction;
    - consequent right ventricular hypertrophy;
    - VSD;
    - 'Overriding aorta': the aorta is above VSD (receives blood from LV and RV).
  - Transposition of the great arteries (4%).
  - Truncus arteriosus (1%): common arterial trunk (receives and mixes deoxygenated and oxygenated blood).
  - Single ventricle (free mixing of deoxygenated and oxygenated blood).

Complications of cynanosis result from a combination of chronic hypoxaemia and secondary erythrocytosis:

- Increased red cell turnover, consequent iron deficiency.
- Hyperviscosity with risk of stroke, thromboembolism and thrombocytopenia.
- Increased urate and risk of renal stones.
- Clubbing and acne.
- Risk of cerebral abcesses.

For locations of ASDs and VSDs, see Figure 13.28. For a clinical summary of VSD, ASD and tetralogy of Fallot, see Table 13.53.

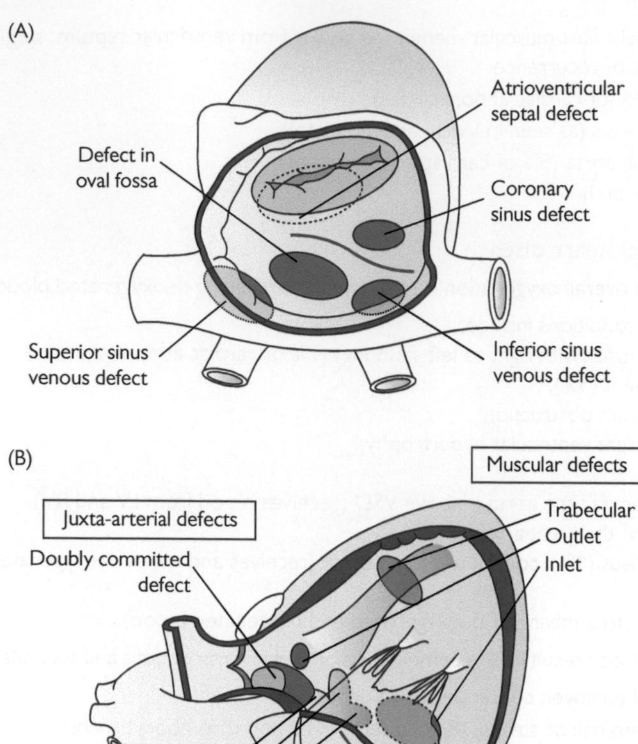

Figure 13.28 Locations of (A) ASDs and (B) VSDs.

Table 13.53 Clinical summary of VSD; ASD and Tetralogy of Fallot (ToF)

Abnormality	Signs	Heart sounds	Murmur	ECG	CXR	Natural history	Treatment
VSD (large)	Thrusting apex (volume overloaded)	Single S2 (loud P2)	Systolic murmur left sternal edge[1]	LV hypertrophy (± RV hypertrophy)	Cardiomegaly. Prominent pulmonary arteries	Progress to pulmonary hypertension and shunt reversal (Eisenmenger's)	Surgical closure or catheter device closure (if VSD in muscular septum)
ASD secundum	RV heave	Fixed splitting of S2	ESM pulmonary	RAD[2], RV hypertrophy and partial RBBB	Mild cardiomegly. Prominent pulmonary arteries	Atrial arrhythmias/ RV failure or signs of pulmonary HTN occur in adulthood. Paradoxical emboli may be the first presentation	Transcatheter device closure is treatment of choice. In the few cases where this is not possible: traditional surgical closure
Tetralogy of Fallot	Clubbing Cyanosis RV heave	Single S2	ESM pulmonary	Sinus, RAD and RV hypertrophy. RBBB following surgical correction	Pulmonary oligaemia. Right-sided arch (25%)	Right ventricular outflow obstruction worsens and R to L shunting increases: cyanosis	Ideally primary repair: closure of VSD and transannular patch enlargement of RVOT. May require initial shunt[3]

[1]A small VSD may result in a loud murmur, as the large pressure difference across a small defect creates a high velocity, turbulent jet.
[2]ASD primum defects (also known as atroventricular septal defect [AVSD]) usually have a significant VSD component. Consequently there is volume overload of the LV and usually *left*, rather than right, axis deviation.
[3]The first shunt to deliver blood into the pulmonary artery, distal to RV outflow tract obstruction/pulmonary atresia was the Blalock–Taussig shunt. This shunt directs blood from the subclavian to the ipsilateral pulmonary artery.

Multiple choice questions

Questions

1. A 65-year-old gentleman presents with meticillin-sensitive *Staphylococcus aureus* (MSSA) prosthetic valve endocarditis 6 months post-mitral valve replacement. Which of the following is the best treatment option?
   A. Complete a 4-week course of vancomycin, rifampicin and gentamicin.
   B. Complete a 6-week course of vancomycin and rifampicin, and discontinue gentamicin after 2 weeks.
   C. Complete at least a 6-week course of flucloxacillin and rifampicin, and discontinue gentamicin after 2 weeks.
   D. Perform a redo mitral valve replacement (MVR) and complete at least a 6-week course of flucloxacillin and rifampicin, and discontinue gentamicin after 2 weeks, timed from the commencement of antibiotics.
   E. Perform a redo MVR and complete at least a 6-week course of flucloxacillin and rifampicin, and discontinue gentamicin after 2 weeks, timed from the date of surgery.

2. A 27-year-old woman, who is 34 weeks into a pregnancy complicated by severe hypertension, presents to the Emergency Department with central 'tearing' chest pain, ischaemic ECG and a weak left radial pulse. Her CXR is unremarkable, other than a slightly widened mediastinal contour. You suspect acute aortic dissection. What imaging strategy will you select?
   A. Immediate transfer to the catheter laboratory for an emergency angiogram.
   B. Transthoracic ECHO by the cardiology registrar who has confirmed he can probably be there within the next hour.
   C. Contrast-enhanced CT aorta.
   D. Cardiac MRI scan in a cancelled slot the same afternoon.
   E. No imaging. Thrombolyse immediately and emergency transfer to cardiothoracic centre.

3. A right-heart catheterisation is performed on a 15-year-old girl with exertional dyspnoea (Table 13.54). What is the correct diagnosis?
   Investigations:
   A. Patent ductus arteriosus.
   B. Ventricular septal defect.
   C. Pulmonary embolus.
   D. Atrial septal defect.
   E. Tetralogy of Fallot.

Table 13.54

Chamber	Pressure (mmHg)	Oxygen saturation (%)
RV	24(sys) 8(diast)	72
PA	35(sys) 14(diast)	90
LV	120(sys) 12(diast)	94
Aorta	100(sys) 60(diast)	94

4. An ECG is shown, which displays QT prolongation, U waves and tall P waves. What is the diagnosis?
   A. Hyperkalaemia.
   B. Hypokalaemia.
   C. Hypercalcaemia.
   D. Hypocalcaemia.
   E. Hypothermia.

5. A 76-year-old man, with no previous medical history is admitted following an episode of syncope after climbing some stairs. When he is examined by the medical doctor in the medical admissions unit, the doctor correctly ascertains that he has clinically severe aortic stenosis. Which of the following is not a marker of severe aortic stenosis on clinical examination?
   A. Slow rising pulse.
   B. Late peaking carotid pulse.
   C. Long ejection systolic murmur.
   D. Loud ejection systolic murmur, which radiates to the carotids.
   E. Signs of left heart failure.

6. Which of the following is not seen in acute rheumatic fever, complicating Group A beta-haemolytic streptococcal pharyngitis?
   A. Migratory polyarthritis.
   B. An apical mid-diastolic murmur.
   C. Chorea.
   D. Prolonged PR interval on ECG.
   E. Vasculitic rash over the buttocks and backs of the legs.

7. Which of the following is not a recognised risk factor for sudden cardiac death in hypertrophic cardiomyopathy (HCM)?
   A. Reduced ejection fraction.
   B. Failure to raise the systolic blood pressure by ≥25 mmHg on exercise testing.
   C. Family history of sudden cardiac death in a first degree relative below the age of 45 years.
   D. Unexplained syncope.
   E. Septal thickness greater than 30 mm.

8. You see a 65-year-old man in clinic. He has a history of myocardial infarction (2 years ago) and moderate systolic heart failure on ECHO. He is NYHA III. He has a third heart sound and bibasal end-inspiratory crepitations. His HR is 61 bpm and BP of 128/86 mmHg. His current medication is aspirin 75 mg, ramipril 10 mg, bisoprolol 5 mg and furosemide 80 mg all once a day (OD). His potassium is 4.7 mM and his renal and liver function are normal. What is the most important adjustment to his medication?
   A. Increase bisoprolol to 7.5 mg OD.
   B. Divide furosemide to be taken 40 mg twice daily (BD).
   C. Increase ramipril to 12.5 mg OD.
   D. Add in spironolactone 25 mg OD.
   E. Add in atorvastatin 10 mg OD.

9. A 35-year-old gentleman presents with sudden syncope while seated. His younger brother passed away suddenly 5 years ago aged 25, although he says he is unclear regarding the cause. His ECG shows downsloping ST-segment elevation in leads V1–3. Which of the following is most correct?
   A. He has a diagnosis of hypertrophic cardiomyopathy and should have an ICD implanted.
   B. He has a diagnosis of Brugada syndrome, and should start β-blockers and consider having an ICD implanted.
   C. He has a diagnosis of catecholaminergic polymorphic ventricular tachycardia and should start β-blockers.
   D. He has a diagnosis of Brugada syndrome, which affects sodium channels and causes myocardial disarray.
   E. He has a diagnosis of Brugada syndrome and should consider having an ICD implanted.

10. A 68-year-old woman presents with a 5-week history of weight loss, fever and muscle aches. On physical examination she has a mid-diastolic murmur at the apex and an echocardiogram reveals a mobile, well-circumscribed mass arising in the left atrium, from the atrial septum. The most likely diagnosis is:
   A. Mitral stenosis.
   B. Infective endocarditis of the mitral valve.
   C. Mitral valve prolapse.
   D. Myxomatous degeneration of the mitral valve.
   E. Left atrial myxoma.

Answers

1. D. This patient has PVE with a known pathogen of MSSA. Trans-oesophageal echocardiography is the first line imaging investigation in PVE (where available). PVE secondary to staphylococci is a class IIa indication for surgery according to the ESC. Flucloxacillin should be given instead of vancomycin given that the patient grew MSSA, and antimicrobial treatment should be given for at least 6 weeks (except gentamicin, which is stopped after 2 weeks). This is timed from the commencement of appropriate antibiotics, unless staphylococci is grown on tissue culture post surgery. (➲ See Management, p. 444 and Tables 13.23 and 13.24.)
2. C. The endocrine milieu of late gestation softens connective tissue and is a risk factor for dissection, as is hypertension. It is right to consider acute dissection in this patient. CXR is normal in ~40% of cases. Acute coronary syndrome (the commonest cardiovascular cause of death in pregnancy) remains a possibility. Dissection should be ruled out before urgent coronary angiography. Contrast CT aortogram is the correct choice for both sensitivity and speed. (➲ See Imaging, Aorta, p. 418 and Table 13.2.)
3. A. PDAs demonstrate a L → R shunt, with a step up in pressure and saturations in the PA (as in this patient). VSDs demonstrate a step-up in pressure and saturations in the RV. ASDs demonstrate a step up in saturations in the low RA (primum defects) or mid ± high RA (secundum defects). Tetralogy of Fallot demonstrate aortic saturations lower than LV saturations due to overriding aorta. (➲ See Invasive cardiology, Haemodynamic measurements, Cases, p. 422.)
4. B. Hypokalaemia – tall P waves, flat/inverted T waves ± ST depression, tall U waves, prolonged PR interval, long QT interval, ± broad QRS. Hypothermia – Osborne J waves, transient Q waves. Hyperkalaemia – absent P waves, tall T waves, broad QRS → sinusoidal QRS (pre-arrest). Hypocalcaemia – long QT interval. Hypercalcaemia – short QT interval. (➲ See Metabolic electrocardiogram abnormalities, p. 417.)
5. D. Neither the amplitude, nor the radiation of the systolic murmur is a marker of severity in aortic stenosis. (➲ See Table 13.19.)

6. E. Answer E. A vasculitic rash on the buttocks and backs of the legs is typical of Henoch–Schonlein purpura, a vasculitis with skin, intestine and renal involvement caused by IgA and C3 deposition. The features described in options A–D are all listed in the criteria for the diagnosis of acute rheumatic fever. (➲ See Table 13.20.)
7. A. Patients with HCM typically have normal or raised ejection fraction. The features described in B–E are all used in the stratification of the risk of sudden death in HCM. (➲ See Table 13.28.)
8. D. This man's HR is well controlled so there is no indication for increasing bisoprolol. Furosemide has no mortality benefit and he does not have symptomatic peripheral oedema. He is on the maximum dose of ACEi (ramipril 10 mg OD). Spironolactone is indicated and has a mortality benefit (RALES trial, N Engl J Med 1999). Statin treatment is also indicated and atorvastatin should be started at 40 mg and titrated up to 80 mg OD. (➲ See Heart failure, Treatment, p. 455, and Tables 13.39, 13.41, 13.42 and 13.45.)
9. E. He has diagnostic criteria for Brugada syndrome (with type 1 ECG pattern: worst prognosis) with two high risk features of SCD (FHx SCD <45 years and syncope). He therefore meets criteria to be considered for ICD implantation (class IIa recommendation HRUK): EP testing may be considered to assess risk of degeneration into VT/VF alongside ambulatory monitoring. There is no proven role for β-blockers in Brugada syndrome; quinidine (inhibits outward sodium channels and stabilises action potential) and isoprenaline (increases intracellular calcium and stabilises action potential) do have a role. Myocardial disarray is noted in hypertrophic cardiomyopathy. (➲ See Channelopathies, p. 476 and Hypertrophic cardiomyopathy, p. 445.)
10. E. Systemic viral-prodrome symptoms are consistent with atrial myxoma and with infective endocarditis. The diagnosis is clinched by a combination of the specific clinical findings of mitral valve obstruction (mid diastolic murmur) and a well-circumscribed mass that arises not from the mitral valve but from the left atrium and the inter-atrial septum. This is typical (80% of myxomas) of the location of a myxoma. (➲ See Cardiac tumours, p. 477, and Table 13.50.)

Chapter 14 **Gastroenterology**

Danny Cheriyan, Charlotte Ford and Stephen Patchett

Investigation of gastrointestinal disease

Oesophagogastroduodenoscopy procedure

- Oesophagogastroduodenoscopy or gastroscopy is a procedure to examine the oesophagus, stomach and duodenum with a thin, flexible endoscope passed via the mouth.
- It typically involves the administration of a local anaesthetic spray into the pharynx or an IV sedative such as midazolam.
- Patients fast for 6 hours prior to the procedure and, if given sedation, should not drive or operate machinery for 24 hours.

Indications

- Diagnostic: heartburn, dyspepsia, dysphagia, weight loss and the investigation of anaemia.
- Acute upper GI bleed: diagnostic and to assess the need for therapeutic intervention (e.g. treatment of actively bleeding duodenal ulcer).
- Therapeutic: foreign body retrieval, dilatation of peptic strictures and stent placement, e.g. for oesophageal malignancy or duodenal obstruction.
- More recent therapeutic advances include radiofrequency ablation (RFA) and endoscopic mucosal resection of Barrett's oesophagus with dysplasia.

Risks

- Sore throat, bleeding, perforation.

Colonoscopy and flexible sigmoidoscopy procedures

Colonoscopy

- Colonoscopy is examination from rectum to caecum with a flexible endoscope passed per rectum.
- It also allows examination of the terminal ileum; important if inflammatory bowel disease is suspected.
- Patients are given full bowel preparation (sodium picosulfate or polyethylene glycol) the day prior to the procedure.
- Colonoscopy usually requires sedation (e.g. IV midazolam) and an opiate (e.g. pethidine or fentanyl).

Flexible sigmoidoscopy

- Sigmoidoscopy is a limited examination of the rectum and sigmoid colon and offers the advantage of a shortened procedure time using little or no sedation.
- There is usually no requirement for large volumes of oral laxatives; a phosphate enema is given to prepare the bowel beforehand.

Indications

- Colonoscopy is indicated in the investigation of diarrhoea, bleeding per rectum, altered bowel habit and iron deficiency anaemia.
- Flexible sigmoidoscopy is used for assessment of acute colitis and for investigation of fresh anorectal bleeding.
- Both colonoscopy and flexible sigmoidoscopy are useful as valuable tools in bowel cancer screening and prevention.

Risks

- Discomfort, bleeding and perforation.
- Though complications are rare, therapeutic procedures such as polypectomy confer added risk.

Endoscopic retrograde cholangiopancreatography procedure

- An advanced endoscopic procedure, which involves the passage of an endoscope via the mouth to the second part of the duodenum.
- Uses a side-viewing scope to facilitate access to the biliary tree or pancreas via the ampulla of Vater.

Indications

- Assessment and treatment of biliary or pancreatic duct obstruction (stones, strictures).
- Acute cholangitis.

Risks

- Approximately 5% risk of pancreatitis.
- Perforation (rare), bleeding (rarely significant).
- Bleeding (rarely significant).

Endoscopic ultrasound procedure

- Endoscopic ultrasound utilises a specialised endoscope with an in-built ultrasound probe to assess pathology within and around the GI tract.

Indications

- Assessment and diagnosis of pancreatic pathology (e.g. suspected pancreatic malignancy or cystic disease), biliary disease, submucosal lesions of upper GI tract and staging of oesophagogastric and rectal malignancy.
- Tissue sampling via fine needle aspiration.
- Therapeutic procedures such as pancreatic cyst drainage.

Oesophageal manometry and pH monitoring

- Oesophageal manometry involves the passage of a thin, pressure sensitive catheter to the lower oesophagus to assess the function of the upper and lower oesophageal sphincter (LOS) and assess oesophageal motility. The normal LOS tone is between 10–30 mmHg.

Indications

- Investigation of dysphagia and non-cardiac chest pain.
- Diagnosis and ongoing assessment of patients with gastroesophageal reflux disease (GORD).

- Preoperative evaluation of patients with GORD in whom fundoplication or alternative surgery is being considered, to select patients likely to benefit.

Video capsule endoscopy

- Involves the patient swallowing a small capsule containing cameras, a light emitting diode and radiofrequency transmitter.
- Images are recorded and transmitted to a device worn around the patient's waist for subsequent evaluation.

Indications

- Video capsule endoscopy (VCE) is used to assess the small bowel for occult GI bleeding and has diagnostic value in inflammatory bowel conditions and small bowel malignancy.
- Advantages are that it is minimally invasive and usually well tolerated.
- At present, it remains a diagnostic test and thus further invasive enteroscopy may be required to confirm a diagnosis histologically or treat pathology.

Risks

- Overall the test is very safe, although a tight stricture anywhere within the GI tract could result in capsule retention or bowel obstruction.

Oral disease

Apthous ulcers

- Aphthous ulcers are painful, round, shallow oral lesions.
- Recurrent aphthous ulceration is the most common cause of non-infective mouth ulceration and is more frequent in children and adolescents than adults.
- Outbreaks tend to be self-limiting.
- The majority of apthous ulcers have no associated systemic disease.
- Associations are recognised with inflammatory bowel disease (IBD), coeliac disease, immunodeficiency and autoimmune conditions (e.g. Behçet's disease and SLE).

Malignant lesions

- Ulcers or lesions in the mouth that do not heal, particularly involving the tongue or lips may be malignant and these require referral (to maxillofacial or plastic surgery units, or oral medicine departments).
- Smoking and alcohol excess increase risk of malignant lesions.
- Many patients have nodal disease at presentation.

Infections of the mouth

Oral candidiasis is a common fungal infection seen in young infants, adults with dentures, diabetics, immunocompromised individuals or patients taking antibiotics and inhaled steroids. Treatment options include oral nystatin suspension (if confined to the oral cavity) or oral fluconazole 50 mg daily (oropharyngeal candidiasis) for 7–14 days.

Common viral infections of the mouth include:

- Herpes simplex virus type 1.
- Coxsackie A virus.
- Herpes zoster.
- Oral manifestations of HIV infection.

Atrophic glossitis

- Inflammatory condition of the tongue with loss of filiform papillae.
- May occur in patients with iron, vitamin B_{12} or folate deficiency.
- The tongue appears smooth and 'glossy', patients may complain of burning with acidic food.

Oesophageal disease

Dysphagia

Dysphagia is the subjective sensation of difficulty in swallowing. Patients may present with difficulty swallowing solids, liquids or both. Typically, mechanical obstruction begins with initial dysphagia to solids and progresses to difficultly with liquids over time; motility disorders often result in dysphagia to both solids and liquids from the outset.

Dysphagia can be classified as:

- Oropharyngeal dysphagia: difficulty initiating swallow, which may be accompanied by coughing, choking, regurgitation or aspiration.
- Oesophageal dysphagia: a sensation of food getting stuck in the oesophagus several seconds after initiating a swallow.

Common causes of dysphagia are shown in Table 14.1.

Table 14.1 Common causes of dysphagia

Cause of dysphagia	Examples
Intrinsic lesion	Benign (peptic) stricture. Malignant stricture. Foreign body. Eosinophilic oesophagitis. Oesophageal ring or web. Zenker's diverticulum.
Extrinsic lesion	Enlarged left atrium in mitral valve disease. Mediastinal mass. Goitre.
Motility disorders	Achalasia. Diffuse oesophageal spasm. Systemic sclerosis.
Neuromuscular disorders	Bulbar palsy. Myasthenia gravis. Stroke. Parkinson's disease.

Investigation

- All patients with new onset dysphagia should be referred for urgent gastroscopy to be performed within 2 weeks.

Eosinophilic oesophagitis

- Eosinophilic oesophagitis (EoE) is a common cause of dysphagia particularly prevalent among adolescents and young adults (1).
- Chronic immune/antigen-mediated oesophageal disease characterised by symptoms related to oesophageal dysfunction and histologically eosinophilic predominant inflammation.
- Food impaction is common.
- Endoscopic features include linear furrowing, circular rings (trachealisation) and stricturing.

Pathogenesis

- Genetic and environmental factors along with adaptive T cell immunity play a role in recruitment of eosinophils and local inflammation.
- Patients often have a history of atopy (e.g. eczema, allergic rhinitis or asthma).

Diagnosis

- Mid-oesophageal biopsies in patients with suspected EoE.
- Biopsies demonstrating high numbers (at least 15 per high power field) of eosinophils in conjunction with a typical history and endoscopic findings are diagnostic.
- A key differential diagnosis is GORD, which may also cause eosinophilic recruitment in the oesophagus.

Management

- Initially acid suppression with proton pump inhibitors (in treatment naïve patients) followed by topical glucocorticoid therapy (e.g. swallowed fluticasone).
- Allergy testing is often advocated in EoE to determine foods that may present a risk for acute allergic reactions and identify EoE triggers.

Patients may present with oesophageal strictures which require therapeutic dilatation.

References

1. Prasad GA, Talley NJ, Romero Y, et al. Prevalence and predictive factors of eosinophilic esophagitis in patients presenting with dysphagia: a prospective study. *Am J Gastroenterol*. 2007;102(12):2627.

Achalasia

Achalasia is a disorder of unknown aetiology causing aperistalsis in the body of the oesophagus and impaired relaxation of the LOS. The pathogenesis is thought to be due to decreased ganglionic cells in the myenteric plexus and degeneration in the vagal fibres of the oesophagus with loss of inhibitory denervation of the LOS. Patients may present at any age with dysphagia to solids and liquids, regurgitation and chest pain.

Investigations

- Gastroscopy is often normal.
- Barium swallow can show oesophageal dilatation, diminished or asynchronous peristalsis, and a tapered distal oesophagus ('bird's beak deformity').
- Oesophageal manometry demonstrates aperistalsis in the distal two-thirds of the oesophagus and impaired relaxation of the LOS (pressure readings of >8 mmHg).

Management

Treatment options for confirmed achalasia depend on the severity of symptoms and patient suitability for intervention.

- *Endoscopic pneumatic dilatation* involves forceful disruption of the muscular fibres of the LOS using a balloon. It carries a significant risk of perforation (2–4%).
- *Laparoscopic myotomy (Heller's myotomy)* involves longitudinal surgical incision of the muscles of the LOS.
- *Peroral endoscopic myotomy (POEM)* is an endoscopic method for performing myotomy of the LOS.
- *Botulinum toxin injection* into the LOS can provide temporary symptomatic benefit (lasting ~6 months), thus requiring repeat procedures. It is generally reserved for patients who are poor surgical candidates.
- *Pharmacological therapy*, such as nitrates or short-acting calcium channel blockers are the least effective in treating achalasia. Their use is limited by side effects (such as headache and dizziness) with nitrates and tachyphylaxis (loss of response) with calcium channel blockers.

Diffuse oesophageal spasm

This is a severe, but rare form of oesophageal dysmotility that typically presents with chest pain and dysphagia in middle-aged patients.

Investigations

- Barium studies may show a 'corkscrew' appearance.
- Oesophageal manometry classically demonstrates >20% simultaneous contractions of the LOS of >30 mmHg amplitude.

Management

- Pharmacological agents including oral nitrates, calcium channel blockers and tricyclic antidepressant agents.

Oesophageal cancer

Historically, the majority of oesophageal cancers have been squamous in origin, but over recent decades there has been a dramatic increase in adenocarcinoma. It presents typically with dysphagia progressing from solids to liquids, with associated weight loss.

Squamous cell carcinoma

- Most frequently arises in the middle or proximal third of the oesophagus.
- Risk factors: smoking, alcohol, foods containing N-nitroso compounds (common in Asia), caustic injury, atrophic gastritis and previous gastrectomy.
- In high incidence areas there is no gender predominance; in low incidence areas the disease is more common in men.

Adenocarcinoma

- Arises from the columnar epithelium of the distal oesophagus usually from within Barrett's metaplasia in patients with long standing GORD.
- Additional risk factors include smoking, excessive alcohol consumption, obesity and male sex.

Investigations

- Gastroscopy.
- CT scan of the thorax and abdomen to stage disease.
- EUS is valuable to stage superficial tumours that may be amenable to endoscopic mucosal resection (EMR) and to biopsy regional lymph nodes.

Management

- Intervention is largely guided by the symptoms and stage of the disease, with only 30% of patients having operable disease at presentation.
- Patients with evidence of metastatic disease are not surgically curable and overall prognosis is poor (5-year survival rates estimated at <10%).
- Palliative chemotherapy and radiotherapy may be appropriate.

Treatment options

- *Surgery (oesophagectomy) with neo-adjuvant or adjuvant chemotherapy and radiotherapy* may be recommended, based on disease staging.
- *EMR* is a potentially curative therapeutic modality for early oesophageal cancers that do not extend beyond the submucosa.

- *Oesophageal stent placement* is useful in patients with dysphagia secondary to malignant lesions. Oesophageal stents placed across the gastro-oesophageal junction (GOJ) often leads to post procedure reflux symptoms.

Gastro-oesophageal reflux disease

Transient and intermittent reflux of gastric contents into the oesophagus is a physiologically normal phenomena and typically asymptomatic. Prolonged reflux that results in mucosal damage or symptoms defines GORD.

Presentation

- Typically heartburn aggravated by bending over and lying down.
- Generally, the severity of symptoms does not correlate well with findings at endoscopy.

Pathophysiology

- Reduced LOS tone can result in the reflux of gastric contents.
- Factors including diet (caffeine, chocolate, alcohol), smoking, medications (nitrates, tricyclic antidepressants, exogenous oestrogen) and pregnancy can reduce LOS tone and exacerbate symptoms.
- Mechanical alteration, e.g. a hiatus hernia may contribute to GORD, particularly if associated with reduced LOS tone.
- Transient LOS relaxations are responsible for the vast majority of GORD in the setting of normal LOS tone. During pharyngeal contraction (swallowing) there is a normal physiological relaxation of the LOS to facilitate the passage of food. Prolonged relaxations and those occurring frequently without swallowing or oesophageal peristalsis may result in significant reflux.

Investigations

- The diagnosis of GORD is usually evident in the clinical history and further investigations are not required in the absence of 'alarm' symptoms such as weight loss, dysphagia, odynophagia, GI bleeding and anaemia.
- NICE have issued guidelines for referral for endoscopy for patients with 'dyspepsia' (Table 14.2). Dyspepsia used to include people with recurrent epigastric pain, heartburn or acid regurgitation, ± bloating, nausea or vomiting.
- *Oesophageal pH monitoring* may be of value to document acid reflux episodes in patients with negative endoscopic findings who are potential candidates for anti-reflux surgery.

Table 14.2 NICE guidelines: investigation of dyspepsia (1)

Symptom and specific features	Recommendation
Dyspepsia (treatment-resistant) age ≥55 years	Non-urgent OGD
Dyspepsia with weight loss, age ≥55 years	Urgent OGD (2 weeks)
Dyspepsia with raised platelet count or nausea or vomiting, age ≥55 years	Non-urgent OGD

Data from NICE (2015), NG12 Suspected cancer: recognition and referral. Available from https://www.nice.org.uk/guidance/ng12

Management

Conservative measures

- Weight loss and elevation of the head of the bed (for nocturnal reflux symptoms).
- Dietary modification avoiding common triggers such as fatty food, caffeine, spicy food and chocolate may be beneficial if there is good correlation with GORD symptoms.
- Tobacco and alcohol should be avoided as they may contribute to reduced LOS tone.

Helicobacter pylori *testing*

- NICE recommend testing for *Helicobacter pylori* in all patients with dyspepsia using a breath test or stool antigen test.
- A 2-week washout period should be left after proton pump inhibitor (PPI) use.

Medical management

For pharmacological agents used to treat GORD or dyspepsia, see Table 14.3.

Table 14.3 Pharmacological agents used in the treatment of GORD/dyspepsia

Drug	Example	Mode of action	Advantages and disadvantages
Antacids	(Aluminium hydroxide) Mucogel® and magnesium trisilicate.	Neutralise gastric pH.	Helpful 'on demand' medication, but have a short duration of action.
Alginate compound preparations and Aluminium hydroxide complex	Gaviscon®. Sucralfate.	Increase viscosity of stomach contents. Some form a viscous gel 'raft' that float on the surface of stomach contents to minimise reflux. Act as a barrier to prevent gastric mucosal injury.	Helpful in treating GORD during pregnancy.
H_2-receptor antagonists	Ranitidine.	Reduce acid by inhibiting the histamine 2 receptor on the gastric parietal cell. Most effective at mediating the rate of basal acid release during fasting and as such are most effective when administered at night.	Tachyphylaxis is commonly seen within a few weeks of use and limits their popularity as maintenance therapy. May result in a rebound acid secretion when discontinued. More suitable as 'on demand' agents, as opposed to a primary method of acid suppression.
Proton pump inhibitors (PPIs)	Omeprazole. Lansoprazole.	Inhibit acid production by irreversibly binding to the hydrogen-potassium ATPase pump.	Generally effective. Maintenance therapy is frequently required. PPIs can take several days to exhibit maximal acid suppression, therefore 'on demand' use may not be effective. Prolonged use of PPIs may result in a rebound acid hypersecretion phenomenon, presumably due to higher levels of gastrin (which is inhibited by gastric acid). The elevated gastrin levels may result in enterochromaffin-like cell hyperplasia.

Surgery

- Anti-reflux surgery is recommended for patients who have symptoms refractory to maximal medical therapy.
- The most common procedure is a laparoscopic Nissen fundoplication.
- This procedure is most beneficial for young patients who have a response to acid suppressant medication, but experience a return of symptoms off medication.

References

1. NICE. Gastro-oesophageal reflux disease and dyspepsia in adults: investigation and management. Clinical guideline CG184, 2014. https://www.nice.org.uk/guidance/cg184.

Barrett's oesophagus

The oesophagus is normally lined with stratified squamous epithelium. In the setting of chronic GORD, the distal oesophagus may undergo a metaplastic change from squamous to columnar epithelium. This metaplastic columnar epithelium is at risk of dysplasia, and therefore prone to malignant transformation with the development of adenocarcinoma.

Risk factors

- Barrett's oesophagus (BO) is seen most frequently in middle-aged males and older adults.
- Specific risk factors include GORD, obesity, and a family history of BO or oesophageal adenocarcinoma.

Diagnosis

- Requires both endoscopic and histological confirmation.
- BO is defined as an oesophagus in which any portion of the normal distal squamous lining has been replaced by metaplastic columnar epithelium, clearly visible (≥1 cm) above the GOJ and confirmed intestinal metaplasia (IMt) from oesophageal biopsies.

Classification and surveillance

- BO is classified into short- and long-segment BO, according to the maximal length of columnar metaplasia from GOJ (see Table 14.4). Long-segment BO has a higher risk of development of adenocarcinoma.

Table 14.4 British Society of Gastroenterology (BSG) recommendations for surveillance in non-dysplastic Barrett's oesophagus (1)

Barrett's segment length	**Interval of endoscopic surveillance**
Short segment Barrett's (<3 cm) with confirmed IMt	Repeat endoscopy in 3–5 years.
Long segment Barrett's (≥3 cm) with confirmed IMt	Repeat endoscopy in 2–3 years.

Data from Fitzgerald RC, et al. British Society of Gastroenterology guidelines on the diagnosis and management of Barrett's oesophagus. *Gut*, 2014 Jan;63(1):7-42.

Dysplasia in Barrett's oesophagus

- Any diagnosis of dysplasia in BO should be confirmed by a second gastrointestinal (GI) pathologist.
- Appropriate management and surveillance should be discussed at a multi-disciplinary conference.

References

1. Fitzgerald RC, et al. British Society of Gastroenterology guidelines on the diagnosis and management of Barrett's oesophagus. *Gut*. 2014;63(1):7–42.

Disorders of the stomach and duodenum

Gastritis

Classification

- Acute gastritis: characterised by acute inflammation with a neutrophilic infiltrate.
- Chronic gastritis: characterised by mononuclear cells and lymphocytes.
  - Further sub-classified as atrophic or non-atrophic gastritis.
- Endoscopically, gastritis can be characterised by its severity, location and whether it is erosive or non-erosive.

Presentation

- Acute gastritis can present with nausea, vomiting, anorexia, bloating, abdominal pain and GI bleeding, although it is frequently asymptomatic.

Treatment

- Remove any precipitating factors and treat with acid-suppression therapy (usually a proton pump inhibitor).
- Patients presenting with signs and symptoms of upper GI haemorrhage require urgent endoscopy ± further therapy.

Helicobacter pylori *infection*

- A Gram-negative, urease-producing bacterium.
- The most common cause of non-atrophic chronic gastritis. HP is most common in the elderly and lower socioeconomic groups.
- Present in approximately 50% of the global population. HP is spread through faecal–oral and oral–oral routes.
- The majority of patients with HP are asymptomatic.
- HP is linked to development of chronic gastritis, peptic ulcer disease, gastric B cell lymphoma and gastric cancer.
- Untreated patients with gastritis due to HP develop chronic gastritis and have a greater risk of duodenal ulcer disease.

Non-invasive tests for *Helicobacter pylori*

HP serology

- Detects IgG antibodies to HP.
- Rapid, simple, relatively inexpensive.
- Useful for initial diagnosis of infection.
- Antibodies may remain indefinitely positive and are, therefore, not useful in assessing response to therapy.

HP faecal antigen

- Highly sensitive and specific.
- Rapid, but relatively expensive.
- Useful to detect active infection and response to therapy.

Urease breath test

- Urease is produced by HP and not normally found in the stomach.
- Carbon-13 or carbon-14 labelled urea is administered orally. If HP is present, the labelled carbon is detectable via a breath test.

- Rapid, highly sensitive and specific, but expensive.
- Useful to detect active infection and response to therapy.

Invasive tests for *Helicobacter pylori*

Invasive testing for HP involves upper endoscopy and biopsy of the gastric mucosa.

Rapid urease test (CLO test)

- Gastric biopsy (typically antral) is added to a urea-containing specimen. HP when present breaks down the urea to release ammonia. This causes a pH-dependent colour change indicating a positive test.
- Rapid, highly sensitive and specific, and inexpensive.
- Bacterial overgrowth (urease producing proteus) and GI bleeding

can produce false-positive results and false-negative results, respectively.

Histology

- Direct visualisation of the organism.
- Highly sensitive and specific, but expensive.

Culture

- Helpful to determine antimicrobial sensitivity in patients with HP, which has been resistant to conventional therapy.

Management

- HP eradication is indicated for:
  - All patients with symptomatic dyspepsia, proven peptic ulcer disease (PUD), atrophic gastritis and gastric mucosa-associated lymphoid tissue (MALToma).
  - Patients with a first-degree family history of gastric cancer or lymphoma.
- Standard first line therapy is a 7-day twice daily course of treatment with a PPI (e.g. omeprazole) and antibiotics (amoxicillin and clarithromycin/metronidazole).

Peptic ulcer disease

Peptic ulcers occur within the GI mucosa of the stomach or duodenum. The term 'peptic' implies a relationship to an acid-bearing area. These lesions penetrate the muscularis mucosa and are usually readily visible at endoscopy. Most peptic ulcers occur in the stomach and proximal duodenum; duodenal ulcers are more common than gastric ulcers. They are more common in men and in the elderly.

Presentation

- Typical symptoms of PUD include epigastric pain (classically soon after eating with gastric ulcers), nausea and vomiting.
- Duodenal ulcers tend to cause pain during periods of fasting.
- Patients may present with complications of a perforated ulcer or upper GI bleed.

Pathogenesis

PUD is the result of an imbalance between factors that protect that GI mucosa and those that damage it.

Protective mechanisms include: the secretion of mucous, bicarbonate and phospholipids, an adequate mucosal blood flow and epithelial cell renewal.

Processes that may damage the gastrointestinal mucosa include: medications (e.g. NSAIDs, aspirin, bisphosphonates), chemotherapy, radiotherapy, infection (HP, cytomegalovirus), ischaemia (shock, vasoconstrictive agents), hyper-secretory states (Zollinger–Ellison syndrome [ZES]) and infiltrative disorders such as Crohn's disease and malignancy.

Investigations

- See Table 14.2 for indications for gastroscopy in patient with dyspepsia.
- Endoscopy should also be strongly considered for patients with dyspepsia who have signs of GI bleeding or a strong family history of upper GI malignancy.
  - If a gastric ulcer is seen, multiple biopsies from the edge and ulcer base are recommended to rule out malignancy, with repeat endoscopy in 6–8 weeks to ensure healing after acid suppression.
  - Uncomplicated duodenal ulcers do not typically require biopsy or follow-up endoscopy after appropriate therapy.
- All patients should be screened for HP and, if positive, receive eradication therapy.

Management

- Acid suppression with PPI.
- HP eradication.
- Stop NSAIDs or aspirin if possible.
- If NSAIDs or aspirin must be continued, then prophylaxis with acid suppression is appropriate.

Further reading

1. Parsons ME, Ganellin CR. Histamine and its receptors. *Br J Pharmacol*. 2006;147(Suppl. 1):S127–35.
2. Sachs G, Shin JM, Vagin O, et al. The gastric H,K ATPase as a drug target: past, present, and future. *J Clin Gastroenterol*. 2007;41(Suppl. 2):S226–42.
3. Wolfe MM & Sachs G. Acid suppression: optimising therapy for gastroduodenal ulcer healing, gastroesophageal reflux disease, and stress-related erosive syndrome. *Gastroenterology*. 2000;118(2 Suppl 1):S9–31.
4. Mejia A, Kraft WK. Acid peptic diseases: pharmacological approach to treatment. *Expert Rev Clin Pharmacol*. 2009; 2:295–314.

Zollinger–Ellison syndrome

ZES is a rare, but important cause of GI mucosal ulceration resulting from acid hypersecretion from a gastrinoma, causing inappropriate hypergastrinaemia in the setting of a low gastric pH (➲ see Chapter 19, Gastrinomas, p. 700). ZES should be considered in patients with severe ulceration of the upper GI tract or ulceration distal to the duodenum.

Investigation

- Fasting plasma gastrin level: elevated if >150 pg/mL; a level >1000 pg/mL is virtually diagnostic.
- Anti-secretory therapy can cause a rise in plasma gastrin and should be stopped for 1 week prior to testing.
- Low acid output states such as atrophic gastritis and pernicious anaemia can also result in hypergastrinaemia.
- A secretin stimulation test can differentiate between a gastrinoma and other causes of hypergastrinaemia. It is, however, cumbersome to perform and, therefore, is rarely done in practice (1).
- Gastric pH measurement: a pH > 3 makes ZES very unlikely.
- Somatostatin receptor scintography and CT may localise the lesion.
- EUS to identify and sample possible gastrinomas around the stomach, duodenum and within the pancreas.

Management

- Symptomatic therapy with acid suppression (PPI).
- The only curative treatment for gastrinoma is surgical resection.
- A multidisciplinary approach is important, particularly in cases of metastatic disease.

References

1. Isenberg JI, Walsh JH, Grossman MI. Zollinger–Ellison syndrome. *Gastroenterology*. 1973;65:140–65.

Gastric neoplasms

Gastric adenocarcinoma accounts for up to 95% of all gastric neoplasms. Less common neoplasms of the stomach include:

- gastrointestinal stromal tumours (GISTs);
- lymphomas;
- neuroendocrine tumours (NETs);
- metastatic disease to the stomach.

Epidemiology and risk factors

- Third most common cause of cancer-related death worldwide and the 10th most common cause of cancer-related mortality in the UK (1).
- Incidence and mortality related to gastric cancer has reduced significantly over the last half century.
- The most important risk factor for gastric adenocarcinoma is *Helicobacter pylori* infection. Additional risk factors include tobacco use, advancing age, male sex, low consumption of fruits and vegetables, and a family history of gastric cancer.

Presentation

- Epigastric discomfort.
- Bloating.
- Early satiety.
- Dyspepsia.
- Advanced lesions may present with nausea, vomiting and weight loss.

Investigations

Gastroscopy and biopsy are the investigations of choice. Further imaging modalities, including EUS and CT, are helpful for staging and to determine an appropriate management strategy.

Management

- A multidisciplinary approach is required, options vary based on tumour stage(2).
- Surgery along with adjuvant or neo-adjuvant chemoradiotherapy is offered to suitable patients with resectable disease.

References

1. Cancer Research UK. Stomach cancer incidence statistics. http://www.cancerresearchuk.org/health-professional/cancer-statistics/statistics-by-cancer-type/stomach-cancer/incidence.
2. Everything NICE says on a topic in an interactive flowchart.http://pathways.nice.org.uk.

Acute upper gastrointestinal bleeding

Upper gastrointestinal (UGI) bleeding can result in haematemesis (vomiting blood) and melaena (passage of dark tarry stools per rectum). NSAIDs and aspirin are frequently implicated in UGI bleeds. Causes are given in Box 14.1.

Box 14.1 Causes of acute upper GI bleeding

Common

- Peptic ulcer (50%).
- Erosions (15–20%).
- Bleeding varices (10–20%).

Less common

- Mallory–Weiss tear (5–10%).
- Reflux oesophagitis (2–5%).

Uncommon

- Gastric neoplasms.
- Hereditary haemorrhagic telangectasia (Osler–Weber–Rendu syndrome) (➲ see Chapter 5, Case 3, p. 120).
- Dieulafoy gastric vascular abnormality.
- Portal gastropathy.
- *Pseudoxanthoma elasticum* (➲ See Chapter 20, Pseudoxanthoma elasticum, p. 749).
- Aortoenteric fistula.

Investigations

- The Blatchford Score (Table 14.5) is calculated pre-endoscopy to risk stratify all patients with an UGI haemorrhage (1).
- UGI endoscopy should be performed within 24 hours for all patients presenting with a Blatchford score of >1.
- A Rockall score should be performed post-endoscopy and predicts mortality (see Table 14.6) (2).

Table 14.5 Blatchford Score for assessment of UGI bleeds

Risk factor at presentation	Threshold and score
Blood urea (mmol/L)	6·5–7·9 = 2 points 8·0–9·9 = 3 points 10·0–25·0 = 4 points >25·0 = 6 points
Haemoglobin for men (g/L)	120–129 = 1 point 100–119 = 3 points <100 = 6 points
Haemoglobin for women (g/L)	100–119 = 1 point <100 = 6 points

Additional markers: pulse ≥100/min = 1 point; presentation with melaena = 1 point; presentation with syncope = 2 points; hepatic disease (known history, or clinical and laboratory evidence, of chronic or acute liver disease) = 2 points; cardiac failure (known history, or clinical and echocardiographic evidence, of cardiac failure) = 2 points.

Reprinted from *The Lancet*, 356, Blatchford, O. et al., A risk score to predict need for treatment for upper gastrointestinal haemorrhage, pp. 1318–1321. https://doi.org/10.1016/S0140-6736(00)02816-6

Table 14.6 Pre- and post-endoscopy Rockall score (maximum score: 7) for upper GI haemorrhage

Risk factor and threshold		**Score**
Age	<60 years	0
	60–79 years	1
	>80 years	2
Shock	None	0
	Pulse >100 + systolic BP>100 mmHg	1
	Systolic BP <100 mmHg	2
Co-morbidity	None Cardiac failure, IHD Renal/liver failure Advanced malignancy	0 2 3 3
Post-endoscopy Rockall Score includes, in addition, the below		
Endoscopic diagnosis/stigmata recent haemorrhage (SRH)		
Endoscopic diagnosis	Mallory–Weiss tear and no SRH.	0
	All other diagnoses.	1
	Malignancy of upper GI tract	2
Major SRH	None or dark spot only.	0
	Blood in UGI tract, adherent clot, visible or spurting vessel	2

Final Rockall score (Maximum score: 11): <3 good prognosis; >8 poor.
Adapted by permission from BMJ Publishing Group Limited. *Gut*, Vreeburg, E. M. et al., Validation of the Rockall risk scoring system in upper gastrointestinal bleeding, 44, pp. 331–335. Copyright © 1999, BMJ Publishing Group Ltd and the British Society of Gastroenterology. http://dx.doi.org/10.1136/gut.44.3.331.
Adapted by permission from BMJ Publishing Group Limited. Rockall, T.A. et al. Risk assessment after acute upper gastrointestinal haemorrhage. *Gut* 38:316–321. Copyright © 1996, BMJ Publishing Group Ltd and the British Society of Gastroenterology. http://dx.doi.org/10.1136/gut.38.3.316

Urgent laboratory investigations

- FBC.
- U&E.
- LFTs.
- Coagulation screen.
- Group and save.

Management

- Assess clinical status and stability of the patient.
- Large bore (16G) IV access; resuscitate appropriately.
- Careful history and examination to determine possible aetiology.
- Plan for endoscopy.

Key points on management of non-variceal bleeding

- Current NICE guidelines (2012) suggest PPI should not be offered routinely pre-endoscopy, since it does not reduce the risk of rebleeding or mortality, although this remains common practice (1,2).

- IV omeprazole should be prescribed post-endoscopy for those with stigmata of recent haemorrhage. (Standard dose of IV omeprazole is 80 mg, followed by 8 mg/hour infusion over 72 hours).
- Endoscopic management of UGI bleeding varies based on findings. Therapeutic modalities include injection of epinephrine, coagulation therapy, clip placement, banding (variceal bleeds) and haemostatic powder application (Hemospray™). Outcomes are superior if >1 therapeutic modality is used.
- If endoscopic therapy fails to control UGI bleeding, interventional radiology for vessel embolisation may be feasible. The final management strategy for UGI bleeds, which are refractory to standard management is surgery. It is also essential to alert the on-call surgical team when a high-risk patient is identified.

Management of variceal bleeding

➲ See Chapter 15, Varices, p. 532.

References

1. Blatchford O, Murray WR, Blatchford M. A risk score to predict need for treatment for upper gastrointestinal haemorrhage. *Lancet*. 2000; 356:1318–21.
2. Vreeburg EM, Terwee CB, Snel P, et al. Validation of the Rockall risk scoring system in upper gastrointestinal bleeding. *Gut*. 1999;44:331–5.

Further reading

1. Sreedharan A, Martin J, Leontiadis GI, et al. Proton pump inhibitor treatment initiated prior to endoscopic diagnosis in upper gastrointestinal bleeding. *Cochrane Database Syst Rev*. 2010;(7):CD005415.

Chronic gastrointestinal bleeding

- Chronic GI bleeding typically presents with iron deficiency anaemia, and occasionally noticeable melaena.
- If OGD and colonoscopy are normal, small bowel evaluation with MR enterography or VCE is helpful in ruling out luminal lesions or small angiodysplastic lesions, which may ooze intermittently.
- Deep enteroscopy may subsequently be required to further evaluate and treat pathology.

Diseases of the small and large intestine

Diarrhoea

- Diarrhoea is the increased frequency of loose or watery stools, which typically results from the combination of decreased fluid absorption and increased gut secretion.
- Acute diarrhoea generally lasts for <14 days, after which it is considered to be persistent, or chronic.
- Diarrhoea can be classified by aetiology as osmotic-, secretory- or motility-related. Motility-related diarrhoea causes increased frequency, rather than true diarrhoea and may be seen in thyrotoxicosis.

For characteristics and causes of osmotic and secondary diarrhoea, see Table 14.7.

Table 14.7 Characteristics and causes of osmotic and secretory diarrhoea

Osmotic diarrhoea	Secretory diarrhoea
• Caused by non-absorbed hypertonic material in gut lumen. • Generally stops with fasting. • Lower volume (< 1L/day). • Examples of aetiology include ingestion of sugars, magnesium, sorbitol, fructose, lactase, polyethylene glycol. • Pancreatic insufficiency and disaccharidase deficiency.	• Increased (net) secretion of fluid and electrolytes into gut lumen. • Does not stop with fasting. • Large volume (>1L/day). • Infections/toxins (e.g. *E. coli*, Cholera, *Salmonella, Shigella*). • Inflammation (ulcerative colitis/Crohn's disease). • Hormone secretion tumours (metastatic carcinoid). • Bile salt-related (after ileal resection).

Investigation and treatment

Acute diarrhoea

- Typically self-limiting and may not require investigation aside from stool microscopy and culture.
- Treatment is supportive management with hydration and electrolyte replacement.

Chronic diarrhoea

- Persistent or chronic diarrhoea warrants investigation and treatment will depend on aetiology.
- A thorough history to evaluate for foreign travel and laxative use is important prior to embarking on invasive investigation.
- Infective causes must be ruled out with stool microscopy, culture (➲ see Chapter 8, Infectious diarrhoea, p. 250 and Table 8.21; Health care-associated *Staphylococcus aureus* infections, p. 239; and *Clostridium difficile* infection, p. 241).
- A flexible sigmoidoscopy with biopsies can assess for mucosal erythema, which may be suggestive an inflammatory or infective aetiology.
- Patients with suspected osmotic diarrhoea and steatorrhoea may require pancreatic assessment with faecal elastase, pancreatic imaging and/or small bowel evaluation (➲ see Chapter 15, Investigations, p. 543).

Constipation

- Constipation is a common and usually benign symptom (e.g. due to low dietary fibre intake). It does not normally require investigation and resolves with lifestyle and dietary advice, although care should be taken to exclude underlying pathology in middle-aged and older populations.
- Medications such as opiates can contribute to slow colonic transit and should be reduced or stopped if possible in patients with constipation.
- Underlying medical conditions, such as hypothyroidism and hypercalcaemia, may result in constipation and should be excluded.
- If lifestyle measures (dietary fibre increase, hydration, exercise) are not sufficient, bulking agents (ispaghula husk) should be tried as first-line medical therapy.
- Osmotic and stimulant laxatives may also be helpful as a short-term therapeutic strategy. Regular use of stimulant laxatives, such as senna may result in tachyphylaxis.

Malabsorption

Malabsorption refers to the impaired absorption of nutrients and can result from defects in the small intestinal membrane transport system to acquired defects in absorptive mucosal surface (Box 14.2).

Box 14.2 Disorders of the small intestine that can result in malabsorption

- Coeliac disease.
- Small bowel bacterial overgrowth.
- Intestinal resection.
- Crohn's disease.
- Whipple's disease (rare).
- Parasitic infections (rare, but endemic to certain areas).

(*Note*: chronic pancreatitis can also result in malabsorption [➲ See Chapter 15, Chronic pancreatitis, p. 543])

Clinical presentation

- Variable, depending on the severity of the condition.
- Greasy, foul smelling stools.

- Weight loss despite adequate caloric intake.
- Patients may have very mild or no symptoms, with the only clue to malabsorption being vitamin deficiencies or anaemia.

Coeliac disease

- Coeliac disease is a gluten-sensitive enteropathy, which is characterised by small bowel mucosal inflammation, crypt hyperplasia, and villous atrophy in response to dietary gluten. Improvement in these features are seen when gluten is eliminated from the diet (1).
- Wheat, barley and rye are common sources of gluten. Distilled alcoholic beverages (including wine) are gluten free, although beer and ale are usually made from gluten-containing grains. Rice, corn and potatoes do not contain gluten.
- Coeliac disease has a strong genetic association with HLA class II genes *HLA DQ2* and *HLA DQ8*. It is more common in Caucasian people of northern European ancestry.

Clinical presentation

- Weight loss, loose stool and signs of nutrient or vitamin deficiencies.
- Non-specific symptoms, such as fatigue, malaise and abdominal bloating.
- Less commonly, dermatitis herpetiformis: an itchy, symmetrical rash with vesicles and crusts on the extensor surfaces of the body.
- Coeliac disease can cause abnormal LFTs and is associated with primary biliary cirrhosis and other autoimmune diseases (e.g. type 1 diabetes mellitus and thyroid disease).

Investigations

- Serological evaluation while on a gluten-rich diet. Immunoglobulin A (IgA) anti-tissue transglutaminase (tTG) antibody is the preferred test for detection of coeliac disease.
- If clinical suspicion for the disease is high, and the anti-tTG antibody is negative, total IgA should be measured. Patients with selective IgA deficiency (more common in patients with coeliac disease compared with general population) may have a false negative result.
- Gastroscopy with duodenal biopsies while on a gluten-rich diet to confirm the diagnosis.

Management

- Most patients with coeliac disease respond well to a gluten-free diet, which should be maintained life-long. Dietician input is critical to successful management.
- Monitor for vitamin and mineral deficiencies that may have resulted from untreated disease.
- Osteopenia may occur due to hyperparathyroidism secondary to vitamin D deficiency. Bone mineral density should be evaluated with a dual energy X-ray absorptiometry (DEXA) scan and treated if required.

References

1. BSG Guidelines on the diagnosis and management of adult coeliac disease. https://www.bsg.org.uk/resource/bsg-guidelines-on-the-diagnosis-and-management-of-adult-coeliac-disease.html.

Further reading

1. Rubin CE, Brandborg L, Phelps PC, Taylor HCJ. Studies of celiac disease. I. The apparent identical and specific nature of the duodenal and proximal jejunal lesion in celiac disease and idiopathic sprue. *Gastroenterology*. 1960;38:28–49.
2. Hopper AD, Hadjivassiliou M, Hurlstone DP, et al. What is the role of serologic testing in celiac disease? A prospective, biopsy-confirmed study with economic analysis. *Clin Gastroenterol Hepatol*. 2008;6:314–20.

Small intestinal bacterial overgrowth

- While the small intestine is not entirely sterile, it typically only contains small concentrations of commensal bacteria that live within or on the mucosal surface of the intestinal lumen.

- Small intestinal bacterial overgrowth (SIBO) is a condition in which these or other non-native bacteria grow to excessive numbers and cause malabsorptive symptoms, excessive fermentation and inflammation. The majority of patients with SIBO have an underlying condition, which results in bacterial proliferation.

For disorders associated with SIBO, see Box 14.3.

Box 14.3 Disorders associated with small intestinal bacterial overgrowth

Stasis or abnormal communication

- Surgically created blind loops (end to side anastomosis).
- Strictures (CD, radiation, surgery).
- Diverticulosis (small intestine).
- Diabetes (decreased gut motility).
- Systemic sclerosis (decreased gut motility).
- Enterocolic fistulas.
- Resection of the ileocaecal valve.

Miscellaneous

- Chronic pancreatitis.
- Chronic liver disease and cirrhosis.
- End stage renal disease.
- Immunodeficiencies.

Clinical presentation

- Abdominal bloating, flatulence and abdominal discomfort.
- Diarrhoea is a common presentation in patients with moderate to severe SIBO and may be related to the deconjugation of bile salts by bacteria.

Investigation

- Carbohydrate breath testing: hydrogen and methane in exhaled air is measured following the ingestion of lactulose, ^{14}C d-xylose or glucose. The bacteria that contaminate the small intestine metabolise these substrates, and thereby produce hydrogen and methane, or ^{14}C (1).
- Jejunal aspirates are rarely performed, but elevated concentration of bacteria is a diagnostic gold standard.
- Typical organisms found in SIBO include bacteriodes, lactobacillus and enterococcus.

Treatment

- Treatment of the underlying aetiology.
- Vitamin and mineral deficiencies should be measured and corrected.
- Antibiotics therapy: not intended to sterilise the small bowel, but rather to restore the balance of commensal flora. Agents that target Gram-negative and anaerobic organisms such as rifaximin, amoxicillin-clavulinic acid, fluoroquinolones and metronidazole are commonly used.

References

1. Khoshini R, Dai SC, Lezcano S, Pimentel M. A systematic review of diagnostic tests for small intestinal bacterial overgrowth. *Dig Dis Sci*. 2008;53:1443–54.

Small intestinal tumours

Tumours of the small intestine are uncommon and may present with abdominal pain, anorexia, diarrhoea, anaemia and rarely obstructive symptoms.

Malignant tumours

- Adenocarcinomas: 50% of malignant tumours of the small bowel. Patients with chronic inflammatory bowel disease are at higher risk.
- Lymphomas: 10–15% of small bowel malignant tumours; may be B or T cell in origin. Patients with coeliac disease are at increased risk of T cell lymphomas of the small bowel or enteropathy associated T-cell lymphomas, although these are rare.
- Neuroendocrine (e.g. carcinoid) tumours of the small intestine (➲ see Chapter 19, Neuroendocrine tumours, p. 700).
- Inherited polyposis syndromes may increase risk of small bowel malignancy (See Box 14.4).

Benign tumours

- Usually incidental findings, include adenomas (have malignant potential), fibromas, leiomyomas and lipomas.

Carcinoid tumours

Carcinoid tumours are the most common type of neuroendocrine tumour arising from serotonin producing cells of the intestine. They produce a variety of peptides and hormones (such as histamine, serotonin and 5-hydroxytryptamine), which are metabolised by the liver. Common GI sites include the stomach, terminal ileum, appendix and rectum. ➲ See Chapter 19, Carcinoid tumours, p. 700, for presentation, investigation and treatment.

Further reading

1. Modlin IM, Kidd M, Latich I, Zikusoka MN, Shapiro MD. Current status of gastrointestinal carcinoids. *Gastroenterology*. 2005;128:1717–51.

Microscopic colitis

Microscopic colitis is a syndrome of chronic watery diarrhoea with characteristic histological features. It occurs more frequently in middle-aged women. The diagnosis is made with colonic biopsies; macroscopic appearances at endoscopy are normal.

Clinical presentation

- Non-bloody diarrhoea, which can be frequent (>5 times per day).
- Abdominal cramping.
- Weight loss, likely due to significant fluid losses.

Investigations

- Colonoscopy with mucosal biopsies.

Treatment

- Medications such as NSAIDS, ranitidine, PPIs and selective serotonin re-uptake inhibitors are associated with microscopic colitis and should be avoided.
- First-line treatment in patients that do not respond to standard anti-diarrhoeal agents is budesonide (1).

References

1. Gentile NM, Abdalla AA, Khanna S, et al. Outcomes of patients with microscopic colitis treated with corticosteroids: a population-based study. *Am J Gastroenterol*. 2013; 108:256–9.

Inflammatory bowel disease, Crohn's disease and ulcerative colitis

- IBD is a disease characterised by chronic, idiopathic inflammation of the intestinal tract.
- Two main subtypes, Crohn's disease (CD) and ulcerative colitis (UC), defined by disease location and histological findings.

- The term indeterminate colitis is used when features are not clearly suggestive of either UC or CD.
- Affects men and women equally, with the peak incidence between 15–25 years. A second peak, though smaller, is seen in between the fifth and seventh decades.
- Smoking is a risk factor for both the development and the severity of CD.
- Patients who smoke have a lower incidence of UC. The reason for this is unclear.

Crohn's disease

CD can affect any portion of the GI tract, from mouth to anus. It classically results in deep ulcerations of the bowel, interspersed with relatively unaffected portions of intestine ('skip' lesions).

Presentation of Crohn's disease

- The commonest site of bowel involvement is the ileocaecal region (~40% of patients).
- CD involving the small intestine typically presents with abdominal pain and weight loss.
- Severe or stricturing disease can result in obstructive symptoms, such as abdominal distension, pain and vomiting.
- Colonic CD usually presents with bloody diarrhoea.

Ulcerative colitis

UC by definition, only affects the colon, with the rectum virtually always being involved.

Presentation of ulcerative colitis

- Typically presents with diarrhoea, which often contains blood and mucous.
- Contiguous inflammation that extends proximally, with varying severity and distance from the anal verge.

Both UC and CD may have associated extra-intestinal conditions such as arthropathies, skin rashes and ocular conditions (see Table 14.8).

Table 14.8 Extra intestinal manifestations (EIMs) in IBD

EIMs that improve with disease activity	EIMs independent of disease activity
Apthous ulceration.	Primary sclerosing cholangitis.
Erythema nodosum.	Pyoderma gangrenosum.
Episcleritis.	Uveitis.
Type 1 peripheral arthropathy (acute self-limiting affecting <5 large joints)*.	Axial arthritis (including sacroilitis)*. Type 2 peripheral arthropathy (prolonged course affecting >5 small joints)*.

* ➲ See Chapter 20, Inflammatory bowel disease-related arthritis, p. 718.

Investigations

Investigations for IBD should be tailored to characterise the subtype, location and severity of disease. Infective causes of diarrhoea that may mimic the presentation of IBD should be excluded.

Laboratory tests

- FBC to assess for anaemia, iron indices, B12 and folate.
- Renal profile to assess for dehydration.
- Markers of inflammation include ESR, CRP and platelet count.
- LFTs: low serum albumin is related to a catabolic state and is a feature of severe disease.

Radiological investigations

- X-ray of the abdomen can provide information regarding bowel wall thickening, disease extent and importantly exclude signs of toxic megacolon.
- Cross-sectional imaging such as CT and MRI are frequently used to delineate disease.
- CT should be used judiciously, as patients are often young at presentation, and may be exposed to a significant cumulative radiation exposure.
- Magnetic resonance enterography (MRE) has proved to be a very useful tool in assessing small bowel disease. In experienced hands, small bowel ultrasonography is also an accurate and safe way of assessing for stricturing and active small intestinal CD.
- VCE has a role in the assessment of small bowel mucosal disease if clinical suspicion remains high despite negative cross-sectional imaging. VCE is contraindicated in stricturing disease due to risk of capsule retention and potential obstruction.

Endoscopic evaluation

- The gold standard for the diagnosis of IBD, providing both a luminal evaluation for extent and severity, and histological specimens for disease characterisation.
- Flexible sigmoidoscopy generally sufficient to evaluate an acute flare in UC.

Treatment

- Aim of treatment is induction and maintenance of remission, as well as effective management of disease relapse.
- Patients with CD who smoke should be advised to stop, as this decreases the rate and severity of relapse.
- Patients with advanced disease are frequently malnourished. Involvement from the nutrition service is, therefore, a critical component of treatment.

For drugs used in the treatment of IBD, see Table 14.9. For acute severe colitis, see Box 14.4 and Table 14.10.

Table 14.9 Drugs used in the treatment of IBD (➲ see Chapter 6, Anti-inflammatory/immunosuppressive therapy, p. 177; Biologics, p. 178, and Tables 6.8 and 6.9, for further details regarding medications)

Drug group	Key points
5-aminosalicylic acid (5-ASAs)	Exact mechanism of action unknown. Act topically, inhibits cytokine, leukotriene and prostaglandin synthesis. Preparations such as mesalazine. Used for mild to moderate colonic disease. Administered orally or rectally (as enema or suppository).
Corticosteroids	Routes of administration include oral, IV and rectal. Mainstay of treatment of acute flares of IBD.
Thiopurines (azathioprine and 6MP)	Take 8–12 weeks to become active. Used for maintenance of remission. Require regular blood monitoring.
Antimetabolites (e.g. methotrexate)	Used in CD. Require blood monitoring.
Calcineurin inhibitors (e.g. ciclosporin)	May be used as rescue therapy for steroid refractory acute colitis.
Biological agents (e.g. infliximab and adalimumab)	See Table 6.9. Licensed for use in moderate to severe CD and UC.

Table 14.10 Acute severe colitis: assessment of severity (Truelove and Witt's criteria 1955) (1)

	Mild	Moderate	Severe
Stool frequency/day	<4	4–6	>6
Temperature (°C)	<36.5	Intermediate	>37.8
Heart rate (bpm)	<90	<90	>90
ESR (mm)	<20	20–30	>30
Haemoglobin (g/dL)	>11	Intermediate	<10

Box 14.4 Acute severe colitis

Acute presentation of colitis is a medical emergency and associated with a 30% risk of colectomy, even with medical treatment.

Investigations

- FBC, renal profile, LFTs, CRP, clotting. Group and Save.
- Stool samples for MC&S and *Clostridium difficile* toxin.
- Abdominal X-ray to exclude toxic megacolon (radiological evidence of colonic dilatation >6 cm primarily involving the ascending or transverse colon).
- An unprepared flexible sigmoidoscopy is indicated to assess mucosal inflammation. N.B. toxic megacolon must be excluded before a flexible sigmoidoscopy due to the risk of perforation.

Treatment

- IV hydrocortisone 100 mg QDS.
- Supportive IV fluids.
- Venous thromboprophylaxis with low molecular weight heparin.
- Stop anticholinergics, opiates, antidiarrhoeal medications.
- Initiate strict stool chart.
- Day 3 is critical and rescue therapy should be initiated if any of the following are present: persistent colonic dilatation of AXR, CRP >45, stool frequency >8.
- Options for rescue therapy include a biological agent (commonly infliximab) or ciclosporin (2).
- Refer for surgical review as routine and if no clinical improvement is seen with rescue therapy colectomy is indicated.

Surgery

- Patients with severe colitis (UC or CD) who do not respond to steroids are likely to require surgery.
- Surgery remains the necessary intervention in patients who develop fulminant colitis despite maximal medial therapy, and for those that develop complications of chronic IBD, such as strictures, abscess formation or perforation.
- While surgery is curative for UC, CD may relapse in other remaining areas of the small or large intestine.

References

1. Truelove SC, Witts LJ. Cortisone in ulcerative colitis: final report on a therapeutic trial. *Br Med J*. 1955;2:1041–8.
2. Travis S, Satsangi J, Lemann M. Predicting the need for colectomy in severe ulcerative colitis: a critical appraisal of clinical parameters and currently available biomarkers. *Gut*. 2001;60:3–9.

Further reading

1. Mowat C, Cole A, Windsor A, et al. Guidelines for the management of Inflammatory bowel disease in adults. *Gut.* 2011;60:571–607.
2. Trost LB, McDonnell JK. Important cutaneous manifestations of Inflammatory bowel disease. *Postgrad Med J.* 2005;81:580–5.

Gastrointestinal infections

➲ See Chapter 8, Intra-abdominal infections, p. 249 and Table 8.21.

Colorectal cancer

- The vast majority (>95%) of colorectal cancer (CRC) are adenocarcinomas.
- Less common causes of colonic neoplasms include lymphoma, carcionoids and leiomyosarcomas.
- Most CRCs occur sporadically. 10–15% of CRC occurs in patients with hereditary non-polyposis colorectal cancer or Lynch syndrome, and in patients with inherited polyposis syndromes (see Table 14.11).
- Risk factors for CRC include smoking, obesity, a personal history of colonic polyps (adenomas), family history, low vegetable consumption and IBD.

Table 14.11 Inherited polyposis syndromes: key features

Inherited polyposis syndrome	Key features
Familial adenomatous polyposis (FAP)	Germline mutation in adenomatosis polyposis coli gene (APC). Promotes tumour growth in large and small intestine (often duodenal). > 100 colonic adenomas. Nearly 100% risk of CRC if untreated.
Gardner syndrome	Subset of FAP. Colonic polyposis and extracolonic manifestations (fibromas, desmoid tumours, supernumerary teeth, osteomas [particularly in the jaw]).
Cowden syndrome	Multiple harmartomas in a variety of tissues. Gastric, duodenal and colonic polyps. Palmoplantar keratosis. Increased risk of GI, renal, thyroid, breast, endometrial malignancy. Brain tumours.
Peutz–Jeghers syndrome	Autosomal dominant. Multiple hamartomas throughout GI tract. Mucocutaneous pigmentation. Increased risk of GI and non-GI cancer.

Clinical presentation

Many patients with CRC are asymptomatic, which highlights the need for bowel cancer screening in high risk groups.

Common presentations include:

- Altered bowel habit.
- Rectal bleeding.
- Less commonly, obstruction due to an advanced lesion.
- Significant weight loss: a concerning feature and may represent advanced disease.

Investigation

- FBC, microcytic anaemia due to iron deficiency.
- LFTs in the setting of metastatic lesions.
- Modalities to evaluate the colon include colonoscopy and CT (virtual) colonography.

Management

- The treatment of CRC depends on staging (➔ using the TNM classification; see Chapter 10, Staging of cancer, p. 326 and Box 10.1.
- Surgery with post-operative or adjuvant chemotherapy is recommended for stage III and some stage II disease.
- Patients with advanced (stage IV) disease are usually unsuitable for surgery, but may undergo palliative chemotherapy.
- Molecularly targeted therapy such as bevacizumab which targets vascular endothelial growth factor has been shown to be of modest benefit in metastatic disease.
- Obstruction due to CRC may require colonic stenting, either as a palliative measure or as a bridge to surgical resection.

National bowel cancer screening programme

- The NHS UK bowel cancer screening programme (BCSP) aims to reduce mortality from CRC. Faecal occult blood testing is offered to 60–74-year-olds every 2 years; those with a positive test are offered a colonoscopy (1).

References

1. NHS bowel cancer screening (BCSP) programme. https://www.gov.uk/topic/population-screening-programmes/bowel.

Irritable bowel syndrome

Irritable bowel syndrome (IBS) is characterised by an irregular bowel habit (diarrhoea, constipation or both) and abdominal pain, in the absence of objective pathology. Common symptoms also include abdominal bloating and excessive flatus. Stress and psychological factors appear to play a significant role. Rome IV criteria defines IBS as having recurrent abdominal pain for a least 1 day per week in the last 3 months, associated with ≥2 of the following: related to defecation, change in stool frequency, change in stool consistency (1).

Calprotectin is a protein that is released by activated neutrophils. A high level of faecal calprotectin is a reliable surrogate marker for inflammation in the bowel and can help to assess disease activity in IBD. A normal level can support a diagnosis of IBS (2).

Treatment

- Treatment is often individually based, and time should be taken to carefully rule out symptoms that suggest more sinister pathology.
- Education and reassurance are critical to patient improvement and satisfaction.
- Management may include simple dietary advice or referral to a dietician for a FODMAP (fermentable oligosaccharides, disaccharides, monosaccharides and polyols) diet. This is a structured exclusion diet that aims to identify dietary triggers, which may be avoided to alleviate symptoms.
- Pharmacological therapy for IBS includes laxatives, anti-diarrhoeal agents, anti-spasmodics and anti-depressants.
- Amitriptyline, at low dose, may be beneficial in patients with abdominal pain related to IBS.

References

1. National Institute for Health and Clinical Excellence. Irritable bowel syndrome in adults: diagnosis and management. NICE Clinical Guideline 61. London: NICE, 2008. www.nice.org.uk/CG061.

2. Schoepfer AM, Trummler M, Seeholzer P, Seibold-Schmid B, Seibold F. Discriminating IBD from IBS: comparison of the test performance of fecal markers, blood leukocytes, CRP, and IBD antibodies. Inflamm Bowel Dis. 2008;14(1):32.

Further reading (for chapter)

1. Bloom S, Webster G and Marks D. *Oxford Handbook of Gastroenterology and Hepatology*, 2nd edn. Oxford: Oxford University Press; 2012.

Multiple choice questions

Questions

1. A 38-year-old man is admitted with a 3-day history of melaena and abdominal pain. He has a past medical history of a recent sports injury and has been taking regular NSAID analgesia.

   Examination findings:

   HR 110/min.
   BP 105/75 mmHg.
   Appears pale.
   Melaena on PR examination; no other significant findings on examination.

   Blood tests:

   Hb 75 (120–165 g/L).
   WBC 5.1 (4–10 × 10^9/L).
   Plts 320 (150–400 × 10^9/L).
   INR 1.1 (0.8–1.1).
   Urea 15 (2.5–7.8 mmol/L).
   Creatinine 95 (50–111 μmol/L).
   LFTs within normal range.

   Which of the following statements is true?

   A. He should receive an endoscopy within 12 hours of admission.
   B. Rockall score should be calculated at first assessment.
   C. Blood transfusion to Hb>100 g/L will reduce mortality.
   D. He should have a repeat endoscopy prior to discharge.
   E. He should not be prescribed a PPI prior to endoscopy.

2. A 19-year-old Asian man with a history of ulcerative colitis presents with 3 days of diarrhoea with fresh blood. He reports opening his bowels 12 times in 24 hours with significant urgency.

   Examination findings:

   Dry mucous membranes.
   HR 110/min.
   BP 99/55 mmHg.
   Abdomen soft and diffusely tender, no organomegaly, no guarding or peritonism.

   Which of the following is most appropriate in the immediate management of this patient?

   A. Send urgent stool cultures for microscopy, culture and sensitivity (MC&S) and *Clostridium difficile* toxin (CDT).
   B. Commence oral fluids.
   C. Request a CT of the abdomen.
   D. Commence IV hydrocortisone 50 mg four times a day (QDS).
   E. Perform an immediate flexible sigmoidoscopy.

3. A 61-year-old lady presents with a 3-month history of progressive dysphagia initially to solids and now to liquids. She has a nocturnal cough and also describes a few recent episodes of regurgitating undigested food.

   What should be the first line investigation?

   A. Barium swallow.
   B. CT chest and abdomen.
   C. Chest X-ray.
   D. Gastroscopy (OGD).
   E. 24-hour pH manometry.

4. A 25-year-old man presents with a 6-month history of epigastric pain and diarrhoea.

   Blood tests:

   Hb 115 (120–165 g/L).
   Plts 315 (150–400 × 10^9/L).
   Urea 9.1 (2.5–7.8 mmol/L).
   Creatinine 88 μmol/L (50–111μmol/L).
   LFTs: normal range.
   Serum gastrin 2145 pg/mL (normal range <55 pg/mL).
   Gastroscopy: significant ulceration of the stomach, duodenum and jejunum.

   Which of the following is not a feature of ZES?

   A. Severe or resistant ulceration in the absence of *H. pylori* or NSAID use.
   B. Unusual sites of ulceration extending beyond the second part of the duodenum.
   C. Fasting serum gastrin >1000 pg/mL off PPI treatment.
   D. Gastric pH > 3.
   E. A positive secretin provocation test.

5. Which if the following conditions is not associated with small intestinal bacterial overgrowth (SIBO)?

   A. Type 1 diabetes mellitus.
   B. Systemic sclerosis.
   C. Whipple's disease.
   D. Crohn's disease.
   E. Previous small bowel surgery.

6. A 62-year-old woman of Indian origin is reviewed in the Gastroenterology clinic with dyspepsia. This has been resistant to omeprazole 40 mg, which she had taken continuously for the past 6 months.

   Serum gastrin 90 pmol/L (<55).
   Gastroscopy: antral gastritis and two 0.5-cm chronic ulcers visible in duodenal bulb.
   Rapid urease (CLO) test: negative.

   Which of the following is the most likely diagnosis?

   A. Tuberculosis.
   B. *H. pylori* infection.
   C. NSAID use.
   D. Crohn's disease.
   E. Zollinger–Ellison syndrome.

7. Which of the following statements regarding IBS is incorrect?

   A. Stress and psychological factors play a significant role.
   B. A faecal calprotectin may exclude alternative diagnoses such as IBD.
   C. Patients may respond to a FODMAPS diet.
   D. Rome IV criteria are valuable in diagnosis of IBS.
   E. A colonoscopy is usually indicated to exclude alternative pathology.

Answers

1. E. NICE guidelines (2012) suggest PPI should not be offered routinely pre-endoscopy, since it does not reduce the risk of rebleeding or mortality; however, this remains common practice. A Blatchford score should be calculated prior to endoscopy to risk-stratify patients. There is no evidence that transfusion to Hb >100 g/L improves prognosis. Endoscopy should be offered to unstable patients immediately after resuscitation and to all other patients within 24 hours of admission. Repeat endoscopy is not routinely indicated and only performed if there is a high risk of rebleed or concern regarding the adequacy of haemostasis. (➲ See Acute upper gastrointestinal bleeding, p. 503 and Tables 14.5 and 14.6.)
2. A. This patient, who has known ulcerative colitis, most probably has a diagnosis of acute severe colitis with tachycardia and significant stool frequency. Excluding infective diarrhoea is vital, as this will alter further management. IV, not oral fluids, should be prescribed. A CT scan should not be performed unless there is significant clinical suspicion for an intra-abdominal collection or perforation. Hydrocortisone is prescribed at a dose of 100 mg QDS. (➲ See Box 14.4.)
3. D. While this history is highly suggestive of achalasia, patients with dysphagia should be investigated with gastroscopy in the first instance to exclude a malignancy of the upper GI tract. CT chest and abdomen may be indicated to stage an upper GI malignancy, but would not be a preferred first-line investigation. 24-hour pH manometry is a valuable diagnostic test to confirm an oesophageal motility disorder (e.g. achalasia) once an upper GI malignancy has been excluded. Barium swallow can be useful when achalasia is suspected, but unlikely to add anything above manometry studies. (➲ See Oesophageal disease, p. 494, including Dysphagia, p. 494.)
4. D. ZES results from acid hypersecretion from a gastrinoma, causing inappropriate hypergastrinemia in the setting of a low gastric pH. ZES should be considered in patients with severe ulceration of the upper GI tract or ulceration distal to the duodenum. (➲ See Zollinger–Ellison syndrome, p. 502.)
5. C. The majority of patients with SIBO have an underlying condition, which results in bacterial proliferation. (➲ See Small intestinal bacterial overgrowth, p. 508 and Box 14.2.)
6. B. The most likely diagnosis is of a false-negative rapid urease test in a patient with *H. pylori* infection. She should be offered non-invasive *H. pylori* testing while off PPI. PPI treatment is also associated with a modestly elevated serum gastrin. The other diagnoses are less likely causes of duodenal ulceration. (➲ See Disorders of the stomach and duodenum, p. 500, including *Helicobacter pylori* infection, p. 500, and Table 14.3.)
7. E. Colonoscopy is not indicated for a diagnosis of IBS in an uncomplicated patient who fulfils Rome IV criteria. Indications for colonoscopy would include a change in bowel habit, iron deficiency anaemia or rectal bleeding. (➲ See Indications, p. 492 and Irritable bowel syndrome, p. 515.)

Chapter 15 **Hepatology**

Stephen R. Atkinson and Ameet Dhar

Hepatology is a branch of medicine concerned with the study, prevention, diagnosis and management of diseases that affect the liver, gallbladder, biliary tree and pancreas. The term hepatology is derived from the Greek words 'hepatikos' and 'logia', which mean liver and study, respectively.

Anatomy and physiology

The liver, pancreas and biliary tree

Structure of the liver and biliary tree

The liver is the largest internal organ (1.2–1.6 kg), which lies inferior to the diaphragm and lateral to the stomach. It is comprised of four lobes. The liver receives its blood supply from the hepatic artery (25%) and the portal vein (75%). The venous drainage is via the hepatic vein to the inferior vena cava. The main blood vessels and bile ducts enter and leave the liver at the hilum.

Microscopic structure

- The lobule is the basic functional unit.
- Sinusoids are specialised capillaries. They do not have basement membrane, and are lined by fenestrated endothelial cells and hepatic macrophages.
- Hepatocytes are arranged in columns between sinusoids and are separated from them by the space of Disse.
- Stellate cells regulate blood flow through sinusoids, synthesise extracellular matrix and generate fibrosis.

The biliary tree

- Bile is excreted from hepatocytes into biliary canaliculi running between them.

- Canaliculi coalesce to form ductules, which enter bile ducts at the portal tract.
- Bile ducts join to form segmental ducts, which merge to form the right and left bile ducts, which then form the common hepatic duct.
- The gallbladder drains via the cystic duct into the common hepatic duct to form the common bile duct, which drains with the pancreatic duct into the second part of the duodenum via the ampulla of Vater.
- The sphincter of Oddi at the lower end of the common bile duct is tonically contracted, but relaxes in response to neurohormonal stimuli generated by eating, releasing bile and pancreatic juices.

For the macro- and microscopic anatomy of the liver, pancreas and biliary tree, see Figure 15.1.

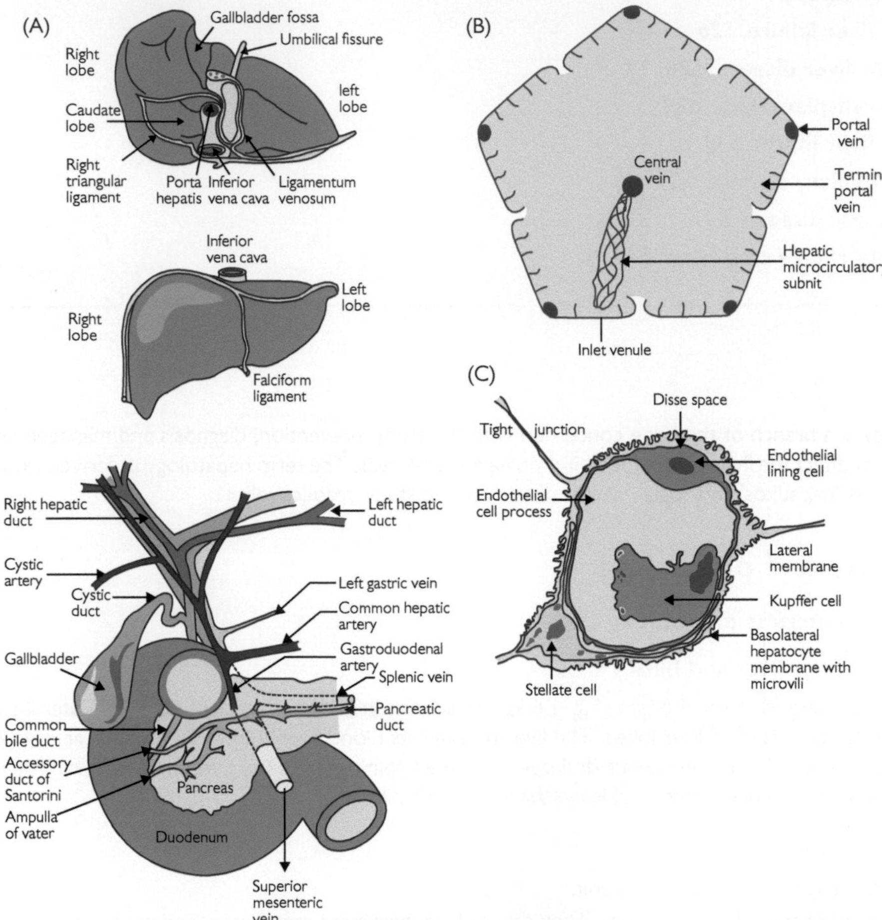

Figure 15.1 Macro- and microscopic anatomy of the liver, pancreas and biliary tree.

Normal hepatic function

- *Energy metabolism includes:*
  - Carbohydrate, protein and lipid synthesis and storage,
  - Degradation, detoxification and secretion of metabolic waste products. Major route for elimination of nitrogenous waste (deamination of amino acids [ammonia excreted by the kidney]).

- *Protein synthesis*, particularly:
  - Coagulation factors (except factor VIII).
  - Albumin.
  - Transport proteins, e.g. transferrin, caeruloplasmin.
  - Acute phase proteins, e.g. C-reactive protein, ferritin.

  Abnormalities in hepatic protein synthesis may be used to assess organ function (e.g. PT, albumin), cause of disease (e.g. α1-antitrypsin deficiency) or indicate underlying disease (e.g. α-FP and HCC).
- *Hormone inactivation and metabolism*, including insulin, glucagon, oestrogens and glucocorticoids. Failure to metabolise oestrogens in chronic liver disease leads to gynaecomastia, paucity of body hair and testicular atrophy in men.
- *Xenobiotic metabolism*: metabolism of toxins and drugs, may be important for elimination or activation, altered liver function may change the pharmacokinetics and side effect profiles of many classes of drugs (➲ See Chapter 3, Metabolism, Excretion, p. 78 and Table 3.16).

Bile

- Bile is important for the digestion of lipids, excretion of metabolic products (e.g. cholesterol, bilirubin), elimination of xenobiotics and neutralisation of gastric acid.

Production

- Increased by gastrin and secretin (~500 mL/day normally).
- Organic solutes (bile acids, phospholipids, cholesterol) are actively transported into the canaliculi; water and electrolytes follow by osmosis.
- Stored and concentrated in the gallbladder, which contracts when stimulated by cholecystokinin (CCK).

Specific components

- Bile acids (10%): critical for emulsification and absorption of dietary lipids. Bile acids are re-absorbed in terminal ileum and return to the liver via the portal vein (enterohepatic circulation).
- Bile pigments (~3%): bilirubin, a potentially toxic product of haem breakdown, is the most important (Figure 15.2). Hepatic conjugation with glucoronic acid (by uridine diphosphoglucuronosyl transferase) increases solubility and permits elimination (via multi-drug resistance protein 2, MRP2).

The pancreas

The pancreas is a retroperitoneal organ, which is macroscopically divided into its head, neck, body, tail and uncinate process. The head lies in the concavity formed by the second and third parts of the duodenum, the remainder stretches superiorly and across the midline to left hypochondrium. The pancreas receives its blood supply from the pancreaticoduodenal arteries and pancreatic branches of the splenic artery; venous drainage is via the splenic and the superior mesenteric veins. Lymphatic drainage is to the coeliac, superior mesenteric, aorto-caval and para-aortic lymph nodes. In the tail, several ductules converge to form the pancreatic duct, which joins the common bile duct at the duodenal papilla.

Microscopic structure

- Endocrine: islets of Langerhans (~1 million) each comprised of four cell types (➲ See Chapter 19, Pathogenesis, p. 671).
- Exocrine: ductal and acinar cells. The majority of the pancreas is arranged in lobules with secretions draining into a ductile.

Normal function of the pancreas

Endocrine and exocrine functions of the pancreas are critical to digestion, absorption and utilisation of nutrients. The endocrine functions of the pancreas are summarised in Table 15.1.

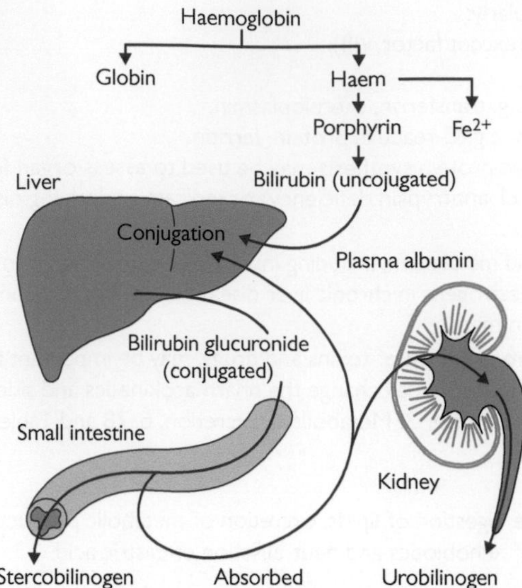

Bilirubin is formed by the breakdown of haemoglobin. In the liver, bilirubin is conjugated with glucuronic acid by hepatocytes, making it water soluble. Conjugated bilirubin is secreted in bile and passes into the gut. Some is taken up again by the liver (the enterohepatic circulation) and the rest is converted to urobilinogen by gut bacteria. Urobilinogen is either reabsorbed and excreted by the kidneys, or converted to stercobilin.

Figure 15.2 The production and excretion of bilirubin.

Reproduced with permission from Gastroenterology. In: *Oxford Handbook of Clinical Medicine*, 10th edn, Wilkinson IB, et al. (Eds). Oxford: OUP. Copyright © 2017 Oxford University Press. DOI: 10.1093/med/9780199689903.001.0001. Reproduced with permission from the Licensor through PLSclear.

Exocrine functions of the pancreas

The pancreas produces ~1.5 L of pancreatic juice per day, which contains:

- Pro-enzymes to degrade proteins (trypsin, elastase), lipids (lipase) and carbohydrates (amylase). Proenzymes are released from acinar cells in response to CCK, and are activated in the duodenum by enterokinase and trypsin.
- Bicarbonate and water to neutralise gastric acid. Bicarbonate is released from ductal cells in response to secretin.

Table 15.1 Major hormones synthesised and released from islets of Langerhans

Hormone	Islet cell source	Stimulus	Action
Glucagon	α cells	↓Insulin secretion. ↓Glucose.	↑Glycogenolysis. ↑Gluconeogenesis.
Insulin	βcells	↑Glucose. ↑Other nutrients (e.g. amino acids, fatty acids). Neurogenic.	↑Glucose uptake. ↑Glycogenesis. ↑Fatty acid synthesis. ↑Amino acid uptake.
Pancreatic polypeptide	PP or F cells	Food intake (mainly protein). Vagal stimulation.	Appetite regulation. ↓Gut motility. ↓Exocrine pancreas secretions (*via* inhibition of insulin action).
Somatostatin	δCells	↑Glucose. ↓Gastric pH.	↓Islet hormones (especially glucagon and insulin).

Further reading

1. Gimson A, Rushbrook S. Gastroenterological disorder, Section 19, Structure and Function of the liver, biliary tract and pancreas. In: Warrell, D.A., Cox, T.M. and Firth J.D. (Eds) *Oxford Textbook of Medicine*, 5th edn. Oxford: Oxford University Press, 2016.

Investigation of the hepatobiliary and pancreatic systems

Blood tests

For blood tests used in the assessment of liver disease, see Table 15.2.

Table 15.2 Blood tests used in the assessment of liver disease

Test	Source	Comments
Bilirubin	Haemoglobin breakdown	Conjugated hyperbilirubinaemia indicates hepatic dysfunction. Used to determine severity and prognosis, and to assess response to treatment.
ALT and AST	Hepatocytes	Intracellular enzymes released from dying hepatocytes. Do not reflect liver function.
ALP and GGT	Biliary epithelium	Found in the bile ducts and elevated in response to injury. Raised GGT is sensitive, but not specific for alcohol abuse.
Albumin	Synthesised by hepatocytes	Often falls in acute and chronic illness and, therefore, does not always reflect liver function. Proteinuria should always be excluded in hypoalbuminaemia.
PT or INR	Clotting factors synthesised in the liver	Reduced synthesis in liver disease leads to prolonged PT/INR. The short half-life of clotting factors makes the PT/INR useful in monitoring liver injury.

Investigation of liver disease

- *Ultrasound* is the first-line imaging modality for hepatobiliary disease.
- *CT and MRI* are used second-line to characterise lesions found on ultrasound, and to provide better anatomical resolution of the pancreas.
- *Endoscopic procedures* include endoscopic retrograde cholangiopancreatogram and endoscopic ultrasound (➲ see Chapter 14, Endoscopic retrograde cholangiopancreatography procedure, p. 492 and Endoscopic ultrasound procedure, p. 492).
- *Liver biopsy* is used to diagnose and assess the severity of hepatic disease. It is usually undertaken percutaneously under US guidance, but in the patients with coagulopathy or ascites the trans-jugular (TJ) route should be used.

Further reading

1. Kaye TL, Guthrie JA. Imaging the liver and biliary tract. *Medicine*. 2015;43(10):562–7. https://www.medicinejournal.co.uk/article/S1357-3039(15)00193-0/fulltext.

Presentations associated with liver disease

Abnormal liver function tests

Liver disease is often asymptomatic, further investigation or consideration of hepatology referral is required for:

- Patients with risk factors or signs of liver disease.
- Significant elevations in LFTs (>2× upper limit of normal [ULN]).
- Persistent abnormalities in LFTs (>6 months).

Initial investigation usually comprises a non-invasive liver screen of blood tests and US. Non-hepatic causes (e.g. alkaline phosphatase in bone disease, alanine aminotransferase [ALT] in muscular injury) should be excluded.

For blood tests used for investigation of abnormal LFTs, see Table 15.3.

Table 15.3 Blood tests used for investigation of abnormal LFTs (non-invasive liver screen)

Test	Abnormality	Relation to liver disease
FBC	Macrocytosis	May indicate alcohol excess.
	Thrombocytopenia	Can suggest hypersplenism related to portal hypertension.
Ferritin	Elevated ferritin	Associated with haemochromatosis, non-alcoholic and alcoholic fatty liver disease.
Copper studies	Serum copper (low) Serum caeruloplasmin (low)	Wilson's disease.
HBV surface antigen	Positivity	HBV infection. If positive perform full HBV serology and DNA level.
HCV IgG	Positivity	Past or chronic HCV infection. If positive perform HCV RNA level.
Immunoglobulins	Elevated IgG Elevated IgM	Autoimmune liver disease, polyclonal expansion in cirrhosis. Primary biliary cirrhosis (PBC).
Anti-mitochondrial antibodies	Positive	M2 pattern in PBC.
Anti-smooth muscle or anti-nuclear antibodies	Positive	Autoimmune hepatitis.
Alpha-1-antitrypsin	Low	Alpha-1-antitrypsin deficiency.

Different patterns of liver biochemistry suggest different causes:

1. Hepatocellular: ALT and aspartate transaminase (AST) raised in excess of other liver enzymes.
2. Cholestatic: ALP and gamma-glutamyl transferase (GGT) raised in excess of other liver enzymes.
3. Isolated hyperbilirubinaemia (other liver biochemistry normal): conjugated (e.g. Gilbert's) or unconjugated (e.g. haemolysis).

For patterns of abnormal LFTs and associated diseases, see Table 15.4.

If a specific cause is not identified, then management may involve:

- Steps directed towards the most likely aetiology (e.g. weight loss for possible non-alcoholic fatty liver disease, abstinence from alcohol, discontinuation of possible causative drugs).
- Liver biopsy (~60% of liver biopsies in this group demonstrate steatosis ± non-alcoholic steatohepatitis).

Jaundice

Biochemically defined as elevated bilirubin (typically >21 μmol/L), clinically apparent > 40 μmol/L. Aetiologies include:

1. *Overproduction of bilirubin*: predominantly unconjugated, rarely >70 μmol/L, caused by increased red cell breakdown (i.e. haemolysis, haematoma dissolution).
2. *Failure of bilirubin conjugation*: either impaired delivery of bilirubin to the liver (e.g. congestive cardiac failure, portosystemic shunting) or enzymatic defects (e.g. Gilberts disease, Crigler–Najjar syndrome).

Table 15.4 Patterns of abnormal LFTs and associated diseases

Abnormality	Putative causes (listed alphabetically)
ALT ≤5× ULN (ALT > AST)	Autoimmune hepatitis. Coeliac disease. Drug-induced liver injury. Haemochromatosis. NAFLD. Viral hepatitis. Wilson's disease.
ALT ≤5× ULN (AST > ALT)	Alcoholic liver disease. Cirrhosis.
ALT ≤5× ULN (extrahepatic)	Haemolysis. Myopathy, strenuous exercise. Thyroid disease.
ALT/AST 5–25× ULN	Acute viral hepatitis. Autoimmune hepatitis. Drug-induced liver injury.
ALT/AST >25× ULN	Acute viral hepatitis. Ischaemic hepatitis. Paracetamol toxicity.

3. *Failure to export bilirubin across the canalicular membrane*: conjugated. Divided into intrahepatic (e.g. viral or alcoholic hepatitis, *MRP2* mutation in Dubin–Johnson syndrome) and extrahepatic (e.g. biliary obstruction). May also occur in non-hepatic conditions (e.g. sepsis).

Gallstones

Uncomplicated gallstone disease

Gallstones are present in ~7% of Western populations. Most gallstones are cholesterol-based; pigment stones form in individuals with chronic haemolysis (e.g. sickle cell disease) or ileal disease. Risk factors include female gender, Caucasian, native American or Hispanic ethnicity, age >40 years, obesity, rapid weight loss and pregnancy.

Clinical presentation

- Biliary colic: right upper quadrant discomfort, may radiate to back and shoulder, classically intermittent.
- Nausea and dyspepsia.
- Incidental finding on US: the majority of patients with gallstones discovered incidentally will remain asymptomatic; 25% experience biliary colic and 1% per year develop complicated disease.
- Gallstone ileus: for presentation and investigations (➔ see Chapter 5, Case 9, 130).

Investigation

- Transabdominal US (sensitivity 84%; specificity 99%). If negative, consider other causes of symptoms.
- If strong suspicion and no alternative cause MRCP is appropriate (CT is less helpful).
- EUS and bile sampling can exclude small gallstones and microlithiasis, respectively.

Complicated gallstone disease

Choledocholithiasis (gallstones in the common bile duct)

Presentation

- Biliary colic and abnormal liver biochemistry ± jaundice.
- May be asymptomatic with abnormal imaging or LFTs.
- May be complicated by acute pancreatitis or cholangitis.

Management

- Definitive management is required; first choice is cholecystectomy, ductal clearance must be established and confirmed first to avoid retained stones.
- ERCP may be used to clear stones, stent (to establish drainage) and perform sphincterotomy (to reduce the likelihood of further stone impaction).

Cholangitis (infected, obstructed biliary tree)

The bacterial infection of static bile results from organisms ascending from the duodenum, usually gram negative bacilli (e.g. *E. coli*, *Klebsiella*); 10–20% are Gram-positive enterococci.

Presentation

- Charcot's triad: right upper quadrant pain, fever and jaundice. May have septic shock.
- Mortality in severe disease nearly 50%.

Investigation

- Blood tests: neutrophilia, conjugated hyperbilirubinaemia, ↑ALP and GGT (usually in excess of the aminotransferases). ALT may be elevated (acute hepatocyte necrosis).
- Imaging: US is first line, but may be negative in ~15%. MRCP is second line (90–95% sensitivity for CBD stones). ERCP remains the gold standard for diagnosing CBD stones.

Management and outcome

- Treat sepsis (fluid resuscitation, blood cultures, antibiotics).
- Restore biliary drainage either endoscopically (ERCP) or by percutaneous transabdominal cholangiography (PTC).
- Most patients improve with conservative measures and biliary drainage may be restored semi-electively.
- Persistent severe sepsis or pain despite conservative measures are indications for urgent biliary drainage. ERCP also allows stone extraction and sphincterotomy.
- PTC is used when clinical condition or anatomy preclude ERCP.

Further reading

1. Clinical Practice Guideline Panel. EASL Clinical Practice Guidelines on the prevention, diagnosis and treatment of gallstones. *J Hepatol*. 2016;65(1):146–81.

Acute liver failure

Acute liver failure (ALF) is defined by hepatocellular injury with hepatic dysfunction and encephalopathy in the absence of pre-existing, chronic liver disease. It may be further categorised into hyperacute, acute and subacute subtypes based upon the duration of illness (<7, 7–21 and 22–180 days, respectively, more than 180 days is not acute). The underlying aetiology is the main determinant of clinical course and outcome.

Common causes include:

1. Drugs: paracetamol, aspirin, statins, flucloxacillin, anti-tuberculous chemotherapy.
2. Toxins: alcohols, *Amanita* toxin.

3. Viral: hepatitis viruses A, B, C, D and E, adenovirus, EBV, CMV, HSV.
4. Immunological: autoimmune hepatitis, haemolysis, elevated liver enzymes and low platelets (HELLP) syndrome.
5. Metabolic: Wilson's disease, acute fatty liver of pregnancy.
6. Vascular: Budd–Chiari, hypoperfusion/ischaemia.

When no caused can be identified, the term 'seronegative' ALF is applied. In the Western world paracetamol toxicity is the most common cause of ALF, while in developing countries viral hepatitis predominates.

Symptoms of ALF may be non-specific (lethargy, malaise, anorexia, nausea and vomiting), or related to liver impairment and inflammation (pruritus related to jaundice, right upper quadrant discomfort). Clinical features include jaundice, hepatic encephalopathy, cerebral oedema and acute portal hypertension (ascites), renal failure (30–50%) and pulmonary oedema (~30%).

Investigations

Laboratory tests

- FBC and coagulation profile. PT is the best marker of liver function and changes are of prognostic significance.
- Liver biochemistry: elevated bilirubin, elevated transaminases (pattern may suggest cause).
- Renal biochemistry: renal failure occurs in 30–50%, it is more frequent in paracetamol poisoning and Wilson's disease.
- Calcium, magnesium, phosphate, glucose and LDH.
- Toxicology screen (including paracetamol and salicylate levels).
- Viral and autoimmune serology (including HIV).
- Arterial blood gases, ammonia and lactate.
- Pregnancy test in females.

Imaging

- US with Dopplers of the main hepatic vessels to exclude vascular pathologies and features of pre-existing liver disease. Contrast-enhanced imaging should be performed with caution due to the risk of contrast nephropathy.

Management

- Close monitoring of biochemical and neurological parameters.
- Pre-emptive discussion and prompt transfer to liver unit for those showing features of worsening liver function.
- Prothrombin time is an important prognostic marker, but patients may develop severe bleeding. Correction of coagulopathy with FFP or prothrombin complex concentrate may be necessitated for procedures or to prevent bleeding.
- Monitoring and correction of physiological parameters (fluid replacement and inotropes).
- Maintenance of nutrition.
- Prompt diagnosis and treatment of sepsis; patients are vulnerable to both bacterial and fungal infections. Sepsis can be difficult to differentiate from the systemic inflammatory response caused by liver injury.

Specific treatments

- NAC for paracetamol toxicity. There should be a low threshold for commencing NAC as the history may be unclear, and NAC may be beneficial in liver failure due to other causes.
- Restoration of venous drainage in Budd–Chari (i.e. with transjugular intrahepatic portosystemic shunt [TIPSS] insertion or anti-coagulation).
- Anti-viral therapies: nucleoside analogues for HBV, aciclovir for HSV.
- Plasma exchange to remove copper in acute Wilson's disease.

Transplantation

Most patients (40-60%) recover with medical therapy; those who deteriorate despite treatment require consideration of liver transplantation. Clinical parameters used in selection for transplantation are the same as those which confer a poor prognosis (Table 15.5). Identification of patients who will do badly is poor (up to 35% of patients listed for transplantation recover spontaneously). One-year survival post-transplantation is >90%.

Further reading

1. McPhail MJ, Kriese S, Heneghan MA. 2015. Current management of acute liver failure. *Curr Opin Gastroenterol.* 2015;31(3):209–14.

Table 15.5 Selection criteria for liver transplantation in ALF (King's college criteria)

Paracetamol-induced ALF	**Non-paracetamol-induced ALF**
Strongly consider if: • Arterial lactate >3.5 mmol/L after early fluid resuscitation. List if: • pH <7.3 or lactate >3.0 mmol/L after adequate volume replacement. • All three of the following criteria are met: • Grade 3 or 4 encephalopathy. • Creatinine >300 μmol/L. • INR >6.5.	List if: • INR >6.5 and encephalopathy present (any grade). • Any three of the following are met: 1. <10 or >40 years of age. 2. Jaundice >7 days before encephalopathy. 3. INR >3.5. 4. Bilirubin >300 μmol/L. 5. Aetiology associated with poor outcome (Wilson's, seronegative, drug-induced liver injury).

Chronic liver disease

Chronic liver disease is characterised by slowly progressive liver injury over time (>6 months, typically many years), leading to the accumulation of fibrosis within the liver and the eventual development of cirrhosis. The major causes (alcohol, chronic HBV and hepatitis C virus [HCV], NAFLD) are discussed in ➲ Hepatobiliary disease, p. 534. Progressive loss of functional hepatocyte mass leads to synthetic dysfunction (hypoalbuminaemia, coagulopathy), failure of metabolic and excretory functions (altered drug metabolism, jaundice), and accumulation of fibrotic tissue leads to portal hypertension and associated complications. The first presentation of chronic liver disease is often with decompensated cirrhosis defined by the development of jaundice, ascites or hepatic encephalopathy.

Clinical examination may reveal features of:

1. Chronic liver disease: leukonychia (hypoalbuminaemia), palmar erythema, spider naevi, and gynaecomastia and paucity of body hair in men.
2. Decompensation: shifting dullness (ascites), jaundice, asterixis (encephalopathy).
3. Portal hypertension: shifting dullness (ascites), caput medusa, splenomegaly.

Ascites

Ascites is defined as the presence of free fluid within the abdomen; in chronic liver disease it develops due to presinusoidal portal hypertension and is associated with:

- Changes in vascular tone: general vasodilatation, raised NO levels.
- Sodium retention (and, therefore, water) due to secondary hyperaldosteronism.
- Decreased ability to excrete free water due to increased antidiuretic hormone (ADH).

Presentation is either symptomatic (e.g. abdominal distension, breathlessness due to diaphragmatic splinting) or as an incidental finding on ultrasound. On examination, shifting dullness (>1–1.5L ascites) or a fluid thrill (tense ascites) may be detectable.

Key investigations when assessing ascites are:

- Abdominal ultrasound with Dopplers to quantify volume, identify appearances of chronic liver disease and portal hypertension, and exclude portal vein thrombosis.
- Fluid should be sampled (tapped) and analysed for WCC to exclude spontaneous bacterial peritonitis (SBP), Gram stain, bacterial culture, and albumin and total protein levels. Fluid LDH, amylase, lipids and cytology may be sent dependent upon appearance and putative causes.
- Calculate serum albumin ascites gradient (SAAG). SAAG = ascitic fluid [albumin] – serum [albumin]; if ≥1.1 g/L suggests ascites secondary to portal hypertension (Table 15.6).

Table 15.6 Interpretation of Serum albumin ascites gradient (SAAG)

High SAAG (≥11 g/L)	Low SAAG (<11 g/L)
Cirrhosis Heart failure Budd–Chiari	Malignancy Tuberculosis Pancreatitis Nephrotic syndrome Autoimmune serositis

The treatment of ascites includes:

- Sodium (<90 mmol/day) and fluid restriction (<1.5 L/day).
- Diuretics: spironolactone (initially 100 mg/day, but up to 400 mg/day), furosemide may be added.

Treatment should target gradual weight loss of 0.5 kg/day (i.e. 500 mL) and patients must be monitored for complications of therapy (hyponatraemia, hyperkalaemia and renal dysfunction). Failure to respond to or inability to tolerate diuretic therapy should trigger consideration of liver transplantation or TIPSS.

Spontaneous bacterial peritonitis

Patients with ascites may develop the complication of SBP due to translocation of bowel organisms into ascites, leading to infection of the fluid. Causative organisms are typically bowel flora (e.g. *E. coli, Klebsiella* sp.), though streptococcal and staphylococcal infections may occur.

SBP may present with fever, abdominal tenderness and an altered mental state, in addition to the clinical features of ascites. SBP must be considered in any patient with ascites with a deterioration in liver function tests. Patients with a low ascitic fluid albumin are at highest risk. Diagnosis is based upon an ascitic fluid WCC >250/mm^3 with >50% neutrophils.

Management entails

- Empirical broad-spectrum antibiotics (e.g. piperacillin-tazobactam, ciprofloxacin), after appropriate cultures have been sent.
- Renal failure and hepatorenal syndrome (HRS) may develop. Early plasma expansion with human albumin solution (HAS) reduces the risk, if this fails IV terlipressin is used.
- Recurrence of SBP approaches 70%, patients surviving an episode should receive antibiotic prophylaxis (lifelong or until liver transplantation).
- A single episode confers a poor prognosis and should prompt consideration of transplantation.

Hepatorenal syndrome

HRS is a cause of kidney injury typically occurring in patients with decompensated cirrhosis.

Contributing pathophysiological factors may include:

- Reduction in effective renal arterial blood volume due to systemic and splanchnic vasodilatation, resulting from the accumulation of vasodilators (e.g. NO).

- Compensatory activation of the renin-angiotensin-aldosterone system and renal vasoconstriction.
- Impaired renal autoregulation resulting in reduced GFR for any given renal perfusion pressure.
- Portal hypertension reducing renal blood flow via excessive sympathetic activation.
- Impaired myocardial contractility.

These factors combine to reduce renal perfusion and thus the GFR, and increase sodium retention. In chronic liver disease, renal impairment is usually slowly progressive (Type 2 HRS), but may be precipitated by an acute event (e.g.GI bleeding, alcoholic hepatitis or sepsis, particularly SBP), leading to a rapidly progressive renal failure within <2 weeks (Type 1 HRS). HRS may develop in patients with fulminant hepatic failure of any aetiology. Hyponatraemia indicates increased risk.

HRS is a diagnosis of exclusion; pre-renal, renal and post-renal causes of kidney injury must be considered and eliminated. Progressively rising creatinine, oliguria, low urinary sodium, inactive urinary sediment and insignificant proteinuria (<500 mg/day) are the classic combination of features found in HRS. Importantly, in HRS the kidneys are histologically normal.

Management principles

- Identify and address acute causes for decompensation of liver function.
- Ensure adequate resuscitation.
- Vasopressors (terlipressin, occasionally noradrenaline in critical care) in combination with albumin in those not responding to initial measures.
- Renal replacement therapy may provide a holding measure to allow recompensation of hepatic function or a bridge to liver transplantation.

Prognosis is poor, without therapy death is virtually inevitable, with therapy 30-day survival is 30–40%, and is inextricably linked to recovery of hepatic function.

Further reading

1. European Association for Study of the Liver. EASL clinical practice guidelines on the management of ascites, spontaneous bacterial peritonitis, and hepatorenal syndrome in cirrhosis. *J Hepatol*. 2010;53:397–417.

Hepatic encephalopathy

Hepatic encephalopathy (HE) is a syndrome of confusion and altered consciousness in patients with advanced liver failure (acute or chronic). It is often reversible, resolving with treatment of precipitants or restoration of liver function.

The pathogenesis has not been fully elucidated, but probably relates to a combination of the development of cerebral oedema, glial cell swelling, impaired cerebral auto-regulation of blood flow and neurotoxin accumulation.

For grading of HE (Westhaven criteria), see Table 15.7.

The diagnosis is made on predominantly clinical grounds. Elevated ammonia is neither sensitive nor specific for HE. Electroencephalograms (EEG) may suggest a metabolic encephalopathy (e.g. generalised slowing, triphasic waves, delta waves).

Key principles of management

- *Exclude alternative explanations for an altered mental status*, particularly sepsis, electrolyte imbalance (e.g. hyponatraemia) and renal failure, intoxication or withdrawal (e.g. alcohol, opiates, benzodiazepines), hypoglycaemia and intracranial pathology (especially subdural haematoma).
- *Identify and manage precipitants*, e.g. sepsis, GI bleeding, constipation, electrolyte disturbances, hepatic vascular occlusion, development of hepatocellular carcinoma (HCC) and portosystemic shunting.

Table 15.7 Grading of HE (Westhaven criteria)

Grade	Features
Minimal	Subtle changes in behaviour and cognition often only detectable using psychometric testing.
Grade 1	Changes in behaviour (euphoria, depression, disinhibition), mild confusion, sleep disturbance (sleep–wake cycle reversal).
Grade 2	Lethargy, moderate confusion, asterixis, easily rousable.
Grade 3	Drowsy, but rousable to voice or pain, incoherence, marked confusion and disorientation.
Grade 4	Coma.

Adapted with permission from Ferenci, P. et al. Hepatic encephalopathy—Definition, nomenclature, diagnosis, and quantification: Final report of the Working Party at the 11th World Congresses of Gastroenterology, Vienna, 1998. *Hepatology* 35(3), 716-721. https://doi.org/10.1053/jhep.2002.31250. © 2003 American Association for the Study of Liver Diseases. Adapted with permission from Wolters Kluwer Health, Inc.: Schiff, E. R. etl al (eds.), Diseases of the Liver, Seventh Edition, © 1993 Lippincott Williams & Wilkins.

- *Specific treatments*:
  - *Lactulose* reduces ammonia levels by acidification of the gut lumen and a reduction in the colonic bacterial load. Titrate to achieve a soft bowel action 2–3 times per day. Additional laxatives may be required.
  - *Antibiotic therapy* to reduce colonic bacterial load, particularly ammonia producing bacteria. Rifaximin is a non-absorbable broad-spectrum antibiotic, which reduces symptoms related to HE and the frequency of relapses in patients with recurrent HE.

Further reading

1. American Association for the Study of Liver Diseases and European Association for the Study of the Liver. Hepatic Encephalopathy in Chronic Liver Disease: 2014. *J Hepatol*. 2014;61:642–59.

Hepatocellular carcinoma

HCC is the most common primary liver cancer. The majority of patients who develop HCC have cirrhosis (~ 90%). African or Asian ethnicity, and a positive family history also confer higher risk. Hepatitis B is oncogenic and patients with chronic HBV may develop HCC in the absence of cirrhosis.

Clinical presentation

The development of HCC is usually asymptomatic until advanced, but the diagnosis should be considered in any patient with chronic liver disease whose hepatic function deteriorates or decompensates. Patients may develop clinical features related to mass effect (e.g. liver capsule pain, obstructive jaundice), vascular invasion causing thrombosis or tumour embolisation, or metastatic disease. Rarely, HCC may present as a pyrexia of unknown origin and occasionally a hepatic bruit may be found.

Due to the vastly increased risk of HCC conferred by cirrhosis, all patients with cirrhosis should be screened for HCC with 6-monthly US. Patients with chronic HCV with advanced liver fibrosis or HBV, and either an active hepatitis or a positive family history for HCC should also be offered screening even in the absence of cirrhosis.

Diagnosis

- *Triple-phase CT*: a patient with HCC may demonstrate a characteristic and diagnostic pattern of contrast enhancement. These changes are: arterial blush (hypervascularity) and late or venous stage washout (less contrast enhancement compared with normal liver), and probably reflect an altered pattern of blood supply to HCC compared with normal liver (arterial blood supply predominates, comparatively little portal blood supply). If present, there is no need for biopsy.
- *Liver biopsy*: a targeted biopsy may be performed where there is diagnostic uncertainty.
- *Alpha fetoprotein* is commonly elevated in HCC, although is not advocated as a screening or diagnostic marker.

Treatment

Treatment of HCC depends upon tumour stage and severity of liver disease. Options include hepatic resection, liver transplantation, RFA, transarterial chemoembolisation of tumours (TACE), systemic chemotherapy or palliation. Prognosis is generally poor and, in spite of treatment, the median survival is only 6 months in patients with cancer-related symptoms or vascular invasion.

Further reading

1. European Association for the Study of the Liver. EASL-EORTC Clinical Practice Guidelines: Management of hepatocellular carcinoma. *J Hepatol*. 2012;56:908–43.

Varices

Varices are dilated veins that develop predominantly at sites of portosystemic anastomosis and decompress the portal system. All patients with a new diagnosis of cirrhosis should undergo upper GI endoscopy to screen for oesophageal varices, with repeat screening endoscopy every 2–3 years.

Risk of bleeding from varices depends on size (positive correlation), appearance (erythema, red wale sign) and location (gastro-oesophageal junction varices are at highest risk due to the thinnest layer of overlying mucosa). Unfavourable appearances (occupying more than one-third of the oesophageal lumen, red wale sign) warrant primary prophylaxis with a non-selective β-blocker (e.g. propranolol) or, if this is not tolerated, variceal band ligation should be considered.

Management of variceal haemorrhage

Variceal haemorrhage has a high mortality (~33%) and presents with features of GI bleeding (haematemesis, melaena, haemodynamic instability).

Management of variceal haemorrhage entails:

- Resuscitation, initially with colloid or crystalloid. Patients with large volume, ongoing blood loss or haemoglobin <8 g/dL should receive transfusion.
- Correction of coagulopathy with blood products where there is active bleeding and evidence of coagulopathy (INR >1.4, platelets <30).
- Terlipressin (1–2 mg bolus followed by 1–2 mg QDS) and broad-spectrum antibiotics improve mortality and reduce the incidence of complications (re-bleeding, infection).
- Urgent upper GI endoscopy within 12 hours, or sooner if ongoing haemodynamic instability despite resuscitation. Oesophageal varices should be treated by endoscopic variceal band ligation, while gastric varices are treated by gluing.

Balloon tamponade (Sengstaken tube) can provide a temporary measure if formal endoscopic therapy is not possible or unavailable. Ongoing or recurrent bleeding soon after endoscopic therapy or in patients with severe decompensated liver disease should trigger consideration of TIPSS.

Further reading

1. Tripathi D, Stanley AJ, Hayes PC, et al. UK guidelines on the management of variceal haemorrhage in cirrhotic patients. *Gut*. 2015;64:1680–704.

Prognostic scoring systems in chronic liver disease

Prognostic scoring systems are widely used in chronic liver disease to assess the severity of disease and guide clinical decision-making.

The Child–Pugh–Turcotte scoring system

Patients are assigned a score for each of five variables, which are then summated to give a score between 5 and 15 (Table 15.8). Group A (5–6 points) are considered well compensated, while groups B (7–9) and C (10–15) signify decompensated disease. Classes A, B and C predict 1-year survival rates of 100%, 80% and 45%, respectively.

Table 15.8 The Child–Pugh–Turcotte scoring system

	1	2	3
Albumin	>35 g/L	28–35 g/L	<28 g/L
Ascites	None	Mild	Moderate or severe
Bilirubin	<34 μmol/l	34–50 μmol/l	>50 μmol/l
Encephalopathy	None	Grade I–II	Grade III–IV
INR	<1.7	1.7–2.3	>2.3

Adapted with permission from Pugh, R. N. H. et al. Transection of the oesophagus for bleeding oesophageal varices. *British Journal of Surgery*. 1973 Aug 1;60(8):646–9. Copyright © 2005, BJS Society Ltd and John Wiley and Sons. https://doi.org/10.1002/bjs.1800600817.

The model for end-stage liver disease score

The model for end-stage liver disease score is widely used to predict short-term survival in chronic liver disease and to assist in transplant listing decisions and organ allocation. It is calculated from the creatinine, bilirubin and INR.

Acute-on-chronic liver failure

Acute on chronic liver failure is defined by a rapid deterioration in hepatic function in patients with cirrhosis. This syndrome is associated with organ failure, renal dysfunction and hepatic encephalopathy, and carries a high risk of short-term mortality (50–90%). It is often precipitated by infection though surgery, bleeding or a drug injury may also be responsible.

Management involves careful screening for and treatment of sepsis, expectant management of complications of hepatic failure, provision of organ support and consideration of liver transplantation.

Liver transplantation

Indications

- Failure to recover liver function in acute liver failure.
- Decompensated chronic liver disease.
- HCC in patients with early disease and good liver function.
- 'Variant' syndromes even when liver function is good, e.g. chronic or recurrent cholangitis in primary sclerosing cholangitis, refractory ascites or hepatic encephalopathy.

The decision to transplant is based primarily upon mortality risk without transplantation and the ability of transplantation to improve quality of life. Patients may be listed electively (chronic liver disease) or urgently (paracetamol toxicity, seronegative hepatitis, acute Wilson's disease or veno-occlusive disease with poor prognostic features). Transplantation treats hepatic dysfunction, but not the underlying disease, and for many indications there is a risk of recurrence (e.g. hepatitis B/C, autoimmune liver diseases and ALD).

Further reading

1. European Association for the Study of the Liver. EASL Clinical Practice Guidelines: Liver transplantation. *J Hepatol.* 2015;64:433–85.

Acute liver injury

Paracetamol poisoning and drug-induced liver injury

Drug-induced liver injury (DILI) is common (~1:10,000 individuals), with up to a third of cases of acute hepatitis and liver failure being caused by drugs. Drugs may induce one of several patterns of liver injury – hepatocellular toxicity, cholestasis, and both macro- or microvesicular steatosis. The pattern of injury may be reflected in the LFTs and help identify the aetiological agent (➲ see Table 3.6). Some drugs, for example, dapsone, methyldopa, sulfonamides and diclofenac, may cause DILI via predominantly immune-mediated mechanisms and be associated with eosinophilia and systemic features, such as fever and rash. DILI may be dose-dependent or independent. Drugs causing dose-dependent hepatotoxicity (e.g. paracetamol) reliably produce toxic metabolites. Innate and adaptive immune mechanisms appear to cause idiosyncratic dose-independent reactions, often accompanied by systemic symptoms (e.g. fever, rash). Female sex, older age, excess alcohol, polypharmacy and co-morbid liver disease have all been described as risk factors for the development of idiosyncratic DILI. Many cases of DILI are subclinical and detected as asymptomatic elevations in liver enzymes.

An accurate and detailed drug history, including herbal, over-the-counter and alternative medicines is vital to identifying putative causes. A non-invasive liver screen, including US to exclude biliary obstruction, is important to exclude non-drug causes of liver injury. Where the diagnosis is unclear, a liver biopsy may be performed; however, there are no histological hallmarks and it can be difficult to distinguish DILI from autoimmune hepatitis.

The most important measure in management is to stop the offending drug. Re-challenge should be avoided due to the risk of more a severe reaction. Liver function should be monitored with serial biochemistry. Patients with severe injury (encephalopathy or INR >1.5), particularly if failing to improve following withdrawal of the offending agent, should be managed in a specialist unit as transplantation may be indicated.

Specific treatments include N-acetylcysteine for paracetamol and levocarnitine for sodium valproate toxicity (➲ see Chapter 3, Paracetamol, p. 83 and Figure 3.3, and Valproate, p. 89, respectively).

Asymptomatic elevations of liver enzymes almost universally resolve (within weeks to months). Most acute liver injury resolve with supportive management. Cholestatic patterns of injury are generally less severe. Aminotransferases >3× ULN and the bilirubin > double normal carry mortality rates as high as 10%.

Further reading

1. Chalsani NP, Hayashi PH, Bonkovsky HL, et al. ACG Clinical Guideline: the diagnosis and management of idiosyncratic drug-induced liver injury. *Am J Gastroenterol*. 2014;109:1–17.

Ischaemic hepatitis

Ischaemic hepatitis arises due to interruption of blood supply to all or part of the liver, and may result from hypotension (e.g. cardiogenic or septic shock) or thrombosis (e.g. sickle cell crisis). The liver's dual blood supply confers protection against vascular occlusion – hepatic artery occlusion typically only produces ischaemic hepatitis if there is co-existent portal vein compromise. Hepatocellular ischaemia leads to widespread necrosis.

The condition is characterised by an early, massive rise in serum transaminases (often ~200 × ULN) and LDH. The precipitating episode is usually clinically apparent. Mild circulatory disturbance may, however, be sufficient in predisposed individuals (e.g. pre-existing congestive hepatopathy or portal hypertension). The diagnosis is clinical and liver biopsy is not usually required.

The clinical course and treatment are determined by the underlying condition. Transaminases peak early (~24 hours) and decline sharply over ~7 days, assuming resolution of the precipitating insult.

Hepatobiliary disease

Alcoholic liver disease

Alcoholic liver disease (ALD) comprises a spectrum of disease in individuals who misuse ethanol (typically >60 g/day in women; >80 g/day in men). Ethanol is metabolised in the liver by alcohol dehydrogenase to acetaldehyde, and then by acetaldehyde dehydrogenase to acetate. This process generates reactive oxygen species, which induce oxidative stress causing hepatocyte necrosis and apoptosis. Chronic ethanol ingestion causes accumulation of intracellular fatty acids and steatosis. Increased gut permeability and lipopolysaccharide in the portal circulation cause neutrophil recruitment leading to steatohepatitis. Inflammation causes hepatocyte injury and produces a fibrotic reaction through activation of hepatic stellate cells. On biopsy alcoholic steatohepatitis is characterised by hepatocyte ballooning, necrosis and apoptosis, combined with steatosis and Mallory–Denk bodies.

Epidemiology

- The development of liver disease is related to lifetime exposure to ethanol.
- Female gender and Hispanic ethnicity increase risk.
- Alcohol speeds up progression of other liver diseases, especially chronic HCV.
- Progression is not universal; 90–100% develop steatosis, 10–35% steatohepatitis, only 8–20% progress to cirrhosis.

Most patients present with cirrhosis or its complications, some may present with abnormal LFTs. A minority of patients present with alcoholic hepatitis, a clinical syndrome of new onset of jaundice with features of liver failure. The Maddrey's discriminant function (mDF), derived using a calculation incorporating the serum bilirubin and PT, is used to assess the severity of disease; severe disease is defined by an mDF >32.

The principle of investigation and management entail

- Screening for and managing:
  - Concomitant causes of liver disease.
  - Complications of cirrhosis.
  - Nutritional deficiencies.
- Excluding biliary obstruction and infection in patients with severe alcoholic hepatitis.
- Achieving and maintaining abstinence is critical.
- Prednisolone may be used in severe alcoholic hepatitis.

Steatosis is reversible, in more advanced disease abstinence prevents progression. In cirrhosis, prognosis is related to the severity of liver dysfunction and continued alcohol consumption, which accelerates progression and decompensation. Patients with severe alcoholic hepatitis have a poor prognosis with 28-day mortality ~25%.

Alcoholic liver disease is the commonest indication for liver transplantation in the Western world. Five-year survival is 72% compared with ~23% in a comparable untransplanted population.

Further reading

1. European Association for the Study of the Liver. EASL Clinical Practical Guidelines: Management of Alcoholic Liver Disease. *J Hepatol*. 2012;57:399–420.

Chronic viral hepatitis

HBV and HCV infection are the commonest causes of chronic liver disease worldwide.

Hepatitis B

The HBV virus is a double-stranded DNA virus comprising a core (nucleocapsid, DNA and polymerase) in a lipid envelope (host-derived containing viral surface antigen). Infection leads to liver damage via two main mechanisms – direct cytopathic effect (minor) and T-cell killing of infected hepatocytes (major). Inflammation caused by the immune response leads to progressive fibrosis and eventually cirrhosis. Patients who develop a profound immune response may develop an acute hepatitis. Hepatitis B is oncogenic (up-regulation of host oncogenes by viral infection) and confers an increased risk of HCC.

Around 300 million individuals are infected worldwide, with 500,000 attributable deaths annually. Transmission of hepatitis B may be horizontal (sexual transmission, injection drug use, health care-associated) or vertical (perinatal). In the developed world, sexual and percutaneous transmission predominate, while in developing countries the majority of new infections are due to vertical transmission from mother to child in the perinatal period and horizontal transmission between children (especially siblings) under 5.

The clinical course of hepatitis B infection is variable:

- Acute hepatitis develops after an incubation period of 1–4 months and typically resolves over 3 months. It is usually subclinical or manifests as constitutional symptoms with a transaminitis.
- Jaundice occurs in the acute phase in a third of patients; fulminant hepatic failure is rare (0.5%).
- Clearance of the virus is defined by undetectable viral surface antigen (HBsAg) and DNA (HBV DNA) with seroconversion to produce surface antibody (anti-HBs IgG).
- Persistence of HBsAg for >6 months defines chronic infection.

- Likelihood of chronic infection is primarily determined by age at time of infection (children infected perinatally have a 90% chance of developing chronic infection, in adults this falls to 5%).

For phases of chronic HBV infection based on the immune system response to the virus, see Table 15.9.

Treatment

Treatment with antivirals should be considered in patients with:

- HBV DNA >2000 IU/mL and serum ALT persistently > ULN.
- Moderate to severe necroinflammation and/or moderate fibrosis.
- Cirrhosis, even if ALT is normal.
- Decompensated cirrhosis and detectable HBV DNA (urgent treatment required).

The aims of treatment are to suppress HBV DNA, normalise ALT levels, and to prevent the development of cirrhosis and HCC. Further assessments include measurement of liver stiffness by Fibroscan and a liver biopsy. Once commenced, treatment is commonly continued indefinitely. Antivirals are most commonly prescribed (either a nucleoside [e.g. lamivudine, entecavir] or a nucleotide analogues [e.g. tenofovir]); interferon may be used in certain situations.

Those not receiving treatment require regular monitoring for development of chronic active hepatitis.

Co-infection with hepatitis D can cause aggressive disease, treatment is challenging (usually with interferon-α).

Further reading

1. European Association for the Study of the LiverEASL Clinical Practice Guidelines: Management of chronic hepatitis B virus infection. *J Hepatol*. 2012;57:167–85.

Hepatitis C

The hepatitis C virus is a small, enveloped, single positive strand RNA flavivirus. There are four common genotypes (1–4) with different geographical distributions and varying responses to treatment. Genotype 1 is most common in Europe and North America. In North Africa and the Middle East genotype 4 is particularly prevalent.

The viral genome includes a protease which cleaves viral polyproteins and is essential in its lifecycle. The HCV RNA polymerase lacks proof-reading capacity and generates a large number of viral quasi-species, which assist in evasion of host immune responses. Hepatic inflammation results from T-cell killing of infected hepatocytes.

Predominant mode of transmission is blood-borne (e.g. infected blood products, sharing contaminated needles for IV drug use or contaminated health-care equipment). Around 216,000 individuals in the UK are chronically infected; injection drug-use is the most important risk factor. Chronic infection develops in 80–100% of exposed individuals.

Affected individuals may present following:

- Screening of at-risk individuals.
- Investigation of clinical, biochemical or imaging evidence of chronic liver disease.
- Investigation of extrahepatic manifestations of HCV infection, e.g. cryoglobulinaemia, glomerulonephritis, porphyria cutanea tarda or lichen planus.

Typically, HCV infection has a long course with disease progressing to cirrhosis after around 30 years. Male sex, older age at time acquisition, viral co-infection, obesity and particularly alcohol are risk factors for more rapid disease progression.

Diagnosis and work-up entails:

- Hepatitis C antibody test. A positive result requires further evaluation by HCV viral RNA load and genotyping (confirms chronic infection).
- Non-invasive estimation of fibrosis (Fibroscan).

Routine liver biopsy is not mandatory but informative regarding fibrosis and inflammation, particularly in those with an abnormal Fibroscan result. The specific treatment is based upon genotype, stage of liver

Table 15.9 Phases of chronic HBV infection based upon the immune response to the virus

Phase	HBsAg	anti-Hbs	HBeAg	anti-HBe	HBV DNA	ALT	Duration	Comments
Immune tolerant phase	+	–	+	–	++++	Normal	10–30 years	High HBV replication and infectivity, no immune response and therefore no inflammation.
Immune reactive phase	+	–	+	–	++	Raised	Typically occurs during second and third decades	An immune response attempts to clear the virus. Viral load falls and ALT rises but wax and wane until seroconversion (eAb production).
Immune control phase	+	–	–	+	±	Normal	Years	Replication is suppressed by immune response. Minimal inflammation and consequently normal liver enzymes.
Immune escape phase (chronic eAg negative hepatitis)	+	–	–	+	++	Raised	Years	Evolution of a variant able to replicate without eAg leads to recurrent hepatitis with higher levels of HBV DNA, necro-inflammation and progressive liver injury.
Resolution	–	+	–	+	–	Normal	Theoretically indefinite	0.5-1% patients per year clear HBsAg. Reactivation may occur especially with immunosuppression.

disease and patient preference. New direct-acting antivirals, with or without pegylated interferon and ribavirin, have revolutionised treatment with cure rates >90% achievable for all common genotypes. The use of interferon is associated with significant physical and psychiatric side effects, including decompensation in patients with cirrhosis, and interferon-free regimens are increasingly available. Liver transplantation prior to treatment should be considered for those with decompensated disease. Post-transplant recurrence is almost invariable and often more aggressive.

Further reading

1. European Association for the Study of the Liver. EASL recommendations on treatment of hepatitis C. *J Hepatol.* 2017;66(1):153–94.

Non-alcoholic fatty liver disease and non-alcoholic steatohepatitis

NAFLD is defined as hepatic steatosis in the absence of an alternative cause (e.g. alcohol, HCV). Patients are classified as having non-alcoholic steatohepatitis (NASH) when there is evidence of inflammation and fibrosis on liver biopsy. The disease results from an excess of hepatocellular lipids causing cellular death and inflammation (steatohepatitis) with resultant fibrosis.

Risk factors for development of NAFLD and NASH include the features of the metabolic syndrome (hypertension, insulin resistance, central adiposity, hypertension and dyslipidaemia).

NAFLD is most prevalent in the Western world, affecting ~20% of the Western population, with NASH in 5%.

Patients may complain of nausea or right upper quadrant discomfort, and may occasionally present with advanced liver disease. Most patients are, however, asymptomatic and discovered incidentally with abnormal liver biochemistry or 'fatty liver' on imaging.

Investigations

Investigations typically reveal:

- Mild elevations in the transaminases (2–4× ULN) and raised ferritin (transferrin saturation is not elevated).
- Hepatic steatosis on imaging.
- Absence of other causes of hepatitis.

Liver biopsy may be required to evaluate diagnostic uncertainty or concerns regarding advanced fibrosis. Management involves achieving weight loss, avoiding other causes of liver injury (e.g. alcohol) and aggressive management of metabolic risk factors.

Further reading

1. European Association for the Study of the Liver. EASL-EASD-EASO Clinical Practice Guidelines for the management of non-alcoholic fatty liver disease. *J Hepatol.* 2016;64:1388–402. http://dx.doi.org/10.1016/j.jhep.2015.11.004.

Autoimmune hepatitis, primary biliary cirrhosis and primary sclerosing cholangitis

For the key features see Table 15.10.

Further reading

1. European Association for the Study of the Liver. EASL Clinical Practice Guidelines: autoimmune hepatitis. *J Hepatol.* 2015;63:971–1004.
2. Chapman R, Fevery J, Kalloo A, et al. Diagnosis and management of primary sclerosing cholangitis. *Hepatology.* 2010;51:660–78.

Haemochromatosis

Hereditary haemochromatosis is an autosomal recessive disorder caused by mutations in the *HFE* gene (chromosome 6) leading to loss of protein function, which modulates intestinal iron uptake. The two

Table 15.10 Key features of autoimmune hepatitis, primary biliary cirrhosis and primary sclerosing cholangitis

Pathogenesis	Onset/associations	Presentation	Investigations	Management/complications
Autoimmune hepatitis				
Immune-mediated chronic active hepatitis of unclear aetiology. Hepatocyte damage is mediated by autoreactive T cells.	Most commonly diagnosed in the 5th decade. Female to male ratio of 4:1. May have a history of autoimmune disease (HLA-DR3 and DR4 strongly associated with AIH in Caucasians).	Spectrum from abnormal LFTs to fulminant hepatitis. Non-specific symptoms such as arthralgia, malaise, nausea and pruritus.	↑ ALT, AST and globulins. Positive autoantibodies (ANA, anti-Sm, anti-soluble liver antigen, anti-LKSM or anti-LC1). Liver biopsy is confirmatory with interface hepatitis and portal lymphocytic cell infiltrates.	Prednisolone and azathioprine. 90% of patients respond to treatment with sustained remission off treatment achieved in 10–40%.
Primary biliary cirrhosis				
Autoimmune liver disease characterised by T-cell mediated destruction of small bile ducts. Biliary ductular obliteration leads to progressive cholestasis and secondary hepatocellular damage and cirrhosis.	Significant female preponderance (95%). Typically diagnosed in the fourth decade. Associated with HLA-DR8 and certain mutations in CTLA-4 (an immunological co-receptor).	Pruritus. Fatigue. Arthralgia. Arthritis. Clinical findings include hyperpigmentation, xanthelasma, excoriation and features of chronic liver disease.	Anti-mitochondrial antibodies are the serological hallmark (seen in 95%). M2 pattern is pathognomonic.	Ursodeoxycholic acid. Management of complications and associated diseases including itch, malabsorption, fat-soluble vitamin deficiency, dyslipidaemia, hypothyroidism and sicca syndrome. Liver transplantation may be required.
Primary sclerosing cholangitis				
Progressive, inflammatory condition affecting the bile ducts causing fibrotic stricturing and cholestasis. Overlap with autoimmune liver disease.	Uncommon (1:100,000) with a slight male preponderance. Usually diagnosed in the fourth to fifth decades. Up to 90% of those affected have evidence of IBD. Associated with HLA-DRw52a.	Abnormal LFTs. Non-specific symptoms include lethargy, and malaise. Later disease may present with cholangitis or chronic liver disease.	Cholestatic LFTs: ↑ ALP/GGT. Markers of autoimmunity (p-ANCA, hypergammaglobulinaemia). MRCP (first line)*: multifocal biliary ductular narrowing with upstream dilatation. ERCP (second line)*: for therapeutic intervention stenting or diagnostic sampling. Liver biopsy to diagnose small duct primary sclerosing cholangitis. * ➲ See Chapter 5, Case 10, p. 131.	Ursodeoxycholic acid can to improve liver biochemistry and may help prevent malignancy. Episodes of cholangitis are treated with antibiotics ± ERCP to improve biliary drainage. Significant risk of cholangiocarcinoma and gallbladder cancer warrants annual screening (MRI/MRCP, US and Ca19-9). Higher risk of colon cancer; annual surveillance with colonoscopy is recommended. Liver transplantation may be indicated for end-stage liver disease.

common causative mutations are *C282Y* and *H63D* (*C282Y* homozygosity accounts for 90% of cases). The resultant increase in iron absorption leads to excess iron deposition in several organs, particularly the heart, liver, gonads and pancreas. Patients may therefore develop cardiomyopathy, chronic liver disease, hypogonadism and (endocrine) pancreatic insufficiency.

Presentation

- Typically in fourth to sixth decade, although later in women due to menstrual blood loss.
- Most often with abnormalities on routine LFTs or screening relatives of affected individuals.
- <25% have end-organ involvement at presentation.
- Fatigue and arthralgia are the most common presenting symptoms.
- Clinical examination may reveal hepatomegaly, features of diabetes, arthropathy due to iron deposition in joints (classically second and third metacarpophalangeal joints, and large joints [➲ see Chapter 20, Haemochromatosis, p. 751]).

Diagnosis

Diagnosis is based upon demonstrating primary iron overload:

- Ferritin >300 μg/L is suggestive, but may be associated with excess alcohol, NAFLD, acute phase response or malignancy.
- Transferrin saturations >45% suggest primary iron overload warranting further investigation.
- HFE genotyping is diagnostic; if inconclusive a liver biopsy may be considered to estimate hepatic iron content.

Patients with serum ferritin <1000 μg/l and normal LFTs have a good prognosis; treat without further evaluation. Patients with a higher ferritin or evidence of liver disease should be considered for a liver biopsy. Symptomatic patients or those with significant iron overload on biopsy should undergo further investigations for evidence of other non-hepatic end-organ damage.

Treatment involves regular venesection, which is typically initiated weekly until iron indices return to normal (ferritin <50 μg/l, transferrin saturation <50%), with maintenance venesection less frequently thereafter. A reduction in dietary iron should also be advised.

With treatment, those without significant liver disease, diabetes or cardiomyopathy have near normal life expectancy. Cirrhosis may improve with treatment, however cardiomyopathy, diabetes and arthropathy are generally irreversible.

Wilson's disease

Wilson's disease is a rare autosomal recessive disorder (1 in 30,000) caused by a mutation in ATP7B (chromosome 13, transport protein responsible for the excretion of copper in bile). Failure of biliary copper excretion leads to copper accumulation, which is predominantly deposited in the liver, eyes and central nervous system.

Presentation

Presentation can be very variable:

- Patients are usually young at diagnosis (first to fourth decades).
- Adolescents typically present with neurological sequelae, rather than liver disease.
- May present with ALF (classically young female patients) and is associated with haemolysis, chronic active hepatitis or asymptomatic biochemical abnormalities.
- Neurological features include dystonia, dysarthria, chorea, tremor and Parkinsonism due to cerebellar and basal ganglia copper deposition. Behavioural and psychiatric symptoms are common.

The classic triad of Wilson's disease is of decreased serum caeruloplasmin, raised 24-hour urinary copper excretion and Kayser–Fleischer rings on slit lap examination (corneal copper deposition; not always present). Neurological features, haemolytic anaemia, elevated copper on liver biopsy and *ATP7B* mutations on genetic analysis may all aid in making a diagnosis.

Treatment

Treatment entails measures to reduce total body copper through reduction in dietary intake and life-long chelation therapy (e.g. penicillamine or zinc acetate). In ALF, dialysis and plasma exchange may be used to rapidly remove copper.

With appropriate treatment the prognosis is generally good; biochemical liver abnormalities and neurological dysfunction tend to improve with successful chelation therapy. For patients with rapidly progressive liver failure mortality is 95% without treatment, although post-transplantation survival is excellent.

Alpha-1-antitrypsin disease

Alpha-1-antitrypsin is a serine protease inhibitor which inhibits neutrophil elastase. Loss of function causes lung disease (➲ see Chapter 11, Bronchiectasis, p. 356). Liver disease is associated with the mutant Z and S alleles (M is wild type), which change the protein conformation and lead to intrahepatocyte polymerisation and damage. Disease may present as chronic active hepatitis or end-stage liver disease. Around half of adults with *PiZZ* genotype (the most severe) have clinically significant liver disease.

No specific therapy is available. Liver transplantation may be performed for decompensated liver disease. Frequently, the lung disease, rather than the liver disease, determines prognosis.

Budd–Chiari syndrome

Budd–Chiari syndrome is veno-occlusive disease causing hepatic venous outflow obstruction at any level between the small hepatic veins and the inferior vena cava. Venous obstruction causes hepatic congestion, ischaemia, distension and dysfunction. Patients frequently have underlying thrombophilia or myeloproliferative disease.

Presentation

- Female preponderance (2:1), often presents in the fourth decade.
- Rapid development of jaundice and ascites and subsequent encephalopathy.
- May follow a more subacute course with progressive development of mild liver biochemical derangements.
- Right upper quadrant pain and hepatomegaly are common.

Doppler US or contrast CT demonstrating hepatic vein or inferior vena caval thrombus are diagnostic. Variants are recognised where obstruction is limited to the small hepatic veins, which may only be diagnosed by liver biopsy.

Treatment entails anticoagulation and consideration of interventional procedures to relieve (angioplasty, stenting) or bypass (TIPPS, surgery) obstruction and resolve portal hypertension. Transplantation is indicated for fulminant Budd–Chiari with anticoagulation to prevent recurrent thrombosis.

Malignant tumours of the hepatobiliary system

For malignant tumours of the hepatobiliary system, see Table 15.11.

Pancreatic disease

Acute pancreatitis

Acute pancreatitis is an acute inflammatory disease, which often produces a profound systemic inflammatory response. Release and activation of proteolytic enzymes within the pancreas leads to auto-digestion. Damaged acinar cells release further trypsinogen and cross-activation of other proteolytic enzymes occurs leading to an exponential increase in pancreatic damage. Spillover of pancreatic enzymes and inflammatory

Table 15.11 Malignant tumours of the hepatobiliary system

Tumour type	Clinical features
Metastatic deposits	Most common malignant liver lesion. Typically multiple. Primary usually GI, breast, lung or melanoma.
Hepatocellular carcinoma	Typically in chronic liver disease (HBV or cirrhosis). Raised α-fetoprotein.
Cholangiocarcinoma	Rare (0.01% incidence), arising from the intra- or extrahepatic bile ducts. Often advanced at presentation with (painless) obstructive jaundice and constitutional symptoms. Diagnosis is made by a combination of imaging (US, CT, MRCP) and ERCP (cytology and therapy). CEA and CA19-9 may be elevated. Local disease may be resected. Chemotherapy, radiotherapy, embolisation and/or ablation with palliation of obstructive jaundice (stenting or bypass) in advanced disease.
Gallbladder cancer	Uncommon. Symptoms tend to mimic gallstone disease. Constitutional symptoms may be present in advanced disease, which may cause obstructive jaundice due to invasion or mass effect. Diagnosis can be made on ultrasound or MRCP. Serum CEA and CA19-9 may be elevated. Local disease is treated by surgical resection whilst advanced disease is treated with radiotherapy ± systemic chemotherapy.

cytokines into the systemic circulation leads to a systemic inflammatory response (SIRS) and multi-organ dysfunction.

Epidemiology

- Incidence is around 30 per 100,000.
- Risk factors: gallstones (most common), alcohol, smoking, hypertriglycerideaemia, drugs (e.g. azathioprine), hypercalcaemia, infections (e.g. mumps, CMV) and toxins (snake, spider or scorpion venom).
- An acute pancreatitis can be initiated by trauma and may also occur post-ERCP.

Presentation is typically with sudden onset abdominal pain, classically epigastric and radiating to the back. Nausea and vomiting are typical. Patients experience abdominal tenderness, with peritonism in severe cases. Rarely, patients with haemorrhagic, necrotising pancreatitis may display ecchymotic lesions in the flanks (Grey–Turner's sign) or peri-umbilical region (Cullen's sign).

The diagnosis is made based upon a typical history with supporting biochemistry and imaging. Serum amylase >3× ULN has good sensitivity and specificity for a diagnosis of acute pancreatitis, but the level may have fallen if presentation is delayed or may not reach this threshold if there is a background of chronic pancreatitis. CT will demonstrate pancreatic oedema, and areas of hypoperfusion and necrosis; US or MRI may be used to identify gallstones. Increasing age, acidosis, WCC, respiratory distress, hypocalcaemia and haemodynamic compromise confer a worse prognosis.

Management principles

- Fluid resuscitation, analgesia and close monitoring.
- Oral nutrition may be poorly tolerated due to nausea, vomiting or ileus, and is withheld to reduce pancreatic stimulation.
- If the condition settles rapidly, oral feeding may resume; prolonged illness necessitates consideration of naso-jejunal or parenteral feeding.
- Infections are common: prophylactic antibiotics are not warranted, but clinical vigilance is required.
- Early ERCP may be considered in patients with severe gallstone pancreatitis, common bile duct obstruction and cholangitis.
- Disease may be complicated by necrotic collections and pseudocyst formation, which can become secondarily infected. These may require drainage (transcutaneously or endoscopically) or by surgery.

Prognosis is related to severity; overall mortality is 5%, rising to ~20% in patients with necrotising disease and almost 50% for those developing multi-organ failure.

Further reading

1. Working Group IAP/APA Acute Pancreatitis Guidelines. IAP/APA evidence-based guidelines for the management of acute pancreatitis. *Pancreatology*, 2013;13(4, Suppl. 2):e1–15. https://www.sciencedirect.com/science/article/pii/S1424390313005255?via%3Dihub.

Chronic pancreatitis

Persistent or recurrent pancreatic inflammation causes progressive patchy architectural distortion, fibrosis and development of foci of calcification. Subsequent loss of exocrine and endocrine tissue ensues. The majority is related to alcohol excess, other causes include cystic fibrosis, pancreatic duct obstruction, autoimmune disease (e.g. SLE), hereditary pancreatitis (autosomal dominant) or idiopathic disease.

Pain (typically epigastric and radiating to the back) is a prominent, but not universal, feature of chronic pancreatitis and can be difficult to manage. It may be continuous or worsened by eating, and is often characterised by exacerbations potentially necessitating hospital admission. Nausea and vomiting may also be present, particularly during exacerbations of disease. Exocrine insufficiency may produce steatorrhoea and clinical features of malabsorption. Endocrine insufficiency and resultant diabetes typically occur late in the disease process.

Investigations

- The diagnosis is based upon demonstration of exocrine insufficiency (clinical features, low faecal elastase) in combination with suggestive imaging changes (calcification and ductal distortion).
- MRCP is the imaging modality of choice. ERCP is reserved for cases where therapeutic intervention is warranted (stricture dilatation, stenting or stone removal).
- In those without a clear risk factor, a family history should be taken and genetic testing for mutations associated with hereditary pancreatitis (CFTR, SPINK-1 and PRSS-1) should be considered.

Management principles

- Modification of risk factors (alcohol abstinence, stopping smoking) and lifestyle advice (small, low-fat meals).
- Pancreatic enzyme supplementation (e.g. Creon®) to treat malabsorption and steatorrhoea. These can also alleviate pain.
- Analgesic agents introduced in a stepwise fashion. The use of tricyclic antidepressants and pregabalin as adjuvant analgesia may reduce opiate requirements.
- Patients with pain and a dominant pancreatic ductal stricture or stone may require an ERCP.
- Surgery for those failing medical treatment (resection or denervation).

Pancreatic malignancy

The vast majority of pancreatic cancers are exocrine (95%), the majority of which are ductal adenocarcinomas. A small number are of endocrine origin. The prognosis is generally poor as patients usually have advanced disease at presentation.

Risk factors for the development of pancreatic malignancy include male gender, age (>45 years), genetic (familial clustering, inherited cancer syndromes such as BRCA1, Peutz–Jehgers and Lynch syndrome), chronic pancreatitis, diabetes, obesity and smoking.

Patients often present with non-specific symptoms of weight loss, malaise and anorexia. Mass effect may lead to obstructive jaundice and abdominal pain radiating to the back. Tumours in the head of the pancreas (~67%) cause jaundice more frequently, back pain is often a feature of tumours in the body or tail Palpation may reveal a mass or hepatomegaly. Courvoisier's sign (palpable non-tender gallbladder) is present in up to 10% of cases.

First-line imaging is usually US. It has good sensitivity for larger tumours and is typically the first investigation in obstructive jaundice. CT should be performed for staging where US suggests cancer, or first line when pancreatic malignancy is considered to be the most likely diagnosis. EUS, PET-CT and even laparoscopy may all be required for accurate staging, particularly if surgery is being considered. Biopsy may be performed during EUS or by percutaneous CT-guided biopsy. CA19-9 has reasonable sensitivity and specificity for large exocrine pancreatic cancers.

Surgery is the only potential curative treatment, although only 20% are suitable at presentation and post-operative 5-year survival is 30% at best. Surgery for head of pancreas tumours classically entails a pancreaticoduodenetomy (Whipple's procedure; removal of the pancreatic head, gallbladder, duodenum, a small segment of jejenum plus partial gastrectomy).

Chemotherapy, with or without radiotherapy, can be offered to those without resectable disease. Biliary interventions such as ERCP and PTC may relieve biliary obstruction and provide symptomatic relief. Median survival is around 12 months.

Multiple choice questions

Questions

1. A 34-year-old man presents to his GP with flu-like symptoms. No specific abnormalities are detected on examination. Blood tests are normal with the exception of his liver function tests which are noted to be abnormal:

    Bilirubin 43 μmol/l (0–21 μmol/L).
    ALT 21 IU/L (0–41 IU/L).
    AST 17 IU/L (0–40 IU/L).
    ALP 84 IU/L (40–129 IU/L).

    He reports consuming 6 pints of cider on a Friday and Saturday night, and recreational marijuana use, otherwise there are no risk factors for liver disease. What is the most likely diagnosis?

    A. Ischaemic hepatitis.
    B. Acute hepatitis A.
    C. Primary sclerosing cholangitis.
    D. Gilbert's disease.
    E. Alcoholic liver disease.

2. A 29-year-old man of Pakistani origin presents with weight loss, fevers and abdominal distension. On examination there is shifting dullness. He undergoes blood tests and a diagnostic ascitic tap.

    Liver function tests demonstrate:

    Bilirubin 23 μmol/l (0–21 μmol/L).
    ALT 12 IU/L (0–41 IU/L).
    AST 10 IU/L (0–40 IU/L).
    ALP 81 IU/L (40–129 IU/L).
    Albumin 22 g/L (35–52 g/L)
    Amylase is 170 IU/L (28–100 IU/L).

    Ascitic fluid:

    Red cell count <50/mm^3.
    White cell count 700/mm^3 (27% neutrophils, 73% monocytes).
    Albumin 19 g/L and Gram stain stain negative.

    What is the likely diagnosis?

    A. SBP.
    B. Tuberculous ascites.
    C. Budd–Chiari.
    D. Pancreatic ascites.
    E. Malignant ascites.

3. A 53-year-old man with known cirrhosis secondary to long-standing alcohol misuse is brought to A&E by his wife. His wife reports recent increasing unsteadiness, falls and confusion, she is unsure whether he is still consuming alcohol.

   He is currently taking vitamin B co-strong, codeine and lactulose. On examination he is disorientated and his GCS is 13, pupils are of normal size, equal and reactive, there is notable bruising over his right temple, no asterixis is demonstrated, although there is a mild tremor with past-pointing on the right hand side. Biochemistry reveals bilirubin 70 μmol/L (0–21 μmol/L), ALT 31 IU/L (0–41 IU/L), AST 67 IU/L (0–40 IU/L).

   What is the next most appropriate step?

   A. EEG.
   B. Arterial ammonia.
   C. CT head.
   D. Blood alcohol concentration.
   E. Naloxone challenge.

4. A 72-year-old woman with known cirrhosis secondary to autoimmune hepatitis presents to A&E reporting a single episode of large volume haematemesis and two episodes of melaena. She last opened her bowels 6 hours ago. On examination she is noted to have pulse rate 94 beats/minute, blood pressure 98/30 mmHg, spider naevi, mild icterus and mild splenomegaly. Her blood tests reveal:

   Hb 9.5 (120–165 g/L).
   Platelets 67 (150–400 × 10^9/L).
   Urea 23 (2.5–7.8 mmol/L).
   Creatinine 102 (50–111 μmol/L).

   In addition to volume resuscitation, what is the next most appropriate step in her management?

   A. Upper GI endoscopy.
   B. High-dose IV proton pump inhibition.
   C. Terlipressin.
   D. Transfusion with packed red cells.
   E. Broad-spectrum antibiotics.

5. A 67-year-old man with a history of chronic congestive heart failure is noted by his GP to have abnormal LFTs. He is currently taking furosemide, rosuvastatin, ramipril, aspirin and clopidogrel. In addition, he had taken 5 days of a 2-week course of co-amoxiclav for a cellulitis of his left leg.

   LFTs:

   Bilirubin 17 μmol/l (0–21 μmol/L).
   ALT 62 IU/L (0–41 IU/L).
   AST 51 IU/L (0–40 IU/L).
   ALP 671 IU/L (40–129 IU/L).

   His last tests 3 months ago were entirely normal.

   Which drug is most likely responsible for his abnormal liver function tests?

   A. Aspirin.
   B. Co-amoxiclav.
   C. Furosemide.
   D. Ramipril.
   E. Rosuvastatin.

6. A 32-year-old woman is referred to hepatology services following a positive hepatitis B test on pregnancy screening bloods.

   Full hepatitis B serology demonstrates:

   HBsAg positive.
   HBcAb IgG positive.

HBV DNA 1,200 copies/mL.
HBeAb positive.
HBeAg negative
ALT 21 (0–33 IU/L).

What is the most appropriate description of the stage of her hepatitis B infection?

A. Acute hepatitis B.
B. Immune tolerant phase.
C. Previous hepatitis B vaccination.
D. Immune control phase.
E. Previous hepatitis B infection.

7. A 34-year-old man is referred to hepatology outpatients with abnormal LFTs. He has a past medical history of diabetes, hypertension and attention-deficit hyperactivity disorder. He reports drinking 13 units of alcohol per week. On examination there are no stigmata of chronic liver disease, his BMI is noted to be 36 kg/m^2.

Blood tests show:

Bilirubin 17 μmol/l (0–21 μmol/L).
ALT 93 IU/L (0–41 IU/L).
AST 60 IU/L (0–40 IU/L).
ALP 102 IU/L (40–129 IU/L).
GGT 242 IU/L (10–71 IU/L).
Ferritin 812 μg/L (30–400 μg/L).
Transferrin saturation 21% (25–45%).
Serum copper 18 μmol/L (11–22).
Caeruloplasmin 0.42 g/L (0.15–0.30) .
Alpha-1-antitrypsin level 0.95 g/L (0.9–1.9).

What is the most likely diagnosis?

A. Haemochromatosis.
B. Non-alcoholic fatty liver disease.
C. Wilson's disease.
D. Alpha-1-antitrypsin deficiency.
E. Alcohol-related liver disease.

Answers

1. D. The presentation is typical of Gilbert's disease; an isolated hyperbilirubinaemia with otherwise normal LFTs. The ALT and AST would be significantly elevated in ischaemic or acute viral hepatitis, while in alcoholic liver disease an elevation of the AST would be anticipated with an AST:ALT ratio of at least 1.5. Primary sclerosing cholangitis would be associated with cholestatic LFTs (elevated ALP and GGT) (➲ see Abnormal liver function tests, p. 523 and Table 15.4).
2. B. There is a low serum albumin ascites gradient (SAAG) ascites (3 g/L). Budd–Chiari and ascites in chronic liver disease (in which SBP could develop) are associated with a high SAAG. There are no features in the history to suggest pancreatic disease and malignancy is usually associated with bloody ascites. The presentation and ethnicity are consistent with tuberculous disease and the predominantly monocytic, low SAAG ascites would be characteristic (➲ see Chronic liver disease, Ascites, p. 528).
3. C. The aetiology of the patient's confusion is probably multifactorial, although with the recent onset of falls, evidence of head injury and findings indicating focal neurology an intracranial pathology should be excluded. Patients with alcohol-related liver disease are at increased risk of subdural haemorrhage due to frequent falls due to intoxication and involutional cerebral changes related to chronic alcohol misuse. Ammonia is neither sensitive nor specific for hepatic encephalopathy (which remains in the differential), an EEG would be helpful, but should be

performed once intracranial disease is excluded and intoxication and/or opiate toxicity have been allowed to resolve (➲ see Chronic liver disease, Hepatic encephalopathy, p. 530).

4. C. This patient has suffered an upper GI haemorrhage. She has chronic liver disease and features of portal hypertension, making a variceal bleed probable. Terlipressin is effective in controlling variceal bleeding and preventing rebleeding. In some studies it has been shown to be as effective as endoscopy. In the absence of contraindications, terlipressin should be administered empirically to patients with suspected variceal haemorrhage. Antibiotics have been shown to reduce morbidity and mortality in the setting of variceal haemorrhage, but their administration is less urgent than that of terlipressin. There is no indication for proton pump inhibition at this stage. In the absence of active bleeding, patients with variceal haemorrhage should be transfused to a target haemoglobin of 8–9 g/dL, over-transfusion has been associated with poorer outcomes. Upper GI endoscopy is clearly indicated. However, in the absence of ongoing haemodynamic instability, despite adequate resuscitation, patients should receive appropriate medical management first (➲ see Chronic liver disease, Varices, p. 532).
5. B. This is a cholestatic picture of liver enzyme abnormalities and is most likely related to recent co-amoxiclav usage. Statins and aspirin/NSAIDs typically cause a hepatocellular pattern of liver injury. Furosemide and ramipril are not typically implicated in drug-induced liver injury (➲ see Acute liver injury, Paracetamol poisoning and drug-induced liver injury, p. 533 and Table 3.6).
6. D. Serology demonstrates eAb seroconversion (HBeAg negative) with low-level HBV DNA and a normal ALT, these are characteristic of the immune control phase. Surface antigen positivity indicates ongoing hepatitis B infection indicating the results are not compatible with previous vaccination or resolved infection. Acute infection is associated with significantly raised HBV DNA and ALT and cAb IgM positivity (➲ see Hepatitis B, p. 535 and Table 15.9).
7. B. This patient has clinical features and blood tests consistent with the metabolic syndrome and NAFLD. The ferritin is often raised in NAFLD and the normal transferrin saturation indicates that there is no primary iron overload. The serum copper profile is normal and does not indicate Wilson's disease, similarly the serum alpha-1-antitrypsin is within normal limits. While the patient does drink alcohol, it is a comparatively small amount, and the AST to ALT ratio is not elevated. Alcohol cessation may improve liver biochemistry, but is unlikely to be the predominant cause of underlying liver disease. (➲ See Wilson's disease, p. 540, Haemochromatosis, p. 538, Alpha-1-antitrypsin disease, p. 541, Non-alcoholic fatty liver disease and non-alcoholic steatohepatitis, p. 538, and Alcoholic liver disease, p. 534).

Chapter 16 **Nephrology**

Behdad Afzali and Refik Gökmen**

Assessment of renal function

One-fifth to one-quarter of the cardiac output is 'seen' by the kidneys every minute. This is the renal blood flow and equates to ~1.2 L/min. Approximately 60% of the blood is plasma in an adult with a haematocrit of 40%. Therefore, the renal plasma flow (RPF), the fraction containing soluble substances, is ~700 mL/min.

The GFR is the amount of filtrate produced by the kidneys per minute (between 90 and 120mL/min in healthy, non-pregnant adults or ~180 L/day). One-fifth of the renal plasma flow is filtered by the glomeruli (the filtration fraction).

*Joint first authors.

Direct and indirect measurements of renal function

Renal function can be measured either directly or indirectly. Direct measurements, such as assessment of the clearance of injected substances, are invasive; therefore, renal function is usually estimated indirectly via surrogate markers, such as serum creatinine and estimated glomerular filtration rate (eGFR). Notably, these formulae have not been validated in a number of demographic groups (e.g. Asian populations) and are unreliable in pregnancy.

There are three important caveats to estimating GFR through these means:

1. All formulae rely on serum creatinine. Creatinine is derived from skeletal muscle and thus is affected by muscle bulk; amputees or those with muscle atrophy, therefore, incorrectly appear to have reduced eGFR.
2. Creatinine concentration represents a balance, *in the steady state*, between creatinine produced from muscle and creatinine cleared by kidneys. Situations causing flux in these opposing forces result in changing creatinines that do not reflect renal function. For example, in acute urinary obstruction causing anuria, serum creatinine usually only increases by approximately 100 μmol/L/day, despite the patient having close to zero renal function requiring immediate intervention. It may take several days before the serum creatinine reaches very high levels.
3. Some creatinine is actively excreted by renal tubules and not just filtered. Therefore, anything interfering with renal excretion of creatinine (e.g trimethoprim) will artefactually appear to cause a drop in eGFR, while true GFR remains unaffected.

As kidney function declines, tubular secretion of creatinine rises. Thus, serum creatinine remains in the normal range until kidney function falls below ~40 mL/min, i.e. until significant renal dysfunction is well established. Hence, early diagnosis of renal failure from creatinine alone is often difficult.

Further reading

1. GFR calculators: serum creatinine and cystatin C (2012) (with SI units). Mdrd.com.
2. NICE. Chronic kidney disease in adults: assessment and management. Clinical guideline CG182. www.nice.org.uk/guidance/cg182.

Renal handling of sodium, potassium and water

Like other solutes, sodium and potassium are freely filtered at the glomerulus; as both ions are critical for cell biology much of the filtered amount is reabsorbed to match the daily ingested amount.

Key points

- Daily renal potassium excretion balances dietary intake (approximately 1.0–1.5 mEq/kg/day). Thus, the kidneys excrete ~10–15% of the daily filtered K^+ load (~10 mEq/kg/day).
- Even less (just < 1%) filtered sodium is excreted on a daily basis.
- These numbers are referred to as the fractional excretion values of K^+ (FE_K) and Na^+ (FE_{Na}).

FE_K is used less commonly in clinical practice than FE_{Na}, with transtubular potassium gradient (TTKG) generally considered a more useful value. It is important to note that fractional excretion is not the same as the urinary concentration or absolute amount of Na^+ or K^+ in the urine.

Renal handling of sodium

Proximal convoluted tubule (60–70% of sodium reabsorption)

The sodium-potassium (Na^+/K^+) ATPase is the key component of renal Na^+ handling, particularly in the proximal convoluted tubule (PCT), the thick ascending loop of Henle (TAL) and the distal convoluted tubule (DCT). These areas correspond to the most metabolically active sites of the nephron.

Key points

- The Na^+/K^+ ATPase is expressed on the basolateral membrane of tubular epithelial cells (Figure 16.1) and actively pumps Na^+ out of the cells, establishing a favourable Na^+ gradient for the influx of Na^+ from the tubular lumen.

- Na^+ co-transporters on the luminal surface transport Na^+ together with other solutes (e.g. phosphate and sulphate, amino acids and glucose) into epithelial cells down the Na^+ concentration gradient, even against the concentration gradient of the co-transported molecules (Figure 16.1).
- Counter-transport of Na^+ against H^+ ions results in reabsorption of HCO_3^- (Figure 16.1B). Thus, approximately two-thirds of filtered Na^+ is reabsorbed at the proximal tubule, together with all of filtered glucose and amino acids and the majority of sulphate, phosphate and bicarbonate.

Loop of Henle (30% of sodium reabsorption)

The sodium potassium 2 chloride ($Na^+/K^+/2Cl^-$) co-transporter (NKCC2) in the medullary thick ascending loop is responsible for re-absorption of a further 30% of luminal Na^+ from the filtrate. This process is driven again by a Na^+ concentration generated by the Na^+/K^+ ATPase favouring movement of Na^+ into tubular cells from the lumen (Figure 16.1C).

Distal convoluted tubule (5–10% of sodium reabsorption)

Sodium reabsorption in the DCT and proximal collecting duct is a hormonally-regulated process involving aldosterone (Figure 16.1D).

Key points

- The Na^+/K^+ ATPase generates a Na^+ gradient favouring movement of Na^+ from the lumen into tubular cells, as is the case elsewhere in the kidney. However, in the DCT the expression of apical sodium channels (the epithelial sodium channel [ENaC]) and sodium-chloride co-transporter (NCCT) are controlled by aldosterone.
- Aldosterone is a steroid hormone and engages intracellular receptors, which initiate gene transcription. Luminal expression of ENaC and NCCT allows entry of Na^+ into DCTs, which accounts for the remainder of Na^+ re-absorption in the nephron.

Renal handling of water

Water reabsorption in the kidney is entirely passive, relying on osmotic gradients for water flow with approximately two-thirds of filtered water reabsorbed in the proximal tubule along with Na^+.

Key points

- Most of regulated water reabsorption from the filtrate occurs in the renal medulla by establishing an osmotic gradient through the counter-current multiplication system, created via the unique structure of the loop of Henle.
- The descending loop of Henle is freely permeable to water, but impermeable to Na^+. The renal medulla is hypertonic relative to the tubular lumen, due to the active extrusion of Na^+ from tubular cells of the thin ascending loop of Henle into the renal medulla via the Na^+/K^+ ATPase (Figure 16.1C). Water therefore passes out of the descending loop of Henle and collecting duct cells down an osmotic gradient (Figure 16.1A) and the luminal concentrations of both Na^+ and urea increase.
- The high Na^+ concentration reaching the TAL (which is freely permeable to Na^+, but not to water) results in movement of Na^+ out of the lumen into the medulla. The high urea concentration reaching the collecting duct cells results in export of urea into the renal medulla. Both these effects contribute to medullar hypertonicity essential for the concentrating ability of the kidney.
- This entire process is dependent on the basolateral Na^+/K^+ ATPase, which requires a supply of oxygen. This explains why hypoxic states (e.g. obstructive sleep apnoea) result in fluid retention and why sudden loss of blood supply to the kidneys causes loss of renal concentrating ability as part of acute tubular necrosis (ATN).

Anti-diuretic hormone

Unlike the loop of Henle, where permeability to water is structurally determined, the permeability of collecting duct cells to water is dependent on the presence of water channels ('aquaporins') in the apical membrane.

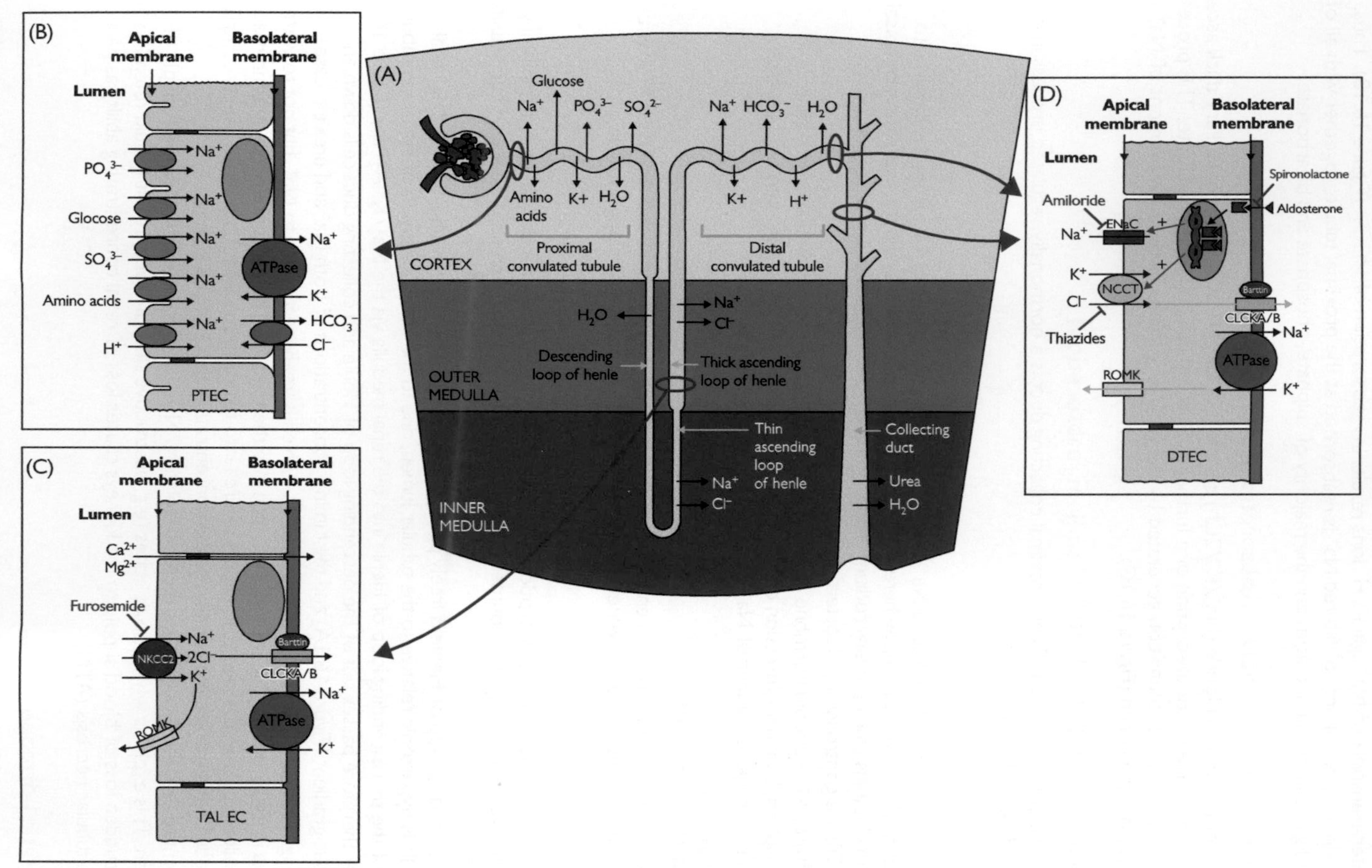

Figure 16.1 Renal handling of sodium.

Key points

- Anti-diuretic hormone (ADH; also known as arginine vasopressin) is produced by the posterior pituitary and binds to arginine vasopressin receptor 2 stimulating fusion of vesicles containing aquaporins with the apical membrane of collecting duct cells.
- Water moves down osmotic gradients, usually from the lumen to the hypertonic renal medulla. Therefore, ADH conserves water and concentrates urine. ADH also increases collecting duct cell permeability to urea, contributing to medullary hypertonicity.

Overall, urinary concentration is largely determined by the need to conserve water and the passive absorption of water along osmotic gradients. In health, urinary volume and concentration ranges from 0.5 L to 3 L per day, and from 50 mOsm/kg to 1200 mOsm/kg.

Renal handling of potassium

Like Na^+, K^+ is freely filtered at the glomerulus, and like Na^+, the majority of K^+ (two-thirds) is reabsorbed in the proximal tubule, with a further 20–25% reabsorbed in the TAL. Once again, the Na^+/K^+ ATPase plays a central role.

Key points

- The main sites at which K^+ reabsorption/secretion are regulated are the initial and cortical portions of the collecting ducts. Although both principal and intercalated cells are intricately involved in K^+ regulation at these sites, a simplified model showing only intercalated cells is depicted in Figure 16.2.
- Bicarbonate ions and hydrogen ions are generated in the intercalated cells through the interaction of carbon dioxide and water, catalysed by carbonic anhydrase. Bicarbonate ions are exchanged for chloride ions (anion exchanger 1; see Figure 16.2).
- Hydrogen ions are excreted and exchanged for K^+, contributing to a reciprocal K^+ reabsorption from the tubular lumen. Hydrogen ions are also pumped out of the cell through a H^+ pump into the lumen.

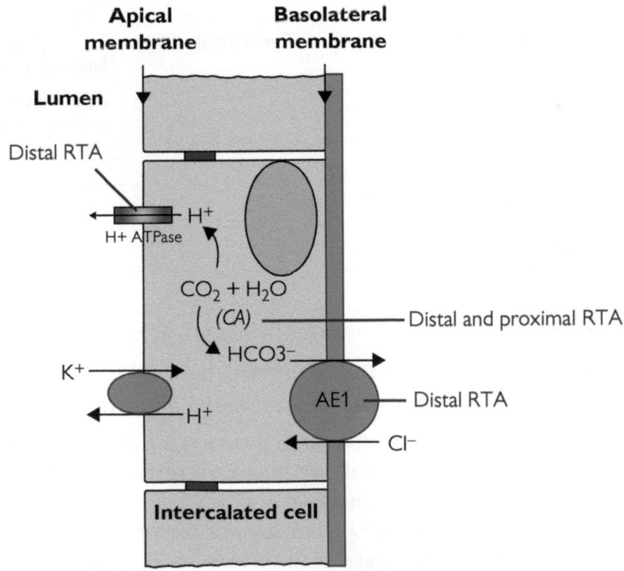

Figure 16.2 Potassium handling in the intercalated cells of the collecting duct. Shown is a simplified diagram of the key transporters and diseases (in blue) arising from mutations in genes encoding key proteins.
AE1, anion exchanger 1; RTA, renal tubular acidosis; CA, carbonic anhydrase.

Further reading

1. Doucet A, Crambert G. *Oxford Textbook of Clinical Nephrology*, 4th edn. Oxford: Oxford University Press.

Acid-base disorders

Enzymatic processes and protein structure are pH dependent; therefore, maintaining proton (H^+) concentration within narrow limits is a physiological priority. A series of buffer systems, which accept protons in lieu of cellular proteins are contributory.

Serum pH is usually maintained between 7.35 and 7.45 (intracellular pH is lower).

Normal daily metabolism generates respiratory acids (CO_2, eliminated through the lungs) and non-respiratory ('metabolic') acids, which are removed from the body by non-respiratory mechanisms, namely the kidneys and liver.

Metabolism generates approximately 1 mEq/kg of protons (H^+) per day. The majority of this metabolic acid load comes from protein catabolism (sulphur-containing amino acids and organophosphates), and a small quantity from by-products of muscle metabolism, e.g. pyruvic and lactic acids.

Physiological handling of dietary acid load

See Table 16.1.

Table 16.1 Series of the key equations (Eqn) for physiological acid handling and buffer systems

Equation	Process	Site	Additional points
1	Sulphur-containing amino acid → $2H^+ + SO_4^{2-}$	Liver	Sulphuric acid generated.
2	$2H^+ + 2HCO_3^- \rightarrow 2CO_2 + 2H_2O$	Extracellular fluid	CO_2 exhaled by lungs.
3	Glutamine → $2NH_4^+ + 2HCO_3^-$	Renal tubular cell	The two bicarbonate ions are required for Eqn 2.
4	$2NH_4^+ + SO_4^{2-} \rightarrow (NH_4^+)_2SO_4^{2-}$	Renal tubule	The sulphate anions (Eqn 1) are filtered by glomeruli. Ammonium sulphate is excreted in the urine.
Buffer system			
5	$H^+ + HCO_3^- \leftrightarrow H_2CO_3 \leftrightarrow CO_2 + H_2O$		
6	$NH_3 + H^+ \leftrightarrow NH_4^+$		

Regulation of pH, buffer systems and the Henderson–Hasselbalch equation

- The major intracellular buffer systems are cellular proteins, haemoglobin and phosphate.
- The major extracellular buffer systems are bicarbonate and ammonia (see Table 16.1, Eqns 5 and 6).

These buffer systems maintain pH within a narrow range provided the change in acid/alkali load is small. They do not, however, remove excess acid/alkali, which require respiratory and renal elimination. The functions of organ systems in regulating pH are shown in Box 16.1.

In essence, respiratory compensation alters P_{CO2}, while renal compensation alters serum bicarbonate concentration. The Henderson–Hasselbalch equation shows the relationship between renal and respiratory function to this end:

$$pH = pKa + log_{10} \frac{[A^-]}{[HA]}$$

where A^- is the conjugate base and HA is the acid.

Box 16.1 Respiratory and renal regulation of acid-base balance

Respiratory regulation of pH

- Regulates P_{CO2}.
- Increases alveolar ventilation if serum pH drops, reducing CO_2 tension.
- Relative rapid mechanism of compensating for excess metabolic acids, but the compensation through this mechanism rarely returns serum pH to normal.

Renal regulation of pH

- Reabsorption of filtered HCO_3^-.
- Generation of new HCO_3^-.
- Secretion of excess acid.
- Relatively slow compensatory mechanism but more likely to return blood pH to normal.

With respect to the HCO_3^-/CO_2 system this can be simplified to:

$$pH = 6.1 + log_{10}\frac{[HCO_3^-]}{(0.03 \times PCO_2)}$$

The Hendersson–Hasselbach equation represents a very important physiologic relationship for both the pulmonary and renal systems, which predicts that the ratio of dissolved CO_2 to HCO_3^-, rather than their actual concentrations, determines hydrogen ion concentration and thus pH.

Renal regulation of acid-base balance

Acid-base disorders represent significant deviations of PCO_2, serum HCO_3^- concentration and pH from the norm.

Acidosis and alkalosis can be either due to respiratory or non-respiratory disorders. Measurement of pH, serum bicarbonate concentration and P_{CO2} is sufficient to determine whether an acid-base imbalance disorder is respiratory or metabolic. (A more practical approach to interpretation of arterial blood gas analysis is discussed in ➲ Chapter 11, Arterial blood gas analysis, p. 384 and Box 11.3).

For important acid–base definitions, see Table 16.2.

Table 16.2 Important acid-base definitions

Parameter	Values
Normal values	
Serum pH	7.35–7.45
Serum HCO_3^- concentration	22–26 mmol/L*
pCO_2	4.8–5.8 KPa (36–44 mmHg)
Important definitions	
Acidaemia	Serum pH <7.35
Alkalaemia	Serum pH >7.45
Acidosis	Relative acid excess**
Alkalosis	Relative alkali excess**

*HCO_3^- is measured as a concentration, so a significant loss of plasma volume, e.g. during a choleric illness, may influence the measured concentration of HCO_3^- in an upward direction, while the patient will still have significant bicarbonate depletion.
**The actual pH depends on rate of development, severity and compensatory mechanisms.

> **Top tips**
>
> - pH is derived from $-\log[H^+]$, since this is a logarithmic scale a lower pH indicates a significantly higher concentration of protons in the extracellular fluid.
> - In a hypothermic individual, physiological changes, including a reduction in pCO_2 (due to increased solubility of CO_2), lead to some alkalinisation of the blood. Warming the patient will reverse this.

Metabolic acidosis

Metabolic acidosis is either due to loss of bicarbonate or excess of metabolic acids. The anion gap is a useful method of differentiating these two causes.

The anion gap

The ionic constituents of the serum are in neutral balance, i.e. anions and cations balance each other out. In practice, however, not all anions (such as proteins and organic acids) are measured. Hence, there appears to be an 'anion gap' (AG), which represents the concentration of unmeasured anions in the serum.

In simplified terms, the AG can be calculated from the formula:

$$AG = \left(\left[Na^+\right] + \left[K^+\right]\right) - \left(\left[HCO_3^-\right] + \left[Cl^-\right]\right)$$

or the shortened form:

$$AG = \left[Na^+\right] - \left(\left[HCO_3^-\right] + \left[Cl^-\right]\right)$$

The normal AG is 8–16 mEq/L.

> **Top tip**
>
> - Serum albumin impacts the AG. Every 10 g/L decline in albumin reduces the normal range of the AG by 4 mEq/L.

Metabolic acidosis with normal anion gap

In patients with a normal AG metabolic acidosis, the primary problem is a loss of bicarbonate from the body. Loss of bicarbonate is nearly completely compensated for by a conservation of chloride. This situation is also known as hyperchloraemic metabolic acidosis. Normal AG metabolic acidosis often arises from:

- GI loss of bicarbonate (including diarrhoea and enteric fistulae).
- Failure of renal conservation of bicarbonate (renal tubular acidosis).
- Drug ingestion (carbonic anhydrase inhibitors, e.g. acetazolamide).
- Excessive administration of normal saline in hospitalised patients.

The causes of a normal AG metabolic acidosis include:

'FUSEDCARS'

- Enteric **F**istula; particularly entero-pancreatic as pancreatic juice is rich in HCO_3^-.
- **U**reteroenteric fistula.
- Excessive IV **S**aline administration.
- **E**ndocrine causes (e.g. hyperparathyroidism).
- **D**iarrhoea.
- **C**arbonic anhydrous inhibitors (e.g. acetazolamide).
- **A**mmonium chloride ingestion.
- **R**enal tubular acidosis.
- **S**pironolactone.

Metabolic acidosis with high anion gap

In high AG metabolic acidosis, the primary acid-base imbalance is an excess of organic acids, which are buffered by serum bicarbonate. The 'extra' acid is represented by an increase in the unmeasured anion (the AG).

A useful mnemonic for causes of a high AG metabolic acidosis is:

'MUDPILES'

- **M**ethanol.
- **U**raemia.
- **D**iabetic ketoacidosis. (Diabetic ketoacidosis is a relatively common condition compared to its less common cousin, alcoholic ketoacidosis.)
- **P**araldehyde poisoning.
- **I**ron toxicity and **I**nfection.
- **L**actic acidosis and **L**iver failure.
- **E**thylene glycol poisoning.
- **S**alicylate toxicity.

Lactic acidosis

Lactic acid is a by-product of anaerobic metabolism. When present in excess (>5 mmol/L), lactic acid causes a high AG metabolic acidosis.

Lactic acidosis and its causes are discussed in ➲ Chapter 12, Lactic acidosis, p. 404 and Box 12.6).

Osmolar gap

In the evaluation of a patient with a high AG metabolic acidosis, calculation of the osmolar gap can be helpful. The osmolar gap is the difference between the measured serum osmolality (by the laboratory) and the calculated one and represents the presence of excess osmotically active molecules in serum (usually of exogenous origin).

$$\text{Osmolar gap} = \text{Measured osmolality} - \text{calculated osmolality}$$
$$\text{Calculated osmolality} = [2 \times Na^+] + \text{glucose} + \text{urea}.$$

The normal osmolar gap is <10 mOsm/kg. Table 16.3 summarises the expected values for the osmolar gap in patients with a high AG metabolic acidosis and demonstrates its value in evaluating cases of suspected poisoning (➲ see Chapter 3, Investigations, p. 80.).

Table 16.3 Expected osmolar gap in high anion gap metabolic acidosis

Normal osmolar gap (<10 mOsm/kg)*	High osmolar gap (≥10 mOsm/kg)
Uraemia	Methanol
Diabetic ketoacidosis	Ethylene glycol
Paraldehyde	Alcoholic ketoacidosis
Iron	
Lactic acidosis	
Salicylate	

* The serum osmolar gap may in fact be slightly increased in ketoacidosis and lactic acidosis.

Top tip

- The osmolar gap is also elevated in poisoning, e.g. ethanol, propylene glycol, acetone and isopropyl ethanol. It is a good idea to calculate it in every unconscious patient in whom the cause is not self-evident.

Clinical aspects of metabolic acidosis

Metabolic acidosis does not usually cause significant systemic upset, unless it is significant (Table 16.4). The symptoms and signs of mild metabolic acidosis are usually related to, and thereby may help to identify, the underlying condition (Box 16.2).

Table 16.4 Sequelae of metabolic acidosis

Organ system	Effects
Cardiac	Hypotension, possibly cardiogenic shock (acidosis is negatively inotropic). Arrhythmias.
Neurological	Headache. Confusion. Coma if severe.
Respiratory	Hyperpnoea. Kussmaul breathing.
Renal	Reduced GFR (vascular constriction and reduced cardiac output). Increased rate of renal decline (in the long-term) in patients with CKD*.
Bone	Bone demineralisation if chronic.
Non-specific	Malaise and muscle weakness. Nausea, vomiting.

NB. The more severe effects are more likely to occur if the acidosis develops rapidly and is severe.
*Treating chronic acidosis with bicarbonate may reduce the rate of renal decline in the long-term in patients with CKD (1).

Box 16.2 Clinical features that may point to the aetiology of metabolic acidosis

History

- Previous history of diabetes mellitus, renal and/or liver disease, GI surgery, fistulating bowel disease.
- Drug history (e.g. salicylate, iron, acetazolamide).
- Ingestion of anti-freeze (ethylene glycol) or methylated spirits.
- Tinnitus and vertigo in salicylate poisoning.
- Visual disturbance or blindness in ethylene glycol ingestion.

Signs

- Hyperaemia of the optic disc in methanol ingestion.
- Reduced pupillary response to light in methanol ingestion.
- Parkinsonism in methanol ingestion.*
- Cranial nerve lesions in ethylene glycol poisoning.

*Methanol can cause haemorrhagic and non-haemorrhagic lesions of the basal ganglia.

Further reading

1. Lee Hamm L, Nakhoul N, Hering-Smith KS. Acid-base homeostasis. *Clin J Am Soc Nephrol.* 2015;10:2232–42.
2. Wagner C, Devuyst O. Renal acid-base homeostasis. In: Turner NN, Lameire N, Goldsmith DJ, et al. (Eds) *Oxford Textbook of Clinical Nephrology*, 4th edn. Oxford: Oxford University Press.

References

1. De Brito-Ashurst I, Varagunam M, Raftery MJ, Yaqoob MM. Bicarbonate supplementation slows progression of CKD and improves nutritional status. *J Am Soc Nephrol.* 2009;20(9):2075–84.

Tubular disorders

Disorders of renal tubules often cause abnormalities of blood and urine biochemistry and may be present before development of symptoms. These conditions are either hereditary or acquired.

Renal tubular acidosis

The general biochemical feature of renal tubular acidosis (RTA) is that of a normal AG metabolic acidosis. There are four forms of RTA. The first two can be primary (hereditary) or secondary (acquired). Type 3 is hereditary and Type 4 is almost always acquired. The secondary causes of Types 1 and 2 RTA are shown in Box 16.3.

Box 16.3 Secondary causes of Type 1 and Type 2 RTA

Type 1 (distal) RTA

- Autoimmune diseases, e.g. Sjögren syndrome, rheumatoid arthritis, SLE.
- Hypercalcaemia.
- Drugs, e.g. ifosfamide, amphotericin B, lithium salts.
- Idiopathic.

Type 2 (proximal) RTA

- Monoclonal gammopathies, e.g. multiple myeloma, amyloidosis.
- Autoimmune diseases, e.g. Sjögren syndrome.
- Drugs, e.g. ifosfamide, carbonic anhydrase inhibitors, tenofovir.
- Heavy metal poisoning, e.g. mercury, lead.
- Idiopathic.

Type 1 (distal) renal tubular acidosis

Pathophysiology

Most mutations causing distal RTA affect the H^+-ATPase (autosomal recessive) or the kidney anion exchanger (AE1; autosomal dominant) in the intercalated cells of the distal renal tubule (Figure 16.3D).

Clinical presentation

Distal RTA results in a failure to excrete H^+ into the tubular filtrate at the distal tubule, meaning that urine pH cannot be acidified below 5.5.

The hallmark of distal RTA is inappropriately alkaline urine in the context of systemic acidosis, where the physiological need should be to excrete excess H^+ at the distal tubule.

Associated features include:

- Hypokalaemia.
- Hypocitraturia.
- Hypercalciuria: calcification of the renal ultrastructure (nephrocalcinosis) and renal stones (nephrolithiasis) are common, as well as osteomalacia from net calcium loss in the urine and chronic acidosis.

Distal RTA has a variable phenotype. Those presenting in childhood have more severe, autosomal recessive phenotypes (failure to thrive, poor growth and renal dysfunction from nephrocalcinosis). Milder forms, usually diagnosed in adulthood, can be found incidentally, e.g. when investigating kidney stones or abnormal kidney function.

A diagnosis of distal RTA is established by a urinary acidification test. Failure to acidify the urine pH < 5.5 following ingestion of an acid load (usually ammonium chloride) confirms the diagnosis of distal RTA.

Distal RTA responds to initiation of oral alkali therapy, usually bicarbonate or citrate salts. Correction of acidosis is usually sufficient to improve hypocitraturia, which in turn reduces the risk of renal stone formation.

Type 2 (proximal) renal tubular acidosis

Proximal RTA is due to incomplete bicarbonate reabsorption in the PCT. Diseases causing global proximal tubular dysfunction can cause proximal RTA as part of Fanconi syndrome, the most common presentation of proximal RTA. Primary forms of proximal RTA are rare, but include mutations in the sodium bicarbonate co-transporter (NBC1), which also includes an ophthalmic phenotype (Figure 16.3A).

Clinical presentation

In general, proximal RTA is more severe than distal RTA, especially if presenting with Fanconi syndrome, and includes normal AG metabolic acidosis and osteomalacia.

- The metabolic acidosis is often self-limiting due to the 'threshold' effect. The proximal tubules retain some ability to reabsorb bicarbonate, reducing the filtrate bicarbonate concentration to a threshold level, usually ~15 mEq/L, resulting in complete reabsorption of filtered bicarbonate. Thus, the urinary acidification test can be 'paradoxically' normal in patients with proximal RTA.
- Patients universally have hypokalaemia due to hyperaldosteronism (from volume contraction) and high delivery of bicarbonate to the distal tubule. The urine calcium level is also high (one of the causes of osteomalacia).
- Normal urinary levels of citrate prevent renal stone formation and nephrocalcinosis.

Management

- Alkali therapy: patients often require large quantities of alkali therapy daily, even more so when suffering from intercurrent illnesses.
- Potassium supplementation: as tubular bicarbonate concentrations rise above the threshold level, more bicarbonate reaches distal tubules causing potassium wasting.
- Thiazide diuretics: help to increase bicarbonate reabsorption from the proximal tubule by volume contraction. This can worsen hypokalaemia, so thiazides are usually prescribed with further potassium supplementation.
- Vitamin D therapy: to improve bone health and calcium/phosphate balance.

Type 3 (mixed proximal and distal) renal tubular acidosis

This rare form of RTA is caused by inheritance of a mutation in carbonic anhydrase type II (CA II) and is seen in infants, most often in North Africa and the Middle East. The syndrome is inherited in an autosomal recessive manner and, because CA II is expressed in multiple organs, presents as a multisystem disorder called the Guibaud–Vainsel syndrome. Salient features include cerebral calcification, mental retardation and osteoporosis (see Figure 16.3A and D).

Type 4 renal tubular acidosis (hypoaldosteronism)

This form of RTA is either from absolute deficiency of aldosterone or resistance to its actions on the renal tubules. The former commonly accompanies hyporeninaemia, typically in long-standing diabetes, but also occurs in the context of adrenal failure. Aldosterone resistance can be either hereditary or acquired. Most acquired forms arise from chronic use of potassium sparing diuretics, e.g. amiloride, or chronic tubulointerstitial disease.

Hereditary forms, termed pseudohypoaldosteronism type I, present as severe salt wasting and hyperkalaemia, features of true hypoaldosteronism, but with high serum levels of renin and aldosterone. Pseudohypoaldosteronism type I can be caused by several different mutations including mutations of the ENaC (that is targeted by amiloride) or the mineralocorticoid receptor, autosomal recessive and dominant conditions, respectively. The former can present with a severe paediatric phenotype during neonatal life (see Figure 16.3E).

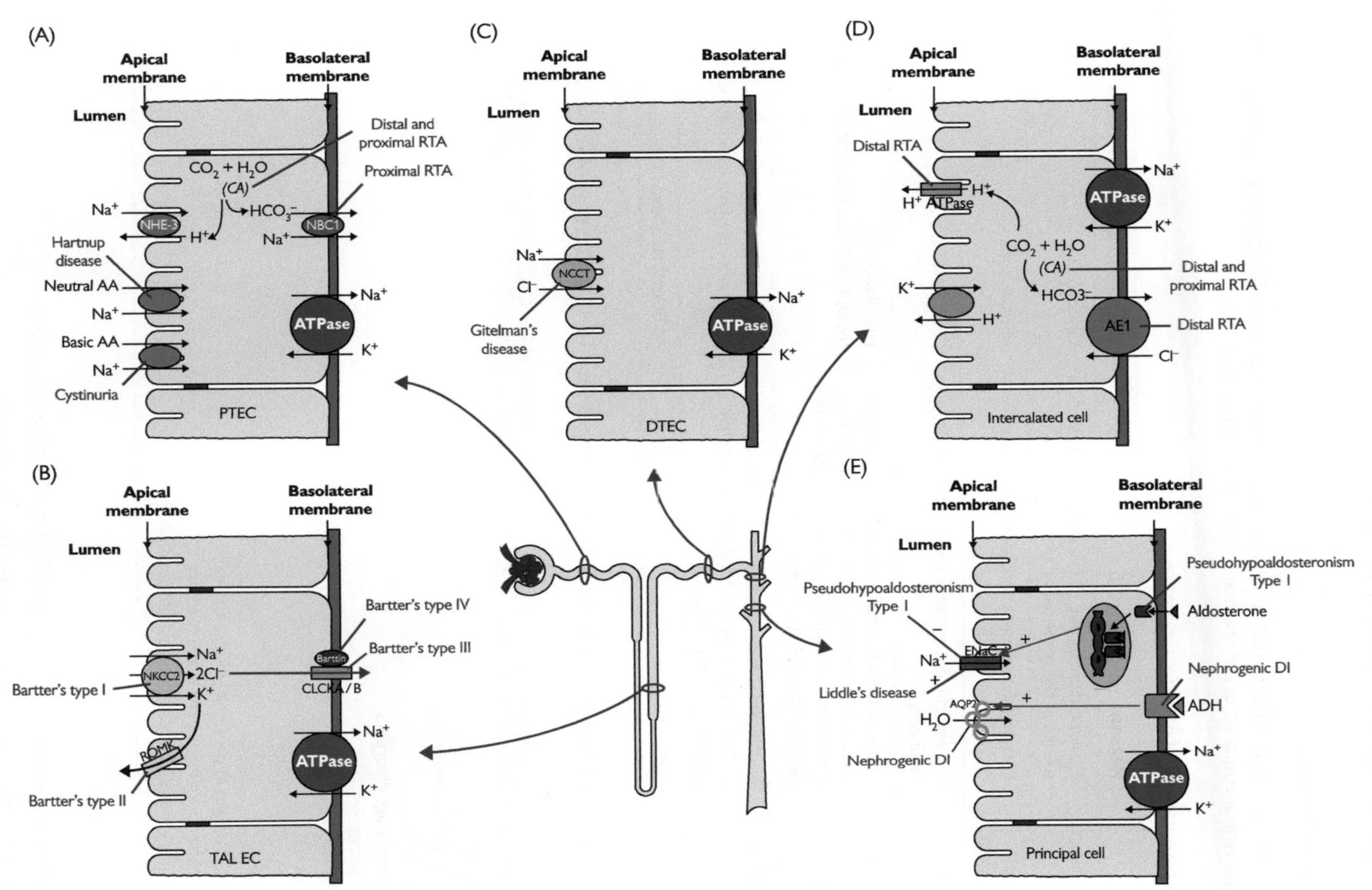

Figure 16.3 Primary causes of solute wasting kidney diseases.

Further reading

1. Walsh S. Approach to the patient with renal tubular acidosis. In: Doucet A, Crambert G. (Eds). *Oxford Textbook of Clinical Nephrology*, 4th edn. Oxford: Oxford University Press.

Fanconi syndrome

Fanconi syndrome is generalised proximal tubular dysfunction and therefore affects many functions of the PCT. It presents with a combination of the features shown in Table 16.5.

Table 16.5 Presentations of Fanconi syndrome

Presentation	Reason	Biochemical abnormalities
Polyuria, polydipsia and dehydration	Osmotic diuresis due to failure to reabsorb solutes in the proximal tubule.	Glycosuria.
Rickets in children; osteomalacia in adults	Loss of calcium and phosphate in the urine.	Phosphaturia.
Growth retardation	Rickets; chronic acidosis; underlying disease, e.g. cystinosis.	Phosphaturia.
Weakness, paralysis	Hypokalaemia (caused by high Na^+ delivery to distal tubule resulting in Na^+/K^+ exchange and type 2 RTA) or hypophosphataemia (failure to reabsorb phosphate in proximal tubule).	Hypokalaemia, hypophosphataemia, phosphaturia.
Incidental proteinuria	Usually sub-nephrotic levels due to failure to reabsorb amino acids or spillover of systemic proteins, e.g. myeloma.	Amino aciduria, dipstick proteinuria, nephrotic syndrome.
Incidental acidosis	Type 2 RTA.	As described above.

The exact presentation and age of onset depends on the cause (Box 16.4) and severity of disease.

Box 16.4 Causes of Fanconi syndrome

Hereditary

- Cystinosis (the commonest).
- Wilson disease.
- Glycogen storage disorders.
- Fructosaemia.
- Galactosaemia.
- Tyrosinaemia.

Acquired

- Drugs, e.g. tenofovir, gentamicin, tetracycline.
- Heavy metal poisoning, e.g. lead and mercury.
- Monoclonal gammopathies, e.g. myeloma, amyloidosis.

Investigations

These aim to determine the degree and type of PCT dysfunction and include:

- Urine chemistry: amino acids, glucose, phosphate, bicarbonate.
- Serum chemistry: bicarbonate, glucose, phosphate, calcium, potassium, sodium and proteins.

Underlying cause is usually directed by the history at presentation.

Management

- Treat the underlying cause, where possible.
- Aim to normalise serum biochemistry, e.g. treatment of RTA, free access to water, supplementation of phosphate and/or vitamin D, and prescription of potassium salts.
- Consider curative options, e.g. liver transplantation in Wilson's disease.

Further reading

1. Cherqui S, Courtoy PJ. The renal Fanconi syndrome in cystinosis: pathogenic insights and therapeutic perspectives. *Nat Rev Nephrol*. 2017; 13(2): 115–31.

Cystinuria and Hartnup's disease

These two conditions are caused by mutations in amino acid transporters in the PCT.

Cystinuria

Cystinuria is a relatively common autosomal recessive disease with a prevalence of 1 per 7000 of the worldwide population. It is caused by mutations in transporters for dibasic amino acids (cystine, ornithine, arginine and lysine), resulting in failure to reabsorb these amino acids from the tubular filtrate.

High levels of cystine are poorly soluble in acidic urine, causing cystine stones, which account for 1% and 6–8% of renal calculi in adults and children, respectively. Occasionally, patients have recurrent UTIs or chronic kidney disease (CKD) from chronic stone disease. Ophthalmic manifestations include corneal deposits of cystine (crystals visible on slit lamp examination) and pigmentary retinopathy.

The diagnosis can be made by very high urinary cystine concentrations, the presence of hexagonal urinary crystals (which may be visible) and imaging studies (cystine stones are radio-opaque).

Cystinuria is managed by minimising the risks of further stone formation, through adequate daily hydration to reduce urinary cystine concentrations and alkalinisation of urine to pH >7. In severe, resistant cases, cystine can also be chelated with penicillamine.

Hartnup's disease

Hartnup's disease is caused by mutations in the transporter for neutral amino acids (e.g. tryptophan) expressed in the PCTs and intestines. This condition does not have a renal phenotype other than amino aciduria, but does have features of tryptophan deficiency.

Tryptophan is needed to make serotonin, melatonin and niacin, so patients present with a pellagra-like dermatosis and neurological disease, such as cerebellar ataxia, nystagmus and tremor.

A high protein diet is required, especially one supplemented with nicotinamide, a metabolite of niacin. Patients should avoid sunlight.

Further reading

1. Pereira DJ, Schoolwerth AC, Pais VM. Cystinuria: current concepts and future directions. *Clin Nephrol*. 2015; 83(3):138–46.

Bartter and Gitelman syndromes

Bartter syndrome

Bartter syndrome is rare and caused by mutations in several transporters in the TAL. There are 5 types of Bartter syndrome, although type V is extremely rare.

Pathophysiology

Mutations in TAL transporters result in failure of the concentrating function of the TAL. The phenotype is of chronic loop diuretic use (renal salt wasting): volume depletion, hypokalaemia and hyperchloraemic metabolic alkalosis secondary to increased delivery of Na^+ to the distal nephron where exchange for K^+ and H^+ occurs. (See Figure 16.3B.).

Presentation

Many patients present early in life (especially as neonates or children) with:

- Polyuria.
- Polydipsia.
- Salt craving.
- Constipation.
- Growth retardation.
- Electrolyte abnormalities (in addition to those mentioned above), including hypercalciuria, causing nephrocalcinosis and hypomagnesaemia.
- Systemic features, such as fever and diarrhoea (caused by an excess prostaglandin E production).

Phenotypes depend on the severity of the gene mutation. Severe electrolyte disturbances can cause cardiac arrhythmias. Also, barttin (Cl^- channel β-subunit) is crucial for renal Cl^- reabsorption and inner ear K^+ secretion, so patients with type IV Bartter syndrome have sensorineural deafness.

Gitelman syndrome

Gitelman syndrome is closely related to Bartter syndrome and is caused by mutations in the sodium chloride co-transporter in the distal tubule.

Presentation

As NCCT is the same transporter targeted by thiazide diuretics, the presentation resembles chronic thiazide use, namely volume depletion and hypokalaemia. The presentation is usually later and less severe than Bartter syndrome. The pathognomonic feature of Gitelman syndrome is severe hypomagnesaemia, although patients can also present with mild hypomagnesaemia. Muscle weakness and fatiguability may occur. The mechanism for underlying renal magnesium wasting in Gitelman syndrome has not yet been fully elucidated.

Treatment for Bartter and Gitelman syndromes

- Generally supportive, with:
  - sodium, potassium, calcium and magnesium supplementation;
  - antagonism of aldosterone and angiotensin II (e.g. angiotensin converting enzyme inhibitor [ACE-i]);
  - treatment of growth retardation with growth hormone.
- Indomethacin to limit prostaglandin secretion in the kidneys in Bartter syndrome.
- End-stage kidney disease (very rare) can be effectively 'cured' by renal transplantation (assuming the donor is not an affected relative).

Tubular diseases of aldosterone biology

These syndromes suggest hyperactive or deficient mineralocorticoid activity, but without significant perturbations in mineralocorticoid levels. They are due to mutations in transporters within the kidneys. There are two key syndromes.

Liddle syndrome

This is caused by an abnormality of a subunit of the ENaC, which prevents ENaC recycling from the cell surface. ENaC activity is enhanced, causing excess sodium reabsorption from the lumen (see Figure 16.3E). Patients have severe hypertension together with hypokalaemia and metabolic alkalosis, features that would suggest hyperaldosteronism. It can be treated with ENaC inhibitors, such as amiloride or triamterene, but is resistant to spironolactone since the condition is not driven by aldosterone.

Pseudohypoaldosteronism type I

This condition, in contrast, is aldosterone resistance, in the presence of normal serum levels of mineralocorticoids. Specifically, patients have salt wasting, hypovolaemia/hypotension and hyperkalaemia. There are two forms, a severe autosomal recessive form (caused by loss of function mutations in ENaC; see Figure 16.3E) and a more benign autosomal dominant version (caused by mutations in the mineralocortoicoid receptor). Both are treated with a high salt diet ± fludrocortisone/carbenoxolone.

Nephrogenic diabetes insipidus (NDI)

NDI renders the kidneys resistant to ADH, resulting in failure to reabsorb water in the collecting ducts (Figure 16.3E) (➲ see Chapter 19, Diabetes insipidus, p. 688, Box 19.4, and Tables 19.8 and 19.9).

Glomerular diseases

There are a number of different ways to classify glomerular disease:

1. Mode of presentation
   a. Nephrotic syndrome.
   b. Nephritic syndrome.
   c. Non-nephrotic proteinuria.
   d. Rapidly progressive glomerulonephritis.
   e. Asymptomatic microscopic haematuria.
   f. CKD.
2. Aetiology:
   a. Primary glomerular disease:
      i. IgA nephropathy.
      ii. Primary focal segmental glomerulosclerosis (FSGS).
      iii. Minimal change disease.
      iv. Idiopathic membranous nephropathy.
      v. Hereditary nephritides.
      vi. Other primary glomerulopathies.
   b. Secondary glomerular disease, for example:
      i. Immune complex deposition: post-infectious glomerulonephritis (GN).
      ii. SLE.
      iii. Mixed essential cryoglobulinaemia.
      iv. Plasma cell dyscrasias: light chain deposition disease, amyloidosis.
3. Histopathological findings (mainly on light microscopy):
   a. Diffuse: involving >50% of glomeruli.
   b. Focal: involving <50% of glomeruli.
   c. Segmental: involving part of the glomerulus.
   d. Global: involving the entire glomerulus.
   e. Membranous: thickening of the glomerular capillary wall.
   f. Proliferative: increased number of cells in glomerulus, which may be infiltrating inflammatory cells.
   g. Crescentic: accumulation of inflammatory cells in Bowman's space often compressing the glomerulus.

   For causes of glomerular disease, see Table 16.6.

Table 16.6 Causes of glomerular disease by mode of presentation

	Nephrotic syndrome	Acute nephritic syndrome	Asymptomatic microscopic haematuria	Rapidly progressive glomerulonephritis
Primary	Minimal change disease. Focal and segmental glomerulosclerosis. Membranous nephropathy. Mesangiocapillary GN.	IgA nephropathy. Mesangiocapillary GN. Post-infectious GN.	IgA nephropathy. Post-infectious GN. Alport's syndrome. Thin basement membrane.	Anti-glomerular basement membrane (GBM) disease. Idiopathic crescentic GN.
Secondary	HIV-associated nephropathy (HIVAN). Renal amyloidosis. Light chain deposition disease. SLE with type 5 lupus nephritis. Secondary membranous nephropathy. Diabetic glomerulosclerosis. Secondary FSGS.	SLE. Infective endocarditis. Cryoglobulinaemia. Henoch–Schönlein purpura. ANCA-associated systemic vasculitis. Shunt nephritis.		ANCA-associated systemic vasculitis and pauci-immune GN. SLE.

Further reading

1. Turner N. Mechanisms of glomerular injury: overview. In: Doucet A, Crambert G. (Eds). *Oxford Textbook of Clinical Nephrology*, 4th edn. Oxford: Oxford University Press.

Nephrotic syndrome

Nephrotic syndrome is caused by failure of the glomerular filtration barrier, mostly because of injury to podocytes or the slit diaphragm. Nephrotic syndrome may be accompanied by reduced GFR (either acute kidney injury [AKI] or CKD), and with microscopic haematuria or red cell casts. There is a significantly increased risk of venous thrombosis, due to loss of anticoagulant factors, such as antithrombin II in the urine, increased platelet aggregation and endothelial dysfunction.

Causes

Common glomerular diseases causing nephrotic syndrome include:

- Minimal change disease.
- FSGS.
- Membranous nephropathy.
- Mesangiocapillary GN.
- HIV-associated nephropathy.
- Renal amyloidosis.
- Light chain deposition disease.
- SLE with type 5 lupus nephritis.
- Diabetic glomerulosclerosis.

Diagnosis

Nephrotic syndrome is defined by:

1. Proteinuria >3.5 g/24 hours (equivalent to urine protein/creatinine ratio >350 mg/mmol).
2. Hypoalbuminaemia (<35 g/L).

3. Oedema.
4. Hyperlipidaemia/hypercholesterolaemia.

Management

- Salt and fluid restriction.
- Loop diuretics.
- Anti-proteinuric drugs: ACE inhibitors/angiotensin receptor blockers.
- Anticoagulation in selected patients.

Further reading

1. Bierzynska A, Saleem M. Recent advances in understanding and treating nephrotic syndrome. F1000Res. 2017 Feb 9;6:121. doi: 10.12688/f1000research.10165.1. eCollection 2017

Acute nephritic syndrome

Glomerulonephritis itself is a spectrum of disease. When combined with hypertension, oedema and oliguria, GN can be classed as 'nephritic' syndrome. Underlying GN is suggested by the combination of impaired renal function, and blood and protein in the urine.

Mechanisms of glomerular injury

Most glomerulonephritides are caused either by immune injury directed at glomerular antigens, or by circulating antigens or antigen-antibody complexes deposited in glomeruli.

Examples of injury caused by in situ antigen-targeting include anti-GBM disease and anti-PLA2R membranous nephropathy.

- Anti-GBM antibodies target the NC1 domain of the $\alpha3$ chain of type IV collagen, a component of the GBM.
- Anti-PLA2R antibodies form local immune complexes that cause epithelial cell injury. Thus, immune complex deposits seen in membranous nephropathy (MN) are sub-epithelial, whereas entrapment of circulating immune complexes, such as in lupus nephritis and infective endocarditis are sub-endothelial.

Ongoing immune injury is mediated by complement fixation and recruitment of inflammatory cells. Ensuing inflammatory mediators, proteases and cytokines disrupt the filtration barrier, and impair glomerular filtration.

Further reading

1. Woywodt A, Chiu D. The glomerulus and the concept of glomerulonephritis. Doucet A, Crambert G. (Eds). *Oxford Textbook of Clinical Nephrology*, 4th edn. Oxford: Oxford University Press.

Specific glomerular diseases

Minimal change nephropathy

Minimal change nephropathy (or minimal change disease [MCD]) is the underlying cause of nephrotic syndrome in 90% of children below six, but only the third most common cause in adults, after MN and FSGS. In adults, MCD is associated with certain drugs (including NSAIDs) and malignancies (e.g. lymphomas). Significant AKI related to intravascular volume depletion may be encountered, and renal or deep vein thrombosis are recognised complications.

The pathogenesis is not fully eludicated, but are likely to involve some or all of disordered T cell immunity, a circulating factor capable of inducing proteinuria and disordered podocyte function.

Diagnosis

There is normal glomerular appearance on light microscopy and negative immunofluorescence. On electron microscopy, however, diffuse effacement of podocyte foot processes are evident.

Treatment

- MCD responds to steroid treatment in up to 90% of adults within 12 weeks.
- 50–75% of adults will go on to have a relapse; options for frequent relapses include calcineurin inhibitors (ciclosporin and tacrolimus) or cyclophosphamide.
- Treatment resistance may prompt re-examination of the diagnosis, especially as sampling error can result in FSGS incorrectly being labelled as MCD.

The long-term prognosis is excellent for most MCD responsive to steroids, if free of relapses.

Further reading

1. Niaudet P, Meyrier A. Minimal change disease: clinical features and diagnosis. In: Doucet A, Crambert G. (Eds). *Oxford Textbook of Clinical Nephrology*, 4th edn. Oxford: Oxford University Press.
2. Niaudet P, Meyrier A. Minimal change disease: treatment and outcome. In: Doucet A, Crambert G. (Eds). *Oxford Textbook of Clinical Nephrology*, 4th edn. Oxford: Oxford University Press.

Focal and segmental glomerulosclerosis

FSGS is a histopathological description referring to a spectrum of idiopathic and secondary diseases affecting the kidney in a similar way.

Pathogenesis and genetics

Although the cause of primary FSGS is unknown, it can recur sometimes immediately after transplantation, suggesting a circulating permeability factor may be responsible.

Mutations in some podocyte proteins are associated with steroid-resistant nephrotic syndrome and childhood-onset FSGS, including *NPHS1* (nephrin), *NPHS2* (podocin), *ACTN4* (alpha-actinin 4) and *TRPC6*. Afro-Caribbean people also have increased susceptibility to FSGS, either alone or in association with hypertension or HIV infection. This risk is at least partly related to variants in apolipoprotein L1 (*APOL1*), which confers protection against *Trypanosoma brucei* infection.

Presentation

Primary FSGS commonly presents with nephrotic syndrome, nephrotic- or sub-nephrotic-range proteinuria. Renal impairment and progression to ESRD are common.

Diagnosis

There are five histological variants of FSGS: collapsing, tip, cellular, perihilar and not otherwise specified. The collapsing variant carries a particularly poor prognosis, while the tip variant may be expected to have a better response to steroids and a better overall prognosis.

Secondary FSGS

Secondary FSGS results from various kidney insults leading to a common pattern of glomerular injury related to haemodynamic stress and glomerular hyperfiltration. This may be related to reduced relative nephron number, e.g. in obesity, reflux nephropathy and renal dysplasia, or other glomerular diseases with glomerular obsolescence, e.g. diabetic nephropathy, HIV, pre-eclampsia, sickle cell nephropathy or membranous nephropathy.

Treatment of secondary FSGS

- Identification and management of the underlying cause if possible.
- ACE inhibitors or angiotensin receptor blockers (ARBs) which can reduce proteinuria and slow the decline in GFR.
- Specific disease-modifying treatment may be considered, particularly if primary FSGS is associated with nephrotic syndrome, e.g. with prolonged high-dose steroids, calcineurin inhibitiors and/or cyclophosphamide.

Further reading

1. Meyrier A, and Niaudet P. Primary focal segmental glomerulosclerosis: clinical features and diagnosis. In: Doucet A, Crambert G. (Eds). *Oxford Textbook of Clinical Nephrology*, 4th edn. Oxford: Oxford University Press.
2. Meyrier A, Niaudet P. Primary focal segmental glomerulosclerosis: treatment and outcome In: Doucet A, Crambert G. (Eds). *Oxford Textbook of Clinical Nephrology*, 4th edn. Oxford: Oxford University Press.

Membranous nephropathy

Membranous nephropathy (MN) is a common glomerular disease, and the leading cause of nephrotic syndrome in white Caucasian adults. Idiopathic MN often has auto-antibodies directed against the glomerular antigen M-type phospholipase A2 receptor (PLA2R). Causes of secondary MN include:

- Autoimmune diseases:
  - SLE.
  - Rheumatoid arthritis.
  - Sarcoidosis.
  - Crohn's disease.
- Infectious diseases:
  - Hepatitis B and C.
  - Syphilis.
  - Filariasis, hydatid cysts, schistosomiasis.
- Drugs:
  - Gold, penicillamine.
  - NSAIDs;
  - Captopril.
- Malignancies.

The association with underlying malignancy increases with age, with >10% of patients over 60 expected to have a malignancy, which may not manifest for many years after the diagnosis.

Diagnosis

Histologically immunoglobulin (usually IgG) and C3 deposition along the capillary walls or outer aspect of the GBM is evident. Light microscopic features include thickening of the basement membrane and 'spikes' on silver staining; sub-epithelial deposits are seen on electron microscopy.

Management

The clinical course of MN is highly variable. Approximately one-third remits spontaneously and one-third progresses to end-stage kidney disease. Abnormal kidney function and heavy proteinuria (>10 g/ 24 hours), or persistent proteinuria >1 year after presentation, are poor prognostic indicators and should prompt consideration of disease-modifying treatment.

Specific treatments

- Immunosuppressive therapy has tended to involve alternating months of steroids and alkylating agents (cyclophosphamide or chlorambucil).
- Data suggest that alternative agents, such as mycophenolate mofetil or rituximab may be equally effective in some patients (1,2).

Key references

1. Chan TM, Lin AW, Tang SC, et al. Prospective controlled study on mycophenolate mofetil and prednisolone in the treatment of membranous nephropathy with nephrotic syndrome. *Nephrology* (Carlton). 2007;12(6):576.
2. Dahan K, Debiec H, Plaisier E, et al. Rituximab for severe membranous nephropathy: a 6-month trial with extended follow-up. *J Am Soc Nephrol*. 2017;28(1):348.

Further reading

1. Cattran DC, Reich HN. Membranous glomerulonephritis: overview. In: Doucet A, Crambert G. (Eds). *Oxford Textbook of Clinical Nephrology*, 4th edn. Oxford: Oxford University Press.
2. Cattran DC, Reich HN. Membranous glomerulonephritis: clinical features and diagnosis. In: Doucet A, Crambert G. (Eds). *Oxford Textbook of Clinical Nephrology*, 4th edn. Oxford: Oxford University Press.
3. Cattran DC, Reich HN. Membranous glomerulonephritis: treatment and outcomes. In: Doucet A, Crambert G. (Eds). *Oxford Textbook of Clinical Nephrology*, 4th edn. Oxford: Oxford University Press.

Mesangiocapillary glomerulonephritis

Mesangiocapillary glomerulonephritis (MCGN), also known as membranoproliferative nephritis, is a histological description of a pattern of glomerular injury that has a number of causes.

Histologically, splitting or 'double-contouring' of the GBM, with interposition of mesangial cell cytoplasm between the endothelium and GBM, is evident. Historically, subtypes of MCGN have been classified according to findings on electron microscopy. However, most cases of MCGN are now known to be either immune complex or complement-mediated. This distinction is likely to be more clinically relevant.

Conditions associated with a mesangiocapillary pattern of injury

1. Immune complex-mediated diseases:
   - Chronic infections.
   - Auto-immune diseases.
   - Idiopathic: MCGN types I, II, III.
   - Paraprotein deposition diseases: light chain deposition, cyroglobulinaemia.
2. Complement mediated diseases:
   - Dense deposit disease (MCGN type II).
   - C3 glomerulopathy.
   - Atypical haemolytic uraemic syndrome (HUS).
3. Conditions without immunoglobulin or complement deposition:
   - Chronic and healed thrombotic microangiopathies.
   - Antiphospholipid syndrome.
   - Radiation nephritis.

For electron microscopic subtypes and associations, see Table 16.7.

Table 16.7 Electron microscopic subtypes and associations

	Type I	**Type II (dense deposit disease)**	**Type III**
Histology	Subendothelial deposits.	Widespread ribbon-like intramembranous deposits.	Subendothelial + subepithelial deposits (membranous change).
Secondary causes	Cryoglobulinaemia (HCV related or mixed essential cryoglobulinaemia unrelated to HCV). Shunt nephritis and other infections.		
Complement	Low C4.	Low C3. C3 nephritic factor.	
Associations		Partial lipodystrophy*.	

*The association between partial lipodystrophy and MCGN type II is a common MRCP topic.

Further reading

1. Salvadori M, Rosso G. Reclassification of membranoproliferative glomerulonephritis: identification of a new GN: C3GN. *World J Nephrol*. 2016;5(4):308–20.
2. Masani N, Jhaveri KD, Fishbane S. Update on membranoproliferative GN. *Clin J Am Soc Nephrol*. 2014;9(3):600–8.

IgA nephropathy

IgA nephropathy is the commonest primary glomerulonephritis in the world. Peak incidence is in the second and third decades of life.

The aetiology of IgA nephropathy is not fully understood. Tissue injury is caused by deposition of abnormally glycosylated IgA1 immune complexes in the mesangium, subsequent mesangial cell activation, and cytokine and growth factor production. Although some families with multiple affected members have been identified, IgA nephropathy is best considered a sporadic disease with likely contribution from both genetic and environmental factors. Although most cases are idiopathic, IgA nephropathy can be associated with liver cirrhosis, coeliac disease, IBD, rheumatic conditions and Henoch–Schönlein purpura (HSP).

Histopathological findings are mesangial cellular proliferation and matrix expansion, with IgA deposition in the mesangium.

Clinical presentation

IgA nephropathy has a variable presentation:

- Asymptomatic microscopic haematuria ± mild proteinuria.
- Recurrent macroscopic haematuria, typically within 1–3 days of an upper respiratory tract infection ('sympharyngitic haematuria').
- CKD from longstanding undiagnosed disease.
- Rarely, AKI with oliguria, which may be associated with a crescentic pattern of injury on biopsy.

Prognosis

- Most patients with isolated haematuria and no proteinuria have low risk of progression, while those with renal impairment at presentation, heavy proteinuria, or tubulo-interstitial fibrosis or glomerulosclerosis on biopsy are at risk of progressive renal impairment.
- Persistent proteinuria of >1 g/24 hours and/or hypertension carries a 50% risk of ESRD at 10 years.
- Overall renal survival is 50–80% at 20 years.

Management

Supportive measures for all patients:

- BP management.
- Renin-angiotensin system blockade with ACE-I or ARBs.

Current evidence supports the use of steroids in a subgroup of patients with deteriorating kidney function, persistent proteinuria, and evidence of active disease (such as proliferative or necrotizing changes) on kidney biopsy (1).

References

1. Lv J, Xu D, Perkovic V, et al. Corticosteroid therapy in IgA nephropathy. *J Am Soc Nephrol*. 2012;23(6):1108.

Further reading

1. Lai KN, Tang SC, Schena FP, et al. IgA nephropathy. *Nat Rev Dis Primers*. 2016;2:16001.

Tubulo-interstitial kidney disease

Acute interstitial nephritis

Acute interstitial nephritis (AIN) is a common cause of AKI. Common causes of AIN include:

- Drugs: the most common cause of AIN. Examples include antibiotics (penicillins, cefalosporins, rifampicin, sulfonamides), NSAIDs, proton pump inhibitors, allopurinol, antiretrovirals, diuretics.
- Infections, including ascending pyelonephritis, tuberculosis and leptospirosis.
- Autoimmune disease, including tubulo-interstitial nephritis and uveitis (TINU) syndrome.
- Idiopathic.

AIN can rarely occur with systemic symptoms, such as fever, arthralgia and a rash. If biopsied, characteristic features include an inflammatory cell infiltrate in the interstitium, which may be eosinophil-rich and include granulomata.

Treatment of drug-induced AIN is withdrawal of the likely agent, plus corticosteroid therapy if the AIN is severe (dialysis-dependent AKI) or if no improvement is seen 10 days after withdrawal of the inciting agent.

Chronic tubulo-interstitial kidney disease

Untreated AIN, or prolonged exposure to the causative agent, can progress to chronic tubulo-interstitial disease. Histologically this is characterised by varying tubular atrophy, interstitial fibrosis and inflammation.

Specific causes

- Chronic drug exposures: NSAIDs, calcineurin inhibitors, chemotherapeutic agents, lithium.
- Aristolochic acid: 'Chinese herb nephropathy' and Balkan endemic nephropathy.
- Reflux nephropathy and chronic pyelonephritis.
- Sarcoidosis.
- Tuberculosis.
- Auto-immune diseases: Sjögren syndrome, which classically initially presents as type 1 RTA.
- Genetic conditions: cystinosis, Dent disease, primary hyperoxaluria.
- Metabolic: chronic hypokalaemia.

Treatment is supportive and involves withdrawal of the causative agent wherever possible.

Renovascular disease

Atherosclerotic renal artery stenosis (RAS) is common, affecting 50% of those with atherosclerotic vascular disease elsewhere (coronary, carotid or peripheral). Up to 5% may also have fibromuscular dysplasia (FMD) causing RAS. FMD is typically seen in younger female patients.

RAS can be associated with a number of syndromes:

- Hypertension, often 'resistant' to treatment.
- Progressive CKD: ischaemic nephropathy.
- Recurrent flash pulmonary oedema.

Investigations

- Biochemical features may include mild hypokalaemia (secondary hyperaldosteronism) and at most mild proteinuria.
- Asymmetric kidneys on US imaging.
- Doppler ultrasonography can help detect RAS in experienced hands.
- Nuclear medicine MAG3 imaging can be useful: uptake of the radioactive tracer is slowed with RAS. This can be accentuated by administrating captopril.
- CT angiography and MR angiography are almost equivalent in sensitivity and specificity.
- The gold standard investigation is digital subtraction intra-arterial angiography.

Management

The key principle of management is careful attention to cardiovascular risk factors.

Treatment of significant RAS by angioplasty and stenting does not necessarily result in improved BP control or preservation of kidney function, likely because atherosclerosis is a systemic process, rather than a single anatomical stenosis.

Endovascular intervention may still be contemplated in a small subgroup, such as those with poorly controlled BP on ≥4 anti-hypertensives, or those with rapidly declining kidney function.

Further reading

1. Ritchie J, Green D, Chrysochou C, and Kalra PA. Renal artery stenosis: clinical features and diagnosis. In: Turner NN, Lameire N, Goldsmith DJ, et al. (Eds) *Oxford Textbook of Clinical Nephrology*, 4th edn. Oxford: Oxford University Press.
2. Ritchie J, Green D, Chrysochou C, Kalra PA. Renal artery stenosis: management and outcome. In: Turner NN, Lameire N, Goldsmith DJ, et al. (Eds) *Oxford Textbook of Clinical Nephrology*, 4th edn. Oxford: Oxford University Press.

Systemic diseases and the kidney

Diabetes

Diabetic nephropathy is the commonest cause of ESRD in the Western world. Although the incidence of ESRD from diabetes is falling, most likely because of renoprotective strategies (e.g. renin-angiotensin system blockade), the increasing incidence of diabetes overall has resulted in an increasing prevalence of ESRD which varies from 18%–30% in all people with diabetes.

Diabetic nephropathy occurs in both Type 1 and Type 2 diabetes; renal disease accounts for 21% of deaths in Type 1 and 11% of deaths in Type 2 diabetes. Nephropathy almost always occurs in association with other microvascular disease (retinopathy and neuropathy) in Type 1 diabetes; this association is not as close in Type 2 diabetes.

Risk factors for development of significant diabetic nephropathy include a family history of diabetes in first degree relative, ethnicity (e.g. African Americans, South Asians and Pima Indians are at increased risk), hypertension, poor glycaemic control, smoking and early glomerular hyperfiltration. Obesity is not an independent risk factor for development of kidney disease.

Pathogenesis of diabetic nephropathy

Diabetic nephropathy results from interplay between genetic predisposing factors and metabolic and haemodynamic pathways. Key mediators of progressive renal injury are thought to be:

- Glomerular hyperfiltration: maladaptive hyperfiltration is evidenced by the benefits of blockading the renin-angiotensin system. Sodium-glucose co-transporter-2 (SGLT2) inhibitors such as canagliflozin and empagliflozin may also have beneficial effects through vasoconstriction of afferent glomerular arterioles.
- Hyperglycaemia and advanced glycation end products (AGEs): hyperglycaemia itself can cause mesangial expansion and increased matrix production; exposure to AGEs enhances expression of type IV collagen and TGF-β by glomerular endothelial and mesangial cells and increases protein kinase C activity, all of which are implicated in renal fibrosis and glomerulosclerosis.

Diabetic nephropathy has five stages:

1. Renal hypertrophy and glomerular hyperfiltration: GFR may be 20-50% above normal.
2. Normalisation of GFR with early histological changes: clinically silent disease.
3. Microalbuminuria (albumin level in urine is detectable by laboratory testing but not by urine dip [<300mg/24h; albuminuria – albumin excretion >300mg/day] or urine albumin/creatinine ratio <30mg/mmol), commonly accompanied by hypertension.
   Persistent microalbuminuria:
   - Typically develops 5–15 years following diagnosis of Type 1 diabetes and is prevalent in 40% of patients after 30 years of diagnosis.
   - Is present in a quarter of patients with Type 2 diabetes 10 years after diagnosis.
4. Overt diabetic nephropathy: increasing proteinuria, falling GFR.
5. ESRF.

The rate of progression from no nephropathy to microalbuminuria to macroalbuminuria to elevated creatinine or ESRD is 2-3% per year for each stage.

Pathological hallmarks of diabetic kidney disease on renal biopsy are:

- Nodular intercapillary sclerosis (Kimmelstiel-Wilson nodules) or diffuse glomerular sclerosis.
- Mesangial expansion and GBM thickening.
- Interstitial fibrosis and atherosclerosis and arterial/arteriolar hyalinosis.

Management

The renal care for diabetic patients involves both the monitoring for and the treatment of established nephropathy. Patients with diabetes should have annual assessment of urine albumin creatinine ratio.

Microalbuminuria

- The threshold for microalbuminuria is >2.5mg/mmol in men and >3.5mg/mmol in women.
- If microalbuminuria is detected, tests should be repeated within 3-4 months; microalbuminuria is confirmed if two of three specimens are positive in the absence of an alternative diagnosis e.g. urinary tract infection.
- Microalbuminuria requires further investigation if there is: hypertension which is resistant to treatment, heavy proteinuria (albumin creatinine ratio > 100 mg/mmol), haematuria, rapid deterioration of GFR, or the patient is systemically unwell. Alternative aetiology is likely if microalbuminuria occurs in absence of retinopathy.

Management to retard progression of renal impairment

- Strict BP control: this is the key intervention, with a target of <130/80 mmHg; tighter target of < 120/75 in patients with proteinuria >1g/day). Blockade of the renin-angiotensin system with either ACE inhibitors or ARBs has anti-proteinuric and renoprotective effects, independent of controlling the BP.
- Strict glycaemic control, which also helps prevent development of proteinuria and clinically evident diabetic nephropathy in patients up to CKD Stage 3 (➲ see Chronic kidney disease, p. 585 and Tables 16.12 and 16.13).
- Reduction of cardiovascular risk: (as with other forms of CKD) through smoking cessation, weight management, increasing activity and managing dyslipidaemia.

The prognostic significance of proteinuria

While heavy proteinuria is a marker of increased risk for rapid decline in kidney function, progression can also be seen without proteinuria. Both microalbuminuria and higher levels of proteinuria are important markers of increased cardiovascular risk: patients with proteinuria are more likely to succumb to cardiovascular disease than progress to ESKD.

Further reading

1. Qi C, Mao X, Zhang Z, Wu H. Classification and differential diagnosis of diabetic nephropathy. *J Diabetes Res*. 2017; 2017:8637138.

Systemic lupus erythematosus

The pathophysiology, clinical features and management of SLE, a multisystem autoimmune disease is discussed in Chapter 20 (➲ Systemic lupus erythematosus, p. 729).

Renal involvement occurs in approximately 50% of patients with SLE, and therefore, screening for renal disease (urinalysis and assessing kidney function) is a crucial part of their long-term management. Renal involvement can range from asymptomatic microscopic haematuria and proteinuria with normal kidney function, to nephritic or nephrotic syndrome and rapidly progressive glomerulonephritis with AKI. Approximately 10% of patients with SLE progress to ESRD.

Investigation

- Serological evaluation for lupus nephritis (➲ see Chapter 20, Drug-induced lupus, p. 730, Diagnosis, p. 731 and Table 20.8).
- While anti-dsDNA titres and complement levels can correlate with disease activity, kidney biopsy is almost always required to establish a diagnosis of lupus nephritis and to assess severity.

Diagnosis

- On renal biopsy, the key pathological changes seen in lupus nephritis all result from glomerular deposition of circulating or locally-derived immune complexes, which fix complement and recruit inflammatory cells and release inflammatory cytokines.
- A 'full house' of immunoglobulin, C3 and C1q deposition is seen in the mesangium or sub-endothelial space. Membranous-like change is associated with sub-epithelial deposits.
- According to the International Society of Nephrology/Renal Pathological Society[1], lupus nephritis can be classified as follows:
    - Class I: Mesangial deposits identifiable on electron microscopy ('minimal mesangial lupus nephritis').
    - Class II: Mesangial proliferative lupus nephritis.
    - Class III: Less than 50% of glomeruli involved ('focal lupus nephritis').
    - Class IV: Greater than 50% of glomeruli involved ('diffuse lupus nephritis').
    - Class IV-S: Less than 50% of glomerular surface area involved ('diffuse segmental lupus nephritis').
    - Class IV-G: Greater than 50% of glomerular surface area involved ('diffuse global lupus nephritis').
    - Class V: Deposits in the subepithelium ('membranous lupus nephritis').
    - Class VI: Greater than 90% glomerular damage ('advanced sclerosing lupus nephritis').

Treatment

Treatment of severe lupus nephritis aims to induce remission using high-dose corticosteroids and cyclophosphamide, followed by maintenance treatment with mycophenolate mofetil (MMF) or azathioprine. Class V nephritis responds less well to treatment, but steroids and MMF are commonly used (➲ see Chapter 20, Treatment, p. 731).

Further reading

1. Zampeli E, Klinman DM, Gershwin ME, Moutsopoulos HM. A comprehensive evaluation for the treatment of lupus nephritis. *J Autoimmun*. 2017;78:1–10.

Systemic vasculitis and the kidney

Small vessel vasculitides often cause glomerular injury, and can present as oliguric AKI or progressive CKD and include:

1. Antineutrophil cytoplasmic antibody (ANCA) associated vasculitis:
    a. GPA (formerly called Wegener's granulomatosis).
    b. Microscopic polyangiitis (MPA).
    c. Renal-limited vasculitis.
    d. Eosinophilic granulomatosis with polyangiitis (formerly called Churg–Strauss syndrome).
2. Henoch-Schönlein purpura.
3. Cryoglobulinaemic vasculitis.

[1]Adapted from *Kidney International*, 93(4), Bajema IM, Wilhelmus S, Alpers CE, et al., Revision of the International Society of Nephrology/Renal Pathology Society classification of lupus nephritis: clarification of definitions, and modified National Institutes of Health activity and chronicity indices, pp. 789–796 (2018). DOI: 10.10216/j.kint.2017.11.023. Epub 2018 Feb 16. PMID: 29459092

Polyarteritis nodosa is a rare small- and medium-vessel vasculitis, which may be associated with HBV and can have renal manifestations, such as microaneurysms, in segmental renal arteries and distal ischaemic changes or infarction. Glomerular changes are not typically seen.

Anti-neutrophil cytoplasmic antibody-associated vasculitis

This group of disorders usually presents in older adults and are discussed in ➲ Chapter 20, Small and medium vessel vasculitis, p. 735). The clinical features include renal involvement, ranging from asymptomatic urinary abnormalities to rapidly progressive glomerulonephritis.

Diagnosis

ANCAs are directed against intracellular antigens, and are classically differentiated on immunofluorescence according to binding patterns, which are either cytoplasmic (C-ANCA) or perinuclear (P-ANCA) (see Table 6.5).

- C-ANCA is usually directed against neutrophil and monocyte proteinase 3 (PR3).
- P-ANCA is usually directed against myeloperoxidase (MPO).

ANCAs are probably directly pathogenic, causing activation of neutrophils and monocytes, and endothelial injury.

GPA is more commonly associated with C-ANCA, and eosinophilic granulomatosis with polyangiitis and MPA are more often associated P-ANCA.

Renal histopathology in all ANCA-associated kidney disease typically shows a focal segmental necrotising crescentic glomerulonephritis. Granulomata may also be present. Immunofluorescence or immunohistochemistry is classically pauci-immune (lack of immune deposits), unlike conditions such as anti-GBM disease and lupus nephritis.

Treatment

Induction of remission is achieved with high-dose steroids and a cytotoxic agent (usually cyclophosphamide). Maintenance treatment is with azathioprine after a minimum of 3 months if remission has been achieved.

Anti-CD20 monoclonal antibody (rituximab) is an alternative to cyclophosphamide in select patients. Plasma exchange is also used at the outset if there is AKI with serum creatinine >500 μmol/L or requiring dialysis, or concomitant pulmonary haemorrhage. Without treatment, AAV has a high mortality.

Further reading

1. Smith ML. Pathology of antineutrophil cytoplasmic antibody-associated pulmonary and renal disease. *Arch Pathol Lab Med.* 2017;141(2):223–231.
2. Jayne D. The patient with vasculitis: overview. In: Turner NN, Lameire N, Goldsmith DJ, et al. (Eds) *Oxford Textbook of Clinical Nephrology*, 4th edn. Oxford: Oxford University Press.
3. Harper L, Jayne D. The patient with vasculitis: treatment and outcome. In: Turner NN, Lameire N, Goldsmith DJ, et al. (Eds) *Oxford Textbook of Clinical Nephrology*, 4th edn. Oxford: Oxford University Press.

Plasma cell dyscrasias and dysproteinaemias

Plasma cell dyscrasias or dysproteinaemias can affect the kidneys in a number of ways including:

- Myeloma cast nephropathy.
- Light and heavy chain deposition disease.
- Amyloidosis.
- AKI related to other manifestations, including hypercalcaemia.

Myeloma cast nephropathy

This is the most common cause of kidney injury seen in patients with multiple myeloma. Freely filtered immunoglobulin light chains complex with uromodulin (Tamm–Horsfall protein) and precipitate in the distal tubule, causing obstruction, rupture of the tubular basement membrane and inflammation. Histologically, it is characterised by proteinaceous casts on microscopy, which appear 'fractured' in appearance and accompanied by an inflammatory infiltrate. Not all species of light chain cause this mode of injury; some may cause light chain deposition disease or amyloidosis.

Monoclonal immunoglobulin deposition diseases

Characterised by glomerular deposition of immunoglobulin and nodular glomerulosclerosis on light microscopy (Congo red negative), it shares morphological features with diabetic glomerulosclerosis (Kimmelstiel–Wilson nodules). Light chain deposition disease is the most common form.

Amyloidosis

Amyloidosis is a group of conditions in which fibrils of beta-pleated sheets of protein deposit abnormally in extracellular tissues. The abnormal protein that binds serum amyloid P protein can be a monoclonal light chain, causing primary (AL) amyloidosis, or a serum amyloid A protein, causing secondary (AA) amyloidosis.

Hereditary or genetic forms such as transthyretin are classed as AH amyloidosis.

The clinical features and management of amyloidosis is discussed in ➲ Chapter 9, Amyloidosis, p. 304.

Renal involvement in amyloidosis usually manifests as nephrotic syndrome. Renal biopsy shows amorphous deposits in glomerular mesangial and capillary walls, with orange-red staining with Congo red, which shows apple-green birefringence with polarised light. Immunohistochemistry can distinguish between AL and AA amyloidosis.

Further reading

1. Sethi S, Fervenza FC, Rajkumar SV. Spectrum of manifestations of monoclonal gammopathy-associated renal lesions. *Curr Opin Nephrol Hypertens*. 2016;25(2):127–37.

Scleroderma renal crisis

Up to 50% of patients with systemic sclerosis (➲ see Chapter 20, Systemic sclerosis, p. 733) have renal disease in the form of reduced GFR, proteinuria or hypertension. For the majority, renal disease follows a benign course.

Scleroderma renal crisis is a life-threatening syndrome, which manifests as AKI, hypertension (though up to 10% may be normotensive) and bland urine (no haematuria or proteinuria). Microangiopathic haemolytic anaemia, hypertensive encephalopathy or heart failure can also occur in association with the hypertension.

Risk factors for scleroderma renal crisis include:

- Diffuse cutaneous systemic sclerosis.
- Recent exposure to glucocorticoids.
- Anti-RNA polymerase III auto-antibody.

Diagnosis of scleroderma renal crisis

Renal biopsy findings may show a thrombotic microangiopathy, with 'onion skin' intimal thickening of intrarenal vessels, ultimately leading to occlusion of the vascular lumen. Although these changes are not specific to scleroderma renal crisis, they are highly suggestive of the diagnosis in the appropriate clinical setting.

Management and prognosis

- BP control is important, usually with an ACE-i; often starting with a short-acting ACE-I (e.g. captopril), with an aim to reduce systolic BP by 10% each day.
- Prostacyclin (epoprostenol) infusions may be used, but are of unproven benefit.
- 25% of patients require dialysis; 50% of these will be long-term. Patients who present in renal crisis with normal BP are at greatest risk of mortality or of needing chronic renal replacement therapy.

Further reading

1. Lynch BM, Stern EP, Ong V, et al. UK Scleroderma Study Group (UKSSG) guidelines on the diagnosis and management of scleroderma renal crisis. *Clin Exp Rheumatol*. 2016;34[Suppl. 100(5)]:106–9.

Rheumatoid arthritis

For renal complications of rheumatoid arthritis ➲ see Chapter 20, Rheumatoid arthritis, p. 705 and Box 20.1.

Thrombotic microangiopathies: thrombotic thrombocytopenic purpura/ haemolytic uraemic syndrome

Thrombotic microangiopathies are a group of conditions characterised by:

- Intravascular haemolysis; direct antiglobulin test (Coombs test) negative.
- Low platelets.
- Tissue ischaemia.

Pathological findings in the kidneys and elsewhere include microthrombi and endothelial cell swelling and detachment.

Causes include:

1. TTP.
2. Diarrhoea-associated ('typical') haemolytic uraemic syndrome (D + HUS).
3. Atypical haemolytic uraemic syndrome (aHUS).
4. DIC.
5. Malignant hypertension.
6. Antiphospholipid antibody syndrome.
7. Drugs, e.g. calcineurin inhibitors tacrolimus and ciclosporin.
8. HIV infection.

Thrombotic thrombocytopenic purpura

Most cases of TTP are characterised by deficient metalloproteinase ADAMTS-13 activity, which cleaves multimers of vWF. The cleaved polypeptides are part of the normal haemostatic response. In TTP, abnormally large vWF multimers cause platelet activation and aggregation, forming platelet-rich thrombi and systemic microangiopathy. In most people, reduced ADAMTS-13 activity comes from auto-antibodies against ADAMTS-13.

Clinical features

Classic pentad of:

1. Fever.
2. Microangiopathic haemolytic anaemia (fragments on blood film signifying haemolysis).
3. Thombocytopenic purpura.
4. AKI.
5. Neurological involvement: confusion, fits, encephalopathy.

Treatment is with plasma exchange, to restore ADAMTS-13 activity. Platelet transfusions are avoided, except in life-threatening haemorrhage.

Haemolytic uraemic syndrome

The combination of AKI with thrombocytopenia and evidence of intravascular haemolysis should prompt evaluation for possible HUS. Renal impairment is more common with HUS than with TTP. Diarrhoea-associated HUS is caused by infection with *Shiga* toxin-forming organisms, most notably *E. coli* O157:H7, *Shigella dysenteriae* type 1, *Salmonella, Campylobacter* and *Yersinia* spp. Treatment is supportive, with no role for plasma exchange.

Atypical haemolytic uraemic syndrome

Disorders of uncontrolled activation of the alternative pathway of complement, which may result from genetic mutations in complement genes, including complement factor H (CFH), membrane cofactor protein, and deletion of *CFHR1* and *CFHR3* (associated anti-CFH antibodies). aHUS commonly recurs after renal transplantation, usually leading to graft loss. Treatment commonly involves plasma exchange. Novel complement inhibitors, including humanised anti-C5 monoclonal antibody (eculizumab [see Table 3.4]), are promising agents for treating aHUS, whether de novo or recurrent in a renal transplant, and potentially for prevention recurrence post-transplantation.

Further reading

1. Noris M, Goodship T. The patient with haemolytic uraemic syndrome/thrombotic thrombocytopenic purpura. In: Turner NN, Lameire N, Goldsmith DJ, et al. (Eds) *Oxford Textbook of Clinical Nephrology*, 4th edn. Oxford: Oxford University Press.

Hepatorenal syndrome

A differential diagnosis for AKI in patients with chronic liver disease includes:

- Sepsis.
- Pre-renal AKI: GI blood loss, diuretic use.
- Nephrotoxins causing acute tubular necrosis, including drugs toxic to both liver and kidneys e.g. paracetamol in overdose.
- Glomerulonephritis associated with viral hepatitis: cryoglobulinaemia and type I MCGN with HCV.
- Hepatorenal syndrome (➔ see Chapter 15, Hepatorenal syndrome, p. 529).

HRS is a potentially reversible syndrome in patients with cirrhosis, ascites and liver failure, consisting of impaired renal function, marked abnormalities in cardiovascular function, and intense over-activity of endogenous vasoactive systems.

Further reading

1. Cárdenas A, Ginès P. The patient with hepatorenal syndrome. In: Turner NN, Lameire N, Goldsmith DJ, et al. (Eds) *Oxford Textbook of Clinical Nephrology*, 4th edn. Oxford: Oxford University Press.

HIV

The kidneys are significant reservoirs for HIV within infected hosts. Patients with HIV are susceptible to a range of kidney diseases. Morbidity associated with renal injury is now a major factor in the management of patients with HIV.

HIV increases risk for both AKI and CKD and the pathological entities described in Table 16.8 may be responsible, together or in isolation.

Table 16.8 Causes of kidney injury in HIV infection

Pre-renal	Volume depletion.	Sepsis. Heart failure. Liver cirrhosis (e.g. from concurrent HCV).
	HIV-associated microangiopathy.	
Renal	Drug nephrotoxicity.	HIV-specific drugs (e.g. tenofovir). Other drugs used in the management of HIV (e.g. co-trimoxazole).
	HIVAN.	
	Immune complex-mediated GN.	
Post-renal	Obstruction.	Crystalluria (e.g. protease inhibitors). Malignancy.

HCV, hepatitis C virus; HIVAN, HIV-associated nephropathy.

HIV-associated nephropathy

This is a unique entity occurring almost exclusively in Afro-Caribbeans, in which patients with advanced HIV present with heavy proteinuria and rapidly declining renal function. Hypertension and oedema are common, but not always present.

A histological diagnosis is usually required as approximately 50% of patients presenting with features consistent with HIVAN have an alternative diagnosis on biopsy. The histological lesion is usually FSGS in which the glomerular tuft is seen to collapse ('collapsing variant of FSGS').

Other than general renal care prescribed for all patients with renal injuries, HIVAN is usually treated with antiretroviral therapy (➲ see Chapter 7, Antiretroviral therapy, p. 220 and Table 7.12), although the renal prognosis still remains relatively poor.

Further reading

1. Saraladevi Naicker S, Paget G. HIV and renal disease. In: Turner NN, Lameire N, Goldsmith DJ, et al. (Eds) *Oxford Textbook of Clinical Nephrology*, 4th edn. Oxford: Oxford University Press.

Inherited kidney disease

Autosomal dominant polycystic kidney disease

ADPKD is the most common inherited kidney disease, affecting between 1 in 400 to 1 in 1000, accounting for approximately 5% of all end-stage kidney disease (ESKD) in developed countries.

Mutations in two different genes can cause ADPKD:

- *PKD1* (polycystin-1): responsible for approximately 85% of cases. Most people with *PKD1* mutations have kidney failure by age 70.
- *PKD2* (polycystin-2): responsible for approximately 15% of cases. Fewer than 50% of individuals with *PKD2* mutations have kidney failure by 70.

Polycystin-1 is a membrane-signalling receptor that complexes with polycystin-2, a calcium-permeable channel. This polycystin complex is a mechanosensor in the cilia of renal collecting duct epithelial cells, sensing flow in the tubular lumen, and regulating cell proliferation, adhesion, differentiation and maturation to form and maintain tubular structure. It is thought that cyst formation is dependent on a 'second hit', with somatic inactivation or mutation of the normal allele.

Clinical features

Extrarenal manifestations of ADPKD include;

- Cystic liver disease: cysts in the liver are common, but rarely have functional impact. In a minority of patients, massive enlargement of the liver can cause pain and mechanical problems, necessitating combined liver-kidney transplantation.
- Intracranial aneurysms: berry aneurysms of intracranial arteries affect approximately 6% of patients with no family history of aneurysms, and 16% of those with a known family history. Aneurysms occur with both *PKD1* and *PKD2* mutations.
- Cysts in other organs: pancreatic cysts are common. Ovarian cysts are not associated with ADPKD.
- Cardiac manifestations: mitral valve prolapse is found in up to 25% of patients. Aortic root dilatation and aortic regurgitation are also described.
- Diverticular disease.

Complications of ADPKD

- Hypertension.
- Progressive renal impairment: high total kidney volume, as assessed by MRI, suggests an increased risk of rapid decline in kidney function.
- Cyst haemorrhage: presenting with acute onset pain and/or haematuria.
- Cyst infection.
- Kidney stone disease.

Treatment

Cystogenesis involves signalling via cAMP, which is increased in collecting duct epithelial cells through the action of vasopressin (ADH) via the vasopressin 2 receptor. The vasopressin receptor antagonist tolvaptan slows cyst growth and may delay progression to ESKD.

Future therapies may include antagonism of mechanistic (formerly mammalian) target of rapamycin (mTOR) and somatostatin analogues.

Further reading

1. Ong ACM, Sandford R. Autosomal dominant polycystic kidney disease: overview. In: Turner NN, Lameire N, Goldsmith DJ, et al. (Eds) *Oxford Textbook of Clinical Nephrology*, 4th edn. Oxford: Oxford University Press.

Autosomal recessive polycystic kidney disease

Autosomal recessive polycystic kidney disease presents in infancy and childhood, and always involves both kidney and liver disease. Liver disease is varied, but commonly includes congenital hepatic fibrosis or non-obstructive intra-hepatic biliary duct dilatation (➲ Caroli disease [see Chapter 5, MCQ 6, p. 143 and Answer to MCQ 6, p. 145]). The condition is caused by mutations in the *PKHD1* gene (polyductin).

Alport syndrome

This syndrome arises from a variety of genetic defects leading to abnormalities in the basement membrane in the glomeruli, cochlea and eye. The classical triad is:

- Progressive renal impairment.
- Sensorineural hearing loss.
- Ocular abnormalities, such as anterior lenticonus and white or yellow perimacular flecks.

80% of cases are X-linked, caused by mutations in *COL4A5* (the α5 chain of type IV collagen). A smaller proportion has an autosomal recessive mode of inheritance, caused by mutations in the *COL4A3* and *COL4A4* genes. Rarely, patients with Alport syndrome develop post-transplant anti-GBM nephritis, as the wild-type α5 chain of type IV collagen in the allograft is recognized as non-self and elicits an immune response.

Tuberous sclerosis

Tuberous sclerosis complex (TSC) is autosomal dominant and associated with hamartoma formation in multiple organs (➲ see Chapter 17, Tuberous sclerosis, p. 637). Angiomyolipomas (AMLs) and cysts are commonly seen in the kidneys. The incidence of renal cell cancers is increased (see Table 10.2).

TSC is caused by mutations in the *TSC1* or *TSC2* genes, encoding the tumour suppressor genes tuberin and hamartin respectively. The *TSC2* gene is adjacent to *PKD1*; deletions inactivating both genes cause combined TSC and ADPKD, but with cysts typically diagnosed in infancy or childhood, and an earlier progression to ESRD.

Von Hippel-Lindau disease

This autosomal dominant disease also leads to cyst formation of the kidneys and pancreas, and is associated with renal cell carcinoma (➲ see Chapter 17, Von Hippel-Lindau disease, p. 637).

Fabry disease

Fabry disease is a multisystem X-linked lysosomal storage disorder caused by deficiency of the enzyme α-galactosidase A, with resultant lysosomal accumulation of the substrate globotriaosylceramide (GL-3). Clinical features include:

- Painful acroparaesthesias (a painful burning or tingling sensation in extremities).
- GI symptoms of diarrhoea, abdominal pain, early satiety, nausea.
- Progressive renal impairment.
- Cardiac dysfunction (including cardiomyopathies and arrhythmias).
- Cutaneous lesions, e.g. classic angiokeratomas.

Early enzyme replacement therapy may protect kidney function and prevent other complications.

Congenital nephrotic syndrome

A number of genetic mutations can cause congenital or childhood nephrotic syndrome and FSGS, including in the genes *NPHS1*, *NPHS2*, *ACTN4* and *TRPC6*.

Drugs and the kidney

Important drugs with renal actions include:

- Diuretics: all diuretics block sodium absorption at one site along the nephron (see Table 16.9).
- ACE-I and ARBs: cause selective vasodilatation of the efferent glomerular arteriole, reducing glomerular hypertension. They should be prescribed with caution in CKD due to the risk of hyperkalaemia, although their use is not contraindicated.

Table 16.9 Diuretics and the kidney

Class	Examples	Mode of action	Clinical use	Adverse effects
Loop diuretics	Furosemide Bumetanide	Block type 2 Na^+ K^+ $2Cl^-$ (NKCC2) transporter in thick ascending limb of loop of Henle (responsible for reabsorption of ~25% of filtered Na^+) (see Figure 16.1C).	Volume overload: more potent natriuretics than thiazides. Limited use in hypertension (unless also volume overloaded). Also cause Ca^{2+} loss.	↓K^+. Metabolic alkalosis.
Thiazide diuretics	Bendroflumethiazide Hydrochlorothiazide Metolazone Indapamide	Block Na^+ Cl^- cotransporter in apical membrane of DCT tubular cells (responsible for ~5–7% of Na^+ reabsorption) (see Figure 16.1D).	Effective in hypertension. Can be useful adjuncts to loop diuretics to aid diuresis.	↓K^+. ↑urate. Impaired glucose tolerance. ↑Ca^{2+}.
Potassium-sparing diuretics	Amiloride Triamterene	Block epithelial Na^+ channel (ENaC) in late DCT and collecting duct (see Figure 16.1D).	Mitigate ↓K^+ seen with other diuretics.	↑K^+.
Mineralocorticoid antagonists	Spironolactone Eplerenone	Block mineralocorticoid receptor in collecting duct (also heart, vasculature, brain) (see Figure 16.1D).	Evidence base in treatment of heart failure. Useful adjunct in treatment of hypertension. Mitigate ↓K^+ seen with other diuretics.	↑K^+.
Carbonic anhydrase inhibitors	Acetazolamide	Block luminal carbonic anhydrase in proximal tubule, inhibit reabsorption of filtered HCO_3^- (see Figures 16.2 and 16.3).	Little efficacy as a diuretic: limited use. Prophylaxis and treatment of altitude sickness.	Metabolic acidosis. Worsening hypercapnia in those with lung disease.

- NSAIDs: decrease renal prostaglandin production, and thereby limit the capacity for glomerular auto-regulation. They are also important causes of both acute and chronic interstitial nephritis. Selective COX-2 inhibitors have not been found to be safer.
- Tenofovir: this nucleotide analogue is an effective component of anti-HIV treatment, but can cause AKI and the proximal tubular Fanconi syndrome.

Acute kidney injury

AKI is common, both in the community and in hospitalised patients. AKI significantly increases morbidity and mortality, both in the short and long term. AKI can be classified as shown in Table 16.10.

Table 16.10 The RIFLE (A) and AKI network (B) criteria for classification of AKI

A	**RIFLE criteria**	
	Creatinine criteria	**Urine output criteria**
Risk	↑>1.5 × from baseline	< 0.5 mL/kg/hour for >6 hours
Injury	↑>2 × from baseline	< 0.5 mL/kg/hour for >12 hours
Failure	↑>3 × from baseline or acute increase >44.2 µmol/L (0.5 mg/dL) if creatinine >350 µmol/L (>4 mg/dL)	< 0.3 mL/kg/hour for >24 hours or anuria >12 hours
Loss	Irreversible AKI or persistent AKI >4 weeks	
End-Stage	End-stage renal disease >3 months	
B	**AKI network criteria**	
	Creatinine criteria	**Urine output criteria**
Stage 1	↑>1.5 × or >26.4 µmol/L (0.3 mg/dL)	<0.5 mL/kg/hour for >6 hours
Stage 2	↑>2 × from baseline	<0.5 mL/kg/hour for >12 hours
Stage 3	↑>3 × from baseline or treatment with RRT	<0.3 mL/kg/hour for >24 hours or anuria >12 hours

RRT, renal replacement therapy.
Adapted from: Bellomo R. et al. Acute renal failure – definition, outcome measures, animal models, fluid therapy and information technology needs: the Second International Consensus Conference of the Acute Dialysis Quality Initiative (ADQI) Group. *Critical Care*, 8(4):R204–12. © Bellomo et al; licensee BioMed Central Ltd. 2007.
Adapted from: Mehta, R. L. et al. Acute Kidney Injury Network: report of an initiative to improve outcomes in acute kidney injury. *Crit Care*, 11(2):R31.© Mehta et al.; licensee BioMed Central Ltd. 2007.

AKI definitions underline the importance of establishing a patient's baseline level of kidney function, and the need to avoid using eGFR in the acute setting, as eGFR calculations assume a steady state (➲ see Direct and indirect measurements of renal function, p. 550).

The aetiology of AKI can be subdivided into pre-renal (due to hypoperfusion), renal (intrinsic) and post-renal (see Figure 16.4).

Acute kidney injury management principles

Management of AKI is supportive (paying particular attention to volume status, sepsis and nephrotoxins), while identifying and treating the underlying cause. The hard indications for dialysis are shown below in the section on RRT. The ECG features of hyperkalaemia and its emergency management are outlined in Tables 16.11A and 16.11B, respectively.

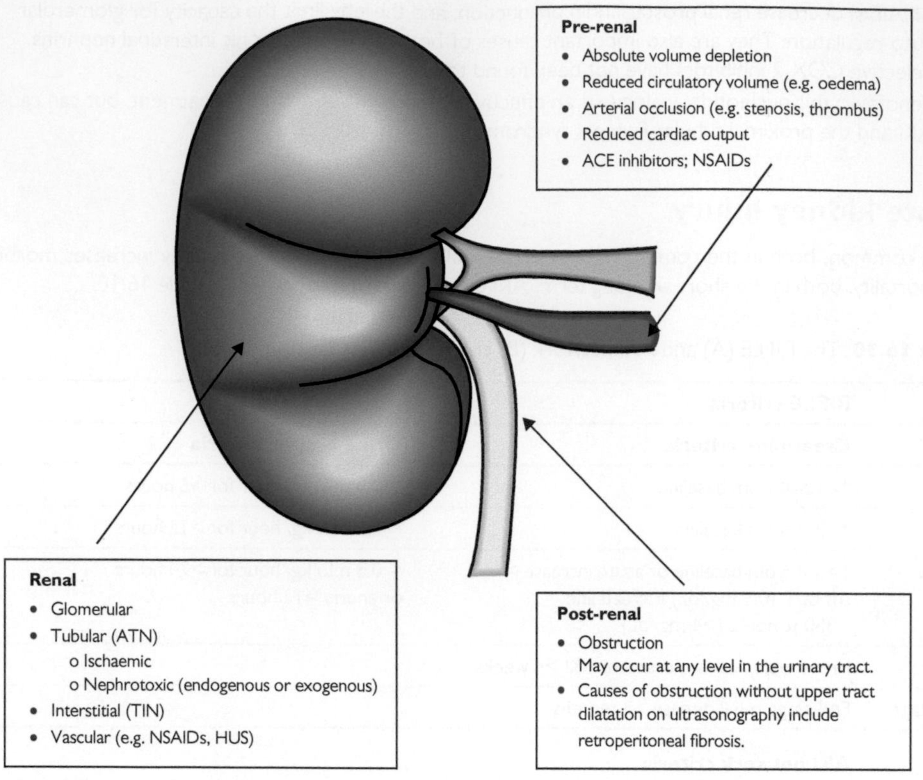

Figure 16.4 Causes of acute kidney injury (AKI).
Reproduced with kind permission of Olivia Bessant.

Table 16.11A ECG features of hyperkalaemia

Stage	ECG change
1	T waves peaked.
2	P waves widened then lost. PR segments lengthened.
3	QRS lengthened. AV block. Sinus bradycardia. Sine waves.
4	Asystole or pulseless electrical activity (PEA); sometimes ventricular fibrillation (VF).

Table 16.11B Emergency management of hyperkalaemia

The following treatments can be initiated in the order shown, until the desired effect is achieved. It is important to remember to also look for the underlying cause, if possible.

Rationale	Treatment
Stabilise cardiac potential to prevent asystole or VF	IV calcium gluconate 10 mL of 10% IV over 10 minutes*.
Shift potassium from the serum into cells**	IV insulin and glucose. IV sodium bicarbonate.
Eliminate potassium from the body	IV diuretics to encourage renal loss of potassium***. Haemodialysis/haemofiltration.
Prevent further potassium absorption to the body	Discontinue any potassium containing IV drips, including parenteral feeding. Discontinue oral drugs that contribute (e.g. oral potassium supplements). Calcium resonium (polystyrene sulfonate) given orally (in conscious patients) and/or rectally (in the unconscious patient).
Treat underlying causes, if apparent	
Measure potassium levels again	Potassium leaks back out of cells and so rebound hyperkalaemia is exceptionally common. Repeated measuring of K^+ is essential. In life-threatening hyperkalaemia, the patient should be monitored one to one with constant ECG tracing and repeated serum K^+ assessment.

*Some sources may suggest that IV calcium is contraindicated when digoxin toxicity is suspected as the cause of hyperkalaemia. This 'stone heart' syndrome is most likely untrue (1); nevertheless, it is important to recognise that the hyperkalaemia associated with digoxin poisoning may be refractory to standard therapies until digoxin levels fall.
** These are temporary measures. The potassium gradually leaks back out of cells again, so it is essential to also eliminate the potassium from the body.
***Contraindicated if the patient is anuric, e.g. ESKD or has suspected urinary tract obstruction.

References

1. Levine M, Nikkanen H, Pallin DJ. The effects of intravenous calcium in patients with digoxin toxicity. *J Emerg Med.* 2011; 40(1):41–6.

Further reading

1. Molitoris BA, Levin A, Warnock DG, et al. Improving outcomes from acute kidney injury. *J Am Soc Nephrol.* 2007; 18(7):1992.
2. Rose BD. *Pathophysiology of Renal Disease*, 2nd edn. New York, NY: McGraw-Hill.
3. Kidney Disease: Improving Global Outcomes (KDIGO) Acute Kidney Injury Work Group. KDIGO Clinical Practice Guideline for Acute Kidney Injury. *Kidney Int Suppl.* 2012; 2:1.

Chronic kidney disease

The overall population prevalence of CKD has been found to be 10–12% in most epidemiological studies in North America, Europe and Australia.

For CKD classification, see Table 16.12.

The suffix 'p' can be used to denote the presence of significant proteinuria (urine protein/creatinine ratio >100 mg/mmol, e.g. stage 3Bp). This emphasises the important risks of proteinuria, of both progressive decline in kidney function, and of cardiovascular disease.

Table 16.12 CKD classification

Stage	eGFR
1	>90 + urinary or structural abnormalities indicating presence of kidney disease.
2	60–89 + urinary or structural abnormalities indicating presence of kidney disease.
3A 3B	45–59 30–44
4	15–29
5	<15 or on dialysis.

Adapted from *Kidney International Supplements*, 3, Kidney Disease: Improving Global Outcomes (KDIGO) CKD Work Group. KDIGO 2012 clinical practice guideline for the evaluation and management of chronic kidney disease, pp. 1–150 (2013). Copyright © 2013, with permission from International Society of Nephrology. Published by Elsevier Inc. All rights reserved. https://doi.org/10.1038/kisup.2012.73.

Table 16.13 Common presentations of kidney diseases by type

Kidney disease	Clinical presentation
Diabetic kidney disease	Asymptomatic abnormalities on urinalysis (proteinuria); proteinuric CKD; nephrotic syndrome.
Glomerular diseases	
Proliferative GN	Nephritic syndrome; asymptomatic abnormalities on urinalysis (haematuria and proteinuria); systemic disease may be present (e.g. rash, arthritis, pulmonary symptoms).
Non-inflammatory	Nephrotic syndrome; asymptomatic abnormalities on urinalysis (proteinuria).
Vascular diseases	
Large vessels	Hypertension; CKD; asymptomatic radiological abnormalities.
Medium-sized vessels	Hypertension; CKD; asymptomatic abnormalities on urinalysis (proteinuria).
Small vessels	Hypertension; CKD; asymptomatic abnormalities on urinalysis (proteinuria).
Tubulointerstitial diseases	
Tubulointerstitial nephritis (TIN)	Kidney disease with urinary tract symptoms; tubular syndromes; asymptomatic abnormalities on urinalysis (pyuria, tubular cells); asymptomatic radiological abnormalities; urine concentrating defect.
Non-inflammatory	Tubular syndromes; asymptomatic abnormalities on urinalysis (proteinuria; pyuria; tubular cells; granular casts); asymptomatic radiological abnormalities.
Cystic diseases	Urinary tract symptoms; asymptomatic abnormalities on urinalysis; asymptomatic radiological abnormalities; asymptomatic CKD; subarachnoid haemorrhage; hypertension.
Diseases in kidney transplants	
Acute rejection	Deterioration in renal function; pain if severe.
Chronic rejection	Hypertension; CKD; asymptomatic abnormalities on urinalysis (pyuria; proteinuria).
Drug toxicity	Hypertension; CKD.
Transplant glomerulopathy	Asymptomatic abnormalities on urinalysis (proteinuria); donor-specific antibodies may be present.
Recurrent disease	Nephrotic syndrome; asymptomatic abnormalities on urinalysis (haematuria; proteinuria); AKI; CKD.

Causes

In the developed world, the most common causes of CKD are:

1. Diabetes.
2. Hypertension and renovascular disease.
3. Chronic glomerulonephritis.
4. Reflux nephropathy.
5. Adult polycystic kidney disease.

For common presentations of kidney diseases by type, see Table 16.13.

Management principles

- Identification and treatment of the underlying cause.
- Management of cardiovascular risk and risk factors for progression of CKD:
  - Smoking cessation.
  - Weight loss and exercise.
  - Management of dyslipidaemia.
  - BP control: the most important risk factor for progression irrespective of cause.
  - Reduction of proteinuria with RAS blockade if possible.
- Management of complications of CKD (typically in stage 4 or 5 CKD):
  - Hypertension and fluid overload.
  - Correction of anaemia with recombinant human erythropoietin and IV iron. The target haemoglobin level is 100–120 g/L.
  - Management of renal bone disease.
  - Correction of acidosis with sodium bicarbonate (shown to slow progression of CKD).
- Education and planning for future treatment:
  - Shared decision-making regarding RRT modalities or conservative management.
  - Establishment of access for haemodialysis (HD) or peritoneal dialysis (PD).
  - Work-up for transplantation.

Patients with any degree of kidney dysfunction have hugely increased risk of cardiovascular disease.

- Most patients with stage 1–3 CKD do not progress to end-stage kidney disease, but die instead from cardiovascular disease.
- Cardiovascular disease is the commonest cause of death in patients with ESKD.

As such, particular attention to cardiovascular risk parameters is essential. Anaemia is a risk factor for morbidity, mortality and hospitalisation in patients with CKD; conversely, restoration of normal levels of Hb in patients with CKD also results in adverse cardiovascular outcomes. The arguments for and against different Hb targets and the optimal way to achieve those are beyond the scope of this chapter.

Renal bone disease

The kidneys play a key role in regulation of calcium and phosphate. CKD, thus, perturbs bone and mineral metabolism (➲ See Chapter 1, Bone and calcium metabolism, p. 1, Magnesium and phosphate: role, regulation and pathology, p. 6, Box 1.1 and Figure 1.1).

Further reading

1. Levey AS, Eckardt KU, Tsukamoto Y, et al. Definition and classification of chronic kidney disease: a position statement from kidney disease: improving Global Outcomes (KDIGO). *Kidney Int*. 2005; 67(6):2089.
2. Abboud H, Henrich WL. Clinical practice. Stage IV chronic kidney disease. *N Engl J Med*. 2010; 362(1):56.

Renal replacement therapy

Modes of RRT include:

1. Continuous RRT modalities used in ICU setting: continuous venovenous haemofiltration (CVVH), continuous venovenous haemodiafiltration (CVVHDF), slow low-efficiency dialysis (SLED), slow continuous ultrafiltration (SCUF) (➲ see Chapter 12, Acute kidney injury, p. 401 and Box 12.4).
2. HD.
3. PD.
4. Transplantation.

Choice of RRT in AKI depends on cardiovascular stability, comorbid conditions, and local availability of expertise and RRT facilities.

Absolute indications for starting RRT in any setting are:

1. Hyperkalaemia refractory to medical management, especially in anuric patients.
2. Metabolic acidosis refractory to medical management.
3. Volume overload (pulmonary oedema) with inadequate response to diuretics.
4. Uraemic complications: pericarditis, encephalopathy.
5. Poisoning, including lithium and ethylene glycol.

Haemodialysis

The key principle in HD is *diffusion* of solutes across a semi-permeable membrane, with the diffusion gradient determined by the composition of dialysate fluid. This differs from haemofiltration (HF), where solutes cross the membrane by *convection*, together with fluid, which crosses the membrane owing to a transmembrane pressure gradient. As large amounts of fluid are removed with HF, replacement fluid is needed. In chronic HD, the transmembrane pressure is set to achieve a prescribed volume of fluid removal (ultrafiltration) in each session.

Key requirements for haemodialysis

- Vascular access.
- Anticoagulation.
- A dialysis membrane in the form of a dialyser and dialysate.

Modifiable variables

- Time and frequency of treatment. Increasing total dialysis time results in improved clearance and improved biochemical parameters.
- Blood flow: this is often dependent on the quality of vascular access, with arterio-venous fistulas being preferable to tunnelled haemodialysis catheters.
- Dialysate composition and flow rate: dialysate sodium, bicarbonate, potassium and calcium levels can be chosen according to the specific needs of the patient.
- Dialyser size and type: increasing the surface area of the dialysis membrane increases solute clearance. Different membranes have different pore sizes, allowing differential clearance of small and medium sized molecules.

Peritoneal dialysis

PD exploits the ability of the peritoneum to function as a semi-permeable membrane in bringing about clearance of water, solutes and small molecules.

Key principles

- Clearance of water (ultrafiltration) depends on the PD fluid being hyperosmolar relative to plasma and extracellular fluid.
- The key osmoles used are either glucose or glucose polymers, such as icodextrin.

- The two alternative forms of PD are continuous ambulatory peritoneal dialysis (CAPD), where patients manually perform 3–5 fluid exchanges in a 24-hour period, and automated peritoneal dialysis (APD), where most of the exchanges are performed by a machine overnight.
- A daytime dwell of PD fluid can be programmed, typically in order to achieve the desired amount of ultrafiltration for the day.

The choice between HD and PD, or between home-based or satellite unit-based treatments, depends on a number of factors. It is the role of the renal MDT to help guide patients and their carers through these choices.

Transplantation: matching, HLA, the alloresponse, mechanisms of immunosuppression

The treatment of choice for many patients with ESKD is transplantation; indeed, living donor kidney transplantation before the need for dialysis (pre-emptive transplantation) can be seen as the gold standard treatment. Deceased donor kidney transplantation is also highly successful, and an increasing proportion of kidney transplants are taking place from donation after circulatory death (DCD) donors as opposed to donation after brain death (DBD) donors.

The alloresponse

The immune response to the transplanted kidney is complex (➲ See Chapter 6, Transplantation immunology, p. 170).

Immunosuppression

Modern transplant immunosuppression involves induction treatment, followed by maintenance immunosuppression. Throughout, the key aim is to maintain a balance between effective suppression of the alloresponse and minimise toxicity associated with long-term immunosuppression. For commonly used immunosuppressive agents, see Table 16.14.

Table 16.14 Commonly used immunosuppressive agents in renal transplantation

Drug	Mechanism	Notes	Specific adverse effects
Tacrolimus, ciclosporin	Calcineurin inhibitors (CNI): block T cell activation downstream of the T cell receptor.	Tacrolimus is now more commonly used.	Progressive fibrosis and scarring. Renal vasoconstriction and hypertension. Tremor (Tac>CyA). Peripheral neuropathy. Thrombotic microangiopathy. Diabetes (Tac>CyA). Hirsutism, gum hypertrophy (CyA).
Sirolimus	Inhibitor of mTOR (mammalian target of rapamycin): regulatory kinase mediating cytokine-dependent cell proliferation. Everolimus is an alternative mTOR inhibitor.	Theoretical advantages in preventing long-term CNI toxicity, and in promoting a tolerogenic immune profile. The mTOR signalling pathway is important in many cancers: anti-cancer effects.	Delayed wound healing. Proteinuria. Pneumonitis. Mouth ulcers.

continued

Table 16.14 *continued*

Drug	Mechanism	Notes	Specific adverse effects
Mycophenolate mofetil (MMF)	Anti-proliferative: active metabolite mycophenolic acid inhibits purine nucleotide synthesis.	Main adjunct to CNIs in most settings.	GI toxicity: nausea, vomiting, diarrhoea. Myelosuppression. Teratogenic.
Azathioprine	Anti-proliferative: active 6-thioguanine metabolites (purine analogues) incorporate into DNA and block replication.	The advent of azathioprine and prednisolone made transplantation possible in the 1950s.	Myelosuppression. Particular increase in skin cancer risk. Interaction with allopurinol.
Corticosteroids	Pleiotropic inhibition of inflammatory responses: inhibition of lymphocyte signalling and trafficking.	Some immunosuppressive regimes involve steroid-avoidance, minimisation or early withdrawal. Corticosteroids also form an important part of the treatment of acute rejection.	Diabetes. Osteoporosis. Hypertension. Hyperlipidaemia.
Basiliximab	Monoclonal antibody directed against IL2 receptor (CD25): IL2R is present on activated T cells.	Non-depleting antibody. Commonly used for induction.	
ATG (anti-thymocyte globulin)	Polyclonal antibody directed against T cell antigens.	Depleting antibody. Used both in induction and treatment of steroid-refractory or vascular rejection.	Serum sickness-type reaction.
Alemtuzumab	Humanised monoclonal anti-CD52: present on many cells of the immune system, including T cells, B cells and monocytes.	Depleting antibody. Used for induction. May allow lower exposure to CNIs in the long term.	
Belatacept	Co-stimulation blocker: fusion protein consisting of Fc domain of human IgG1 + extracellular portion of co-stimulatory molecule CTLA-4.	May have a role in long-term immunosuppression regimes to avoid use of CNIs.	Long term efficacy and safety not fully characterised.
Eculizumab	Humanised monoclonal anti-C5: terminal component of complement cascade.	Use in the treatment of acute antibody-mediated rejection, particularly in the context of HLA-incompatible transplantation.	Particular risk of infection with encapsulated micro-organisms including *N. meningitides*.
IV immunoglobulin	Poorly understood, and likely multi-factorial: up-regulation of inhibitory Fc receptors, increased clearance of antibody etc.	Use in the treatment of antibody-mediated rejection.	Systemic febrile reaction. Acute kidney injury.

CyA, ciclosporin; Tac, tacrolimus.

Complications of transplantation

The main factors to consider in the long-term management of kidney transplant recipients are:

- Risk of ongoing immune injury to the transplant: acute and chronic rejection, cell- and antibody-mediated.
- Risk of recurrent primary disease: notable in primary FSGS and some forms of glomerulonephritis.
- Infectious complications.
- Increased malignancy risk: this includes post-transplant lymphoproliferative disorder (PTLD), which may be Epstein–Barr virus driven, and increased risk of solid tumours and skin malignancies.
- Increased cardiovascular and metabolic risk.

Infectious complications

These differ with time since transplantation: hospital-acquired and post-operative infections predominate in the first month; viral and opportunistic infections increase in importance after the first month; chronic viral infections, and EBV and BK virus in particular, are important beyond 6 months.

- CMV can cause significant morbidity and mortality in kidney transplant recipients. The highest risk of CMV disease is in CMV seronegative recipients who receive a kidney from a seropositive donor. Prophylactic treatment of all recipients, or monitoring for CMV DNA replication combined with pre-emptive treatment of those with viral replication, are alternative strategies.
- *Pneumocystis jurovecii* (prophylaxis with co-trimoxazole typically continues for 12 months post-transplantation).
- BK virus; a polyoma virus that can cause a progressive nephropathy in kidney transplant recipients and lead to graft loss. No effective specific treatments exist. Management includes monitoring for BK viraemia and reduction of immunosuppression where possible, to facilitate viral clearance.

Further reading

1. Levy J, Brown E, Lawrence A (Eds). *Oxford Handbook of Dialysis*, 4th edn. Oxford: Oxford University Press, 2016.
2. MacPhee I, Fronek J (Eds). *Handbook of Renal and Pancreatic Transplantation*. Oxford: Wiley-Blackwell, 2012.

Multiple choice questions

Questions

1. A 22-year-old man presents with a short history of ankle swelling. He appears otherwise well. Clinical examination reveals bilateral ankle oedema.

   Relevant clinical investigations:

   Serum albumin 20 g/L (35–50 g/L).
   Lipid profile: total cholesterol 8.6 (1.0–5.0 mmol/L).
   Triglycerides 2.2 (0.5–2.0 mmol/L).
   Urinary protein 5 g/L.
   Renal biopsy: membranous nephropathy.

   Which of the following is not a recognized cause of membranous nephropathy?

   A. Systemic lupus erythematosus.
   B. Snail fever.
   C. Lymphoma.
   D. Hartnup's disease.
   E. Crohn's disease.

2. A 3-year-old child is brought to see you by her parents for poor growth. For a long time her parents tell you she has been persistently thirsty, drinks a lot of water and passes urine very frequently. She has blonde hair and blue eyes. She has features of rickets on clinical examination, confirmed on radiographic studies. Slit lamp examination of the corneas shows crystals.

   Biochemistry:
   - Na^+ 137: 135–145 mmol/L.
   - K^+ 2.8: 3.5–5.0 mmol/L.
   - Cl^- 121: 96–108 mmol/L.

   Arterial blood gas:
   - pH 7.21: 7.34–7.45.
   - HCO_3^- 5.1: 22–26 mmol/L.
   - Anion gap 10: 8–16 mEq/L.

   Urinalysis:
   - Glucose 2+.
   - Protein 1+.

   Which of the following is the most likely diagnosis?

   A. Wilson's disease.
   B. Myeloma.
   C. Cystinosis.
   D. Lead poisoning.
   E. Galactosaemia.

3. A 26-year-old female presents with a short history of ankle swelling. On closer questioning she has a history of recurrent joint swelling, episodic fever and reports occasional 'dark urine'. On examination, you notice a butterfly rash and ankle swelling. BP is recorded as 145/90 mmHg and urinalysis reveals 3+ protein.

   A renal biopsy is carried out and shows diffuse thickening of the glomerular basement membrane affecting every glomerulus and sub-epithelial deposits of C1q, C3, IgG and IgM.

   Which of the following is the most likely diagnosis?

   A. Idiopathic membranous nephropathy.
   B. Anti-GBM disease.
   C. Lupus nephritis class I.
   D. Lupus nephritis class III.
   E. Lupus nephritis class V.

4. A 31-year-old male presents unwell with ESKD and is commenced on haemodialysis. He reports a long history of recurrent episodes of 'red urine', particularly following upper respiratory tract infections. He has an uncle who also had renal failure and was previously on dialysis. He has had 'problems with his vision' in the past and has always been 'a little hard of hearing'.

   Physical examination is largely unremarkable. He undergoes formal audiometric evaluation and is confirmed to have sensorineural deafness. His mother is willing to donate a kidney and he receives a live related transplant from her. Post-operative care is routine and there are no immediate complications.

   Six months post-transplant he is rushed into hospital acutely unwell with AKI complicated by pulmonary oedema and hyperkalaemia. A transplant kidney biopsy shows a crescentic nephropathy with linear deposition of IgG and C3.

   What is the most likely diagnosis?

   A. Alport syndrome with hyperacute antibody-mediated transplant rejection.
   B. Alport syndrome with chronic transplant rejection.
   C. Alport syndrome with antiglomerular basement membrane disease.
   D. Recurrent lupus nephritis.
   E. Thin basement membrane disease.

5. A 22-year-old female on haemodialysis is rushed into the Emergency Department unwell. She is unconscious and unable to communicate. Airway is patent and she is breathing spontaneously. BP is within normal range. An ECG shows a sinus bradycardia with heart rate of 30 beats/minute.

   Arterial blood gas:

   pH 7.21: 7.35–7.45.
   pO_2 10.2: 10–14 kPa.
   HCO_3^- 11: 22–26 mmol/L.
   Na^+ 138: 135–145 mmol/L.
   K^+ 7.8: 3.5–5.0mmol/L.

   Which of the following should be the first treatment initiated?

   A. IV insulin and glucose.
   B. Calcium resonium (polystyrene sulfonate) administered rectally as the patient is unconscious.
   C. IV calcium.
   D. IV adrenaline.
   E. IV 8.4% sodium bicarbonate.

6. A 25-year-old male Londoner presents having noticed that his urine is dark red in colour. He reports a 2-day history of sore throat, fever and muscle pains. His blood pressure is 150/88 mmHg, urine dip shows 3+ blood, 2+ protein. Blood tests show a serum urea level of 8.8 (2.5–7.8 mmol/L), creatinine 148 (50–111 mmol/L). He undergoes a biopsy and there are no proliferative lesions in the glomeruli.

   Which is the most likely diagnosis?

   A. IgA nephropathy.
   B. Post-streptococcal glomerulonephritis.
   C. Infective endocarditis.
   D. Granulomatous polyangiitis.
   E. HIV seroconversion illness.

7. A 19-year-old woman is referred to the acute medical take with a short history of an episode of bloody diarrhoea 2 weeks ago. She recalls having eaten some sausages at a barbeque the day prior to developing these symptoms. She has since experienced increasing nausea and malaise with some ankle swelling. She also reports difficulty passing urine. She has a past medical history of menorrhagia and chronic back pain for which she takes NSAIDs.

   Bedside observations:

   Afebrile.
   HR 122 beats/minute.
   BP 160/95 mmHg.

   Examination findings:

   Pale with 'puffy eyes' and evidence of petechiae over legs.
   Fine crepitations at both lung bases.
   Appendicectomy scar.

   Bloods:

   WBC 7.6 (4–10 × 10^9/L).
   Hb 84 (120–165 g/L).
   Platelets 65 × 109/L (150–400 × 10^9/L).
   INR 1.0 (0.8–1.1).
   APTT ratio 1.1 (1.0–2.5).
   Na^+ 132 (133–146 mmol/L).
   K^+ 6.1 mmol/L (3.5–5.3 mmol/L).
   Urea 24 mmol/L (2.5–7.8 mmol/L).
   Creatinine 540 (50–111 μmol/L).

   Urinalysis:

   3+ Blood.
   1+ protein.

Which is the most likely diagnosis?

A. Analgesic nephropathy.
B. Post-streptococcal glomerulonephritis.
C. Henoch–Schönlein purpura.
D. IgA nephropathy.
E. Haemolytic-uraemic syndrome.

8. A 65-year-old Afro-Caribbean woman presents with a few months' history of progressive tiredness and shortness of breath on exertion. She complains of recent back pain and has been using increasing amounts of analgesia. She has a history of hypertension controlled with amlodipine alone and sickle cell trait. Physical examination is unremarkable.

Blood tests:

Hb 84 (120–165 g/L).
WBC 4.1 (4–10 × 10^9/L).
Platelets 142 (150–400 × 10^9/L).
Na^+ 138 (133–146 mmol/L).
K^+ 4.8 (3.5–5.3 mmol/L).
Urea 18 (2.5–7.8 mmol/L).
Creatinine 320 (50–111 μmol/L).
Bilirubin 12 (0–21 μmmol/L).
ALP 140 (30–130 μ/L).
ALT 40 (7–56 μ/L).
Albumin 32 (25–50 g/L).
Total protein 90 (60–80 g/L).
Corrected calcium 2.15 (2.1–2.7 mmol/L).
Phosphate 0.8 (0.8–1.5 mmol/L).

Urinalysis:

Protein 2+.

Which of the following investigations is most likely to provide the underlying diagnosis?

A. Haemoglobin electrophoresis.
B. Renal tract US scan.
C. Immunoglobulins and serum protein electrophoresis.
D. Skeletal survey.
E. Blood film.

9. Which one of the following statements is correct regarding secondary causes of glomerular disease?

A. HIV infection is most commonly associated with membranous nephropathy.
B. FSGS is commonly a manifestation of underlying malignancy in the elderly.
C. Rheumatoid arthritis is associated with AL amyloidosis.
D. NSAID use can be associated with minimal change nephropathy.
E. HCV infection is commonly associated with IgA nephropathy.

10. A 58-year-old man is seen in CKD clinic with stable stage 4 chronic kidney disease. He has recorded BP readings at home of between 140/82 and 165/98 mmHg. He has a mild degree of peripheral oedema. Past medical history included diabetes and a history of peripheral vascular disease. His current medications are ramipril 10 mg OD, amlodipine 5 mg OD, furosemide 40 mg OD, lansoprazole 30 mg OD, aspirin 75 mg OD, atorvastatin 40 mg OD, linagliptin 5 mg OD and insulin.

Blood tests:

Hb 98 (120–165 g/L).
MCV 90 (0–99fL).
Ferritin 320 (20–500 mg/L).
Transferrin saturation 32% (16–45%).
Na^+ 139 (133–146 mmol/L).

K^+ 4.8 (3.5–5.3 mmol/L).
HCO_3 18 (22–26 mmol/L).
eGFR 21 mL/min (compared with 23 mL/min 12 months previously).
Corrected calcium 2.27 (2.1–2.7 mmol/L).
Phosphate 1.6 (0.8–1.5 mmol/L).
PTH 170 (15–65 ng/L).
HbA1C 8.0%.

Which one of the following regarding the management of his CKD is correct?

A. Treatment with an ACE-I is absolutely contraindicated with this level of kidney function.
B. Correction of anaemia with an erythropoiesis stimulating agent (erythropoietin) improves symptoms, but has no impact on mortality.
C. Plans should be made for the initiation of dialysis as soon as possible.
D. Correction of the metabolic acidosis with oral sodium bicarbonate may slow the progression of his CKD.
E. The raised PTH level is likely to be a consequence of primary hyperparathyroidism given the normal serum calcium.

Answers

1. D. Hartnup's disease is a genetic condition leading to amino aciduria. Snails are edible and delicious and 'snail fever' is another name for schistosomiasis, a recognised cause of membranous nephropathy (➲ see Membranous nephropathy, p. 569 and Hartnup's disease [under Cystinuria and Hartnup's disease], p. 563).
2. C. This is a classical presentation for infantile cystinosis causing Fanconi syndrome (➲ see Fanconi syndrome, p. 562, Box 16.4 and Table 16.5).
3. E. This patient has classical features of lupus, with evidence of membranous change in the kidneys and deposition of a 'full-house' pattern on immunofluorescence (➲ see Systemic lupus erythematosus [under Systemic diseases and the kidney], p. 574).
4. C. Patients with Alport syndrome have abnormal collagen in the kidneys. Exposure of their immune system to normal collagen for the first time generates antibody formation against GBM post-transplantation (➲ see Inherited kidney disease, Alport syndrome [under Inherited kidney disease], p. 581).
5. C. The first treatment for life threatening hyperkalaemia is to stabilise cardiac muscles with IV calcium. Subsequent treatments are to lower serum potassium (➲ see Acute kidney injury management principles [under Acute kidney injury], p. 583 and Tables 16.11A and 16.11B).
6. A. This 'sympharyngitic' presentation is typical for IgA nephropathy. No specific features are given that would be suggestive of the alternative diagnoses. The lack of proliferative lesions argues against post-infectious GN, which remains one of the leading causes of acute GN in developing countries, but not the UK (➲ see IgA nephropathy, p. 571).
7. E. The presentation of presumed AKI together with anaemia and thrombocytopenia should always prompt the possibility of a thrombotic microangiopathy. In conjunction with a history of bloody diarrhoea, this presentation is in keeping with diarrhoea-associated ('typical' or D+) haemolytic uraemic syndrome (➲ see Thrombotic microangiopathies: thrombotic thrombocytopenic purpura/ haemolytic uraemic syndrome [under Systemic diseases and the kidney], p. 578).
8. C. The underlying diagnosis is most likely to be multiple myeloma since there is renal impairment in association with a large globulin fraction and possible features of bone marrow suppression. The serum calcium is normal, as is often the case (➲ see Plasma cell dyscrasias and dysproteinaemias [under Systemic diseases and the kidney], p. 576).

9. D. The most common glomerular manifestations of HIV infection are HIV-associated nephropathy (HIVAN), a collapsing variant of FSGS, and an immune complex-mediated glomerulonephritis (➲ see HIV, p. 579 and Table 16.8). Underlying malignancy is associated with membranous nephropathy (➲ see Membranous nephropathy, p. 569). Rheumatoid arthritis is associated with secondary (AA) amyloidosis (➲ see Box 20.1). HCV infection is associated with cryoglobulinaemic vasculitis and mesangiocapillary glomerulonephritis, as well as with membranous nephropathy. (➲ see Membranous nephropathy, p. 569, Mesangiocapillary glomerulonephritis, p. 570 and Table 16.7). NSAID use has been described as a cause of minimal change nephropathy (➲ see Minimal change nephropathy, p. 567).
10. D. ACE-Is and ARBs can be problematic in advanced CKD owing to hyperkalaemia, but their use is not contraindicated. Correction of anaemia reduces cardiovascular mortality, as well as improving quality of life. Although patient education and preparations are ideally instituted well in advance, the majority of patients with CKD commence RRT once the eGFR is below 10 mL/min. Secondary hyperparathyroidism is associated with the deficiency of active vitamin D in kidney disease; the serum calcium does not necessarily fall below the normal range. A *normal* PTH level in association with a *high* serum calcium is suggestive of primary hyperparathyroidism (➲ see Chronic kidney disease, p. 585).

Chapter 17 **Neurology**

Robert Adam, Charles Marshall* and Jonathan Birns*

Clinically oriented neuroanatomy and localisation

Clinical neurological localisation is dependent upon sound knowledge of the functional anatomy of the nervous system. Neurological pathology may involve the CNS, which comprises the brain and the spinal cord, spinal roots, nerves, ganglia and plexuses, the neuromuscular junction (NMJ) and muscles. Clinical patterns of symptoms and signs (syndromes) can be used in order to isolate clinico-anatomical regions of interest.

Cortical syndromes

Frontal lobes

- Contain somatotopically organised motor regions posteriorly (homunculus).
- More anterior parts are dedicated to the integration of sensory inputs and cognitive networks (that are formed with the basal ganglia and the thalamic nuclei), which lead to important roles in 'executive function' (including planning and decision making), emotional expression, problem solving, memory, language, judgment and sexual behaviour.
- Broca's area (inferior frontal gyrus) is involved in speech production.

* Joint first authors.

Temporal lobes

- Involved in processing sensory input to enable retention of visual memories, language comprehension and emotion association.
- Contain the hippocampus playing a key role in the formation of explicit long-term memory.
- Involved in auditory processing:
  - Primary auditory cortex receives sensory information from the ears and secondary areas process the information into meaningful units such as speech and words.
- Wernicke's area, which spans the region between temporal and parietal lobes, plays a key role (in tandem with Broca's area) in speech comprehension.
- Functions of the left temporal lobe include low-level perception and extend to comprehension, naming and verbal memory.
- Visual temporal lobe areas interpret the meaning of visual stimuli and establish object recognition:
  - Ventral parts are involved in high-level visual processing of complex stimuli such as faces (fusiform gyrus) and scenes (parahippocampal gyrus):
    - Anterior parts of this 'ventral stream' are involved in object perception and recognition.

Parietal lobes

- Involved in sensory integration, spatial attention/representation and language.
- Damage leads to:
  - Hemisensory loss and neglect.
  - Spatial disorientation.
  - Astereognosis (inability to identify an object by active touch of the hands without other sensory input).
  - Agraphaesthesia (disorientation of the skin's sensation across its space, e.g. difficulty recognising a written number or letter traced on the skin).
  - Dysphasia.
  - Dyscalculia (difficulty in learning or comprehending mathematics).
  - Constructional apraxia.
  - Anosognosia (deficit of self-awareness).

Parietal lobe syndromes

Gerstmann syndrome

- Associated with lesions affecting the dominant (usually left) angular and supramarginal gyri.
- Characterised by:
  - Dysgraphia (deficiency in the ability to write).
  - Dyscalculia.
  - Finger agnosia (inability to distinguish the fingers on the hand).
  - Left-right disorientation.

Balint's syndrome

- Simultanagnosia (inability to perceive the visual field as a whole).
- Oculomotor apraxia (difficulty in fixating the eyes).
- Optic ataxia (inability to move the hand to a specific object by using vision).

Occipital lobes

- Visual processing centre of the brain containing the primary visual (striate) cortex and many extrastriate regions specialised for tasks such as visuospatial processing, colour differentiation and motion perception.
- Bilateral lesions of the occipital lobe can lead to cortical blindness (Anton's syndrome).

Extrapyramidal tracts

These are found in the reticular formation of the pons and medulla, and target neurons in the spinal cord involved in reflexes, locomotion, complex movements and postural control. These tracts are modulated by various parts of the CNS, including the nigrostriatal pathway, the basal ganglia, the cerebellum, the vestibular nuclei and different sensory areas of the cerebral cortex. The basal ganglia are important in the initiation of movement and the maintenance of stereotyped movements. Postural control, resting muscle tone, automatic associated movements (such as swinging the arms while walking) and emotional motor expression (smiling, frowning, laughing, crying, etc.) are all functions of the basal ganglia.

Cerebellum

The cerebellum plays an important role in motor control. It may also be involved in some cognitive functions such as attention and language, regulating fear and pleasure responses. The cerebellum does not initiate movement but contributes to coordination, precision and timing. It receives input from sensory systems of the spinal cord and from other parts of the brain, and integrates these inputs to fine-tune motor activity.

Cerebellar damage produces disorders in fine movement, equilibrium, posture and motor learning. The main clinical syndromes consist of ataxia, which affects gait, limb coordination, speech (dysarthria) and eye movements. Deficits are observed with movements on the same (ipsilateral) side of the body as the lesion.

The limbic areas

The subcortical limbic brain contains structures which are relatively primitive in terms of the evolution of the mammalian brain. Correspondingly, they subserve more primal functions of motivation, emotion, learning and memory. Structures are heavily interconnected and incorporate the following.

Diencephalic structures

- Hypothalamus:
  - Centre for the limbic system.
  - Connected with:
    - The frontal lobes, septal nuclei and the brainstem reticular formation via the medial forebrain bundle.
    - The hippocampus via the fornix.
    - The thalamus via the mammillothalamic fasciculus.
  - Regulates a great number of autonomic and endocrine processes.
- Mammillary bodies:
  - Receive signals from the hippocampus via the fornix and project them to the anterior thalamic nuclei.
  - Involved in memory processing.

Subcortical structures

- Septal nuclei: set of structures considered a 'pleasure zone' that lie in front of the lamina terminalis.
- Amygdala: located deep within the temporal lobes and related to a number of emotional processes, especially fear.
- Nucleus accumbens: involved in reward, pleasure and addiction.

Cortical structures

- Orbitofrontal cortex: region in the frontal lobe involved in the process of decision-making.
- Piriform cortex: part of the olfactory system.
- Entorhinal cortex: region of the temporal lobe playing an important role in memory formation and consolidation.
- Hippocampus and associated structures: playing a vital role in the consolidation of new memories.
- Fornix: white matter structure connecting the hippocampus with other brain structures, particularly the mammillary bodies and septal nuclei.

Focal limbic syndromes are rare, but a growing number of autoimmune syndromes are recognised specifically to affect these structures, e.g. NMDA-R (N-methyl-D-aspartate receptor) and VGKC (voltage-gated potassium channel) antibodies are now recognised as likely pathogens in the limbic encephalitides, which cause some or all of fever, seizures, mood/psychotic disturbances and abnormal movements.

Brainstem and cranial nerves

There are three main functions of the brainstem:

1. Conduction:
   - Ascending sensory pathways from the body include the spinothalamic tract (for pain and temperature sensation) and the dorsal column, fasciculus gracilis and cuneatus tracts (for touch, proprioception and pressure sensation).
   - Upper motor neurons descend to synapse in the spinal cord.
2. Cranial nerves III–XII emerge from the brainstem to supply the face, head and viscera.
3. Integrative functions involved in cardiovascular and respiratory control, pain regulation, alertness, awareness and consciousness.

Brainstem syndromes

Lateral medullary (Wallenberg's or posterior inferior cerebellar artery) syndrome

- Clinical manifestation resulting from occlusion of the posterior inferior cerebellar artery (PICA), or one of its branches or of the vertebral artery resulting in infarction of the lateral part of the medulla oblongata.
- Characterised by loss of pain and temperature sensation on the contralateral side of the body and ipsilateral side of the face.
- Clinical symptoms include dysphagia, dysarthria, ataxia, facial pain, vertigo, nystagmus, Horner's syndrome (➲ see Chapter 18, Horner's syndrome: interruption of the sympathetic pathway, p. 651 and Table 18.2), diplopia and possibly palatal myoclonus.

Weber's syndrome

- Midbrain infarction resulting in ipsilateral III nerve palsy and contralateral weakness.

Benedikt's syndrome

- Paramedian midbrain syndrome characterised by the presence of a III nerve palsy, and contralateral ataxia and tremor.

Spinal cord

The spinal cord extends from the foramen magnum to the conus medullaris at the level of L1–2. It conveys information between the central and peripheral nervous systems, but is considered part of the CNS. It is made of 31 segments that each contain sensory and motor nerve roots which merge to form the spinal nerves. The dorsal roots are fascicles of axons in the spinal cord that receive sensory information from the skin, muscle and visceral organs. Ventral roots carry efferent fibres that arise from motor neurons whose cell bodies are found in the ventral (anterior) horns of the grey matter of the spinal cord.

For incomplete lesions of the spinal cord, see Figure 17.1A–C.

Central cord syndrome

See Figure 17.1A.

- Most common form of cervical spinal cord injury, characterised by loss of power and/or sensation in arms and hands.
- Lesions above T6 may cause spinal shock (➲ see Chapter 12, Spinal shock, p. 396 and Table 12.2).
- May result from neck trauma or cervical spondylosis.
- Most common incomplete spinal cord injury syndrome:
  - After an incomplete injury, signals to and from the body are reduced, but not necessarily entirely blocked.

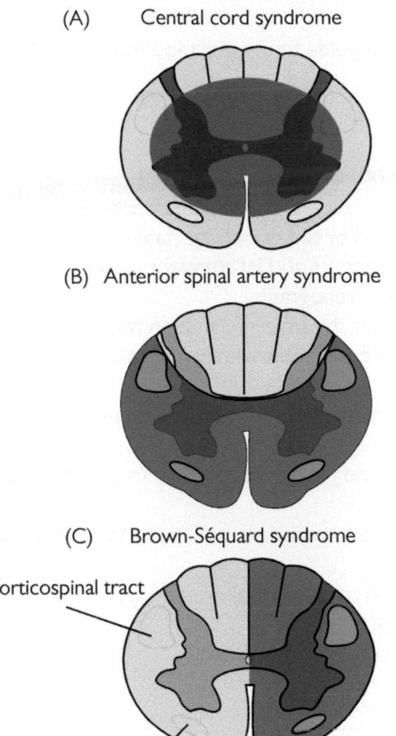

Figure 17.1 (A) Central cord syndrome. (B) Anterior spinal artery syndrome. (C) Brown–Séquard syndrome.

Anterior spinal artery syndrome

See Figure 17.1B.

- Primary blood supply to the anterior portion of the spinal cord is interrupted, causing ischaemia and/or infarction in the anterior two-thirds of the spinal cord.
- Characterised by loss of motor function below the level of injury, loss of sensation carried by the anterior columns of the spinal cord (pain and temperature), and preservation of sensation carried by the posterior columns (fine touch and proprioception).

Brown–Séquard syndrome

See Figure 17.1C.

- Results from a lesion affecting the dorsal column-medial lemniscus and corticospinal tract.
- Characterised by loss of motor function (hemiparaplegia) and loss of vibration sense, fine touch, proprioception and two-point discrimination ipsilateral to the spinal injury, and by loss of pain and temperature sensation contralateral to the injury. The axons of posterior columns decussate at the medulla, while those of the spinothalamic tract decussate within one to two spinal segments above their point of entry.

Neurological investigations

Imaging

➲ See Chapter 5, Introduction and guide to imaging modalities, p. 111.

- Skull X-ray:
  - Useful for bony lesions or fractures.
- CT:
  - Provides rapid acquisition of high resolution whole brain imaging.
  - Useful for imaging the skull vault and the brain parenchyma.
  - Information can be enhanced by the use of injectable contrast medium which can be used to enhance the appearance of tumours and inflammatory lesions as well as to outline vascular structures in CT angiography and venography.
  - CT perfusion imaging enables dynamic information regarding blood flow in the brain by recording the presence of contrast in brain areas with respect to the time of injection.
- MRI:
  - Useful for high resolution imaging of the central and peripheral nervous system and muscles.
- Nuclear medicine:
  - Specific neurotransmitters and their transporters can be radiolabelled and emission is recorded by a gamma camera.
    - Particularly useful in movement disorders (➲ see Movement disorders, p. 616).
  - FDG PET:
    - Useful in the identification of areas of altered metabolism.
- US and Doppler flow imaging:
  - Used to image the arterial supply of the brain.

Neurophysiology

Electroencephalogram

The EEG is commonly obtained using a bipolar 'montage' of scalp electrodes to record the 'surface EEG' consisting of excitatory and inhibitory post-synaptic potentials (excitatory post-synaptic potentials [EPSPs] and inhibitory post-synaptic potentials [IPSPs]). The resultant trace is used to facilitate the diagnosis of epilepsy and other disorders of consciousness including differentiating causes of encephalopathy.

Nerve conduction studies

- Used to identify whether abnormal nerve function is due to slow conduction (suggestive of demyelination, and therefore inflammatory aetiologies) or reduced (even blocked) conduction amplitudes (suggestive of axonal damage).
- Used to diagnose focal mononeuropathies (e.g. median or ulnar neuropathies) and to identify the likely site of compression or damage (i.e. at the wrist or elbow, respectively).
- Less common uses include:
  - Acute Guillain–Barré syndrome. N.B. Nerve conduction studies (NCS) changes may lag behind the clinical syndrome by up to 2 weeks.
  - Motor neurone disease: sensory studies are normal, but motor neuropathy and denervation are found.
- F wave studies:
  - A strong electrical stimulus (supramaximal stimulation) is applied to the skin surface above the distal portion of a nerve so that the impulse travels both distally (orthodromic) and proximally (antidromic); when the antidromic stimulus reaches a cell body, a small portion of the neurons backfire and an orthodromic wave travels back down the nerve and the reflected stimulus evokes a small, second action potential (F wave).
  - Used to identify proximal problems at the dorsal root ganglion.

Electromyogram

- Technique for evaluating and recording the electrical activity produced by skeletal muscles.
- Used in primary muscle disease (e.g. myopathy/myositis) or in disease secondary to abnormal motor transmission (e.g. myasthenia gravis).
- Surface electromyogram (EMG):
  - Records muscle activity from the surface above the muscle on the skin.
  - >1 electrode (usually 2) are needed because EMG recordings display the voltage difference between separate electrodes.
  - Limitations include surface electrode recordings being:
    - restricted to superficial muscles;
    - influenced by the depth of the subcutaneous tissue at the site of the recording.
- Intramuscular EMG:
  - Performed using a variety of different types of recording electrodes including:
    - Monopolar needle electrode:
      - Fine wire inserted into a muscle with a surface electrode as a reference or two fine wires inserted into a muscle referenced to each other.
    - Concentric needle electrode:
      - Incorporates a fine wire, embedded in a layer of insulation that fills the barrel of a hypodermic needle, that has an exposed shaft serving as the reference electrode and an exposed tip serving as the active electrode.
- Single fibre EMG:
  - Designed to have very tiny recording areas allowing for the discharges of individual muscle fibres in a motor unit to be discriminated.
    - Sensitive test for dysfunction of the NMJ caused by drugs, poisons or diseases such as myasthenia gravis.
- Pathologic abnormalities include:
  - Fasciculation potential:
    - Involuntary activation of a motor unit within a muscle.
  - Fibrillations:
    - Represent the isolated activation of individual muscle fibres, usually as the result of nerve or muscle disease.

Brainstem auditory-evoked responses

- Reflect neuronal activity in the auditory nerve, cochlear nucleus, superior olive and inferior colliculus of the brainstem.

Visual-evoked responses/potentials

- Reflect the speed of transmission of a visual stimulus to an occipital surface electrode.
- Useful in diagnosing primary CNS demyelination such as that seen in multiple sclerosis (MS).

Somatosensory-evoked potentials

- Used in the evaluation of the peripheral nervous system and the large-fibre sensory tracts in the CNS, specifically for:
  - Localisation of the anatomic site of somatosensory pathway lesions.
  - Identification of impaired conduction caused by axonal loss or demyelination.
  - Confirmation of a non-organic cause of sensory loss.

Cerebrospinal fluid examination

LP, usually performed under local anaesthesia, with or without imaging guidance (fluoroscopy/CT), is used to examine both CSF pressure and constituents. Normal CSF pressure is 0–20 cm H_2O. Usual constituents analysed include protein, glucose, and red and white cell counts. High protein levels are indicative of inflammation. White cell counts >5 × 10^9/L are considered abnormal, and suggest infection or inflammation. Raised white cell counts are usually differentiated into polymorphs and monocytes. High polymorph counts are suggestive of infection or malignancy. Monocytosis is suggestive of acute bacterial infection. Bacterial consumption lowers CSF glucose levels whereas in viral infection (or inflammation), CSF glucose levels are normal. Viral and/or bacterial PCRs are often used to try to identify/exclude infectious candidates. Specific preparations may be required to look for fungal infection, e.g. India ink for cryptococci (➲ see Chapter 8, CSF studies, p. 244 and Table 8.16).

Additional commonly used CSF assays include protein electrophoresis for oligoclonal bands (evidence of primary CNS inflammation/demyelination). Less common tests include autoantibodies, 14-3-3 protein levels in Creutzfeldt–Jakob disease, metabolites such as lactate in mitochondrial diseases and pterins (heterocyclic compounds composed of a pteridine ring system) to exclude inborn errors of metabolism.

In the unconscious patient or where raised CSF pressure is suspected (i.e. in the presence of blurred optic discs), brain imaging must be initially performed to minimise the risk of LP, which might otherwise precipitate descent of brain matter through the foramen magnum (coning). For the CSF pressure reading to be meaningful, the patient must be supine; the needle most often being inserted at the L4/5 interspace.

Stroke

Stroke is defined as a rapid onset of focal neurological deficit lasting more than 24 hours, with no apparent cause other than disruption of blood supply to the brain. A TIA refers to a similar presentation that resolves within 24 hours, although the majority resolve within 1 hour. Stroke is the third commonest cause of death and single largest cause of adult disability worldwide. The prevalence of stroke increases with age, but 25% of strokes occur in those under the age of 65. While the majority of strokes are associated with classical vascular risk factors, including hypertension, diabetes mellitus, dyslipidiaemia and cardiac disease, less common causes such as arterial dissection, vasculitis and recreational drug misuse have increased importance in younger individuals. Overall risk also varies with ethnicity, with higher rates in Afro-Caribbean populations.

Diagnosis

Based on clinicoradiographic stroke assessments, the triad of Where? What? and Why? are crucial to inform on:

- Anatomy: Where is the lesion?
- Pathology: What is the lesion?
- Aetiology: Why has this occurred?

Vascular supply of the brain

The blood supply to the brain is delivered by two internal carotid arteries and two vertebral arteries which anastomose at the base of the brain to create the circle of Willis (Figure 17.2). The carotid arterial system supplies the anterior two thirds of the brain (anterior circulation) and the vertebrobasilar arterial system supplies the posterior third of the brain (posterior circulation). For each system, there are three components: the extracranial arteries, the major intracranial arteries and the small superficial and deep perforating arteries. Communications can occur between cerebral arteries at the circle of Willis, via anastomoses between the branches of the external carotid artery and the intracerebral circulation, and via anastomoses between cerebral vessels on the brain surface. This can be important in providing a protective role in patients with arterial occlusion.

Understanding the basic knowledge of the arterial supply and neuroanatomy of the brain helps to identify stroke symptoms secondary to damage to specific vascular territories (Figure 17.3 and Table 17.1).

- Anterior cerebral artery (ACA) supplies the anterior and superior medial frontal lobe.
- Middle cerebral artery (MCA) supplies the posterior and inferior frontal lobes, parietal lobe, superior and lateral temporal lobes, and internal capsule, basal ganglia (putamen, globus pallidus, caudate nucleus) and corona radiata.

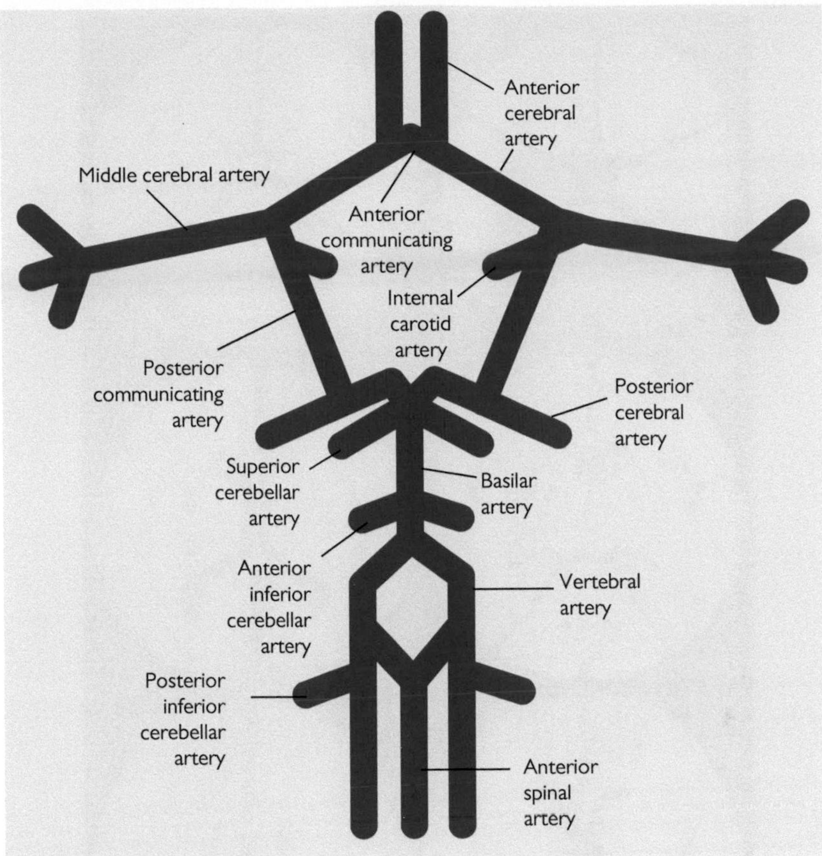

Figure 17.2 Arterial blood supply of the brain.

- Posterior cerebral artery (PCA) formed from a continuation of the basilar artery supplies the inferior temporal lobes, occipital lobes and thalamus.

The somatosensory homunculus and motor homunculus are pictorial representations of the anatomical divisions of the somatosensory and motor cortices, respectively, with each showing how much of its respective cortex innervates certain body parts. Different parts of the homunculus have different arterial vascular supply with lower limb structures having predominant ACA supply, upper limb and face having predominant MCA supply, and tongue sensorimotor function and swallowing having predominant PCA supply.

Three boundary zones or watershed areas, with limited if any collateral supply, exist in the brain that are particularly prone to ischaemia in the face of reduced blood flow. They are the:

- Anterior watershed between the superficial territories of the MCA and ACA in the fronto-parasagittal area.
- Posterior watershed between superficial territories of the MCA and PCA in the parieto-occipital area.
- Internal watershed between superficial perforating artery and deep lenticostriate artery territories supplying the deep-brain structures (basal ganglia, thalamus, centrum semiovale and corona radiata).

Pathology and pathophysiology

15% of strokes are haemorrhagic, while 85% are ischaemic, with differentiation requiring brain imaging. There are various causes of haemorrhagic stroke:

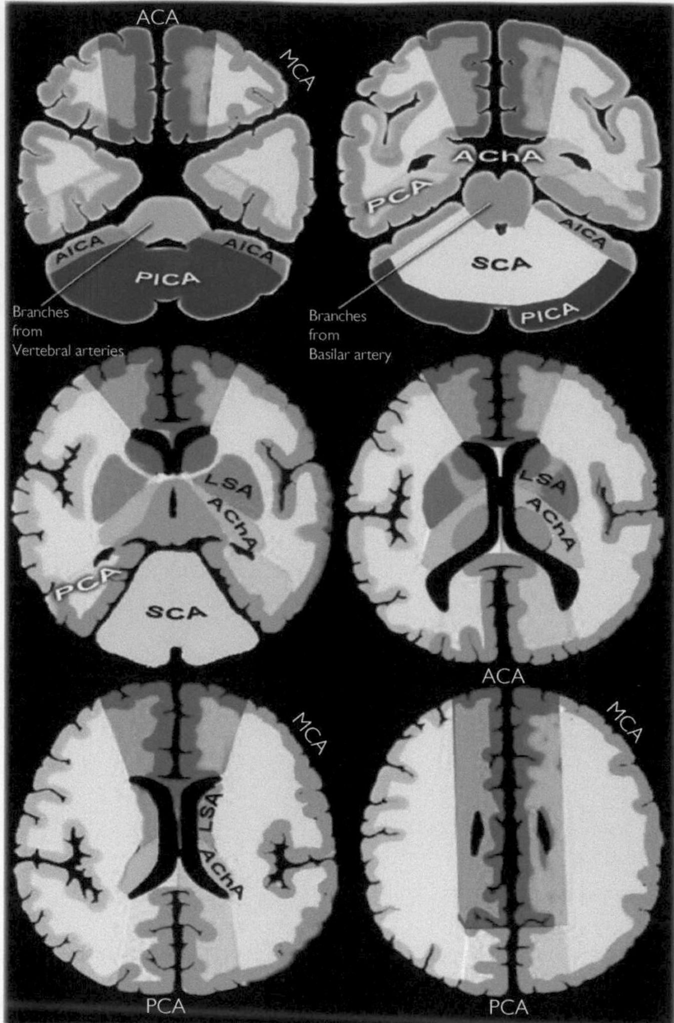

Figure 17.3 Vascular territories of the brain.

MCA, middle cerebral artery; AICA, anterior inferior cerebellar artery; PICA, posterior inferior cerebellar artery; AChA, anterior choroidal artery; SCA, superior cerebellar artery; LSA, lenticostriate artery; PCA, posterior cerebral artery; ACA, anterior cerebral artery.

Reproduced with permission Radiology Assistant. http://www.radiologyassistant.nl/

- Anatomical factors:
  - Lipohyalinosis and microaneurysms in small vessel disease.
  - Arterio-venous malformations (AVMs).
  - Amyloid angiopathy.
  - Saccular aneurysms:
    - Occurring particularly along the Circle of Willis where communicating vessels link the main cerebral vessels.
    - Multiple in approximately 25% of patients, predominantly when there is a familial pattern.
    - Major cause of subarachnoid haemorrhage (SAH).
  - Venous sinus thrombosis.
- Haemodynamic factors:
  - Hypertension.

Table 17.1 Stroke syndromes

Vascular territory	Stroke symptoms
Anterior cerebral artery territory	Motor deficit with leg predominating over arm. Other frontal lobe features include urinary incontinence, lack of motivation, disinhibition and aphasic syndromes with reduced spontaneous output or mutism.
Middle cerebral artery territory	Motor/sensory deficit with the face/arm affected more than leg, homonymous hemianopia, dyspraxia, visuospatial neglect, dysphasia (if dominant hemisphere affected).
Posterior cerebral artery territory	Macular sparing homonymous hemianopia, cortical blindness, amnesic disorder (involvement of temporal lobes), visuospatial dysfunction.
Verterbrobasilar artery territory	Nausea, diplopia, vertigo, nystagmus, ataxia, hemiplegia, quadriplegia, hemianopia, coma.

- Haemostatic factors:
  - Antiplatelet, anticoagulant and thrombolytic drugs, haemophilia, thrombocytopenia.
- Other factors:
  - Intracerebral tumours, alcohol, recreational drugs (cocaine, amphetamines), vasculitis.

The mechanism of ischaemic stroke is the occlusion of a CA by in-situ thrombus formation or an embolus from a proximal source, and less commonly by low flow distal to an occluded or highly stenosed artery. In ischaemic stroke, brain tissue receiving little or no blood flow is known as the ischaemic core and is comprised of cells that die rapidly. The ischaemic core radiates outward from the occluded area and, typically, 1.9 million neurons are lost every minute. Surrounding the ischaemic core is the ischaemic penumbra (tissue that is functionally impaired and at risk of infarction, but that may be saved if reperfused). Indeed, if perfusion is not restored to the penumbra, any tissue not receiving sufficient collateral arterial supply will undergo infarction; as such, the defining principle of acute ischaemic stroke therapy is to salvage the ischaemic penumbra and thereby reduce the extent of tissue infarction and improve clinical outcome.

The major underlying causes of ischaemic stroke are:

- Large vessel atherothromboembolism (45%).
- Cardiac embolism (25%).
- Small artery microatheroma (25%).
- Non-atheromatous disease, e.g. dissection, vasculitis (5%).
- Haematological disorders, e.g. thrombophilia (<5%).

Small vessel disease and lacunar stroke

Occlusion of small penetrating arteries (typically of diameter <400 μm) results in development of lacunar infarction (<1.5 cm in diameter). Four main lacunar stroke syndromes exist:

- Pure motor hemiparesis (50%); unilateral pyramidal weakness involving face, arm and leg.
- Pure hemisensory loss (5%); unilateral sensory loss involving face, arm and leg.
- Hemisensorimotor loss (35%); unilateral pyramidal weakness and sensory loss involving face, arm and leg.
- Ataxic hemiparesis (10%); combination of unilateral pyramidal weakness and ataxia affecting arm and/or leg.

Management

All stroke patients should be admitted to and managed on a stroke unit for multidisciplinary optimisation of hydration, nutrition, continence, pressure care, mobility, oxygenation and BP, glycaemic and lipid control, and minimisation of venous thromboembolism and post-stroke seizures. No specific medical treatment exists for haemorrhagic stroke, but IV, and intra-arterial thrombolysis and thrombectomy exist as hyperacute ischaemic stroke therapies.

Secondary prevention

- Lifestyle modification:
  - Weight loss.
  - Cessation of use of cigarettes, ethanol and recreational drugs.
- Management of high BP, diabetes mellitus (DM) and hyperlipidaemia (➲ see Chapter 13, Hypertension, Investigations, Table 13.12, and Management, p. 432 and Tables 13.13, 13.14, 13.15, 13.16 and 13.17; Chapter 19, Management, p. 673 and Table 19.3; and Chapter 1, Lipids and atherosclerosis, p. 20 and Figures 1.5, 1.6 and 1.7).
- Anti-thrombotic drug therapy for ischaemic stroke:
  - Antiplatelet agents for large/small artery aetiology:
    - Clopidogrel as first line agent.
  - Anticoagulation for cardioembolic aetiology (e.g. atrial fibrillation [➲ See Chapter 13, Disease classification system of supraventricular tachycardias, p. 468 and Table 13.48.).
- Carotid endarterectomy for patients with symptomatic carotid artery stenosis.

Further reading

Intercollegiate Stroke Working Party. National clinical guideline for stroke. 2016. Partyhttps://www.strokeaudit.org/SupportFiles/Documents/Guidelines/2016-National-Clinical-Guideline-for-Stroke-5t-(1).aspx.

Epilepsy

Epilepsy is a disorder of the brain characterised by an enduring predisposition to generate seizures (transient occurrence of signs and/or symptoms due to abnormal excessive or synchronous neuronal activity in the brain). The predisposition to neuronal hyperexcitability, and therefore seizures, may be generated by one or more abnormalities of:

- Sodium channels:
  - Multi-subunit structures (incorporating α and β subunits) that undergo conformational modifications, when stimulated by a change in transmembrane voltage, to regulate sodium influx to a cell, leading to depolarisation from its resting intracellular potential (approximately –70 mV).
  - Sodium channel blockers (e.g. sodium valproate; zonisamide) reduce the opportunity for depolarisation and other drugs achieve a similar effect by stabilising the channel in its resting (closed) state (e.g. phenytoin; carbamazepine), binding to the inactive state (e.g. lamotrigine), increasing slow inactivation (e.g. lacosamide) or prolonging the inactive state (e.g. rufinamide).
- Calcium channels:
  - T-type low voltage-sensitive Ca^{2+} channels that contribute to burst firing are targets for ethosuximide.
  - L-, P- Q- and N- type Ca^{2+} channels are targets for lamotrigine, topiramate and gabapentin.
- Potassium channels:
  - Responsible for the repolarisation of the plasma membrane after the Na^{+}-induced depolarisation phase.
  - Direct activation limits the firing of action potentials by hyperpolarising the neural membrane.
  - KCNQ2-5 channels are a target for retigabine.
  - Mutations have been identified in benign neonatal familial convulsions.
- γ-aminobutyric acid physiology (with GABA being the most important and prominent inhibitory neurotransmitter in the brain):
  - $GABA_A$ agonists stimulate receptor-mediated Cl^{-} fluxes, enhancing hyperpolarisation and inhibiting action potentials.
  - Valproate, gabapentin and vigabatrin increase GABA synthesis and turnover and inhibit breakdown.
- Glutamatergic ion channels:
  - Felbamate, topiramate and ketamine are antagonists at glutamatergic NMDA-Rs that are non-selective cationic channels.

    - Topiramate is an antagonist at α-amino-3-hydroxy-5-methyl-4-isoxazolepropionic acid (AMPA) glutamate receptors that are non-selective cationic channels.

Many of these mechanisms are interdependent, e.g. voltage-dependent T-type Ca^{2+} channels control burst firing of thalamocortical projections under the hyperpolarising influence of $GABA_B$ receptors, which stimulate K^+ channel opening.

Secondary epilepsy

Symptomatic seizures occur in the presence of recognised insults:

- Metabolic, e.g. electrolyte/glucose disturbance.
- Infectious, e.g. meningitis, encephalitis.
- Autoimmune, e.g. vasculitis, limbic encephalitis, Rasmussen's encephalitis (affecting a single cerebral hemisphere and characterised by frequent and severe seizures, hemiparesis, encephalitis and dementia).
- Cerebral structural damage: lowers seizure threshold. Causes include:
    - Surgery, trauma, subarachnoid/subdural haemorrhage, abnormal vasculature, e.g. AVM, cavernoma:
        - blood is particularly epileptogenic, especially when it contacts the cortical surface.
    - Tumours:
        - benign and malignant, whether primary or metastatic.
    - Demyelination.

Classification

Seizures may emerge from an abnormal 'focus' within the brain and thereby lead to symptoms dependent upon their origin, e.g. temporal lobe seizures may be associated with memory disturbance, *déjà vu* and/or hallucinatory phenomena, and frontal lobe seizures may lead to stereotypic motor and behavioural disturbances. Such focal seizures may lead to secondary generalised seizures. When focal seizures cause reduced or lost awareness, they are termed focal dyscognitive (or complex partial) seizures. Seizures may appear to arise in the whole brain in a simultaneous manner, such that a primary 'focus' is not easily determined (Figure 17.4).

Diagnosis

Based on history (as examination is usually unremarkable).

- Prodromal symptoms are often used to distinguish seizure from other causes of loss of consciousness and include metallic tastes, *déjà vu*, 'rising' gastric sensations, 'a sense of impending doom'.
- Urinary incontinence and/or tongue biting are common, but not diagnostic.
- Head turning, eye deviation and focal limb onset suggest an epileptic onset substrate.
- Automatisms or odd stereotyped behaviours suggest frontal lobe seizures.
- Headache, fever and psychosis may suggest autoimmune aetiology, including cerebral vasculitis/ limbic encephalitis.
- Post-ictal prolonged confusion and disorientation are suggestive of a generalised seizure (and less likely due to syncope in which disorientation is usually brief).

Investigations include:

- Serum biochemistry:
    - To investigate for metabolic abnormalities, e.g. hyponatremia.
    - Lactate and prolactin levels may increase, but are not reliably sensitive.
- Brain imaging:
    - Indicated in new onset seizures in adults.
- CSF examination if seizures are accompanied by the manifestations of systemic illness:
    - e.g. herpes simplex virus HSV DNA detection by PCR in suspected HSV encephalitis.
    - e.g. increased protein and white cell counts, and evaluation of NMDA-R and VGKC antibodies in autoimmune encephalitis.

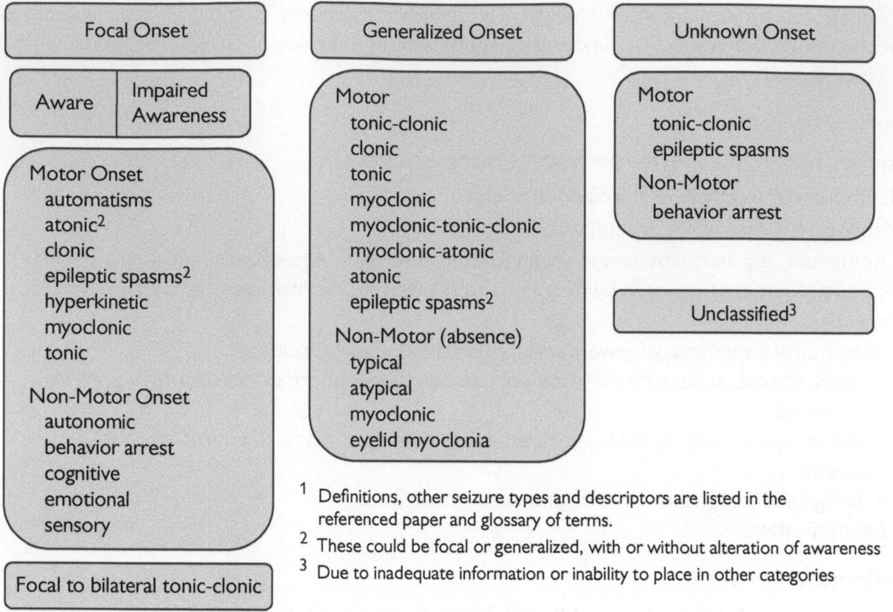

Figure 17.4 ILAE proposal for revised terminology for organization of seizures and epilepsies 2017.
Reproduced from R.S. Fischer and M. Saul. The 2017 ILAE Classification of Seizures. *Epilepsia*, a journal of the International League against Epilepsy. Distributed under the terms of the Creative Commons Attribution-ShareAlike 4.0 International License (CC BY-SA 4.0). https://creativecommons.org/licenses/by-sa/4.0/.

- EEG:
  - May be normal inter-ictally.
  - May be abnormal in patients not having seizures due to structural brain abnormalities, metabolic derangement and/or drugs (both prescribed and recreational).
  - Routine scalp EEG is particularly useful in patients:
    - With idiopathic generalised epilepsy to identify an interictal 'signature' of abnormality.
    - With structural lesions where anatomical foci may be revealed to be relevant by the presence of corroborative electrical abnormalities.
    - Immediately following an apparent generalised event when there is a higher likelihood of EEG abnormality (although the absence of such abnormality is a poor surrogate for non-epileptic events).
  - Additional techniques used to facilitate EEG interpretation include:
    - Recording of sleep and awake EEG.
    - Photic stimulation and hyperventilation:
      - to attempt to provoke epileptiform electrical activity.
    - Prolonged recordings, which may be 'ambulatory'.
    - Sleep-deprived EEG.
    - Video-telemetry.
    - Invasive intracranial EEG (using brain surface or deep electrodes) in patients in whom surgery is being considered.
- Advanced functional imaging (including ictal single-photon emission computed tomography (SPECT)/functional MRI):
  - To identify a seizure focus and/or assess the normal brain functions of potential surgical targets.

Treatment

See Table 17.2.

Table 17.2 Drug choice for management of epilepsy

	First line	Second line	Adjunctive therapy	Additional options
Generalised seizures				
Tonic-clonic	Sodium valproate.	Lamotrigine, carbamazepine or oxcarbazepine.	Clobazam, lamotrigine, levetiracetam, sodium valproate or topiramate.	
Absence	Ethosuximide or sodium valproate.	Lamotrigine.	Two of lamotrigine, ethosuxamide or sodium valproate.	Clobazam, clonazepam, levetiracetam topiramate or zonisamide.
Absence with other seizures	Sodium valproate.	Lamotrigine or topiramate.	Two of topiramate, lamotrigine, sodium valproate.	
Myoclonic	Sodium valproate.	Levetiracetam or topiramate.	Two of levetiracetam, sodium valproate or topiramate.	Clobazam, clonazepam, piracetam or zonisamide.
Tonic/atonic	Sodium valproate.		Sodium valproate plus lamotrigine.	Rufinamide or topiramate.
Focal seizures				
	Carbamazepine or lamotrigine.	Levetiracetam, oxcarbazepine or sodium valproate.	Carbamazepine, clobazam, gabapentin, lamotrigine, levetiracetam, oxcarbazepine, sodium valproate or topiramate.	Eslicarbazepine acetate, lacosamide, phenobarbital, phenytoin, pregabalin, tiagabine, vigabatrin or zonisamide.

Management of epilepsy in pregnancy

Anti-epileptic medications are a major cause of teratogenicity and fetal malformations, and minimising this risk is a vital part of epilepsy management in women of childbearing age. Fetal toxicity is generally dose-related, and therefore efforts should be made to minimise anti-epileptic exposure. In some cases, it is appropriate to consider cessation of anti-epileptic agents during the first trimester (when the risk to the fetus is greatest) and then restart in the third trimester (when the risk of seizures is greatest).

Sodium valproate is most strongly associated with malformations and neurodevelopmental problems and, as such, should be a drug of last resort in fertile women. Other older anti-epileptics, such as phenytoin, carbamazepine and phenobarbital are all associated with a significantly increased risk of teratogenicity and, therefore, newer anti-epileptics are preferred. Lamotrigine has been well studied in pregnancy and, although it does still carry a small dose-dependent risk to the fetus, is generally the medication of choice. Pregnancy can reduce serum lamotrigine levels, and these should therefore be monitored and the dose increased when necessary. Levetiracetam has less extensive pregnancy data, but appears to be safe. All women with epilepsy should be given daily folic acid during the preconception period and while pregnant to reduce the risk of neural tube defects. Many anti-epileptic drugs induce infantile vitamin K deficiency, and the neonate should receive supplementation at birth and again at 28 days.

Status epilepticus

Status epilepticus is defined as a seizure lasting >30 minutes, but which should be suspected after 5 minutes. The first line anti-epileptic therapy has to be considered after or during attendance to managing the patient's airway (breathing and circulation are usually only affected as a result of airway compromise). As there may be clenched teeth and movement, obtaining airway and IV access can be difficult. Nasopharyngeal airways may be more practical than oral (Guedel) airways and the route of drug administration may have to be rectal or buccal in the first instance. A reasonable protocol for the drug management of status epilepticus includes:

1. Benzodiazepines:
   - Diazepam can be given orally, rectally or IV.
   - Midazolam is available for buccal use, but can also be given IM or IV.
   - Lorazepam is an effective agent of appropriate onset and offset.
2. Phenytoin or sodium valproate or levetiracetam (all available IV).
3. Consideration of an additional agent (another of the above and/or phenobarbital).
4. General anaesthesia (traditionally with thiopental, but increasingly with propofol and/or midazolam).

Prognosis

The prognosis of epilepsy is highly variable. Many patients will have easily managed seizures that respond to simple monotherapy. Refractory epilepsy (not responding to ≥2 anti-epileptic drugs) carries a poorer prognosis. Uncontrolled epilepsy carries a significant mortality risk, due to sudden unexpected death in epilepsy (SUDEP) and an increased risk of traumatic injury and complications such as aspiration pneumonia. Status epilepticus has a significant (up to 20%) 30-day mortality.

Further reading

1. Fisher RS, Acevedo C, Arzimanoglou A, et al. ILAE Official Report: a practical clinical definition of epilepsy. *Epilepsia*. 2014; 55:475–82.

Multiple sclerosis and related diseases

Multiple sclerosis

Pathogenesis/pathophysiology

MS is an autoimmune inflammatory disease in which autoreactive lymphocytes attack and damage oligodendrocytes. It therefore causes demyelination of the CNS and optic nerves, which have oligodendrocyte-derived myelin, but does not affect the other cranial or peripheral nerves that have Schwann cell myelin. T-cells and macrophages infiltrate lesions, with demyelination and subsequent remyelination. This leads to a clinical pattern of relapse and remission. When axonal degeneration supervenes, a progressive pattern of disability emerges.

Environmental risk factors

- Cigarette smoking.
- Latitudinal gradient.
  - Higher prevalence further from the equator:
    - Migrants acquire the MS risk of their destination if they move before the age of 14.
- Putative association with Epstein–Barr virus infection in view of increased EBV seropositivity and incidence of prior infectious mononucleosis.

Genetic risk factors

- Female gender.
- No Mendelian heritability, but increased risk in family members:
  - A monozygotic twin sibling has a 35% risk of MS.
  - In common siblings, MS risk is 5%.

- Genome-wide association studies have revealed specific major histocompatibility complex alleles, regulators of T-cell function and genes related to vitamin D metabolism to be implicated as genetic risk factors.

Clinical features

MS can cause myriad neurological symptoms, dependent on lesion location. The commonest presenting syndrome is optic neuritis, with painful, acute monocular visual loss with loss of colour vision. Other frequent manifestations include spinal cord syndromes, ataxia, diplopia, hemiparesis and vertigo. Uhtoff's phenomenon (exacerbation of symptoms with a rise in temperature) and Lhermitte's phenomenon (tingling down the spine and arms on neck flexion) are characteristic (but not pathognomonic).

There are four distinct temporal patterns in MS:

1. The commonest is relapsing-remitting multiple sclerosis (RRMS), characterised by episodes of acute neurological deterioration with subsequent recovery.
2. Most patients with RRMS eventually develop secondary progressive multiple sclerosis (SPMS), with gradual neurological decline without discrete relapse episodes.
3. A minority of patients (<10%) have primary progressive multiple sclerosis (PPMS), with a progressive neurological decline without any history of relapses.
4. Relapsing-progressive MS (relapses superimposed upon gradual progression) is also described.

Diagnosis remains clinical, but is supported by results of imaging (MRI being first line), CSF and neurophysiological (e.g. visual-evoked potential [VEP]) investigations. Patients' clinical events (attacks) are disseminated in 'time' and 'space' (i.e. due to anatomically disparate lesions).

Management

Infection may be associated with a deterioration of pre-existing symptoms ('pseudo-relapses') or it may trigger new lesions (true relapses). Active infection should be excluded and treated before specific MS treatment is commenced. Urinary infection is most common in view of frequent bladder dysfunction in MS. Steroids (e.g. methylprednisolone 1 g IV daily for 3 days/500 mg PO daily for 5 days) may speed the rate of recovery from an acute relapse, but do not affect the ultimate outcome of the relapse; hence, they are generally used only for relapses that impair function.

For symptomatic treatments for MS, see Table 17.3; for disease-modifying treatments, see Table 17.4

Multiple sclerosis in the pregnant patient

- Decreased rate of relapse in first and second trimesters.
- Increased rate of relapse in third trimester and post-partum period.
- Corticosteroids can be used to treat relapses.
- Minimal evidence exists about the safety of disease-modifying therapies and these are often suspended during pregnancy.

Other neuroinflammatory disorders

Neuromyelitis optica (Devic's disease)

- Severe, often bilateral optic neuritis.
- Spinal cord syndrome with longitudinally extensive transverse myelitis (lesion extends over multiple vertebral levels).
- Often associated with antibodies to aquaporin-4.
- Anti-myelin oligodendrocyte glycoprotein (MOG) antibodies may account for some aquaporin seronegative cases.
- Treatment comprises steroids, steroid-sparing agents (e.g. azathioprine, mycophenolate mofetil [MMF]), plasmapheresis and sometimes cyclophosphamide or rituximab.

Table 17.3 Symptomatic treatments for MS

Symptom	Treatments available	Beneficial effects	Side effects/complications
Spasticity	Physiotherapy.	Reduce muscle spasms and maintain range of movement.	
	GABAergic agents (e.g. baclofen, gabapentin, pregabalin).	Promote muscle relaxation.	Sedation and generalised hypotonia (head drop, impaired mobility, etc.). (intrathecal baclofen pumps can be used to deliver the drug locally, with reduced systemic side effects).
	α2 adrenergic agonists (e.g. tizanidine).		
	Benzodiazepines (e.g. diazepam, clonazepam).		
	Botulinum toxin.	Temporary weakening/paralysis of specific muscles/muscle groups.	Unwanted weakness due to spread/wrong site of injection; development of neutralising antibodies.
	Cannabinoid preparations (e.g. nabiximols).	Licensed only for patients in whom multiple other agents have failed.	Dizziness, drowsiness and disorientation.
Bladder and bowel symptoms that include urgency, frequency and urge incontinence, urinary retention and constipation	Anticholinergic drugs (e.g. oxybutynin/solifenacin).	Improve symptoms of over-activity.	May worsen incomplete voiding and cognition.
	Catheterisation.	Incomplete voiding leads to frequent urinary tract infections, and can be managed with intermittent self-catheterisation (ISC) or suprapubic catheters.	Prophylactic antibiotics may be required.
	Intravesical botulinum toxin injections.	May be combined with ISC for very problematic bladder over-activity.	
	Various.	Constipation can be managed with a combination of laxatives, enemas and biofeedback techniques.	
Depression	➲ See Chapter 22, Antidepressants, p. 781 and Table 22.2.		
Poor mobility	Physiotherapy and occupational therapy.	Important in maintaining mobility, balance and posture. Functional electrical stimulators can be used for foot-drop.	
	Walking aids.	Often required; include sticks, crutches, walking frames and wheeled walkers, as well as wheelchairs (powered/unpowered) and mobility scooters.	
	Fampridine (4-aminopyridine).	Shown to increase walking speed.	
Fatigue	Modafanil. Methylphenidate. Amantadine. Physiotherapy, e.g. graded exercise programmes.	Some reduction in daytime somnolence.	
Neuropathic pain	See Chapter 10, Management of neuropathic pain, p. 340.		

Table 17.4 Disease modifying treatments for MS

Preparation	Name	Indication	Mode of action	Efficacy	Side effects
Intra-muscular/ sub-cutaneous injectable – daily/weekly dependent upon preparation	Interferon-β (IFNβ)	Active RRMS (at least 2 relapses in previous 2 years).	Reduces the number of inflammatory cells that cross the blood brain barrier.	Annual relapse rate ↓ by ~1/3.	Injection site reactions, flu-like symptoms, depression, hepatotoxicity, development of neutralising antibodies.
SC daily injection	Glatiramer acetate		A polymer of amino acids found in myelin basic protein which may act as a decoy for immune targeting of myelin.	Relapses requiring hospital admission ↓ by 50%. Benefit on long-term disability less clear.	Injection site reactions, fever, flu-like symptoms.
Oral	Fingolimod	RRMS in patients who have failed injectables or are unable to take them.	Sphingosine analogue that causes sequestration of lymphocytes in lymph nodes and prevents CNS invasion.	Annual relapse rate ↓ by ~60%.	Macular oedema, hepatotoxicity, heart block (initiation requires cardiac monitoring).
	Teriflunomide	Active RRMS (at least 2 relapses in previous 2 years) but not highly active or rapidly evolving severe RRMS.	Blocks proliferation of stimulated lymphocytes.	Annual relapse rate ↓ by 17–36%.	Diarrhoea, nausea, vomiting, increased levels of alanine aminotransferase, paraesthesiae/ dysaesthesiae, infections, alopecia.
	Dimethyl fumarate	Active RRMS, but not highly active or rapidly evolving severe RRMS.	Promotes anti-inflammatory activity and can inhibit expression of pro-inflammatory cytokines and adhesion molecules.	Relapse ↓ by 50%.	Flushing, abdominal pain, diarrhoea, nausea.
IV monoclonal antibody infusion	Natalizumab	Highly active RRMS.	Humanised monoclonal antibody against the cell adhesion molecule α4-integrin.	Relapse ↓ by 68%.	Risk of progressive multifocal leukoencephalopathy that is dependent on Creutzfeldt-Jakob virus antibody status and treatment duration.
	Alemtuzumab	Highly active RRMS.	Humanised monoclonal antibody that binds to CD52, a protein on the surface of mature lymphocytes.	Relapse ↓ by 70%.	Immune thrombocytopenic purpura, thyroid autoimmunity, malignancy.

Acute disseminated encephalomyelitis

- Often post-infectious (especially mycoplasma).
- Widespread CNS demyelination.
- No dissemination in time ('monophasic').
- Treatment with steroids (after exclusion of infectious encephalitis). Intravenous immunoglobulin or plasmapheresis may also be beneficial.
- A minority go on to develop MS.

Neurosarcoidosis

- Most frequently presents with cranial neuropathies, meningeal disease or pituitary involvement.
- Parenchymal involvement of the CNS is also seen, which can mimic MS and can occur in the absence of systemic manifestations of sarcoidosis.
- PET scanning is increasingly used in diagnosis.
- Serum and CSF angiotensin-converting enzyme levels are poorly sensitive.
- Treatment is with steroids, steroid-sparing agents (e.g. azathioprine, methotrexate, MMF), and sometimes with anti-TNF agents (e.g. infliximab).

Behçet's disease

➲ See Chapter 20, Behçet's disease, p. 742 .

CNS lupus

➲ See Chapter 20, Systemic lupus erythematosus, p. 729 and Tables 20.7 and 20.8.

- Demyelination and CNS vasculitis may occur.
- Associated antiphospholipid syndrome (APLS) (➲ see Chapter 20, Antiphospholipid syndrome, p. 732) can cause thromboembolic stroke and cerebral venous sinus thrombosis.
- Treatment is as for severe non-neurological systemic lupus erythematosus (SLE).

CNS vasculitis

- Causes multiple areas of cerebral infarction.
- May occur as part of a systemic vasculitis (usually anti-neutrophil cytoplasmic antibody positive).
- When it occurs as a primary CNS vasculitis, diagnosis is extremely difficult, and may require brain biopsy.
- Treatment is generally with steroids and cyclophosphamide/rituximab.

Further reading

1. Polman CH, Reingold SC, Banwell B, et al. Diagnostic criteria for multiple sclerosis: 2010 Revisions to the McDonald criteria. *Ann Neurol*. 2011; 69:292–302.

Movement disorders

Parkinson's disease

Idiopathic Parkinson's disease is the 2nd most prevalent neurodegenerative disease (after Alzheimer's disease), affecting 2% of the population aged >60 years. Monogenic causes are rare, but an increasing number of candidate genes are recognised, which probably interact with multiple environmental exposures to contribute to the prevalence of the disease.

Parkinson's disease is due to degeneration of dopaminergic neurons in the nigrostriatal pathway. Abnormal accumulation of a protein, α-synuclein, bound to ubiquitin, occurs in the damaged cells, forming cellular inclusions called Lewy bodies. This particularly occurs in the ventral pars compacta of the substantia nigra.

Presentation and classification

Bradykinesia is the sine qua non of Parkinson's disease and, for confident diagnosis, this feature should be combined with ≥1 of rigidity, resting tremor and/or postural instability. A combination of motor and non-motor, dopaminergic and non-dopaminergic symptoms and signs are also seen. Parkinson's disease classically presents asymmetrically, so very symmetrical initial presentations suggest alternative causes (e.g. essential tremor, dystonic tremor, drug induced tremor, vascular Parkinsonism, normal pressure hydrocephalus). Later in the disease duration, the signs may appear more symmetrical.

- *Early presentation:*
  - Anxiety – may precede motor symptoms by decades.
  - Olfactory decline/anosmia – an early but non-specific sign.
  - Rapid eye movement (sleep) behavioural disorder (REM-BD) – strongly predictive of future neurodegenerative pathology.
  - Cognitive impairment – often of frontostriatal executive dysfunction.
- *Middle presentation*:
  - Tremor:
    - Classically a resting tremor, 'pill-rolling' in nature, involving the thumb and index finger with a frequency of 3–5 Hz.
    - Typically asymmetric, often unilateral initially, but commonly later involving the contralateral limb.
    - May also affect the legs, chin, lips and trunk.
    - Exacerbated by stress/emotion.
    - Masked by deliberate movement.
    - Revealed by distraction manoeuvres, e.g. asking the patient to move the contralateral limb or perform simple cognitive tasks such as counting back from 100.
  - Rigidity – increased tone described as 'cog-wheeling' and felt as a ratcheting throughout the range of movement, often at the wrist or elbow, with a similar frequency to the tremor.
  - Bradykinesia:
    - Breakdown of fine finger movements, difficulty with gait initiation or rising from a chair, a short stride length and/or a 'festinant' (hurrying) gait.
    - Arm swing is often reduced on the (more) affected side and patients turn 'en bloc'.
- *Late presentation:*
  - Worsening of symptoms and spread to involve the contralateral limbs.
  - Cognitive problems become more apparent with poor memory and visual hallucinations.
  - Systemic symptoms such as constipation, dysphagia, sleep disorder and autonomic failure (especially orthostatic hypotension and thermodysregulation) become as important and disabling (or more so) than the motor disability.

Investigations

The diagnosis of movement disorders remains clinical but neurotransmitter-labelled imaging studies and other investigations may be useful in certain situations:

- *L-DOPA challenge*: patients are assessed before and after a large dose of levodopa (200-400 mg), using a validated measure, such as a timed walk and/or unified Parkinson's disease rating scale (UPDRS) score. Improvement with levodopa, though not diagnostic of Parkinson's disease, is a useful guide to the likely efficacy of dopaminergic therapy.
- *DaTSCAN*: an ioflupane (^{123}I) radioisotope is injected into patients. A gamma camera produces SPECT images, which demonstrate the isotope's high affinity for the dopamine transporter, particularly in the striatum. Patients with Parkinson's disease may demonstrate either unilaterally or bilaterally reduced uptake. Dopaminergic drugs can influence the scan and it must therefore be interpreted in this context. Other presynaptic dopamine labelling isotopes are also available. Where DaTSCAN is unavailable, ^{18}F-FDG PET CT is sometimes used for similar purposes.

- *MIBG scan*: there is some evidence that metaiodobenzylguanidine (MIBG) scans can help differentiate between idiopathic Parkinson's disease and other Parkinsonian syndromes, as a result of a correlation between nigrostriatal degeneration and autonomic dysfunction.

Prognosis

55% of patients die within 10 years of diagnosis, with pneumonia being the commonest cause of death. Of the patients that survive:

- 68% have postural instability (predictors include age, non-tremor-dominant motor phenotype and comorbidity).
- 46% have dementia (predictors include age, motor impairment, 'posterior-cortical' cognitive deficits and *MAPT* [microtubule-associated protein tau] genotype).
- 23% are free of postural instability/dementia.

Management

Drug therapy

Dopaminergic therapies

The most effective treatment for Parkinson's disease is replacement of lost endogenous dopamine. This may be achieved by administration of levodopa in concert with a peripheral dopa decarboxylase inhibitor (either carbidopa or benserazide) to prevent its peripheral breakdown. Normally, this is achieved by oral medication. Later in the disease when fluctuations in symptoms become problematic ('on-off' phenomena with a switch between mobility and immobility with end-of-dose or 'wearing off' [worsening of motor function]), duodenal administration has been shown to provide more steady plasma levels and an improved clinical state.

Alternatively, there are various dopamine agonists (e.g. bromocriptine, cabergoline, pergolide, ropinirole, pramipexole) available in oral form. These agents are associated with a susceptibility to impulse control disorders. Patients are therefore counselled of the dangers of pathological gambling, extramarital affairs, compulsive hoarding/collecting and punding. A related problem is dopamine dysregulation syndrome in which patients seek ever higher and more frequent doses of their dopaminergic drugs despite no apparent clinical benefit. Transdermal (rotigotine) and SC (apomorphine) dopamine agonists have been developed in order to try to provide a steady state drug level and also to avoid problems for patients with dysphagia. The 'ergot'-derived dopamine agonists, bromocriptine, cabergoline and pergolide have been associated with pulmonary, retroperitoneal and pericardial fibrotic reactions, and cardiac valvulopathy. Patients taking cabergoline or pergolide should undergo echocardiography prior to starting treatment, within 3–6 months of initiating treatment and subsequently at 6–12-month intervals.

Monoamine oxidase inhibitors (e.g. rasagiline, selegiline) and the catechol-o-methyl transferase (COMT) inhibitor (entacapone) are additional agents often used in later Parkinson's disease when wearing off phenomena begin to occur.

Non-dopaminergic therapies

- Amantadine:
  - Weak agonist at the NMDA-R that increases dopamine and norepinephrine release.
- Anticholinergics, e.g. trixhexyphenidyl/benzhexol, orphenadrine, procyclidine:
  - Useful for treatment of tremor.
  - Considerable anticholinergic side effect burden.

Treatment of non-motor symptoms

- Antidepressants for mood disorder (➔ see Chapter 22, Antidepressants, p. 781 and Table 22.2.
- Laxatives for constipation.
- Anti-salivary agents for sialorrhoea, e.g. anticholinergics, hyoscine.

- Fludrocortisone (a mineralocorticoid), midodrine (α1-receptor agonist) and droxidopa (amino acid prodrug of norepinephrine that crosses the blood–brain barrier) for symptomatic orthostatic hypotension.
- Cholinesterase inhibitors (e.g. rivastigmine, galantamine and donepezil) for dementia.
- Neuroleptics for hallucinations or psychosis, taking care to avoid excessive dopamine antagonism that may worsen Parkinson's disease symptoms; hence, quetiapine is most commonly employed.

Non-drug therapy

Deep brain stimulation

Patients who have a profound motor disturbance (especially motor fluctuations or intractable tremor) may benefit from surgical intervention. Deep brain stimulation (DBS), particularly of the subthalamic nucleus but also of the globus pallidus interna (GPi) and ventro-intermediate nucleus of the thalamus, has been used very successfully in treating marked tremor and dyskinesia.

Multidisciplinary team support

- Parkinson's disease specialist nurses.
- Physiotherapists and occupational therapists (who may provide walking aids, handrails and other adaptations).
- Speech and language therapists to manage dysphagia and dysarthria.
- Psychiatrists/psychologists to assist with progressive dementia.

Other Parkinsonian syndromes

Parkinson's disease with dementia

Cognitive impairment is an expected part of the progression of Parkinson's disease. Common features include hallucinations, REM-BD and memory impairment. This may be difficult to differentiate from comorbid Alzheimer's and/or vascular dementia.

Dementia with Lewy bodies

Dementia with Lewy bodies (DLB) should be considered when cognitive disturbance presents early in the disease process, particularly if present before the motor disorder. There is often exquisite sensitivity to levodopa with dyskinesias and hallucinations at very low doses. DLB and Parkinson's disease with dementia may not be distinct pathological entities, but merely reflect the temporal and spatial distribution of Lewy body deposition in the brain.

Multiple system atrophy

Early autonomic involvement (postural hypotension, urinary incontinence and male impotence) and/or cerebellar symptoms/signs with Parkinsonism should provoke consideration of this diagnosis. Parkinsonism (MSA-p) or cerebellar signs (MSA-c) may predominate. Cognition is often preserved. The response to levodopa is often poor. Head drop is common. The primary neuropathology is of α-synuclein inclusions.

Progressive supranuclear palsy (Steele–Richardson–Olszewski syndrome)

The hallmark of this clinical syndrome is frequent falls and axial rigidity associated with a vertical, supranuclear gaze palsy. Levodopa response is variable. Imaging may reveal the 'hummingbird' or 'penguin' appearance of the brainstem on MRI. The primary neuropathology is of tau protein deposition.

Corticobasal degeneration

- Parkinsonism.
- Alien hand syndrome (hand movement without the patient being aware of what is happening).
- Apraxia (ideomotor apraxia and limb-kinetic apraxia).

- Aphasia.
- Associated with the deposition of abnormal tau protein in the brain.
- Overlap with progressive supranuclear palsy (PSP) and frontotemporal dementia (FTD).

Atypical parkinsonism

- Neuroacanthocytosis.
- Brain iron accumulation syndromes, e.g. pantothenate kinase-associated neurodegeneration.
- Genetic forms of Parkinson's disease, e.g. with mutations in leucine rich repeat kinase (LRRK), phosphatase and tensin-holding homologue-induced putative kinase (PINK) and Parkin genes.

Other hypokinetic movement disorders

Dystonia

- Involuntary muscle contraction and spasm of opponent muscle groups.
  - Generalised dystonias:
    - Rare.
    - Associated with specific genetic abnormalities.
    - Treatment may be symptomatic, with GABAergic agents and anticholinergics, and with DBS of the GPi in refractory cases.
  - Focal dystonias:
    - Often 'task specific' (provoked by specific muscle activity), e.g. writer's cramp, embouchure dystonia (musicians), laryngeal dystonia.
    - May be unrelated to activity, e.g. cervical and oromandibular dystonia, hemifacial spasm, blepharospasm.
    - Often treated with botulinum toxin to affected muscle groups.

Hyperkinetic movement disorders

Idiopathic essential tremor

- Bilateral, fine, 4–6 Hz postural tremor worse on attempted fine manipulation (e.g. tying neck ties/ doing up buttons).
- Improved by alcohol, benzodiazepines and β-blockade.
- Worsened by anxiety/stress.
- Often a strong family history.
- Initially usually involves the hands; may later spread to involve the head/neck and face (titubation).
- Many patients have some dystonia.

Dystonic tremor

- May often resemble the tremor of either Parkinson's disease and/or essential tremor (ET).
- May be relieved/reduced by touching the affected body part or muscle.

Orthostatic tremor

- Lower limb tremor (bilateral) that occurs on standing.

Rubral (Holmes) tremor

- Due to damage to the red nucleus or its surrounding structures.

Huntington's chorea

A rare autosomal dominantly inherited triplet repeat (CAG) disorder, which shows anticipation (➲ see Chapter 2, Anticipation, p. 47 and Table 2.2, and Trinucleotide repeat disorders, p. 49 and Table 2.4). The degree of severity and early age of onset show positive correlation with the degree of expansion. The main symptoms are of a choreiform movement disorder with associated cognitive and neuropsychiatric abnormalities. Treatments include typical (e.g. haloperidol) and atypical (e.g. olanzapine and aripiprazole) neuroleptics, mood stabilisers/antidepressants and tetrabenazine.

Headache

The brain itself is not sensitive to pain, because it lacks nociceptors, but intracranial nociceptive structures include:

- Large intracranial vessels.
- Dura mater.
- Peripheral terminals of the trigeminal nerve.
- The trigemino-cervical complex:
  - caudal trigeminal nucleus;
  - dorsal horns of C1/2.

Primary headache syndromes

Migraine

Genetic associations suggest a potential role of ion channels, e.g. familial hemiplegic migraine with mutations in *CACNA1A* calcium and *SCN1A* sodium channel genes. Clinical features include:

- Episodic headache, often unilateral and/or throbbing, and retro-orbital and/or temporal in location.
- Sensory sensitivity:
  - photophobia;
  - phonophobia;
  - kinesiophobia;
  - osmophobia.

Triggers include:

- Barometric pressure/humidity.
- Sleep (lack or excess).
- Dietary intake, e.g. cheese, caffeine, alcohol.
- Stress (either excess or in periods of relief).
- Physical exertion.
- Loud noise.
- Bright light.
- Hormonal changes such as puberty, menses and menopause.

Migraine with aura involves:

- Visual fortifications, e.g. zig-zags, flashing lights, scintillating scotomata;
- Tinnitus.
- Other sensory disturbance.
- Weakness; ataxia; dysphasia.

Management involves:

- Patient education/use of diaries.
- Lifestyle adjustment.
- Regulation of environmental factors.

- Avoidance of specific triggers.
- Awareness of increased stroke risk in women who also smoke and use oestrogen-containing contraceptives.
- Avoidance of analgesia overuse.
- Acute treatment:
  - NSAIDs, e.g. aspirin, ibuprofen;
  - paracetamol;
  - ergotamine;
  - triptans, e.g. sumatiptan, naratriptan, rizatriptan, zolmitriptan, eletriptan.
  - anti-emetics:
    - antihistamines, e.g. prochlorperazine, cyclizine;
    - dopaminergic blockade, e.g. metoclopramide, domperidone;
    - serotonin antagonists, e.g. ondansetron.
- Prophylactic treatments:
  - Considered when headaches occur more than 3–4 times per month.
  - Side effects must be weighed against possible benefits for the available pharmacologic agents that include:
    - β-blockers, e.g. propranolol;
    - tricyclic antidepressants, e.g. amitriptyline, dosulepin, nortriptyline;
    - neuromodulators, e.g. pizotifen, topiramate, sodium valproate, gabapentin, pregabalin.

Tension headache

- Commonly occurs comorbidly with migraine.
- Classified as episodic or chronic.
- Simple analgesics are often effective.
- Amitriptyline is often an effective preventative.

Trigeminal autonomic cephalalgias

Cluster headache

- Prevalence 1:1000.
- Male preponderance.
- More common in smokers.
- Associated with severe, but frequent short-lived episodes of retro-orbital, 'boring' pain (usually seconds).
- Bouts of activity and inactivity, e.g. 1–2 episodes lasting a few weeks per year.
- Associated trigeminal/other cranial nerve dysautonomic symptoms including:
  - red/watery eye;
  - rhinorrhoea;
  - ptosis;
  - unilateral photophobia/phonophobia.
- Acute management involves use of oxygen and triptans.
- Prophylaxis may be achieved with verapamil (for prolonged therapy) and corticosteroids (during bouts).

Paroxysmal hemicrania

- Similar phenomenology to cluster headache.
- Short, but frequent attacks.
- Responds to indomethacin.
- No gender bias.

Short-lasting unilateral neuralgiform headache with conjunctival injection and tearing and short-lasting unilateral neuralgiform headache with cranial autonomic symptoms

- Short, but frequent attacks.
- Rarely occurs as a phenomenon secondary to posterior fossa/pituitary lesions.
- Prevented by antiepileptics, e.g. lamotrigine, topiramate, carbamazepine, gabapentin.

Primary sex headache

- Precipitation by sexual excitement.
- Bilateral at onset.
- Prevented or eased by ceasing sexual activity before orgasm.

Primary stabbing headache

- Short-lived jabs of pain, lasting seconds or minutes.
- No associated cranial autonomic features.
- Recurring at irregular intervals (hours to days).

Chronic daily headaches

Arise from multiple aetiologies including:

- Analgesia overuse.
- Chronic migraine.
- Chronic tension-type headache.
- Hemicrania continua.
- Chronic paroxysmal hemicranias.
- Short-lasting unilateral neuralgiform headache with conjunctival injection and tearing.
- Hypnic headache.

Secondary headache

Secondary headaches may relate to relatively benign pathology (such as during febrile illnesses due to common viral infections), but may also be indicative of more sinister underlying pathology. Headache 'red flags' include:

- New onset in a patient >50 years.
- Vomiting: may suggest raised intracranial pressure (ICP).
- Morning headaches: may suggest raised ICP or CO_2 retention.
- Visual obscurations: may suggest raised ICP and/or pituitary pathology.
- Fever, neck stiffness, purpuric rash.
- Focal neurological symptoms.
- 'Thunderclap' headache reaching maximal intensity within 5 minutes – may suggest SAH.

Specific causes of secondary headache include:

- SAH.
- Reversible cerebral vasocontriction syndrome:
  - Association with pregnancy and the post-partum period.
  - Causes thunderclap headache.
  - Vasospastic changes on imaging.
- Posterior reversible encephalopathy syndrome:
  - May be caused by malignant hypertension, eclampsia and immunosuppressants, e.g. tacrolimus.
  - Characterised by:
    - Headache, confusion, seizures and visual loss.
    - Altered signal occipito-parietally on MRI.
  - Not always posterior, nor reversible, nor associated with encephalopathy.

- Giant-cell arteritis: ➲ see Chapter 20, Giant cell arteritis, p. 740.
- Meningitis: ➲ see Chapter 8, Meningitis, p. 244 and Tables 8.15, 8.16, 8.17.
- Idiopathic intracranial hypertension:
  - Increased prevalence in women of childbearing age.
  - Often presents with morning headaches ± intermittent scotomata.
  - Associated with:
    - Weight gain/high body mass index.
    - Chiari malformation (downward displacement of the cerebellar tonsils through the foramen magnum).
    - Polycystic ovarian syndrome.
  - Blurred optic discs on fundoscopy.
  - Investigations include:
    - CT/MR-venography to exclude venous sinus thrombosis.
    - Lumbar puncture:
      - diagnostic if CSF opening pressure >20 cmH_2O in the absence of a structural cause.
  - Management options include:
    - lumbar puncture;
    - acetazolamide;
    - topiramate;
    - weight loss;
    - lumbar-peritoneal/ventriculo-peritoneal shunting.

Further reading

1. Headache Classification Committee of the International Headache Society. The International Classification of Headache Disorders, 3rd edition. *Cephalalgia*. 2013;33:629–808.

Neuro-oncology

Metastatic disease

Metastatic disease to the CNS is more common than primary CNS tumours. Metastases may be single or multiple, and may present with seizures, focal deficits, raised ICP or haemorrhage. Tumours commonly metastasising to brain include lung, breast, kidney and melanoma. Treatment depends on the underlying tumour and the size, number and location of metastases, and may include surgery, radiotherapy and chemotherapy. Prognosis is poor with median survival being approximately 9 months.

Malignant meningitis involves diffuse infiltration of the meninges by metastatic tumour and may cause headache, raised ICP, cranial neuropathies and radiculopathies. Diagnosis is with contrast-enhanced MRI showing meningeal enhancement and CSF demonstrating malignant cells.

Primary central nervous system tumours

- Astrocytoma:
  - Grade 1 – pilocytic astrocytoma; mostly in children; curable with surgery.
  - Grade 2 – diffuse astrocytoma; often transforms into higher grade tumours; median survival 4 years.
  - Grade 3 – anaplastic astrocytoma; median survival 1.6 years.
  - Grade 4 – glioblastoma multiforme; median survival 0.7 years.
  - Although grade 2–4 tumours are generally not curable, survival improves with combined resection and radiotherapy, and in glioblastoma multiforme, adjuvant chemotherapy with temozolomide is often used.
- Meningioma:
  - Tumour of the dura.
  - Generally benign and curable with resection but a minority have atypical features and require adjuvant radiotherapy.

  - Asymptomatic meningiomas are commonly found incidentally on imaging and can often be managed conservatively with periodic surveillance.
- Primary CNS lymphoma:
  - B-cell lymphoma.
  - Can be sporadic or associated with immunosuppression (especially HIV).
  - Treated with chemotherapy and radiotherapy.
  - Median survival is approximately 18 months.
- Acoustic neuroma:
  - Benign tumour of the myelin-forming Schwann cells of the vestibular division of the vestibulocochlear nerve.
  - Usually occurs spontaneously, but present in 90% of patients with neurofibromatosis (NF) type 2.
  - Primary symptoms are hearing loss, tinnitus and dysequilibrium.
  - Larger tumours may compress cranial nerves V, VII, IX and X, and/or the cerebellum causing focal deficits and/or increase ICP.
  - Treatment is by surgery or radiotherapy, and often results in substantial or complete hearing loss in the affected ear.
- Other tumour types including oligodendroglioma, ependymoma, developmental tumours and germ cell tumours.

Paraneoplastic neurological syndromes

Paraneoplastic syndromes are not due to the local presence of cancer cells, but are mediated by humoral factors secreted by tumour cells or by an immune response. A number of anti-neuronal antibodies, directed against antigens present in both neurons and tumour cells, have been identified in patients with paraneoplastic neurological syndromes, suggesting a role in their aetiopathogenesis (Table 17.5). Paraneoplastic neurological syndromes may be the presenting feature of a tumour and their recognition may lead to cure of a very early-stage cancer. Management is with treatment of the underlying tumour, and with immunotherapy for anti-NMDA-R antibody encephalitis (with steroids, IVIG and plasmapheresis [and rituximab and cyclophosphamide as 2nd line therapy]) where the antibody has been shown to be causative.

Muscle disease

Presentation

- Presents with weakness.
- 'Negative' symptoms include stiffness, rigidity and fatigue.
- 'Positive' symptoms include muscle cramps, twitches or 'rippling' and discoloured urine (indicating the presence of products of muscle breakdown).

Investigation

Serum tests

- Systemic causes of weakness, e.g. anaemia, electrolyte/endocrine disturbance.
- Creatine kinase (CK):
  - Wide variation in the normal range; higher in men and in black people.
  - Elevated after:
    - Intense periods of exercise.
    - Rhabdomyolysis following prolonged immobilisation.
    - Denervation.
    - Drug ingestion (especially statins).
    - Muscle disease when the magnitude of increase is instructive:
      - Five-fold rise is suggestive of an inflammatory myopathy (myositis).
      - Modest (< four-fold) rises in toxic and degenerative conditions.

Table 17.5 Anti-neuronal antibodies and associated paraneoplastic neurological syndromes

Anti-neuronal antibody	Associated paraneoplastic neurological syndrome	Associated causal tumour type
Anti-Hu	Paraneoplastic cerebellar degeneration (PCD) Encephalomyelitis Subacute sensory neuropathy (SSN)	Small cell lung carcinoma (SCLC)
Anti-Yo	PCD	Ovary Breast
Anti-Ri	Cerebellar ataxia Opsoclonus (rapid, involuntary, multivectorial [horizontal and vertical], unpredictable, conjugate, fast eye movements)/ myoclonus (brief, involuntary muscle twitching) syndrome Brainstem encephalomyelitis	Breast Fallopian tube SCLC Neuroblastoma
Anti-CV2	PCD Limbic encephalitis* Encephalomyelitis Sensory neuropathy	SCLC Sarcoma
Anti-PNMA2	PCD Limbic encephalitis* Brainstem encephalomyelitis Sensory neuropathy	Various cancers including testicular
Anti-amphiphysin	Stiff person syndrome PCD Encephalomyelitis SSN	Breast cancer SCLC
Anti-Recoverin	Retinopathy	SCLC
Anti-Tr	PCD	Hodgkin's disease
Anti-SOX1	PCD Lambert–Eaton myasthenic syndrome (➲ see Lambert-Eaton myaesthenic syndrome, p. 632)	SCLC
Anti-NMDA	Anti-NMDA-R encephalitis	Teratoma

*Limbic encephalitis is characterised by subacute development of short-term memory deficits, and by headache, irritability, sleep disturbance, delusions, hallucinations, agitation, seizures and psychosis.

- Lactate:
  - Blunted rise after exercise in glycolytic or glycogenolytic disorders.
- Ammonia:
  - Amplified increase after exercise in glycolytic or glycogenolytic disorders.

Genetic testing

- Increasingly available.
- May become a 'first-line' investigation.

Neurophysiology

EMG may be helpful in discriminating between denervation (due to motor neuropathy), NMJ disorders (e.g. myasthenia gravis) and primary muscle disease. However, the myopathic pattern of fibrillations, positive sharp waves and complex repetitive discharges is less helpful in distinguishing between types of myopathic process.

Muscle biopsy

- Often crucial in making the diagnosis.
- Moderately involved muscles are usually chosen as severely atrophic muscles often do not yield specific diagnostic changes.
- Enzymic stains, immunohistochemistry and electron microscopy may be helpful.

Inflammatory muscle disease

Idiopathic myositis

Idiopathic myositides include dermatomyositis, polymyositis and inclusion body myositis. All of these conditions share the key features of predominantly proximal muscle wasting and weakness. Their specific clinical features and management are discussed in ➲ Chapter 20, Table 20.6. They are caused by separate pathological mechanisms, but distinguishing one from another, or from other conditions, can be difficult.

Autoimmune-associated myositis

- SLE.
- Rheumatoid arthritis.
- Mixed connective tissue disease.
- Sjögren's syndrome.

Infection-associated myositis

- Viral (HIV, EBV, CMV, HTLV-1).
- Bacterial (staphylococcus, Lyme disease, tuberculosis).
- Parasitic (nematodes, protozoa).

Other diseases associated with myositis

- Vasculitis.
- Sarcoidosis.

Drug-induced muscle disease

Drugs commonly associated with myopathy include:

- **L**ipid lowering agents, e.g. statins, fibrates, nicotinic acid, ezetimibe.
- **S**teroids.
- **D**rugs of abuse, e.g. alcohol, heroin, cocaine.
- **C**olchicine, chloroquine.
- **H**ydroxychloroquine.
- **A**miodarone.
- **P**erhexiline.

Muscular dystrophies

- Result from multiple genetic abnormalities affecting muscle protein components in the sarcolemma, nuclear envelope, sarcomere, enzymes and/or extracellular matrix.
- Some syndromes are related to single identified gene disorders, whereas others are due to multiple different mutations (genotypes) that lead to a similar phenotype.
- Symptoms and signs include:
  - Progressive muscular wasting/imbalance/immobility.

  - Gowers' sign:
    - Patient has to use his/her hands and arms to 'walk' up his/her own body from a squatting position due to lack of hip and thigh muscle strength.
  - Waddling gait.
  - Calf muscle pseudohypertrophy.
  - Scoliosis.
  - Respiratory difficulty.
  - Cardiomyopathy.
- Diagnosis is facilitated by the results of muscle biopsy, increased CK, EMG and genetic testing.
- Treatment is supportive with no curative therapies available.

Xp21 dystrophies

Duchenne muscular dystrophy (DMD) and Becker muscular dystrophy are X-linked recessive conditions caused by dystrophin gene mutations at locus Xp21. Dystrophin is responsible for connecting the cytoskeleton of each muscle fibre to the underlying basal lamina and its absence permits excess calcium to penetrate the sarcolemma, increasing intracellular oxidative stress. Muscle fibres then undergo necrosis and are ultimately replaced with adipose and connective tissue.

DMD has an incidence of 1 per 3600 male infants, while Becker muscular dystrophy occurs in 1.5–6 per 100,000 male births. Symptoms in DMD usually appear before the age of 6, while symptoms in Becker muscular dystrophy usually appear at age 8–25 years. Life expectancy in DMD is <40 years (although improved from yesteryear due to improved ventilatory support). Becker muscular dystrophy has a less severe reduction in dystrophin correlating with a reduced severity of phenotype, with calf muscle pseudohypertrophy being common and cardiomyopathy sometimes being the first presentation.

Emery–Dreifuss muscular dystrophy

- Caused by mutations in the *LMNA* or *EMD* genes that encode for lamin A, lamin C and emerin protein components of the nuclear envelope, respectively.
  - Emerin is highly expressed in cardiac muscle where it localises to adherens junctions within intercalated discs to function in mechanotransduction of cellular strain and in beta-catenin signalling:
    - Emerin mutations result in cardiac conduction abnormalities and dilated cardiomyopathy.
- Patients normally present in childhood and the early teenage years.
- Clinical signs include:
  - Muscle weakness and wasting, starting in the distal limb muscles and progressing to involve the limb-girdle muscles.
  - Cardiac conduction defects and arrhythmias.
- Three subtypes are distinguishable by their pattern of inheritance:
  - X-linked (most common);
  - autosomal dominant;
  - autosomal recessive.

Congenital muscular dystrophies

- Onset at birth.
- Symptoms include muscle weakness, joint deformities and shortened lifespan.
- Problems may be restricted to skeletal muscle, or muscle degeneration may be paired with effects on the brain and other organ systems.

Limb girdle muscular dystrophies

- Dominant limb girdle muscular dystrophies (LGMD1) and recessive (LGMD2) forms.
- Multiple genes and proteins identified.
- All show a similar distribution of muscle weakness, affecting both upper arms and legs.

Facioscapulohumeral dystrophy

- Autosomal dominant inheritance.
- Associated with truncation of non-coding region of chromosome 4.
- Facial weakness precedes upper limb (shoulder) girdle weakness.
- Often distal weakness in the lower limbs with foot drop. Proximal leg weakness is a late feature.
- Symptoms usually develop in early adulthood.

Oculopharyngeal muscular dystrophy

- Recessive and dominant forms.
- Age at onset is 40–70 years.
- Symptoms affect muscles of the eyelids, face and throat, followed by pelvic and shoulder muscle weakness.
- Rare cause of late-onset ophthalmoplegia.
- May mimic myasthenia gravis.

Myotonic dystrophy

Myotonic dystrophy (dystrophia myotonica, myotonia atrophica) is an autosomal-dominant, chronic, slowly progressing, highly variable, inherited multi-systemic disease. It is characterised by:

- wasting of the muscles (muscular dystrophy);
- distal weakness;
- myotonia with difficulty in releasing handgrip;
- frontal balding;
- myopathic facies;
- cognitive impairment;
- somnolence;
- cataracts;
- endocrine problems:
  - type 2 diabetes mellitus;
  - thyroid dysfunction;
  - testicular atrophy.
- cardiac problems:
  - cardiomyopathy;
  - cardiac conduction defects.

There are two main types:

- Myotonic dystrophy type 1 (MD1) – also called Steinert disease.
  - The affected *DMPK* (dystrophia myotonica protein kinase gene) (➔ see Chapter 2, Anticipation, p. 47 and Table 2.2, and Trinucleotide repeat disorders, p. 49 and Table 2.4) on the long arm of chromosome 19 encodes myotonic dystrophy protein kinase, a protein involved in regulating the production and function of important structures inside muscle cells by interacting with other proteins, e.g. inhibition of myosin phosphatase that itself plays a role in muscle contraction/relaxation.
  - Has a severe congenital form, a milder childhood-onset form and an adult-onset form.
  - Most often affects the facial muscles, levator palpebrae superioris, temporalis, sternocleidomastoids, distal muscles of the forearm, hand intrinsic muscles and ankle dorsiflexors.
- Myotonic dystrophy type 2 (MD2) – also called proximal myotonic myopathy (PROMM).
  - The affected *ZNF9* gene on chromosome 3 encodes the zinc finger domain-containing ZNF9 protein believed to function as an RNA-binding protein.
  - Rarer than MD1 and usually with milder signs and symptoms.

DM1 is a trinucleotide repeat disorder with an expansion of the cytosine-thymine-guanine (CTG) triplet repeat in the *DMPK* gene. *DMPK* alleles with >37 repeats are unstable (normal between 5 and 37 repeats), and additional trinucleotide repeats may be inserted during cell division in mitosis and meiosis. Consequently, children inheriting *DMPK* alleles, which are longer than their parents', are more likely to have an earlier onset and display a greater severity of the condition, a phenomenon known as anticipation (➲ see Chapter 2, Anticipation, p. 47 and Table 2.2, and Trinucleotide repeat disorders, p. 49 and Table 2.4).

DM2 is a tetranucleotide repeat disorder with an expansion of the cytosine-cytosine-thymine-guanosine (CCTG) tetranucleotide repeat in the *ZNF9* gene. The repeat expansion for DM2 is much larger than for DM1, ranging from 75 to >11,000 repeats. Unlike DM1, the size of the repeated DNA expansion in DM2 does not make a significant difference in the age of onset or disease severity, and displays only mild anticipation, in contrast to DM1.

Motor neurone disease

- Progressive neuronal degenerative disease leading to severe disability and death.
- Several different clinical subtypes:
  - Amyotrophic lateral sclerosis (ALS):
    - Most common.
    - 5–10% of cases are familial, mostly of autosomal dominant inheritance:
      - 40% involve a mutation of the *C9ORF72* (chromosome 9 open reading frame 72) gene associated with development of FTD-ALS.
      - 20% involve a mutation of the copper/zinc superoxide dismutase (*SOD1*) gene on chromosome 21.
      - 3–5% involve a mutation of the fused in sarcoma (*FUS*) gene on chromosome 16.
      - May involve a mutation of transactive response DNA-binding protein (TARDBP) on chromosome 1.
    - Upper and lower motor neurone involvement of bulbar structures (nerves, tracts and muscles [including those of the tongue, pharynx and larynx] connected to the medulla) and upper and lower limbs.
    - Dominant bulbar weakness is termed 'progressive bulbar palsy' (PBP).
    - Approximately 50% of patients die within 30 months of symptoms beginning.
  - Primary lateral sclerosis (PLS):
    - exclusive upper motor neurone involvement;
    - tends to progress more slowly.
  - Progressive muscular atrophy (PMA):
    - involves only lower motor neurons.

Investigations

Clinical history and examination may be sufficient for diagnosis with classical bulbar weakness, wasting and fasciculations (including of the tongue). However, less clear-cut cases can be supported by a modest rise in CK and EMG changes consistent with denervation. MRI of the spine/brainstem is often performed to rule out multi-level compressive/degenerative disease as a mimic of motor neurone disease (MND) (for example, mixed upper and lower motor neurone signs could be due to multilevel radiculo-myelopathy). Increasingly, genetic testing is used first line.

Management

The treatment of MND is supportive. A modest survival improvement has been demonstrated with riluzole (delaying the requirement for ventilation and/or tracheostomy and extending life by about 2–3 months). Multidisciplinary clinics are commonly employed to address the needs of patients with MND with:

- Speech therapists assessing and treating bulbar dysfunction (including discussions around altered diet and/or alternative feeding routes such as via gastrostomy).

- Physiotherapists and occupational therapists extending useful motor function with appropriate exercises and walking aids.
- Respiratory/palliative care physicians facilitating decisions regarding ventilatory support.

Neuromuscular junction disorders

Myasthenia gravis

- Typified by 'fatigable' muscle weakness:
  - Muscle weakness becomes more prominent with repetitive muscle contraction.
  - Symptoms become more obvious as the day progresses.
- May be localised:
  - Commonly to eyes, bulbar muscles or both (oculobulbar myasthenia).
  - Causes fatigable ophthalmoplegia (resulting in diplopia), ptosis, dysarthria and dysphagia.
  - Weight loss is a common sequel of bulbar involvement.
- May be generalised:
  - Affecting limb muscles and leading to respiratory compromise.
  - May cause 'myasthenic crisis' where emergent respiratory support is required.

Pathophysiology

Myasthenia gravis is an autoimmune disorder. IgG antibodies against the acetylcholine receptor in the muscle membrane are detectable in 75% of patients. These antibodies bind to the receptor leading to blockade and cross-link muscle surface AChRs increasing their rate of internalisation, or bind complement leading to destruction of the muscle end-plate. Loss of voltage-gated Na^+ channels at the end-plate leads to reduced muscle membrane depolarisation and an increase in the threshold necessary to intiate a muscle action potential.

20–25% of patients are anti-AChR antibody negative (seronegative myasthenia gravis [SNMG]) and IgG antibodies to muscle specific kinase (MusK) are found in >50% of ocular/generalised SNMG patients. MusK is a receptor tyrosine kinase expressed selectively in skeletal muscles that helps to cluster post-synaptic proteins, including AChR, at the NMJ. Anti-MusK antibodies may activate complement inducing lysis of the post-synaptic membrane.

Treatment

In mild, especially ocular myasthenia, acetylcholinesterase inhibitors are used to treat the symptoms. Pyridostigmine is the most common choice. Cholinergic side effects of this treatment (e.g. diarrhoea) may be managed with propantheline bromide.

Immunosuppression/immunomodulation is used to reduce AChR antibody production. Those with mild disease are treated with low doses of corticosteroid, e.g. prednisolone. More severe disease may require higher doses of corticosteroid, but caution is advised as high-dose steroid therapy may be associated with an initial deterioration in symptoms. Refractory disease can be treated with steroid-sparing immunosuppressants including methotrexate, azathioprine, ciclosporin and MMF, and rituximab in severe disease. In acute, severe episodes of 'myasthenic crisis' (which may be triggered by drugs [➲ see Chapter 3, Patients with myasthenia gravis, p. 74], intercurrent illness or be idiopathic) IVIG is the mainstay of therapy. Plasmapheresis (to remove the antibody) has not been found to be superior to IVIG.

Congenital myasthenia

- Inherited neuromuscular disorder with pre-synaptic, synaptic or, more commonly, post-synaptic NMJ defects.
- >50% of mutations affect genes encoding AChR subunits.

Lambert–Eaton myasthenic syndrome

- Rare, autoimmune disorder.
- Antibodies are formed against presynaptic voltage-gated calcium channels impairing release of acetylcholine by the presynaptic terminal of the NMJ.
- Associated with underlying malignancy in 60% of cases, most commonly Small cell lung carcinoma (SCLC).
- Characterised by weakness, typically proximally, and fatigue.
- 75% of patients have disruption of autonomic nervous system function.
- Weakness is often relieved temporarily after exertion, e.g. improvement of power on repeated hand grip (Lambert's sign).
- If present, treatment of an underlying malignancy often relieves symptoms; other treatments used include steroids, azathioprine, IVIG, pyridostigmine and 3,4-diaminopyridine.

Tetanus

Tetanus toxin binds to peripheral nerve terminals, is taken up by endocytosis and transported within axons and across synaptic junctions until it reaches the CNS, where it becomes rapidly fixed to gangliosides at presynaptic inhibitory motor nerve endings. The toxin blocks the release of the inhibitory neurotransmitters glycine and GABA across the synaptic cleft. This results in generalised muscular spasms of jaw muscles (trismus), facial muscles (resulting in an appearance called risus sardonicus), and chest, neck, back and abdominal muscles, and buttocks; back muscle spasms often cause arching, called opisthotonus. Spasm of respiratory muscles may cause respiratory compromise. There may be autonomic dysfunction in severe cases with heart rate and BP lability, arrhythmia, fever, profuse sweating, peripheral vasoconstriction and ileus. Muscle rupture and rhabdomyolysis may complicate extreme cases.

Treatment is in a critical care setting to allow cardiorespiratory monitoring and mechanical ventilation, if required. Therapeutic paralysis with neuromuscular blocking agents is necessary in severe cases. Tetanus immunoglobulin should be administered. Even with treatment, the mortality rate is about 10% and is higher in unvaccinated people and people >60 years of age.

Botulism

Botulism is caused by the toxin produced by the bacterium *Clostridium botulinum*. The toxin inhibits acetylcholine release across synapses, leading to paralysis that typically starts with the muscles of the face and then spreads towards the limbs. In severe forms, botulism leads to paralysis of respiratory muscles, causing respiratory failure, necessitating critical care support. If patients survive the acute phase of illness, recovery is usually complete.

Neuropathy

Patterns and causes of peripheral neuropathy

Neuropathies may involve sensory and/or motor nerves with symptoms including:

- Sensory disturbance:
  - Lack of sensation (numbness).
  - Altered sensation, e.g. paraesthesiae.
  - Excess or inappropriate sensation, e.g. hyperalgesia or allodynia.
- Pain:
  - Large fibre damage causes shooting pains.
  - Small fibre neuropathies cause burning or stinging pain.
- Weakness:
  - Focal weakness, e.g. a foot drop in common peroneal nerve palsy.
  - More global weakness in peripheral neuropathies.

Neuropathies may appear focal initially but present in multiple locations later (multifocal neuropathy), or they may involve nerves in a generalised fashion. In the latter case, a 'length-dependent' pattern is classical, and causes a 'glove and stocking' distribution of sensory and/or motor loss. Autonomic disturbance may affect bladder, bowel and/or sexual function, as well as reduced sweating or tear production.

For causes of small fibre neuropathy, see Table 17.6 and for causes of motor neuropathy, see Table 17.7.

Table 17.6 Causes of small fibre (predominantly sensory) neuropathy

Category	Example
Idiopathic (~30%)	
Hereditary	Fabry's disease; hereditary sensory and autonomic neuropathies; familial amyloid.
Metabolic	Diabetes mellitus; hyperlipidaemia.
Toxic	Alcohol; metronidazole; highly active antiretroviral therapy (HAART).
Infective	HIV; leprosy; botulism.
Autoimmune	Associated with monoclonal gammopathy of unknown significance (MGUS), sarcoidosis, SLE, inflammatory bowel disease.

Table 17.7 Causes of motor neuropathy

Inherited	Acquired
Distal hereditary motor neuropathy	Motor neurone disease; ➲ see Motor neurone disease, p. 630.
Spinal muscular atrophy	Monomelic atrophy (Hirayama disease) and other idiopathic focal motor neurone disorders.
Bulbospinal muscular atrophies	Acute motor axonal neuropathy.
Tay–Sachs disease (hexosaminidase A deficiency)	Multifocal motor neuropathy with conduction block.
	Paraneoplastic motor neuropathy.
	Brachial amyotrophy.
	Metabolic causes including diabetic mellitus and porphyria.
	Infective causes including poliomyelitis, West Nile virus and Central European encephalitis.
	Toxins including lead and dapsone.
	Compressive neuropathies, e.g. median nerve (carpal tunnel syndrome), common peroneal nerve.

Inflammatory neuropathies

Acute inflammatory demyelinating polyneuropathy (Guillain–Barré syndrome)

- Incidence 1–2/100,000 (most common cause of acute neuromuscular weakness in the developed world).
- Usually a monophasic illness.
- May be triggered by infection:
  - Most commonly identified agent is *Campylobacter jejuni*.
  - Other bacteria (e.g. mycoplasma pneumonia, haemophilus influenza) and viruses (e.g. CMV, HIV) are implicated.

    - Immune responses to ganglioside-like epitopes on the surface of triggering infectious agents cross-react with gangliosides displayed on nerve cells, resulting in macrophage-mediated attack of either the Schwann cell or the axolemma.
- Classical history is of a preceding infectious illness followed by onset of distal sensory loss 1–2 weeks later.
- Sensory loss may progress and spread proximally.
- Motor involvement may occur.
- Deep tendon jerks are typically lost.
- Cranial nerve involvement may occur with severe demyelination.
- Severe axonal damage may result with patients requiring ventilatory support, inotropic support (when there is autonomic instability) and tube feeding (as swallowing is often impaired).
- Diagnosis is made clinically but a raised CSF protein and abnormal NCS (e.g. slowed conduction velocities with prolonged F-wave and distal latencies) are supportive.
- Anti-GM2 ganglioside antibodies may follow CMV infection and are associated with a predominantly sensory neuropathy.
- IgG anti-GM1 ganglioside antibodies, axonal involvement and advanced age are poor prognostic indicators.
- Specific treatment options include IVIG and plasma exchange.

Guillain–Barré syndrome variants

- Miller–Fisher syndrome
    - Triad of ataxia, areflexia and ophthalmoplegia causing a proximal/descending pattern of nerve involvement.
    - IgG anti-GQ1b ganglioside antibodies are found in 90–95% of patients.
- Axonal variants:
    - Acute motor axonal neuropathy.
        - Associated with anti-GD1a and anti-GalNAcGD1a ganglioside antibodies.
    - Acute motor and sensory axonal neuropathy.

Chronic inflammatory demyelinating polyneuropathy

- Relapsing and remitting nerve dysfunction causing sensorimotor disturbance.
- No clear infectious triggers.
- Less severe than Guillain–Barré syndrome.
- Autonomic dysfunction is unusual.
- Diagnosis requires evidence (from NCS) of demyelination in at least two nerves.
- CSF protein level may be high.
- Nerve roots may be enlarged or enhance with gadolinium on MRI.

Chronic inflammatory demyelinating polyneuropathy (CIDP) variants include:

- Multi-focal motor neuropathy with conduction block:
    - affects men > women;
    - associated with anti-GM1 ganglioside antibodies.
- Multi-focal acquired demyelinating sensory and motor neuropathy (Lewis–Sumner syndrome).
- Sensory ataxic CIDP.
- Distal acquired demyelinating sensory neuropathy.
- Chronic relapsing axonal neuropathy.

CIDP treatment options include:

- steroids (if not motor predominant);
- IVIG;
- cyclophosphamide;
- plasma exchange.

Investigations

- NCS:
  - Helpful in delineating the type of nerve damage, e.g. demyelinating or axonal.
- EMG:
  - Useful in motor neuropathy as muscle will demonstrate changes secondary to denervation or conduction block.
- Nerve biopsy:
  - Reserved for when other diagnostic options have failed.
  - Usually from a sensory nerve identifiably and recently affected (using neurophysiology) or from a nerve that will not cause major disability when damaged, such as the sural nerve.
- Imaging:
  - To identify focal nerve damage, particularly in sites less amenable to neurophysiology or biopsy, such as the brachial plexus.

Neurogenetic diseases

Neurogenetic disorders often have a family history, but may occur in the absence of a family history due to:

- anticipation;
- new mutations;
- incomplete penetrance;
- non-paternity;
- autosomal recessive inheritance;
- heteroplasmy (presence of >1 type of organellar genome [e.g. mitochondrial DNA] within a cell or individual);
- failure to recognise the condition in other family members.

Diagnostic genetic testing should only be undertaken after careful counselling about the possible implications of a positive test. It is best to establish which family members would want to know about the result before it is available. Presymptomatic testing is typically performed only after consultation with a geneticist (➲ see Chapter 2, Box 2.2, and Chapter 25, Screening, p. 844, Boxes 25.3, 25.4 and 25.5 and Figures 25.1 and 25.2).

Ataxias

- Early-onset ataxias (<20 years old) are generally autosomal recessive.
  - Friedreich's ataxia:
    - Trinucleotide repeat expansion in Frataxin gene (➲ see Trinucleotide repeat disorders, p. 49 and Table 2.4).
    - Ataxia with axonal neuropathy, pes cavus and cardiac abnormalities.
  - Ataxia telangiectasia:
    - Ataxia with cutaneous and ocular telangiectasia and immunodeficiency.
- Late onset ataxias (>20 years old) are generally autosomal dominant spinocerebellar ataxias classified as:
  - Autosomal dominant cerebellar ataxia type I (ADCA 1):
    - Ataxia with complex neurological features, e.g. pyramidal and/or extrapyramidal features, cognitive impairment, neuropathy.
    - Includes SCA types 1, 2, 3, 12 and 17 (polyglutamine diseases characterised by trinucleotide repeats with a disease-associated protein [e.g. ataxin-1 in SCA1; ataxin-3 in SCA3] containing a large number [usually >35] of repeats of glutamine residues [➲ see Autosomal dominant disorders, p. 47 and Table 2.4]).
  - ADCA type II:
    - Ataxia with retinopathy.
    - Includes SCA type 7.
  - ADCA type III:
    - Pure ataxia (sometimes with mild pyramidal features).
    - Includes SCA type 6.

Neuropathies

- Charcot–Marie–Tooth (CMT) disease (hereditary motor and sensory neuropathy) is mostly autosomal dominant with a prevalence of 1 in 2500. It causes mixed motor and sensory neuropathy, typically with deformities such as pes cavus, and management focuses on foot care, orthotics and genetic counselling. It is classified as:
  - CMT 1 – demyelinating:
    - Slow conduction on NCS.
    - Most commonly due to a duplication of the *PMP22* gene on chromosome 17 (CMT 1a); other genes include *MPZ* and *EGR2*.
  - CMT 2 – axonal:
    - Reduced amplitudes on NCS.
    - Most commonly due to mitofusin 2 mutations.
  - CMT X:
    - X-linked mutation in the connexin 32 gene.
    - Affects males more than females.
    - Can be axonal or demyelinating.
- Hereditary neuropathy with liability to pressure palsies (HNPP):
  - Due to a deletion of the *PMP22* gene.
  - Causes frequent pressure palsies (e.g. common peroneal, median and ulnar nerves) with a background CMT-like neuropathy.
- Pure hereditary sensory neuropathies (HSN), motor neuropathies (HMN) and sensory-autonomic neuropathies (HSAN).

Muscular dystrophies

➲ See Muscular dystrophies, p. 627.

Mitochondrial disorders

- Usually maternally inherited due to mitochondrial DNA mutations, but can be autosomal recessive or dominant due to nuclear DNA contributions to mitochondrial function.
- Often show heteroplasmy with variable phenotype due to uneven distribution of abnormal mitochondria between cells.
- Key investigations include:
  - Serum CK and lactate.
  - Mitochondrial DNA analysis.
  - MRI brain.
  - EMG.
  - Muscle biopsy: shows cyclo-oxygenase-negative muscle fibres and 'ragged red fibres' (muscle fibres with clumps of diseased mitochondria accumulating in the subsarcolemmal region on modified Gömöri trichrome staining).
  - Enzyme analysis of muscle tissue for respiratory chain defects.
- Cause a wide-range of neurological syndromes, classically with sensorineural deafness and myopathy. Recognised syndromes include:
  - Mitochondrial encephalomyopathy with lactic acidosis and stroke-like episodes (MELAS).
  - Myoclonus epilepsy with ragged red fibres (MERRF).
  - Chronic progressive external ophthalmoplegia (CPEO).
  - Kearns–Sayre syndrome with ophthalmoplegia, pigmentary retinopathy, ataxia and cardiac arrhythmia.
  - Leber's hereditary optic neuropathy.

Neurocutaneous syndromes

Disorders characterised by multiple hamartomas of the central and peripheral nervous system, eye, skin, and viscera (➔ see Chapter 5, Case 13, p. 136).

- Neurofibromatosis type 1 (affects 1:3000):
  - Autosomal dominant inheritance.
  - NF1 gene on chromosome 17.
  - Diagnostic criteria based on the presence of ≥2 of:
    - ≥6 café-au-lait spots (diameter >5 mm in pre- and >15 mm in post-pubertal individuals).
    - ≥2 neurofibromas of any type or ≥1 plexiform neurofibroma.
    - Freckling in the axilla or inguinal regions.
    - ≥2 Lisch nodules (pigmented hamartomatous nodular aggregates of dendritic melanocytes) of the iris (occur in ~95% of cases).
    - Optic glioma.
    - A distinctive bony lesion, e.g. dysplasia of sphenoid bone or thinning of long bone cortex.
    - A first-degree relative with NF type 1.
- Neurofibromatosis type 2 (affects 1:40,000):
  - Autosomal dominant inheritance.
  - *NF2* gene on chromosome 22.
  - Diagnostic criteria are met by an individual who has bilateral acoustic neuromas or a first-degree relative with NF type 2 and either unilateral acoustic neuroma or two of the following:
    - neurofibroma;
    - meningioma;
    - glioma;
    - schwannoma;
    - juvenile posterior subcapsular lenticular opacity.
- Tuberous sclerosis (affects 1:10,000):
  - Autosomal dominant inheritance.
  - Associated with:
    - Cognitive impairment.
    - Epilepsy.
    - Adenoma sebaceum (cutaneous hamartomas) around the nose and cheeks.
    - Shagreen patches (areas of pigmented thick leathery skin, usually on the lower back or nape of the neck or scattered across the trunk or thighs).
    - Ash-leaf spots (hypomelanic macules).
    - Subungual harmatomas.
    - Subependymal nodules (SENs) and subependymal giant cell astrocytomas (SEGAs).
    - Retinal astrocytomas.
    - Visceral hamartomas, e.g. renal angiomyolipoma (➔ see Chapter 16, Tuberous sclerosis, p. 581).
- Von Hippel–Lindau disease (affects 1:32,000):
  - Autosomal dominant inheritance, but 20% of cases are due to de novo mutations.
  - Mutation in the von Hippel–Lindau tumour suppressor gene on chromosome 3.
  - Characterised by retinal and CNS haemangioblastomas, phaeochromocytomas, multiple cysts in the pancreas and kidneys, and an increased risk of malignant transformation of renal cysts into renal cell carcinoma.

Dementia and movement disorders

- Early-onset Alzheimer's disease (➔ see Chapter 22, Dementias, p. 791 and Table 22.7).
- Frontotemporal dementia:
  - Familial in up to 30% of cases, mostly with the behavioural variant.

- Genetic variants include:
  - Tau-positive FTD with Parkinsonism caused by mutations in the *MAPT* gene on chromosome 17.
  - Frontotemporal lobar degeneration with TAR DNA binding protein 43 (TDP43)-positive inclusions (FTLD-TDP) due to a:
    - Mutation in the *GRN* (granulin) gene on chromosome 17;
    - Mutation in the *VCP* (valosin-containing protein) gene on chromosome 9 with patients presenting with a complex picture of multisystem proteinopathy that can include ALS, inclusion body myopathy, Paget's disease of bone and FTD;
    - Hexanucleotide repeat expansion in intron 1 of C9ORF72 as the cause of chromosome 9p21 ALS-FTD.
- Familial cases of Parkinson's disease can be caused by mutations in the *LRRK2, PARK2, PARK7, PINK1* or *SNCA* genes.
- Huntington's chorea (➲ see Huntington's chorea, p. 621).

Neurological complications of systemic disease

Cardiovascular disease

- Embolic stroke (➲ see Stroke, p. 604, Figures 17.2, 17.3 and Table 17.1).
  - Cardioembolism from arrhythmia (e.g. atrial fibrillation), cardiomyopathy, valve disease, structural heart disease (e.g. patent foramen ovale, atrial myxoma) or cardiac surgery.
  - Embolism from disease of the aorta and/or carotid and vertebral arteries.
- Spinal cord ischaemia resulting from embolism or aortic dissection or surgery (➲ see Spinal cord, p. 600 and Figure 17.1).
- Post-cardiac surgery delirium.
- Hypoxic-ischaemic brain injury after cardiac arrest:
  - Early brain CT findings include diffuse swelling with effacement of the basal cisterns, ventricles and sulci, attenuation of the gray–white matter interface, hypodensity of the cortical grey matter and basal ganglia, and focal areas of infarction in watershed areas.
  - Brain MRI findings include widespread hyperintensity initially involving the basal ganglia, followed by the cortex and subcortical white matter, cerebellum and hippocampus.
  - Generalised electrical or burst suppression and post-anoxic status epilepticus EEG patterns carry a poor prognosis.

Gastrointestinal disease

- Encephalopathy in severe hepatic failure, due to the accumulation of toxins including ammonia and amino acids, characterised by fluctuating delirium, asterixis and apraxia, and stupor and coma in severe cases.
- Non-Wilsonian hepatolenticular degeneration, characterised by Parkinsonism, dystonia and cognitive decline, in cases of chronic liver disease with manganese deposition in the basal ganglia.
- Neurological manifestations of malabsorption syndromes (e.g. coeliac disease) and/or deficiencies of vitamins or trace elements (e.g. vitamins B1, B_{12}, D and E and copper) that may include neuropathy, myelopathy, encephalopathy and ataxia.

Haematological disease

- Anaemia may cause non-specific symptoms including fatigue and (pre)syncope, but may be an important indicator of underlying aetiologies that have neurological sequelae (e.g. vitamin B12 deficiency, sickle cell disease).
- Leukaemias may cause a range of neurological features related to direct infiltration, cerebral haemorrhage due to thrombocytopenia, infections due to impaired immunity, and hyperviscosity.

- Plasma cell dyscrasias are associated with spinal cord compression due to vertebral myeloma, cranial neuropathies due to meningeal infiltration, and demyelinating peripheral neuropathies.
- Coagulation disorders may cause both arterial stroke (e.g. APLS) and venous sinus thrombosis (e.g. factor V Leiden, protein C/S deficiencies).
- Bleeding disorders such as haemophilia and disseminated intravascular coagulation can lead to haemorrhagic stroke.
- Thrombotic thrombocytopenic purpura causes neurological symptoms in many patients, including fluctuating consciousness, seizures, encephalopathy, and both ischaemic and haemorrhagic strokes.

Endocrine disease

- Hyperthyroidism causes tremor, myopathy, upper motor neurone features, agitation, fever and (rarely) encephalopathy.
- Hypothyroidism has neurological complications including lethargy, impaired attention and myxoedema coma, as well as ataxia, myopathy and polyneuropathy.
- Diabetes mellitus is an important cause of peripheral neuropathy and diabetic amyotrophy.
- Acute dysglycaemia (<2.7 mmol/L or >22.2 mmol/L) can cause transient focal neurological symptoms that can mimic TIA/stroke and a depressed level of responsiveness.
- Pituitary tumours may present with headache and visual disturbance (especially bitemporal hemianopia) and, in the case of pituitary apoplexy, with thunderclap headache and sudden bilateral visual loss.

Renal disease

- Uraemia may cause encephalopathy acutely, characterised by irritability, confusion, disorientation, asterixis, myoclonus, seizures and coma, and a distal predominantly sensory neuropathy chronically, that may be reversible when the uraemia is corrected.
- Dialysis may cause encephalopathy both acutely, due to haemodynamic and osmotic shifts (dialysis disequilibrium syndrome), or chronically due to the aluminium content of the dialysate.

Electrolyte disturbance

- Hyponatraemia can cause encephalopathy, seizures and coma. When hyponatraemia is corrected too rapidly, central pontine myelinolysis may occur with demyelination, primarily in the central pons and midbrain, with pseudobulbar palsy, quadriparesis, oculomotor abnormalities and occasionally locked-in syndrome (characterised by quadriplegia and anarthria while consciousness, cognition and vertical eye movement are preserved). Prognosis is variable, but some patients recover well despite severe clinical and radiological involvement.
- Hypo- and hyperkalaemia can both cause severe muscle weakness, either primarily or as part of a periodic paralysis syndrome.
- Hypocalcaemia causes paraesthesiae, tetany and seizures.
- Hypomagnesaemia is an important cause of eclamptic seizures.

Immunosuppression

- Acute infection with HIV may cause meningitis, meningoencephalitis or Guillain–Barré syndrome.
- Chronic HIV infection may be complicated by distal polyneuropathy, CIDP, myelopathy and/or dementia.
- Complications of immunosuppressive drugs include tremor, encephalopathy, seizures, neuromuscular disorders, visual disturbance and CNS malignancy.
- Graft versus host disease can cause myasthenia, neuropathy and myositis.

Toxic insults to the nervous system

For neurological side effects of prescribed medicines, see Table 17.8.

Table 17.8 Neurological side ffects of prescribed medications

Neurological symptom	Implicated medication
Encephalopathy	Valproate, lithium, neuroleptics, tricyclic antidepressants, opiates, anticholinergics, histamine receptor antagonists, benzodiazepines.
Memory disturbance	Chemotherapy agents, antiepileptics (especially topiramate), anticholinergics, antidepressants, corticosteroids.
Confusional state	Barbiturates, benzodiazepines, anti-Parkinsonian agents, antidepressants, corticosteroids, abrupt withdrawal of drugs.
Movement disorder (including acute dystonia, Parkinsonism and tardive dyskinesia)	Metoclopramide, neuroleptics, tricyclic antidepressants, selective serotonin reuptake inhibitors.
Tremor	Lithium, antiepileptics (especially valproate), immunosuppressants, sympathomimetics, levodopa.
Seizure	Antipsychotics, lithium, antimicrobial agents, theophylline, aminophylline, caffeine, cocaine, lidocaine, methylphenidate, chemotherapy agents, opiates.
Impairment of neuromuscular transmission	Antibiotics (especially aminoglycosides), quinidine, chloroquine, penicillamine, β-blockers, phenytoin, neuroleptics, muscle relaxants.
Neuropathy	Antibiotics (especially metronidazole; nitrofurantoin; isoniazid), chemotherapy agents (especially cisplatin; vinca alkaloids), statins, amiodarone, hydralazine, gold, chloroquine, colchicine, allopurinol, tacrolimus, ciclosporin, antiretrovirals.
Myopathy	Statins, amiodarone, corticosteroids, zidovudine, chloroquine.

Ethanol

- Acute intoxication is associated with stupor, coma, psychosis, amnesia and cerebellar dysfunction.
- Chronic abuse causes:
  - ataxia;
  - dementia;
  - neuropathy;
  - myopathy;
  - Wernicke–Korsakoff syndrome (with apathy, confusion, amnesia, ataxia and ophthalmoplegia) in the presence of thiamine deficiency:
    - if untreated, Wernicke's encephalopathy progresses to Korsakoff's syndrome with dense anterograde amnesia.
- Withdrawal of alcohol causes delirium tremens, with fluctuating confusion, hallucinations, psychosis, tremor and seizures (➲ see Chapter 22, Misuse of alcohol and other substances in relation to psychiatry, p. 794 and Table 22.8).
- Contaminants in alcohol may be extremely toxic, e.g. methanol (causing optic neuropathy and cerebral oedema) and ethylene glycol (causing seizures and cranial neuropathies).

Recreational drugs

➲ See Chapter 3, Recreational drugs, p. 92 and Table 3.20.

Environmental toxins

- Heavy metals, e.g. lead, arsenic, mercury:
  - May cause seizures, psychosis, cognitive impairment and encephalopathy.

- Lead intoxication also causes a motor neuropathy.
- Organophosphates (found in pesticides):
  - Exert cholinergic effects due to inhibition of acetylcholinesterase that include mydriasis, confusion and ataxia.
  - Chronic exposure may cause neuropathy, ataxia and quadriparesis.
- Carbon monoxide:
  - May lead to headaches, dizziness and confusion at low concentrations.
  - May result in seizures, coma and hypoxic brain injury at higher levels.
  - May cause a chronic encephalopathy with dystonia due to basal ganglia necrosis.

Ethical and legal principles in neurology

Capacity and deprivation of liberty

Loss of capacity is frequently encountered in neurology and can be impaired at any of the four stages: understanding information (e.g. in receptive dysphasia), retaining information (e.g. with impairments of memory or attention), weighing the information (e.g. with executive dysfunction) or communicating a decision (e.g. with expressive dysphasia). Capacity should be carefully assessed for each decision independently, taking into account cognitive and neuropsychological assessments (➲ see Chapter 22, Mental Capacity Act and Mental Health Act, p. 795 and Table 22.9, and Chapter 27, Capacity, p. 882).

When a patient lacks capacity, decisions should be made by their clinicians in their best interests (taking into account consultees' representation of their wishes), unless the patient has a Lasting Power of Attorney (LPA) for health and welfare decisions. If there is no appointed LPA, and no family or friends available to act as consultees, an independent mental capacity advocate (IMCA) should be appointed. When a patient lacks capacity to choose whether to remain in hospital or another care facility, Deprivation of Liberty Safeguards apply under the Mental Capacity Act 2005 (➲ see Chapter 27, Autonomy, p. 883).

Driving

Discussions about driving should be an important part of many neurological consultations (Table 17.9). If patients drive despite advice to the contrary and do not inform the Driver and Vehicle Licensing Agency

Table 17.9 Driving regulations for persons with neurological disorders

Diagnosis	DVLA patient recommendations for car and motorcycle licenses
Epilepsy or multiple unprovoked seizures	Must stop driving and inform DVLA. Review license issued. May normally drive after 12 months seizure-free (including auras and myoclonic jerks).
Withdrawal of epilepsy medication	Must not drive during withdrawal and for 6 months after last dose.
First unprovoked seizure	Must inform DVLA. Driving prohibited for 6 months.
Provoked seizure	Must inform DVLA. Decision about safety to drive depends on the cause.
Syncope	May drive if typical vasovagal syncope with prodrome occurring only while standing; otherwise DVLA must be informed.
Chronic disorders, e.g. MS, MND, Parkinson's disease	Must inform DVLA. Review license may be issued.
Stroke/TIA	Must not drive for 1 month. Must inform DVLA if there are residual symptoms at 1 month, especially visual, cognitive or impaired limb function. In case of multiple TIAs, must inform DVLA and not drive for 3 months.

(DVLA) of their neurological condition, a doctor has a duty to breach confidentiality to disclose any relevant medical information (➲ see Chapter 27, Disclosure in relation to fitness to drive, p. 885 and Box 27.1).

Further reading

1. DVLA. Neurological disorders: assessing fitness to drive. 2016. https://www.gov.uk/guidance/neurological-disorders-assessing-fitness-to-drive.
2. Brainstem death (➲ see Chapter 12, Brainstem death, p. 405).

Multiple choice questions

Questions

1. A 66-year-old hypertensive, diabetic man presents to A&E with sudden development of right-sided weakness. On examination, he has weakness of the right arm and leg, with weakness and sensory loss in the left side of the face, left-sided ataxia and a Horner's syndrome. Which vascular territory is likely to be involved?
   A. Anterior inferior cerebellar artery.
   B. Middle cerebral artery.
   C. Anterior cerebral artery.
   D. Posterior cerebral artery.
   E. Posterior inferior cerebellar artery.
2. A 40-year-old woman presents with leg weakness, urinary frequency and dysaesthesia, developing over 72 hours. On examination, she has 3/5 weakness in her legs, with brisk reflexes, upgoing plantars and a sensory level at T8. MRI of her spinal cord shows inflammatory change extending through most of the thoracic cord. Which investigation is most likely to be diagnostic?
   A. CSF oligoclonal bands.
   B. Aquaporin 4 antibodies.
   C. MRI brain.
   D. Visual-evoked potentials.
   E. Serum B12.
3. An 18-year-old woman has had several episodes where she has lost consciousness. Which of the following would be least compatible with a diagnosis of vasovagal syncope?
   A. Occurring only while standing.
   B. Jerks while unconscious.
   C. Prodromal symptoms.
   D. Tongue-biting.
   E. Feeling unsettled afterwards.
4. A 42-year-old man presents with numbness and weakness in his legs, developing gradually over the previous 48 hours. He has no past medical history, except for a recent episode of gastroenteritis. On examination, he has grade 3/5 weakness at the hips and knees, and grade 2/5 at the ankles. He is areflexic in both arms and legs, with sensory loss up to the waist. Which of the following is most likely to confirm the diagnosis?
   A. Nerve conduction studies.
   B. MRI lumbar spine.
   C. EMG.
   D. Acetylcholine receptor antibodies.
   E. Ganglioside antibodies.

5. A 68-year-old woman has a 6-month history of deteriorating speech difficulty, with occasional coughing while eating. On examination, she is dysphonic, with stiff, slow tongue movements, a brisk jaw jerk, and some wasting of the dorsal interossei in her hands. Which of the following is the most likely diagnosis?
   A. Progressive non-fluent aphasia.
   B. Myasthenia gravis.
   C. Syringobulbia.
   D. Posterior fossa tumour.
   E. Motor neurone disease.

6. A 75-year-old woman with Parkinson's disease has responded very well to levopdopa/carbidopa 250 mg TDS, but has recently been finding that the effect wears off 1 hour before the next dose is due. Which is the most appropriate change to her treatment?
   A. No change.
   B. Add pramipexole.
   C. Increase dose of levodopa.
   D. Add entacapone.
   E. Add apomorphine.

7. A 20-year-old woman comes to clinic complaining that she has the same bad feet as the rest of her family. On examination, she has pes cavus, with distal sensory loss. Nerve conduction studies show slowing of conduction velocities. Which investigation is most likely to be diagnostic?
   A. Nerve biopsy.
   B. Oral glucose tolerance test.
   C. Testing for duplication of *PMP22* gene.
   D. Serum B12.
   E. Testing for mutation in mitofusin 2 gene.

8. A 30-year-old man with juvenile myoclonic epilepsy (JME) has been seizure-free on valproate since age 22. He tells you in clinic that he stopped taking his valproate just over a year ago, and has remained seizure-free in this time, but has noticed occasional jerks in the mornings. What is the correct advice to give him about driving?
   A. He has been seizure-free for over a year so he does not need to do anything.
   B. He must inform the DVLA that he stopped his medication, but can continue to drive.
   C. He must inform the DVLA about his jerks and stop driving until he has not had any for a year.
   D. He must stop driving for 6 months while his medication is restarted.
   E. He can continue to drive as long as he avoids sleep-deprivation.

9. A 28-year-old man presents with recurrent headaches. He describes episodes of severe pain localised around the right eye, lasting for up to an hour at a time, and associated with watering of the eye and stuffiness of his nose. Which of the following is most appropriate as a prophylactic therapy?
   A. Oxygen.
   B. Sumatriptan.
   C. Amitriptyline.
   D. Verapamil.
   E. Propranolol.

10. A man in his seventies has noticed difficulty climbing the stairs and hand weakness over the last year. On examination he has wasting of his quadriceps and forearm muscles, with normal reflexes and sensation. His CK is mildly elevated. What is the most likely diagnosis?
   A. Peripheral neuropathy.
   B. Inclusion body myositis.
   C. Cervical myelopathy.
   D. Limb girdle muscular dystrophy.
   E. Amyotrophic lateral sclerosis (ALS).

Answers

1. E. The description is of the lateral medullary syndrome of Wallenberg. It is caused by a stroke in the territory of the PICA (➲ see Lateral medullary (Wallenberg's or posterior inferior cerebellar artery) syndrome, p. 600).
2. B. Longitudinally extensive myelitis is highly unusual in multiple sclerosis, and suggests a diagnosis of neuromyelitis optica, which is caused by antibodies to aquaporin-4 in a majority of cases (➲ see Neuromyelitis optica [Devic's disease], p. 613).
3. D. Tongue-biting would be a red flag for epilepsy. Jerks are common during vasovagal syncope and can be quite dramatic. Most people with vasovagal syncope describe taking a while to return to feeling normal afterwards, but without significant somnolence or confusion, as are seen in postictal states (➲ see Epilepsy, p. 608).
4. A. The diagnosis is likely to be Guillain–Barré syndrome . Nerve conduction studies would be expected to show conduction slowing with prolonged F-wave latencies and possibly conduction block. Occasionally, they are normal early in the course of the illness, in which case they should be repeated for diagnostic confirmation. Ganglioside antibodies are sometimes found in Guillain–Barré syndrome, but are not a particularly valuable diagnostic test. Neuroimaging may exclude a spinal cord syndrome (in which areflexia may be found acutely), but are unlikely to reveal a diagnosis. Areflexia in the arms effectively rules out a cauda equina syndrome (➲ see Acute inflammatory demyelinating polyneuropathy (Guillain–Barré syndrome), p. 633).
5. E. A neurodegenerative disorder is likely given her age and slow progression over 6 months. The presence of upper and lower motor neurone features makes motor neurone disease the most likely diagnosis (➲ see Motor neurone disease, p. 630).
6. D. Entacapone is a COMT inhibitor, which potentiates the action of levodopa, and is therefore particularly useful for 'wearing-off'. Increasing levodopa or adding a dopamine agonist, such as pramipexole would be useful if she has an inadequate response to her levodopa dose, although the latter should be used with caution in older patients. Apomorphine is given by SC infusion in patients with severe motor fluctuations (➲ see Parkinson's disease, Management, p. 618).
7. C. The clinical and investigative features are consistent with Charcot–Marie–Tooth 1 disease in which duplication of the *PMP22* gene may be diagnostic (➲ see Neuropathies, p. 636).
8. C. Restarting valproate would be likely to stop the jerks, and prevent further seizures (of which he is at high risk). See Table 17.9 delineating the driving regulations for persons with neurological disorders, including epilepsy.
9. D. The history is suggestive of cluster headache for which verapamil is a prophylactic therapy (➲ see Cluster headache, p. 622).
10. B. Inclusion body myositis typically occurs in the seventh and eighth decades, and causes insidious development of muscle weakness, especially in the forearms and quadriceps (see Table 20.6). A peripheral neuropathy is unlikely with normal reflexes and no sensory signs (➲ see Neuropathy, p. 632). Cervical myelopathy causes upper motor neurone features. Limb girdle muscular dystrophy presents earlier in life with proximal weakness (➲ see Muscular dystrophies, p. 627). A pure lower motor neurone disease is a possible differential diagnosis, but ALS requires the presence of upper motor neurone features (➲ see Motor neurone disease, p. 630).

Chapter 18 **Ophthalmology**

Anupam Chatterjee and David Bessant

Ocular anatomy

For basic ocular anatomy, see Figure 18.1.

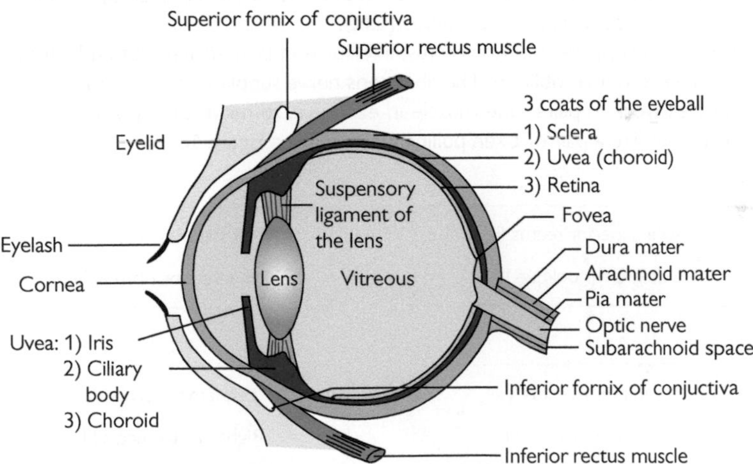

Figure 18.1 Diagram of basic ocular anatomy.

Reproduced with permission from Ophthalmology. In *Oxford Handbook of Clinical Specialties*, Tenth Edition, Baldwin A. et al. (Eds.). Oxford, UK: OUP. Copyright © 2016 Oxford University Press. DOI: 10.1093/med/9780198719021.001.0001. Reproduced with permission of the Licensor through PLSclear.

The eye is one of the most complex organs in the body, so appreciating its anatomy is important in understanding the diseases that affect it. The most important structures are:

- Eyelids: keep moisture inside and foreign objects out of the eye.

- Cornea: transparent layer at the front of the eye, which must be clear and regular in shape to give good vision and is continuous with the sclera posteriorly.
- Conjunctiva: layer of clear tissue covering the sclera. When it gets inflamed it becomes red.
- Sclera: dense, fibrous tissue that forms the white, outermost layer of the eye and is continuous with the cornea.
- Uveal tract: a vascular layer within the sclera that comprises of three parts, the iris, the ciliary body and the choroid. Inflammation of this layer is referred to as uveitis.
- Lens: normally clear and transparent. In conjunction with the cornea it focuses images onto the retina. The lens is held in position by the suspensory ligament (the zonular fibres) that passes to the ciliary body.
- Vitreous: transparent gel that fills the cavity between the lens and the retina. It adheres to the retina and can tear the retina if it detaches, sometimes leading to retinal detachment.
- Retina: light-sensitive tissue which contains photoreceptor cells (rods and cones) and ganglion cells, whose axons project via the optic nerve to the lateral geniculate body. The neural retina is supported by the retinal pigment epithelium, which contains numerous melanin granules to absorb light and prevent reflection. If this layer is damaged melanin may be released resulting in pigmented retinal lesions (e.g. retinitis pigmentosa, chorioretinitis).

Eye movements

Most adults with eye movement disorders of recent onset have significant eye muscle, nerve or brain pathology. A longstanding eye movement disorder may be due to a childhood squint.

Causes include:

- Palsies of the ocular motor nerves.
- Thyroid eye disease.
- Myasthenia gravis.
- Complex eye movement problems from brainstem disease.

Six extraocular muscles are involved in eye movements and they are innervated by the IIIrd (oculomotor), IVth (trochlear) and VIth (abducens) cranial nerves (CN).

The oculomotor nerve supplies superior rectus, inferior rectus, medial rectus and inferior oblique. The trochlear nerve supplies superior oblique. The abducens nerve supplies lateral rectus.

Extraocular muscles work in pairs, one muscle in each eye, to move the eyes in a particular direction. They are yoked together like a pair of oxen pulling a plough (see Figure 18.2).

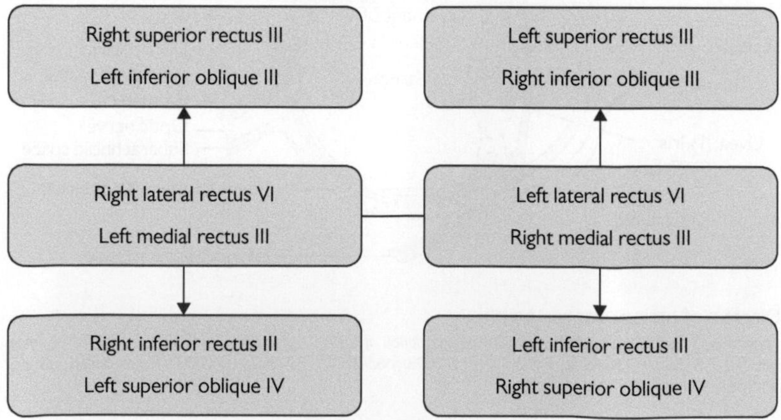

Figure 18.2 Cardinal positions of gaze, muscles involved and cranial nerves supplying them. Patient's eye movements are displayed from the doctor's perspective (i.e. patient's right eye is on the left side).

Palsies of the ocular motor nerves

Oculomotor (IIIrd) nerve palsy

- A complete IIIrd CN palsy causes the eye to deviate laterally (exotropia) and downwards, adopting a 'down and out' position, and resulting in horizontal ± vertical diplopia. An ipsilateral ptosis will occur due to concomitant denervation of the levator palpebrae superioris muscle.
- Partial IIIrd nerve palsies can mimic other types of strabismus and be difficult to diagnose.
- It is important to note that parasympathetic fibres controlling pupil constriction run along the outside of the IIIrd nerve. Hence, external compression of the IIIrd nerve may lead to pupillary dilation (e.g. due to a posterior communicating artery aneurysm).

For causes of CN III palsy, see Table 18.1.

Table 18.1 Causes of CN III palsy

Aetiology	Examples
Vascular, pupil sparing	Microvascular infarction. Giant cell arteritis.
Compressive (may involve pupil)	Posterior communicating artery aneurysm. Internal carotid artery aneurysm. Meningioma, parasellar tumour.
Brainstem infarction	Weber's, Benedikt's syndrome (➲ see Chapter 17, Brainstem syndromes, p. 600).
Brainstem demyelination	Multiple sclerosis.
Trauma	
Congenital	

Other lesions may mimic a IIIrd nerve palsy: myasthenia gravis, orbital mass/inflammation (e.g. GPA).

Trochlear (IVth) nerve palsy

- The superior oblique muscle is supplied by the IVth CN, which intorts (rotates inwards) and depresses the eye (primarily in the adducted position).
- A IVth CN palsy therefore presents as vertical diplopia that is worse on down-gaze.
- To compensate for this, patients tilt their head away from the affected side and lower their chin.
- Late presentation of congenital IVth nerve palsies is common.
- Head trauma may result in unilateral or bilateral superior oblique nerve palsies.
- Other causes: compression, ischaemia, inflammation.

Abducens (VIth) nerve palsy

- The VIth CN supplies the lateral rectus muscle, which abducts the eye.
- A VIth CN palsy results in horizontal diplopia that worsens both, while looking towards the affected side and in the distance (the eyes diverge for distance and converge for near vision).
- The affected eye is deviated inwards (esotropia) with limitation of abduction.
- Ischaemia (e.g. due to diabetes, hypertension, temporal arteritis) is the commonest cause.
- Other causes: compression, inflammation, trauma.
- Raised intracranial pressure can result in downward displacement of the brainstem, causing stretching of the VIth nerve and unilateral or bilateral VIth nerve palsy (a false localising sign).

Other ocular motility disorders

Nystagmus

Nystagmus describes an involuntary movement of the eyes away from fixation followed immediately by either: a fast (jerk nystagmus) or slow (pendular nystagmus) counter movement.

- It may be congenital or acquired. Acquired nystagmus is most often caused by abnormalities of vestibular input. Congenital nystagmus may be due to poor visual acuity (sensory nystagmus).
- Nystagmus is also classified according to its direction of movement, e.g. downbeat, upbeat.
- Causes of acquired nystagmus include: lesions of the brainstem, Arnold–Chiari malformation.

Internuclear ophthalmoplegia

Internuclear ophthalmoplegia is caused by a disorder of the medial longitudinal fasciculus (MLF), which permits conjugate eye movement by connecting the contralateral paramedian pontine reticular formation (PPRF)-abducens nucleus complex to the ipsilateral IIIrd nerve. If the right MLF is affected, the right eye will be unable to adduct completely when the patient looks to the left side. The left eye that is abducted will also experience simultaneous horizontal jerk nystagmus. Abduction of the right eye will be entirely normal. Causes include demyelination, vascular disease, trauma and brainstem tumours. Control of horizontal eye movements is shown in Figure 18.3.

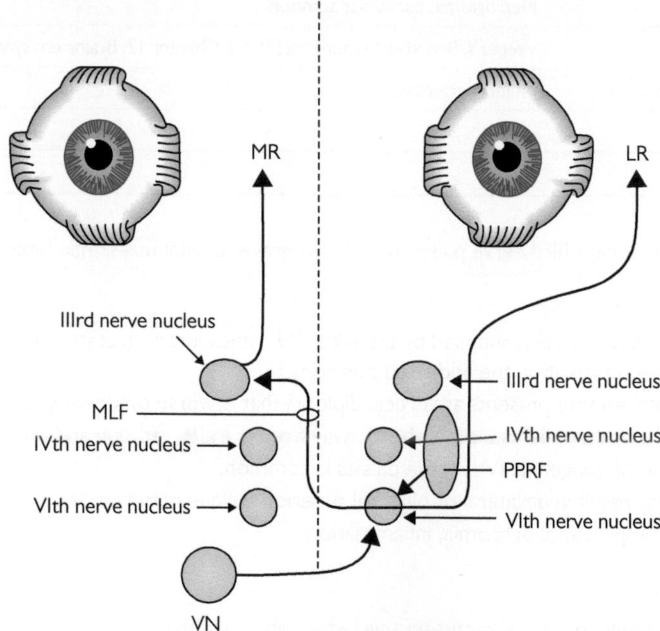

Figure 18.3 Control of horizontal eye movements. LR, lateral rectus; MLF, medial longitudinal fasciculus; MR, medial rectus; PPRF, paramedian pontine reticular formation; VN, vestibular nucleus.

Myasthenia gravis

➲ See Chapter 17, Myasthenia gravis, p. 631.

This autoimmune disease can cause ocular motility defects that resemble a cranial neuropathy. Myasthenia should be considered if:

- Symptoms are variable in nature (typically worse towards the end of the day).

- Presentation is atypical or 'complex' (not fitting the pattern of a specific cranial nerve defect).
- Ptosis is present, especially if this is bilateral (➲ see Ptosis).

Dysthyroid eye disease

➲ See Chapter 19, Dysthyroid eye disease, p. 681.

- There is a risk of sight loss due to:
- Optic nerve compression.
- Corneal exposure.

Therefore, any patient complaining of blurred vision should have an urgent ophthalmic review.

Ptosis

Ptosis is a drooping upper eyelid. It does not refer to lower eyelid sagging, which can occur in a facial nerve palsy.

Ptosis can occur in isolation or together with a range of other clinical signs such as pupil abnormalities, eye movement disorders and anhydrosis. It is important to note that both the levator palpebrae superioris muscle (levator muscle) (innervated by the IIIrd CN) and Muller's muscle (which has sympathetic innervation) help to raise the upper lid, hence ptosis may occur when either one of these muscles or their nerve supply is affected.

Causes

Congenital

Usually a long history and unchanging:

- Poor development of the levator muscle causes a congenital ptosis. Typically unilateral and results in absence of an upper lid skin crease (usually 8–10 mm from the upper lid margin).
- Marcus Gunn 'jaw-winking' ptosis, the droopy eyelid rises when the jaw is opened due to an aberrant connection between the motor branches of the trigeminal nerve innervating the external pterygoid muscle and the fibres of the oculomotor nerve. This condition is usually diagnosed in small children and affects only one eyelid.

Aponeurotic/mechanical

- Involutional: ageing and weakness of the levator muscle (frequently bilateral).
- Dermatochalasis: excess eyelid skin, sometimes treated for cosmetic reasons.

Neurological

- IIIrd CN palsy: unilateral (➲ see Oculomotor (IIIrd) nerve palsy, p. 647 and Table 18.1).
- Horner's syndrome: a unilateral partial ptosis in association with a constricted pupil (miosis) and hemifacial loss of sweating (anhydrosis) (➲ see Horner's syndrome: interruption of the sympathetic pathway, p. 651, Table 18.2 and Figure 18.4).

Systemic

- Myasthenia gravis causes variable/fatigable ptosis (➲ see Myasthenia gravis [under Eye movement], p. 648)
- Myotonic dystrophy: for clinical features (➲ see Chapter 17, Myotonic dystrophy, p. 629).

Pseudoptosis

- Shrinking of eyeball: microphthalmos/pthisis bulbi.
- Contralateral proptosis.

Treating ptosis

Treat underlying medical condition

Surgical repair involves tightening the levator muscles in order to lift the eyelid.

Pupils

Movements of the pupil are controlled by the parasympathetic and sympathetic nervous systems.

The pupils constrict (miosis) when the eye is illuminated (parasympathetic activation, sympathetic relaxation) and dilate (mydriasis) in the dark (sympathetic activation, parasympathetic relaxation). When the eyes accommodate (focus for near vision) they also converge and the pupils constrict. The pupils are normally equal in size, but 20% of people may have physiological anisocoria (unequal pupils – typically ≤1 mm difference), with no associated disease.

The parasympathetic fibres reach the eye through the IIIrd CN from the Edinger–Westphal nucleus (in the midbrain). The sympathetic supply consists of three neurons.

The first order neuron descends from the hypothalamus to synapse in the cervical spinal cord (C8–T2 level). The second order (preganglionic) neuron exits the spinal cord and travels in the cervical sympathetic chain through the brachial plexus, over the pulmonary apex and synapses in the superior cervical ganglion. The third order (postganglionic) neuron travels along the internal carotid artery into the cavernous sinus. Here, the oculosympathetic fibres join the first division of the trigeminal nerve to enter the orbit (See Table 18.2).

For the sympathetic pathway to the eye, see Figure 18.4.

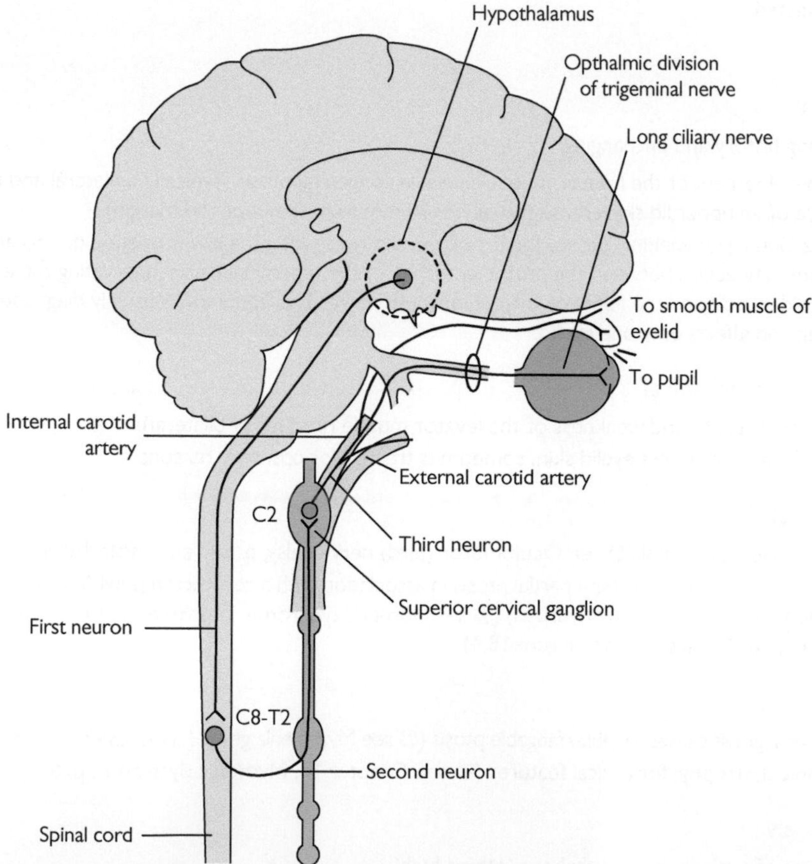

Figure 18.4 Sympathetic pathway to the eye.

Diagnosis

- Determine which pupil is abnormal.
- Search for associated signs.

Disorders of the pupil may result from:

- Ocular disease.
- Disorders of the controlling neurological pathway.
- Pharmacological action.

Diseases of the eye which cause irregularity of the pupil and alter its reaction include:

- Ocular inflammation where posterior synechiae may give the pupil an irregular appearance.
- The sequelae of intraocular surgery.
- Blunt trauma to the eye, which may rupture the sphincter muscle causing irregularity, or fixed dilation (traumatic mydriasis).

Constricted pupils

Horner's syndrome: interruption of the sympathetic pathway

The sympathetic pathway may be affected by a multitude of pathologies due to its extended course (see Table 18.2).

Table 18.2 Differential diagnosis of Horner's syndrome

	Anatomical location	**Possible causes**
First order neuron Absence of sweating in the entire half of the body	Brainstem.	Stroke, tumour, demyelination.
	Spinal cord.	Syringomyelia, tumour, trauma.
Second order neuron Preganglionic: absence of sweating in the face, typically in V_1 division	Lung apex.	Pancoast's tumour.
	Neck.	Tumour in cervical nodes, surgery, trauma, common carotid dissection.
Third order neuron Postganglionic	Internal carotid artery.	Dissection.
	Cavernous sinus.	Thrombus, tumour.
	Orbit.	Tumour.
Congenital	Iris colour may be altered when compared with the fellow eye (heterochromia).	

Clinical findings

- Miosis: a small pupil on the affected side. This is more noticeable in the dark when the fellow, normal pupil, dilates more than the affected pupil.
- Ptosis: usually partial on the affected side.
- Anhydrosis: lack of sweating on the affected side if the sympathetic pathway is affected proximal to the base of the skull.
- Enophthalmos: an apparent recession of the globe into the orbit.

Argyll Robertson pupils

Bilateral small, irregular pupils showing light-near dissociation (they accommodate, but do not react to light). Classically caused by neurosyphilis (➲ see Chapter 7, Syphilis, p. 199, Tables 7.6, 7.7 and 7.8, and

Figures 7.5 and 7.6), and occasionally by diabetic neuropathy. Management is related to the underlying disease.

Bilateral miosis may also occur in coma, and in patients taking pilocarpine for glaucoma or receiving morphine.

Dilated pupils

IIIrd cranial nerve palsy

Compressive IIIrd nerve lesions can cause a dilated pupil. Coma associated with dilation of the pupil may result from the increased pressure on the IIIrd nerve due to an intracranial mass (e.g. a haematoma) (➲ see Oculomotor (IIIrd) nerve palsy, p. 647 and Table 18.1).

Adie's tonic pupil

This describes a unilateral (80% of cases), mydriatic pupil presenting typically in otherwise healthy young adults, especially women (F:M 2:1).

The affected pupil is:

- Enlarged.
- Poorly reactive to light.
- Slow to constrict, with sustained miosis on accommodation.
- Supersensitive to dilute pilocarpine (0.1%).

Occasionally, it is associated with diminished deep tendon reflexes (Holmes–Adie syndrome) and autonomic nerve dysfunction. Believed to occur due to denervation of parasympathetic fibres. Often occurs following a viral illness (e.g. Herpes zoster ophthalmicus).

Dilated pupils may also be caused by drugs, both topical (tropicamide; atropine) and systemic (cocaine or amphetamines).

Relative afferent pupillary defect

Normally, each illuminated pupil promptly becomes constricted. The opposite pupil also constricts consensually. With the majority of ocular diseases that impair vision, such as cataract or diabetic maculopathy, the pupils respond normally.

When the optic nerve (or the entire retina, e.g. central retinal artery occlusion) is damaged, the sensory (afferent) stimulus sent to the midbrain is reduced. When a light is moved away from the unaffected eye and shone on the affected eye the pupil, responding less vigorously, dilates from its prior constricted state. This response is a relative afferent pupillary defect (RAPD; Marcus Gunn pupil).

Visual pathway and visual field defect

Visual fields overview

The visual field of each eye can be divided into four quadrants by the vertical and horizontal midlines, both of which intersect at the point of fixation. The field to the right of the vertical midline travels to the left side of the brain (and vice versa; see Figure 18.5). The fields above and below the horizontal midline travel to the temporal and parietal lobes, respectively. Neurological pathology tends to obey the vertical midline, whereas glaucoma and retinal occlusive disease obey the horizontal midline. Each eye is tested independently, either by confrontation or automated testing.

Determining the cause of visual field loss

- Was the onset sudden, rapid or slow?
- Where is the field loss?
- Does it affect one eye or both?
- Are there any associated neurological or ophthalmic symptoms?

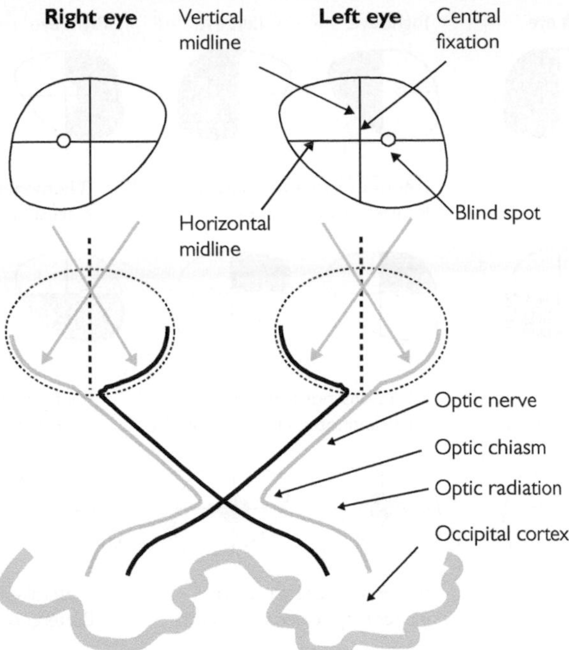

Figure 18.5 The visual field and associated visual pathways.

Confrontation visual field testing

- The examiner should sit facing the patient at a distance of 1 m. Each eye should be assessed separately. The patient should cover or close one eye and look directly at the examiner's eye opposite. The examiner also closes their fellow eye.
- The target must be equidistant between the examiner and patient.
- Starting at the top outer quadrant, a target object (e.g. fingers or hatpin) is moved in from the periphery and the patient is instructed to state when they first see the object and, as it moves towards the centre, whether it disappears.
- The process is repeated in each quadrant and for each eye separately.
- If a defect is detected, that area can be re-examined to define it further.

For visual field defects with location of pathology, see Figure 18.6.

Lesions at the level of the retina or optic nerve

Lesions before the chiasm produce a field defect in the affected eye only.

Retinal disease

- Retinal detachment: tends to be fairly rapid in onset and may be preceded by floaters and flashes. Field loss does not necessarily respect the horizontal or vertical midlines. May follow trauma or be associated with high myopia.
- Central retinal artery occlusion: causes sudden complete loss of vision in one eye. Branch retinal artery occlusions will cause loss of the upper or lower visual field (an 'altitudinal' defect), or just one quadrant of the field. In the acute phase (4–6 weeks), the affected retina will look pale and poorly

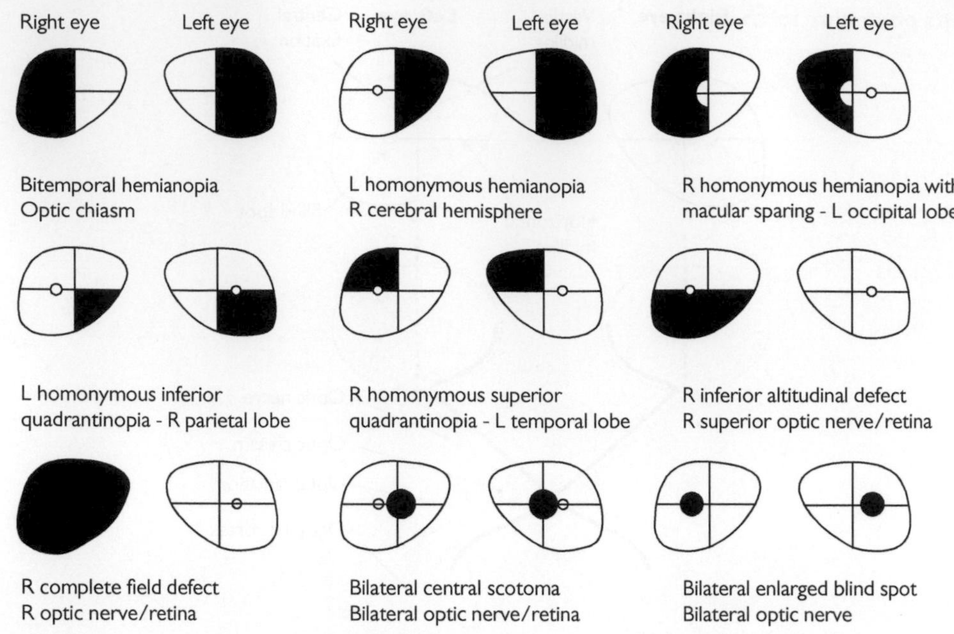

Figure 18.6 Visual field defects with location of pathology. Patient's visual fields are displayed from the doctor's perspective (i.e. patient's right eye is on the left side).

supplied with blood vessels. Subsequently, optic atrophy will develop associated with attenuated retinal arteries.

- Central retinal vein occlusion: presents suddenly, like arterial occlusion, but multiple haemorrhages can be seen scattered throughout the fundus.

Optic nerve disease

Defects from damage to the optic nerve tend to be central, asymmetrical and unilateral. May be associated with an afferent pupillary defect (➲ see Relative afferent pupillary defect, p. 652). Visual acuity is often affected. Causes include:

- Optic neuritis.
- Ischaemic optic neuropathy.
- Glaucoma.
- Trauma.

Lesions just before the chiasm can occasionally produce a central scotoma in one eye and a small defect in the upper temporal field of the fellow eye (junctional scotoma) as the decussating fibres from the inferior nasal retina loop back into the contralateral optic nerve after decussating (anterior chiasmal syndrome, e.g. meningioma).

Lesions at the chiasm

- These classically produce a bitemporal hemianopia.
- If encroaching on the chiasm from below (e.g. pituitary tumours), the defect is worse in the upper visual fields.
- If compression occurs from above (e.g. craniopharyngioma), the lesion is worse in the lower quadrants.

Lesions posterior to the chiasm

These produce homonymous field defects; a lesion in the right optic tract produces a left visual field defect and vice versa. Lesions in the optic radiations cause complete (left or right) homonymous hemianopia without macular sparing. This is seen following a stroke affecting the middle cerebral artery territory. The more posterior the lesion affecting the visual pathways is, the more congruous the visual field defect will be.

- Lesions in the temporal radiation cause congruous homonymous superior quadrantinopia, e.g. tumours.
- Lesions in the parietal radiation (rare) cause homonymous inferior quadrantinopia.
- Lesions in the anterior occipital, visual cortex (common) produce a contralateral homonymous hemianopia. Macular sparing may occur when visual cortical infarction is caused by a posterior cerebral artery occlusion if the posterior occipital (macular) cortex has a dual blood supply from both the middle and the posterior cerebral arteries.
- Lesions in the posterior occipital cortex may produce a congruous homonymous macular defect e.g. blunt injury to the occiput.
- Injury to both occipital lobes (e.g. bilateral strokes or trauma) may lead to a state of cortical blindness.

Optic nerve abnormalities

The optic nerve is comprised of axons that originate in the ganglion cell layer of the retina and project to the lateral geniculate body in the midbrain. These axons are heavily myelinated and, once damaged, do not regenerate.

Optic atrophy has many possible causes, the frequency of which depends on the age of the patient. In younger patients, optic atrophy is most commonly due to demyelination, whereas in those >50 years of age an ischaemic cause is more likely.

Clinical examination

- Visual acuity: optic neuropathy frequently presents with loss of central vision, leading to reduced visual acuity.
- Pupillary reactions: a relative afferent pupillary defect may be present.
- Colour vision: may be reduced.
- Visual fields: some lesions (e.g. a pituitary tumour) may give rise to peripheral visual field loss with relatively well preserved visual acuity.
- Fundoscopy: optic disc changes may include:
  - total pallor;
  - temporal pallor (sometimes seen in demyelination, toxic neuropathy and nutritional deficiency);
  - bow-tie pallor (compression of the optic chiasm);
  - cupping (glaucomatous optic atrophy).

Causes of a swollen optic disc

- Papilloedema (swelling secondary to raised intracranial pressure – usually bilateral).
- Papillitis (swelling due to inflammation = optic neuritis).
- Malignant hypertension.
- Ischaemic optic neuropathy.
- Diabetic optic neuropathy.
- Central retinal vein occlusion.
- Intraocular inflammation.

Papilloedema

See Figure 18.7.

- Visual acuity is normal initially, but may be reduced in late stage.
- Normal colour vision.
- No RAPD.
- Headache: worse in the morning.

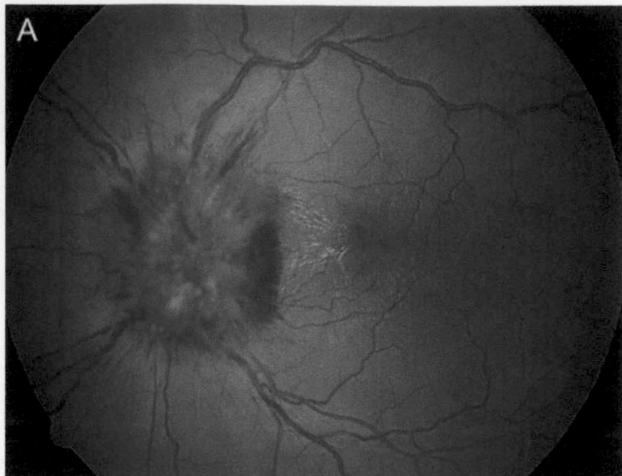

Figure 18.7 (see colour plate section) Papilloedema. The optic disc appears hyperaemic, with blurred margins, splinter haemorrhages, and engorged, dilated surrounding veins. There is early development of tiny hard exudates tracking along the maculopapular bundle.
Courtesy of Brian R. Younge, MD, Mayo Clinic, Rochester, Minnesota. Used with permission.

Investigations

- BP.
- CT scan/MRI to rule out space-occupying lesion.
- If no space-occupying lesion then proceed to lumbar puncture (elevated opening pressure may indicate idiopathic intracranial hypertension).

Optic neuritis

Inflammatory – most commonly due to demyelination (multiple sclerosis):

- Sudden loss of vision with recovery over 6–12 weeks.
- Painful eye movements.
- Reduced visual acuity.
- Impaired colour vision.
- RAPD.
- Visual field defect: variable.
- Optic disc may be normal or swollen.
- Visually-evoked responses (VERs) show increased latency.

Other causes include infections, e.g. syphilis, TB, viral (e.g. HSV, VZV).

Optic atrophy

For causes of optic atrophy, see Table 18.3 and Figure 18.8.

Table 18.3 Causes of optic atrophy

Aetiology	Examples
Inherited	Leber's hereditary optic neuropathy.
Glaucoma	
Inflammatory	Demyelination. Sarcoidosis. Wegener's granulomatosis.
Vascular (ischaemic) optic neuropathy	Arteritic (giant cell arteritis). Non-arteritic.
Retinal	Central retinal artery occlusion. Retinitis pigmentosa.
Compressive optic neuropathy	Optic nerve glioma or meningioma. Chiasmal compression, e.g. pituitary adenoma, craniopharyngioma. Dysthyroid eye disease.
Toxic optic neuropathy	Drugs (e.g. ethambutol), tobacco, alcohol.
Nutritional	B12 deficiency.
Trauma	

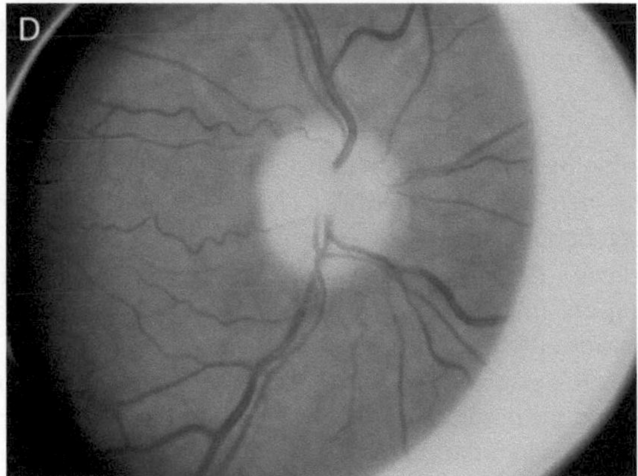

Figure 18.8 Optic atrophy: marked pallor of the optic disc.

Reproduced with permission from Neuro-ophthalmology: Disorders of Visual perception, Pupils, and Eyelid. In Flemming K.D. and Jones Jr L.K. (Eds.). *Mayo Clinic Neurology Board Review: Clinical Neurology for Initial Certification and MOC.* Rochester (MN), US: Mayo Clinic Scientific Press. Copyright © 2017; used with permission of Mayo Foundation for Medical Education and Research, all rights reserved.

Arteritic anterior ischaemic optic neuropathy

Giant cell arteritis may cause occlusion of the posterior ciliary arteries supplying the optic nerve.

Untreated, this can cause sudden sequential and, therefore, bilateral blindness. Giant cell arteritis is discussed in ➲ Chapter 20, Giant cell arteritis, p. 740.

Non-arteritic anterior ischaemic optic neuropathy

The mechanisms involved in the development of optic disc ischaemia are unclear and may include local arteriosclerosis, with or without thrombosis, embolisation from a remote source, vasospasm or some combination of these processes.

- Patients usually aged between 45–65 years.
- Altitudinal visual field defect.
- Visual loss of variable degree.
- Swollen optic disc with oedema/splinter haemorrhages.
- Normal ESR and CRP.
- Hypertension.

Retinal abnormalities

Diabetic eye disease

Pathophysiology

Diabetic retinopathy affects 40% of the diabetic population and is the commonest cause of blindness among working-age adults. Diabetic retinopathy results from prolonged hyperglycaemia and hypertension, so the degree of retinopathy is highly correlated with:

- Duration of diabetes.
- Blood glucose levels.
- BP levels.

Pregnancy can impair blood glucose control and thus worsen retinopathy.

In type 1 diabetes <2% of patients have retinopathy at diagnosis, while 98% are affected after 25 years. In contrast 21% of type 2 diabetics have retinopathy at diagnosis.

As patients are asymptomatic until they have advanced retinopathy or maculopathy, the National Screening Committee (NSC) recommends annual retinopathy screening by digital retinal photography.

Diabetic retinopathy classification by National Screening Committee[1]

- *No retinopathy – R0*: patients are expected to return for annual screening.
- *Background retinopathy – R1*: early signs of localised retinal ischaemia include microaneurysms (dots) and blot haemorrhages. Requires annual screening.
- *Pre-proliferative retinopathy – R2*: more widespread ischaemia, which leads to the development of fluffy 'cotton wool spots' (micro-infarcts), venous dilation/beading/loops and intraretinal microvascular abnormalities (IRMA). Usually screened every 4–6 months.
- *Proliferative retinopathy – R3*: extensive ischaemia leads to the release of vascular endothelial growth factor (VEGF) and the development of new vessels, on the inner (vitreous) surface of the retina, which may extend into the vitreous cavity with subsequent vitreous haemorrhage. Neovascularisation is often accompanied by preretinal fibrous tissue that, along with the vitreous, can contract, resulting in tractional retinal detachment. Neovascularisation may also occur on the iris (rubeosis iridis) leading to neovascular glaucoma. Vision loss with proliferative retinopathy may be severe. Requires urgent ophthalmological referral (for review within 2 weeks).

Diabetic maculopathy

Diabetic maculopathy – M1: is caused by oedema from leaking capillaries ± ischaemia due to capillary loss. It is the most common cause of vision loss due to diabetic eye disease and may occur irrespective of the severity of retinopathy. The presence of hard exudates (discrete, yellow particles within the macula) suggests chronic oedema. Routine ophthalmic review is indicated (within 13 weeks).

[1] Adapted with permission from Harding, S., R. et al. Grading and disease management in national screening for diabetic retinopathy in England and Wales. *Diabetic Medicine* 20:965. Copyright © 2003, Diabetes UK and John Wiley and Sons. https://doi.org/10.1111/j.1464-5491.2003.01077.x

Diagnosis of diabetic retinopathy

- Fundoscopy: confirms the diagnosis.
- Colour fundus photography: to grade the level of retinopathy.
- Fluorescein angiography: to determine the extent of ischaemia.
- Optical coherence tomography: to assess severity of macular oedema and treatment response.

Treatment of diabetic retinopathy

- Control of blood glucose and BP.
- For clinically significant macular oedema, focal laser treatment ± intraocular injection of anti-VEGF drugs (ranibizumab [Lucentis®], aflibercept [Eylea®]).
- Proliferative diabetic retinopathy with high-risk characteristics (new vessels on the optic disc, vitreous or pre-retinal haemorrhage, rubeosis or neovascular glaucoma) should be treated with pan-retinal laser photocoagulation. This treatment significantly reduces the risk of severe vision loss.
- Vitrectomy can help preserve and often restore lost vision in patients with persistent vitreous haemorrhage or tractional retinal detachment.

See Figures 18.9–18.11 for images of diabetic retinopathy and maculopathy.

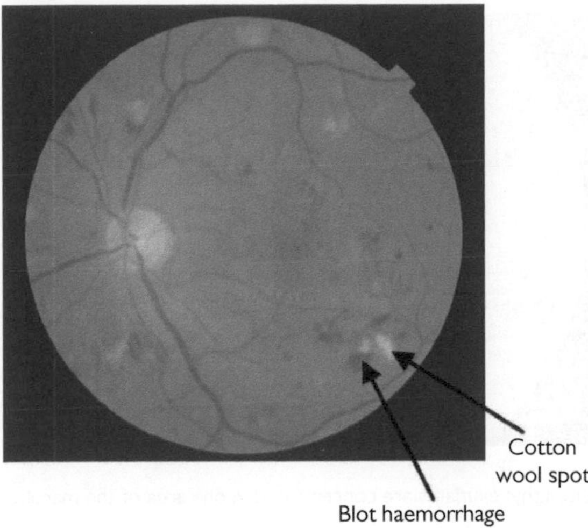

Figure 18.9 (see colour plate section) Pre-proliferative diabetic retinopathy. Cotton wool spots and blot haemorrhages are indicated.

Reproduced with permission from Leigh R. Pre-proliferative and proliferative retinopathy. In *Diabetic Retinopathy Screening to Treatment*, Dodson, P. (Ed). Oxford, UK: Oxford University Press. Copyright © 2008 Heart of England Retinal Screening Centre. DOI:10.1093/med/9780199544967.003.0007.

Retinal vascular events

See Figure 18.12.

Retinal vein occlusion

Retinal vein occlusion (RVO) is one of the most frequent causes of blindness after diabetic retinopathy. If it happens at the optic nerve it is called a central retinal vein occlusion (CRVO); if at a branch it is referred to as branch retinal vein occlusion (BRVO). 90% of CRVO occurs in those aged >50 years. In 30% of cases CRVO is ischaemic and may result in rubeotic glaucoma leading to pain and blindness in the affected eye. BRVO accounts for some 30% of all retinal vein blockages.

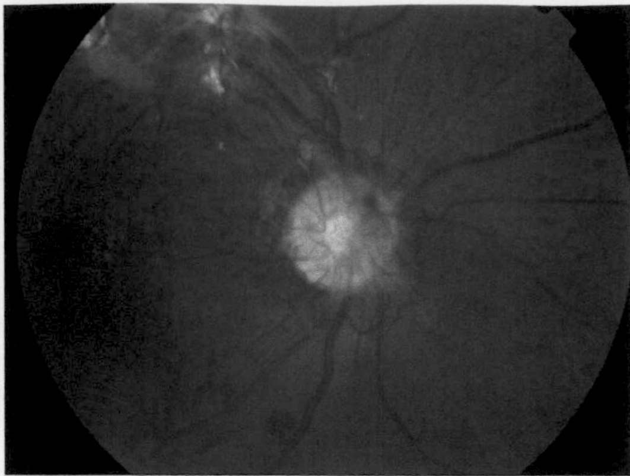

Figure 18.10 (see colour plate section) Proliferative diabetic retinopathy. New vessels have formed all over the optic disc. They are fine, looping, and aimless.

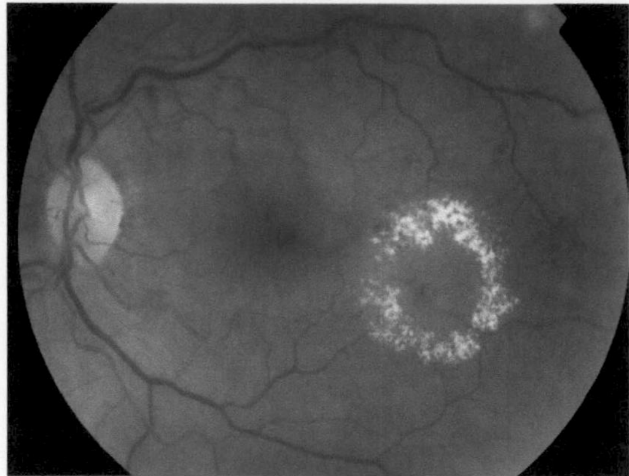

Figure 18.11 Diabetic maculopathy: exudates are concentrated in one area of the macula and beginning to impinge into the fovea.

Symptoms

Blurring of vision or visual loss, typically suddenly, but sometimes gradually due to the development of macular oedema.

Risk factors of RVO

- Hypertension.
- Diabetes mellitus.
- Bleeding or clotting disorders.
- Vasculitis.
- Use of oral contraceptives.
- Primary open-angle glaucoma or close-angle glaucoma.

Treatments

- Identify and treat any underlying medical problems.

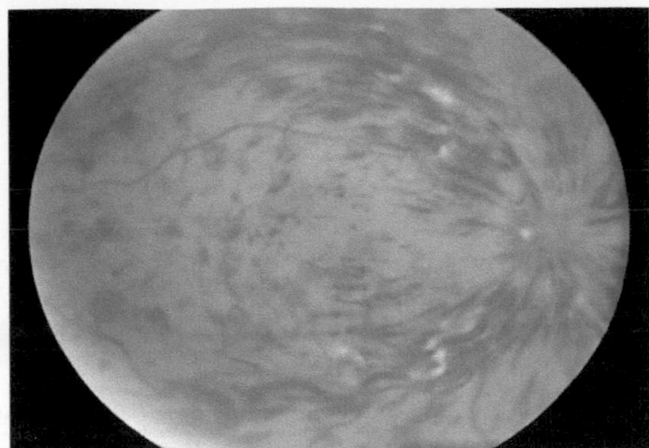

Figure 18.12 (see colour plate section) Central retinal vein occlusion. Profuse flame haemorrhages have formed between the nerve fibres in all quadrants. Cotton wool spots representing microinfarcts are often also present.
Reproduced with permission from Frith P. The eye in general medicine. In *Oxford Textbook of Medicine*, Fifth Edition, Warrell D. A. et al. (Eds.). Oxford, UK: OUP. Copyright © 2013 Oxford University Press. Reproduced with permission of the Licensor through PLSclear.

- Intra-vitreal anti-VEGF drugs (ranibizumab [Lucentis®], aflibercept [Eylea®]) to treat macular oedema.
- Laser treatment for neovascularisation.

Central retinal artery occlusion

Central retinal artery occlusion (CRAO) is a blockage of the central retinal artery. This is a very serious condition that requires emergency treatment. If it occurs in one of the branches of the central retinal artery, it is a branch retinal artery occlusion (BRAO).

Symptoms of CRAO

Sudden loss of vision in the affected eye.

Risk factors of CRAO

About 75% of CRAO have hypertension or blocked coronary arteries. Risk factors include:

- Smoking.
- Hypertension.
- Hypercholesterolaemia.
- Diabetes mellitus.
- Coronary heart disease.
- History of stroke.

Treatment

Emergency diagnosis and treatment of vision loss by lowering the eye pressure with ocular massage, anterior chamber paracentesis and medication in the first few hours can sometimes restore vision.

Retinal detachment

Retinal detachment is separation of the neurosensory retina from the underlying retinal pigment epithelium. Retinal detachment should be suspected in any of the following:

- Sudden increase or change in floaters or photopsia (flashes).
- Curtain or veil across the visual field.
- Any sudden, unexplained loss of vision.
- Vitreous haemorrhage that obscures the retina.

Risk factors

- Myopia.
- Previous cataract surgery.
- Ocular trauma.
- Proliferative diabetic retinopathy.
- Sickle cell retinopathy.
- Severe uveitis, especially in Vogt–Koyanagi–Harada disease and choroidal hemangioma.

Treatment is surgical; refer urgently to an ophthalmologist.

Retinitis pigmentosa

Retinitis pigmentosa (RP) is a slowly progressive, bilateral degeneration of the retina and retinal pigment epithelium that frequently leads to severe loss of vision. It can be caused by many different genetic mutations. Transmission may be autosomal recessive, autosomal dominant, X-linked or mitochondrial. RP may occur as part of a syndrome (see Figure 18.13 and Table 18.4).

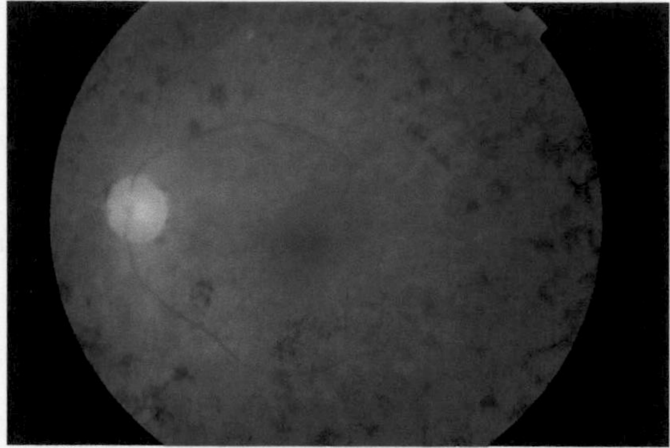

Figure 18.13 (see colour plate section) Retinitis pigmentosa: Peripheral retinal pigmentation classically occurs in a 'bone-spicule' pattern (like the branches of a tree) although it may also take the form of multiple small black spots.
Reproduced with permission from Imaging Service Moorfields Eye Hospital.

Symptoms and signs

Symptoms include night blindness and loss of peripheral vision. Central vision may also be affected in advanced cases. The development of cataracts and cystoid macular oedema can contribute to the loss of vision.

The typical fundoscopic features of RP are:

- Hyperpigmentation in a bone-spicule configuration in the mid to peripheral retina.
- Narrowing of the retinal arterioles.
- Waxy yellow appearance of the disc.

The diagnosis should be suspected in patients with poor night vision or a family history of RP. Diagnosis is made by fundoscopy and confirmed by electrophysiological assessment, which demonstrates loss of retinal function, predominantly affecting rod photoreceptors. The rods are more numerous in the periphery of the retina and function in scotopic (low light) conditions. Cone photoreceptors that mediate colour vision and are more numerous in the macula are relatively spared. Other retinopathies that can simulate RP should be excluded; they include retinopathies associated with syphilis, rubella, chloroquine or thioridazine.

Family members should be screened to establish the hereditary pattern. Patients may wish to seek genetic counselling before having children. Presently, RP is untreatable (with the exception of restricting phytanic acid intake in Refsum disease), but experimental gene therapy offers the possibility of treatment in the future.

Table 18.4 Syndromes associated with RP

Syndrome	Clinical features	Inheritance
Usher syndrome	Congenital neurosensory deafness.	Autosomal recessive.
Refsum disease	Deafness. Cerebellar ataxia. Peripheral neuropathy. Cardiomyopathy. Ichthyosis. Palpable peripheral nerves.	Autosomal recessive (disorder of phytanic acid metabolism).
Lawrence–Moon–Bardet–Biedl syndrome	Deafness. Polydactyly. Short stature. Learning disability. Hypogonadism. Renal disease. Diabetes.	Autosomal recessive.
Kearns–Sayre syndrome	Chronic progressive external ophthalmoplegia (bilateral symmetrically reduced eye movements and ptosis). Cardiac conduction defects. Cerebellar syndrome.	Mitochondrial.

Macular degeneration

Age-related macular degeneration (ARMD) is the leading cause of permanent vision loss in the elderly.

Risk factors include:

- Age.
- Family history.
- Smoking.
- Cardiovascular disease.
- Hypertension.
- Obesity.

ARMD can be classified as dry or wet:

- *Dry ARMD* (non-exudative or atrophic): 85% of ARMD. Funduscopic changes include drusen, areas of chorioretinal atrophy, and pigmentary changes to the retinal pigment epithelium.
- *Wet ARMD* (exudative or neovascular): accounts for 80–90% of severe vision loss caused by AMD. Funduscopic changes include retinal oedema and localised elevation, detachment of the retinal pigment epithelium, and exudates in and around the macula.

Diagnosis of ARMD is confirmed by fluorescein angiography, and optical coherence tomography.

Treatment

Wet ARMD is treated with intravitreal anti-VEGF drugs (ranibizumab [Lucentis®], aflibercept [Eylea®]). Dietary supplements according to the AREDS2 trial for unilateral wet or high-risk dry ARMD (1).

References

1. AREDS2 Research Group. Lutein/zeaxanthin and omega-3 fatty acids for age-related macular degeneration. The Age-Related Eye Disease Study 2 (AREDS2) Controlled Randomized Clinical Trial. *J Am Med Ass.* 2013; 309(19):2005–15 .

Cataract

Cataracts occur when changes in the lens of the eye cause it to become less transparent, and are a common, usually age-related, cause of vision loss.

Risk factors

- Diabetes.
- Drug induced, e.g. steroids, statins.
- Traumatic.
- Previous eye injury or inflammation.
- Family history (primarily for congenital cataracts).

Symptoms

- Blurred or double vision.
- Glare and sensitivity to bright lights.
- Colours appear faded.
- Difficulty reading or driving (especially at night).

Treatment

Surgery involves replacing the cataract with an artificial intraocular lens (IOL).

Choroidal tumours

Naevus/melanoma

As malignant transformation is rare, choroidal naevi rarely require treatment. Depending on its appearance, patients with a choroidal naevus should have their eyes examined every year.

If the choroidal naevus has orange pigmentation, is leaking fluid, or has a thickness of ≥2 mm it may be (or may become) a malignant choroidal melanoma.

If the choroidal naevus looks suspicious, further examination may include the use of US, specialised photography or an intraocular angiogram.

Choroidal metastases

The choroid is the most common ocular site for metastatic disease, owing to abundant vascular supply. The primary cancers that most commonly lead to choroidal metastases include breast cancer (45%) and lung cancer (25%). Bilateral, multifocal metastases are most often secondary to breast cancer, whereas unilateral metastasis are more commonly found with lung cancer. These generally appear as a yellow sub-retinal mass associated with sub-retinal fluid.

Red eye

Red eye is the main sign of ocular inflammation or infection. The cause of red eye can be diagnosed through a detailed history and careful eye examination. Recognising the symptoms that indicate the need for an urgent referral to an ophthalmologist is essential.

Symptoms necessitating an urgent referral

- Moderate-to-severe eye pain.
- Photophobia (intolerance of bright lights).
- Ciliary injection (redness in a ring around the iris), suggesting inflammation.
- Reduced vision.
- Seeing coloured haloes around point sources of light.

- Copious purulent discharge.
- Corneal involvement (ulcer).
- Known or suspected eye trauma.
- Recent ocular surgery.
- Pupillary distortion or abnormal reaction.
- Herpes simplex or herpes zoster.
- Proptosis.
- Contact lens wear (increased risk of corneal ulcer).
- Chemical burns: these are an ophthalmic emergency and should be immediately irrigated for at least 10 minutes with saline or running water before any steps are taken. Common agents include cement, plaster powder and oven cleaner, all of which are alkaline. They should be referred even if there are no residual symptoms.

An initial eye examination can be carried out with a pen torch, but a slit lamp examination is preferable for detecting keratitis and uveitis. Treatment is based on the underlying cause.

Differential diagnosis

Non-urgent

Usually superficial conditions that tend to cause a gritty, burning sensation. Causes include:

- Conjunctivitis – the most common.
- Blepharitis: chronic inflammation of the eyelids.
- Subconjunctival haemorrhage.
- Inflamed pterygium/pingueculum (sunlight-induced growth of fibrous tissue on the cornea/conjunctiva).
- Dry eyes.
- Allergy to environmental factors.
- Episcleritis: a mild, inflammatory disorder not associated with eye complications. It responds to topical medications, such as anti-inflammatory drops.

Urgent

Pain is more severe and aching in nature, often with blurred vision and photophobia. Causes include:

- *Acute glaucoma*: older patients (>50 years). A sudden increase in eye pressure, extremely painful with blurring of vision, hazy cornea and a fixed dilated pupil.
- *Keratitis*: inflammation of the cornea. A white ulcer may be visible.
- *Uveitis*: inflammation of the uvea, which includes the iris, ciliary body, and choroid (see Figure 18.1). Circum-corneal injection, miosis, irregular pupil (synechiae) (➲ see Uveitis).
- *Scleritis*: localised scleral erythema and frequently severe pain. A serious inflammatory condition that can result in permanent vision loss. 30–40% of patients have an underlying systemic autoimmune condition (e.g. rheumatoid arthritis, Wegener's granulomatosis) (➲ see Scleritis, p. 666).
- *Hyphaema*: blood filling the anterior chamber, causing a horizontal fluid level.

Uveitis

Uveitis can be classified based on which part of the eye is affected:

- Anterior uveitis (the most common form) affects the anterior segment of the eye and is often referred to as iritis.
- Intermediate uveitis is inflammation of the ciliary body and anterior vitreous.
- Posterior uveitis is inflammation of the choroid (choroiditis), retina (retinitis) or optic nerve head (papillitis).

Most uveitis is idiopathic; however, it may be due to systemic autoimmune disorders (e.g. sarcoidosis), infection (e.g. TB), trauma or neoplasia. Symptoms may develop over hours or days (acute uveitis), or more gradually (chronic uveitis). The major causes of visual loss in people with uveitis are cystoid macular oedema, secondary cataract, and secondary glaucoma due to inflammation of the trabecular (drainage) meshwork.

Clinical features

- Pain in one or both eyes (pain may be worse when contracting the ciliary muscle).
- Red eye (not always present).
- Diminished or blurred vision (although vision may be normal initially, but become impaired later).
- Photophobia.
- Floaters.
- An unreactive or irregular-shaped pupil due to synechiae (adhesions between the iris and lens) from previous episodes.

Treatment

- For non-infectious uveitis, topical or oral corticosteroids are used to reduce inflammation and prevent adhesions in the eye. A mydriatic drug (e.g. cyclopentolate 1%) is given in conjunction to paralyse the iris sphincter muscle. This relieves pain and prevents the formation of synechiae.
- For infectious uveitis (bacterial, viral, fungal or parasitic), an appropriate antimicrobial drug, as well as corticosteroids and cycloplegics are used.
- People with severe or chronic uveitis ± co-existing systemic disease, may also be given immunosuppressive drugs, TNF inhibitors, disease-modifying antirheumatic drugs (DMARDs) or immunosuppressants, depending on locally agreed shared care guidelines.

Behçet's disease

➲ See Chapter 20, Behçet's disease, p. 742.

Ocular involvement

70% of patients have anterior segment iridocyclitis with hypopyon, or posterior segment involvement with retinal vasculitis. Symptoms include periorbital pain, redness, photophobia and blurred vision. Ophthalmoscopy shows venous engorgement, retinal haemorrhages, yellow–white exudates deep in the retina, white focal retinal infiltrates, retinal oedema and optic disc oedema with hyperaemia.

In most cases, the ocular symptoms follow the oral and genital ulcers by 3–4 years, although ocular disease is the initial manifestation in 20%.

Sarcoidosis

➲ See Chapter 11, Sarcoidosis, p. 351 and Figure 11.2.

- Involvement of the eyes and adnexa occurs in 25–54% of patients.
- Anterior uveitis is the most common ocular manifestation of sarcoidosis, but posterior uveitis occurs in 25–30% of patients with ocular sarcoid. Approximately 20% of patients with ophthalmic sarcoid have involvement of the orbit or lacrimal gland, presenting with proptosis, ptosis or ophthalmoplegia.
- Heerfordt syndrome: uveitis, parotid enlargement and occasionally papilloedema.
- Löfgren syndrome: erythema nodosum, bilateral hilar adenopathy, arthralgia, anterior uveitis.

Scleritis

See Figure 18.14.

Scleritis may be localised, nodular or diffuse. It may involve the anterior (visible segment) ± posterior segments of the eye, and usually manifests with redness of the eye and severe eye pain.

Anterior scleritis (90% of cases)

- Non-necrotising (75% of cases):
  - Usually unilateral.

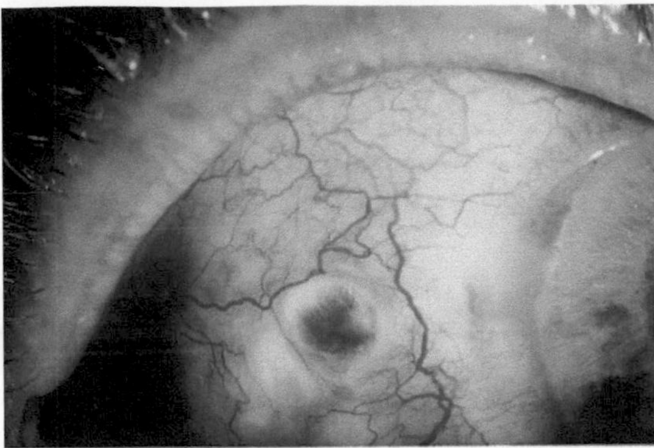

Figure 18.14 (see colour plate section) Scleritis demonstrating scleromalacia. Vasculitis results in focal ischaemia, with translucency and thinning of the sclera, which may perforate.

 - Hyperaemia of superficial and deep episcleral vessels; does not blanch with vasoconstrictors.
 - Anterior uveitis may be present.
 - Tenderness of globe.
- Necrotising (15% of cases): may occur in rheumatoid arthritis:
 - Most severe form (may be painless).
 - 75% will eventually have visual impairment.
 - Avascular necrosis leading to areas of scleral thinning with bluish-grey discolouration and eventually scleral melting with ectasia and choroidal herniation.

Posterior scleritis (10% of cases)

- Involves sclera posterior to the equator. Eye may be white.
- Ophthalmoscopy may reveal exudative retinal detachment, macular oedema, optic disc oedema, but may also show no abnormality.

Investigation and treatment

- Investigation for systemic associations such as rheumatoid arthritis.
- Systemic non-steroidal anti-inflammatory drugs.
- Systemic immunosuppression (corticosteroids ± other immunosuppressant drugs and biologics, e.g. TNF inhibitors).

Multiple choice questions

Questions

1. A 66-year-old Caucasian gentleman presents with a 5-day history of horizontal diplopia that worsens when he looks to the right. The diplopia disappears when he covers either one of his eyes. He is a known hypertensive and takes amlodipine 5 mg OD. On examination his right eye does not abduct fully. Pupils are equal and reactive. No other ocular abnormalities are noted. His BP is 184/85 mmHg. A random blood sugar taken was within normal limits. Which of the following statements is most likely?
 A. He has a microvascular right VIth CN palsy that should resolve within 3 months. He requires a higher dose of anti-hypertensive medication.

B. He has a microvascular right VIth CN palsy due to giant cell arteritis. An urgent ESR is required.
C. He may have a compressive right VIth CN palsy and requires urgent CT brain/orbits.
D. He has a microvascular right VIth CN palsy that should resolve within 6 months. The raised systolic BP may be secondary to 'white coat syndrome'.
E. He has a restrictive right VIth CN palsy that should resolve within 3 months. Investigation for thyroid eye disease should be initiated.

2. A 22-year-old male university student presents with a unilateral left-sided ptosis. He mentions that 3 days earlier he was playing rugby and was involved in quite a rough tackle and that his symptoms have appeared since then. He is in good health and on no medication. On examination, the ptosis is mild and the pupil is smaller on the affected side. His BP is 122/83 mmHg. A random blood sugar taken was within normal limits. Which of the following statements is most likely?
   A. This gentleman has always had a congenital ptosis but the recent trauma has brought his attention to it.
   B. It is likely that trauma has caused ecchymosis and swelling of his upper lid causing a pseudo-ptosis.
   C. He has a left IIIrd nerve palsy that requires urgent imaging to rule out posterior communicating artery aneurysm.
   D. This gentleman has avulsed the levator muscle from its aponeurosis and requires referral to oculoplastics.
   E. This gentleman has Horner's syndrome and requires urgent imaging to rule out a carotid dissection.

3. An 82-year-old male with a history of hypertension presents to A&E with sudden painless loss of vision in the right eye. On examination his visual acuity is 6/60 in the right eye; 6/6 in the left eye, with inferior visual field loss and the presence of an RAPD in the right eye. Fundoscopy revealed no significant retinal pathology in the affected eye. Which of the following statements is most likely?
   A. This gentleman is experiencing an evolving retinal detachment that requires urgent referral to ophthalmology.
   B. This gentleman has suffered a hemi-retinal vein occlusion and requires investigation of vascular risk factors.
   C. This gentleman is experiencing anterior ischaemic optic neuropathy and requires urgent ESR/CRP bloods to be sent off.
   D. This gentleman has suffered a vitreous haemorrhage secondary to diabetic retinopathy and requires urgent referral to ophthalmology.
   E. This gentleman has suffered an artery occlusion affecting the lower half of the retina and requires urgent referral to the local TIA service.

4. A 24-year-old diabetic patient presents with new vessels on her right optic disc and a small vitreous haemorrhage. Her retinopathy is best managed by:
   A. Intravitreal anti-VEGF injections.
   B. Tight blood sugar and BP control.
   C. Laser photocoagulation of the new vessels.
   D. Pan-retinal photocoagulation laser.
   E. Macular grid laser.

5. A 31-year-old man with a history of ankylosing spondylitis presents with unilateral eye pain, blurred vision and photophobia. On examination, there is unilateral pupil constriction and circumcorneal redness. Which of the following is the treatment of choice?
   A. Ofloxacin eye drops.
   B. Pilocarpine eye drops and oral acetazolamide.
   C. Oral prednisolone.
   D. Dexamethasone and cyclopentolate eye drops.
   E. Oral non-steroidal anti-inflammatory medication.

Answers

1. A. This gentleman has uncontrolled hypertension that is likely to have contributed to a right microvascular VIth CN palsy. An urgent ESR should be taken because giant cell arteritis is a rare, but possible cause of microvascular disease. His symptoms should resolve within 3 months. If they are still present after this time, investigation with MRI brain/orbits should be undertaken. He must not drive with diplopia. He could, however, continue with one eye patched if the other eye still meets the DVLA visual requirements (Box 18.1) (➲ see Abducens (VIth) nerve palsy, p. 647).

Box 18.1 DVLA visual standards for driving

1. In good daylight, driver must be able to read the registration mark fixed to a vehicle registered under current standards at a distance of 20 m.
2. The visual acuity must be at least Snellen 6/12 with both eyes open or in the only eye if monocular.
3. They must possess a visual field of at least 120° on the horizontal (at least 50° to the left and to the right). In addition, there should be no significant defect in the binocular field that encroaches within 20° of the fixation above or below the horizontal meridian.

Adapted from Assessing fitness to drive – a guide for medical professionals, https://www.gov.uk/guidance/assessing-fitness-to-drive-a-guide-for-medical-professionals. 2018.

2. E. With the history of trauma, it is likely that carotid dissection has disrupted the sympathetic nervous supply to Muller's muscle resulting in a unilateral partial ptosis, small pupil and anhydrosis (patients rarely complain of anhydrosis, but this history may be elicited with direct questioning). He requires urgent imaging and appropriate referral (➲ see Ptosis, p. 649).
3. C. Giant cell arteritis may cause occlusion of the posterior ciliary arteries supplying the optic nerve (➲ see Optic nerve abnormalities, p. 655 and Table 18.3).
4. D. Patients with proliferative diabetic retinopathy require urgent pan-retinal photocoagulation laser (within two weeks). Pan-retinal laser treatment reduces VEGF levels, which would remain elevated if the new vessels were treated directly. Tightening blood sugar control and BP control can actually worsen the retinopathy in the short term, although there is long-term benefit. Macular grid laser and anti-VEGF (Lucentis®) injections are appropriate for diabetic macular oedema (maculopathy) (➲ see Diabetic eye disease, p. 658).
5. D. The diagnosis is anterior uveitis (iritis). Treatment is with topical steroids to reduce inflammation and dilating drops to prevent adhesions between the lens and iris (synechiae). Early referral to an ophthalmologist is important (➲ see Uveitis, p. 665).

Chapter 19 **Diabetes and Endocrinology**

Chitrabhanu Ballav, Sophie A. Clarke* and John Wass*

Diabetes mellitus

Pathogenesis

The endocrine pancreas comprises of one million islets of Langerhans that form 1% of the pancreatic mass. The islets are multicellular clusters of α, β, δ and PP cells secreting glucagon, insulin, somatostatin and pancreatic polypeptide, respectively. β cells form 65–80% of islet cells and secrete insulin at high glucose concentrations. Insulin acts on peripheral tissue receptors to increase glucose uptake from the circulation. α cells make up 15–20% of islet cells and secrete glucagon when plasma glucose levels fall. High glucagon and low insulin levels favour release of glucose from the liver by glycogenolysis and gluconeogenesis.

Diabetes mellitus (DM) is characterised by chronic hyperglycaemia from defects in insulin secretion, insulin action or both. This leads to dysfunction of organs including the eyes, kidneys, nerves and blood vessels. Typical osmotic symptoms of hyperglycaemia include thirst and polyuria. Patients may also present with dehydration and infections. Currently 2.9 million people (4.5% of adults) in the UK have diabetes.

Presentation and classification

Type 1

10% of adults have diabetes mellitus; prevalence 1 per 1000.

- Patients typically present with weight loss before the age of 40 years, with a peak age of onset at 10–14 years. They are ketosis prone, and may present with ketoacidosis (➲ see Diabetic ketoacidosis, p. 677).
- Results from absolute lack of insulin secretion following destruction of β cells in pancreatic islets by autoantibodies.
- Autoantibodies are detectable in 80–90% of newly diagnosed patients and are directed against cytoplasm of islet cells, insulin and most commonly glutamic acid decarboxylase (GAD 65).
- Other autoimmune disorders (e.g. coeliac disease, hypothyroidism and Addison's disease) occur more commonly in patients with type 1 diabetes.
- Major genetic susceptibility is associated with HLA class II alleles. 85% of patients with type 1 diabetes do not, however, have a family history in first-degree relatives, although there is a 30% risk if both parents are affected, with 30–70% concordance for identical twins.
- Treatment is with life-long insulin.

* Joint first authors.

Type 2

90% of adults with diabetes.

- This heterogeneous group of disorders develops when insulin secretion fails to control chronic hyperglycaemia due to reduced insulin sensitivity.
- Diagnosis is usually made in patients above 40 years of age, although South Asians may be diagnosed as young as 25 years.
- Obesity is the most potent risk factor, and results from complex interactions between environmental factors and multiple diabetogenic genes. People with a positive family history are two to six times more likely to develop type 2 diabetes. Type 2 diabetes is six times more common in South Asians and three times more common in people with African/African-Caribbean origin.
- Treatment is started with diet, lifestyle and oral agents like metformin.

Other causes of diabetes

- Monogenic diabetes (maturity onset diabetes of the young [MODY]) is the commonest variant resulting from inherited or spontaneous mutations in a single gene.

MODY is suspected when:

- Patients develop diabetes under the age of 6 months.
- There is significant family history of diabetes.
- There is mild to moderate fasting hyperglycaemia (5.5–8 mmol/L) without ketoacidosis.
- Features of insulin resistance (e.g. obesity or acanthosis nigricans) are absent in patients labelled as type 2 diabetes.
- There is persistent C-peptide secretion 3 years after diagnosis in absence of autoantibodies in patients labelled as type 1.

For genetic causes of diabetes, see Table 19.1.

Table 19.1 Genetic causes of diabetes

Disorder (% of cases)	Mutation in gene encoding/ chromosome	Features and management
MODY 1 (10%)	Hepatocyte nuclear factor-4α (HNF-4α) on chromosome 20	Treated with sulfonylurea initially; may need insulin with disease progression.
MODY 2 (32%)	Glucokinase on chromosome 7	Slightly elevated fasting blood glucose often identified on screening and rarely requires treatment.
MODY 3 (52%)	HNF-1α on chr. 12	Diabetes develops in late teens or early twenties and responds well to sulfonylurea.
MODY 5	HNF-1β on chr. 17	Most common phenotype is renal cysts and diabetes syndrome (RCAD).
Neonatal diabetes	Monogenic with mutations in more than 15 genes reported	Diabetes occurring in the first 6 months of life.

- Pancreatic diabetes: following pancreatitis, surgery, trauma, neoplasia or destruction of pancreas in haemochromatosis and cystic fibrosis.
- Gestational diabetes mellitus (GDM): ➲ see Chapter 23, Gestational diabetes, p. 799 and Table 23.2.
- Associated with endocrinopathies including Cushing's syndrome, acromegaly, glucagonoma, hyperthyroidism, polycystic ovarian syndrome.

Diagnosing diabetes mellitus

Diagnosis of DM is dependent on the plasma glucose level after an overnight fast (fasting) or following an oral glucose tolerance test (OGTT), which includes a fasting glucose level plus a glucose 2 hours after 75 g oral glucose (Table 19.2).

Table 19.2 Diagnosis of diabetes mellitus

Diabetes mellitus confirmed	Impaired glucose tolerance (IGT)	Impaired fasting glucose (IFG)
Fasting glucose ≥ 7.0 mmol/L	Fasting plasma glucose <7.0 mmol/L and 2-hour plasma glucose 7.8–11 mmol/L.	Fasting plasma glucose 6.1–6.9 mmol/L and 2-hour plasma glucose <7.8 mmol/L.
2 hours post-OGTT glucose ≥11.1 mmol/L		
Random glucose ≥11.1 mmol/L		
HbA1c ≥6.5% (48 mmol/mol) if symptoms present for >2 months		

Glycosylated haemoglobin (HbA1c):

- Is a measure of non-enzymatic glycosylation of the haemoglobin within red blood cells.
- Correlates well with mean blood glucose (BG) levels over the previous 8–12 weeks (the life span of a red blood cell).
- May not be reliable in conditions like haemoglobinopathies (reduced RBC lifespan), pregnancy, chronic kidney disease (CKD), chronic liver disease, anaemia, and in diagnosis of pancreatic or type 1 diabetes. In some of these instances fructosamine levels are more reliable.

Prognosis

Patients with type 1 diabetes have shorter life span, with men living 11 years less and women 13 years less than those without diabetes. Mortality is also increased in type 2 diabetes, and depends on the age of diagnosis. Cardiovascular disease is the major cause of death (44% in type 1 and 52% in type 2). The other major cause of death is kidney disease (21% in type 1 and 11% in type 2). For every 1% increase in HbA1c, risk of death from a diabetes-related cause increases by 21.

Management

Lifestyle changes and dietary advice

Recommended for people who are overweight (BMI >25kg/m^2), impaired fasting glucose (IFG) or impaired glucose tolerance (IGT), in addition to those with confirmed diabetes.

For antidiabetic medication, see Table 19.3.

Insulin

Insulin treatment is essential in type 1 diabetes and in type 2 diabetes once there is β-cell failure.

- Depending on duration of action insulin may be short acting (duration of action 2–4 hours, e.g. insulin aspart, glulysine), intermediate acting (6–8 hours, e.g. isophane insulin), or long acting (12–24 hours, e.g. insulin glargine, detemir, degludec). Short-acting insulin is used with meals and for IV infusion during hyperglycaemic emergencies, and for management of glucose levels during surgery.
- Analogue insulin is less hypoglycaemic and therefore preferred over human insulin.

Table 19.3 Antidiabetic medication

Class of anti-diabetics with examples	Mechanism of action	Features
Biguanides (e.g. metformin)	Increases insulin sensitivity in liver and muscle and decreases hepatic glucose output.	Weight neutral. Has glycaemia independent cardiovascular benefit. Often the initial treatment in type 2 diabetes. Avoided in renal impairment (dose reduction for CKD stage 3, stopped when CKD stage 4). Gastrointestinal side effects like bloating, nausea and diarrhoea are common.
Sulfonylureas (e.g. gliclazide, glibenclamide)	Increases insulin secretion by binding to K-ATP(SUR) channels on β-cells.	Causes weight gain. Risk of hypoglycaemia (caution: vulnerable patients, e.g. elderly).
Thiazolinedinediones (e.g. pioglitazone)	Increases insulin sensitivity by activating peroxisome proliferator activator receptor (PPAR-γ), in turn increasing expression of glucose transporters.	Pioglitazone may cause fluid retention (caution: heart failure) and osteoporotic fractures.
Incretin based drugs 1. Glucagon-like peptide-1 (GLP-1) analogues – SC injections (e.g. exenatide, liraglutide). 2. Di-peptidyl peptidase 4 (DPP4) inhibitors (e.g. sitagliptin, linagliptin)	Incretin hormones (e.g. GLP1), are released by the gut in response to oral nutrients. They increase food induced insulin secretion, but are quickly degraded by enzymes called dipeptidyl peptidase IV (DPP IV).	Causes weight loss. GLP1 analogues are used in patients with BMI ≥35. Caution: if history of pancreatitis and pancreatic malignancy. DPP IV inhibitors are oral agents that prolong the action of endogenous GLP1. Linagliptin is the only DPP-4 inhibitor, which may be used in renal impairment. Side effects include nausea, vomiting.
α-Glucosidase inhibitors (e.g. acarbose)	Taken with food, inhibits enzymatic degradation of complex carbohydrates reducing intestinal absorption.	Rarely used as can give rise to uncomfortable postprandial fullness, flatulence and diarrhoea.
Sodium glucose co-transporter 2 (SGLT2) inhibitors (e.g. empagliflozin, dapagliflozin, canagliflozin)	Inhibits glucose re-absorption from kidneys facilitating loss of glucose in urine.	Urinary infections may be a concern. Contraindicated in renal impairment.
Meglitinides (e.g. repaglinide)	Weakly binds to K-ATP(SUR) on β-cells and increases insulin secretion.	Used to control post-prandial blood glucose.

NICE guidance on glucose management in type 2 diabetes

NICE recommends individualised HbA1c goals for patients. Metformin is started after diagnosis unless contraindicated (e.g. poor renal function, eGFR<30 mL/min/1.73m^2) or not tolerated for GI side effects. While on a single drug, goal for HbA1c is 48 mmol/mol (the goal is higher, 53 mmol/mol if a hypoglycaemia-inducing drug like sulfonylurea is selected as first treatment). Usually, a second or a third drug should be added if the HbA1c increases above 58 mmol/mol. For patients started on metformin, choices for second drug include DPP-4 inhibitors, pioglitazone, sulfonylurea or SGLT2-inhibitors.

Insulin is indicated when HbA1c goals are not achieved with three drugs (or two drugs when patients are not on metformin). GLP-1 analogue treatment may be used instead of insulin in patients with a BMI >35 kg/m^2, or if insulin has serious impact on occupation (e.g. driving restrictions for driving group 2 vehicles [1]). When starting patients on insulin, human insulin (like neutral protamine Hagedorn [NPH] insulin) is used and may be changed to analogue insulin (Lantus®), if hypoglycaemia or inadequate control is a problem.

NICE guidance on management of type 1 diabetes

Patients should be started on basal bolus insulin (long-acting basal insulin levemir alongside bolus of short-acting insulin for meals) at diagnosis. Use of continuous SC insulin infusion (CSII, or insulin pumps) is recommended early for patients with recurrent hypoglycaemia, impaired hypoglycaemia awareness and inability to achieve HbA1c of 8.5% (69 mmol/mol) with multiple daily injections.

Reference

1. https://www.gov.uk/guidance/diabetes-mellitus-assessing-fitness-to-drive

Further reading

1. Definition and diagnosis of diabetes mellitus and intermediate hyperglycaemia: Report of a WHO/IDF consultation (January 2006). https://www.who.int/diabetes/publications/Definition%20and%20diagnosis%20of%20diabetes_new.pdf.
2. Diabetes in the UK 2012 (April 2012). *Key statistics on Diabetes*. London: Diabetes UK.
3. NICE. Type 1 diabetes in adults: diagnosis and management. NICE guideline NG28. Type 1 diabetes, August 2015. https://www.nice.org.uk/guidance/ng17 and Type 2 diabetes in adults: management. NICE guideline CG28 (December 2015). https://www.nice.org.uk/guidance/ng28.

Complications of diabetes

Diabetes complications can be microvascular, like retinopathy, nephropathy or neuropathy, or macrovascular, like hypertension, peripheral vascular disease, coronary artery disease and cerebrovascular disease. Tighter control of blood glucose delays the onset and reduces the frequency of microvascular complications in diabetes. Cardiovascular complications do not correlate with hyperglycaemia and their benefit in preventing macrovascular complications remain controversial.

Diabetic eye disease

➲ See Chapter 18, Diabetic eye disease, p. 658 and Figures 18.9, 18.10 and 18.11.

Diabetic renal disease

➲ See Chapter 16, Diabetes, p. 573.

Diabetic neuropathy

➲ See Chapter 17, Neuropathy, p. 632 and Tables 17.6 and 17.7.

Neuropathy affects 40% of patients with diabetes. Hyperglycaemia leads to abnormal polyol metabolism and oxidative stress causing abnormal glycation of nerve cell proteins. Ischaemia secondary to vasoconstriction leads to nerve cell loss, abnormal nerve conduction and patchy regeneration. Neuropathy may be sensory, motor or autonomic.

Peripheral sensory neuropathy

Commonly affects the toes, with loss of temperature, pain and joint position sense, and dysaesthesia. The most common sign in diabetic distal polyneuropathy is loss of ankle reflexes. Painful neuropathy is treated with duloxetine, or amitriptyline if duloxetine is contraindicated. Pregabalin is used as second line agent either alone or in combination with amitriptyline. Opioids like tramadol are often required as add-on treatment.

Autonomic neuropathy

Common in diabetes and suggestive features include postural hypotension, gustatory sweating, anhidrosis, urinary retention/overflow incontinence, diarrhoea and reduced pupillary light reflex. Specific problems of autonomic neuropathy include:

- Erectile dysfunction: affects 40% of males with diabetes.
- Gastroparesis: affects 30–40% of patients with diabetes and presents with nausea, vomiting, early satiety, post meal bloating and upper abdominal pain. Correction of electrolyte abnormalities, good

glycaemic control and discontinuation of agents delaying gastric emptying like GLP1 agonists are the recommended management strategies. Treatment with gastric prokinetic agents like metoclopramide or erythromycin may be necessary.

Diabetic foot

Diabetic foot pathology is the result of a combination of peripheral vascular disease and neuropathy, and affects 5–10% of patients with diabetes.

1. Neuropathic ulcers: warm foot with intact pulses, reduced sensation with ulceration and callus formation at pressure points. Local necrosis and osteomyelitis may be present.
2. Ischaemic (often neuro-ischaemic): cold foot and absent peripheral pulses.

Charcot foot

➲ See Chapter 20, Charcot joint, p. 750.

Infected foot

Common in patients with diabetic foot ulcers. Beta-haemolytic streptococci and *Staphylococcus aureus* are the most common pathogens. When deep soft tissue collections are present, imaging is required to rule out osteomyelitis.

Management

In addition to local wound management, off-loading of pressure ulcers, management of vascular insufficiency and antibiotics if there is evidence of infection are important.

Macrovascular disease

Cardiovascular (CV) diseases including ischaemic heart disease, strokes and peripheral vascular disease are responsible for 44% and 52% of death in people with type 1 and type 2 diabetes, respectively. Patients with diabetes have a two-fold increased risk of strokes, and the risk of MI is similar to that of a non-diabetic after a previous MI. As diabetes predisposes to cardiovascular disease, it is recommended that high risk patients (e.g. patients with hypertension, Asian, etc.) with normal HbA1c should undergo OGTT, to exclude early changes of altered glucose homeostasis.

- Management of hyperglycaemia, including early initiation of insulin does not reduce the overall risk of macrovascular complications. A 1% reduction of HbA1c is associated with a 15% relative risk reduction in non-fatal MI, but has no benefit on stroke or all-cause mortality.
- Albuminuria is the strongest predictor of CV events and can be used alongside risk engines (like the United Kingdom Prospective Diabetes Study [UKPDS]) for accurate estimation of risk in asymptomatic diabetic patients.
- Among oral antidiabetics, the agent of choice for modest benefit on risk of MI is metformin; sulfonylureas reduce the risk, but are associated with weight gain and hypoglycaemia. Empagliflozin, and possibly other SGLT2 inhibitors are the only other antidiabetics that may have glucose independent cardiovascular benefit.
- Lipid modification (➲ see Chapter 1, Lipids and atherosclerosis, p. 20 and Figures 1.4, 1.5, 1.6, 1.7 and Box 1.2).
- CV risk reduction strategies like anti-hypertensives and statins are recommended in type 2 diabetes. Statins should be used to reduce total and LDL cholesterol levels (recommended levels: TC ≤4mmol/L, LDL C ≤2 mmol/L). The protective effect of HDL is lost in diabetes; therefore, treatment aimed at increasing HDL levels is not useful. BP should be maintained at <140/85 (<130/80 with coexistent renal disease). Anti-hypertensive drugs acting on the renin–angiotensin–aldosterone system are preferred for their additional benefit with albuminuria.
- Antiplatelet drugs (e.g. aspirin) are recommended for secondary, but not for primary prevention.
- Myocardial revascularisation strategies in diabetes is challenging, because of more diffuse atherosclerosis in the epicardial vessels and higher rate of restenosis following percutaneous

coronary intervention. In diabetic patients with multivessel disease CABG is preferred over PCI. In PCI, drug-eluting stents are preferred over bare metal stents.

Further reading

1. Ryden L, et al. The task force on diabetes and cardiovascular diseases of the European Society of Cardiology (ESC) and of the European Association for the Study of Diabetes (EASD). *Eur Heart J*. 2007; 28:88–136.

Emergencies in diabetes

Diabetic ketoacidosis

Diabetic ketoacidosis (DKA) presents acutely with dehydration, nausea, abdominal pain and weight loss. It may be the first presentation of type 1 diabetes, or may be precipitated by inadequate insulin replacement, intercurrent infection, MI or stroke in these patients. Mortality is high unless managed appropriately. In DKA there is relative or absolute insulin deficiency, with low peripheral glucose uptake and increased hepatic gluconeogenesis and glycogenolysis. Raised counter-regulatory hormones like epinephrine, cortisol and glucagon favour lipolysis. The fatty acids are used by hepatocytes as an alternate source of energy. Acidic intermediates and ketone bodies are by-products of fatty acid metabolism.

Features include:

1. Hyperglycaemia: capillary BG >11mmol/L.
2. Ketonaemia: blood ketones >3 mmol/L or urine ketones > ++.
3. Acidosis: venous pH <7.3, bicarbonate <15mmol/L.

Fixed rate IV insulin infusion should be commenced immediately. Fluid replacement is with isotonic 0.9% sodium chloride supplemented with potassium to maintain levels around 5.5 mmol/L.

Aims of treatment in the first 6 hours include:

1. ↓ Blood ketone level by 0.5 mmol/L/hour.
2. ↑ Venous bicarbonate level by 3 mmol/L/hour.
3. ↓ Blood glucose level by 3 mmol/L/hour.

IV insulin may be replaced with SC insulin once the patient is clinically stable and blood ketones <0.3 mmol/L.

Hyperglycaemic hyperosmolar state

Hyperglycaemic hyperosmolar state (HHS) is usually seen in the elderly, has a higher mortality than DKA and may be associated with MI, stroke or peripheral arterial thrombosis.

- Less acute presentation over days with hypovolaemia, high plasma osmolality >320 mOsm/kg (sodium and urea typically high), and marked hyperglycaemia without significant ketonaemia or acidosis. Intensive fluid replacement with isotonic 0.9% sodium chloride (typically 3–6 L/12 hours) is the cornerstone of management.
- Correction of hyperglycaemia should be gradual (↓ blood glucose typically <5 mmol/hour). A fixed rate insulin infusion is started only if there is ketonaemia or BG level has stopped falling with IV fluid.
- Prophylactic anticoagulation is recommended.

Hypoglycaemia

Hypoglycaemia is defined as BG <4 mmol/L and is more common in diabetes, especially with insulin treatment. Warning symptoms like sweating, palpitations, tremor, peri-oral tingling and feeling hungry occur with BG levels between 3 and 4 mmol/L. These symptoms are often lost in long-standing diabetic patients, making them more vulnerable to severe hypoglycaemia (when help is required to recover, e.g. resultant unconsciousness). In type 1 diabetes hypoglycaemia is suspected with HbA1c <6.1% (43 mmol/mol), or when lower than expected from self-monitored levels. Structured education programmes, insulin pumps, pancreas or islet transplant are strategies for managing hypoglycaemia unawareness. Patients with ≥2 episodes (or ≥1 for group 2 drivers) of severe hypoglycaemia in a year must be advised not to drive and to inform the DVLA (➲ see Reference [1], p. 675).

Thyroid

The thyroid gland is composed of two lateral lobes with a mid-line isthmus. It is further subdivided into pseudo-lobules formed of follicles. These consist of follicular cells that synthesise and secrete thyroglobulin and thyroid hormones into the central colloid for storage. Situated between the follicular cells are parafollicular cells (also known as C-cells), which secrete calcitonin. Blood supply is from the superior and inferior thyroid arteries and each follicle is surrounded by a rich capillary network. The thyroid is the only source of thyroxine (T4), which follicular cells synthesise using dietary iodine. They also form smaller amounts of tri-iodothyronine (T3), although the majority of circulating T3 (80%) derives from peripheral de-iodination of T4 by the liver and kidney. Circulating T3 and T4 are bound to plasma proteins (thyroid-binding globulin [TBG], prealbumin and albumin). Only the free or unbound hormone (referred to as fT4 or fT3) is available to tissues. Total hormone levels are dependent on TBG and changes in this can result in apparent changes in thyroid hormone levels, whereas levels of free hormones correlate more closely with the metabolic state.

For conditions affecting TBG, see Table 19.4.

Table 19.4 Conditions that affect TBG

Conditions that raise TBG	Conditions that lower TBG
Pregnancy	Chronic liver disease
Use of oestrogen containing oral contraceptives	Systemic illness
Acute intermittent porphyria	Steroids

Hypothalamic–pituitary–thyroid axis

Control of thyroid hormone release is governed closely by feedback from circulating thyroid hormones:

- Detection of low circulating T3 and T4 results in hypothalamic release of thyrotropin-releasing hormone (TRH).
- TRH causes thyroid-stimulating hormone (TSH) release from the anterior pituitary gland.
- TSH increases iodide uptake from the plasma and stimulates thyroid peroxidase activity, resulting in greater thyroid hormone production.
- Circulating T3 and T4 negatively feedback on both the pituitary gland and hypothalamus, leading to reduced secretion of TRH and TSH.

Thyroid investigations

Blood tests

Given the interaction between the hypothalamus, and pituitary and thyroid glands, TSH will be suppressed in hyperthyroidism where circulating thyroid hormones are increased. Conversely, underactivity of the thyroid gland will be associated with a raised TSH (see Table 19.5).

Table 19.5 Summary of thyroid function test results in disease

Condition	TSH	fT3	fT4
Primary hyperthyroidism, i.e. due to Graves' disease, toxic nodule	↓	↑	↑
Subclinical hyperthyroidism	↓	↔	↔
Primary hypothyroidism	↑	↓	↓
Secondary hypothyroidism, i.e. due to pituitary failing to secrete TSH	↓	↓	↓
Failure of peripheral conversion	↔	↓	↔

Antibodies are useful in determining the cause of thyroid dysfunction and include TSH receptor antibodies (more commonly associated with hyperthyroidism in Graves' disease) and thyroid peroxidase (TPO) antibodies (seen in Hashimoto's thyroiditis).

Imaging

Ultrasound

US is used to determine thyroid size and to characterise any nodules that may have been identified on examination. Fine needle aspiration cytology may be performed to distinguish between benign and malignant nodules if there are any suspicious features on US (➲ see Thyroid nodules, p. 682).

Scintigraphy

Radiolabelled iodine or sodium pertechnetate may be used to quantify cellular metabolic activity in nodules. Results of uptake scan include:

- Homogenous increase in uptake: Graves' thyrotoxicosis.
- Increased uptake in a nodule with normal/reduced uptake in the remaining gland (hot nodule): toxic nodule.
- Reduced uptake in a nodule implies metabolically inactive (cold nodule): suspicious of malignancy.
- Homogenous reduced uptake: thyroiditis.

Computed tomography

CT provides additional anatomical information, and is especially useful when assessing a retrosternal or retrotracheal thyroid gland.

Thyrotoxicosis

Thyrotoxicosis results from exposure to excess thyroid hormones. It is 10 times more common in women than in men. It may result from over-activity of the thyroid gland itself (hyperthyroidism) or excess thyroid hormone production due to another stimulus.

Causes of hyperthyroidism

- Intrinsic over-activity of the thyroid gland is the most common cause.
  - Graves' disease: over-stimulation of thyroid from stimulating autoantibodies to TSH receptors.
  - Toxic nodules with autonomous function (solitary or multiple).
- Excessive thyroid stimulation.
  This is rare. Causes include pituitary thyrotroph adenoma, pituitary thyroid hormone resistance and trophoblastic tumours producing hCG with homology to TSH.
- Non-hyperthyroid causes:
  - Ectopic thyroid tissue (e.g. metastatic thyroid carcinoma).
  - Surreptitious use of exogenous thyroid hormone.
  - Transient thyrotoxic phase in inflammation of the thyroid or thyroiditis (➲ see Thyroiditis, p. 682).

Irrespective of its aetiology, the signs and symptoms of thyrotoxicosis result from both the direct effects of excess thyroid hormone production and the resulting increased sympathetic drive.

Symptoms of thyrotoxicosis

Hypermetabolism results in weight loss, increased appetite, heat intolerance, palpitations (atrial fibrillation and supraventricular tachycardia), diarrhoea and anxiety.

- Tiredness, weakness and lethargy may result from skeletal myopathy. More rarely, chorea and periodic paralysis (a painless paralysis, more common in men and the Asian population) are described.
- Oligomenorrhoea and altered sexual function (reduced libido) may occur.

Signs of thyrotoxicosis

- Hyperdynamic circulation with warm peripheries, bounding, fast pulse, palmar erythema and sweatiness of the skin.
- Fine tremor.
- Hyper-reflexia.
- Hair loss.
- Onycholysis.

Investigations in a patient presenting with thyrotoxicosis

- TSH, fT4, fT3 levels and thyroid antibodies (see Table 19.5).
- A radionucleotide uptake scan may be performed where toxic nodule or toxic goitre is suspected.

Management

- The metabolic effects of hyperthyroidism should be controlled with either β-blockers or, where contraindicated, calcium channel blockers. Propranolol (a non-selective β-blocker) is often preferred at a dose of 20–80 mg TDS.
- Antithyroid medications:
  - Thionamides (e.g. carbimazole and propylthiouracil [PTU]) inhibit thyroid peroxidase, necessary for thyroid hormone synthesis.
  - A higher daily dose is used initially with gradual down-titration according to fT3, fT4 and TSH every 2–3 months.
  - Alternatively, a 'block and replace' regime may be used, whereby antithyroid medications are given to completely suppress endogenous thyroid hormone production, with thyroxine given alongside this to ensure sufficient levels of T4.
  - In pregnancy, TSH level is suppressed (➲ see Chapter 23, Hyperemesis gravidarum, p. 806 and Table 23.4). However, high level of free T4 or T3 is treated to reduce risk of early miscarriage. In the first trimester, PTU is recommended because of uncertain risk of teratogenicity with carbimazole. While clinical practice may differ, current guidelines advise switching to carbimazole, thereafter due to the reported, although low, risk of hepatotoxicity with PTU (although this risk is the same across the whole of pregnancy). While both PTU and carbimazole can be used while breastfeeding, PTU is favoured due to its lower concentration in breastmilk.
  - Important side effects include agranulocytosis, seen in 0.1–0.5% of patients, typically presenting with fever and oropharyngeal infective symptoms. Obstructive jaundice and rarely fulminant liver failure can occur with PTU. Patients should be provided with written information regarding the above.

Once the patient has been rendered biochemically euthyroid, further definitive treatment will depend on the underlying cause and may include radioactive iodine therapy (RAI) or surgery.

For thyrotoxic storm, see Box 19.1.

Graves' disease

Graves' disease is an autoimmune condition associated with hyperthyroidism, orbitopathy, goitre and pretibial myxoedema. It results from TSH receptor antibodies stimulating TSH receptors, leading to increased thyroid hormone production and stimulating thyroid growth. It is the commonest causes of thyrotoxicosis in iodine replete areas, with a prevalence of 100–200 per 100,000 population. Genetic susceptibility is evidenced by the presence of familial disease clusters, and strong monozygotic twin concordance (20–40%). Specific genes in the HLA region on chromosome 6 interact with environmental stimuli, to result in the condition. Patients with Graves' disease present with symptoms of thyrotoxicosis, ocular manifestations and pretibial myxoedema.

Box 19.1 Thyrotoxic storm

- This is a rare life-threatening condition due to overwhelming hypermetabolism.
- Patients present with high fever, tachycardia, diarrhoea, vomiting and rarely altered consciousness/coma.
- May be precipitated by acute illness (e.g. infection), or following RAI or surgery.
- Treatment is often in a high-dependency setting. Supportive measures include cooling and fluid resuscitation often via central access. A full septic screen should be performed and broad spectrum antibiotics started. Emergency sedation may be required. Glucose should be monitored 4-hourly and corrected.

Antithyroid measures include:

- β-blockers and propylthiouracil.
- IV hydrocortisone to prevent conversion of T4 to T3.

Lugol's iodine after the first dose of PTU. This blocks iodination in the thyroid gland, and thus further production of thyroid hormone.

Dysthyroid eye disease

Dysthyroid eye disease (TED) is a potentially serious complication of Graves' disease. It is more common in women and in those who smoke, and precedes the onset of thyrotoxic symptoms in 20% of patients. Deposition of glycosaminoglycans, lymphocytic infiltration and periorbital fat deposition results in localised swelling of the extra-ocular muscles causing eyelid retraction, proptosis (forward protrusion of the orbit), exophthalmos (as evidenced by visible sclera below the iris) and complex ophthalmoplegia. Sight-threatening complications of TED may include corneal ulceration and compressive optic neuropathy.

Management of TED

- Acute TED presenting with loss of acuity or colour vision is an emergency, and requires urgent ophthalmology review. Initial treatment includes systemic steroids. Orbital decompression may become necessary.
- If corneal exposure occurs, adequate lubrication is essential, as well as taping of the eyelids during sleep.
- Residual strabismus or lid retraction following medical treatment may require surgical correction.
- All patients should be referred to the ophthalmology clinic.
- Patients should be advised to stop smoking.
- While TED is not an absolute contraindication for RAI, ophthalmology colleagues should be closely consulted prior to its administration. Short course of steroids and avoiding post-treatment hypothyroidism can prevent progression of eye disease, after treatment.

Pretibial myxoedema

Pretibial myxoedema is caused by deposition of hyaluronic acid in the dermis. The lesions are typically raised, waxy and yellow brown, often associated with hyperhidrosis. Prominent hair follicles give it the classical *peau d'orange* appearance. While rare, they are more common in patients who have thyroid acropachy or TED. Treatment includes compressive bandaging and topical steroids in severe cases.

Goitre

The term goitre refers to any enlargement of the thyroid gland, and may be multinodular or a simple smooth goitre.

Causes of goitre

- A physiological smooth goitre is often found in pregnancy, as well as in areas where iodine deficiency is endemic. Patients may be euthyroid, hypo- or hyperthyroid.
- Pathological causes of a diffuse goitre include syndromes resulting in thyroiditis and medication (e.g. amiodarone [➔ see Amiodarone and its effect on the thyroid gland, p. 684] and lithium).
- Multinodular goitres may be non-toxic or toxic (30% of goitres).

Investigations

- TSH and free thyroid hormones to assess thyroid status.
- Flow-volume loop to assess for tracheal obstruction (➲ see Flow volume loops, p. 378 and Figure 11.4), and CT scan to look for tracheal compression.

Management

- Hyperthyroidism should be treated with antithyroid medication (➲ see Management, p. 680).
- Definitive surgical intervention may be warranted where significant obstruction is found, as evidenced by symptoms (shortness of breath or persistent cough, particularly when recumbent) or flow-volume loop/imaging.

Thyroid nodules

Thyroid nodules are usually benign (90%) including colloid nodules, follicular adenomas or nodules with lymphocytic infiltration. Malignant nodules include papillary cancers (75%), follicular (15%), medullary (5%) and others (lymphoma, anaplastic and metastasis). Approach to thyroid nodules include:

- Clinical characterisation assessing size, consistency, lymphadenopathy, severity of compressive symptoms.
- Biochemical tests to check thyroid status.
- US characterisation: US-guided fine needle aspiration is recommended for most nodules.
- Thyroid uptake scan (➲ see Scintigraphy, p. 679).
- Cytological classification: benign nodules may need to be re-assessed after a few months. Suspicious or malignant nodules should be referred for surgical assessment.
- Surgery is necessary for nodules larger than 4 cm, if they are rapidly growing or if there is suspicious or malignant cytology.
- Calcitonin level is raised in medullary thyroid cancer (MTC). MTC may be part of MEN2 (➲ see MEN2, p. 701). Familial MTC is common and patients should undergo testing for re-arranged during transfection (RET) proto-oncogene.

Thyroiditis

Thyroiditis refers to any inflammatory process affecting the thyroid gland and typically results in an acute hyperthyroid phase, with subsequent hypothyroid stage.

Post-partum thyroiditis

This may present as transient hyperthyroidism, transient hypothyroidism or transient hyperthyroidism followed by hypothyroidism. Patients may have a painless goitre or no obvious thyroid swelling. It occurs within 1 year post-partum, although the majority of patients present within the first 6 months following delivery. It has strong association with type 1 diabetes. 50% of patients with high TPO antibody develop post-partum thyroiditis, suggesting a possible role of autoantibodies.

De Quervain's thyroiditis (subacute thyroiditis)

De Quervain's thyroiditis usually occurs after a viral upper respiratory tract infection. Patients complain of fever and a painful thyroid gland, which may or may not be enlarged. Characteristically, there is an initial hyperthyroid phase, followed by a hypothyroid phase. Investigations show reduced uptake on radioisotope scan and a raised ESR. Treatment includes NSAIDs (ibuprofen 400 mg TDS with proton pump inhibitor cover) and steroids if necessary (prednisolone 40 mg OD reducing over a 4-week period). β-blockers can be used to control the initial thyrotoxic symptoms. Antithyroid medications are not indicated as symptoms result from thyroid hormone release, as opposed to excess thyroid hormone synthesis.

Suppurative infections

Suppurative infections may cause an acute thyroiditis (organisms include staphylococcal and streptococcal infections, tuberculosis and fungal infections). Patients present with symptoms of sepsis, along with a diffusely enlarged, tender goitre that is usually the predominant symptom. Patients may present with symptoms and signs of either hyper- or hypothyroidism, or be euthyroid. Treatment includes antibiotics and steroids, as well as monitoring of thyroid function.

Riedel's thyroiditis

Riedel's thyroiditis is rare and caused by a chronic fibrosing process, leading to a characteristic 'woody' sensation on palpation of the thyroid gland. It is associated with fibrosis of other structures including salivary glands and bile ducts (sclerosing cholangitis) and retroperitoneal fibrosis. Patients are euthyroid. Surgery may be required for symptomatic management.

Other chronic causes of thyroiditis

- Hashimoto's thyroiditis is an autoimmune condition, whereby lymphocytes and plasma cells infiltrate follicles, resulting in damage to the follicular membrane, and hyperplasia. An irregularly textured goitre results. TPO antibodies are found in >90% of patients and patients typically present with hypothyroidism.
- Atrophic thyroiditis is thought to represent end-stage thyroid disease and is seen in patients who are TPO antibody positive, without the presence of a palpable goitre.
- Management for both Hashimoto's and atrophic thyroiditis includes replacement of T4 and monitoring of any nodules for suspicious change.

Hypothyroidism

Hypothyroidism is caused by reduced levels of circulating thyroid hormones. It is more common in women than men with prevalence of 2% and 0.2%, respectively. In iodine-replete areas, autoimmune disease is the commonest cause of hypothyroidism.

Causes

- Primary hypothyroidism (pathology affecting the thyroid gland itself):
  - Autoimmune hypothyroidism (Hashimoto's thyroiditis, atrophic thyroiditis).
  - Post-radiation.
  - Iodine deficiency.
  - Drugs, e.g. lithium and amiodarone.
  - Infiltrative processes (e.g. sarcoidosis and amyloidosis).
  - Congenital defects, e.g. failure of thyroid gland formation.
- Secondary hypothyroidism: this is rare, occurring in 1:20,000 to 1:80,000 of the general population. It results from hypothalamic-pituitary dysfunction leading to a failure of TSH production. Causes include:
  - Pituitary mass lesions – these can result in pituitary apoplexy, interruption of hypothalamic–pituitary circulation and can disrupt function of pituitary thyrotrophs.
  - Other central lesions affecting hypothalamic-pituitary circulation, e.g. meningiomas, craniopharyngiomas, metastatic lesions.
  - Infiltrative processes, e.g. sarcoidosis, lymphocytic hypophysitis.
  - Radiation therapy targeted at the hypothalamus or pituitary.

Symptoms and signs

- General: lethargy, fatigue and cold intolerance.
- Cardiovascular: bradycardia and hypotension.
- Gastrointestinal: constipation is common and weight gain is typical despite reduction in appetite.
- Dermatological: alopecia, dry skin, and coarsening of hair.
- Neuropsychiatric: slowing of cognition and low mood.

Investigations

- Thyroid function tests: raised TSH and low fT4 in primary hypothyroidism; both TSH and fT4 low in secondary hypothyroidism (➲ see Thyroid investigations, p. 678 and Table 19.5).
- Elevated cholesterol level.

Management

- Thyroid hormone replacement requires levothyroxine treatment. A typical starting dose is 50mcg OD. The dose should be adjusted according to TSH and fT4, aiming for a normal TSH in primary hypothyroidism, and normal fT4 in secondary hypothyroidism. Thyroxine dose is increased in pregnancy by 25–50%.
- Caution should be used in elderly patients and those with a cardiac history, as a sudden increase in metabolic rate could result in cardiac decompensation.

For myxoedema, see Box 19.2.

Box 19.2 Myxoedema

- Rare, life-threatening state of decompensated hypothyroidism.
- More common in elderly and often precipitated by acute insult, e.g. infection, myocardial infarction.

Signs and symptoms

- General: hypothermia.
- Neuropsychiatric: preceding depression, hallucinations and delusions ('myxoedema madness'). Seizures occur in up to 20% of patients.
- Cardiovascular: bradycardia with low voltage complexes on ECG.
- Respiratory: pleural effusions, hypoventilation due to reduced respiratory drive.
- Metabolic: hypoglycaemia (resulting from hypothyroidism itself or concomitant adrenal insufficiency) along with evidence of renal impairment.

Management

Typically takes place in an intensive care setting.

- Slow rewarming, aiming for no more than 0.5°C/hour.
- Oxygen to maintain saturations >94% and IV fluids to correct hypovolaemia.
- Low threshold for hydrocortisone 100 mg QDS IM or continue IV if hypoadrenalism suspected.
- Thyroid replacement: either NG or IV replacement of T4 and T3, switching to oral levothyroxine once the patient has sufficiently recovered. Protocol varies and is done under the supervision of a senior endocrinologist.

Amiodarone and its effect on the thyroid gland

A large proportion of amiodarone is comprised of iodine (37% by weight), and it is structurally very similar to thyroxine, T4. It has a variable half-life ranging up to 100 days. Total iodine stores may remain elevated for up to 9 months after discontinuation of the drug. Due to its similarity to thyroxine, up to 20% of patients taking amiodarone experience thyroid dysfunction.

During the first month of treatment with amiodarone, serum T4 levels rise by 20–40% as amiodarone prevents entry of T4 and T3 into peripheral tissues. Amiodarone also inhibits deiodination, reducing peripheral conversion of T4 to T3, and thus leading to lower levels of circulating T3. Pituitary TSH typically rises over this time due to reduction in iodination. As well as these initial changes, more persistent dysfunction may be seen.

Amiodarone-induced thyrotoxicosis

Type 1 amiodarone-induced thyrotoxicosis (AIT)

This typically affects patients with pre-existing thyroid dysfunction and is seen in areas of low iodine intake. It results from excess thyroid hormone synthesis due to the high iodine content of amiodarone. A goitre is frequently present. Radioiodine uptake scan is normal. This, like thyrotoxicosis in Grave's disease, is treated with carbimazole or propylthiouracil.

Type 2 AIT

This is the result of a destructive thyroiditis, caused by the toxic effects of amiodarone in patients with a previously normal thyroid gland. Damage to follicular cells results in release of preformed thyroid hormone leading to thyrotoxicosis. Radioiodine uptake is reduced. Treatment with glucocorticoids (e.g. prednisolone) reduces the conversion of T4 to T3 and reduces inflammation.

Amiodarone-induced hypothyroidism

The Wolff Chaikoff effect describes the phenomenon whereby a large iodine load prevents iodine organification necessary for thyroid hormone synthesis. Hence, amiodarone, with its large iodine content, inhibits thyroid hormone synthesis and can result in hypothyroidism. Following diagnosis of amiodarone-induced hypothyroidism (AIH) (by the exclusion of other causes including autoimmune disease), amiodarone should be discontinued if possible, and thyroid hormone replacement started. Even where amiodarone is stopped, supplemental thyroxine will be necessary initially due to the long half-life of amiodarone.

Further reading

1. Narajana S, Woods D, Boos C. Management of amiodarone-related thyroid problems. *Ther Adv Endocrinol Metab.* 2011; 2(3):115–26.

Pituitary gland

The pituitary gland lies in the pituitary fossa and is composed of the anterior pituitary gland (adenohypophysis) and posterior pituitary gland (neurohypophysis). Surrounding structures include the optic chiasm and III, IV and VIth cranial nerves, which lie in the cavernous sinuses laterally. Pituitary adenomas account for around 10% of all intracranial tumours and are benign lesions. They may be functioning or non-functioning. Due to the anatomy of the pituitary fossa, both may present with symptoms including headache, visual field defect (bitemporal hemianopia; ➲ see Chapter 18, Lesions at the chiasm, p. 654 and Figure 18.6) and can cause ophthalmoplegia if extending into the cavernous sinus laterally.

Hormones from the anterior pituitary gland are regulated by hormones secreted from the hypothalamus, and include prolactin, growth hormone, adrenocorticotrophic hormone (ACTH), the gonadotrophins (luteinising hormone [LH] and follicular-stimulating hormone [FSH]), and TSH. The posterior pituitary (neurohypophysis) is a continuation of the pituitary stalk at the base of the hypothalamus and contains the axonal ends of neurons projecting from the hypothalamus. The neurohypophyseal hormones, vasopressin and oxytocin, are produced in the hypothalamus and are transported down these unmyelinated axons to the posterior pituitary, where they are stored and, subsequently, released into the systemic circulation.

Functioning anterior pituitary tumours

Where pituitary adenomas derive from hormone-secreting cells of the anterior pituitary, they will result in distinct clinical pictures (see Table 19.6).

Table 19.6 Syndromes resulting from functioning anterior pituitary adenomas

Secretory cell	Hormone	Pathology from adenoma of secretory cell
Lactotroph	Prolactin	Prolactinoma
Somatotroph	Growth hormone (GH)	Acromegaly
Corticotroph	Adrenocorticotrophic hormone (ACTH)	Cushing's disease
Thyrotroph	Thyroid-stimulating hormone (TSH)	Thyrotrophinoma
Gondaotrophs	Luteinising hormone (LH), follicle stimulating hormone (FSH)	Tumours secreting LH/FSH in isolation are rare and are not typically associated with a specific pathological pattern

Data from Wass, J. and Owen, K. (eds.). *Oxford Handbook of Endocrinology and Diabetes*, Third Edition, 2014, Oxford, UK: Oxford University Press

Prolactinoma

Prolactinomas typically present with galactorrhoea (in both men and women), reduced libido, oligomenorrhoea and erectile dysfunction.

Differential diagnoses for raised prolactin level include:

- Pregnancy/breastfeeding.
- Hypothyroidism.
- Medications (including dopamine receptor antagonists, e.g. metoclopramide, domperidone, and antidepressants including TCA and SSRIs).
- Stress.
- Polycystic ovarian syndrome (PCOS); an important differential in a woman presenting with oligo- or amenorrhoea, although typically PCOS causes only minimal increases in prolactin.
- Raised prolactin can also be due to the 'stalk effect', whereby a pituitary tumour causes displacement of the pituitary stalk, removing the negative impact of dopamine on prolactin release.

Clinical examination should include visual field and cranial nerve assessment, as well as assessing for other causes of hyperprolactinaemia (e.g. acne and hirsutism in PCOS).

Investigations

These are important to ensure other anterior pituitary hormones are functioning normally, and to exclude a macroadenoma (>10 mm in size).

- Pituitary hormone profile (LH and FSH with corresponding oestrogen/testosterone, TSH and fT4 to ensure that TSH is appropriate for fT4 level, 09.00 hours cortisol with ACTH, and insulin-like growth factor 1 [IGF1]).
- Formal visual field assessment via Ophthalmology referral if any concerns regarding field defect.
- MRI pituitary to assess lesion size.

Management

- Dopamine agonists (e.g. bromocriptine, cabergoline): suppress prolactin levels and typically shrink prolactinomas. Cabergoline is taken once weekly and is relatively well tolerated. Side effects include dizziness, fatigue and rarely behavioural change (e.g. disinhibition); cardiac and retroperitoneal fibrosis have been described. Patients should be given written information about these side effects, and should also be advised to stop the medication immediately should they become pregnant.
- Surgery: only rarely required when lesions have failed to respond to medical treatment.

Acromegaly

Acromegaly is the clinical syndrome resulting from growth hormone excess. Causes include:

- Pituitary adenomas (99% cases): macroadenomas (pituitary lesion >10mm in size) account for 75% of cases at presentation.
- Ectopic growth hormone (GH)/GH-releasing hormone (GHRH) secretion: this is very rare; examples include GHRH-secreting tumours of the hypothalamus and GHRH secretion by neuroendocrine tumours, e.g. carcinoid tumours or small cell lung cancers.

Symptoms and signs

These result from the tumour itself and the excess GH/IGF1 secretion.

For clinical features of acromegaly, see Box 19.3.

Acromegaly may be part of MEN1 with associated symptoms and signs of parathyroid adenoma and pancreatic lesions (➲ see MEN1, p. 700).

Investigations

- IGF-1 to confirm growth hormone excess. IGF-1 is released by the liver in response to GH secretion, but unlike GH, does not show diurnal variation.

Box 19.3 Clinical features of acromegaly

Clinical features due to excess GH/IGF1

- Soft tissue overgrowth: enlarged, swollen hands and feet, macrognathia (enlarged jaw), coarsening of facial features, macroglossia and carpal tunnel syndrome.
- Hyperhidrosis and skin tags are common.
- Pituitary gigantism in children. Adults do not grow taller (as their epiphyses have already fused).
- Hypertrophic arthropathy of the knees, ankles and hips (➲ see Chapter 20, Acromegaly, p. 750).
- Hypertension.
- Dilated cardiomyopathy.
- Sleep apnoea: due to macroglossia and enlargement of pharynx and larynx soft tissues.
- Insulin resistance, which may progress to diabetes (found in 10–15% of cases).
- Increased risk of neoplasia, particularly colon, stomach and uterine leiomyomata.

- OGTT confirms the diagnosis of GH excess with failure to suppress GH to <0.6 μg/L.
- Pituitary hormone profile should be performed.
- Imaging: pituitary MRI. If no pituitary lesion is identified, further investigations, including CT chest/ abdomen/pelvis to determine the source of excess GH secretion.

Management

- Surgical removal of pituitary lesion (first line) via the trans-sphenoidal approach is often curative. Medical treatment (second line) includes somatostatin analogues (octreotide or lanreotide) and dopamine agonists (cabergoline and bromocriptine) when GH levels remain high after surgery.
- Radiotherapy if there is residual tumour after surgery and medical treatment is unavailable, unsuccessful or not tolerated.
- Pegvisomant (an injectable GH receptor antagonist) may be used in patients who fail to respond to the above measures.

Cushing's syndrome

Cushing's syndrome is the result of excess corticosteroid, which may be endogenous or exogenous. Endogenous causes may be either ACTH-dependent (stimulating excess production of cortisol) or ACTH-independent (due to intrinsic pathology affecting the adrenal gland itself).

For causes of Cushing's syndrome, see Table 19.7.

Table 19.7 Causes of Cushing's syndrome

Pseudo-Cushing's (clinical symptoms and signs in the absence of excess cortisol)	Exogenous steroid excess	Endogenous cortisol excess	
		ACTH-dependent	**non-ACTH-dependent**
Alcohol	Prescribed: inhaled/ topical/oral preparations.	Pituitary adenoma (Cushing's disease).	Adrenal adenoma (accounts for 10% of Cushing's syndrome).
Severe depression	Non-prescribed (e.g. anabolic steroid use).	Ectopic ACTH secretion (e.g. bronchial carcinoid).	Adrenal carcinoma.
		Ectopic corticotrophin-releasing hormone (CRH) secretion (e.g. phaeochromocytoma).	

Signs and symptoms

- Weight gain, with centripetal obesity, supraclavicular and interscapular fat pad.
- Hirsutism, stria (pink/purple), thin skin, bruises.
- Characteristic round, plethoric face.
- Proximal myopathy.
- Hypertension.
- Glucose intolerance, which may progress to DM.
- Oligomenorrhoea in women.
- Mood changes with irritability and low mood common.

Investigations

- Biochemical investigations:
  - The first step is to confirm endogenous hypercortisolism: overnight dexamethasone suppression test (1 mg dexamethasone taken at midnight, followed by measurement of cortisol level at 09.00 hours the following morning), 24-hour urine collection for free cortisol excretion, midnight cortisol and/or the low dose dexamethasone suppression test (0.5 mg six-hourly [completely suppresses cortisol secretion at 48 hours in normal subjects]).
  - Basal ACTH level to distinguish between ACTH-dependent and -independent causes. Raised basal ACTH levels may be secondary to pituitary or ectopic secretion.
  - In most pituitary adenomas:
    - A high dose dexamethasone suppression test (1 mg six-hourly for 48 hours [completely suppresses cortisol secretion at 48 hours]).
    - Corticotropin-releasing hormone (CRH) test (iv CRH) will result in an exaggerated rise in ACTH and cortisol level.
- Radiological investigations:
  - If ACTH dependent:
    - MRI pituitary.
    - Inferior petrosal sinus sampling if no lesion identified on MRI.
    - CT chest/abdomen/pelvis to identify ectopic source of ACTH if MRI and inferior petrosal sinus sampling unable to identify ACTH secreting lesion.
- Adrenal imaging to look for cortisol secreting adrenal lesions if ACTH independent.
- Osteoporosis screening, including DEXA scan may be required (➲ see Chapter 20, Osteoporosis, p. 724 and Figure 20.2).

Management

- Stop contributing medications if possible, or introduce alternative medication.
- Bone protection where necessary (➲ see Chapter 20, Treatment, p. 725 and Figure 20.2).
- Pituitary adenoma (Cushing's disease) requires surgical intervention with careful follow-up to assess for recurrence. Adrenal enzyme inhibitors (e.g. metyrapone) may be used pre-operatively to reduce circulating cortisol levels.
- Ectopic ACTH or CRH: surgical removal of the causative tumour. Where this is not possible, metyrapone may be used.
- Adrenal pathology, e.g. adrenal adenoma, adrenal carcinoma: treatment is with surgical removal of lesions.

Diabetes insipidus

Diabetes insipidus (DI) is characterised by passing large volumes (>3 L/day) of dilute urine (osmolality < 300 mOsm/kg) and is the result of either failure to produce ADH (central or cranial diabetes insipidus), or a failure of the distal convoluted tubules and collecting ducts of the kidneys to respond to ADH (nephrogenic diabetes insipidus; ➲ see Figure 16.3E). Patients present with polyuria, polydipsia, nocturia, enuresis and volume depletion (when access to water is restricted).

For causes of diabetes insipidus, see Table 19.8.

Investigations

Table 19.8 Causes of diabetes insipidus

Cranial diabetes insipidus	Nephrogenic diabetes insipidus
Trauma.	Drug induced, e.g. lithium, demeclocycline, amphotericin B.
Tumours, e.g. craniopharyngiomas.	Metabolic: hypercalcaemia, hypokalaemia.
Inflammatory processes, e.g. sarcoidosis, lymphocytic hypophysitis.	Renal failure with tubular dysfunction, sickle cell nephropathy.
Infections, e.g. meningitis.	Hereditary (mutations in the receptor for ADH or in aquaporin 2).
Vascular insufficiency, e.g. in Sheehan's syndrome (panhypopituitism secondary to pituitary infarction due to massive blood loss at delivery).	
Idiopathic.	

- Confirm polyuria with 24-hour urinary collection.
- Exclude other causes including diabetes mellitus, hypercalcaemia and renal failure.
- Water deprivation test to confirm diagnosis and distinguish between cranial and nephrogenic DI (see Box 19.4 and Table 19.9).

Box 19.4 Water deprivation test

Diagnosis of DI is confirmed if serum osmolality is >300 mOsm/kg and urine osmolality <300 mOsm/kg after 8-hour fluid deprivation. To distinguish between cranial and nephrogenic DI: IM desmopressin (2 μg) is given at 8 hours, and paired serum and urine osmolality is repeated hourly over the next 4 hours.

Partial DI

- Partial cranial or nephrogenic diabetes insipidus occurs when ADH secreted is insufficient to concentrate urine adequately. False positive and false negative results with water deprivation test may be as high as 30%, and additional investigations (e.g. sodium levels, prolonged water deprivation test) may be necessary to confirm the diagnosis.
- Psychogenic polydipsia should be suspected if plasma osmolality continues to be normal after 8 hours of fluid deprivation (<300 mOsmol/kg), or if a slight increase in plasma osmolality is followed by an increase in urine osmolality (>300 mOsmol/kg).

Table 19.9 The urine osmolality (mOsmol/kg) interpretation following water deprivation test

Diagnosis	After 8 hours fluid deprivation	After desmopressin
Cranial DI	<300	>800
Nephrogenic DI	<300	<300
Primary polydipsia	>800	No change
Partial DI/polydipsia	300–800	<800

Management

- Adequate fluid replacement is vital to prevent severe dehydration and hypernatraemia.
- A low salt diet.
- Desmopressin replacement for cranial DI (intranasal spray, sublingual tablets or rarely IM injections).
- Thiazide diuretics (mild volume contraction results in increased salt and water reabsorption in the proximal parts of the nephron, so much less filtrate reaches the collecting duct).
- NSAIDs (e.g. indometacin) may be used for nephrogenic DI.
- Correction of any underlying secondary causes of nephrogenic diabetes mellitus.

Further reading

1. Bichet DG. Approach to the patient with polyuria. In: Turner NN, Lameire N, Goldsmith DJ, et al. (Eds) *Oxford Textbook of Clinical Nephrology*, 4th edn. Oxford: Oxford University Press.

Hypopituitarism

Hypopituitarism results from complete or partial deficiency of anterior and/or posterior pituitary hormones. It follows a characteristic order, where loss of GH and gonadotrophins precede loss of TSH and ACTH production. Clinical presentation is often insidious.

Causes

- Congenital empty sella.
- Pressure from pituitary tumours.
- Post-irradiation.
- Post-surgery.
- Pituitary infarction (e.g. apoplexy after a hypotensive episode with subsequent bleeding into usually a previously unknown pituitary tumour [if postpartum, known as Sheehan's syndrome]).

Symptoms and signs

- GH deficiency: fatigue, low mood and difficulty concentrating.
- ACTH deficiency: fatigue, nausea, weight loss, hypoglycaemia.
- Gonadotrophin deficiency: loss of libido, amenorrhoea.

Investigations

- Baseline bloods including pituitary function (09.00 hours cortisol, LH/FSH, oestradiol, testosterone, TSH and fT4, prolactin).
- Dynamic function tests including:
  - Insulin tolerance test (ITT) or glucagon test to confirm GH and ACTH reserve. Hypoglycaemia and glucagon should both lead to an increase in cortisol and GH where the pituitary is functioning.
  - GnRH stimulation is rarely used to assess gonadotrophins. It does not distinguish pituitary from hypothalamic pathology.

Management

- Hormone replacement therapy is essential. ACTH deficiency is treated with hydrocortisone replacement in a regime similar to that in adrenal insufficiency (e.g. 10 mg on waking, 5 mg at midday and 5 mg at 18.00 hours, ➲ see Management, p. 695). Similarly, the resulting secondary hypothyroidism is treated with levothyroxine (➲ see Hypothyroidism, Management, p. 684) and gonadotrophins with oestrogen or testosterone.
- It is important to replace or confirm ACTH reserve before commencing thyroxine as the resulting increase in metabolism could otherwise precipitate an Addisonian crisis.

- In adults, replacement of GH (subcutaneously) will often relieve symptoms of low mood and fatigue. The Quality of Life Assessment of Growth Hormone Deficiency in Adults (QoL-AGHDA) questionnaire is used to determine severity of symptoms and a score of ≥11, along with biochemical demonstration of GH insufficiency, is used to demonstrate the need for replacement (1).

Reference

1. National Institute for Clinical Excellence (NICE) (2003) Human growth hormone (somatropin) in adults with growth hormone deficiency. NICE Technological appraisal guideline TA64. 2016. https://www.nice.org.uk/guidance/ta64.

Hyponatraemia

Defined as serum sodium <135 mmol/L, hyponatraemia may be acute or chronic. Symptoms include subtle changes in cognition to severe, life-threatening neurological disturbances.

Causes

Pathological causes of hyponatraemia can be thought of as resulting in:

1. Hypovolaemic hyponatraemia: this results from sodium and water loss and may be:
   - Renal: diuretics, mineralocorticoid deficiency (e.g. Addison's disease, congenital adrenal hyperplasia [CAH]), renal failure.
   - Extra-renal: GI loss (vomiting, diarrhoea).
2. Euvolaemic hyponatraemia: syndrome of inappropriate antidiuretic hormone (SIADH), primary polydipsia.
3. Hypervolaemic (dilutional) hyponatraemia: heart failure, cirrhotic liver disease, hypothyroidism.

Other important causes include medications, e.g. ACE-i, SSRIs, thiazide diuretics.

Symptoms and signs

- Nausea, vomiting.
- Alteration in cognition with confusion, seizures and coma.
- Signs of underlying pathology, e.g. hyperpigmentation in Addison's disease.

Investigations

- Fasting lipids and serum protein levels. Hyperlipidaemia and hyperproteinaemia (e.g. in multiple myeloma) can cause pseudohyponatraemia due to relative expansion of plasma volume.
- Serum urea and electrolytes and liver function tests to exclude salt losing states.
- Cortisol levels (to rule out hypoadrenalism) and thyroid function.
- Paired plasma and urine osmolality.

Management

- Chronic mild asymptomatic hyponatraemia does not usually need treatment.
- Stop any contributing medications, e.g. ACE-i, aldosterone receptor blockers, SSRIs, thiazide diuretics.
- In severe hyponatraemia aim to increase sodium level gradually (typically at less than 12 mmol/L over 24 hours). Rapid change in sodium could result in the irreversible and life threatening central demyelination (➲ see Chapter 17, Electrolyte disturbance, p. 639) so frequent monitoring of sodium levels (e.g. 2–4 times over 24 hours) is recommended.
- Where severe symptoms are present (vomiting, confusion, seizures, reduced consciousness), admission to a high dependency setting and hypertonic saline should be considered (1.8% or 3% saline may be used according to an agreed protocol).
- Hypovolaemic hyponatraemia is treated with IV normal saline.
- Hypervolaemic hyponatraemia is managed by cautious fluid restriction, and may be as strict as 750–1000 mL per 24 hours if necessary.

- Demeclocycline or vasopressin antagonists, e.g. tolvaptan, may also be used in resistant hyponatraemia.

Syndrome of inappropriate antidiuretic hormone

ADH secretion from the posterior pituitary is stimulated by increased plasma osmolality, as detected by hypothalamic osmoreceptors. It acts on the collecting ducts to increase water permeability, and thus results in plasma dilution and concentration of urine.

In SIADH, ADH levels are not suppressed by low plasma osmolality, leading to inappropriate concentration of urine.

SIADH is diagnosed when:

- Serum osmolality is low.
- Urine osmolality is high (>100 mOsm/kg despite low serum osmolality).
- Urine sodium frequently >40 mmol/L.
- There are no other causes of increased sodium loss (i.e. renal dysfunction).

Causes of SIADH

- Malignancy: small cell cancer of lung, head and neck cancers.
- Infections: bacterial or viral.
- CNS disease: stroke, space occupying lesions, e.g. abscess, post-trauma or surgery.
- Drugs: antiepileptics, SSRI.
- Idiopathic.

Management of SIADH includes fluid restriction and where persistent, ADH antagonists, e.g. tolvaptan, may be considered (see Table 3.4).

Further reading

1. Spasovski G, Vonholder R, Allolio B, et al. Clinical practice guideline on diagnosis and treatment of hyponatraemia. *Eur J Endocrinol*. 2014; 170:G1–G47.
2. Levy A. Pituitary disease: presentation, diagnosis, and management. *J Neurol Neurosurg Psychiat*. 2004; 75(Suppl 3):iii47–52.

Adrenal gland

Anatomy and physiology

The adrenal glands comprise an outer cortex and inner medulla. The cortex synthesises steroid hormones utilising cholesterol and has three components:

- Zona glomerulosa: secretes mineralocorticoids including aldosterone following stimulation by angiotensin II (the final stage of the renin-angiotensin-aldosterone pathway) (see Figure 19.1).
- Zona fasciculata: secretes glucocorticoids and small amounts of adrenal androgen dehydroepiandrosterone (DHEA). ACTH controls both cortisol and adrenal androgen secretion. ACTH is released from the anterior pituitary gland when stimulated by hypothalamic CRH. Demonstrating a circadian rhythm, cortisol and adrenal androgen levels peak in the morning.
- Zona reticularis: secretes adrenal steroids including DHEA and androstenedione. Peripherally, adrenal androgens are converted to testosterone and its active metabolite, dihydrotestosterone.

The adrenal medulla is composed of chromaffin cells. It synthesises catecholamine from tyrosine following sympathetic stimulation.

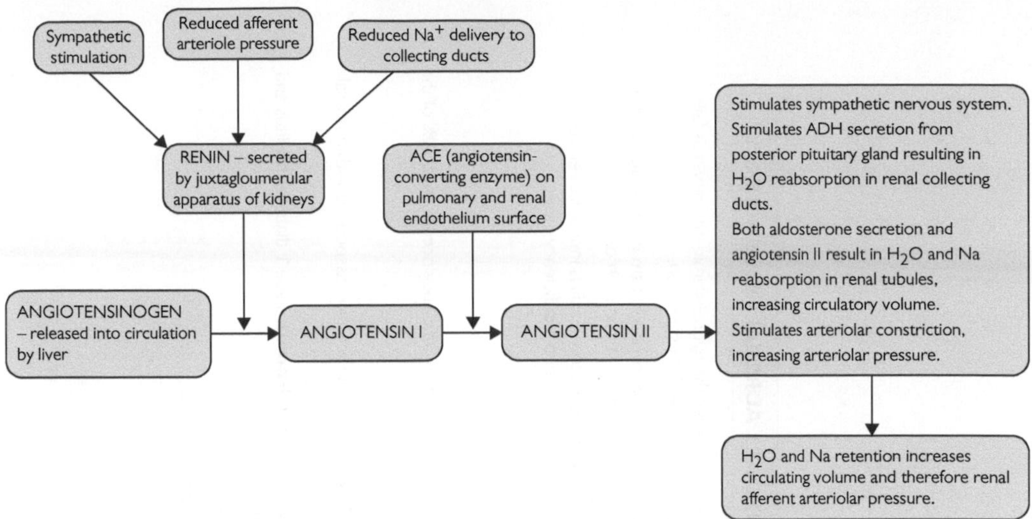

Figure 19.1 The renin–angiotensin pathway.

Adrenal insufficiency

Adrenal insufficiency may be primary, due to pathology affecting the adrenal gland itself (Addison's disease), or secondary due to failure of the pituitary or hypothalamus (see Figure 19.2).

Symptoms and signs

These vary depending on the hormones affected. Glucocorticoid deficiency results in fatigue, nausea, muscle weakness, fasting hypoglycaemia and hyperpigmentation. Hyperpigmentation occurs due to negative feedback leading to increased ACTH, stimulating melanocytes. It is not seen in secondary hypoadrenalism. Where mineralocorticoid deficiency occurs (primary adrenal insufficiency) symptoms include dizziness, anorexia and weight loss. Typical electrolyte imbalances may be seen (hyponatraemia, hyperkalaemia). Adrenal androgen insufficiency is most obviously seen in women where the adrenal cortex is the primary source of androgen precursor, resulting in reduction of axillary/pubic hair and reduced libido in women.

Investigations

Biochemistry shows hyponatraemia and hyperkalaemia and low 09.00 hours cortisol. Where adrenal insufficiency is suspected, a short Synacthen® test should be performed:

- Short Synacthen® test: 250 μg Synacthen® (tetracosactide) is given IM/IV. Cortisol levels are taken at baseline, and 30 and 60 minutes. Thresholds of cortisol level for detecting adrenal insufficiency is specific to the assay being used. Low cortisol levels lead to high ACTH from loss of feedback inhibition. ACTH should also be measured if secondary hypoadrenalism is suspected. Very low ACTH levels and loss of other trophic hormones from anterior pituitary make the diagnosis of secondary hypoadrenalism more likely.
- Long Synacthen® test (to differentiate between primary and secondary adrenal insufficiency) is rarely used due to improvements in ACTH measurements.
- Further investigations for primary adrenal insufficiency include renin and aldosterone levels, adrenal antibodies and imaging of the adrenal glands.
- Full pituitary profile and imaging of the pituitary gland should be performed in cases of secondary adrenal insufficiency.

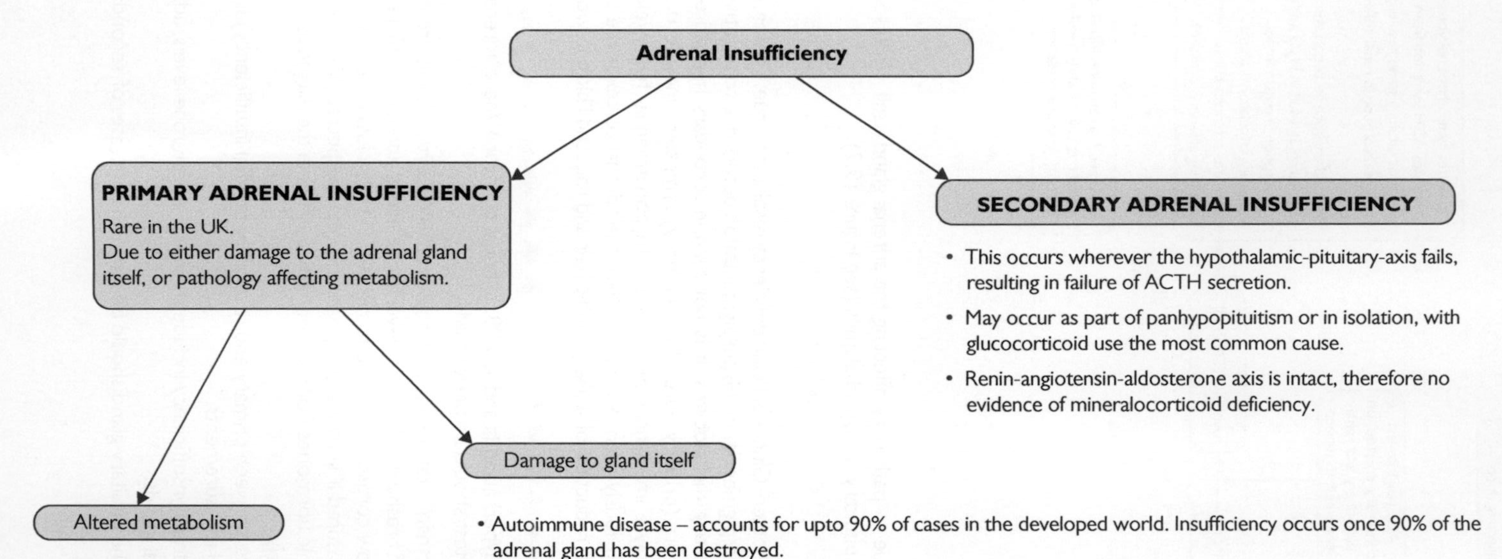

Figure 19.2 Adrenal insufficiency.

Management

- Glucocorticoid replacement: hydrocortisone is typically given in three divided doses (a common starting regime is 10 mg on waking, 5 mg at midday and 5 mg in the evening).
- Mineralocorticoid replacement: this is done using fludrocortisone and aims to prevent hyponatraemia, dehydration and hyperkalaemia. Postural BP and plasma renin activity are used to monitor response as the resulting decrease in renal perfusion is detected by the juxtaglomerular apparatus in mineralocorticoid deficiency. Renin is released in response and is therefore typically elevated (see Figure 19.1).
- All patients should have a medical alert badge and be aware of steroid sick day rules.

The medical emergency of Addisonian crisis is outlined in Box 19.5.

Box 19.5 Acute adrenal insufficiency: Addisonian crisis

This medical emergency carries a high mortality and should be considered in any patient presenting with profound shock, particularly in patients with a history of longstanding steroid use, or other autoimmune conditions.

Management

- IV fluids (0.9% sodium chloride).
- An initial bolus 100 mg hydrocortisone IV is usually followed by IM hydrocortisone.
- High doses of hydrocortisone have a mineralocorticoid effect and, therefore, concomitant administration of fludrocortisone is not required.
- Once the patient is able to tolerate oral medications, high dose oral steroid (hydrocortisone) TDS is started.
- Fludrocortisone is added once glucocorticoid stores are sufficient.

Primary hyperaldosteronism

Primary hyperaldosteronism accounts for 10% of all patients with hypertension, with a prevalence of up to 4% of the total population. Patients present with hypertension and hypokalaemia, although potassium may be normal at presentation.

Causes

- Bilateral adrenal hyperplasia is the commonest cause, typically presenting in adulthood. The cells in the zona glomerulosa are more sensitive to angiotensin II and, therefore, the aldosterone release is greater than expected for the level of renin or angiotensin II.
- Aldosteronoma (Conn's syndrome) is more common in women, and age of onset is between 30 and 60 years.
- Adrenal carcinoma (rare).

Symptoms and signs

- Hypertension (especially if <40 years old).
- Weakness due to hypokalaemia.
- Polydipsia and polyuria due to inability to concentrate urine.

Investigations

- Electrolytes: hypokalaemia is often seen.
- Elevated aldosterone and suppressed renin with ratio of ≥800, off antihypertensives with a typical clinical picture confirms diagnosis.
- CT, MRI or adrenal vein sampling may be used to localise the site of the lesion.

Management

- Where a unilateral adenoma is identified and found to be functioning, surgical removal is performed.
- In patients with adrenal hyperplasia, or if surgery is not possible, medical management is initiated with spironolactone or eplerenone.

Phaeochromocytoma and paraganglionoma

Phaeochromocytomas are rare catecholamine secreting tumours originating from adrenal tissue. Paragangliomas also secrete catecholamines, but originate from distal neural crest derivatives, and are found extra-adrenally (most commonly in the head or neck).

Symptoms and signs

Characteristically presents with episodic symptoms:

- sweating;
- palpitations;
- headache;
- feeling of apprehension;
- abdominal pain and nausea.

Investigations

- Confirm catecholamine excess with urinary metanephrines.
- CT/MRI for localisation.
- MEN IIa and IIb, von Hippel–Lindau's syndrome and neurofibromatosis type 1 may be associated with phaeochromocytomas. Investigations should be performed if indicated.

Management

- α-blockade, e.g. with phenoxybenzamine, followed by beta-blockade. It is imperative that α-blockade is instigated first to prevent unopposed alpha adrenergic stimulation, which could result in life-threatening hypertensive crisis.
- Surgery is curative.
- Long-term follow up is recommended to assess for recurrence.

Congenital adrenal hyperplasia

CAH are autosomal recessive conditions, resulting from defects in enzymes necessary for aldosterone and cortisol synthesis. The commonest cause is 21, hydroxylase (21OH) deficiency. Low cortisol and aldosterone leads to increased ACTH secretion and subsequent adrenal hyperplasia. Steroid precursors that would normally be used to synthesise cortisol, in the absence of 21OH activity, are used to make testosterone, leading to testosterone and androstenedione excess.

For clinical adrenal hyperplasia, see Table 19.10.

Table 19.10 Clinical adrenal hyperplasia

	Presentation	**Investigations**	**Management**
Classical CAH	Diagnosed in neonate. Virilisation and cliteromegaly in females. Profound volume loss and hyponatraemia due to lack of aldosterone.	Measurement of 17-hydroxyprogesterone (17OHP; steroid precursor). ACTH, renin and androgens.	Small doses of glucocococorticoids - to ensure adequate replacement and suppress excess ACTH. Mineralocorticoids to maintain circulating volume. Antiandrogens, e.g. cyproterone acetate.
Non-classical CAH	Usually partial 21OH deficiency leads to adequate cortisol and aldosterone synthesis, but androgen excess with acne and hirsutism.		

Reproductive endocrinology

Male reproductive endocrinology

The testes are responsible for spermatogenesis and androgen synthesis, and comprise several seminiferous tubules surrounded by interstitial tissue. They have a volume of approximately 15–20 mL each and are suspended by the spermatic cord (composed of the sympathetic nerves, testicular arteries and testicular veins). Leydig cells within the interstitial tissue produce testosterone when stimulated by pituitary LH. Sertoli cells and epithelial cells in the seminiferous tubules are responsible for spermatogenesis. The seminiferous tubules drain into the rete testis, which ultimately drains seminiferous fluid into the epididymis.

Androgen production and spermatogenesis

Testosterone is required for the development of sexual characteristics, as well as spermatogenesis. Hypothalamic stimulation results in pulsatile GnRH secretion, and subsequent FSH and LH secretion by the anterior pituitary gland. LH acts on Leydig cells stimulating production of testosterone. Androgens negatively feedback on LH release directly, and subsequently indirectly negatively feedback on GnRH secretion.

Gynaecomastia

Gynaecomastia is the finding of breast tissue enlargement, defined as the presence of >2 cm breast tissue. It occurs in approximately 30% of men under the age of 30 years of age, and results from conditions where oestrogen predominates. This may be due to a lack of testosterone, reduction in the action of testosterone, or increased oestrogen production or action (see Table 19.11).

Table 19.11 Causes of gynaecomastia

Physiological	Reduction in testosterone production/action	Increased oestrogen production/action	Drugs
Puberty: transient gynaecomastia.	Primary hypogonadism, e.g. Klinefelter's.	Obesity: ↑ peripheral aromatisation.	Androgen inhibitors, e.g. spironolactone.
Neonates: affects up to 90% male neonates due to maternal hormone transfer.	Secondary hypogonadism, e.g. Kallman's.	Tumours producing oestrogens or androgens: adrenal or testicular tumours.	Oestrogen containing medications, e.g. digoxin.
Idiopathic.	Peripheral androgen resistance.	Liver cirrhosis: ↓ oestrogen metabolism and ↑SHBG.	Other medications, including ACEI, TCA.
	Chronic kidney disease.	Hyperthyroidism.	

Investigations

- Full hormonal profile including oestradiol, testosterone, sex hormone-binding globulin (SHBG), hCG (elevated in some testicular tumours), TSH, LH, FSH.
- Imaging: testicular US, imaging of the breasts may be necessary depending on the history.

Management

The underlying cause must be identified and treated where possible. Gynaecomastia causing significant physical or psychological problems, may be treated with anti-oestrogenic agents, such as tamoxifen. Referral for reduction mammoplasty may be considered in long-standing cases.

Hypogonadism

In men, this refers to a failure of testosterone production. It is classified as either primary (due to conditions affecting the testes directly) or secondary.

Primary hypogonadism

Testosterone production is reduced, despite normal hypothalamic and pituitary function. Investigations show a low testosterone with appropriately raised LH and FSH.

Causes include Klinefelter's syndrome (see Box 19.6), cryptorchidism (undescended testes), orchitis, testicular trauma, chronic illness (including chronic renal failure and liver cirrhosis), chemotherapy and radiotherapy.

Box 19.6 Klinefelter's syndrome (47, XXY)

Most common inherited cause of primary hypogonadism. Features include small, firm testes, gynaecomastia, cognitive dysfunction and tall stature. Patients may present in adulthood with gynaecomastia, reduced libido, erectile dysfunction and infertility.

Investigations

Low testosterone, elevated FSH and LH (due to negative feedback), raised SHBG and oestradiol, azoospermia.

Management

Testosterone replacement therapy, fertility services (intracytoplasmic sperm injection has been successful).

Secondary hypogonadism

Hypothalamic or pituitary dysfunction results in testicular failure due either to structural damage, or conditions affecting hypothalamic/pituitary function. Testosterone will be low, and LH/FSH will be normal or low. Causes include systemic illness, infiltrative disease (e.g. sarcoidosis), tumours and Kallman's syndrome.

- *Kallman's syndrome* results from a failure of GnRH neurons to migrate to the hypothalamus during embryonic development. It may affect males and females, and clinical features include anosmia and hypogonadism. Biochemistry will reveal low testosterone, LH and FSH in males, and MRI may show absence of the olfactory bulbs. Administration of GnRH restores pituitary function. Management includes testosterone replacement and exogenous gonadotrophins for the purposes of fertility.
- *Prader Willi syndrome* includes features such as short stature, learning disabilities and developmental delay, obesity and hypogonadism. The majority of cases result from deletion of the region of paternally inherited chromosome (chr. 15). It may also result from chromosomal non-disjunction leading to both copies of chr. 15 being inherited from the mother. Management requires an MDT approach, and may include growth hormone therapy, genetic counselling and management of diet.

Female reproductive endocrinology

The ovaries are retroperitoneal structures lying on either side of the uterus. They are supplied by bilateral ovarian arteries, originating from the aorta, and drained by the left and right ovarian veins to the left renal vein and inferior vena cava, respectively. The nerve supply lies within the suspensory ligament of the ovary.

For a summary of the menstrual cycle, see Table 19.12.

Menstrual disorders

Primary amenorrhoea refers to patients who have not experienced menstruation by the age of 16 years old. It may result from reproductive structural abnormalities, hypothalamic–pituitary disorders or from chromosomal disorders leading to an absence of menstruation. The causes are given in Table 19.13.

Other causes include congenital adrenal hyperplasia (➲ see Congenital adrenal hyperplasia, p. 696 and Table 19.10) and androgen insensitivity syndrome.

For Turner's syndrome, see Box 19.7.

Secondary amenorrhoea refers to patients who have previously menstruated who experience cessation of menstruation for >6 months. It may result from pathology affecting the ovaries, the uterus or the hypothalamic–pituitary axis (Table 19.14). Systemic disorders may also alter hypothalamic–pituitary function and thus cause secondary amenorrhoea.

Table 19.12 Summary of the menstrual cycle

Day of cycle	Hormone changes	Ovarian cycle	Uterine cycle
Day 0–4			*Menstruation*
Day 4–14	LH/FSH stimulate follicular maturation. Oestradiol is secreted from maturing follicle.	*Follicular phase:* Maturation of dominant follicle into Graafian follicle (mainly FSH driven).	*Proliferative phase:* Laying down new endometrial layer (oestrogen driven).
Day 14	GnRH surge followed by LH surge just before ovulation.	*Ovulation*	
Day 14–28	Progesterone secreted from corpus luteum. LH/FSH levels fall off.	*Luteal phase:* post-ovulation corpus luteum (LH/FSH helps formation of corpus luteum).	*Secretory phase:* endometrium receptive to implantation (progesterone supported) .

Table 19.13 Causes of primary amenorrhoea

Structural disorders	Hypothalamic-pituitary disorders	Chromosomal disorders
Imperforate hymen.	Kallman's syndrome (➲ see Secondary hypogonadism, p. 698).	Turner's syndrome.
Congenital absence of vagina, cervix or uterus.	Pituitary disorders.	

Box 19.7 Turner's syndrome

Affects 1 in 2500 births. Karyotype 45 XO.

Features include short stature, high arched palate, wide spaced nipples and webbed neck. Also associated with hypothyroidism, renal abnormalities and coarctation of the aorta.

Management includes hormone replacement therapy and monitoring and treatment of any complications.

Table 19.14 Causes of secondary amenorrhoea

Ovarian pathology	Hypothalamic-pituitary dysfunction	Uterine disorders
Polycystic ovarian syndrome: characterised by hyperandrogenism, oligomenorrhoea, raised BMI.	Hyperprolactinaemia: increased prolactin released from the anterior pituitary gland. Associated with galactorrhoea and pituitary mass.	Adhesions.
Premature ovarian failure: raised gonadotrophins, oestrogen deficiency.	Panhypopituitism, e.g. from infiltrative disorder or pituitary mass.	
	Infiltrative disorder of hypothalamus.	
	Weight loss or excessive exercise resulting in hypothalamic dysfunction.	

Management of secondary amenorrhoea requires the identification and treatment of any underlying cause.

Further reading

1. Holt R, Hanley N. Reproductive endocrinology. In *Essential Endocrinology and Diabetes*, 5th edn, pp. 99–127. Oxford: Blackwell Publishing, 2007.

Neuroendocrine tumours

These rare tumours originate from neuro-epithelial tissue and are characterised by the production of peptide hormones in response to nervous stimulus.

Carcinoid tumours

May be associated with MEN1, NF1, von Hippel–Lindau syndrome and tuberose sclerosis. Symptoms include diarrhoea, flushing, bronchoconstriction and right-sided heart lesions, and only occur with lung carcinoids, or once they have metastasised to the liver (thus releasing serotonin into the systemic circulation). Urinary 5-hydroxyindoleacetic acid (5HIAA) will be raised. CT/MRI or specialised scans, like octreotide scanning, may be used to localise the lesion (➲ see Chapter 10, Radiographic scintigraphy, p. 321, and Chapter 5, Case 15, p. 138). Management includes resection of the primary lesion, somatostatin analogues (e.g. octreotide), radiotherapy, chemotherapy and embolisation.

Insulinomas

Symptoms include those of hypoglycaemia and weight gain, with eating resolving symptoms. Diagnosis requires the demonstration of hypoglycaemia (serum glucose <2.2 mmol/L) with raised insulin and C-peptide (indicating endogenous insulin secretion), with the absence of urinary sulfonylurea metabolites. Endoscopic US or MRI may identify the lesion. Surgical excision is often curative.

Gastrinomas

25% are associated with multiple endocrine neoplasia 1 (*MEN1*) (➲ see MEN1), most occur sporadically. Typically localised in the pancreas, they may also arise from the duodenum or distant sites. Diagnosis is dependent on raised gastrin levels in the presence of raised gastric acid. Treatment includes reduction of gastric acid secretion (with PPI and H2 blockers), but ultimately surgical resection may be required. Zollinger–Ellison syndrome occurs due to the continuous production of gastrin resulting in multiple ulcers. For investigations and management ➲ see Chapter 14, Zollinger-Ellison syndrome, p. 502.

Glucagonomas

These arise from pancreatic α cells and are associated with necrolytic migratory erythema. They typically metastasise and are often incurable at diagnosis. Plasma glucagon will be raised. Endoscopic US and CT is used for localisation. Surgery can be curative, although the majority will not be amenable to surgery. Somatostatin analogues (e.g. octreotide) provide symptomatic relief and parenteral nutrition can aid symptoms.

VIPomas

These present with refractory, profound secretory diarrhoea and electrolyte imbalances. Surgery offers the only curative option and some symptomatic relief.

Somatostatinomas

These extremely rare tumours occur in the duodenum or head of the pancreas. Patients may present with symptoms of malabsorption, weight loss or obstructive jaundice due to gallstone. Diagnosis requires raised somatostatin levels. Management is rarely curative, but surgery can improve symptoms.

Multiple endocrine neoplasia

These inherited conditions are characterised by the finding of endocrine neoplasms in combination.

MEN1

Prevalence is estimated at approximately 1 per 30,000 of the population. It is autosomal dominant and is characterised by the finding of the '3 Ps'.

- **P**arathyroid adenomas (primary hyperparathyroidism is the most common presenting feature, being found in >90% of patients).
- Anterior **p**ituitary adenomas (typically prolactinomas or those secreting GH resulting in acromegaly).
- **P**ancreatic neuroendocrine tumours (gastrinomas [predominate], insulinomas).

Diagnosis depends on the finding of *two* out of three of the above types of tumours, or one of the above tumours in the presence of a positive family history of MEN1.

Management often involves surgical excision of individual lesions and genetic counselling. Gastrinomas account for much of the associated mortality and morbidity, but symptoms may be improved by both medical (e.g. PPIs) and surgical treatments. Screening is more difficult for the first degree relatives of patients without an identified genetic mutation. They should be offered annual screening with hormonal profiling and imaging as appropriate. Hormones to be checked include:

- Calcium and PTH: to assess for parathyroid tumours.
- Gastrin: to assess for gastrinoma.
- Fasting glucose and insulin: to assess for insulinoma.
- Prolactin/IGF1 as appropriate: to assess for pituitary lesion.

MEN2

This results from a mutation in the RET proto-oncogene and is characterised by the finding of *medullary thyroid cancer*.

- MEN2a:
  - Medullary thyroid cancer.
  - Phaeochromocytoma.
  - Parathyroid neoplasia.
- MEN2b:
  - Medullary thyroid cancer.
  - Phaeochromocytoma.
  - Marfanoid habitus.
  - Mucosal neuromas.

Treatment includes total thyroidectomy for medullary thyroid carcinoma along with alpha- and beta-blockade, and surgical removal of any phaeochromocytomas. Genetic analysis is crucial in identifying any at-risk offspring.

Multiple choice questions

Questions

1. You see a patient in clinic who has noticed an eccentric thyroid swelling. On examination, you find features consistent with hyperthyroidism. You suspect that she may have a toxic nodule. Which of the following investigations will be most helpful?
   A. TSH receptor antibodies.
   B. Thyroid ultrasound scan.
   C. Fine needle aspiration of the nodule.
   D. Technetium uptake scan of the thyroid.
   E. CT scan of the neck.

2. A 68-year-old gentleman was found at home drowsy and confused. On examination, his chest was clear and heart sounds were normal. There was no focal neurology. Bloods done at the A&E were as follows:

   Haemoglobin: 17.2 g/dL (13.0–18.1)
   WCC: 5.2 × 10^9/L (3.7–11).
   Platelets: 536 × 109/L (150–450).
   Na: 150 mmol/L (136–145).
   K: 5.5 mmol/L (3.5–5.1).
   Urea: 12 mmol/L (3.2–7.4).
   Creatinine: 184 μmol/L (63–111).
   Glucose: 34 mmol/L (fasting: 4–6).
   Bicarbonate: 20 mmol/L (22–26).
   Ketones: 0.3 mmol/L (<0.5).
   HbA1c: 10% (86 mmol/mol) (<42).
   ECG: no evidence of ischaemia.
   Urine dip: glucose +++, nitrites –, protein ++.

   What is the most important step in management of this gentleman?

   A. IV isotonic 0.9% sodium chloride.
   B. IV hypotonic 0.45% sodium chloride.
   C. IV fixed-rate insulin infusion.
   D. IV antibiotics.
   E. Perform venesection.

3. A 48-year-old African gentleman was diagnosed with type 2 diabetes 4 years ago. He has smoked 10 cigarettes/day for the past 10 years and has a family history of type 2 diabetes. On examination, he has a BMI of 35, his BP is 150/90 mmHg and has background retinal changes in both eyes. He has a HbA1c of 7.9% (IFCC 63 mmol/mol). His albumin-creatinine ratio is 45 mg/mmol. Other blood investigations are as follows:

   Total cholesterol: 6 mmol/L.
   LDL cholesterol: 3 mmol/L.
   HDL cholesterol: 0.9 mmol/L.
   Triglyceride: 4 mmol/L.
   Urea 5 mmol/L (3.2–7.4).
   Creatinine: 120 μmol/L (63–111).
   eGFR: 20 mL/min.

   Which of the following is the strongest predictor of risk of MI in this gentleman?

   A. History of smoking.
   B. His blood pressure.
   C. His albumin-creatinine ratio.
   D. His BMI.
   E. His HbA1c.

4. A 31-year-old lady presents with polyuria and polydipsia. Her medical history is otherwise unremarkable and she is not on any medications. Her physical examination is normal.

   Routine blood tests:

   Hb: 13.8 g/dL (13.0–18.1).
   WCC: 4.2 × 10^9/L (3.7–11).
   Platelets: 3.6 × 10^9/L (150–450).
   Na: 143 mmol/L (135–145).
   K: 3.8 mmol/L (3.5–5.1).
   Urea: 3 mmol/L (3.2–7.4).

Creatinine: 62 μmol/L (63–111).
Corrected Ca: 2.25 mmol/L (2.1–2.55).
Glucose (fasting): 6.5 mmol/L (4–6).

Urine output: 4.5 L/day.
She had a water deprivation test.

After 8 hours:
Plasma osmolality: 310 mOsm/kg (275–295).
Urine osmolality: 126 mOsm/kg.

4 hours following desmopressin injection:
Plasma osmolality: 286 mOsm/kg (275–295).
Urine osmolality: 824 mOsm/kg.

The next best investigation is:

A. Psychological assessment.
B. Pituitary MRI.
C. Renal biopsy.
D. OGTT.
E. Visual fields.

5. A 51-year-old man presents with a 6-month history of reduced libido and erectile dysfunction. On examination, you find him to have a raised BMI of 35 kg/m^2, with central obesity. There are no striae present. Testicular examination is unremarkable.

Blood tests reveal the following:
Testosterone is 4.0 nmol/L (6.7–25.8).
FSH is 1 IU/L (2–12).
Prolactin 130 mU/L (54–381).
TSH 6.0 mU/L (0.35–4.9).

Random cortisol 390 nmol/L (>500 at 09.00 hours) and random glucose 11 mmol/L (fasting 4–6).

What investigations should be performed next?

A. Urgent MRI pituitary.
B. OGTT, full pituitary profile.
C. DEXA scan to ensure adequate bone mineralisation.
D. Prostate-specific antigen (PSA).
E. OGTT, full pituitary profile, DEXA scan.

6. A 45-year-old patient was found by her partner at home unconscious. On arrival of paramedics, her capillary blood glucose was 1.9 mmol/L. She was given high dose dextrose and brought to A&E.

Her partner stated that she had recently been more difficult and described her as being increasingly 'moody' and agitated. On more than one occasion, he has come home to find her slurring her words and drowsy. She has abused alcohol in the past and he thinks she may have started drinking again.

Before seeing the patient, you review her results on the hospital system. You note that her calcium is 2.75 mmol/L (2.1–2.55). A urine pregnancy test is negative.

Which of the following would confirm your clinical suspicion for an underlying unifying diagnosis?

A. The finding of a palpable thyroid nodule.
B. Evidence of bilateral galactorrhoea.
C. Potassium of 3.0 mmol/L.
D. Albumin of 35 g/L.
E. TSH 2.0 mU/L.

Answers

1. D. This is the only way of confirming activity within the thyroid gland. (➲ See Thyroid, Thyroid investigations, p. 678 and Table 19.5.)
2. A. The gentleman has hyperosmolar hyperglycaemia. This is not DKA as blood ketones are low and he is not acidotic. Intensive fluid management is the most important feature of management. (➲ See Emergencies in diabetes, DKA and hyperglycaemic hyperosmolar state, p. 677.)
3. C. Albumin-creatinine ratio (as a measure of albuminuria) in people with diabetic nephropathy is one of the strongest predictor of cardiovascular disease. (➲ See Diabetes mellitus, Macrovascular disease, p. 676.)
4. B. These results are in keeping with cranial DI. (➲ See Diabetes insipidus, p. 688, Box 19.4 and Tables 19.8 and 19.9.)
5. E. This patient has hypogonadotrophic hypogonadism with an elevated random glucose. Diabetes mellitus is associated with hypogonadism and this should be investigated, as well as any biochemical evidence of pituitary pathology. DEXA scan to assess bone mineralisation in any patient with hypogonadism is important. (➲ See Hypogonadism, p. 697.)
6. B. The clinical scenario in this question suggests an underlying diagnosis of MEN1 (insulinoma, prolactinoma and hyperparathyroidism as suggested by the recurrent hypoglycaemic episodes, galactorrhoea and hypercalcaemia respectively). (➲ See MEN1, p. 700.)

Chapter 20 **Rheumatology**

Elena Nikiphorou, Anna Nuttall* and Rupa Bessant*

Rheumatoid arthritis

Pathogenesis

Immune dysfunction in rheumatoid arthritis (RA) results in a surge of inflammatory cells, synovial vascularity and increased intra-articular fluid volume. The deeper hypercellular layer of synovium is known as 'pannus'. The destructive process in RA develops at the junction between the synovium, articular cartilage and subchondral bone, and results in porotic bone and erosions.

- Dendritic cells express Toll-like receptors, which bind to foreign and self-antigens, initiating auto-inflammation through the adaptive system.
- B cells, macrophages, fibroblast-like synoviocytes and osteoclasts are activated by up-regulation of T-helper 1 cells by:
  - Class II MHC molecules on APCs.
  - CD80 and CD86 on APCs, binding onto CD28 on T cells, resulting in co-stimulation.
- Mechanisms of B cell involvement in RA include:
  - Auto-antibody production (rheumatoid factor [RF] and anti-cyclic citrullinated peptide [anti-CCP]). RF is an immunoglobulin (usually IgM) with antibody specificity for the Fc region of IgG.
  - T cell co-stimulation, production of pro-inflammatory cytokines.
  - Antigen presentation of T cells.
  - Development of immune complexes (Fc receptor-complement activation; ➲ see Chapter 6, Humoral mediators of the adaptive immune system, p. 150, and Complement, p. 150).

* Joint first authors.

Synovial joint involvement in rheumatoid arthritis

The principal target of RA is the synovial joint. Bone, cartilage, synovium, synovial fluid (SF), tendons, ligaments and entheses (points at which tendons/ligaments join to the bone) are all important components of a synovial joint.

Synovial fluid analysis

Helps to differentiate between infective, crystal-related or other forms of inflammatory arthritides:

- Macroscopic appearance of synovial fluid:
  - Normal: straw-coloured and viscous; forms a 'string' of fluid.
  - Inflammatory (e.g. RA): yellow or green; viscosity is decreased (no string sign).
  - Haemarthrosis: a bloody aspirate; causes include trauma, tuberculous arthritis, coagulation disorders and anticoagulation therapy.
- Microscopic appearance of effusions:
  - Cell count:
    - Inflammatory – high WCC (>1000 cells/mm^3 [>1.0 × 10^9/L]); predominantly neutrophils and lymphocytes >50% polymorphonuclear cells.
    - Septic – very high WCC (>50,000 cells/mm^3 [50 × 10^9/L]), but may occur in rheumatoid, crystal and reactive arthritides (ReA); usually >90% polymorphonuclear cells.
    - Non-inflammatory: WCCs <1000/mm^3.
  - Crystals:
    - Monosodium urate (gout): needle-shaped, negatively birefringent on polarised microscopy.
    - Calcium pyrophosphate (pseudogout): rhomboid, positively birefringent on polarised microscopy.
- Microbiology:
  - Gram stain, acid-fast methods, and bacteriological, fungal and mycobacterial cultures are important in suspected infection (inoculation into blood culture bottles improves sensitivity). Longer incubation periods (usually 4 weeks) are required if fastidious or slow-growing organisms are suspected. PCR analysis (including bacterial 16S rDNA if recent antibiotic use) can be undertaken. Antimicrobial therapy is guided by sensitivity testing.
- Glucose level may be very low in septic arthritis (e.g. tuberculosis). Low levels may also be seen in RA.

Presentation and classification

RA is the commonest chronic inflammatory joint disease, with a prevalence of 1% in the industrialised world. Disease expression is multifactorial, precipitated by environmental trigger(s) occurring in genetically susceptible individuals:

- The shared epitope of the HLA-DRB1*04 cluster is found in >80% patients with RA.
- Cigarette smoking is associated with a higher risk and severity of RA.

For classification criteria for RA, see Table 20.1.

Clinical features

Symptoms

- Typically insidious onset, with pain, swelling and stiffness affecting ≥1 joint.
- Sub-acute onset in ~one-third of patients with systemic manifestations (fatigue, weight loss, malaise). In elderly patients, a more acute presentation can occur.
- 'Inactivity stiffness': worse in the morning and after periods of immobility.
- Joint involvement: classically symmetrical. Predominantly affects proximal interphalangeal (PIP), metacarpophalangeal (MCP) joints, wrists, metatarsophalangeal (MTP) joints, knees and hips; sparing of distal interphalangeal (DIP) joints.

Table 20.1 The 2010 American College of Rheumatology/European League Against Rheumatism classification criteria for RA (adapted from Aletaha et al., 2010 [2])

	Score
A. Joint involvement:	
• 1 large joint	0
• 2–10 large joint	1
• 1–3 small joints (with or without involvement of large joints)	2
• 4–10 small joints (with or without involvement of large joints)	3
• >10 joints (at least 1 small joints)	5
B. Serology (at least 1 test result is needed for classification):	
• Negative RF and negative ACPA	0
• Low-positive RF or low-positive ACPA	2
• High-positive RF or high-positive ACPA	3
C. Acute-phase reactants (at least 1 test result is needed for classification):	
• Normal CRP and normal ESR	0
• Abnormal CRP or Abnormal ESR	1
D. Duration of symptoms:	
• <6 weeks	0
• ≥6 weeks	1

Target population (who should be tested?): Patients (1) who have ≥1 joint with definite clinical synovitis (swelling); (2) with the synovitis not better explained by another disease. Classification criteria for RA (score-based algorithm: add score of categories A–D: a score of ≥6/10 is needed for classification of a patient as having definite RA).
ACPA, anticitrullinated protein antibody.
Adapted by permission from BMJ Publishing Group Limited. *Annals of the Rheumatic Diseases*, Aletaha, D. et al. 2010 Rheumatoid arthritis classification criteria: an American College of Rheumatology/European League Against Rheumatism collaborative initiative, 69, 9, pp. 1580–1588. http://dx.doi.org/10.1136/ard.2010.138461.

Clinical manifestations

- Soft-tissue swelling over the joints with tenderness.
- Joint deformities: swan-neck and boutonniere in the fingers, Z-thumb, ulnar deviation at the MCP joints, radial deviation of the wrist joint, over-riding and hammer toes.
- Rheumatoid nodules (~20% of patients):
  - Firm, mobile and usually over pressure points.
  - Consist of fibrinoid necrosis and palisading histiocytes.
- Muscle weakness (due to disuse atrophy), tenosynovitis and bursitis.

For complications and extra-articular manifestations of RA, see Box 20.1.

Diagnosis

Laboratory

- FBC: normochromic, normocytic or hypochromic microcytic anaemia, thrombocytosis, neutropenia associated with Felty's syndrome (see Box 20.1).
- Inflammatory markers (ESR and CRP): elevated, especially in acute flares.
- Auto-antibodies (RF and anti-CCP): anti-CCP has greater sensitivity and specificity than RF. Anti-CCP can be detected several years prior to onset of RA.
- Renal, liver and bone biochemistry: to exclude other pathologies and prior to institution of medical treatments.

Box 20.1 Complications and extra-articular manifestations of rheumatoid arthritis

- *Skin*: palmar erythema, leucocytoclastic vasculitis, Raynaud's phenomenon.
- *Bone*: osteoporosis and avascular necrosis.
- *Haematological*: anaemia, leucopaenia, thrombocytosis, lymphoma (2–3-fold increase in incidence, especially in long-standing RA). Felty's syndrome (triad of splenomegaly, pancytopaenia [most frequently neutropaenia] and RA).
- *Respiratory*: interstitial lung disease, pleurisy, pleural thickening, pleural effusions, lung nodules, bronchiectasis, Caplan's syndrome (pulmonary nodulosis and pneumoconiosis).
- *Cardiac*: inflammatory pericardial effusions, nodule formation in the heart (rare); ischaemic heart disease and stroke.
- *Ocular*: scleritis, episcleritis, scleromalacia perforans and sicca symptoms due to secondary Sjögren's syndrome.
- *Renal*: membranous glomerulonephritis, NSAID-induced tubulointerstitial nephritis and analgesic nephropathy (papillary necrosis); pauci-immune necrotising glomerulonephritis; secondary AA amyloidosis (a life-threatening complication in longstanding disease).
- *Neurological*:
  - Entrapment neuropathies, e.g. carpal tunnel syndrome, sensorimotor neuropathy and mononeuritis multiplex.
  - Atlanto-axial subluxation – a life-threatening complication of RA. In milder cases, presents with cervical or occipital pain and headache without neurological deficit, but in more severe cases, with cervical myelopathy leading to paraesthesia, weakness and upper motor neurone signs in the limbs, and bladder and bowel sphincter dysfunction. Flexion-extension radiographs of the cervical spine and MRI are used for diagnosis.

Synovial fluid analysis in RA

➲ See Synovial fluid analysis, p. 706.

- Undertaken if diagnostic uncertainty or to exclude other pathology, e.g. septic arthritis.

Imaging tests

- Plain film radiography.
- Joint US examination.
- MRI of small joints of the hands and feet may help (e.g. peri-articular osteopaenia, erosions, joint space narrowing), where plain films and US have been unremarkable.

Prognosis

Early diagnosis (Table 20.1) and treatment with newer and better synthetic and biologic disease-modifying anti-rheumatic drugs (DMARDs) has transformed the outcome of patients with RA. Comorbidity may contribute to functional decline and mortality, especially cardiovascular disease, malignancy and infections.

Poor prognostic indicators

- Female gender.
- Smoking.
- Presence of the shared epitope HLA-DRB1*04 cluster.
- RF positivity with high titres (especially IgA RF) and anti-CCP.
- High disease activity score (DAS) on presentation:
  - DAS is a composite score of the swollen and tender joint counts, the visual analogue scale of patients' assessment of their general health, and either ESR or CRP.
  - A DAS based on 28 joints (DAS-28) is used to guide treatment (➲ see Biologic DMARDs, p. 709).

- High inflammatory markers.
- Insidious onset.
- Constitutional symptoms.
- Early erosions.
- Presence of nodules.
- Poor functional state at 1 year and social deprivation.

Management

An MDT approach is required (physiotherapy, occupational therapy, podiatry and chiropody), with good patient education and counselling. DMARDs and pain relief (e.g. simple analgesics and NSAIDs) are required. Surgical intervention (e.g. arthrodesis and joint replacement) can improve pain and joint function. A more aggressive early treatment therapy in RA in a 'step down' approach is applied.

Glucocorticoids

- Effective for acute symptom control.
- Can be administered:
  - Orally.
  - Intra-articularly, provided septic arthritis has been excluded.
  - Intra-muscularly or intravenously.
- Long-term toxicity limits their use. Caution should be undertaken if comorbidities, e.g. diabetes, osteoporosis and psychiatric illness.

DMARD therapy

Combination DMARD therapy is more effective than monotherapy.

The two main groups of DMARDs are synthetic and biologic. Monitoring of bloods (especially FBC, LFTs) and symptoms is required. Screening for infections (including TB) is essential prior to initiation of treatment due to the immunosuppressive effects of DMARDs. Lifestyle advice including diet, travel and vaccination guidance enables an informed decision to be made.

Synthetic DMARDs

- Conventional synthetic DMARDs (csDMARDs):
  - Methotrexate, a competitive inhibitor of dihydrofolate reductase (DHFR), is the first-line DMARD (1, 2). DHFR catalyses the conversion of dihydrofolate to the active tetrahydrofolate. Folate is needed for nucleoside thymidine production (required for DNA synthesis) and for purine and pyrimidine base biosynthesis. In RA, methotrexate has further inhibitory actions on T- and B-cell function.
  - Methotrexate is often used in combination with sulfasalazine, hydroxychloroquine and leflunomide.
  - Ciclosporin, azathioprine, penicillamine and gold salts are rarely used currently, mainly due to their toxicity.
- Targeted synthetic DMARDs (tsDMARDs):
  - Janus kinase (JAK) inhibitors (e.g. baracitinib, tofacitinib) are targeted small molecule oral systemic DMARDs.

Biologic DMARDs

Biologic DMARDs comprise a group of recombinant proteins targeted against specific molecules or molecular interactions. The use of biologic DMARDs is limited by their high costs. Biosimilar DMARDs have been introduced in recent years as a more cost-effective therapy and are being increasingly used instead of bio-original DMARDs. Treatment with biologics is initiated if there is evidence of active disease (DAS 28 >5.1) and patients have failed treatment with two DMARDs, one being methotrexate (unless specifically contraindicated) (2).

- Biologic DMARD use mandates a careful screening process prior to treatment initiation including screening for:
  - Mycobacterial infections: if active, requires treatment. Prophylactic anti-TB therapy for those with potential latent disease (e.g. past history of TB or abnormal CXR).
  - Hepatitis B and C and HIV: hepatitis B vaccination is offered to high risk patients. Furthermore, influenza (including vaccines generated for specific strain outbreaks) and pneumococcal vaccinations are given prior to biologic DMARDs (unless contraindicated).
  - Malignancy: caution is warranted in patients with previous malignancy and premalignant conditions (e.g. Barrett's oesophagus, cervical dysplasia). The risk for specific skin cancers (e.g. malignant melanoma) should be discussed, and preventative skin care and surveillance offered. Anti-tumour necrosis factor (TNF) treatment must be discontinued if malignancy is confirmed.
- Anti-TNF therapy is contraindicated in patients with:
  - Multiple sclerosis and used with caution with other demyelinating diseases.
  - NYHA grade 3 or 4 cardiac failure (see Table 13.39) and used with caution in patients with mild cardiac failure (NYHA grade 1 or 2).
- TNFα inhibitors: the most widely used biologic DMARDs; include two anti-TNF-α antibodies, infliximab (chimeric human-murine monoclonal antibody) and adalimumab (recombinant human monoclonal antibody), and a recombinant human TNF receptor fusion protein, etanercept. Etanercept and adalimumab are administered SC; infliximab is administered IV. They produce rapid and sustained symptom improvement, as well as retarding joint destruction and radiological progression.
- B-cell depletion/anti-CD20: rituximab is an anti-CD20 (receptor on B cells) monoclonal antibody used if anti-TNF therapies fail or cannot be used.
- Other agents (may be used as a first line biologic agent in RA, or if TNF-α inhibitors fail):
  - T cell co-stimulatory blocker, abatacept – a fusion protein that binds to CD80 and CD86 receptors on APC, thereby, selectively blocking their interaction with CD28 on T cells.
  - IL-6 receptor antibody, tocilizumab – strongly suppresses CRP production, therefore masking infection; contraindicated in diverticular disease.

References

1. British Society of Rheumatology (BSR) guidelines: https://www.rheumatology.org.uk/practice-quality/guidelines.
2. NICE. Rheumatoid arthritis in adults: management. Clinical guideline CG79. https://www.nice.org.uk/guidance/ng100.

Psoriatic arthritis

Pathogenesis

Genetic factors

- Family history of psoriasis or psoriatic arthritis (PsA) in 40% of patients.
- Increased frequency of psoriasis and PsA in monozygotic and dizygotic twins.
- HLA associations:
  - Increased frequency of HLA-B13, B17, B27, B38, B39, DR4, DR7 and Cw6.
  - HLA B22 may be protective.
- Links with chromosome 16q (*22-A*) class I MHC chain-related gene A, and TNF-α and TNF-β polymorphisms on chromosome 6 associated with progressive, erosive disease.

Immunological factors

- Predominance of T cytotoxic (CD8+) cells in SF and entheses.
- Pro-inflammatory cytokines (e.g. TNF-α and interleukins) increased in the synovium and SF (pattern similar to RA).

Environmental factors

- Higher levels of antibody to streptococcal organisms.
- Altered balance between CD4 and CD8+ T cells or a viral trigger may predispose to psoriasis and PsA in patients with HIV.
- Stress may trigger PsA.

PsA pathophysiology is largely centred around the enthesis (unlike in RA, where it is mainly in the synovium).

Presentation and clinical manifestations

Joint inflammation in PsA ranges from peripheral disease to axial (Table 20.2) (1), synovium and soft tissue involvement, enthesitis, osteolysis and new bone formation. The skin disease usually predates the arthropathy, often by many years.

Patterns of PsA based on Moll and Wright classification system are shown in Table 20.2.

Table 20.2. Patterns of PsA based on Moll and Wright classification system

Type	Characteristic features
Symmetric polyarthritis*	Multiple, symmetric involvement of small or large joints, similar to RA. More erosive joint damage, independent from the frequency of the polyarthritis. Female predominance.
Asymmetric oligoarthritis*	The most common presenting type. <5 small or large joints affected on either side of the body. Male predominance.
Distal arthritis	Involvement of the DIP joints.
Arthritis mutilans	Destructive and deforming; subluxation of joints and telescoping of digits. Generally long-standing disease. Female preponderance.
Spondyloarthropathy	Includes sacroilitis and spondylitis, can be asymmetrical. HLA B27 link stronger with bilateral sacroiliitis.

* Commonest presentations.

Reprinted from *Seminars in Arthritis and Rheumatism*, 3, Moll, J. M., Wright, V., Psoriatic arthritis, pp. 55-78. Copyright © 1973 with permission from Elsevier. https://doi.org/10.1016/0049-0172(73)90035-8.

Diagnosis and classification

Classification of CASPAR study criteria for PsA are presented in Box 20.2.

Box 20.2 Classification of psoriatic arthritis (CASPAR) study criteria for PsA

Musculoskeletal inflammation (inflammatory arthritis, enthesitis or back pain). Plus ≥3 of the following:

1. Skin psoriasis (current or previous, or a positive family history if the patient not affected).
2. Nail lesions.
3. Dactylitis.
4. Negative RF.
5. Juxta-articular bone formation on radiography.

Reproduced with permission from Taylor, W. et al., Classification criteria for psoriatic arthritis: development of new criteria from a large international study. *Arthritis & Rheumatology*, 2006;54:2665–73. Copyright © 2006, American College of Rheumatology and John Wiley and Sons. https://doi.org/10.1002/art.21972.

- *Dactylitis* ('sausage digit'): uniform swelling of soft tissues between the MCP and interphalangeal joints, with the appearance of diffusely swollen digital tufts.
- *Nail lesions:* have a strong association with arthropathy (especially DIP joints). ➲ See Chapter 21, Clinical features, p. 759.
- In the absence of psoriasis, PsA sine psoriasis should be considered with nail lesions, distal and asymmetric joint involvement, dactylitis, a positive family history of psoriasis and presence of HLA-Cw6.
- *Enthesitis* can involve the pelvic bones, Achilles tendon and plantar fascia. Marked osteitis or synovitis may be present in the immediately adjacent tissues.
- *Tenosynovitis* can occur, e.g. flexor tendons of the hands.
- *Uveitis*: typically presents with a painful, red eye ± blurred vision (➲ see Chapter 18, Uveitis, p. 665).

Investigations

- *Laboratory investigations*: In PsA, laboratory investigations are not diagnostic, but may suggest an underlying inflammatory process e.g. ↑ESR and a leukocytosis (Table 20.3).
  - *Immunological tests*: low titres of RF and, without exposure to anti-TNF therapies, anti-nuclear (ANA) and anti-double stranded (DNA) antibodies can be seen in PsA. HLA antigens may help support the diagnosis of PsA.
- *Radiographic tests*:
  - Joint erosions.
  - Joint space narrowing.
  - Bony proliferation (e.g. periarticular and shaft periostitis). Can occur at the entheses, particularly around the pelvis and calcaneum resulting in ankyloses of a joint.
  - Spur formation.
  - Osteolysis (e.g. 'pencil in cup' deformity and osteolysis of terminal phalanges).
  - Ankylosis.
  - Spondylitis.
  - Soft tissue swelling.

For laboratory anomalies in PsA, see Table 20.3.

Table 20.3 Laboratory abnormalities seen in PsA

Test	Result	Significance
Hb	Low	Anaemia of chronic disease; prolonged NSAID use.
WCC	High	Leucocytosis indicative of inflammation/infection.
ESR/CRP	High	Inflammation/infection. Correlates with disease activity.
Urate	High	Metabolic changes/increased skin cell turnover.*
Immunoglobulins	High	Inflammation. Increased IgA associated with spondyloarthropathy.

*An acute monoarthritis necessitates exclusion of gouty arthritis, even with an established underlying diagnosis of PsA.

Management

PsA requires an integrated, MDT approach (➲ see Rheumatoid arthritis, Management, p. 709).
Medical treatments include:

- *NSAIDs*: the first line of treatment, especially in axial disease.
- *Corticosteroids*: may exacerbate skin disease.

- *Synthetic DMARDs*: methotrexate is the first line treatment for skin and joints in PsA. Other DMARDs include sulfasalazine, leflunomide and ciclosporin. Hydroxychloroquine can exacerbate the skin lesions. The British Society of Rheumatology (BSR) suggests treatment with ≥2 DMARDs, for at least 6 months (of which ≥2 months is at standard target dose [unless intolerance or toxicity limits the dose]) prior to the introduction of anti-TNF agents.
- *Biologic DMARDs*: include anti-TNF agents, JAK1/3 inhibitor (tofacitinib), PDE4 inhibitor (apremilast), IL-12/23 inhibitor (ustekinumab) and IL-17 inhibitor (secukinumab, ixekizumab):
    - Improve all facets of the disease, including skin, joints and entheses.
    - May further potentiate the risk of specific skin cancers; caution is needed in patients previously treated with PUVA (➲ see Biologic DMARDs, p. 709).
    - Annual skin checks by a consultant dermatologist are recommended.

Prognosis

Poor prognostic factors in PsA include:

- Polyarticular presentation.
- High inflammatory markers (ESR).
- Presence of HLA B27, B39 and DQw3.
- Anti-CCP positivity.

Crystal arthritis

Gout

Risk factors for gout include hyperuricaemia, male gender, obesity and rapid weight loss. Secondary hyperuricaemia is caused by reduced excretion (more commonly) or overproduction of uric acid.

Causes of hyperuricaemia (➲ see Chapter 1, Causes of hyperuricaemia, p. 32).

Presentation and clinical manifestations

Acute gout

- History:
    - Usually monoarticular, typically first MTP joint (podagra: gout affecting the great toe).
    - Weight-bearing joints (e.g. knees), elbows, wrists and small joints of the hand.
    - Tenosynovitis.
    - Usually self-limiting attacks lasting up to a week.
    - Systemic manifestations: malaise, low grade fever.
- Clinical manifestations:
    - Hot, swollen, painful joint(s) often with overlying/surrounding erythema.
    - Desquamation of skin overlying the affected joint.
    - Bursitis (typically olecranon or pre-patellar bursae).

Chronic gout

- History:
    - Polyarticular presentation; may be monoarticular.
    - Gradual increase in frequency and duration of attacks.
    - Tophus formation (deposits of urate crystals, lipids, proteins and calcium).
    - Joint destruction and deformity resulting from repeated attacks.

- Clinical manifestations:
  - As for acute gout, but with deformity and impaired function of joints.
  - SC tophi are found at the elbows, knees, dorsal aspect of MCP joints, pinna of the ear and Achilles tendon. Tophi can also occur in other organs. A creamy, thick discharge may extrude through the skin, and infection may ensue.

Diagnostic tests

- Laboratory:
  - Leucocytosis can occur in acute gout.
  - Elevated inflammatory markers.
  - Biochemistry may indicate underlying cause (e.g. raised urea/creatinine, LFTs and bone profile).
  - Serum urate level can be normal during an acute attack (unlike chronic gout).
- Synovial fluid analysis (➲ see Synovial fluid analysis, p. 706):
  - SF examination should be undertaken promptly to avoid disintegration of the crystals.
  - Exudate from gouty tophi can also be analysed under polarised light microscopy.
  - Septic arthritis should be excluded as crystal arthropathy and sepsis can co-exist.
- Imaging tests: plain radiographs.
- Acute gout: non-specific soft tissue swelling; often unremarkable.
- Chronic gout may show:
  - Erosions with periosteal bone formation ('erosion with overhanging margin').
  - Tophi near joints: appear eccentric and nodular, ± calcification. They can erode the cortex of the bone. The classic 'punched out lesion' with a sclerotic border is seen when a tophus erodes the joint.

Prognosis

Chronic tophaceous gout may be progressive, with development of renal calculi, in those with long-standing hyperuricaemia, persistent risk factors and poor drug compliance.

Management

Patient education and dietary advice is important to ensure understanding of risk factors for hyperuricaemia. Patients should be screened and treated for comorbidities, e.g. hypertension, diabetes.

Acute gout

- NSAIDs: traditionally indometacin, other NSAIDs are also effective.
- Colchicine: lower dose is better tolerated (less likely to cause diarrhoea).
- Glucocorticoids:
  - Oral steroids, e.g. prednisolone 20–50 mg daily for 5–10 days (or longer, as indicated).
  - Intra-articular if only one or two joints are affected.
  - IM in polyarticular gout.
  - Rarely, IV administration required.
- Other: simple analgesics, topical ice, rest.

Chronic gout

As for acute gout, but additional medication for patients with >2–3 gout attacks, or after one attack in those with gouty tophi, renal insufficiency, uric acid stones and on diuretics.

The following agents can be commenced 2–4 weeks after an acute attack:

- Uricostatic agents: inhibitors of xanthine oxidase enzyme, which inhibits production of urate from hypoxanthine and xanthine.
  - Allopurinol, febuxostat (if allopurinol contra-indicated or ineffective), thiopurinol, oxipurinol.
  - Lower dose allopurinol (if high dose not tolerated) in combination with benzbromarone.

- Uricosuric agents: second line in those intolerant or resistant to allopurinol. They promote renal excretion of uric acid crystals and therefore increase risk of stone formation.
  - Sulfinpyrazone, probenecid, benzbromarone.
- Other:
  - Uricolytic agents (forms of urate oxidase, e.g. uricozyme and rasburicase). High risk of antibody formation and infusion reactions.
  - Colchicine: long-term prophylactic treatment (lower doses than for acute attacks).
  - Losartan, fenofibrate and statins have a weak uricosuric effect. Useful adjuvants in patients who may benefit from their therapeutic hypotensive and lipid-lowering effects.

Surgical intervention for extensive joint destruction.

Pseudogout

Pseudogout results from excessive deposition of calcium pyrophosphate dehydrate (CPPD) crystals in joints, and may cause an acute or chronic arthropathy.

CPPD disease presentations and diagnostic criteria are shown in Table 20.4.

Table 20.4 CPPD disease presentations and diagnostic criteria

Description	Presentation and clinical manifestations
Pseudogout	Usually a monoarthropathy (e.g. knee, shoulder, wrist); rarely in smaller joints. Acute pain, swelling, overlying erythema; mimics septic arthritis. Attacks usually self-limiting (last longer than gout). Systemic manifestations similar to gout with fever and malaise. Can be severe in elderly, with hypotension and confusion.
Pseudorheumatoid	Polyarthritic presentation with synovitis, large joint symptoms and generalised stiffness.
Pseudo-osteoarthritis: • with attacks • without attacks	Acute on chronic symptoms ± synovitis. Pain and stiffness are the commonest manifestations.
Asymptomatic	Incidental chondrocalcinosis on plain radiographs.
Pseudoneurotrophic	Rare, can result in severe joint destruction ± neuropathy. Association with tertiary syphilis.
Tophaceous CPPD deposits Spinal CPPD deposits: 'crowned dens syndrome' deposits around the atlanto-axial joint; spinal stenosis; cervical myelopathy. Tendon and bursa deposits	Tophaceous deposits can occur in tendons, bone and bursae. Spinal deposits tend to occur in the ligamentum flavum and can result in cord compression. In the crowned dens syndrome, acute attacks of neck pain may be associated with malaise and low grade temperature.

Data from Rosenthal AK, Ryan LM. In *Arthritis and Allied Conditions*. Koopman, WJ (Ed) (14th edition). Philadelphia: Williams and Wilkins pg. 2348–71, 2001.

Diagnostic tests

Laboratory

- As for gout (➲ see Diagnostic tests, p. 714), but need to exclude associated electrolyte and metabolic abnormalities, including haemachromatosis, hypothyroidism, hyperparathyroidism, hypomagnesaemia, hypercalcaemia, hypophosphataemia, Wilson's disease, gout and diabetes mellitus.

Imaging tests: plain radiographs

- Acute pseudogout: unremarkable or show non-specific soft tissue swelling.
- Chronic pseudogout: chondrocalcinosis commonly in medial and lateral menisci of the knee, triangular fibrocartilage of the wrist and symphysis pubis.
- Joint space can be narrowed, with subchondral cyst formation and relative paucity of osteophytes (unlike osteoarthritis).
- Spinal disease: subchondral cysts in the facet joints and disc calcification.

Management

Underlying causes should be identified and treated.

Acute peudogout

- NSAIDs.
- Simple analgesics.
- Glucocorticoids: usually intra-articular.

Chronic pseudogout

As for acute pseudogout, plus:

- Colchicine: usually lower daily dose than gout.
- Glucocorticoids: short course of oral steroids; intra-articular with monoarthropathy.
- Surgery (joint replacement) if extensive cartilage loss.

Reactive arthritis

Reactive arthritis (ReA) describes an aseptic inflammatory condition of the joints, which is triggered by an extra-articular infectious agent (Box 20.3). They are classically Gram-negative obligate or facultative intracellular aerobic bacteria, which invade the mucosae, have lipopolysaccharide as part of their outer membrane and contain virulence factors, which alter host immune responses. Reiter's syndrome refers to ReA associated with urethritis and/or eye inflammation.

Box 20.3 Common organisms involved in ReA

Enteric bacteria

- *Salmonella* (various serovars).
- *Shigella (flexneri, dysenteriae, sonnei)*.
- *Yersinia (enterocolitica, pseudotuberculosis)*.
- *Campylobacter (jejuni, coli, Clostridium difficile, Escherichia coli* 0157).

Urogenital bacteria

- *Chlamydia trachomatis* (persists in host for years).
- *Mycoplasma genitalium*.
- *Ureaplasma urealyticum*.

Respiratory bacteria

- Group A beta haemolytic streptococcus.
- Chlamydia pneumonia.

Presentation

Clinical features

History

- Usually young people affected (25–35 years).
- Inflammatory-type back pain and peripheral joint oligoarthritis (usually lower limbs) within 6 weeks of relevant infection.
- History of enteric (e.g. diarrhoea) or genitourinary (e.g. dysuria) symptoms.
- Systemic symptoms: malaise, lethargy, loss of appetite, etc.

Examination

- Monoarticular or polyarticular presentation (usually of large joints), ± synovitis.
- Dactylitis.
- Positive sacroiliac stress test.
- Plantar fasciitis and enthesitis (usually in lower limbs); can become crusty and confluent. May be difficult to discriminate from pustular psoriasis.
- Keratoderma and pustulosis on palms and soles.
- Balanitis (if urogenital).
- Erythema nodosum.

Classification criteria

ReA is classified using major and minor criteria (1).
Major criteria include:

- Arthritis and two of the following: asymmetrical presentation, mono- or oligoarthritis, and mainly affecting the lower limbs.
- Prior symptomatic infection, with either one or two of the following, each starting 3 days to 6 weeks before the arthritis: enteritis (diarrhoea for ≥1 day), urethritis (dysuria or discharge for ≥1 day).

Minor criteria include:

- A triggering infection proven by urethral or cervical swab for *Chlamydia trachomatis* or a positive urine ligase reaction, or enteric pathogens associated with ReA identified by stool cultures, and
- Ongoing synovial infection indicated by positive immunohistology or PCR for chlamydia.

ReA is defined as definite if two major criteria and a relevant minor criteria are satisfied. ReA is probable if there are only two major criteria, or one major and ≥one minor criteria.

Diagnosis

Laboratory

- Raised inflammatory markers (ESR/CRP).
- IgA can be elevated.
- RF and ANA negative.
- HLA B27 positive in 60–90% of patients with ReA.
- Urogenital smear may be negative, even if high suspicion of infection.
- Urinalysis for leucocytes; culture may be negative (sterile pyuria).
- Antibodies (IgG, IgA, IgM) to relevant organisms can be raised.

Synovial fluid analysis

- Undertaken to rule out septic or crystal arthritis.
- Inflammatory cell infiltrate; no organisms grown.

Imaging

- Plain film radiographs:
  - Sacroiliitis: frequently unilateral.
  - Enthesophytes: appear eroded (bone appearance smooth in diffuse idiopathic skeletal hyperostosis [DISH] enthesophytes).
  - Peripheral arthritis: mostly non-erosive.
- MRI: high signal uptake on T2-weighted sequences at sacroiliac joints (SIJs), sites of entheses (peripherally) ± synovitis and at corners of vertebrae (Romanus lesions) as with ankylosing spondylitis (AS).

Prognosis

ReA is usually mild and self-limiting; ~75% achieve remission by 2 years. A relapsing-remitting or an aggressive chronic progressive course occurs in 15%. HLA B27 presence predicts more severe disease.

Management

Management includes patient education, screening and counselling for sexually transmitted diseases and HIV, and slit-lamp examination to exclude uveitis.

Medical treatment

- Antibiotics, e.g. 3-month course of lymecycline for urogenital ReA; 10-day (or longer) course of doxycycline.
- Pain relief, e.g. NSAIDs, simple analgesics.
- Glucocorticoids: intra-articular or short oral course in peripheral joint disease.
- Synthetic DMARDs: sulfasalazine and methotrexate in chronic disease.
- Biologic DMARDs: although not licensed, chronic ReA has been successfully treated with anti-TNF.

Reference

1. Braun J, Kingsley G, van der Heijde D, et al. On the difficulties of establishing a consensus on the definition of and diagnostic investigations for reactive arthritis. Results and discussion of a questionnaire prepared for the 4th International Workshop on Reactive Arthritis, Berlin, Germany, July 3–6, 1999. *J. Rheumatol*. 2000; 27(9):2185–92.

Inflammatory bowel disease-related arthritis

Pathogenesis

Inflammatory bowel disease-related arthritis, otherwise known as enteropathic arthritis, describes an inflammatory arthritis affecting the peripheral joints or the axial skeleton (spondyloarthropathy [SpA] type) in patients with IBD, such as Crohn's disease or ulcerative colitis. An impairment of gut-mediated immunity and increased bowel permeability allowing entry of bacteria into the circulation is thought to play a key role. CD4 Th1 cell and macrophage activation, IL-12, IL-15, IL-16, IL-18, TNFα and IFNγ are all implicated in the inflamed mucosa of Crohn's patients, but this immunopathological link with the joints/entheses remains to be established. SpA is associated with HLA B27.

Presentation and clinical manifestations

Peripheral arthritis

History

- Usually transient, migratory and non-deforming.
- Knee and ankle joints most commonly affected.
- Acute flares are generally self-limiting and subside within 6 weeks; recurrences are common.
- Intestinal symptoms (abdominal pain, altered bowel habit, passing blood per rectum) usually antedate or coincide with joint flares.

Clinical manifestations

- Hot, swollen, painful joint(s) often with overlying/surrounding erythema.
- Systemic manifestations (e.g. malaise, lethargy, low-grade fever, loss of appetite).

Spondyloarthropathy

History

- Inflammatory spinal pain (first part of the day, associated stiffness, improves with exercise and anti-inflammatories).
- Alternating buttock pain.
- Features of enthesopathy, e.g. at Achilles tendon insertion site.
- Dactylitis.
- Sacroiliitis does not correlate with the onset or exacerbation of IBD and may antedate for years the onset of colitis/ileitis.

Clinical manifestations

- As for AS (➲ see Presentation and clinical manifestations, p. 720):
  - Positive sacroiliac stress test.
  - Features of dactylitis and enthesopathy.

Extra-articular manifestations common to both peripheral arthritis and spondyloarthropathy

- Eyes: anterior uveitis, episcleritis, marginal keratitis.
- Mucocutaneous: aphthous ulcers, urethritis, cervicitis.
- Skin: erythema nodosum, pyoderma gangrenosum.

Investigations

Laboratory

- Raised inflammatory markers: may reflect either active joint disease or active IBD, or both. Peripheral arthritis and SpA can flare without raising the acute phase response.
- Anaemia of chronic disease.
- Tests reflecting malabsorption: e.g. low vitamin B12 and folate; coeliac screen; low albumin with protein-losing enteropathy.

Imaging tests

- Enteropathic SpA features are similar to those found in all SpAs (➲ see Radiological, p. 722).
- Peripheral joint space narrowing and erosions on X-rays; synovitis (on US/MRI).

Management

Patient education, physiotherapy and close liaison with a gastroenterologist are pertinent to the management of enteropathic arthritis.

Medical treatments

- NSAIDs are effective for the joint symptoms, but can aggravate IBD and worsen anaemia. Simple analgesics are preferred, e.g. paracetamol, codeine.
- Glucocorticoids (oral, IV, IM or intra-articular) in severe polyarticular disease are very effective.
- Bisphosphonates, e.g. pamidronate infusions for spinal osteitis-related pain and osteoporosis.
- Mesalazine has weak activity against enteropathic SpA.
- Synthetic DMARDs (e.g. methotrexate, sulfasalazine) for peripheral arthritis. In enteropathic arthritis sulfasalazine, which is also helpful for IBD, may be considered instead of a traditional 5-ASA (mesalazine). Similarly, azathioprine is beneficial for both IBD and peripheral arthritis.

Biologic DMARDs: anti-TNF agents (adalimumab, infliximab) are effective for IBD and for joint symptoms.

Surgery

Surgical intervention for severe destructive arthropathy.

Prognosis

Severe SpA has a worse outcome. Anti-TNF treatment can decelerate the destructive process and may lead to remission.

Ankylosing spondylitis

Pathogenesis

A complex interplay of genetic, immunological and environmental factors contribute to the aetiology of AS.

Genetic factors

- The precise role of HLA B27 in the pathophysiology of AS remains unexplained.
- Monozygotic concordance rate ~70%.
- First degree relatives have an ~10% risk of developing the disease, whereas only 1–5% of HLA B27 individuals develop AS suggesting that other factors are involved.

Immunological factors

- HLA B27 may not behave like other class I molecules: its heavy chains can form homodimers without the beta-2-microglobulin light chain ('HLA B27 misfolding') that, following recognition by lymphocytes, can be involved in the pro-inflammatory response.
- In the spine, inflammation results in calcification and bone formation at entheses with fibrocartilage as a target tissue. Syndesmophytes (bony bridges between vertebrae) can develop and may merge to form a 'bamboo spine'.

Environmental factors

- Infection, specifically *Klebsiella*, has been linked with the onset of AS.

Presentation and clinical manifestations

History

- Insidious onset usually before the age of 45 years.
- Inflammatory back pain, especially in lower back with alternate buttock pain (sacroiliitis). Systemic symptoms (fatigue, malaise, lethargy, low grade fever).
- Enthesitis, e.g. plantar fasciitis may precede the onset of AS for many years.
- Dyspnoea, which can be related to:
  - Reduced chest expansion.
  - Lung fibrosis (classically apical).
  - Cardiovascular system involvement (➲ see Disease classification system of bradycardias, p. 465).
- Previous/current inflammatory eye disease, e.g. uveitis (painful, red eye).

Examination

- Restricted spinal movements, especially at the lumbar and cervical regions, leading to deformities, e.g. kyphosis and complete loss of movement.
- Evidence of enthesitis.
- Peripheral joint arthritis/synovitis.
- Reduced chest expansion.

- Extra-articular manifestations:
  - Eye involvement: anterior uveitis.
  - Cardiovascular involvement:
    - Valvular lesions: classically aortic regurgitation due to aortitis of the ascending aorta.
    - First- to third-degree block due to fibrosis of the conduction system (➲ see Chapter 13, Electrocardiography, p. xxx).
  - Pulmonary involvement: although rare, lung fibrosis can occur in the upper lobes with subsequent invasion by aspergillus (➲ see Chapter 5, Case 1, p. 118 and Causes of fibrosis, p. 123). Poor thoracic expansion (partly due to thoracic spine ankylosis) and ventilatory difficulty in lung infection or cardiac disease contribute to the morbidity and increased mortality rate seen in patients with AS.
  - Renal involvement: amyloidosis in long-standing disease.
  - Neurological involvement: e.g. due to spinal fractures, atlanto-axial subluxation causing cervical myelopathy, cauda equina syndrome.
  - Metabolic bone disease: e.g. osteopaenia and osteoporosis in long-standing disease.

Diagnosis

For modified NY criteria for AS, see Box 20.4.

Box 20.4 Modified New York criteria for AS

Diagnosis

Clinical criteria

- Low back pain and stiffness for >3 months; improves with exercise, but not relieved by rest.
- Limitation of motion of the lumbar spine in both the sagittal and the frontal planes.
- Limitation of chest expansion relative to normal value, corrected for age and sex.

Radiological criterion

- Sacroiliitis grade >2 bilaterally or sacroiliitis grade 3–4 unilaterally (see Table 20.5).

Grading

- *Definite*: AS if radiological criterion present with ≥1 clinical criterion.
- *Probable*: AS if three clinical criteria present or if the radiological criterion is present without any signs or symptoms fulfilling the clinical criteria.

Adapted with permission from van der Linden, S. et al. Evaluation of diagnostic criteria for ankylosing spondylitis. A proposal for modification of the New York criteria. *Arthritis & Rheumatology*, 1984 Apr;27(4):361–8. https://doi.org/10.1002/art.1780270401.

For sacroiliitis grading, see Table 20.5.

Table 20.5 Sacroiliitis grading

Grade	Radiological criterion
0	Normal.
I	Blurring of the margins.
II	Minimal sclerosis with some erosions.
III	Definite sclerosis on both sides of joint.
	Severe erosions with pseudowidening of joint space ± ankyloses.
IV	Complete ankyloses.

Reproduced with permission from Geijer, M. et al. The validity of the New York radiological grading criteria in diagnosing sacroiliitis by computed tomography. *Acta Radiologica*, 2009;50 (6): 664–73. https://doi.org/10.1080/02841850902914099.

Investigations

Laboratory investigations

- HLA B27 in > 90% of Caucasians with AS; 50–80% in other ethnic groups (normal prevalence in the UK population ~8%).
- Raised ESR (may be normal).
- Anaemia of chronic disease (normocytic, normochromic).
- Raised IgA.

Radiological

- Pelvis:
  - Blurring of sub-chondral bone plate of SIJs.
  - Erosions and sclerosis of bone adjacent to SIJs (usually iliac side first).
  - SIJ ossification.
  - Bony ankyloses (late stage).
  - Symphysis pubis sclerosis/erosion/ankylosis (late).
- Spine:
  - Vertebral squaring ± small marginal syndesmophytes (early).
  - Erosions/sclerosis at vertebral body corners (Romanus lesions; late).
- Peripheral skeleton:
  - Hips: enthesophytes (around femoral head); diffuse concentric joint space narrowing; bony ankylosis.
  - Peripheral joints: periarticular bone proliferation (osteoperiostitis); enthesopathy, e.g. at the insertion of the Achilles tendon to the calcaneous bone.

Plain film radiographs of SIJs and spine in early AS can be normal. MRI may detect early AS changes and bone oedema.

Osteoporosis is a common complication of AS, largely confined to the axial skeleton, with a greater prevalence in men, in patients with syndesmophytes, cervical fusion, peripheral joint involvement, increasing age and disease duration. In late AS, extraspinal bone may obscure osteoporotic vertebrae, leading to artifactually increased lumbar BMD measurements obtained by DEXA scanning. More accurate investigations (e.g. quantitative CT or DEXA scanning of lateral aspect of L3 vertebra) are required in the presence of syndesmophytes.

Management

Main objective is to achieve symptom control and maintain movement and functional ability, monitoring for extra-articular disease.

Medical treatments

- NSAIDs: slow-release preparation, especially if night pain and morning stiffness are severe.
- Additional analgesics, e.g. paracetamol/codeine.
- Corticosteroid injections: indicated for enthesitis, and intra-articular for peripheral and SIJ involvement.
- Synthetic DMARDs: e.g. sulfasalazine and methotrexate for peripheral inflammatory joint disease. They are ineffective for axial disease.
- Biologic agents:
  - Anti-TNFs: adalimumab, certolizumab pegol, etanercept, golimumab and infliximab for severe active AS in patients with inadequate response, or unable to tolerate NSAIDs (1).
  - IL-17 inhibitor: secukinumab.

Surgery

- Osteotomy, fusion of unstable segments and laminectomies in severe spinal disease to improve symptoms, functional ability, raising eyeline and improving lung ventilation.

Prognosis

Poor indicators include:

- Polyarticular presentation with synovitis.
- High inflammatory markers.
- Anaemia.
- Hip involvement.
- Osteoporosis.
- Cardiovascular and respiratory disease.

References

1. NICE. TNF-alpha inhibitors for ankylosing spondylitis and non-radiographic axial spondyloarthritis. Technology appraisal guideline TA383. https://www.nice.org.uk/guidance/ta383.

Bone diseases

Bone constantly undergoes modelling to adapt to changing biomechanical forces, and remodelling to maintain bone strength and homeostasis. The remodelling process consists of resorption of old bone and formation of new bone by an interrelated four-phase cycle involving osteoclasts and osteoblasts. For the interaction between osteoblasts and osteoclasts, see Figure 20.1.

- *Activation:* colony stimulating factor-1 (CSF-1) driven recruitment of osteoclast precursors (of macrophage/monocyte lineage) from the circulation. A transmembrane osteoblast protein RANKL of the TNF family binds RANK receptors on the surface of the osteoclasts thus activating them. This process is negatively regulated by osteoprotegenerin (OPG) also found on the surface of osteoblasts, which acts as a decoy receptor for RANK.
- *Resorption:* osteoclasts release acid from plasma-membrane derived vesicles leading to dissolution of hydroxyapatite. The organic matrix is resorbed by matrix metalloproteinases and cysteine proteinases such as cathepsin K.

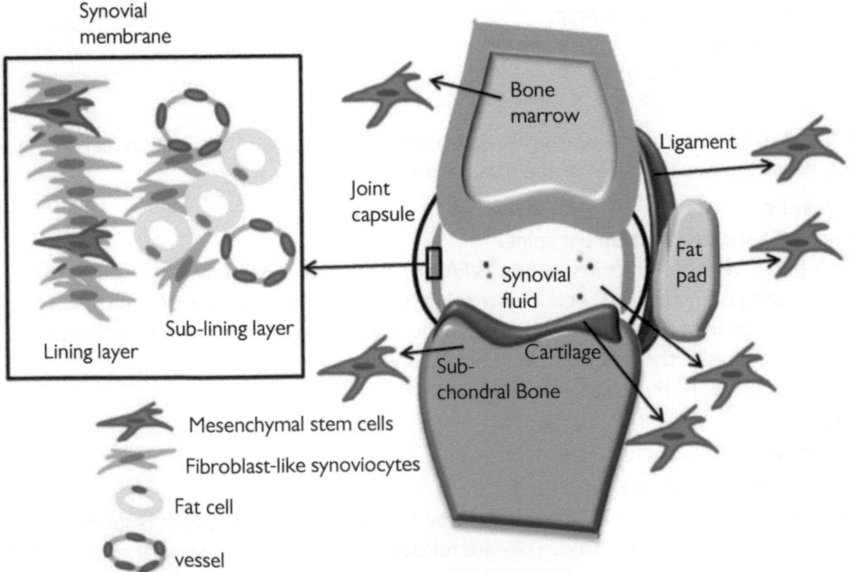

Figure 20.1 Interaction between osteoblasts and osteoclasts.

- Reversal: bone resorption transitions to bone formation.
- Bone formation: osteoblasts synthesise new collagenous organic matrix and mineralise it with calcium and phosphate. Osteoblasts within the matrix undergo apoptosis or become osteocytes, which maintain bone structure, and secrete sclerostin, which inhibits osteoblast function. Each bone remodelling cycle results in production of a new osteon.

Osteoporosis

A skeletal disorder characterised by compromised bone strength predisposing to an increased risk of fracture. The WHO definition is BMD that lies ≥2.5 standard deviations (SD) below the average value for young healthy women.

Risk factors

- Age.
- Familial/hereditary (e.g. maternal hip fracture).
- Smoking, excessive alcohol.
- Poor nutrition/low BMI.
- Sedentary lifestyle/prolonged immobilisation.
- Early menopause, >1 year of amenorrhoea.
- Male hypogonadism.
- Medical conditions: RA, Cushing's disease, untreated hyperthyrodism, Type I diabetes mellitus, hyperparathyrodism, malabsorbtion, multiple myeloma, organ/bone marrow transplant, pregnancy.
- Drugs: steroids, antiepileptics, antioestrogens, antiandrogens, selective serotonin reuptake inhibitors, depo-progesterone contraception, long-term low molecular weight heparin.

Clinical features

History of fracture, risk factors as above. Vertebral fractures can be painless, height loss may be apparent.

Investigations

- DEXA of hip, lumbar spine or wrist:
  - Osteoporosis: T-score ≤–2.5.
  - Osteopenia: –2.5 < T-score ≤–1.
  - Normal BMD: T score >–1.

Sclerotic old vertebral fractures, osteoarthritis, AS, metal plates and aortic calcification may give falsely high BMD values, which are not indicative of the true bone fragility.

- Spinal imaging:
  - X-ray of the thoracic and lumbar spine.
  - DEXA-based vertebral fracture analysis (VFA) for subclinical vertebral fractures. This low radiation lateral imaging of the thoracic and lumbar spine helps to identify vertebral fractures, up to two-thirds of which are asymptomatic. These patients are at increased risk of further fracture and have a better response to therapy (even with BMD between –1 and –2.5).
- Calcium, phosphate, PTH, alkaline phosphatase, Vitamin D.
- TFTs, U&Es.
- Myeloma and coeliac screen.
- LH, FSH, oestrogen, testosterone.
- Bone turnover markers in serum and urine can be used to monitor treatment response and guide retreatment following drug holidays. They are released when N- and C-terminal extensions of procollagen are removed by specific proteases during its conversion to collagen in osteoblasts. Laboratories most commonly measure:
  - Bone formation marker: serum type 1 N-terminal procollagen.
  - Bone resorption markers: serum collagen type 1 cross-linked C-telopeptide (CTX) and urinary collagen type 1 cross-linked N-telopeptide (NTX).

Treatment

For the fracture risk assessment tool to evaluate fracture risk and a guide to management, see Figure 20.2.

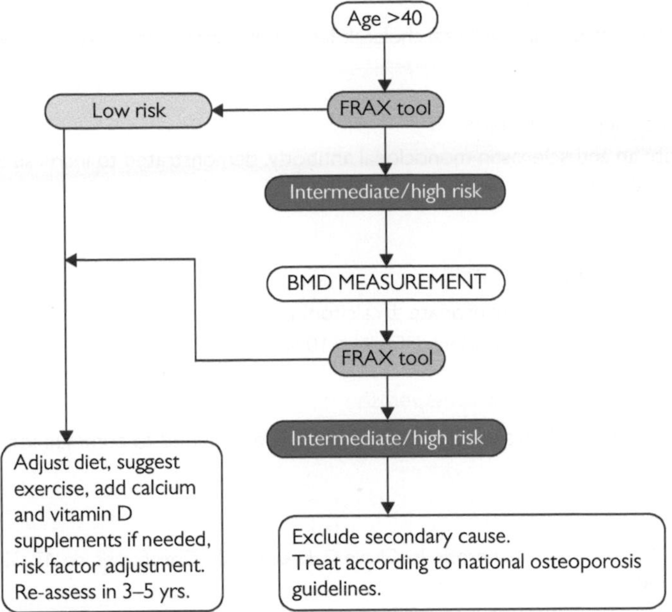

Figure 20.2 Fracture risk assessment tool (FRAX) to evaluate fracture risk and guide management

Antiresorptive

1. Oral bisphosphonates reduce fracture risk significantly, e.g. weekly alendronic acid for 5 years followed by a drug holiday. Alendronic acid is incorporated into bone mineral surfaces inhibiting osteoclast farnesyl pyrophosphate synthase, thus preventing cell resorptive activity and accelerating apoptosis. Atypical subtrochanteric fragility fractures are seen with long-term bisphosphonate use. They have poor oral absorption, poor compliance and a high incidence of upper GI side effects.
2. IV bisphosphonates: 3 years of yearly zoledronic acid prevents vertebral fractures and increases BMD. Side effects include a transient acute phase response with first infusion (myalgia, arthralgia, fever). Osteonecrosis of the jaw (ONJ) is a rare complication. Hypocalcaemia can occur with inadequate Vitamin D replacement.
3. Strontium ranelate has an increased cardiac risk (in addition to VTE risk) and use is restricted to patients with no known cardiovascular risk factors who cannot tolerate other treatments.
4. Denosumab is a humanised IgG2 monoclonal antibody to RANKL (see Table 3.4) for primary and secondary osteoporosis prevention. Safe with renal impairment. Side effects: infections, rashes, ONJ. Hypocalcaemia, with inadequate vitamin D replacement.

Anabolic

Teriparatide is a recombinant PTH administered by SC daily injection for 18–24 months. Intermittent PTH has an anabolic effect favouring bone formation. Teriparatide is reserved for patients with severe osteoporosis and recurrent fractures. Contraindications include Paget's disease, history of bone cancer and hypercalcaemia.

Hormonal

1. Hormone replacement therapy (HRT): protects against BMD loss, but breast cancer, cardiovascular and VTE risks exist. Best considered in women with premature menopause.

2. Raloxifene: a selective oestrogen receptor modulator licenced for vertebral fracture prevention only. Prevents breast cancer, can cause hot flushes and VTE.

Vitamin D replacement

Aim for >50 nmol/L by replenishing with oral cholecalciferol or IM ergocalciferol in patients with malabsorption.

Future therapies

- Odanacatib: a cathepsin K inhibitor.
- Romosozumab: an anti-sclerostin monoclonal antibody, demonstrated to increase BMD in post-menopausal women.
- RANK inhibitors.

Treatment of acute vertebral fracture

- Medically with analgesia, IV pamidronate ± calcitonin.
- Kyphoplasty/vertebroblasty considered if pain >10 weeks.

Treatment of glucocorticoid-induced osteoporosis

Prevention is required if steroid treatment of >5 mg/day is anticipated to continue for >3 months with a T score <–1.5.

Further reading

1. Clark E, Clunie G. Diagnosis of osteoporosis. In: Clunie G, Keen R (Eds) *Osteoporosis*, pp. 17–32. Oxford: Oxford University Press, 2007.

Paget's disease

Pathogenesis

A focal disorder of bone remodelling in men and women >40 years. Increased bone resorption by multinucleated osteoclasts, followed by accelerated osteoblast action and haphazard collagen deposition, results in enlarged disorganised mosaic bone structure lacking lamellar pattern. Familial clustering of Paget's disease is recognised.

Clinical features

- Frequently asymptomatic.
- Bone pain, deformity, pathological fractures, osteoarthritis.
- Deafness.
- Change in skull shape, headache, dental problems (mandibular involvement).
- Spinal claudication.
- Complications: secondary hyperparathyroidism, hypercalcaemia/hypercalciuria (due to immobility), gout, high output cardiac failure (rare), sarcoma.

Investigations

- Raised ALP.
- Raised bone resorption markers (NTX, CTX).
- Check PTH, calcium, phosphate, vitamin D.
- Radiography: plain radiograph (patchy sclerosis and lucency with coarse trabecular pattern), isotope bone scan, MRI.

Treatment

- Asymptomatic patients with low complications risk can be monitored.
- IV zoledronic acid is the gold-standard treatment (single infusion can induce remission).
- Oral bisphosphonates and intravenous pamidronate.

Osteomalacia and rickets

➲ See Chapter 1, Bone and calcium metabolism, p. 1, Figure 1.1 and Box 1.1.

Osteogenesis imperfecta

A genetic (mainly autosomal dominant [AD]) disturbance of collagen 1 production. The Sillence classification includes nine genetically defined subtypes: Type I is the mildest, Type II is lethal, Type III is severe with short stature and characteristic facies, the rest are moderate to severe. Most patients present with blue-grey sclerae, deafness, poor growth, bone deformity and fractures early in life. Multidisciplinary management includes IV bisphosphonates to increase BMD, surgical management of fractures and deformities, physiotherapy and occupational therapy.

Osteomyelitis

➲ See Chapter 8, Osteomyelitis, p. 258 and Tables 8.23 and 8.24.

Connective tissue disease

Inflammatory myopathy

For clinical features, pathogenesis and management of inflammatory myopathies, see Table 20.6.

Table 20.6 Clinical features, pathogenesis and management of inflammatory myopathies

Type of myositis	Polymyositis (PM)	Dermatomyositis (DM)	Inclusion body myositis (IBM)
Demographics Female:male Age (years)	2:1 40–60 Higher prevalence in black individuals.		1:3 >50
Pathogenesis	CD8+ cytotoxic T-cell driven process to muscle, nuclear and cytoplasmic autoantigens. Suggested triggers include viruses (e.g. HIV, parvovirus), drugs (e.g. penicillamine, phenytoin) and malignancies (8%).	CD4+ T cell driven humorally-mediated microangiopathy causing capillary damage with resulting ischaemic muscle injury.	Primarily a degenerative disorder with a likely secondary cytotoxic inflammatory component causing myofibre necrosis.
Clinical findings	Proximal symmetrical muscle weakness affecting the upper and lower limbs, and neck. Myalgia during the active phase. Respiratory muscle and myocardial involvement. Swallowing can be affected.		Insiduous, often asymmetrical muscle weakness with prominent wrist flexor, finger flexor, and knee extensor involvement. Thenar and hypothenar eminence is spared (unlike MND). Loss of manual dexterity is common. 60% have dysphagia; dysphonia and facial weakness can occur.
	Anti-synthetase syndrome (30% of PM): Defined by the presence of the anti-synthetase autoantibodies and ≥1 of: interstitial lung disease, inflammatory myopathy and small joint symmetrical inflammatory polyarthritis.	1. Cutaneous manifestations (can precede muscle involvement): • Heliotrope rash (violaceous oedematous affecting eyelids). • Gottron's papules over MCP and PIP joints and extensor surfaces. Histologically vasculitic, raised psoriaform plaques.	

continued

Table 20.6 *continued*

Type of myositis	Polymyositis (PM)	Dermatomyositis (DM)	Inclusion body myositis (IBM)
	Other common features include Raynaud's phenomenon, fever and mechanic's hands (thickened, cracked skin on the palms and radial surfaces of fingers [especially index]).	• Erythematous rash: ♦ on face, neck and chest ('V sign'); on shoulders and back ('shawl sign'); • Nail-fold changes: periungal telangiectasia and infarcts, rugged cuticles. 2. Amyopathic DM with cutaneous ± ILD features only can occur. It is associated with anti-CADM-140 antibody. 3. Respiratory muscles may be involved. 4. Extra-myopathic features (present in 50% of patients): fever, weight loss, arthritis, ILD, dysphagia, cardiac involvement, calcinosis. 5. Malignancy is found in 20% of patients including ovarian, lung, GI. It is often temporally unrelated to myositis onset. Associated with anti-p155/140, anti-TIF1-γ and anti-MDA5 antibodies.	
Diagnostic criteria (Bohan and Peter 1975 [1])	3/4 of: 1. Objective symmetrical proximal muscle weakness ± dysphagia and respiratory muscle weakness. 2. Raised CK. 3. Positive EMG findings. 4. Positive muscle biopsy.		
		DM: plus one of the cutaneous manifestations listed above.	
Investigations	Exclude other causes of muscle weakness/raised CK levels: • Recent strenuous exercise and use of anabolic steroids. • Statins can cause an immune-mediated necrotising myopathy with antibodies to HMGCR. • Higher CK values may be a normal variant in black individuals. • Check: TFTs (hypo/hyperthyroidism), Vitamin D and bone profile (osteomalacia). • Myasthenia gravis, muscular dystrophy, myotonic dystrophy, inherited metabolic myopathies, rhabdomyolysis. General investigations: • CK (raised in acute disease; normal/low once muscle damage is complete). • Troponin T/I. • ESR, CRP (often raised in the acute phase). • LFTs (AST and ALT will be raised reflecting muscle breakdown). • U&Es (usually normal unlike in rhabdomyolysis). • EMG (diagnostic short-duration, polyphasic motor unit potentials with spontaneous fibrillation potentials). • CXR, PFTs ± mammography and HRCT/PET scans to exclude underlying malignancy (esp. in men >50 and women >60 years with DM) and ILD, and baseline prior to immunosuppressives. Bedside spirometry in acute disease. • MRI of affected areas is useful diagnostically and helps target muscle biopsy.		CK <X12 upper limit of normal (modest elevation compared to PM/DM). Myopathic EMG.

Table 20.6 *continued*

Type of myositis	Polymyositis (PM)	Dermatomyositis (DM)	Inclusion body myositis (IBM)
Biopsy	Fibre necrosis, degeneration, regeneration, and an inflammatory cell infiltrate.		Endomysial inflammation with myofibre eosinophilic cytoplasmic inclusions and rimmed vacuoles containing β amyloid and ubiquitin.
	Endomysial CD8+ T cells surrounding healthy myofibrils. Necrosis of Type I and II muscle fibres with phagocytosis and evidence of regeneration.	CD4+ injury to capillaries and perifascicular myofibers which undergo atrophy and fibrosis.	
Antibodies	Myositis specific antibodies against: • Specific tRNA synthetases including: ◆ anti-Jo-1 (histidyl; 25% of patients with PM); ◆ anti-PL12 (alanine); ◆ anti-PL7 (threonine). • Helicase proteins: nuclear Mi-2 antibodies. • Components of the signal recognition particle (SRP): ◆ Patients usually have a more acute onset and may have poor response to treatment. ◆ Predict poor prognosis with cardiac involvement. ◆ Little extramuscular disease.		Negative.
	Myositis associated antibodies confer overlap with other CTDs: • PM/Scl and anti-Ku antibodies in PM/SSc overlap. • Anti-nRNP Abs are a diagnostic requirement for mixed connective tissue disease (MCTD). • Anti Ro antibodies in overlap with SLE or SjÖgren's syndrome.		
Treatment	Pulse IV corticosteroids for induction and/or tapering oral regime for maintenance. DMARDs are steroid sparing, cyclophosphamide, rituximab and IVIG for severe/resistant cases.		None shown to be effective.
		DM: UV protection and topical corticosteroids.	

Reference

1. Bohan A. History and classification of polymyositis and dermatomyositis. *Clin Dermatol*. 1988; 6(2):3–8.

Systemic lupus erythematosus

Pathophysiology

Systemic lupus erythematosus (SLE) is a heterogeneous autoimmune systemic disorder which results from a combination of genetic, environmental and hormonal factors. Over 90% of patients are women (high oestrogen state is a trigger), with disease onset often at childbearing age.

SLE is a B-cell-driven disease triggered by disordered clearance of apoptotic cell material. Polymorphisms in opsonins have been linked with SLE. Flares occur with increased apoptosis and immune activation states, e.g. infections, stress and UV light.

Clinical presentation

Cutaneous and renal manifestations (➲ see Chapter 21, Cutaneous lupus erythematosus, p. 769 and Table 21.10, and Chapter 16, Systemic lupus erythematosus, p. 574, respectively).

For revised classification criteria for SLE, see Table 20.7.

Table 20.7 1997 Revised Classification Criteria for SLE (American College of Rheumatology, Arthritis & Rheumatism, September 1997). Criterion: ≥4 is diagnostic.

Criterion	Definition
1. Malar rash	Fixed erythema over the malar eminences, spares the nasolabial folds.
2. Discoid rash	Erythematous raised patches with adherent keratotic scaling and follicular plugging. May be an isolated dermatological presentation, 35% are ANA positive, only 6.5% progress to SLE.
3. Photosensitivity	Skin rash as a result of sunlight exposure.
4. Oral ulcers	Oral or nasopharyngeal ulceration, usually painless.
5. Arthritis	Synovitis involving ≥2 peripheral joints, tenosynovitis is also common. Arthritis: erosive or Jaccoud's (deformities without erosions resulting from recurrent synovitis and inflammation of the joint capsule. The deformities are usually reducible but may later become fixed).
6. Serositis	Pleuritis, pericarditis, peritonitis.
7. Renal disorder	Renal histology consistent with immune complex-mediated glomerulonephritis. Proteinuria >0.5 g/24 hours or 3+ on dipstick, raised urine protein:creatine ratio, cellular casts.
8. Neuropsychiatric disorder	CNS and PNS involvement: aseptic meningitis, seizures, psychosis, anxiety, headache, cognitive dysfunction, myelopathy, mono/polyneuropathy.
9. Haematological disorder	Haemolytic anaemia, lymphopaenia, thrombocytopenia.
10. Immunologic disorder	Anti-dsDNA Ab, anti-Sm Ab, APL Ab, low C3/C4, false positive VDRL.
11. ANA	Positive titre.

Additional manifestations

- Ophthalmic: orbital inflammation, keratitis, scleritis, ischaemic optic neuropathy.
- Vasculitis: skin, internal organ (e.g. GI).
- Raynaud's phenomenon.

Disease complications

- Cardiovascular disease.
- Infections from immunosuppression and neutropenia.
- Macrophage activation syndrome (MAS):
  - Histocyte phagocytosis of normal haematopoietic elements in the bone marrow and peripheral organs leads to a profound inflammatory response characterised by fever, hepatosplenomegaly, lymphadenopathy and CNS dysfunction.
  - Laboratory features: pancytopenia, elevated CD25 and CD163 cells, deranged LFTs, disseminated intravascular coagulation (with low fibrinogen causing low ESR despite persistently raised CRP), high ferritin and raised triglycerides.
  - A rare complication with high mortality rate. Also occurs in juvenile idiopathic arthritis (JIA) and adult-onset Still's disease.

Drug-induced lupus

- Triggered by drugs including hydralazine, methyldopa, phenytoin, penicillamine, procainamide, isoniazid.
- Presents with fever, serositis, arthralgia and rashes. Renal and CNS involvement are rare.
- Anti-histone antibody positive, anti-dsDNA negative.

Diagnosis

- ANA: Hep2cell nucleus immunofluorescence after exposure to SLE patient sera. A homogenous pattern usually signifies dsDNA binding. The titre indicates the dilution at which fluorescence is still present, titres >1:160 are significant.
- Extractable nuclear antigens (ENAs): can be extracted from the nucleus with saline and display a speckled nuclear immunofluorescence. Anti-dsDNA antibodies are an example of anti-ENA antibodies. Subtype analysis includes iodine immunoassay, immunofluorescence against DNA-rich mitochondria of single cell organism *Crithidia luciliae* and ELISA.

For common SLE-associated anti-ENAs, see Table 20.8.

Table 20.8 Common SLE associated anti-ENAs. SLE can present with multiple antibodies developing to neighbouring antigenic foci

Autoantibody	Target antigen (ENA)	Sensitivity; specificity	Clinical relevance
Anti-dsDNA	DNA	60%; 99%	Associated with lupus nephritis (cross reaction with glomerular basement membrane proteins). Titres correlate with disease activity.
Anti-Ro	Ribonuclearproteins (RNP)	30–50%; low specificity	Cross the placenta to cause neonatal lupus. 2% risk of congenital heart block, 20% if previous child affected. Associated with subacute cutaneous lupus and Sjögren's syndrome.
Anti-La	RNP	10–15%; low specificity	Secondary Sjögren's syndrome, photosensitivity, neonatal lupus.
Anti-Smith (anti-Sm)	Small nuclear RNPs, similarities with EBV proteins	20–30%; >90%	CNS, renal lupus, vasculitis, lung and pericardial involvement.
Anti-nRNP (Anti-U1RNP)	Nuclear RNP	30–40%; low specificity	Associated with MCTD.
Anti-C1q	Complement component C1q	45%; 72%	Low complement, lupus nephritis, hypocomplementaemic urticarial vasculitis.

Other blood tests

- FBC (cytopaenias), haemolytic screen if Hb falls (haptaglobulins, bilirubin, LDH, blood film).
- ESR (raised in active disease, falls in MAS).
- CRP (normal, moderate rise with serositis or arthritis).
- U&Es, urine dipstick, urine PCR; if abnormal, proceed to renal biopsy (➔ see Chapter 16, Systemic lupus erythematosus, p. 574).
- C3, C4 (complement falls during flares).

Treatment

- Mild disease:
    - Arthralgia and mucocutaneous involvement: antimalarials and intermittent low-dose steroids.
- Moderate disease:
    - Internal organ involvement or significant skin disease: azathioprine or mycophenolate mofetil (MMF).
    - Methotrexate for inflammatory arthritis.
    - Steroids help induce remission and treat flares.

- Severe disease:
  - Renal lupus: MMF or azathioprine.
  - CNS lupus:
    - Initiation therapy: Corticosteroids (usually IV methylprednisolone), cyclophosphamide (highly potent with fast onset).
    - Maintenance therapy: MMF or azathioprine.
  - Monoclonal antibodies:
    - Rituximab (anti-CD20): used in renal, haematological and cerebral lupus.
    - Belimumab: an anti-Blys ligand (important in B cell differentiation and proliferation); especially indicated for mucocutaneous involvement and arthritis.
    - Newer agents emerging include atacicept (anti-Blys and APRIL).

Prognosis

Death is often caused by early cardiovascular disease, infections and end-organ damage (most commonly renal).

Antiphospholipid syndrome

Antiphospholipid syndrome (APLS) is an autoimmune hypercoagulable state characterised by venous, arterial and small vessel thrombosis, and/or pregnancy morbidity in the presence of antiphospholipid (aPL) antibodies. 30-40% of patients with SLE carry aPL antibodies, only 10% of these patients have APLS. 50% of APLS is primary. The diagnosis requires the presence of aPL antibodies on two occasions, 12 weeks apart, together with one clinical feature.

Clinical features

- *Vascular thrombosis*: deep vein thrombosis/pulmonary embolism, thrombotic cerebrovascular accident, cerebral venous sinus thrombosis, hepatic and renal vein thrombosis, myocardial infarction, avascular necrosis of bone and retinal vascular occlusions. Cutaneous findings include livedo reticularis, skin ulceration and purpura due to superficial vascular thrombi.
- *Pregnancy morbidity* (can be isolated without other thrombotic risk):
  - >3 consecutive miscarriages at <10 weeks gestation.
  - Preterm birth (<34 weeks gestation) due to severe pre-eclampsia, eclampsia or placental insufficiency.
  - ≥ 1 late-term (>10 weeks gestation) spontaneous pregnancy losses.
- Thrombocytopenia is not part of the criteria, but is commonly present.
- Catastrophic APLS is characterised by multiple small vessel thromboses that can lead to multi-organ failure with high mortality rates.

Antiphospholipid antibodies

Antiphospholipid antibodies (APLA) target phospholipid-rich membrane of cells such as platelets and endothelium.

- Lupus anticoagulant (LA) is a functional test: a positive test refers to the ability of aPL to cause prolongation of *in vitro* clotting assays, such as activated partial thromboplastin time and dilute Russell viper venom test, which is not reversed when the patient's plasma is diluted 1:1 with control platelet-free plasma. In contrast, such mixing studies do correct the clotting abnormality associated with factor deficiencies. Confirmatory studies are performed to document the phospholipid dependence of the inhibitor (adding phospholipids reverses the clotting prolongation, which is due to aPL).
- Positive anti-cardiolipin antibodies (IgM or IgG). These bind domain 1 of β2 glycoprotein1 pentomers causing their dimerisation on a phospholipid membrane. This results in enhanced clotting through platelet and endothelial activation and thrombotic cytokine production.
- Positive anti-β2 glycoprotein1 antibodies (anti-β2 GP1 IgM or IgG).

Differential is with other pro-coagulable states such as malignancy, protein C and S deficiency, vasculitis, thrombotic microangiopathies (thrombotic thrombocytopenic purpura, haemolytic uraemic syndrome, disseminated intravascular coagulation, haemolysis, elevated liver enzymes and low platelets), and heparin-induced thrombocytopenia (➲ see Chapter 9, Thrombophilia, p. 291 and Table 9.13).

Treatment

- Primary prevention: aspirin for patients with aPL antibodies and SLE (aPL antibodies without SLE or thrombotic history does not warrant prophylaxis).
- Secondary prevention: heparin, warfarin or new oral anticoagulants (e.g. rivaroxaban).
- Pregnancy morbidity is preventable with heparin and aspirin treatment.
- Immunosuppression has no role.

Systemic sclerosis

Pathophysiology

An autoimmune disorder characterised by skin and internal organ fibrosis, and endothelial dysfunction of unknown aetiology. Inflammatory, immunological and microvascular triggers result in massive fibroblast activation and extracellular matrix deposition.

Clinical features and treatment

- Skin: three stages – oedematous, indurative and (after ~3 years) atrophic. Findings include sclerosis, sclerodactyly, calcinosis, telangiectasia, classic systemic sclerosis (SSc) facies with nasal thinning, microstomia (reduced mouth opening) and thin lips with increased furrowing. The extent of skin involvement determines the subtypes:
  - Limited cutaneous SSc (previously 'CREST'): skin fibrosis distal to the elbows and knees, and the face.
  - Diffuse cutaneous SSc: skin fibrosis extending proximal to the elbows and knees, often involving the chest and abdomen, as well as the face. DMARDs (e.g. MMF, methotrexate) can produce modest results.
  - Morphoea: patches of skin sclerosis, no internal organ involvement; ANA negative. Linear morphoea often affects extremities in children and may cause limb deformities. Face and scalp involvement can extend to underlying bone with *en coup de sabre* ('sword strike injury') appearance, and ocular deformities.
  - SSc sine scleroderma: internal organ involvement without skin disease.
- *Raynaud's phenomenon and digital ischaemia*: digital vasospasm results in the sequential blanching (white), cyanotic (blue) and hyperaemic (red) triphasic changes. Complicated by digital ulcers and gangrene. Treatment includes:
  - Calcium channel blockers, ACE inhibitors, SSRIs (e.g. fluoxetine).
  - Digital ischaemia and necrosis require IV prostacyclin (epoprostenol).
  - Surgery is best avoided unless infection/pain are intractable.
  - Digital ulcer infections are treated with antibiotics.
  - Sildenafil aids ulcer healing. Bosentan (ET A/B receptor antagonist) can prevent ulcer formation by decreasing systemic vascular resistance.
- *GI tract*:
  - Oesophageal involvement is invariable. Symptoms include dyspepsia, dysphagia, and dry cough and hoarse voice due to acid reflux. Treatment is symptomatic with proton pump inhibitors and domperidone.
  - Stomach telangiectasia ('watermelon stomach') causes low Hb. Treated with argon laser therapy. Gastroparesis can occur.
  - Small bowel involvement may result in stagnation and pseudo-obstruction with bacterial overgrowth, bloating, diarrhoea and malabsorption (requiring rotating antibiotics and parenteral nutrition).
  - Colonic fibrosis and smooth muscle atrophy causes constipation. Anal sphincter dysfunction results in incontinence.

- *Pulmonary*:
  - Non-specific interstitial pneumonia (NSIP) type lung fibrosis can be mild to extensive. Associated with anti-scl-70 antibody against topoisomerase I. IV cyclophosphomide can produce modest improvement.
- *Pulmonary arterial hypertension (PAH)*:
  - Associated with anti-centromere antibody.
  - Pulmonary arterial pressure >25 mmHg on pulmonary angiography is diagnostic; echocardiogram is used for screening.
  - Differentials: PH secondary to thromboembolic disease, pulmonary fibrosis, left ventricular failure.
  - Treatment: sildenafil, bosentan and SC prostacyclin (epoprostenol).
- Cardiac: conduction defects (may cause sudden death), myocarditis, pericardial effusions.
- Renal: ➲ see Chapter 16, Scleroderma renal crisis, p. 577.

Mimicking conditions

1. Generalised morphoea: large confluent areas of induration involving ≥2 anatomical sites.
2. Nephrogenic SSc: skin changes similar to SSc following administration of gadolinium-based contrast.
3. Toxic-oil syndrome.
4. Chronic graft versus host disease may resemble morphoea.
5. Diabetic cheiroarthropathy (➲ see Diabetic cheiroarthropathy (limited joint mobility syndrome), p. 750).
6. Scleredema adultorum (of Buschke): a complication of types I and II diabetes mellitus. Firm non-pitting oedema involving the head, neck, shoulders and trunk, with sparing of the hands and feet.

Sjögren's syndrome

Pathophysiology

An autoimmune condition characterised by dysfunction and destruction of exocrine glands, mainly salivary and lacrimal. Can be primary or secondary to other autoimmune disorders (e.g. SLE, RA, SSc). Patients are positive for anti-Ro (65%), anti-La (50%) antibodies, ANA and RF (>99%). There is a 5% lifetime risk of NHL including MALT lymphoma.

Clinical features

- Fatigue, keratoconjuctivitis sicca, xerostomia with poor dentition, parotid swelling, arthralgia and non-erosive arthritis.
- Complications include mononeuritis multiplex, CNS demyelination, purpuric skin rashes, ILD, lymphoma and cryoglobulinaemia.
- Associated with primary biliary cirrhosis (PBC) and distal (Type I) RTA.

Investigations

- ANA, ENA (Ro and La), RF, anti-mitochondrial antibodies (with PBC).
- Immunoglobulins (polyclonal expansion), ESR (raised due to high immunoglobulins), cryoglobulins (may be present).
- US of salivary glands ± biopsy, salivary flow <0.1 mL/min (normal 0.3–0.5 mL/min), parotid sialography, positive Schirmer's test (<5 mm/5 min).

Treatment

- Surveillance for dental disease and lymphoma.
- Artificial tears/ophthalmic lubricants, saliva sprays and stimulants for symptomatic relief.
- Mild disease: hydroxychloroquine. Moderate to severe: methotrexate, rituximab and corticosteroids.

Mixed connective tissue disease

Clinical features of mixed connective tissue disease (MCTD) include a combination of SLE, SSc and PM in the presence of a positive anti-nRNP antibody with one diagnosis dominating initially. Pulmonary hypertension is the commonest cause of death. Treatment is directed against specific disease manifestations.

Eosinophilic fasciitis

Pathogenesis

A rare, localised fibrosing disorder of the fascia. The aetiology and pathophysiology are unclear. May be associated with aplastic anaemia or haematological malignancies.

Clinical features

- Often preceded by excessive physical activity.
- Skin involvement:
  - Symmetrical swelling, induration and thickening of the skin and subcutaneous fascia (the latter not involved in SSc).
  - Spares the digits (unlike SSc).
  - Sequential stages of skin involvement: blotchy erythema, peripheral hyperpigmented non-pitting oedema (*peau d'orange*), woody induration.
  - Venous guttering on limb elevation due to connective tissue tethering.
  - Raynaud's and visceral involvement are not found (unlike SSc).
- Inflammatory arthritis of hands and wrists (40% of cases), and joint contractures.
- Carpal and tarsal tunnel syndrome.

Investigations

- Eosinophilia (~66% of patients only).
- Hypergammaglobulinaemia (~75% of cases).
- Bone marrow biopsy to exclude associated malignancy.
- ESR is raised.
- ANA +ve in one-third of cases.
- MRI findings are characteristic and help target biopsy.
- Histology: thickened collagen bundles with inflammatory cells (including eosinophils).

Treatment

Corticosteroids with DMARDs (methotrexate, azathioprine, ciclosporin and cyclophosphamide) as steroid-sparing agents.

Vasculitis

Small and medium vessel vasculitis

Eosinophilic granulomatosis with polyangiitis (previously Churg–Strauss syndrome)

Pathogenesis

A rare systemic eosinophilic necrotising granulomatous polyangiitis of unknown aetiology. 50% is P-ANCA positive against neutrophil myeloperoxidase.

Diagnosis

The ACR 1990 classification criteria[1] is used with 99.7% specificity and 85% sensitivity if ≥4/6 criteria are present:

1. Asthma: late onset, often poorly controlled.
2. Eosinophilia >10%.
3. Mono/polyneuropathy.
4. Pulmonary infiltrates: transient/migratory, due to eosinophilic pneumonia and/or alveolar haemorrhage.
5. Paranasal sinus abnormality.
6. Extravascular eosinophils on biopsy.

Clinical features

- Occurs in all ages and both sexes.
- Systemic: fever, arthralgia, weight loss, myalgia.
- Respiratory: asthma is universal, nasal polyps, cough, wheeze, dyspnoea.
- Cutaneous: purpuric rash, cutaneous granulomata ~50%.
- Neurological: peripheral neuropathy, mononeuritis multiplex ~75%.
- Cardiac: endomyocardial disease with heart failure and arrhythmia ~50%.
- Renal: pauci-immune focal segmental glomerulonephritis.

Investigations

- ANCA.
- FBC for eosinophilia ($>1.5 \times 10^9$/L).
- ESR and CRP (raised).
- Urinalysis, U&Es, urine protein creatinine ratio.
- CXR, ECG, echocardiogram.
- Nerve conduction studies.
- Granulomata on biopsy of affected organ.

Treatment

- Corticosteroids (tapering dose), adding azathioprine, methotrexate or MMF.
- Cyclophosphomide with organ-threatening disease.
- Rituximab if ANCA positive.

Granulomatosis with polyangiitis (previously Wegner's granulomatosis)

Pathogenesis

Granulomatous necrotising polyangiitis. >90% C-ANCA positive against proteinase 3. Anti-PR3 antibodies are thought to activate neutrophils inducing release of lysosomal enzymes into the microvasculature.

Clinical features

- Average age of onset is 50 years, slightly more common in males.
- Systemic: fever, arthralgia, weight loss, myalgia.
- Ear, nose, and throat (ENT): nasal crusting (commonest symptom), sinusitis, epistaxis, perforated septum, deafness, tracheal stenosis.
- Pulmonary: cavitating lesions cause cough, haemoptysis, dyspnoea.

[1] Data from Hunder GG, Arend WP, Bloch DA et al. (1990), The American College of Rheumatology 1990 criteria for the classification of vasculitis: Introduction. *Arthritis & Rheumatology*, 33: 1065–1067, American College of Rheumatology.

- Cutaneous: purpuric rash, ulcers.
- Peripheral neuropathy.
- Renal: segmental necrotising pauci-immune crescentic glomerulonephritis.
- Others:
  - orbital pseudotumour;
  - scleritis;
  - GI involvement (vasculitis, ischaemia, ulceration, perforation).

Investigations and treatment

As for EGPA: ➲ See Investigations and treatment, p. 736.

Microscopic polyangiitis

Pathogenesis

Pauci-immune necrotising polyangiitis. P-ANCA against MPO found in 75% of patients and thought to be pathogenic.

Clinical features

- Systemic: fever, arthralgia, weight loss, myalgia.
- Pulmonary: cavitating lesions cause cough, haemoptysis, dyspnoea. Alveolar haemorrhage is very common (if renal involvement present exclude anti-glomerular basement membrane disease), ILD.
- ENT: 20% of patients, similar to granulomatosis with polyangiitis.
- Renal: virtually uniform, may be asymptomatic. Renal-limited MPO disease is well described. Histology as in GPA (➲ see Chapter 16, Systemic vasculitis and the kidney, p. 575).
- Cutaneous: purpuric rash, digital ischaemia, livedo reticularis.
- Neurological: sensorimotor neuropathy, mononeuritis multiplex in 60%.

Investigations and treatment

As for EGPA: ➲ See Investigations and treatment, p. 736.

Polyarteritis nodosa

Pathogenesis

Necrotising systemic polyangiitis causing microaneurysm formation (especially at vessel bifurcations), aneurysmal rupture, thrombosis, and consequently organ ischaemia or infarction. Associated with HBV infection. Absence of ANCA is a diagnostic requirement.

Clinical features

- Occurs in all ages, slight male predominance.
- Spares pulmonary and glomerular vessels (unlike ANCA positive vasculitidies).
- Systemic: fever, arthralgia, weight loss, myalgia.
- Cutaneous: purpura, livedo reticularis, subcutaneous nodules, ulcers.
- Neurological: Peripheral motor and/or sensory neuropathy. Mononeuritis multiplex (e.g. wrist/foot drop).
- Renal: ischaemia (causes hypertension or renal failure), renal haemorrhage (➲ see Chapter 16, Systemic vasculitis and the kidney, p. 575).
- Other complications: testicular and mesenteric ischaemia, stroke, retinal vasculitis.

Investigations

- Raised CRP, ESR.
- LFTs, HBV serology.
- Urinalysis, U&Es.
- Angiography for aneurysms – gold standard for imaging diagnosis.
- Biopsy of affected organ.

Treatment

- As for EGPA: ➲ See Investigations and treatment, p. 736.
- Antivirals ± plasma exchange for HBV.
- Polyarteritis nodosa does not relapse once treated.

Kawasaki disease

Pathogenesis

A childhood (rarely adult) inflammatory panarteritis. Has a predilection for coronary arteries leading to thrombosis, vascular occlusion and scarring. Infectious aetiology suggested.

Clinical features

Febrile illness, polyarthralgia, cervical lymphadenopathy, conjunctival congestion, oral mucosal inflammation, palm and sole erythema, truncal polymorphous (not vesicular) rash.

Investigations

- Raised ESR, CRP, WCC.
- Ischaemic ECG changes.
- Echocardiogram: pericardial effusion.
- Coronary angiography.

Treatment

- Acute: high-dose aspirin and intravenous immunoglobulin.
- Maintenance: lower dose aspirin.
- Good prognosis, mortality 0.1%.

Henoch–Schönlein purpura

Pathogenesis

A systemic disease caused by an immune-mediated small vessel vasculitis. Seasonal peaks driven by preceding infection e.g. upper respiratory tract (streptococci, mycoplasma or viral). Perivascular IgA1 and C3 deposition in skin and kidney is characteristic.

Clinical features

Most frequent in children; incidence in adults is 13 per million.

The 1990 ACR classification criteria require ≥2/4 of:

- Palpable purpura: non-thrombocytopenic, in dependent areas (lower extremities and buttocks).
- Bowel angina: diffuse abdominal pain, worse post-prandial, bloody diarrhoea.
- Age onset <20 years.
- Histology: granulocytes in artery/venule walls.

Additional features

- Arthralgia/arthritis may precede the rash.
- Renal: in up to 80% of adults causing haematuria/proteinuria. Biopsy shows diffuse proliferative (± crescentic) glomerulonephritis with mesangial IgA deposits.
- Rarer complications: orchitis, pancreatitis, CNS involvement.

Prognosis

Complete recovery in 90%. Can recur, especially with renal involvement.

Investigations

- Urinalysis, U&Es, renal biopsy.
- Skin biopsy: leucocytoclastic vasculitis with IgA deposits.
- Infection screen to determine the precipitating cause.

Treatment

- NSAIDs in mild cases.
- Corticosteroids if more severe disease.
- Cyclophosphamide, followed by azathioprine for glomerulonephritis.

Cryoglobulinaemic vasculitis

Pathogenesis

Small vessel vasculitis caused by cryoglobulinaemic deposits. Cryoglobulins are immunoglobulins that undergo reversible precipitation at low temperatures (<37°C).

- Type I monoclonal cryoglobulinaemia is associated with haematological malignancies.
- Types II and III (80%) are mixed, caused by monoclonal and polyclonal RFs (usually IgM).
  - They form immune complexes with polyclonal IgG Fc regions and activate complement causing vascular damage.
  - Produced in autoimmune conditions with abnormal immunoglobulin expansion (e.g. SLE, Sjögren's syndrome, RA).
  - HCV is the commonest cause worldwide.
- Essential cryoglobulinaemia (<10%): no underlying cause.

Clinical features

- Systemic: fever, arthralgia, weight loss, myalgia.
- Cutaneous: rash, purpura, Raynaud's phenomenon.
- Neurological: peripheral neuropathy, mononeuritis multiplex.
- Renal involvement.

Investigations

- Viral serology: HCV, HBV, HIV, cytomegalovirus.
- Cryoglobulin detection: sample transported warm, serum refrigerated for 3–7 days to detect the cryoprecipitate.
- Urinalysis, U&Es, renal biopsy (membranoproliferative glomerulonephritis with intracapillary thrombi containing cryoprecipitate).
- Skin biopsy.
- RF present in 70%, hypocomplementaemia.
- Screen for haematological malignancies.

Treatment

- Treat the underlying cause, e.g. HCV.
- Internal organ involvement: as for EGPA: ➲ See Investigations and treatment, p. 736.
- Rituximab.
- Plasmapheresis for life-threatening cases.

Cutaneous leucocytoclastic angiitis (urticarial vasculitis)

Pathogenesis

Small vessel vasculitis characterised by leukocytoclasis (neutrophil degeneration), vascular damage (caused by nuclear debris from infiltrating neutrophils) with immune complex deposition and vessel fibrinoid necrosis. 50% of cases are secondary to medications, infections, systemic vasculitis, autoimmune disorders (e.g. SLE, Sjögren's syndrome) or malignancy; 50% are idiopathic.

Hypocomplementaemic urticarial vasculitis (HUV) is characterised by positive C1q antibody, low C3/C4 and systemic involvement (see Clinical features, below), and is associated with SLE in >50% of cases, unlike the normocomplementaemic urticarial vasculitis (NUV) form.

Clinical features

- Palpable purpura, especially in dependent areas.
- Urticarial lesions: distinct from simple urticarial: last >24 hours, painful rather than pruritic, leave a pigmented mark.
- HUV systemic features: fever, fatigue, arthralgia/arthritis, serositis, glomerulonephritis or interstitial nephritis, uveitis, conjunctivitis or episcleritis, angioedema-like lesions and Raynaud's phenomenon.

Investigations

- Exclude underlying infection, autoimmune disease, malignancy, systemic small vessel vasculitis.
- Complement levels and C1qAb.
- Skin biopsy.

Treatment

- Treat the underlying cause if found.
- Skin limited disease: topical corticosteroid treatment only.
- Severe skin or systemic disease: immunosuppression with corticosteroids ± DMARDs.

Large vessel vasculitis

Giant cell arteritis

Giant cell arteritis (GCA) is the commonest systemic vasculitis. It affects large vessels, particularly the aorta and its extracranial branches.

Pathogenesis

Thought to be a response to endothelial injury in temporal arteries, causing dendritic cell activation and CD4+ T cell recruitment. Histology demonstrates segmental granulomatous inflammation, giant cells, fragmented elastic lamina, mixed inflammatory infiltrate and neovascularisation.

Clinical features

- Age >50 years.
- PMR symptoms in 50% of patients (➲ see Polymyalgia rheumatica, p. 742).
- Temporal headache, usually unilateral, due to temporal artery involvement. Temporal artery tenderness, swelling and loss of pulsation.
- Visual disturbance: sudden and complete, or with transient warning episodes, bilateral or unilateral, permanent in up to 60%. Due to posterior ciliary and ophthalmic artery involvement. Fundoscopy reveals ischaemic optic neuropathy.
- Jaw and lingual claudication.
- Rarer complications:
  - MI, stroke.
  - Aortic: aneurysms, dissection, rupture.
  - Subclavian, axillary, renal, iliac and femoral artery involvement.
- A paraneoplastic aetiology needs to be excluded.

Investigations

- FBC: microcytic anaemia, thrombocytosis.
- Raised ESR, CRP.
- Temporal artery biopsy:
  - Skip lesions, therefore large section required.
  - 80% sensitive pre-steroid treatment; 20% after 1 week of treatment.
- Imaging:
  - Temporal artery US scan (hypoechoic halo around artery ± segmental stenosis/occlusion).
  - FDG-PET highlights activity in the larger affected vessels, cranial arteries are too small to be visualised.

Treatment

- Symptoms respond rapidly (within hours) to high-dose oral corticosteroids (60 mg). Tapered down over 24 months.
- Ocular symptoms: IV methylprednisolone for 3 days at induction.
- Leflunomide or methotrexate for refractory disease.
- IL-6 inhibitor tocilizumab.

Further reading

1. Bhaskar Dasgupta B, Borg FA, Hassan N, et al. BSR and BHPR Guidelines for the management of giant cell arteritis. *Rheumatology* (Oxford). 2010; 49(8):1594–7.

Takayasu arteritis (TA)

Pathogenesis

A rare, systemic, inflammatory large-vessel granulomatous necrotising vasculitis of unknown aetiology, which affects women of childbearing age. Vessel skip lesions can be stenotic, occlusive or aneurysmal. Involves the aorta and its primary branches.

Clinical features

- Age <40 years.
- Systemic: fever, arthralgia, weight loss, myalgia.
- Proximal stenosis may cause:
  - Claudication of extremities.
  - Decreased brachial arterial pulse, >10 mmHg BP difference between arms.
  - Bruits over subclavian arteries or abdominal aorta.
  - Subclavian steal syndrome.
- Hypertension due to renal artery stenosis.
- Mesenteric ischaemia.
- MI, stroke.
- PAH.
- Ischaemic retinopathy.

Investigations

- Anaemia, raised ESR, CRP. Inflammatory markers may not correlate with the degree of vessel wall inflammation.
- Angiography is the investigation of choice (➲ see Chapter 5, Case 8, p. 128).
- Magnetic resonance angiography (MRA), FDG-PET will highlight affected vessels.

Treatment

- Corticosteroids: achieve high remission rates.
- Steroid-sparing agents: azathioprine, methotrexate, MMF and cyclophosphamide.
- Biologics in resistant cases (anti-TNFα agents, tocilizumab, rituximab).
- Stenting/surgical intervention for chronic vascular lesions.

Polymyalgia rheumatica

Pathogenesis

A common chronic inflammatory condition of unknown aetiology. Shoulder and hip girdle bursitis thought to underlie the clinical presentation.

Clinical features

- Age >50 years.
- Proximal limb girdle myalgia and morning stiffness >1 hour; usually rapid in onset.
- Systemic: fever, weight loss.
- 15% have GCA symptoms.

Investigations

- Raised ESR, CRP, anaemia.
- Exclude other autoimmune conditions and malignancy (can be paraneoplastic).

Treatment

Prednisolone starting at 15 mg OD tapered over 18–24 months. Methotrexate can be added.

Behçet's disease

Pathogenesis

A systemic vasculitis affecting veins and arteries of all sizes. Highest prevalence in Turkey, Japan and the silk route. Associated with HLA-B51.

Clinical features

Age of onset 20–40 years with a 4:1 female:male ratio.

Diagnostic criteria

Oral ulceration ≥3 times in 12 months plus two of the following:

- Recurrent painful genital ulceration: scrotal or labial, heals with scarring.
- Eye lesions: anterior or posterior uveitis, can cause blindness. A hypopyon may be present (➔ see Chapter 18, Behçet's disease, p. 666).
- Skin lesions: erythema nodosum, pseudofolliculitis, acneiform and papulopustular lesions.
- Positive pathergy test is characteristic: hyper-reactivity to minor skin trauma after 48 hours.

Other systems affected

- Nervous system
  - Acute meningoencephalitis with brain stem involvement, pyramidal tract lesions, cerebral venous sinus thrombosis and intracranial aneurysms.
  - Chronic progressive neuro-Behçet's disease, presents with dementia, ataxia and dysarthria.
  - CSF neutrophilia (as opposed to CSF lymphocytosis in most neuroinflammatory conditions).
- Vascular disease
  - Peripheral venous thromboses have an inflammatory, rather than thrombotic pathogenesis. Thrombi adhere to the vessel and do not cause pulmonary emboli.

- ◆ Arterial involvement is rare. It is similar to Takayasu arteritis with vessel occlusion and aneurysms. Pulmonary artery involvement presents with haemoptysis and can be fatal in anticoagulated patients.
- Musculoskeletal
  - ◆ Arthralgia and arthritis.
- Gastrointestinal
  - ◆ Indistinguishable from IBD lesions.

Differential diagnosis

Differential diagnosis includes herpetic viral ulcers, syphilis, IBD, MAGIC syndrome (overlap of Behçet's with replapsing polychondritis).

Investigations

Mild inflammatory response, *HLA-B51* genotyping, organ-specific imaging.

Treatment

- Topical steroids for orogenital ulcers ± steroid asthma inhaler for oral ulcers.
- Colchicine improves arthritis, erythema nodosum and orogenital ulceration.
- Azathioprine, methotrexate, cyclophosphamide, anti TNFα agents and steroids for more serious cases.
- Anticoagulation for venous thrombi is not indicated. They resolve with immunosuppression.

Relapsing polychrondritis

Pathogenesis

A rare condition characterised by recurrent episodes of cartilage inflammation and destruction. Peak age of onset is 50 years with an equal sex distribution. Relapsing polychrondritis (RP) is associated with HLA-DR4, other autoimmune conditions and haematologic malignancy.

Clinical features

McAdam's diagnostic criteria[2]: 3/6 *or* positive cartilage biopsy plus ≥1 of the following criteria required:

- Recurrent auricular chondritis: pain, redness and swelling of ear(s), sparing the lobule(s). Can lead to:
  - ◆ Floppy pinna ('cauliflower' deformity).
  - ◆ Conductive hearing loss from stenosis of the external auditory canal or Eustachian tube chondritis.
- Arthritis: non-erosive, sero-negative, asymmetric.
- Nasal chondritis: distal nasal septum, can cause saddle nose deformity.
- Ocular inflammation: e.g. scleritis, uveitis.
- Respiratory tract chondritis: laryngeal, tracheal and bronchial cartilage is replaced by collapsible fibrotic tissue causing airway obstruction, leading to inspiratory stridor and expiratory wheeze.
- Cochlear and/or vestibular damage: e.g. tinnitus, hearing loss.
- Other features include:
  - ◆ Purpura, cerebral vasculitis, aortitis.
  - ◆ Systemic: fever and weight loss.

Relapsing polychondritis leads to high disability, but low mortality (secondary to respiratory or cardiovascular compromise, or infections).

Investigations

There is no specific test for RP.

- CRP, ESR (may be raised).
- Biopsy of affected structures.

[2] Reproduced with permission from McAdam, L. P. et al., Relapsing polychondritis: prospective study of 23 patients and a review of the literature. *Medicine*, 55(3): 193–215. Copyright © 1976 Williams & Wilkins Co.

- CT chest (thickening, stenosis and calcification of airways).
- Lung function studies (flow-volume curves: extra-thoracic obstruction [➲ see Chapter 11, Flow volume loops, p. 378 and and Figure 11.4]).

Treatment

- Corticosteroids.
- DMARDs, e.g. methotrexate, azathioprine.
- Cyclophosphamide with organ-threatening disease.

Age-related rheumatological diseases

Juvenile idiopathic arthritis

JIA is defined as arthritis of unknown aetiology with onset before age 16 and persisting for ≥6 weeks with no other identified cause.

Presentation and clinical manifestations

The International League of Associations for Rheumatology has classified JIA as follows:

- Systemic onset JIA.
- Oligoarticular JIA.
- Polyarticular JIA (RF negative).
- Polyarticular JIA (RF positive).
- Juvenile psoriatic arthritis.
- Enthesitis-related arthritis.
- Undifferentiated arthritis.

Clinical manifestations vary from mono/oligoarthritis to widespread polyarthritis; systemic symptoms (e.g. fever, malaise); SpA with sacroiliitis and extra-articular manifestations (e.g. uveitis); enthesitis, psoriatic rashes, dactylitis.

Systemic onset JIA (Still's disease) may present acutely, with spiking fevers, evanescent rash, myalgias and arthralgias. Generalised lymphadenopathy, hepatosplenomegaly, polyserositis, anorexia, weight loss and growth abnormalities are common. Rarely a myocarditis, coagulopathy, MAS, CNS, eye, pulmonary and renal disease, and later, amyloidosis can develop.

Diagnosis and investigations

Laboratory

- FBC: haemoglobin may be low, normocytic normochromic or microcytic; WCC normal or mildly elevated, platelets raised (acute phase response).
- Raised ESR/CRP (often only mildly).
- RF, dsDNA and HLA B27 are helpful in classification; raised ANA (higher risk of iritis).
- Serology: for suspected viral/bacterial triggers.

Synovial fluid analysis

- Straw-coloured fluid, high WCC, sterile culture.

Imaging

- MRI to define the joint anatomy.

Management

- Pharmacologic treatment:
  - NSAIDs, synthetic DMARDs (methotrexate, sulfasalazine, hydroxychloroquine).
  - Biologic DMARDs (anti-TNF, IL-6 receptor antibody, IL-1 receptor antagonist [anakinra]).
  - Glucocorticoids for acute flares (oral, intra-articular or parenteral).

- Multidisciplinary approach (➲ see Management, p. 709) should include academic counselling.
- Surgery: including for micrognathia and joint replacement.

Prognosis

~40% JIA proceeds to arthritis in adulthood; ~40–50% have severe functional limitations.

Osteoarthritis

Pathogenesis

Osteoarthritis (OA), a chronic degenerative joint disorder, can be of primary or secondary aetiology. Genetic, environmental and risk factors (including age, obesity, joint malalignments and occupation) contribute to development of OA. Altered expression of matrix metalloproteinases (MMPs) and tissue inhibitors of MMPs lead to excessive proteolysis.

- *Macroscopic changes*: cystic bone degeneration, cartilage loss, osteophyte formation at joint margins.
- *Microscopic changes*: flaking and fibrillation of articular cartilage with altered vascularity and cellularity of the subchondral bone result in sclerosis and new bone formation.

Presentation and clinical manifestations

The symptoms of OA are worse after activity (unlike inflammatory arthritides), and improve with rest. Early morning stiffness, if present, is short-lived and localised to the affected joints.

- Family history, especially in the 'nodal generalised' OA.
- Secondary causes of OA include: joint trauma, inflammatory/crystal arthritis, metabolic/endocrine disease (e.g. diabetes, haemachromatosis, acromegaly, hyperparathyroidism, alkaptonuria).

Clinical findings on examination

- Bony enlargement at the DIP and PIP joints (Heberden's and Bouchard's nodes).
- Carpometacarpal (CMC) joint involvement.
- Valgus/varus deformities (e.g. at knees and ankles).
- Joint crepitus and restriction of movement, e.g. hip internal rotation.

Diagnosis and investigations

The diagnosis of OA is made on clinical and radiological grounds. SF analysis may identify co-existent crystal disease (➲ see Synovial fluid analysis, p. 706). Plain radiographs can show:

- Joint space narrowing.
- Subchondral changes: sclerosis and cysts.
- Bone collapse/attrition.
- Osteophyte formation.
- Osseous ('loose') bodies.
- Crystal deposition, e.g. chondrocalcinosis in CPPD.

MRI useful if surgery is being considered, or in secondary OA when alternative joint pathology co-exists.

Management

Management focuses on pain relief, limiting progression and preservation of function.

- Intra-articular glucocorticoids injections for symptomatic, inflamed joints, e.g. knees or CMC joints.
- Glucosamine and chondroitin sulphate supplements may lead to symptomatic relief.
- Patient education should include appropriate advice regarding muscle strengthening exercises (± physiotherapy input) and, if relevant, weight loss. Occupational therapy is helpful (e.g. splints for malalignment). OA can be progressive necessitating surgical intervention (e.g. arthroscopy, osteotomy, partial/total arthroplasty).

Monoarthropathy

Differential diagnosis

Differential diagnosis of a painful, hot, swollen joint includes:

1. *Septic arthritis*. Always to be excluded first:
   - Risk factors include: immunosuppression, diabetes, malignancy, extremes of age, septic focus elsewhere, recent instrumentation, alcoholism, IVDU, pre-existing joint disease and prosthetic joint.
   - Arises from direct inoculation, haematogenous or contiguous spread.
   - Causes of septic arthritis: see Table 20.9. *Staphylococcus aureus* and streptococci account for ~90% of cases.

Table 20.9 Common organisms which cause septic arthritis

Organism	Examples	Association
Bacterial	Staph. *aureus*	Healthy adults, pre-existing arthritis, prosthetic joints.
	Streptococcal spp.	Healthy adults, splenic dysfunction.
	Neisseria gonorrhoea	Young sexually active adults.
	Gram-negative spp.	Trauma, IVDU, immunosuppression.
Mycobacterial	M. *tuberculosis*	Immunosuppression, endemic area travel.
Fungal	*Blastomyces dermatitidis*;	Immunosuppression.
	Candida albicans	
Spirochaete	*Borrelia burgdorferi*	Tick bite history.

- Site:
  - Monoarticular >80%, of which >50% involves the knee joint.
  - Oligoarticular or polyarticular: associated with pre-existing arthritis.
- Investigations:
  - Blood cultures are positive in 33%; joint aspirate culture positive in 70%.
  - SF analysis: ➲ see Synovial fluid analysis, p. 706.
  - Blood tests show raised CRP, ESR, WCC.
  - Imaging:
    - Plain radiography: often normal at presentation; screen for osteomyelitis or pre-existing joint disease.
    - CT and MRI: especially for joints difficult to examine: hip, SIJ.
- Treatment:
  - Analgesia.
  - Parenteral antibiotics is guided by SF microscopy; 6 weeks treatment, initially 2 weeks IV.
    - Gram-positive cocci: flucloxacillin or clindamycin; vancomycin if MRSA risk.
    - Gram-negative bacilli: third-generation cephalosporin.
    - No organisms identified: treat in clinical context.
  - Orthopaedic assessment: for joint washout and management of prosthetic joint (may require removal).
  - DMARDs are often discontinued.
  - Anti-TNFα agents are withheld for 12 months.
- Prognosis:
  - 11% mortality, 50% in patients with RA.

    - 70% functional impairment.
    - Poor joint outcome: *Staph. aureus* infection, increasing age, pre-existing joint damage or arthritis, prosthetic material.
2. *Crystal arthritis*: gout or pseudogout.
3. *Flare/new presentation of an inflammatory arthropathy*: e.g. RA, spondyloarthropathies.
4. *Osteoarthritis flare*: swollen weight-bearing joint (e.g. knee) with minimal pain and erythema.

Further reading

1. Coakley G, Mathews C, Field M, et al. on behalf of the British Society for Rheumatology Standards, Guidelines and Audit Working Group. BSR & BHPR, BOA, RCGP and BSAC guidelines for management of the hot swollen joint in adults. *Rheumatology*. 2006; 45(8):1039–41.

Hypermobility syndromes

In hypermobility syndromes, joints have a greater range of movement, allowing for age, gender and ethnicity. Hypermobilty is caused by hereditary variability or defects in collagen structure, ranging from mild benign to severe cases that affect cardiovascular and autonomic function, and cause structural impairment to skin and joints.

The Beighton score[3] quantifies hypermobility using a 9-point system, 1 point for each hypermobile site (on right and left): little finger passive dorsiflexion to >90°, thumb passive dorsiflexion to the flexor aspect of the forearm, elbow hyperextension >10°, knee hyperextension >10°; plus 1 point for forward flexion of the trunk with knees fully extended allowing the palms to rest flat on the floor.

Ehlers–Danlos syndrome

The classification of Ehlers–Danlos syndrome (EDS) was revised in 2017. This is likely to evolve as new genes are identified (1). See Table 20.10.

Marfan syndrome

Pathogenesis

An autosomal dominant disorder caused by mutation in *fibrillin-1* gene on chromosome 15q21.1. Prevalence is 1:5000, incidence 1:20,000, 25% arise from new mutations.

Fibrillins are glycoproteins secreted by fibroblasts, they self-assemble into microfibrils and associate with elastin in the elastic fibres. Microfibrils and elastic fibres are organised into tissue-specific architectures that reflect the mechanical demands of individual organ systems.

- Skin: microfibrils extend from the basement membrane of the dermal/epidermal junction into the reticular dermis, where they run parallel to the epidermis together with elastic fibres. This loosely organised network confers pliability to the skin.
- Eyes: parallel bundles of microfibrils anchor the lens and adjust its thickness by conducting tension from the ciliary body.
- Aorta: microfibrils associate with elastin in the tunica media to form concentric lamellae that separate individual vascular smooth muscle cell layers and confer elasticity to the aortic wall.

Clinical features

- Skeletal system:
    - Pectus carinatum.
    - Pectus excavatum.
    - Arm span to height ratio >1.05.

[3] Data from Beighton PH Horan F. Orthopedic aspects of the Ehlers-Danlos syndrome. *The Journal of Bone and Joint Surgery. British volume*. 1969; 51: 444–453.

Table 20.10 Classification of hypermobile, classical and vascular EDS (other subtypes include kyphoscoliotic, arthrochalasia and dermatosparaxis)

Name (previous type)	Major criteria	Minor criteria	Inheritance	Affected protein and gene mutation
Hypermobile (type 3)	Diagnostic criteria: Presence of criteria 1, 2 *and* 3: 1. Generalised joint hypermobility Beighton score: >4 (>50 years) or >5 (≤ 50 years). 2. ≥ 2 of: ◆ Systemic manifestations of a more generalised connective tissue disorder. ◆ Positive family history. ◆ Musculoskeletal complications. 3. Exclusion of alternative diagnoses including other subtypes of EDS.		AD	TNXB, COL3A1
Classical (types 1 & 2)	• Skin hyperextensibility and atrophic scarring. • Joint hypermobility.	• Easy bruising. • Soft, doughy skin. • Skin fragility (or traumatic splitting). • Molluscoid pseudotumours. • SC spheroids. • Hernia (or history thereof). • Epicanthal folds. • Complications of joint hypermobility (e.g. subluxation). • Family history (first degree relative).	AD	Procollagen type V COL5A1, COL5A2
Vascular (vEDS) (type 4)	• Family history of vEDS with causative variant in COL3A1. • Arterial rupture at a young age. • Spontaneous colon perforation. • Uterine rupture during the third trimester. • Carotid-cavernous sinus fistula (CCSF) formation.	• Bruising: non-traumatic and/or at unusual site. • Thin, translucent skin with increased venous visibility. • Characteristic facial appearance. • Spontaneous pneumothorax. • Acrogeria. • Talipes equinovarus. • Congenital hip dislocation. • Small joint hypermobility. • Tendon and muscle rupture. • Keratoconus. • Gingival recession and gingival fragility. • Early-onset varicose veins.	AD	Procollagen type III COL3A1

AD, autosomal dominant.

Data from Malfait F et al., The 2017 international classification of the Ehlers-Danlos syndromes. *American Journal of Medical Genetics Part C: Seminars in Medical Genetics*, 175(1):8–26. doi: 10.1002/ajmg.c.31552.

 - Thumb sign (positive when the entire distal phalanx of the flexed thumb extends beyond the ulnar border of the palm [Steinberg's sign]) and wrist sign (positive when the tip of the thumb covers the entire fingernail of the fifth finger when wrapped around the contralateral wrist).
 - Scoliosis >20°.
 - Elbow hyperextension >10°.
 - Pes planus.
 - Protrusio acetabulae.
- Dura:
 - Lumbosacral dural ectasia by CT or MRI.
- Ocular system:
 - Ectopia lentis.
- Cardiovascular manifestations: emphasised by Ghent nosology (2010) (1):
 - Dilatation of ascending aorta involving at least sinuses of Valsalva.
 - Dissection of ascending aorta.

Differential diagnosis

Congenital contractual arachnodactyly (*fibrillin-2* mutation, similar skeletal features, without ocular or cardiovascular manifestations), homocystinuria, EDS.

Management

- Annual echocardiogram to monitor aortic root size. Elective aortic root/arch repair when the diameter is >50 mm.
- Treat hypertension to reduce the risk of aortic dilatation.
- Annual ophthalmology assessment for myopia, lens dislocation, retinal detachment.
- Orthopaedic surgery for severe scoliosis.
- Genetic testing.

Reference

1. Loeys BL, Dietz HC, Braverman AC, et al. The revised Ghent nosology for the Marfan syndrome. *J Med Genet.* 2010; 47:476–85.

Pseudoxanthoma elasticum

A rare autosomal recessive condition characterised by progressive calcification and fragmentation of elastic fibres, affecting the skin, retina and cardiovascular system.

Pathogenesis

Caused by mutations in the *ABCC6* gene on chromosome 16, encoding an ATP-binding transporter on the mitochondrial-associated membrane. This gene is mainly expressed in the liver and kidney, the pathological manifestations are due to the resulting metabolic disorder.

Clinical features

Diagnosed from early childhood to seventh decade of life. 2:1 female:male ratio.

- Cutaneous: affects the lateral aspect of the neck and other crease areas. Small yellow papules in a cobblestone or 'plucked chicken' pattern. Skin later becomes lax and hangs in folds. Acneiform lesions, brown macules and granulomatous nodules can occur.
- Gastrointestinal: mucosal involvement with upper or lower GI bleeding.
- Ocular: angioid streaks (grey or brown curvilinear bands radiating from the optic disc) are fissures in the calcified Bruch's membrane. Choroidal neovascularisation may cause retinal haemorrhages.
- Cardiovascular: claudication, renal artery stenosis, ischaemic heart disease, mitral valve prolapse.

Treatment and prognosis

Mortality and morbidity dependent on the extent of systemic involvement. Treatment involves minimising cardiovascular risk, regular ophthalmology follow-up with laser photocoagulation to prevent haemorrhages, avoiding NSAIDs and warfarin, high impact exercise and a high calcium diet.

Rheumatological manifestations of other diseases

Diabetic cheiroarthropathy (limited joint mobility syndrome)

Pathogenesis

Occurs with long standing type I (more commonly) and type II diabetes mellitus. Range of movement of tendon sheaths is limited. The pathogenesis is thought to involve glycosylation of skin collagen, decreased collagen degradation, micro-angiopathy of dermal and SC blood vessels and diabetic neuropathy.

Clinical features

- Painless loss of hand function.
- Swelling of the fingers with thick, tight, waxy skin.
- Pathognomic 'prayer sign': pressing palms together retains a gap between opposed palms and fingers.
- Flexion contractures of the fingers at advanced stages.
- Differential diagnosis includes Dupuytren's disease, SSc, tendon rupture.

Treatment

Good diabetic control, physiotherapy.

Charcot joint

Pathogenesis

A progressive destruction of bones and soft tissues of weight bearing joints with resultant pathological fractures, joint dislocations and deformities. Due to sensory or autonomic neuropathy complicating conditions such as diabetes mellitus, syphilis, chronic alcoholism and spinal cord injury (➲ see Chapter 17, Neuropathy, p. 632 and Table 17.6). A combination of unperceived trauma to an insensate foot with continuing ambulation, and abnormal blood flow leads to osteopaenia and eventually sclerotic changes.

Clinical features

Range from mild swelling to significant deformity with instability and acute inflamed joint. Pain does not correlate with the extent of the disease. Concomitant vascular disease (both micro- and macrovascular) and skin ulceration (requiring exclusion of osteomyelitis) are often present.

Investigations

Early radiographic findings reveal joint effusion, joint space narrowing, soft tissue calcification and fragmentation of subchondral bone. Later there is destruction of articular surfaces, osteophytosis, intra-articular loose bodies, dislocations and erosions.

Treatment

Podiatry, good footwear, surgery for severe deformity.

Acromegaly

The general clinical features and management of acromegaly are discussed in ➲ Chapter 19, Acromegaly, p. 686 and Box 19.3.

Musculoskeletal symptoms

- Generalised arthralgia, including lumbar spine pain.
- Carpal tunnel syndrome.
- Proximal muscle weakness.

Clinical musculoskeletal findings

- Signs of osteoarthritis, often in non-weight-bearing joints.

Radiological findings

Widening of joint spaces due to cartilage, synovial and soft tissue hypertrophy. Most frequently seen in knees, MCPs and interphalangeal joints. Other changes include early osteophytes, DISH-like hyperostosis and enlarged base and tufts of terminal phalanges.

Haemochromatosis

Clinical features and management: ➲ see Chapter 15, Haemochromatosis, p. 538.

Clinical musculoskeletal symptoms and findings

- Pain, stiffness and enlargement, typically of the second and third MCP joints, without evidence of synovitis.
- Pseudogout episodes in knees, wrists, intervertebral discs and symphysis pubis.

Radiological findings

- Joints affected: MCPs, mid-carpal and radiocarpal, elbows and glenohumeral. This distribution is not typical for OA.
- Joint space narrowing, subchondral cysts and sclerosis with prominent hook-like osteophytes.
- Chondrocalcinosis is often evident.

Treatment

- Venesection does not improve the arthropathy.
- Simple analgesia with NSAIDs and physiotherapy.

Multiple choice questions

Questions

1. A 68-year-old man with background of ischaemic heart disease presents with left-sided temporal headaches and intermittent visual loss over 3 days, fever, pain on chewing and bilateral shoulder stiffness. Your acute management will include:
   A. Blood tests to include CRP, ESR, FBC, ophthalmology review, temporal artery biopsy, prednisolone 60 mg daily, reducing dose over 6 months.
   C. CT brain, carotid artery Doppler, ECG, echocardiogram.
   D. ANCA, ESR, CRP, MRI and MRA brain.
   A. Prednisolone 30 mg daily tapered over 4 weeks with omeprazole and Vitamin D.
   E. Blood tests to include CRP, ESR, FBC, ophthalmology review, temporal artery biopsy, admit for 3 days of IV methylprednisolone followed by prednisolone 60 mg daily reducing dose over 24 months.

2. A 58-year-old man with known excessive alcohol consumption and clinical evidence of a deforming arthritis and multiple soft tissue swellings, developed a large olecranon bursa. His past medical history includes a previous GI bleed and history of kidney stones. Routine blood tests showed elevated acute phase proteins and a leucocytosis. Rheumatoid factor result pending. X-rays showed erosive changes over two of the MCP joints.

   The bursa has been aspirated. What do you expect the fluid to show?

   A. Inflammatory cell infiltrate only.
   B. Inflammatory cell infiltrate with negatively birefringent crystals under polarised light.
   C. Inflammatory cell infiltrate with positively birefringent crystals under polarised light.
   D. Non-inflammatory cell infiltrate with gram positive stain.
   E. Non-inflammatory cell infiltrate with gram negative stain.

3. A 45-year-old man presents with right hip pain. A plain pelvic radiograph demonstrates an area of patchy sclerosis with trabecular coarsening in the left pubic ramus. Blood tests demonstrate normal calcium, ALP 560 (40–129 IU/L), Vitamin D 25 nmol/L (<50 nmol/L is insufficient). The likely diagnosis and appropriate treatment are:

   A. Paget's disease, patient to have one zoledronic acid infusion after Vitamin D is replaced to >50 nmol/L.
   B. Paget's disease, to start monthly IV zoledronic acid treatment for 1 year after Vitamin D is replaced to >50 nmol/L.
   C. Vitamin D deficiency with Looser's zones, to start IM ergocalciferol.
   D. Osteosarcoma requiring surgical excision.
   E. Plasmacytoma requiring radiotherapy.

4. A 40-year-old woman recently treated for ovarian cancer presents with proximal muscle weakness, an erythematous rash on the face and chest, abdominal distension and shortness of breath. Investigations show CK 15,000 IU/L, AST 150 IU/L (10–35 IU/L), ANA negative, pleural effusions on CXR and ascites on abdominal US scan.

   The likely diagnosis is:

   A. Polymyositis with SLE overlap causing the rash and serositis.
   B. Dermatomyositis secondary to ovarian cancer with malignant ascites and pleural effusions.
   C. Rhabdomyolysis secondary to cancer recurrence.
   D. Mixed connective tissue disease.
   E. Chemotherapy induced muscle necrosis and serositis.

5. A 36-year-old woman with SLE has a 2-month history of increased arthralgia, rashes and fevers. Which investigation set is most useful in assessing disease activity?

   A. CRP, ESR, C4, ANA.
   B. ESR, FBC, dsDNA antibody level, C3.
   C. dsDNA antibody level, ANA, U&E, ESR.
   D. Urine PCR, CRP, ESR, anti-CCP Ab level.
   E. ANA, ANCA, C3, C4, C1q Ab.

6. A 48-year-old woman managed with hydroxychloroquine for Sjögren's syndrome presents with a 1-month history of night sweats, fevers and cervical lymphadenopathy. Blood tests reveal ESR 100 mm/hr, CRP 90 mg/L, positive ANA 1:1000, Ro positive, La positive, RF positive, monoclonal band on serum electrophoresis. The likely diagnosis is:

   A. Infection in an immunosuppressed patient.
   B. Lymphoma.
   C. New diagnosis of SLE overlap.
   D. Mixed connective tissue disease.
   E. Kikuchi disease.

7. A 29-year-old woman was diagnosed with APLS after an axillary vein thrombosis and positive lupus anticoagulant on two occasions 12 weeks apart. She is on warfarin and aspirin and would like to consider pregnancy. Your advice is:
   A. Pregnancy is absolutely contraindicated.
   B. Stop warfarin as soon as pregnancy is confirmed, but continue aspirin.
   C. Stop aspirin as soon as pregnancy is confirmed, but continue warfarin.
   D. Change warfarin to SC heparin as soon as pregnancy is confirmed, continue aspirin.
   E. Change warfarin to SC heparin as soon as pregnancy is confirmed, stop aspirin.

8. A 37-year-old woman presents with proximal muscle weakness, Raynaud's phenomenon, and arthralgia with joint swelling. Investigations reveal ANA 1:1000, anti-nRNP antibody, CK 560 IU/L, ESR 56 mm, CRP 60 mg/L. What is the diagnosis?
   A. SLE.
   B. Polymyositis.
   C. Dermatomyosistis.
   D. Mixed connective tissue disease.
   E. Rheumatoid arthritis.

9. A 50-year-old man presents with a fever, arthralgia, left-hand paraesthesia, shortness of breath and cough on the background of a 3-year history of asthma. On examination, he has a purpuric rash on his arms, a wheeze on auscultation and reduced sensation in median nerve distribution on the left arm. Chest radiograph shows patchy shadowing at the right base, bloods reveal an eosinophilia 3.1×10^9 /L (normal range 0.0–0.4), raised ESR, CRP, and positive ELISA against neutrophil myeloperoxidase (P-ANCA). The likely diagnosis is:
   A. Infective exacerbation of asthma, carpal tunnel syndrome, reactive rash.
   B. Eosinophilic granulomatosis with polyangiitis (EGPA, previously Churg–Strauss syndrome).
   C. Henoch–Schonlein purpura complicating a viral chest infection with exacerbation of asthma.
   D. Granulomatosis with polyangiitis (GPA, previously Wegner's granulomatosis).
   E. Microscopic polyangiitis.

10. A 35-year-old female patient presents with a 5-year history of widespread arthralgia, recurrent joint subluxations and history of poor skin healing. Her Beighton score is 7/9, she has increased skin stretch over her elbows and widened scars on her knees. On examination she is of average build, there is no evidence of synovitis, her cardiovascular examination is normal. Blood testing by the GP (which includes inflammatory markers and RF) is unremarkable.

    The likely diagnosis is:
    A. Pseudoxanthoma elasticum.
    B. Ehlers–Danlos syndrome, hypermobile type 3.
    C. Ehlers–Danlos syndrome, vascular type 4.
    D. Marfan syndrome.
    E. Osteogenesis imperfecta.

Answers

1. E. BSR guidelines recommend IV methylprednisolne for visual involvement followed by a slow reducing course of high dose prednisolone (➲ see Giant cell arteritis, p. 740).
2. B. The most likely diagnosis here is gout (➲ see Crystal arthritis, p. 713).
3. A. The radiographic features are pathognomic of Paget's disease. Osteosarcoma causes a dense central medullary lesion with a prominent periosteal reaction and surrounding. A plasmacytoma causes a lytic lesion (➲ see Paget's disease, p. 726).

4. B. Dermatomyositis is commonly associated with ovarian cancer, when conventional ANA testing is negative (Table 20.6).
5. B. Flares of SLE are commonly associated with increased ESR, pancytopenia, rising dsDNA antibody level and a fall in C3 (➲ see Systemic lupus erythematosus, Diagnosis, p. 731, Other blood tests, p. 731 and Table 20.8).
6. B. Sjögren's syndrome carries a 5% lifetime risk of NHL (➲ see Sjögren's syndrome, p. 734). Kikuchi disease is a self-limiting necrotising lympadenitis with negative auto-immune serology.
7. D. Warfarin is highly teratogenic after 6 weeks gestation. Heparin and aspirin are safe and used to prevent obstetric complications (➲ see Treatment [under section Antiphospholipid syndrome], p. 733).
8. D. This patient has features of myositis, Raynaud's and synovitis in the presence of anti-nRNP antibody (➲ see Mixed connective tissue disease, p. 735).
9. B. Late onset asthma, eosinophilia, mononeuropathy and pulmonary infiltrates fulfil 4/6 on the diagnostic criteria for EGPA. Henoch–Schonlein purpura does not cause eosinophilia and the rash distribution is in dependent areas. GPA causes upper respiratory symptoms without eosinophilia, patients are C-ANCA positive. MPA patients have no history of asthma or eosinophilia (➲ see Eosinophilic granulomatosis with polyangiitis (previously Churg–Strauss syndrome), p. 735).
10. B. ➲ See Hypermobility syndromes, pp. 747–749, and Table 20.10. Hypermobile EDS is characterised by arthralgia, joint hypermobility and subluxations in the absence of systemic findings.

Chapter 21 **Dermatology**

Jennifer Crawley and Donal O'Kane**

Structure of the skin

The skin is the largest organ in the body and consists of three distinctive layers, namely the epidermis, the dermis and the subcutaneous tissue or subcutis.

Epidermis

The epidermis is the outermost layer of the skin. It is composed predominantly of keratinocyte cells, which differentiate as they migrate from the immature basal cell layer, and stratum basale through the stratum spinosum, stratum granulosum and finally stratum corneum. It also contains:

- Melanocytes, which produce melanin and help protect the skin against the harmful effects of ultraviolet radiation.
- Langerhans cells, involved in immune surveillance.
- Merkel cells, which have a sensory function.

Epidermal thickness varies greatly depending on site, from 0.1 mm on the eyelids up to 1.5 mm on the palms and soles.

Dermis

The dermis is located below the epidermis and composed predominantly of collagen (which provides skin architecture and tensile strength) and elastic fibres, which provide elasticity and resilience. The dermis also houses blood vessels, lymphatics, nerves and skin appendages including hair follicles, sebaceous glands and sweat glands.

Subcutaneous tissue

This layer is composed predominantly of adipose cells, loose connective tissue, blood vessels and nerves.

For structure of the skin, see Figure 21.1, and for functions of the skin see Table 21.1.

* Joint first authors.

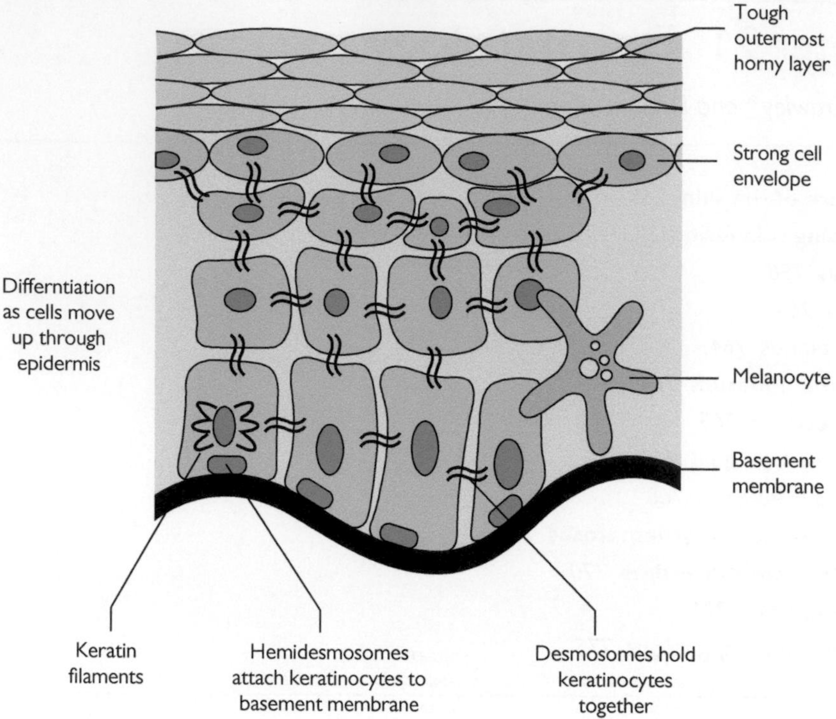

Figure 21.1 Structure of the skin.

Reproduced with permission from Structure and function of the skin. In: Burge S, et al. (Eds) *Oxford Handbook of Medical Dermatology*, 2nd edn. Oxford: OUP. © 2016 Oxford University Press. Reproduced with permission of the Licensor through PLSclear.

Table 21.1 Functions of the skin

Skin function	**Key points**
Barrier	The stratum corneum is composed of tightly packed dead keratincoytes (corneocytes) bound together by a lipid-rich extracellular matrix. It functions as a physical barrier to the outflow of fluids and electrolytes, and the inflow of micro-organisms and toxins.
Immune defence	Skin provides the first line of defence against invading pathogens via the structural integrity of the stratum corneum, antimicrobial peptide production by keratinocytes, antigen detection by Langerhans cells, and cytokine release by keratinocytes, lymphocytes and macrophages.
Thermoregulation	The rich dermal blood supply has an important role in temperature regulation via vasodilation and vasoconstriction. Sweating helps to cool the body.
Restricts UV damage	The combination of the compact stratum corneum and melanin production by melanocytes limits UV penetration through the skin.
Vitamin D production	Dermal synthesis is a major source of vitamin D, resulting from exposure of the cholesterol precursor 7-dehydrocholesterol to UVB.
Sensation	Skin allows sensory perception of heat, pain, touch, vibration and pressure.

Describing skin lesions

Morphology

The morphology is the description of individual lesions (Table 21.2).

Table 21.2 Morphology of skin lesions

Term	Appearance	Example
Macule	Change in colour or consistency of the skin without any elevation.	Junctional naevus.
Papule	Raised dome-shaped lesion <5 mm diameter.	Compound naevus.
Nodule	Raised dome-shaped lesion >5 mm diameter.	Nodular melanoma.
Vesicle	Raised fluid-filled lesion <5 mm diameter.	Herpes simplex.
Bulla	Raised fluid-filled lesion >5 mm diameter.	Bullous pemphigoid.
Pustule	Raised pus-containing cavity.	Acne.
Plaque	Circumscribed, plateau-like elevation of the skin.	Psoriasis.
Erosion	Superficial circumscribed loss of epidermis.	Pemphigus vulgaris.
Ulcer	Circumscribed loss of skin extending into the dermis or below.	Venous ulcer.
Targetoid	'Bulls-eye' configuration.	Erythema multiforme.

Arrangement

This reports how individual lesions are related to one another.

- Linear: arranged in a line, e.g. scabies burrows.
- Annular: arranged in a ring, e.g. dermatophyte infections.
- Reticular: net-like arrangement, e.g. livedo reticularis.
- Discrete: individual lesions separated by normal skin.
- Coalescing: individual lesions merging together.
- Grouped: multiple similar lesions together in one area, e.g. varicella zoster.

Distribution

Distribution describes areas of the body involved.

- Generalised: universal distribution, which can be mild (scattered) or severe (diffuse).
- Extensor: distributed on extensor surfaces (e.g. anterior knee), e.g. psoriasis.
- Flexural: distributed on flexor surfaces (e.g. posterior knee), e.g. atopic eczema.
- Symmetrical: suggestive of endogenous cause, e.g. atopic eczema, psoriasis.
- Asymmetrical: suggests external cause, e.g. contact eczema, infection, trauma.
- Dermatomal: following a nerve root distribution, e.g. herpes zoster.
- Photosensitive: affecting sun exposed sites, such as face, 'V' of neck, dorsal hands.
- Palmoplantar: distribution on palms and soles, e.g. palmoplantar psoriasis.
- Köbnerised: in certain disorders new skin lesions (with the same clinical and histological characteristics) can develop at a site of cutaneous injury (including surgical scars). This process is termed the Köbner phenomenon. For conditions associated with Köbner's phenomenon, ➲ see Box 21.2.
- Follicular: arising from hair follicles, e.g. bacterial folliculitis.

See Table 21.3 for a systematic approach to skin lesion recognition.

Table 21.3 A systematic approach to skin lesion recognition

Morphology	Arrangement	Distribution	Possible diagnosis
Vesicles	Grouped	Dermatomal	Herpes zoster (shingles)
Erythematous nodules	Discrete	Extensor shins	Erythema nodosum
Scaly plaques	Annular	Assymetric on body	Tinea corporis
Violaceous papules	Grouped	Flexor wrists	Lichen planus
Pustules	Discrete	Palmoplantar	Palmoplantar pustular psoriasis

Psoriasis

Psoriasis is a chronic, non-infectious inflammatory skin condition. It affects approximately 2% of the UK population. In psoriatic plaques the epidermis is hyperproliferative with elongation of the rete ridges. The dermis contains an inflammatory cell infiltrate of both CD4 +ve and CD8 +ve T cells, in addition to tortuous and dilated blood vessels. Despite the strong familial tendency, it does not follow a Mendelian pattern of inheritance. Family history is positive in 30% of patients. Psoriasis is a polygenic disorder and the aetiology is multifactorial. Both environmental and genetic factors interact to produce the clinical features of psoriasis.

Predisposing or exacerbating factors

- Trauma; psoriasis exhibits Köbner phenomenon.
- Infections including streptococcus and HIV.
- Alcohol.
- Drugs, including β-blockers, lithium and anti-malarial drugs.
- Stress.
- Abrupt withdrawal of steroid treatment (topical or oral).

Box 21.1 Conditions associated with Köebner's phenomenon

- Psoriasis.
- Lichen planus.
- Vitiligo.
- Lichen nitidus.
- Erythema multiforme.
- Grannuloma annulare.
- Darier's disease.
- Hailey–Hailey disease.
- Pityriasis rubra pilaris.
- Kaposi sarcoma.
- Necrobiosis lipoidica.
- Morphoea.
- Elastosis perforens sirpiginosa.
- Pellagra.
- Kyrle disease.

Clinical features

Psoriasis is a clinical diagnosis. Typical features include:

- Skin
  - Well-demarcated, raised erythematous plaques with silvery scale.
  - Lesions may be single, or multiple and scattered.
  - A symmetrical distribution on extensor surfaces, scalp, umbilicus, groin and natal cleft.
  - Köbner phenomenon may be apparent.
- Nails
  - Pitting: psoriatic pits are large, deep and irregularly scattered within the nail plate.
  - Onycholysis: apparent splitting of the nail with distal nail plate detachment.
  - Subungual hyperkeratosis: thickening of the nail plate.
- Joints
  - ➲ See Chapter 20, Psoriatic arthritis, p. 710 and Tables 20.2, 20.3 and Box 20.2.
  - ~20% of patients with psoriasis subsequently develop psoriatic arthritis.
  - Nail, scalp or groin psoriasis indicate a higher risk of psoriatic arthritis.

Clinical subtypes

Psoriasis can exist as a spectrum of different cutaneous manifestations and different variants can coexist in any one particular individual at any one time.

Common clinical presentations of psoriasis include:

1. Chronic plaque psoriasis.
2. Guttate psoriasis: small, symmetrical and superficial scaly papules scattered over the body, especially the trunk, commonly triggered by streptococcal infections.
3. Hyperkeratotic palmoplantar psoriasis.
4. Flexural psoriasis, mainly affecting intertriginous areas.
5. Pustular psoriasis, either limited to the palms and soles or generalised.
6. Erythrodermic psoriasis: generalised erythema and scaling, which carries a significant risk of sepsis and, in severe cases, cardiovascular compromise (see Box 21.2).

Box 21.2 Erythroderma

Erythroderma is a potentially life-threatening condition with presents with erythema and scaling involving at least 90% of the skin surface area.

Common causes

- Psoriasis.
- Eczema.
- Drugs.
- Malignancy.

Assessment should entail a detailed history (including personal and family history of skin disease, and a drug history) and examination (e.g. psoriatic nail changes). Laboratory tests should include investigation for eosinophilia ± skin biopsy.

Management priorities

- Replacement of fluids and electrolytes.
- Monitoring body temperature.
- Treatment of secondary infections/sepsis.
- Treatment of the underlying condition.

Disease severity

Disease assessment tools are used to establish disease severity and functional status.

- *Psoriasis Area and Severity Index (PASI)*: the PASI is an objective assessment of the severity of psoriasis. It includes redness, scaling, thickness and area of involvement. Maximum score is 72.
- *Dermatology Life Quality Index (DLQI)*: this questionnaire provides a subjective measure of the impact that any dermatological condition can have on a patient's life. Social and psychological problems are commonly associated with psoriasis.

Management

There is no curative treatment for psoriasis; management is directed at disease control. The treatment choice is determined by disease severity, response to therapy, coexisting psoriatic arthritis and patient preference. In the majority of patients, psoriasis is a non-life-threatening disease, but psychosocial morbidity is considerable. Consideration of the psychological impact of the disease is an essential component of care.

Topical treatments

- Emollients are applied at least twice daily to maintain skin hydration, and minimise itch and tenderness. They can also be used as alternatives to soap, which can dry the skin and aggravate itch.
- Vitamin D analogues (e.g. calcitriol and calcipotriene) inhibit proliferation and promote differentiation of keratinocytes. They are used as monotherapy as well as in combination with other treatments (e.g. topical steroids). There is a small risk of skin irritation and hypercalcaemia if applied to >40% body surface area.
- Salicylic acid (a keratolytic agent) can be used alone or with a topical steroid.
- Topical steroids are used short term during flares. They have anti-inflammatory and anti-proliferative effects. A rebound flare may occur if withdrawn abruptly, and they are associated with risk of skin atrophy with prolonged use.
- Coal tar has antimicrobial, anti-inflammatory and antipruritic effects, and an antiproliferative effect, which may be due to suppression of DNA synthesis. Can stain hair, skin and clothing, and cause skin irritation.
- Dithranol is a cytotoxic agent, which inhibits a variety of cellular functions reducing keratinocyte proliferation. Skin irritation and staining are common.

Photo (chemo) therapy

- Indications include moderate to severe psoriasis not controlled by topical treatments.
- Photo(chemo)therapy can be used as monotherapy or in combination with other treatments.
- Narrow-band ultraviolet B (UVB) is the optimal irradiation. It is commonly given three times weekly for ~6 weeks. Guttate psoriasis responds well to phototherapy, especially to UVB.
- Psoralen (topical or oral) plus ultraviolet A (PUVA) penetrates deeper than UVB and is usually given twice weekly for ~6 weeks.
- Acute side effects of phototherapy include erythema, blistering or a burning sensation.
- The major long-term risk is of carcinogenesis. Alternative treatments should be considered for those who have had 150 treatments with PUVA or 350 with UVB.

Systemic treatments

Indications for escalation to a systemic agent include severe psoriasis and psoriasis resistant to topical treatments and photo (chemo) therapy.

- Retinoids (e.g. acitretin) are vitamin A derivatives, which inhibit epidermal proliferation. Given as an oral daily dose they can be used in combination with UVB/PUVA. Common side effects include dry skin and chelitis. They are highly teratogenic so are generally only used in men or post-menopausal women. Serum lipids and LFTs should be monitored while on treatment.

- Methotrexate[1] is a folic acid antagonist, which inhibits epidermal proliferation and also has immunosuppressive effects. Given as a once-weekly dose (oral or SC).
- Ciclosporin[1] has an immunosuppressive agent via the inhibition of T cell function.

Biological therapies

➲ See Chapter 20, Biologic DMARDs, p. 709, for screening required and the risks of the biological agents.

- Indications include severe psoriasis with previous failure of conventional systemic agents.
- New onset psoriasis is a recognised complication of anti-tumour necrosis factor (TNF) agents. Allergic reactions are commoner with infliximab as it is a chimeric human-murine antibody.
- The formation of antidrug antibodies over time can result in loss of efficacy.

For biological agents used in the treatment of psoriasis, see Table 21.4.

Table 21.4 Biological agents used in the treatment of psoriasis

Name	Mechanism of action	Route	Frequency
Infliximab	Chimeric human-murine TNF-α antibody	IV	6–8 weekly
Adalimumab	Human TNF-α antibody	SC	Fortnightly
Etanercept	TNF receptor fusion protein	SC	Once/twice weekly
Ustekinumab	Human IL12 and IL23 antibody	SC	12-weekly
Secukinumab	Human IL17A antibody	SC	Monthly

Further reading

1. NICE. Psoriasis: The assessment and management of psoriasis. Clinical guideline CG153.London: NICE, 2012. https://www.nice.org.uk/guidance/cg153.
2. Psoriasis Association. http://www.psoriasis-association.org.uk.

Eczema

Atopic eczema (AE), also known as atopic dermatitis, is a chronic, inflammatory, itchy skin condition affecting 20% of children, with ~10% of cases persisting into adulthood. A defect in epidermal barrier function appears to be the primary pathogenic mechanism, including defects in the filaggrin protein (which is important in keratinocyte adhesion). The resultant increase in barrier permeability allows irritants and antigens to penetrate the skin and trigger skin inflammation.

Predisposing or exacerbating factors

- Infection, typically bacterial (e.g. *Staphylococcus aureus*) and viral infections (e.g. herpes simplex virus).
- Irritants, such as frequent use of soaps and detergents.
- Contact allergens (much more common than food allergens).
- Stress.

Clinical features

- Commonly localised to elbow and knee flexures, wrists and hands, but can be generalised in severe cases.
- Itchy, erythematous papules and patches with fine scale and secondary excoriations.
- Skin is often inflamed and vesicular. Crusted lesions can be seen in the acute setting.

[1] ➲ See Table 6.8 and Chapter 20, Management, p. 712, for mode of action, complications and monitoring.

- Lichenification (skin thickening with accentuation of skin markings) occurs in the chronic setting.
- Honey-coloured crusting is typical of secondary bacterial infection, commonly *Staph. aureus*.
- Punched-out painful erosions, often with systemic upset, are characteristic of eczema herpeticum (secondary infection with herpes simplex virus).

Diagnostic criteria for atopic eczema are shown in Table 21.5.

Table 21.5 Diagnostic criteria for atopic eczema

Major (essential)	Minor (≥3 required)
Itchy skin in the past 12 months	History of flexural involvement.
	History of generally dry skin.
	Visible flexural eczema.
	Symptoms beginning under age 2*.
	Personal history of atopic disease**.

*Not used in children under 4.
**If under 4, family history sufficient.
Reproduced with permission from Williams, H.C. et al., UK working party's diagnostic criteria for atopic dermatitis. III. Independent hospital validation. *British Journal of Dermatology*, 131:3, 406–16. https://doi.org/10.1111/j.1365-2133.1994.tb08532.x. © British Association of Dermatologists.

Other types of eczema

These can be grouped into endogenous and exogenous types.

Endogenous

- Seborrheoic eczema: typically involves scalp, eyebrows, nasolabial folds, and less commonly sternum, upper back and axillae. The commensal yeast *Malassezia furfur* is implicated in the pathogenesis.
- Stasis eczema: eczematous change on the lower legs associated with venous insufficiency. More severe cases can trigger a generalised eczema.
- Discoid eczema: coin-shaped eczematous patches with overlying crusting, often on limbs.

Exogenous

- Contact irritant: triggered by a direct cytotoxic effect from the agent in contact with the skin.
- Contact allergic: a delayed cell-mediated immune reaction (Type IV hypersensitivity [➲ see Chapter 6, Type IV hypersensitivity, p. 162]). Diagnosed by patch testing, which involves exposing skin to the suspected allergen for 48 hours to induce an eczematous reaction.

Assessing disease severity

Eczema is typically graded as mild, moderate or severe. Severity scales used for eczema include:

- Six Area Six Sign Atopic Dermatitis (SASSAD) index: grades intensity of eczema at six body sites.
- Eczema Area and Severity Index (EASI): grades severity and extent of eczema in four body regions.
- Patient-Orientated Eczema Measure (POEM): a self-assessment questionnaire which grades itch, sleep disturbance, bleeding, weeping, cracking, flaking and dryness.
- Dermatology Life Quality Index (DLQI): measures the impact a patient's skin disease has had on their quality of life in the previous week.

Management

The mainstay of treatment for contact irritant and allergic eczema is the identification and avoidance of the causative agent. There is no cure for atopic eczema and treatment is aimed at disease control. Important initial steps include patient education and avoidance of triggering factors. Careful consideration should also be given to the psychological impact of the disease.

Topical treatments

- Soap substitutes.
- Emollients are the mainstay of eczema treatment. They should be applied frequently (at least BD), with improvement in skin hydration and barrier function.
- Topical steroids: disease severity dictates steroid choice, with steroid strength usually reduced as eczema improves to prevent a rebound flare. Potent steroids are generally avoided on skin folds and the face due to the risk of skin atrophy. Twice weekly maintenance treatment with a moderate potency steroid is typically used to prevent relapses. For the topical steroid treatment ladder, see Table 21.6.

Table 21.6 The topical steroid treatment ladder

Eczema severity	Features	Steroid potency
Mild	Dry skin, infrequent itch, little impact on quality of life.	Mild.
Moderate	Dry erythematous skin, frequent itch, moderate impact of daily activity and sleep.	Moderate.
Severe	Widespread dry erythematous skin, incessant itch, severe impact on daily activities and sleep.	Potent (or very potent).

- Topical calcineurin inhibitors (e.g. tacrolimus) are non-steroidal immunomodulating agents used second-line for mild-moderate eczema. They do not cause atrophy and are therefore particularly useful on the face and in skin folds.

Photo (chemo) therapy

- Indications include moderate or severe disease not controlled by topical treatments.
- Narrowband UVB is generally first-line. PUVA treatment regimens mirror those used in psoriasis (➲ see Photo (chemo) therapy, p. 760).

Systemic

- *Managing bacterial infections* is typically achieved with oral antibiotics, with topical antimicrobials reserved for localised infection. Eczema herpeticum is managed with systemic antivirals (e.g. acyclovir) and cessation of topical steroids.
- *Antihistamines* may be useful for controlling pruritus in acute flares. Sedating agents (e.g. hydroxyzine) are more effective than non-sedating antihistamines (e.g. cetirizine).
- *Systemic steroids* (e.g. oral prednisolone) may abort an acute flare of eczema. These are typically combined with a reducing course of topical steroids to prevent a rebound flare.
- *Azathioprine*[1] can be a useful agent.
- *Methotrexate*[1] has comparable efficacy to azathioprine in the management of eczema.
- *Ciclosporin*[1] can be used as a short-term or intermittent long-term treatment option when other systemic agents are contraindicated.

[1] ➲ See Chapter 6, Anti-inflammatory/immunosuppressive therapy, p. 177 and Table 6.8 for mode of action and monitoring.

Further reading

1. National Eczema Society. http://www.eczema.org.

Lichen planus

Lichen planus (LP) is an inflammatory skin disorder of unknown cause affecting 1% of individuals, most commonly between the ages of 30–50 years and in women more than men. It is characterised histologically by a band of lymphocytes, which attack basal epidermal keratinocytes.

Clinical features

- Skin: LP classically presents with itchy, violaceous papules and plaques. Fine white lines may be visible on the surface (Wickham's striae). The lesions commonly involve distal sites, although a more generalised distribution and Köbnerisation can be seen.
- Nails: involvement of the nails is seen in up to 10% of patients with LP, commonly with longitudinal ridging and thinning, but hyperkeratosis and onycholysis are also reported.
- Scalp (lichen planopilaris): involvement of the hair follicles on the scalp can result in a scarring alopecia.
- Oral and genital LP: Wickham striae and erosions are often observed on mucous membranes.

Precipitants

- Hepatitis C.
- Medications (e.g. ACE inhibitors, β-blockers and hydroxychloroquine).

Diagnosis

LP is usually a clinical diagnosis. A skin biopsy may be required if the diagnosis is unclear.

Management

The majority of classical skin lesions of LP resolve within 1–2 years, but may be more persistent when involving other sites. LP is a self-limiting disorder, treatment largely focuses on inducing remission and controlling pruritus.

- Steroids are useful for controlling acute flares administered in topical, intra-lesional or oral form, depending on distribution and severity.
- Photo(chemo)therapy (both UVB and PUVA) can be used in similar regimes as utilised in eczema and psoriasis (➲ see Photo (chemo) therapy, p. 760).
- Steroid-sparing agents, such as hydroxychloroquine, oral retinoids, ciclosporin and methotrexate may be used, depending on chronicity and clinical picture.

Further reading

1. Le Cleach L, Chosidow O. Lichen planus, *N Engl J Med.* 2012; 366:723–32.

Erythema nodosum

Erythema nodosum (EN) is a panniculitis (inflammation of sub-cutaneous fat) and is thought to represent a delayed hypersensitivity reaction to infection, medication or underlying disease, although in one-third of cases a trigger is unidentifiable. EN is more common in women, and between the age of 20 and 40 years.

Clinical features

EN presents with tender, erythematous nodules symmetrically distributed on the shins, and less commonly, on the thighs and forearms.

Diagnosis

The diagnosis of EN is made clinically. A skin biopsy is only required if the diagnosis is uncertain. Further investigations should be guided by the history and examination and may help identify the underlying trigger.

For common causes and associations of EN, see Box 21.3.

Box 21.3 Common causes and associations of erythema nodosum

- Idiopathic.
- Streptococcal (most common infective cause).
- Other infections (*Campylobacter, Salmonella*, viral upper respiratory tract infections).
- Sarcoidosis.
- Inflammatory bowel disease.
- Drugs (oral contraceptive pill, penicillin, tetracyclines, sulfonamides).
- Tuberculosis.
- Behçet's disease.

Management

EN is a self-limiting disease. Treatment is, therefore, largely symptomatic and includes leg elevation/compression (if lower limbs involved) and NSAIDs. The underlying cause should be sought and treated where possible, and potentially causative medication discontinued. Systemic steroids can be useful when infection has been excluded. Oral colchicine is useful in refractory cases, especially in the context of Behçet's disease.

Skin infections

See Table 21.7.

Table 21.7 Dermatological manifestations of common bacterial, viral and fungal infections and infestations

Bacteria	Presentation	Clinical features
Streptococcus	Cellulitis	Tender, warm, erythematous and oedematous skin, most commonly seen on the lower leg. A portal of entry may be evident (➲ see Chapter 8, Cellulitis, p. 254).
	Erysipelas	More superficial involvement of the dermis than cellulitis so the involved skin is further raised and well-demarcated (➲ see Chapter 8, Cellulitis, p. 254).
	Scarlet fever	Predominant in children, sore throat and fever, diffuse erythema with overlying papules ('sandpaper rash'), facial flushing and strawberry tongue, linear petechiae in folds (Pastia's lines).
	Erythema marginatum	Erythematous macules, which spread centrifugally with central clearing. Associated with acute rheumatic fever (➲ see Chapter 13, Rheumatic heart disease, p. 439 and Table 13.20).
Staphylococcus	Folliculitis	Peri-follicular papules and pustules. Painful boils with deeper infection.
	Impetigo	Honey-coloured crusting and ooze. Blisters may be present. Face and extremities are most commonly involved.
	Scalded skin syndrome	Tender erythema, flaccid blisters and peeling. Commonly starts peri-orally and in the flexures, before becoming more generalised. Seen most frequently in neonates and immunosuppressed adults.

continued

Table 21.7 *continued*

Virus	Presentation	Clinical picture
Herpes simplex (➲ see Chapter 7, Herpes simplex virus, p. 206 and Box 7.2)	Herpes labialis	Primary and recurrent vesicular eruptions with subsequent crusting of oral and genital mucosa (commonly caused by HSV1 and HSV2, respectively).
	Eczema herpeticum	Punched out painful lesions.
	Herpetic whitlow	Recurrent painful vesicular lesions commonly seen on a digit.
Varicella zoster (VZV)	Chickenpox	Primary VZV infection presents with a prodrome of fever and pharyngitis, followed by an itchy vesicular rash developing on the face, and subsequently trunk and extremities.
	Shingles	Reactivation of VZV can occur any time after primary infection. Prodrome of pain/ tingling followed by painful grouped vesicles within a dermatome.
HIV	Skin involvement present in 80-90% of patients with HIV and can be present at any stage of the disease (➲ see Chapter 7, Candidiasis, Kaposi's sarcoma and other skin manifestations, p. 215, Figures 7.12, 7.13 and Table 7.11).	
Pox virus	Molluscum contagiosum	Dome-shaped papules with an umbilicated punctum. Generally persist for years with no systemic symptoms and then self-resolve. Seen in young children and immunosuppressed (such as HIV infection).
Parapox virus	Orf	Isolated targetoid nodule, commonly on a finger, transmitted by direct contact with infected sheep/goats.
Human papilloma (➲ see Chapter 7, Human papilloma virus, p. 205)	Viral warts	Infects keratinocytes of skin and mucous membranes (over 100 subtypes). Typical skin lesions are hyperkeratotic papules which coalesce into plaques.
Parvovirus B19		Presents as erythema infectiosum, typically in children (malar erythema ['slapped cheeks'], reticular rash on the body, pharyngitis and coryzal symptoms).
Measles		Prodromal symptoms include Koplik's spots on the buccal mucosa which are pathognomonic. Facial erythematous macular rash becomes generalised. Respiratory complications and encephalitis are rare sequalae. (Incubation period is ~10 days).
Other	**Presentation**	**Clinical picture**
Fungi	Tinea	Dermatophyte infections of the skin (e.g. tinea corporis [body], tinea capitis [scalp]). Present as asymmetric, erythematous, scaly patches of skin with a leading edge, which can progress to a kerion (raised, spongy lesion).
	Pityriasis versicolor	Caused by malassezia yeast. Asymptomatic macules (light brown in pale skin and hypopigmented in darker skin), with a fine scale predominantly on the trunk.
Infestations	Scabies (*Sarcoptes scabiei*) (➲ see Chapter 7, Scabies, p. 204)	Itchy (worse at night) papules and burrows (represent an intra-epidermal tunnel and are diagnostic). Finger-webs, wrists, axillae, umbilicus and male genitalia are commonly involved.

Bullous pemphigoid

Bullous pemphigoid (BP) is the most common autoimmune blistering disease. It rarely presents before 60 years of age, although its incidence (13 cases per million per year) increases with age. In BP, autoantibodies target two basement membrane antigens (BP180 and BP230) resulting in complement activation, inflammatory cell recruitment and subsequent sub-epidermal blister formation.

Clinical features

Non-bullous phase

A prodromal non-bullous phase commonly precedes the bullous phase and can last weeks to months. This phase varies from intractable itch with no rash to widespread urticated papules and plaques.

Bullous phase

Tense, itchy 1–3-cm fluid-filled (clear or haemorrhagic) blisters form on inflamed or normal skin, accompanied by erosions and crusting. Lesions heal without scarring. The trunk, flexural extremities and skin folds are commonly involved, oral mucous membrane involvement (erosions) is seen in 30%. Localised disease is also common.

Precipitants and associations of bullous pemphigoid

- Neurological diseases including dementia, Parkinson's disease and multiple sclerosis. (Similarities between antigens of the skin and the nervous system may be responsible for these associations.)
- Solid organ and lymphoproliferative malignancies.
- Other skin conditions including burns, trauma, psoriasis and lichen planus. Inflammation at the dermal–epidermal junction leading to exposure of BP antigens may explain these associations.
- Medications such as diuretics (bumetanide and furosemide), antibiotics (penicillin and ciprofloxacin) and ACE-i.

Diagnosis

Diagnosis is based on clinical findings, but skin biopsy may reveal histological hallmarks of sub-epidermal blistering and, importantly, immunofluorescence demonstrating linear deposits or IgG and/or C3 along the basement membrane.

Differential diagnosis

As the non-bullous phase is non-specific, the differential diagnosis may include eczema, urticaria and scabies. In the bullous phase, the differential diagnoses includes other immunobullous disorders, infections (e.g. bullous impetigo), bullous drug reactions and insect bites.

For diagnosis and clinical features of immunobullous skin diseases, see Table 21.8.

Table 21.8 Immunobullous skin diseases

Diagnosis	Clinical features
Mucous membrane pemphigoid (MMP)	Can affect any mucous membrane surface with inflammation, erosions and scarring (differentiates MMP from BP).
Pemphigoid gestationis	Tense sub-epidermal blisters on the abdomen, which become more extensive during late pregnancy or early post-partum period.
Dermatitis herpetiformis	Intensely itchy papules and vesicles over limb extensors and buttocks. Associated with coeliac disease (➲ see Chapter 14, Coeliac disease, p. 508).
Pemphigus	An immunobullous disorder characterised by erosions and flaccid blisters.
Linear IgA disease	Sub-epidermal disorder resulting in grouped or annular vesicles in a 'string of pearls' configuration.
Epidermolysis bullosa acquisita	A rare sub-epidermal blistering disorder, which can present with acquired skin fragility or closely mimic BP.

Management

BP is a self-limiting disorder which tends to resolve over months to years. It has a significant mortality of 11–48% in the first year, which is attributed to co-morbidities and treatment-related complications. The goals of therapy are to control symptoms and blister formation, while minimising adverse effects of treatment. Specific treatments include:

- Wound dressings to cover eroded skin.
- Topical steroids are considered first-line in BP, especially for localised disease.
- Antibiotics (e.g. tetracyclines also have an anti-inflammatory effect).
- Oral steroids (e.g. prednisolone [initiated at 0.3 mg/kg/day depending on extent of disease]) can be used and gradually reduced after blistering is minimal/absent.
- Immunosuppressive steroid-sparing agents such as azathioprine, methotrexate and mycophenolate mofetil may be used in refractory disease.

Pemphigus vulgaris

Pemphigus vulgaris (PV) is an immunobullous disorder characterised by erosions and flaccid blisters. IgG antibodies target antigens on the surface of keratinocytes, either desmoglein 3 alone (mucous membrane involvement only) or both desomglein 3 and desmoglein 1 (skin also involved). Mean age of onset for PV is 50–60 years, with an incidence of ~1–5 cases per million.

Clinical features

- Mucous membranes: all patients with PV have painful mucosal membranes erosions. The oral cavity is the predominant mucous membrane involved, with the conjunctiva, nose, oesophagus and genitals less commonly affected.
- Skin: half of patients with PV will have skin involvement and any cutaneous site may be affected. Blisters characteristically have a thin roof and rupture easily resulting in painful erosions, which ooze and bleed easily, in contrast to intact blisters. Blistering can be induced by exerting pressure on perilesional skin due to lack of keratinocyte cohesion (Nikolsky sign). As skin involvement is superficial, any lesions which do heal do not scar.

Variants of pemphigus are given in Table 21.9.

Table 21.9 Variants of pemphigus

Variant	Key point
Pemphigus foliaceus	Superficial variant of PV with no mucous membrane involvement.
Drug-induced pemphigus	Triggered by D-penicillamine and, less commonly, by ACE-i.
IgA pemphigus	Rare variant triggered by IgA rather than IgG antibodies.
Paraneoplastic pemphigus	Severe oral disease associated with malignancy.

Diagnosis

The diagnosis of PV is based on clinical findings, biopsy of skin and mucous membranes to identify IgG antibodies, and blood sampling to identify circulating antibodies. The characteristic staining pattern of IgG around the periphery of adjoining keratinocytes gives a classical 'chicken-wire' appearance.

Management

The goal of treatment is to induce remission and minimise treatment-related morbidity:

- Potent topical steroids are occasionally sufficient for localised disease (skin or mucous membranes).

- Oral steroids (e.g. prednisolone) at sufficient dose (e.g. 40–60 mg/day) may achieve rapid disease control.
- Steroid-sparing agents such as azathioprine, mycophenolate mofetil are commonly required.

Common causes of blistering are given in Box 21.4.

Box 21.4 Common causes of blistering

- Stevens-Johnson syndrome.
- Toxic epidermal necrosis.
- Genetic conditions:
  - Epidermolysis bullosa.
- Immunobullous conditions:
  - Bullous pemphigoid.
  - Pemphigus vulgaris.
  - Pemphigus foliaceus.
  - Dermatitis herpetiformis.
  - Epidermolysis bullosa acquisita.
- Drug-induced.
- Infection:
  - Staphylococcal scalded syndrome.
  - Bullous impetigo.
  - Cellulitis.
- Arthropod bites.

Cutaneous lupus erythematosus

Cutaneous lupus erythematosus (CLE) is an autoimmune inflammatory skin disorder that can be associated with systemic lupus erythematosus or occur independently. The pathogenesis is unclear, but appears to be a complex interplay between genetic and environmental factors (including ultraviolet radiation). For types of CLE, see Table 21.10.

Table 21.10 Types of cutaneous lupus erythematosus

Variant	Features
Discoid lupus (DLE)	Discoid erythematous scaly plaques with follicular plugging (dilated follicles filled with keratin). Heal with scarring and dyspigmentation (hypo- and hyper-). Involvement of face, scalp (scarring alopecia) and ears is common, but it may be generalised.
Subacute cutaneous lupus (SCLE)	Annular, erythematous plaques with central clearing, typically on the upper trunk, shoulders and arms, with sparing of the face. Lesions typically last longer than ACLE, but do not scar like DLE. 70% of patients with SCLE have a positive anti-Ro antibody (see Table 20.8).
Acute cutaneous lupus (ACLE)	A manifestation of active SLE, presents with bilateral erythema of the cheeks commonly referred to as a 'butterfly rash'. This is typically transient following sun exposure. Involvement of the extensor forearms and hands can be seen, with relative sparing over the joints. ACLE lesions classically clear without scarring.

Associations and precipitants

- SLE: all variants can be seen in association with SLE; acute cutaneous lupus erythematosus (ACLE) is seen exclusively in SLE, whereas discoid lupus erythematosus (DLE) is more commonly an independent disease process.
- Ultraviolet light exposure can induce flares of all subtypes.

- Medications: subacute CLE (SCLE) can be drug-induced (e.g. griseofulvin, diltiazem, NSAIDs and proton-pump inhibitors).
- Smoking is associated with a more active disease course.

Diagnosis

- Made on the basis of clinical examination and histological findings (histology is generally not required when a firm diagnosis of SLE has been made).
- Histology typically reveals basal keratinocyte damage and a band-like inflammatory cell infiltrate in the dermis (upper dermis in ACLE and SCLE; upper and lower dermis in DLE).
- Patients presenting with CLE should undergo investigation for SLE (➲ see Chapter 20, Diagnosis, and Other blood tests, p. 731 and Tables 20.7 and 20.8).

Management

Management of CLE is guided by the presence of systemic disease, disease severity, response to treatment and patient preference (➲ see Chapter 20, Treatment, p. 731):

- Photoprotection.
- Smoking cessation.
- Topical treatment: potent topical steroids (e.g. clobetasol propionate) are the primary treatment for CLE. Intralesional steroids and topical calcineurin inhibitors (e.g. tacrolimus) may also be beneficial.
- Oral antimalarials: hydroxychloroquine is commonly used first line (200 mg OD or BD). Chloroquine and/or quinacrine are typically used if hydroxychloroquine is not tolerated or is ineffective.
- Additional treatment options for refractory cutaneous disease include methotrexate, mycophenolate mofetil, oral retinoids (e.g. acitretin) and IVIGs.
- Cosmetic camouflage and hair pieces (if there is significant alopecia) may be used.

Skin in systemic disorders

Pyoderma gangrenosum

Pyoderma gangrenosum (PG) is a misnomer, it is neither infectious nor gangrenous; PG is instead a chronic, recurrent, inflammatory skin disorder characterised by solitary or multiple painful ulcers with a violaceous or gun-metal grey border. Pathergy (exacerbation at sites of accidental or iatrogenic trauma) may be observed and correlation of clinical and histological findings is required as histology is often non-specific. 50% of cases of PG are associated with an underlying disease (see Box 21.5).

Box 21.5 Causes and associations of pyoderma gangrenosum

- Idiopathic.
- Inflammatory bowel disease.
- Arthritis (seronegative or seropositive).
- Haematological disease (including myelodysplasia, monoclonal gammopathy, hairy cell leukaemia, acute and chronic myeloid leukaemia).
- Rarer associations include diabetes, solid malignancies, autoimmune hepatitis, sarcoidosis.

Treatment

Dependent on any underlying disease, may include topical and systemic steroids, ciclosporin, dapsone and infliximab for refractory disease.

Sarcoidosis

Sarcoidosis is a multisystem granulomatous disease of unknown aetiology. Cutaneous involvement is seen in approximately 25% of cases, and may be the first and only presentation of the disease.

Clinical presentations

- Red-brown papules and plaques occur on the face, lips, neck and upper extremities (the most common presentation). Diascopy (compression of a lesion with a glass slide) produces a yellow-brown 'apple jelly' colour.
- Lupus pernio presents as red-purple plaques and nodules on the nose, ears, cheeks and lips, which may ulcerate. 75% of patients with lupus pernio have associated pulmonary sarcoidosis.
- Subcutaneous sarcoid (Darier–Roussy sarcoid) is characterised by multiple firm nodules most commonly seen on the arms.
- Infiltration of pre-existing scars (or tattoos), which become thickened and red-purple in colour.

Management

Depends on severity and presence of systemic disease. Options include topical steroids or tacrolimus, hydroxychloroquine and methotrexate.

Amyloidosis

Amyloidosis describes the deposition of insoluble amyloid protein within tissues and can affect any organ tissue. Dermatologists may encounter amyloidosis as primary cutaneous disease or as a manifestation of a systemic amyloidosis. Systemic amyloidosis is discussed in ➲ Chapter 9, Amyloidosis, p. 304.

Cutaneous features

- Smooth, waxy papules and plaques commonly on the face (periorbitally), neck and trunk.
- Petchiae and purpura occur with minimal trauma, e.g. periorbital purpura ('raccoon eyes') with Valsalva manouvre.

Porphyria

The porphyria disorders (including porphyria cutanea tarda) are genetic or acquired deficiencies in enzymes involved in haem synthesis. These are discussed in ➲ Chapter 1, Porphyrias, p. 32, Figure 1.10 and Table 1.4.

Drug eruptions

Maculopapular eruptions

Maculopapular drug eruptions represent 95% of cutaneous drug eruptions. The majority represent a delayed T lymphocyte mediated (type IV) hypersensitivity reaction with activation of other inflammatory cells including eosinophils and macrophages. They typically develop approximately 7 days after treatment is commenced (sooner if previously sensitised) and clear within 7–10 days of cessation of the offending drug.

Factors that may lower the threshold for developing an adverse drug reaction include a concurrent viral infection, congenital or acquired immunodeficiency, and multiple medications.

Clinical features

Erythematous blanching macules and papules are commonly observed on the trunk and proximal limbs in a symmetrical pattern and may become more generalised. Pustules and bullae, and purpura on the lower legs are only observed rarely. Maculopapular drug eruptions are usually pruritic in nature.

Common causes of maculopapular drug rashes

- Antibiotics (e.g. penicillins, macrolides, quinolones, sulfonamides).
- Anticonvulsants (e.g. carbamazepine, phenytoin).
- NSAIDs.
- Allopurinol.

Diagnosis

- A typical history and clinical features are usually sufficient to make a diagnosis.
- Eosinophilia supports the diagnosis (more marked in drug reaction with eosinophilia and systemic symptoms [DRESS] syndrome).
- Histology can be useful if the diagnosis is unclear, and typically shows a superficial dermal perivascular inflammatory infiltrate containing eosinophils.

Management

- The definitive management is to identify and stop the causative agent.
- Topical steroids and oral antihistamines are effective measures for symptom control.
- Patients should be advised to seek medical attention if they develop erythroderma, fever, mucous membrane involvement or blisters, as these are associated with progression to severe drug hypersensitivity reactions such as DRESS (➔ see Drug reaction with eosinophilia and systemic symptoms).

Drug reaction with eosinophilia and systemic symptoms

DRESS describes a systemic drug hypersensitivity reaction and typically develops 2–6 weeks after drug initiation. In addition to skin involvement, hepatitis (severe in 10%), myocarditis, interstitial nephritis and pneumonitis may develop. Pathogenesis is poorly understood, but a viral-induced T lymphocyte expansion cross-reacting with the drug has been proposed.

Drugs causing DRESS

- Anticonvulsants (carbamazepine, lamotrigine, phenytoin, valproate).
- Allopurinol (most common cause).
- Vancomycin.
- Dapsone.
- Sulfasalazine.

Clinical features

- Confluent macular erythematous rash, often predominant around hair follicles.
- Face, trunk and extremities initially, then more generalised (typically >50% body surface area).
- Vesicles, blisters and purpura.
- Facial oedema.
- Pyrexia.
- Diffuse lymphadenopathy.

Diagnosis

- Usually made by characteristic clinical findings in a patient prescribed a 'culprit' medication.
- Peripheral eosinophilia and deranged LFTs are typical.
- Histological confirmation may be provided with skin biopsy; features overlap with a maculopapular drug rash, and include a lymphocytic infiltrate at the dermal-epidermal junction and the presence of eosinophils.

Treatment

- Drug withdrawal is important, but may not be sufficient for clinical recovery.
- Systemic steroids are used when systemic involvement is present, these may require continuation for several weeks to prevent relapse.
- Recovery typically occurs over weeks to months.

Acute generalised exanthematous pustulosis

Pathogenesis

Acute generalised exanthematous pustulosis (AGEP) is a rare (3–5 cases per million) T-cell-mediated inflammatory pustular skin eruption; 90% of cases are drug-induced. The median time to onset is 1 day for antibiotics and 11 days for all other causative drugs. AGEP typically resolves spontaneously within 1–2 weeks of stopping the causative drug.

Clinical features

- Macular erythematous rash with numerous overlying non-follicular sterile pustules.
- Typically develops on the face, armpits or groin, and then becomes more generalised over a few hours.
- Facial oedema, petechiae and mucous membrane involvement develop in up to 50% of patients.
- Fever and leucocytosis are generally present.
- Resolution of the pustular eruption is followed by desquamation (peeling of the skin).
- Secondary infection and hypocalcaemia may develop.

Drugs which commonly cause AGEP

- Antibiotics (e.g. penicillins, macrolides).
- Calcium blockers (e.g. diltiazem).
- Antimalarials.
- Terbinafine.
- Anticonvulsants.

Diagnosis

AGEP should be considered when a patient develops a pustular eruption with pyrexia after commencing a new medication. AGEP can be difficult to differentiate from pustular psoriasis clinically. A detailed drug history is essential. A skin biopsy may be useful; necrotic keratinocyes and eosinophils favour AGEP over psoriasis.

Management

Withdrawal of the offending drug is the main priority. Topical steroids and oral antihistamines are effective measures for symptom control. Systemic treatments are not commonly required as rapid resolution is typical.

Stevens–Johnson syndrome and toxic epidermal necrolysis

Stevens–Johnson syndrome (SJS) and toxic epidermal necrolysis (TEN) are severe mucocutaneous reactions characterised by epidermal detachment and necrosis. Both form part of a continuum and are differentiated by the extent of skin detachment, rather than erythema (<10% in SJS, >30% in TEN, and 10–30% in SJS/TEN overlap). Causative medications are identified in approximately 90% of cases of SJS/TEN. Certain factors lower the threshold for developing SJS/TEN, including concomitant infection and HIV, which increases risk 100-fold.

The pathogenesis is likely to reflect a cell-mediated cytotoxic reaction against keratinocytes resulting in cell death.

Common triggers of SJS/TEN

- Allopurinol.
- Sulfonamides.
- Antibiotics (e.g. penicillins, macrolides, quinolones).
- Anticonvulsants (e.g. carbamazepine, lamotrigine, phenytoin).
- NSAIDs (e.g. piroxicam).

Clinical features

- Prodromal symptoms prior to rash (including fever, cough, conjunctivitis).
- Coalescing erythematous macules are typical, with purpuric centres or generalised erythema.
- Flaccid blisters and epidermal detachment develop. Pain is often a predominant feature.
- Nikolsky sign may be positive (extension of areas of skin detachment with lateral pressure).
- Mucous membrane erosions are seen in approximately 90%.
- Complications include skin failure (dehydration, electrolyte imbalance, infection) and multi-organ dysfunction.
- Mortality for TEN can be predicted with the SCORTEN (severity of illness scale for TEN; see Table 21.11) and ranges from 3% for SCORTEN 0–1 to 90% with a SCORTEN of >5.

Table 21.11 SCORTEN for SJS/TEN

Prognostic factor	**SCORTEN**
Age ≥40	1
Malignancy	1
Body surface area detached ≥10%	1
Heart rate ≥120/min	1
Serum urea >10 mmol/L	1
Serum glucose >14 mmol/L	1
Serum bicarbonate >20 mmol/L	1
	7

Adapted from *Journal of Investigative Dermatology*, 115, 2, Fouchard, N. et al., SCORTEN: a severity-of-illness score for toxic epidermal necrolysis, pp, 149–53. https://doi.org/10.1046/j.1523-1747.2000.00061.x

Diagnosis

SJS and TEN are clinical diagnoses. Confirmatory histological findings are of basal layer keratinocyte necrosis progressing to full-thickness epidermal necrosis with epidermal detachment.

Management

- Prompt withdrawal of the offending drug is the mainstay of treatment.
- Patients with TEN are typically managed in an intensive care or burns unit (➔ see Chapter 12, Skin failure and burns, p. 404).
- Supportive care encompasses wound management, eye care, electrolyte and fluid management.
- There is conflicting data on the benefit of systemic steroids, IVIG and ciclosporin.

Further reading

1. British association of Dermatology. http://www.bad.org.uk.
2. Burge S. *Oxford Handbook of Medical Dermatology*, 2nd edn. Oxford: Oxford University Press, 2016.
3. Bessant R. *The Pocketbook of PACES: Oxford Specialty Training Revision Texts*. Oxford: Oxford University Press, 2012, pp. 608–32 and Plates 4–8.
4. Burns DA. *Rook's Textbook of Dermatology*. Oxford: Wiley-Blackwell, 2016.

Multiple choice questions

Questions

1. Which of the following conditions does not display Köbner phenomenon?
   A. Pityriasis rubra pilaris.
   B. Lichen planus.
   C. Erythema marginatum.
   D. Vitiligo.
   E. Necrobiosis lipoidica.
2. Which of the following is true regarding psoriasis?
   A. Guttate psoriasis is commonly triggered by staphylococcus.
   B. Flexural involvement of limbs is predominant.
   C. Topical steroids should be withdrawn abruptly.
   D. The epidermis is hyperproliferative.
   E. Oral retinoids are the first-line systemic agent in young women.
3. Which of the following conditions is not associated with pyoderma gangrenosum?
   A. Hairy cell leukaemia.
   B. Monoclonal gammopathy.
   C. Seronegative arthritis.
   D. Irritable bowel disease.
   E. Chronic active hepatitis.
4. In which of the following conditions is blistering not commonly seen?
   A. Pemphigus vulgaris.
   B. Porphyria cutanea tarda.
   C. Sarcoidosis.
   D. Linear IgA disease.
   E. Staphylococcal scalded skin syndrome.
5. Which of the following is not a cause of scarring alopecia?
   A. Discoid lupus erythematosus.
   B. Alopecia areata.
   C. Lichen planopilaris.
   D. Tinea capitis.
   E. Localised scleroderma.

Answers

1. C. Erythema marginatum does not display Köbner's phenomenon. See Box 21.1.
2. D. The epidermis is hyperproliferative in psoriasis. The psoriatic plaques are symmetrically distributed on the extensor surfaces, scalp, umbilicus, groin and natal cleft. Guttate psoriasis is commonly triggered by streptococcal infections. A rebound flare may occur if topical steroids are withdrawn abruptly. Oral retinoids are highly teratogenic and are therefore used with caution in young women. ➲ See Psoriasis, p. 758.
3. D. Inflammatory bowel disease, not irritable bowel disease, is associated with pyoderma gangrenosum. ➲ See Pyoderma gangrenosum (under Skin in systemic disorders), p. 770 and Box 21.5.
4. C. Sarcoidosis is not a blistering dermatoses. Blistering is seen in all of the other conditions. ➲ See Sarcoidosis, p. 771, Tables 1.4, 21.8 and Box 21.4.
5. B. Alopecia areata is a non-scarring autoimmune condition that leads to small areas of hair loss. Options A, C and D are the three commonest causes of scarring alopecia. ➲ See Lichen planus, p. 764, and Tables 21.7 (tinea capitis), 21.10 (DLE) and Systemic sclerosis, p. 733. Alopecia areata is an autoimmune condition, which presents with non-scarring alopecia. It is associated with other autoimmune conditions such as vitiligo, pernicious anaemia and thyroid disorders.

Chapter 22 **Psychiatry**

Rob Tandy and Kingsley Norton

Psychological aspects of physical illness

Many sufferers from physical conditions experience or exhibit psychological and behavioural features. Three main response modes are described:

- Approach and tackling:
  - Adaptive, when minimising risks to health and supporting adaptation to altered circumstances, e.g. fact-finding about the illness/treatment/unwanted effects.
  - Prejudices recovery in excess by being disproportionately illness-focused, distracting from the patient's focus on other aspects of psychosocial functioning, e.g. role of parent or spouse.
- Avoidance:
  - May be emotionally-protective.
  - May result in withdrawal from investigations/treatment; thus being maladaptive.
- Freezing and capitulating:
  - Reflects extreme passivity, resulting in the patient's non-participation in essential treatment.
  - May be normal as an initial reaction to a frightening and unexpected diagnosis.
  - When prolonged, is maladaptive, unless no realistic hope exists.

Taking into account and being sensitive to the factors below can help inform decisions about the timing of and setting for discussing diagnosis, treatment and prognosis (e.g. a separate appointment, presence of a friend/partner), as well as what level of information to impart:

- Meaning of the symptom/disorder to the patient.
- Psychosocial impact of the symptom/disorder on the patient's life.
- The patient's past experience of illness, treatment and recovery.
- Quality of relationship with the patient and diagnosing/treating doctor.
- Style and content of doctor–patient communication used in breaking the diagnosis.
- Knowledge of the patient's personality and coping strategies.
- Quality of the patient's support system.

To identify the cut-off point between a healthy and a pathological psychological response requires a detailed knowledge of psychopathological phenomena, recognising that some represent a quantitative and others qualitative difference from the healthy spectrum.

Psychopathology

The psychiatrist uses the standard medical approach (history-taking; examination [including mental state]; investigations [including collateral information]; diagnosis; and treatment) to elicit, label and categorise the patient's abnormal experiences and/or behaviour. This involves the psychiatrist interviewing the patient (and significant others in his/her life) to produce a valid statement of the *psychopathology* that is present, before aggregating the symptoms/signs and assigning them to an overarching syndrome or diagnosis, such as affective disorder or schizophrenia, in order to direct treatment. To elicit such psychopathological information in a reliable fashion requires knowledge of the relevant abnormal phenomena, as well as advanced interviewing and communication skills, including observational and listening skills.

Symptoms and signs

The distinction between *symptom* – what is complained of by patient – and *sign* – what is elicited by the clinician – is not usually made. Patients' descriptions of abnormal mental phenomena are taken as symptoms, whether the patient is simply describing their experience or complaining of them. Aggregated symptoms are regarded as indicative of particular mental disorders, descriptions of which follow in later sections.

Form and content of abnormal phenomena

The *form* of mental abnormality refers to its phenomenological 'structure' (e.g. delusion or hallucination), and the *content* to its colouring (e.g. 'persecutory' or 'commenting'). Form is key to diagnosis and, therefore, a main concern of the treating physician. On the whole, the patient is more concerned with the content.

History-taking and mental state examination

Even where patients lack insight and do not complain of symptoms, in order to diagnose and treat, the psychiatrist aims to identify abnormalities of:

- mood;
- thinking;
- perception;
- belief;
- volition;
- movement (behaviour);
- cognitive function.

Abnormal mood

Feelings and *affect* refer to marked, but transitory (emotional) reactions to an event, person or object, whereas *mood* is a more prolonged prevailing state. In health, mood varies according to internal and external world influences. Evidence is sought therefore for differences from the patient's premorbid/normal mood state. The examiner should look for:

- Quality (happy, sad, irritable, etc.).
- Appropriateness to the context.
- Consistency (e.g. sustained low mood).
- Marked diurnal variation.
- Lack of reactivity.
- Blunting or flattening, loss of feeling, degrees of elation.

Abnormal thinking

Abnormal forms of thinking are reflected in observable or reported changes from the patient's usual functioning, particularly, in terms of:

- Rate (accelerated/retarded).
- Flow of associations (thought block/flight of ideas).
- Poverty of thoughts.
- Concreteness.
- Over-inclusiveness.

Abnormal perception

In health, perception makes meaning of sensory input. Hallucinations are perceptions that arise in the absence of external stimuli. Illusions are psychological distortions of perception in the face of actual external stimuli. Pseudo-hallucinations are self-generated perceptions that are perceived by the person as being 'inside their head'. While hallucinations are experienced as concrete, real and in outer objective space, pseudo-hallucinations are located in subjective space/perceived with the inner eye or ear. Hallucinations, representing serious psychopathology, are categorised as auditory; visual; bodily sensation; olfactory; gustatory. (Hypnagogic and hypnopompic hallucinations, occurring on falling into or emerging from sleep, respectively, are not usually psychopathological, i.e. lie within the range of normality).

Abnormal beliefs

A person holding a false, unshakeable idea or belief, which is out of keeping with their educational, cultural and social background, has a *delusion*. There are two sorts – primary and secondary. Primary delusions, pathognomonic of schizophrenia, arise de novo, whereas secondary delusions derive, understandably, from another psychopathological form (e.g. hallucination). Delusions are to be distinguished from *over-valued ideas*, which are intense preoccupations pursued by the patient, but with beliefs that are not unshakable in nature.

Common 'themes' of delusions, include:

- persecution;
- morbid jealousy;
- grandiosity;
- guilt and unworthiness;
- poverty and nihilism;
- hypochondriasis;
- passivity.

Abnormality of volition

Abnormal volition may be associated with disturbance of the patient's experience of *need* (e.g. absence of hunger), *motivation* (e.g. driving patient to find food) and/or *will*. Where the patient has an experience of being controlled (so-called 'passivity' phenomena), there is the possibility that he/she behaves under the influence of pathological beliefs, which can render them a serious danger to self, others and society.

Abnormality of movement

Movement may be speeded up or slowed down, or show various qualitative abnormalities. Abnormalities may be involuntary, voluntary (but carried out unconsciously) and/or else result from (conscious) will. Common technical terms include:

- *Agitation*: physical restlessness and signs of increased arousal (being the physical expression of a subjective mood state e.g. anxiety disorder).
- *Hyperactivity*: relates to a mental state accompanied by increased motor activity (sometimes with aggression, over-talkativeness or uncoordinated activity, e.g. in mania).

- *Hyperkinesis*: may occur in brain damage or epilepsy and may present as explosive anger, outbursts or irritability.
- *Psychomotor retardation*: implies slowness of the initiation, execution and completion of physical activity (frequently accompanying retardation of thought, as part of severe depressive illness).

Impairment of cognitive function

Different domains of cognition may be affected including:

- *Attention*: focusing of consciousness on an experience or subject.
- *Concentration*: maintaining focus.
- *Memory*: short- and long-term, both being affected by impaired attention and concentration.
- *Language*.

Detection of a significant abnormality may dictate more thorough evaluation of the mental state examination or a specialist neuro-psychological opinion, to exclude a physical cause and/or create a valid baseline.

Making a psychiatric diagnosis

Psychiatric diagnoses may be viewed as hierarchical. Diagnosis at a given level excludes symptoms of all higher members in the hierarchy but (potentially) embraces the symptoms of all the lower members:

1. Organic psycho-syndromes: whatever other symptoms are present (psychotic or non-psychotic), when there is evidence of causative physical disease, the diagnosis is 'organic'.
2. Schizophrenia: characterised by typical symptoms (➲ see Schizophrenia, p. 789 and Table 22.6), as long as organic causation is excluded.
3. Bipolar disorder: where both schizophrenic and bipolar symptoms are present, the classification is schizophrenia.
4. Neurotic symptoms (e.g. phobic or obsessive-compulsive symptoms): represent the lowest level and may be present at any level, remaining subordinate to the overarching diagnosis.

Classifying psychiatric disorders

Ideally, classification is based on aetiology. However, causation remains incompletely understood in all major categories. Two categorical classifications are in widespread use:

- International Classification of Diseases (ICD) hails from the WHO, allowing international comparison for epidemiological, clinical and research purposes.
- Diagnostic and Statistical Manual of Mental Disorders (DSM), is time-consuming to apply, being better-suited to research than the clinic.

Psychotropic medications

'Psychotropic' refers to drugs that therapeutically alter a patient's brain/mind. They are categorised according to the syndromes they treat.

Antipsychotics

Typical (e.g. haloperidol, chlorpromazine)

These drugs are proven to be effective. They exert an antagonist effect at dopamine, acetylcholine, adrenaline/noradrenaline and histamine receptor sites, the dominant therapeutic effect being postulated as postsynaptic dopamine D2 receptor antagonism. However, there is no antipsychotic efficacy achieved with drugs that act exclusively at D2 receptors, which in practice imposes a choice of unselective receptor-binding, beneficial drug effects deriving from a combination of dopamine D2 and 5-hydroxytryptamine 2 antagonism.

For the mode and site of action and common side effects of typical antipsychotics, see Table 22.1.

Table 22.1 Mode and site of action and common side effects of typical antipsychotics

Neuro-transmitter activity	Site/pathway	Side effects
Anti-dopaminergic	Tubero-fundibular pathway.	Galactorrhoea, gynaecomastia, menstrual irregularities, reduced libido.
	Nigro-striatal pathway.	Parkinsonism, dystonia, akathisia, tardive dyskinesia.
Anti-cholinergic	Muscarinic sites.	Dry mouth, blurred vision, urinary retention, constipation, confusion.
Anti-adrenergic	Likely peripheral sites.	Postural hypotension, ejaculatory failure.
Anti-histaminergic	Likely central sites.	Drowsiness.

Neuroleptic malignant syndrome can be caused by all classes of antipsychotics (➲ see Table 3.18).

Atypical (e.g. risperidone, olanzapine, quetiapine, clozapine)

So-called *atypical* antipsychotic drugs exhibit an alternative range of receptor activity to *typical*, with differing side effect profiles:

- Clozapine, the most potent molecule, acts at 5-HT2, dopamine D4, dopamine D1, muscarinic, and alpha-adrenergic receptors. This drug can cause:
  - Neutropenia, which is dangerous, but reversible; hence, for physical health reasons a formal, registered Clozapine Monitoring Service is required.
  - Myocarditis and cardiomyopathy.
- Atypical antipsychotic drugs may produce delayed ventricular repolarisation with prolonged QT interval, serious tachyarrhythmia and sudden death syndrome. ECG monitoring is required, both at baseline and regularly throughout treatment (➲ see Chapter 13, Drug-induced VT, p. 472).
- Metabolic effects commonly include significant weight gain, increased risk of diabetes and atherogenic dyslipidaemia (low HDL and raised fasting triglycerides). Use of a partial agonist such as aripiprazole, can be an alternative antipsychotic in patients with metabolic syndrome.

Antidepressants

For the mode of action, side effects and harmful drug interactions of antidepressants, see Table 22.2.

Table 22.2 Mode of action, side effects and harmful drug interactions of antidepressants

Drug class	Neurotransmitter activity	Side effects	Dangerous interactions with other medication
Tricyclics (e.g. amitriptyline, dosulepin and clomipramine)	Post-synaptic inhibition of re-uptake of noradrenaline (NA) and 5HT.	Anti-cholinergic: dried mouth, blurred vision, urinary retention, constipation, QT prolongation on ECG.	
Selective serotonin reuptake inhibitors (e.g. fluoxetine, sertraline and citalopram)	Post-synaptic inhibition of re-uptake of 5HT.	Fewer anti-cholinergic side effects, but nausea and vomiting commoner than with tricyclics.'Discontinuation' effect with sudden cessation <24 hours involving anxiety, irritability, flu-like symptoms and myalgia.	
Type A monoamine oxidase inhibitor (moclobemide)	Selective inhibitor of Type A oxidase systems for both 5HT and NA.	Hypotension, dry mouth, constipation, urinary difficulties, sexual dysfunction, 'hypertensive crisis.	Some cough mixtures and decongestants that contain sympathomimetic molecules.

Serotonin syndrome results from the increased levels of serotonin on the central and peripheral nervous systems, either following initiation of or an increase in the dose of the treatment. It is potentially fatal (➲ see Chapter 3, Selective serotonin reuptake inhibitors, p. 87).

Mood stabilisers

These drugs are used to treat severe affective disorders; moderate to severe mania; prophylaxis of bipolar disorder (main indication); and refractory depression (in combination with an antidepressant).

For the mode of action, side effects and problematic drug interactions of mood stabilisers, see Table 22.3.

Table 22.3 Mode of action, side effects and problematic drug interactions of mood stabilisers

Drug	Site/pathway	Therapeutic dose	Side effects	Interactions with other medication
Lithium carbonate	Precise site(s) not known (lithium is widely distributed).	(0.60–0.75 mmol/L)	NB. Toxic effects occur above 1.5 mmol/L: nausea, diarrhoea, muscle weakness, drowsiness, ataxia, coarse tremor, coma and death. Adverse effects: GI disturbance, polyuria, polydipsia, fine tremor, exacerbation of psoriasis, metallic taste, oedema and weight gain. Induced disorders: nephrogenic diabetes insipidus, hypothyroidism and hyperparathyroidism.	ACE inhibitors, NSAIDs and thiazide diuretics.
Carbamazepine	Inhibition of sodium channels thus reducing glutamate release, lowering turnover of dopamine and NA.		Dizziness, diplopia, drowsiness and ataxia. NB. It is teratogenic.	Induces own metabolism and that of other drugs (e.g. contraceptive pill) on chronic use.

Anxiolytics and hypnotics

Benzodiazepines bind to central gamma-aminobutyric acid (GABA)-A receptors producing desired clinical effects, and are used as:

- anxiolytics;
- hypnotics;
- anticonvulsants;
- muscle relaxants.

Benzodiazepine side effects include:

- dizziness;
- decreased mental acuity;
- drowsiness;
- impairment of short-term memory;
- physiological dependence with a withdrawal state.

Zopiclone is a cyclopyrrolone also acting at GABA-A receptors with side effects similar to those of benzodiazepines.

Psychological treatments

Psychological treatments (sometimes referred to as 'psychotherapies') rely on the quality of the therapist–patient relationship as well the theory, style and content of clinical interaction. Many varieties of psychotherapy exist, ranging from short-term and problem-solving to long-term and exploratory therapies, aimed at changing aspects of personality (Table 22.4).

Selection, care pathways, interactions and contraindications

Counselling may be applied successfully in the first instance, assuming therapist competency and an awareness of the limitations of method. However, some clinical presentations that appear simple turn out to need more in-depth approaches; hence, a range of individualised pathways, so-called 'stepped care', is required. With careful selection and monitored application, psychological and pharmacological interventions can be beneficially combined. N.B. Ongoing addiction/significant dependence upon illicit substances or alcohol, acute psychosis and significant brain damage may be contraindications, with highly specialist services being required.

Where premorbid personality and support network are relatively robust, cognitive behavioural therapy (CBT) is usually the next step to deal with circumscribed symptom targets. However, some patients dislike the discrete focus on cognitions (thought-patterns) or also require attention to their emotional aspects, the latter being provided by longer-term and less-structured therapies. These afford patients greater influence to direct the agenda, developing trust and fostering deeper self-revelation, while allowing the therapist to be more challenging of patients' ill-adapted schemas or defences, and thereby effecting deeper (personality-related) change. These therapeutic approaches are more likely to generate unwanted effects, e.g. over-dependency on therapists; hence, careful matching of modality with patient is required.

Neuroses

Neuroses are *mental disorders without organic cause, delusions or hallucinations, but with insight preserved.* They are characterised by prominent anxiety symptoms and associated with behavioural attempts (from avoidance in phobias to [magical] tackling in obsessive-compulsive disorder) to lessen or remove them. They are categorised as:

- Phobias.
- 'Other' (panic disorder, generalised anxiety, mixed anxiety/depression).
- Obsessive-compulsive disorder.
- Reaction to severe stress/adjustment disorder.

Epidemiology

- Lifetime risk is 1 in 4.
- Female:male ratio is 2:1.
- Peak is in middle age.
- Associated with social disadvantage.
- 75% are 'phobias': social, simple or agoraphobia.

Aetiology

The heritability of generalised anxiety disorder is 30%. There is a shared liability to anxiety and depression, with environmental experiences ('threat' versus 'loss' generally) determining type of neurosis. Genetic factors probably convey non-specific vulnerability to neurotic disorders, exerting their influence during brain development in childhood, or by modifying neurotransmission in adults. Differences in the contribution of

Table 22.4 Main types of psychological therapy: indications and other relevant characteristics

Type of therapy	Patient profile	Theoretical basis	Typical duration	Treatment aims
Cognitive behavioural therapy (CBT)	Anxiety and/or depression; other neurotic syndromes; some psychotic disorders.	Learning theory: replacing learned maladaptive ideas, thoughts or beliefs by more adaptive ones.	Usually short-term (less than 6 months) except where condition is chronic or more complex.	Correcting 'silent assumptions' about self, others and the future.
Dialectical behaviour therapy (DBT)	Self-harming patients with emotionally unstable personality disorder (PD) (borderline type).	Learning theory: problem-solving techniques in combination with mindfulness, using group training and individual therapy approaches.	Skills development and learning of alternative coping behaviours determines length (2+ years).	Equipping patients with alternatives to self-harming to regulate emotions.
Schema-focused therapy	Particularly adapted for treating a range of PDs, including emotionally unstable.	Learning theory: evolved from CBT to include early, maladapative 'schemas' (which are typical beliefs and associated behaviours – more or less transient self-states).	Long-term to identify relevant schemas and their reinforcement, to facilitate experimentation; hence rational change.	Producing change in maladaptive aspects of the patient's personality.
Psychoanalysis-derived therapy (including transference-focused therapy)	Complicated grief and depressive disorders, some PD, e.g. emotionally unstable and avoidant.	Psychoanalysis: deploying concepts of conscious/unconscious mind and recognising the importance of early relationships and that with therapist.	Short-term (e.g. dynamic interpersonal therapy) (4 months), to long-term (1–3 years).	Using individual, group or family methods to identify internal relationship problem and hence insight into working of mind and more conscious choice.
Systemic therapy	Mainly in use for families, with an 'identified' patient.	Systems theory: viewing people, groups (including family) and organisations as arranged in hierarchies with potentially conflicting and/or overlapping roles and objectives.	Usually short-term, up to 1 year.	Identifying and resolving conflicts arising from multi-system membership.
Counselling	Problems with coping with life's developmental challenges, e.g. puberty, parenthood, mid-life, old age, bereavement and serious physical illness.	Proven therapeutic power of warmth, empathy and positive regard.	Usually, short-term and time-limited inputs.	Supporting clients to find solutions and anticipate future difficulties with greater confidence, through identification of unconscious motivation.

genetic factors to different neurotic disorders is less clear, with a partially inherited susceptibility to all types of neurotic disorder being most likely.

Neurochemistry

Ascending noradrenaline (NA) and 5HT pathways, terminating in the limbic and neo-cortex regions, are implicated. NA function produces increased arousal and 5HT is associated with fear and avoidant behaviour. Other neurotransmitters, such as GABA are also mediators of anxiety.

Childhood experiences

Parental separation, maternal death and traumatic events in childhood are associated with later agoraphobia and panic disorder. People who experienced neglect or physical or sexual abuse are more vulnerable to anxiety (and depression) as adults.

Psychological

Panic attacks can be viewed as catastrophic misinterpretations of harmless bodily sensations and lead to automatic assumptions about illness, which increases levels of anxiety; hence, a vicious cycle of panic can develop.

Treatment

Reassurance, education and supportive therapy help in mild cases. Moderate or severe disorders require more intensive and problem-focused interventions:

- Problem-solving skills.
- Making life changes to reduce stress.
- Improving support systems.
- Psychological therapies and/or medication.

A range of psychological approaches exists, being applied according to patient preference, complexity and severity. CBT is especially helpful for:

- Uncomplicated cases.
- Cases of recent onset.
- Where good support systems are present.
- When precipitating factors no longer apply.

Perpetuating interpersonal stressors can be ameliorated via insight-directed, individual or group psychoanalytic therapies.

In cases that are refractory to psychological intervention, the addition of medication should be considered:

- Benzodiazepines are rapidly effective, but can induce dependence.
- Tricyclic antidepressant and SSRI medications, with slower-onset of action, carry less risk of abuse.
- Azapirones (e.g. buspirone, a partial agonist of 5HT1A receptors that does not induce dependence, and is used in the treatment of short- to medium-term anxiety) are effective in generalised anxiety, but not panic disorder.
- Monoamine oxidase inhibitors (MAOI) can be useful, although should not be first-line.
- β-blockers, in the absence of contraindications, help decrease palpitations, tremor and flushing.

Prognosis

Approximately 50% of neurotic disorder patients recover in 3 months, a further 25% within 1 year, the rest remaining chronic. Poorer prognosis is associated with:

- older age;
- co-morbidity;
- physical illness;

- persistent social problems;
- poverty of social support.

The relative risk of death is raised nearly two-fold, accounted for by a marked increase in deaths by suicide and accident.

Personality disorder

Personality disorder (PD) refers to *an enduring pattern of thinking, feeling and behaving (not linked with or limited to episodes of illness or substance misuse/alcohol intoxication), which is maladaptive in a range of personal, interpersonal and social settings*. It can cause considerable personal suffering and/or harm to self and/or others. The pattern is not characteristic of the person's cultural or subcultural background.

Many subtypes have been described, but most show low inter-rater reliability. Certain 'clusters' within PD show greater reliability and validity:

1. Cluster A (odd or eccentric).
2. Cluster B (dramatic or erratic).
3. Cluster C (anxious or inhibited).

In clinical practice, cluster B (subtypes borderline, narcissistic, histrionic and antisocial) is most prevalent and clinically problematic to treat, because of problems with patient engagement in treatment and negative professional response to therapeutic difficulty. As evidence-based treatments for most subtypes do not yet exist, diagnosing of the overarching cluster (A, B or C) is the most clinically relevant step.

Population surveys suggest (approximated) prevalence of any PD to be:

- 5–10% in the general population.
- 20% in the family doctor's waiting room.
- 30% in the psychiatric outpatient/community samples.
- 40% in acute psychiatric wards.
- 50% or higher in forensic in-patient/prison settings.

Aetiology

Genetic

Relevant twin and adoption studies are inconclusive regarding the heritability of PD. Certain personality 'traits', such as impulsivity, do have established genetic links. However, they do not correlate directly with subtypes.

Environment

Parents of PD patients have high rates of psychiatric diagnoses (not necessarily PD), e.g. alcoholism and substance abuse. Emotional abuse/neglect is a potent negative influence, undermining psychosocial adaptation. Sexual and physical abuse is frequently reported in PD patients. Early or repeated separations from parents are damaging, in the absence of protective (interpersonal) factors. Violence, emotional volatility, lack of respect for personal boundaries and emotional cruelty by parents (or others) damages development, simultaneously installing mental models of maladaptive attitudes and behaviour.

Treatment

Multiple approaches have been advocated, reflecting a range of personal/interpersonal difficulties and PD subtype co-morbidity. Experts agree that a strong therapeutic alliance between patient and therapist is crucial to success. In severe cases, multiple agencies, sometimes including the Criminal Justice system, are needed, requiring openness of inter-professional communication and authentic collaboration to maintain clinical focus and effect clinical progress.

Approaches

- Supportive.
- Group and/or individual psychoanalytic.
- Schema-focused.
- Dialectical behaviour.
- Mentalisation-based therapy.
- Family.

Pharmacotherapy may be necessary, but should be kept to a minimum. Mood stabilisers and antipsychotics (dispensed safely where risk of suicide) may be helpful to facilitate affect-regulation and decrease impulsive/destructive activity. In-patient treatment may be required during a crisis, but should be minimised, due to risk of inappropriate dependency on other people/services. Specialist in-patient settings have a place in the clinical management of selected severe cases.

Prognosis

Good quality prospective treatment outcome studies show positive results in expert hands. However, some patients do not benefit, due to disadvantageous (perpetuating) factors – financial/social poverty, ill-health, co-morbid diagnoses – and may require long-term reliance on multi-agency interventions. Overall, therapeutic pessimism is misplaced, with around 50% reaching clinical recovery. However, in the remainder, the suicide rate remains very high.

Affective disorders

Affective disorders represent common psychiatric conditions – in one major study the lifetime prevalence for all affective disorders was 6.1–9.5%, with depressive disorders being the most common. They are characterised by depressed or elevated mood, sometimes associated with 'biological' disturbance (sleep, appetite, libido) and/or psychosocial function impairment. Aetiology is multifactorial, deriving from an interaction of the following established factors:

- *Genetic*: no single mode of inheritance is known. Family studies reveal increased risk of unipolar depression and bipolar disorder in patients' first-degree relatives. Twin studies show high concordance for unipolar depression (40–50% in monozygotic [MZ] twins; 20–25% in dizygotic twins) and for bipolar disorder (40–70% in MZ twins).
- *Neurotransmitter systems*: the 'monoamine hypothesis' proposes that depression is caused by a depletion, and mania by an excess, of central monoamines. Reduced levels of monoamines and their metabolites are found in the cerebrospinal fluid of depressed patients. The pharmacological effect of tricyclic and SSRI antidepressants further supports this hypothesis, such drugs provoking mania in predisposed subjects.
- *Neuro-endocrine*: disturbances of the hypothalamic–pituitary–adrenal axis are reported in depression, with disruption of circadian rhythm of cortisol secretion. Increased secretion of ACTH, cortisol, beta-endorphin and prolactin have been found in depressed patients.
- *Physical illness*: depression is associated with various physical disorders (e.g. Cushing's syndrome, hypothyroidism) and is common following stroke and myocardial infarction. Individuals with one long-term physical health condition are 2–3 times more likely to develop depression than the rest of the population. Physical illness may serve as an adverse life event or chronic stressor, hence predisposing to depression.
- *Psychological*: cognitive theorists propose a triad of learned, negative evaluations of the patient's self, current life situation and future. These promote and maintain the depressed state. Psychoanalytic theories focus on the role of prior loss (e.g. bereavement, chronic ill-health) and an (unconscious) internalisation of consequent (denied) anger, as precursors of depression. Mania is viewed as an (unconscious) defence against the emotional pain of loss.

- *Social*: high expression of critical emotion in the patient's social setting has been shown to increase relapse. Excess negative (e.g. 'loss') life events, including physical illness, occur in the 6 months preceding a depressive episode. Vulnerability factors, such as the lack of a confiding relationship and loss of mother (before the age 11) increase the risk of depression in women.

Clinical features

For categorisation of affective disorders and their characteristics, see Table 22.5.

Table 22.5 Categorisation of affective disorders and their characteristics

Category	Severity	Typical features
Unipolar disorder	Mild depression	Sustained low mood. Anhedonia. Reduced energy. Thoughts that life is not worth living. Absence of suicidal ideation.
	Moderate depression	*In addition*: Diurnal mood variation. Sleep disturbance. Reduced appetite/weight loss. Low libido. Impaired concentration. Suicidal ideation, without plans.
	Severe depression	*In addition*: Hallucinations (usually auditory – critical 'voice'). Mood-congruent delusions (e.g. of own 'badness'). Suicidal activity (may also occur after mood lifts).
Bipolar disorder (Episodes of moderate/severe depression [as above] and at least one episode of mania or vice versa, i.e. with manic episodes dominating)	Mild mania (hypomania)	Elated mood. Increased energy. Over-activity. Pressure of speech. Need for less sleep.
	Moderate mania	*In addition*: Social disinhibition. Hypersexuality. Impaired judgement. Grandiosity.
	Severe mania	*In addition*: Grandiose delusions. Reckless, dangerous or criminal behaviour, congruent with delusional content.

Clinical management

Unipolar disorder

For mild unipolar depression, psychological treatment is first choice. CBT is effective in half of cases. For more complex cases, e.g. where there are perpetuating interpersonal factors or biological features, psychodynamic psychotherapy and/or antidepressant medication are indicated.

For moderate/severe unipolar depression, which may be life-threatening, an antidepressant is first-line treatment, using the lowest tolerated dose. With associated psychotic symptoms, an antipsychotic may be added and rarely electro-convulsive therapy (ECT) may be needed. All antidepressant classes and ECT are now known to promote adult hippocampal neurogenesis, suggesting that this may be an ameliorating factor in depressive states.

Where suicidal ideation or self-neglect are serious, admission to hospital (sometimes compulsorily under Section 2 or 3 of the Mental Health Act [MHA]) may be required. To reduce risk of relapse, drug treatment should be continued for at least 6 months after symptom remission. Long-term treatment emphasises prevention of relapse, via psycho-education, and identifying and reducing relevant risk factors.

Bipolar disorder

For depressive episodes in bipolar disorder, to avoid triggering mania, mood-stabilising drugs (e.g. lithium carbonate) must be considered, in place of SSRI and tricyclic medication. To facilitate early presentation, hence minimising the damaging sequelae of mania, psycho-education for patients and families is imperative. Community psychiatric services' involvement, to optimise compliance with treatment, is usually also indicated. Where mania is severe, there may need to be compulsory hospital admission under the MHA. In addition, antipsychotic medication or ECT may be required, to safeguard the patient and/or others. Although the mechanism of ECT on the brain/mind is complex and ill-understood, and side effects can be serious, it can effect speedy improvement in both severe depression and mania, where other treatments are considered, clinically, to be too slow or ineffective; thus it may be life-saving.

Schizophrenia

Schizophrenia is a severe mental disorder whose precise aetiology is unknown, but which has recognisable subtypes and recognised associations/risk factors. A multifactorial model of aetiology is postulated, deriving from the interaction of established associations.

- *Genetic*: there is no single mode of inheritance, but adopted children share their biological parents' risk (approximately 10%) and MZ twins are 45% concordant.
- *Pre-natal and peri-natal*: approximately 20% of patients have experienced pre- or peri-natal complications, e.g. maternal influenza, pre-eclampsia or fetal distress syndrome.
- *Age/gender*: The wide age of onset (15–45 years) and the male excess is not satisfactorily explained.
- *Structural brain abnormalities*:
  - CT and MRI studies reveal increased lateral ventricular space and reduced cortical grey matter volumes, with marked cyto-architectual changes in limbic and prefrontal areas.
  - Post-mortem studies show lowered brain weights.
  - Histological studies show hippocampal cell abnormalities.
  - Functional brain studies show hypo-frontality (reduced cerebral blood flow to prefrontal cortex) and overactivity elsewhere (e.g. temporal region).
- *Neurotransmitter systems:* clinical effectiveness of some antipsychotic drugs is associated with their affinity for D2 dopamine brain receptors. Other neurotransmitter systems (e.g. glutamate) have also been implicated, without clarity over primacy, i.e. whether clinical effect is mediated directly or indirectly via affecting the dopaminergic system.
- *Social*: relapses are associated with prior adverse life events, including living with families/other people displaying high expressed emotion in the form of critical comments.

Diagnosis

Diagnosis is based on the presence of the following symptoms/signs, for which there is no identifiable organic basis. General criteria for diagnosis are:

- one 'clear' or two 'not clear-cut' symptoms from 1 to 4; or
- two symptoms from 5 to 8, present for at least 1 month.

NB. For a diagnosis of simple schizophrenia, symptom 8 and 9 need to have been present for at least 1 year.

Symptoms/signs

1. Thought echo*, insertion*, withdrawal* and/or broadcasting*.
2. Delusions of passivity, delusional perception*.
3. Auditory hallucinations in running commentary*, third person*, or emanating from a part of the body.
4. Persistent delusions.
5. Persistent hallucinations in any modality.
6. Thought disorder.
7. Catatonic symptoms.
8. Negative symptoms/defect state: paucity of speech, blunting of affect.
9. Significant deterioration in behaviour; aimlessness, social withdrawal (applies only to a diagnosis of simple schizophrenia [➔ see Table 22.6]).

Other terminology

Crow (1) proposed the concept of positive (acute) symptoms (delusions, hallucinations, and thought disorder), and negative (chronic) symptoms (affective flattening, apathy and poverty of speech). Although non-specific, this is commonly used terminology.

Kurt Schneider (2) described a number of 'first rank symptoms', their presence being highly suggestive of schizophrenia. Most of these are asterisked in the symptom list above, but he also included somatic passivity, the experience of being a passive recipient of a bodily sensation imposed from an external agency.

Acute phase schizophrenia

- Prodromal phase preceding frank psychotic symptoms with disturbed affect and perplexity.
- Usually with delusions (persecutory, grandiose, religious or hypochondriacal) and associated disturbed general behaviour, including impaired or bizarre social interaction.
- Hallucinations in any of the five senses are often present, most commonly 'voiced' auditory.
- Thought disorder (with neologisms, incoherence and irrelevant speech) may be present.

Chronic phase schizophrenia

- Acute symptoms may resolve (some patients never relapse) or may not, the course being unpredictable.
- With repeated relapses, 'acute' symptoms tend to last longer or remain.
- Flattening or blunting of affect is present, with a subjective inability to feel or effectively express deep emotion.
- Incongruity of affect represents an emotional response grossly at odds with the setting and/or topic of conversation.
- A 'defect state' may exist, with apathy, paucity of speech, loss of interests and social withdrawal.

Subtypes

For diagnostic sub-categories of schizophrenia, see Table 22.6.

* Schneiderian first-rank symptom.

Table 22.6 Diagnostic sub-categories of schizophrenia

Category	Typical clinical features
Paranoid	Prominent delusions and hallucinations. Some disturbance of affect, speech and volition. Psychosocial functioning may be intact between relapses.
Hebephrenic	Usually early onset (age 15–25). Thought disorder predominates. Marked affect and volition disturbance. Delusions and hallucinations are usually fleeting and fragmentary. Rapid progression to 'residual' category.
Catatonic	General criteria for schizophrenia are fulfilled, with one or more of the following, dominating: • Stupor/mutism. • Excitement. • Posturing. • Negativism.
Undifferentiated	General criteria for schizophrenia may be fulfilled, which do not tally with the identified subtypes.
Residual	A chronic stage, with prominent negative symptoms (and one episode in the previous year meeting criteria for schizophrenia).
Simple	Decline in social and interpersonal functioning, in which negative symptoms develop, but without positive symptoms.

Clinical management

Hospitalisation may be necessary, sometimes with compulsory detention and treatment, under the Mental Health Act 1983, since, lacking insight, the patient may pose a danger to self/others. Community follow-up is required post-discharge, with careful attention to the integration of different treatment elements. Non-clinical issues such as finances, accommodation, and educational and vocational achievements and aspirations may need targeting.

Where a serious criminal act has been committed (related to diagnosis), prolonged admission and complex recovery pathways are entailed. Antipsychotic medication is usually central to recovery of both acute and chronic phases, drugs being administered orally or in injectable form, with close monitoring for side effects (e.g. extra-pyramidal or metabolic). Cognitive behavioural and family therapy interventions can be effective adjuncts. Promoting independence, physical health and personal development are the aims of 'recovery', as well as avoiding inappropriate dependence on services.

References

1. Crow TJ. Molecular pathology of schizophrenia: More than one dimension of pathology? *British Medical Journal*, 1980; 280:66-68.
2. Schneider, K. *Clinical Psychopathology*. New York: Grune and Stratton, 1959.

Dementias

Dementia is *a global deterioration in brain functions in clear consciousness, which is usually progressive and irreversible, ultimately leading to significant impairments in activities of daily living, affecting psycho-social and intellectual functioning.*

- *Cortical dementias* (including Alzheimer's disease [AD] and some cerebrovascular dementias): cause dysphasia, dyspraxia and agnosias (disruption to language, personal functioning and perception).
- *Subcortical dementias*: incorporate cognitive slowness and behavioural changes of apathy and inertia. Causes include cerebral small vessel disease, multiple sclerosis, Huntington's disease, HIV infection and progressive supranuclear palsy.

- *'Cortico-subcortical' dementias*: comprise features of cortical and subcortical dementias. Causes include Lewy body dementia and prion dementia.

For specific dementias, see Table 22.7.

Table 22.7 Specific dementias

Dementia	Pathological features	Aetiology/risk factors	Clinical features
Alzheimer's disease (AD)	Generalised cerebral atrophy, most pronounced in frontal and temporal lobes. Microscopic lesions: amyloid plaques; neurofibrillary tangles; neuronal loss; astrocytosis; microgliosis.	Autosomal dominant inheritance in early onset AD: three genes identified: • beta amyloid precursor protein (*APP*) gene: chromosome 21 • presenilin (*PS*) genes: PS-1 on chromosome 14; PS-2 on chromosome 1. Apolipoprotein E (APOE) polymorphism: APOEε4 allele increases risk by three times in heterozygotes and by 15 times in homozygotes. First degree relative: increases risk 2–6-fold.	Insidious onset. Gradual progression. Short-term memory loss. Progresses over time to loss of other memory types. Dysphasias. Dyspraxias and decline in personal functioning. Behavioural changes including apathy, agitation, wandering and aggression.
Vascular cognitive impairment	Areas of cerebral infarction/haemorrhage. Lipohyalinosis, atheromatosis and/or amyloid angiopathy of cerebral blood vessels. Blood–brain barrier dysfunction. Neural tract disruption. Hypoxia/hypo-perfusion increases formation of AD lesions with reduced elimination of amyloid. Some discrete vascular syndromes – ➲ see Specific vascular syndromes (with no AD overlap), p. 793.	Stroke (15–30% develop dementia 3 months post-stroke). Hypertension. Diabetes mellitus. Hypercholesterolaemia. Cigarette smoking. Alcohol abuse.	Depends on aetiology of vascular cognitive impairment: Post-stroke dementia – cortical and subcortical dementia syndromes, depending on areas of brain affected. Multi-infarct dementia – stepwise deterioration in cognitive function. Strategic infarcts – abrupt onset of cognitive impairment and/or striking behavioural effects. Subcortical vascular cognitive impairment – executive dysfunction (impairment of volition, information processing, planning and purposive action) and gait apraxia.
Dementia with Lewy bodies (DLB)/Parkinson's disease dementia (PDD)	Often identified post-mortem. Lewy bodies: eosinophilic inclusion bodies, found in brainstem nuclei in PD, but also in cerebral cortex in DLB. Degeneration of cholinergic neurones and depletion of acetylcholine. AD type changes. Minor vascular disease in 1/3 cases		Significant functional disability secondary to motor dysfunction, neuropsychiatric symptoms and severity of cognitive impairment. PDD diagnosed when Parkinson's disease present for at least 1 year prior to onset of dementia. DLB diagnosed when dementia and Parkinsonian features occur simultaneously. Fluctuating cognition. Significant variation in attention/alertness. Florid visual hallucinations. Spontaneous Parkinsonian features. Severe neuroleptic sensitivity. REM sleep behaviour disorder.

Reprinted from *Companion to Psychiatric Studies*, Eighth Edition, Johnstone, E. et al. (eds.). Churchill Livingstone.

Specific vascular syndromes (with no AD overlap)[1]

- *CADASIL* (cerebral autosomal dominant arteriopathy with subcortical infarcts and leukoencephalopathy).
- *HCHWA-D* (hereditary cerebral haemorrhage with amyloidosis).
- *Familial British Dementia with amyloid angiopathy.*
- *HERNS* (hereditary endotheliopathy with retinopathy, nephropathy and stroke).
- *Fabry disease*: X-linked recessive lysosomal storage disorder (➲ see Chapter 16, Fabry disease, p. 581).
- *MELAS* (mitochondrial myopathy, encephalopathy, lactic acidosis and stroke-like episodes).

Other causes of dementia[2]

- Inherited:
  - Huntington's disease.
  - Wilsons' disease (hepatolenticular degeneration).
  - Leucodystrophies.
- Acquired:
  - Frontotemporal degeneration (including Pick's disease).
  - Progressive supranuclear palsy.
  - Corticobasal degeneration.
- Infective:
  - HIV-1 infection.
  - Prion dementias (including variant Creutzfeldt-Jakob disease).
  - Whipple's disease (infection with *Tropheryma whippelii*).
  - Subacute sclerosing panencephalitis (complication of childhood measles infection).
  - Herpes encephalitis.
- Inflammatory:
  - Multiple sclerosis.
  - SLE.
  - Cerebral vasculitis.
  - Hashimoto's encephalopathy.
- Neoplastic.
- Traumatic.
- Structural:
  - Hydrocephalus.
  - Subdural haematoma.
- Metabolic/endocrine:
  - Hypothyroidism.
- Deficiency:
  - Vitamin B deficiency.
- Substance-induced:
  - Alcohol (direct effect of alcohol also compounded by other factors, e.g. thiamine deficiency, head injury, hypoglycaemia).

Assessment

- Mini-mental state examination (MMSE):
  - Most commonly used screening scale.

[1] Reprinted from *Companion to Psychiatric Studies*, Eighth Edition, Johnstone, E. et al. (eds.). Churchill Livingstone.

[2] Reprinted from *Companion to Psychiatric Studies*, Eighth Edition, Johnstone, E. et al. (eds.). Churchill Livingstone.

- Assessing several cognitive domains.
- Brief and easily administered; total scoring out of 30.
- Montreal Cognitive Assessment (MoCA):
  - Administered in approximately 10 minutes, assessing several cognitive domains.
  - Total scoring out of 30.
  - Advantage over MMSE in assessing mild cognitive impairment/patients with vascular cognitive impairment/executive dysfunction.

Management

- Diagnosis via demonstration of progressive global cognitive impairment and impact on person's ability to function.
- Use of assessment tools (➲ see Assessment, p. 793).
- Physical examination focusing on vascular/neurological systems.
- Modifying vascular risk factors.
- Exclusion of differential diagnoses: blood tests to screen for reversible causes of memory loss (e.g. hypothyroidism, vitamin B_{12} deficiency).
- Brain imaging.
- Referral to neuropsychologist if unusual features.
- Pharmacological treatment:
  - Cholinesterase inhibitors (e.g donepezil, galantamine, rivastgmine):
    - Effective across severities in AD.
    - Improve cognitive and neuropsychiatric aspects of AD.
    - May be disease-modifying.
  - *N*-methyl-D-aspartate (NMDA) receptor antagonist (memantine):
    - For moderate-to-severe Alzheimer's disease.

Misuse of alcohol and other substances in relation to psychiatry

Definition

Misuse is defined in the ICD-10 as *mental and behavioural disorders caused by psychoactive substance use*, with coding depending on the substance involved[1]. Specific clinical conditions arising from the substance are represented as the following sub-codes:

0 Acute intoxication.
1 Harmful use (i.e. causing damage to physical and mental health).
2 Dependence syndrome.
3 Withdrawal state.
4 Withdrawal state with delirium (e.g. delirium tremens with alcohol).
5 Psychotic disorder.
6 Amnesic syndrome.
7 Residual and late onset psychotic disorder.
8 Other mental and behavioural disorders.
9 Unspecified mental and behavioural disorder.

Dependence is diagnosed if *three or more* indications apply:

- Compulsion to take/difficulty in controlling substance use.
- Characteristic physiological withdrawal state on reduction/cessation.
- Substance use to prevent withdrawal state.

[1] Reprinted from The ICD-10 Classification of Mental and Behavioural Disorders: Clinical descriptions and diagnostic guidelines.

Table 22.8 Alcohol dependence – psychiatric and medical complications

Associated disorders	Clinical consequences
Organic disorders	Blackouts. Delirium tremens (➲ see Ethanol, p. 640.). Withdrawal seizures. Wernicke's encephalopathy. Korsakoff's syndrome. Alcohol-induced dementia.
Psychosis	Alcoholic hallucinosis – rare, caused by chronic alcohol intake producing auditory hallucinations in clear consciousness.
Mood disorders	Chronic alcohol abuse causes severe transient depressive symptoms. Suicide rate in alcoholics is 50% higher than in normal population.
Neurotic disorder	May predispose to alcohol abuse as alcohol may be used to relieve symptoms of anxiety.
Pathological jealousy	Associated with alcoholism although may also be caused by other conditions, e.g. schizophrenia.
Personality disorder	Excessive drinking may be employed to ameliorate interpersonal difficulties. Particular association to dissocial PD. May be underlying genetic predisposition, particularly in those whose biological fathers were alcoholics.

- Increased dose required to achieve previous effect (tolerance).
- Narrowing of activities to focus on substance use.
- Persistent use despite harmful sequelae.

NB. 'Withdrawal' refers to symptoms emerging on reduction or cessation of substances and includes alcohol-related delirium tremens. Characteristic symptoms/signs are delirium, hallucinations, delusions, agitation, autonomic over-activity and seizures.

For psychiatric and medical complications of alcohol dependence, see Table 22.8.

Mental Capacity Act and Mental Health Act

The *Mental Capacity Act 2005* formalises the best practice of 'common law'. It is a legal framework that acts to protect people who have impaired or absent ability to make decisions, e.g. in the context of medical treatment. For consent or refusal to be valid, a patient must:

- Be provided with enough information.
- Act voluntarily.
- Have 'capacity' to take that decision.

Capacity assessment

Five principles guide assessment:

1. Adults are assumed to have capacity unless shown otherwise.
2. All practical steps must be taken to help an individual make a decision.
3. A person is not to be treated as unable to make a decision merely because they make an unwise decision.
4. An act done or decision made on behalf of a patient who lacks capacity must be done in their 'best interests'.
5. … and in the least restrictive way.

An assessment of capacity must be carried out whenever there is concern that a person's decision-making ability may be compromised, because:

- Person's behaviour has raised suspicion of incapacity.
- Someone who knows the patient has raised concerns.
- Patient has been diagnosed with impairment of mind or brain.
- There has already been an established lack of capacity with respect to other decisions.

If the person has an impairment or disturbance of mind or brain, an assessment of their capacity needs to be carried out to determine if they can:

- understand;
- retain;
- weigh up the information; and
- communicate the decision.

NB. Capacity is not 'all or nothing' and is not a test of reasonableness. A person is not to be treated as unable to make a decision merely because they make an unwise decision. People are entitled to make their own decisions based upon their own value systems. The fact that a person has a mental illness does not automatically mean they lack capacity to make a decision about medical treatment. The person's best interests are:

- not strictly defined;
- broader than just medical considerations; and
- dependent upon the individual and their circumstances: physical, psychological, social and spiritual.

The *Mental Health Act (MHA, 1983, revised 2007)* is the current legal framework within which mental health services in England, Wales and Northern Ireland provide care and treatment of mentally ill patients. It makes provision for a wide range of circumstances. In particular, it stipulates (via particular, numbered 'Sections' of the Act) when admission to hospital and/or treatment can be carried out against the patient's will. This is enacted where the mental disorder is of a nature or degree that warrants action to be taken by relevant health care or social services professionals to: safeguard the patient's health (or life) and/or protect others from the patient's aggression/dangerous behaviour, emanating from their mental disorder. The Act makes provision for patients who have committed crimes on account of their disorder of mind, taking into account the appropriate institutional location of such 'offender patients', i.e. whether in prison or in a secure treatment unit. Provision also exists for the challenging of such compulsory detention or treatment by patient or family and for regular review for the use of compulsion at all.

NB. Under the MHA, physical illness is exempt, unless the treatment of the physical illness will improve the symptoms of the mental illness, e.g. delirium/acute toxic confusional state. (In these situations there is the option of using the MCA or MHA and which one is used will be judged on a case-by-case basis.)

For commonly used 'sections' of the MHA, see Table 22.9.

Table 22.9 Commonly used 'sections' of the MHA

'Section'	Purpose	Legal criteria	Length	Other comments
2	To allow compulsory admission/detention of someone with mental disorder.	Person is suffering from a mental disorder of a nature and degree warranting detention in hospital for assessment *and* Detention is in the interests of the person's health and safety or with view to the protection of others.	28 days. Cannot be renewed. If further detention required, application should be made for section 3.	This section is intended for diagnostic assessment; medical treatment requires the patient's consent. Persons detained have a right of appeal to both Mental Health Tribunal and to the hospital managers.
3	To allow compulsory admission/detention of someone with mental disorder. Persons detained may already have been detained under Section 2, 4, 5(2) or 5(4).	Person is suffering from a mental disorder of a nature and degree warranting detention in hospital for assessment *and* Detention is in the interests of the person's health and safety or with view to the protection of others *and* Such treatment cannot be provided to them unless they are detained under this section *and* Appropriate medical treatment is available to them.	6 months. Can be renewed if legal criteria still met, and that treatment cannot be provided, unless the person continues to be detained.	Treatment of the person's mental disorder is permitted, with or without consent for the first 3 months of detention. This covers administration of medication, but more stringent safeguards apply when the proposed intervention is electroconvulsive therapy (ECT).
5(2)	An in-patient decides they no longer want to be assessed/receive treatment or wishes to leave hospital and may need to be assessed under S2 or S3 as above. S5(2) allows a doctor to 'hold' the patient for up to 72 hours to enable S2/S3 assessments to take place.	The view of a doctor that an application ought to be made for the admission of the patient to hospital. The patient must be an inpatient – S5(2) cannot be used in an A&E department.	72 hours	Any compulsory treatment during the 72 hours duration would need to have justification in 'common law' or under the Mental Capacity Act, or with the patient's consent. Possible outcomes: • conversion to S2/S3; • the responsible clinician decides to 'end' the detention; • the person, following assessment by two doctors, is deemed not detainable under S2 or S3.

Multiple choice questions

Questions

1. In personality disorder:
   A. Psychotropic medication is the mainstay of treatment.
   B. Psychological and pharmacological treatments cannot be safely combined.
   C. Multi-professional involvement must be avoided.
   D. Crisis interventions usually suffices.
   E. Clinical recovery is achieved in 50% of cases.
2. Bipolar disorder:
   A. Shows 25% concordance in MZ twin pairs.
   B. May be precipitated by antidepressant medication.
   C. Usually requires in-patient treatment under the Mental Health Act.
   D. Does not respond to ECT.
   E. Tends to show an unremitting course.
3. In paranoid schizophrenia:
   A. Thought disorder predominates.
   B. Motor disturbance is characteristic.
   C. Negative symptoms are prominent.
   D. Remission is unlikely.
   E. Hallucinations are common.
4. In dementia:
   A. Prevalence is not age related.
   B. Alzheimer's disease accounts for 90% of cases.
   C. Post-mortem findings are necessary to make the diagnosis.
   D. Anti-antipsychotics may worsen mental impairment.
   E. Anti-cholinesterase inhibiting drugs have no place in treatment.
5. Dependence on alcohol is characterised by:
   A. Consumption above Government-recommended daily intakes.
   B. Conviction for drink-related driving offences.
   C. The presence of pathological jealousy.
   D. Physical illness associated with high alcohol consumption.
   E. Narrowing of social activities to focus on alcohol consumption.

Answers

1. E. Therapeutic pessimism is misplaced, since 50% make a clinical recovery; successful suicide rate is, however, high in those who do not (➲ see Personality disorder, p. 786).
2. B. As SSRI and tricyclic medication may trigger mania, mood-stabilising drugs should be considered (➲ see Affective disorders, p. 787 and Table 22.5).
3. E. Hallucinations are usually very prominent in acute phases, but psychosocial functioning may be intact between relapses (➲ see Table 22.6).
4. D. Antipsychotic medication can worsen mental impairment and increase risk of cerebrovascular disease, with no hard evidence of long-term benefit (➲ see Dementias, p. 791 and Table 22.7).
5. E. Evidence for any narrowing of activities should be sought, via enquiry into daily routine, since it is an important marker of severity of dependence (➲ see Misuse of alcohol and other substances in relation to psychiatry, p. 794 and Table 22.8).

Chapter 23 **Obstetric Medicine**

Dev Kevat and Lucy Mackillop

Introduction

Numerous major physiological changes occur during a normal pregnancy. These are summarised in Table 23.1.

Obstetric medicine takes into consideration the well-being of both the mother and the fetus. While maternal health should not be compromised, for each management decision the risks and benefits to both mother and fetus must be explained to the mother. The risk to the fetus is frequently dependent on the gestational stage. Pharmacological risks (including teratogenic risks) in pregnancy are discussed in ➲ Chapter 3, Pregnancy, p. 76. The dose of established medications may need to be reviewed during pregnancy (e.g. a 25–50% higher dose of levothyroxine). A multidisciplinary approach involving the obstetric, neonatal and other specialists, e.g. anaesthetists is often required.

Gestational diabetes

Gestational diabetes (GDM) occurs in approximately 8% of all pregnancies. Incidence of GDM is rising due to increasing BMI and maternal age among women of childbearing age.

Women with pre-existing Type 1 and Type 2 diabetes mellitus (DM) should have pre-conception assessment and counselling, and require regular specialist review throughout pregnancy, to adjust medication, and monitor for renal, ophthalmic and other complications.

Patients with pre-existing Type 1 DM often require less insulin in the first trimester, and higher doses thereafter. Patients with pre-existing Type 2 DM commonly need increasing doses of hypoglycaemics as pregnancy progresses.

Pathophysiology

The pathogenesis of GDM is not yet fully understood, one theory suggests development of GDM follows an antigenic insult from the fetus. Insulin requirements in late pregnancy are approximately 3-fold that prior to pregnancy. Women with GDM have insufficient pancreatic β-cell function to meet these demands

Table 23.1 Physiological changes during pregnancy

System	Physiological changes
Cardiovascular	• 25–45% increase in cardiac output through increased heart rate (+10 to 20 beats/minute) and stroke volume. • Peripheral vasodilation. • Decrease in systolic and diastolic BP in first and second trimester, with increase towards pre-pregnancy baseline in the third trimester.
Respiratory	• 20% increase in oxygen consumption. • Compensated respiratory alkalosis. • No change to respiratory rate.
Haematological	• 50% increase in plasma volume over pregnancy causing a dilutional anaemia. • ↑ Red cell mass (which frequently requires iron and folate supplementation). • Rise in MCV for aforementioned causes. • A tendency to a prothrombotic state with: ◆ ↓ in free protein S levels; ◆ ↑ Factor VII, Factor VIII, Factor X, Von Willebrand Factor, fibrinogen and plasminogen activator inhibitor Type 1 (PAI-1).
Renal	• 50% increase in renal blood flow and glomerular filtration rate. • Bladder smooth muscle relaxes; increasing capacity.
Immunological	• Shift away from cell-mediated immunity (Th1 response) to humoral immunity (Th2 response).
Endocrine and Metabolic	• Increase in oestrogen, progesterone, cortisol and prolactin levels. • Decrease in LH and FSH. • Increase in thyroid-binding globulin levels. • Increase in basal metabolic rate (BMR) throughout pregnancy of 15%.
Gastrointestinal	• Increased gut transit time. • Progesterone causes relaxation of lower oesophageal sphincter – may result in GORD.
Dermatological	• Development of stria gravidarum ('stretch marks'). • Hyperpigmentation of abdominal midline/linea nigra, nipples and/or face (melasma/chloasma faciei).

Data from: Bentur Y. Ionizing and nonionizing radiation in pregnancy. In: *Maternal-fetal toxicology*, Second Edition, Koren G (Ed), Marcel Dekker, New York, 1994, p.515; and Guidelines on diagnosis and management of acute pulmonary embolism. Task Force on Pulmonary Embolism, European Society of Cardiology. *European Heart Journal*, 2000; 21:1301.

and are unable to maintain normal blood glucose ranges. In addition, the placental hormones, oestrogen, human placental lactogen and cortisol, predispose to insulin resistance.

GDM is associated with an increased risk of significant complications to mother and baby, largely due to the effects of macrosomnia. These risks may be ameliorated by tight glycaemic control.

Risk factors for gestational diabetes

- Non-white ethnicity.
- A family history of GDM.
- Conditions associated with insulin resistance, such as polycystic ovary syndrome.

Diagnosis

A diagnosis of GDM can be made following a 75-g oral glucose tolerance test performed for at-risk mothers between 24 and 28 weeks.

Mothers suspected to have previous GDM (e.g. with a history of a large baby [>90th centile or 4.5 kg]), as well as those previously diagnosed with GDM, should be advised to self-monitor glucose levels and undergo an additional OGTT early in their pregnancy.

For NICE guidelines for diagnosis of GDM by OGTT, see Table 23.2.

Table 23.2 NICE guidelines for diagnosis of GDM by OGTT

GDM diagnosis (75 g OGTT)	
Fasting	≥5.6 mmol/L
2 hour	≥7.8 mmol/L
Treatment targets	
Fasting	5.3 mmol/L
1 hour post-prandial	7.8 mmol/L
2 hour post-prandial	6.4 mmol/L

Treatment

GDM may be diet controlled, or may require treatment with metformin or insulin therapy. Obstetric units may use a treatment classification to guide decisions regarding the management of a pregnancy (e.g. induction of delivery) as the risk of neonatal complications is higher among women requiring insulin therapy.

Complications

Fetal complications of GDM include:

- Macrosomia.
- Shoulder dystocia.
- Post-partum hypoglycaemia.
- Hyperbilirubinaemia.
- Respiratory distress syndrome with the need for special/intensive care.
- Stillbirth: although rare occurs at an increased rate, the need for induction should be balanced against risks of prematurity.
- History of maternal GDM confers an increased risk of DM in later life.

Maternal complications of GDM include an increased risk of:

- Hypertensive disorders of pregnancy.
- Planned or emergency caesarean section, and instrumental delivery.
- Port-partum haemorrhage.
- Type 2 DM with an absolute 10-year risk of 20–40%.

Management

Lifestyle modification

- Dietary advice: foods of a lower glycaemic index (complex, rather than processed, and simple carbohydrates, vegetables and lean proteins), portion control, smaller meals more frequently.
- Regular moderate activity.

Medical therapies

- Metformin may be used in the second and third trimesters of pregnancy with no increased risk of adverse perinatal outcomes.

- Insulin is the main form of medical therapy; weekly or fortnightly dose titration is used to achieve target blood glucose levels. The major risk of insulin therapy is hypoglycaemia and patients should be counselled appropriately.

Antenatal and post-partum care

- Women with GDM require fetal scanning to monitor growth and well-being. If spontaneous delivery does not occur, delivery is frequently induced between 38 and 41 weeks, depending on maternal and fetal factors.
- Insulin therapy should cease after delivery of the placenta with blood sugar level monitoring continued for at least 24 hours.
- An OGTT or fasting blood glucose should be performed at 6 weeks post-partum and patients counselled about the risk of developing GDM in future pregnancies and Type 2 DM long term.

Obstetric cholestasis

Pathogenesis

Obstetric cholestasis (OC) is multifactorial in pathogenesis with genetic, hormonal and environmental influences. There is a wide ethnic variation in the incidence of OC. Approximately 10% of cases of OC are associated with mutations in the gene encoding multidrug-resistant protein 3 (MDRP3). This affects the function of a phospholipid transporter within the hepatocyte membrane, resulting in elevated bile acid levels and an increased sensitivity to oestrogen. Oestrogen concentrations are greatly increased during pregnancy and this may inhibit the export of the bile salts from hepatocytes.

Clinical features

- Pruritus; onset is commonly in the third trimester and worse at night. Pruritus usually affects palms and soles, but may also be generalised.
- Constitutional symptoms of cholestasis, such as anorexia and malaise.
- Less commonly reported features include abdominal pain, steatorrhoea, pale stools and dark urine.

Diagnosis

A diagnosis of OC is made in patients with pruritus with no alternative identifiable cause, in association with raised bile acids (a key finding) and abnormal LFTs (commonly elevated transaminases and gamma-glutamyl transferase), which resolve post-partum.

It is essential that other causes of abnormal LFTs or elevated bile acids are excluded (➔ see Chapter 15, Abnormal liver function tests, p. 523 and Tables 15.3 and 15.4).

Severe OC disease (bile acids > 40 mmol/L) is associated with an increased risk of fetal complications. Progressive elevation of LFTs, bile acids or development of a coagulopathy may prompt intervention (e.g. delivery). Of note, severity of symptoms (e.g. pruritus) is independent of the degree of elevation of LFTs or bile acids.

Complications

- Fetal distress and stillbirth.
- Premature delivery.
- Meconium passage during delivery.
- Post-partum haemorrhage.

Management

- Close monitoring of LFTs and bile acids (weekly basis).
- Topical treatments for symptomatic relief of pruritus (e.g. calamine lotion and aqueous cream with menthol).
- Oral ursodeoxycholic acid can reduce pruritus.

- Oral Vitamin K may be indicated, particularly when the prothrombin time is elevated (biliary obstruction may ↓ absorption of fat soluble vitamins).
- Rifampicin can be used in combination with ursodeoxycholic acid for patients with severe OC. Its mechanism is by enhancing bile acid detoxification.

Early delivery is dependent on gestation and disease severity, if possible, with symptomatic management until 37 weeks gestation.

Further reading

1. Williamson C, Geenes V. Intrahepatic cholestasis of pregnancy. *Obstet Gynecol*. 2014; 124(1):120–33.
2. Obstructive Cholestasis (Green Top Guideline No 43.) RCOG 2011. https://www.rcog.org.uk/en/guidelines-research-services/guidelines/gtg43/.

Acute fatty liver of pregnancy

Acute fatty liver of pregnancy (AFLP) is a rare, but life-threatening, condition with an incidence of 1 in 7 000–19,000 pregnancies.

Pathogenesis

The pathogenesis of AFLP is unknown, although there is an association with an inherited deficiency of a mitochondrial enzyme that catalyses a reaction in the β-oxidation of fatty acids: long chain 3-hydroxyacetyl coenzyme-A dehydrogenase (LCHAD).

Clinical features and diagnostic criteria

A diagnosis of AFLP is based on the Swansea criteria (see Table 23.3) (1):

Table 23.3 Swansea criteria

Diagnosis of AFLP requires ≥6 of the following in the absence of another explanation		
Clinical		Vomiting
		Abdominal pain
		Polydipsia/polyuria
		Encephalopathy
Biochemical	Hepatic	High bilirubin (>14 μmol/L)
		High AST/ALT (>42 IU/L)
		High ammonia (>47 μmol/L)
	Renal	High uric acid (>340 μmol/L)
		Renal impairment (creatinine >150 μmol/L)
	Endocrine	Hypoglycaemia (<4 mmol/L)
	Haematological	Leucocytosis (>11 × 10^6/L)
		Coagulopathy (PT >14 s or APTT >34 s)
Radiological	Abdominal US	Ascites or bright liver echo
Histological	Liver biopsy	Microvesicular steatosis

Adapted by permission from BMJ Publishing Group Limited. *Gut*, Ch'ng, C. L. et al., Prospective study of liver dysfunction in pregnancy in Southwest Wales, 51, pp. 876–880. Copyright © 2002 BMJ Publishing Group Ltd and the British Society of Gastroenterology. http://dx.doi.org/10.1136/gut.51.6.876.

Hypoglycaemia is caused by impaired hepatic glycogenolysis and portends a poor prognosis. Diabetes insipidus occurs rarely.

Investigations

- Liver biopsy is not usually indicated, since it has a high risk of fulminating coagulopathy. Furthermore, histological confirmation may not influence management since the approach for other potential diagnoses (e.g. HELLP syndrome) remains the same (e.g. supportive care and expeditive delivery).
- Imaging may reveal microvesicular fatty infiltration or evidence of bleeding (e.g. subcapsular haematoma).

Complications

Maternal complications

- Disseminated intravascular coagulation.
- Pancreatitis.
- Acute kidney injury.
- Encephalopathy.
- Wound seroma.
- Death (7%).

Fetal complications

- Increased mortality (10–15%) often through asphyxia.
- Intrauterine growth restriction (IUGR).
- Complications of prematurity.
- LCHAD deficiency.

Management

Management centres around supportive care by an MDT and expedited delivery. Maternal stabilisation should be achieved prior to delivery and may involve:

- Correction of coagulation abnormalities.
- Correction of electrolyte disturbance.
- Treatment of hypoglycaemia.
- Careful management of fluid status.

After delivery, clinicians should be vigilant for the development of haemorrhagic pancreatitis or pseudocysts. In practice, liver transplantation is rarely performed for AFLP, although input from a transplant hepatologist may be required in patients with progressive liver failure.

References

1. Ko HH, Yoshida E. Acute fatty liver of pregnancy. *Canad J Gastroenterol*. 2006; 20(1):25–30.

Peri-partum cardiomyopathy

Peri-partum cardiomyopathy (PPCM) is a rare disorder thought to affect less than 1 in 2000 births in European countries. It is a form of dilated cardiomyopathy defined as:

> An idiopathic cardiomyopathy presenting with heart failure secondary to left ventricular systolic dysfunction, toward the end of pregnancy (e.g. after 36 weeks) or in the months following delivery (e.g. within 5 months) with echocardiogram showing left ventricular ejection fraction <45%, fractional shortening <30%, left ventricular end-diastolic dimension >2.7 cm/m^2 for which no other cause of heart failure is found. (1)

Pathogenesis

The pathogenesis of PPCM is poorly understood with various theories in existence:

- Viral myocarditis seen on endomyocardial biopsy of women with PPCM suggests an abnormal immune response to the small number of fetal cells in the maternal circulation. 'Loss of tolerance' to these cells around the time of delivery may account for the timing of onset of PPCM.
- Significantly increased concentrations of TNF-α (inflammatory cytokine) and Fas/Apo-1 (marker of programmed cell death) have been found in the plasma of women with PPCM, which may play a role.
- Mouse model studies have suggested an increase in prolactin levels is a factor contributing to the development of PPCM.

Clinical features

Typical features and clinical signs of heart failure (see Tables 13.37 and 13.38).

Differential diagnosis

- Myocardial infarction.
- Pulmonary embolism.
- Valvular heart disease.
- Pre-eclampsia.
- Infiltrative diseases.

There is no widely agreed grading system for PPCM, but left ventricular ejection fraction on echocardiogram is generally considered key to assessing severity. This value at presentation also predicts recovery of cardiac function to baseline.

Complications

- Dilated cardiomyopathy.
- Arrhythmias.
- Hypotension.
- Altered mental status.
- Syncope.
- Mural thrombi, which can precipitate systemic and pulmonary emboli.
- Death (mortality 5–32%).

Management

- Requires a highly skilled MDT approach, including obstetric physicians, cardiologists, obstetricians, neonatalogists, specialist nurses and midwives.
- Pharmacological therapy includes vasodilators (e.g. hydralazine) and β-blockers (e.g. metoprolol and carvedilol). Thiazide diuretics (e.g. hydrochlorothiazide) should be used with caution as large fluid shifts may ensue resulting in clinical deterioration. The addition of digoxin can be of value, particularly in women with a greatly diminished ejection fraction. In the post-partum period women may benefit from ACE-i, angiotensin receptor blocker and loop diuretics.
- Anticoagulation with warfarin or low molecular weight heparin should be considered in all women with PPCM to reduce the risk of mural thrombus formation and embolic phenomena.
- Close fetal monitoring is required in all pregnant women, and early or emergency delivery may be required. In the event of irreversible clinical deterioration despite medical therapy, cardiac transplantation may be indicated.

Emerging therapies

Bromocriptine appears to reduce the degree of cardiac dysfunction in patients with PPCM, since a cleaved protein fragment derived from prolactin may be involved in the pathogenesis of PPCM. This benefit is presumably achieved by reducing prolactin levels.

Future pregnancies

PPCM is not an absolute contraindication to future pregnancy, although women who do not recover left ventricular function are advised against further pregnancies due to the high risk of further decompensation and even death in subsequent pregnancy.

References

1. Elkayam U. Clinical characteristics of peripartum cardiomyopathy in the United States: diagnosis, prognosis, and management. *J Am Coll Cardiol.* 2011; 58(7):659–70.

Further reading

1. Nanda S, Nelson-Piercy C, Mackillop L. Cardiac disease in pregnancy. *Clin Med.* 2012; 12(6):553–60.

Hyperemesis gravidarum

Hyperemesis gravidarum (HG) affects between 0.3 and 2% of pregnancies and is characterised by severe and intractable vomiting with onset in the first trimester. It is distinguished from the more common nausea and vomiting of pregnancy (NVP) or 'morning sickness' by its severity (significant electrolyte disturbance and weight loss > 5%).

Pathophysiology

- Higher levels of serum human chorionic gonadotrophin are found in women with HG. HCG may have a stimulatory effect on the secretory processes of the GI tract, or may mimic the effect of TSH acting on the TSH receptor. This action can lead to biochemical hyperthyroidism with suppression of TSH production via negative feedback (➲ see Chapter 19, Thyrotoxicosis, p. 679 and Box 19.1). This effect can be addressed by treating the HG, rather than using anti-thyroid medication.
- *Helicobacter pylori* infection has been implicated as a causative factor for HG with higher rates of infection seen in affected women.
- Oestradiol levels may a play in role in the development of HG with higher levels adversely affecting gastric emptying and GI motility.

Clinical features

- Frequent or intractable vomiting.
- Nausea.
- Hypersensitivity to smells especially of food.
- Hyper-salivation and spitting.
- Anorexia.
- Fatigue and lethargy.

Diagnosis

HG is a diagnosis of exclusion. GI (e.g. peptic ulcer disease, gastritis, small bowel obstruction), endocrine/metabolic (e.g. hyperthyroidism, hyperkalaemia, Addison's disease), infective causes, drug-related causes and other explanations for symptoms should be considered.

For an investigative approach to hyperemesis gravidarum, see Table 23.4.

Clinical features of severe disease

- Degree of dehydration.
- Inability to maintain oral fluid intake.
- Malnutrition, lack of weight gain or weight loss.

Table 23.4 Investigative approach to hyperemesis gravidarum

Investigation	Purpose
Venous or arterial blood gas	Assess for a metabolic alkalosis.
Electrolytes	Exclude hypokalaemia, hyponatremia.
Renal function	Exclude acute renal impairment.
Albumin	Assess nutritional status.
Calcium	Exclude hypercalcaemia as an alternative cause, which may suggest hyperparathyroidism.
Full blood count	Exclude anaemia, infection.
Glucose	Exclude hyperglycaemia or a new diagnosis of diabetes.
Thyroid function tests	Exclude hyperthyroidism.
Urine dipstick and culture	Assess for ketonuria, infection.
Helicobacter pylori antibody or breath testing	Exclude *H. pylori* infection.
Transvaginal/abdominal US	Recognised association between HG and molar and multiple pregnancies.

Complications of hyperemesis gravidarum

HG causes significant morbidity in pregnant women. In the UK, deaths from HG have resulted from hypokalaemia, aspiration pneumonia and the rare complication of Wernicke's encephalopathy.

Maternal complications

Gastrointestinal

- Vitamin deficiencies (e.g. B1, B6 and B12).
- Malnutrition.
- Mallory–Weiss tears.
- Oesophageal rupture.
- Aspiration pneumonia.

Psychological/psychiatric

- Depression.
- Anxiety.
- Insomnia.

Neurological

- Wernicke's encephalopathy.
- Central pontine demyelination on correction of hyponatremia.
- Peripheral neuropathy due to vitamin deficiencies.

Haematological

- Thrombosis due to dehydration.
- Anaemia.

Fetal complications

Fetal complications occur more commonly if maternal weight gain during pregnancy is <7 kg. These complications include:

- IUGR.
- Small for gestational age at birth.
- Premature birth (<37 weeks).
- Low APGAR at birth.

HG is associated with increased rates of induction of birth and caesarean section.

Management

General measures

- Rehydration with intravenous fluid therapy.
- Correction of electrolyte abnormalities.
- Vitamin supplementation including thiamine and multivitamins.
- Nutritional intake may be improved by eating smaller meals and avoiding fatty and spicy foods.
- Anti-emetic medications and therapies.
- Psychosocial support.

Medical therapies

The relevant risks of anti-emetics prior to prescribing should be discussed. A combination of therapies is often needed. The following have demonstrated clinical efficacy:

- ginger (*Zingiber officinale*);
- metoclopramide;
- promethazine;
- pyridoxine (B6);
- droperidol and diphenhydramine;
- ondansetron;
- corticosteroids.

Considerations in severe hyperemesis gravidarum

- Enteral feeding or total parenteral nutrition may be indicated.
- Early delivery particularly if fetal growth is reduced or symptoms severe.
- Termination of pregnancy (at an appropriate gestation) in women with severe and intractable HG, which is not responding to treatment.

Further reading

1. Ismail S, Kenny L. Review on hyperemesis gravidarum. *Best Pract Res Clin Gastroenterol*. 2007; 21(5):755–69.

Gestational hypertension

Gestational hypertension (GH) or pregnancy-induced hypertension (PIH) affects 8–10% of all pregnancies.

Pathophysiology

Abnormal cytotrophoblast invasion of spiral arterioles leads to reduced placental perfusion, resulting in widespread endothelial dysfunction with decreased production of nitric oxide and prostacyclin, which have a relaxing effect on endothelium. In contrast, endothelin and thromboxane levels are increased.

The physiological increase in cardiac and renal output in a normal pregnancy is balanced by a decrease in vascular sensitivity to angiotensin II, thereby maintaining BP at normotensive levels. Women with GH are thought to have enhanced responsiveness to angiotensin II with consequent hypertension.

Risk factors

- Previous history of essential hypertension, pre-eclampsia or GH.
- Diabetes (Type 1, Type 2, gestational).
- Obesity (BMI >35 kg/m^2).
- Pre-existing underlying renal or vascular disease.
- Multifetal pregnancy.
- Age >40 years or pregnancy interval >10 years.

Clinical features

- Women may be asymptomatic.
- Headache.
- Visual disturbance.

All women with GH should be assessed for other signs and symptoms suggestive of pre-eclampsia.

Diagnosis

GH is defined as an elevated BP (>140/90 mmHg on two occasions at least 4 hours apart) after 20 weeks gestation. By definition, the BP of women with PIH returns to normal levels post-partum.

GH should be distinguished from pre-existing or chronic hypertension.

Disease classification

Current NICE guidelines describe two categories of GH[1]:

- Hypertension: diastolic blood pressure >109 mmHg, systolic blood pressure 140–159 mmHg.
- Severe hypertension: diastolic blood pressure ≥ 110 mmHg, systolic blood pressure ≥ 160 mmHg.

Complications

Major fetal complications of GH:

- IUGR.
- Pre-term delivery.

Major maternal complications of GH:

- Renal dysfunction.
- Placental abruption.
- Haemorrhagic stroke and/or hypertensive encephalopathy (rare).

Approximately 25% of women with GH develop pre-eclampsia. A history of PIH increases the long-term risk of developing essential hypertension and cardiovascular disease.

[1] Adapted from © NICE (2019) CG133 Hypertension in pregnancy: the management of hypertensive disorders during pregnancy. Available from https://www.nice.org.uk/guidance/cg133. All rights reserved. Subject to Notice of rights NICE guidance is prepared for the National Health Service in England. All NICE guidance is subject to regular review and may be updated or withdrawn. NICE accepts no responsibility for the use of its content in this product/publication.

Management

Surveillance

- Close monitoring of BP, initiating treatment when indicated to reduce the risk of hypertensive crisis in the mother.
- Monitoring growth and well-being of the fetus.
- Assessing symptoms and diagnosing complications, e.g. pre-eclampsia.

For management of gestational hypertension, see Table 23.5.

Table 23.5 Management of gestational hypertension

	GH	Severe GH
Admit	Do not routinely admit.	Yes.
Treat with medication	Yes, if BP remains above 140/90 mmHg. Oral labetalol first-line agent. Target: 135/85mmHg.	Yes, oral labetalol first-line agent. Target: diastolic 80–100 mmHg, systolic <150 mmHg.
Frequency of monitoring	Once or twice a week until BP <135/85 mmHg.	Every 15–30 min until BP is <160/110 mmHg.
Test for proteinuria	At each visit using reagent strip reading device or urinary protein:creatinine ratio.	Daily using reagent strip or reading device or urinary protein:creatinine ratio.
Blood tests	Measure FBC, LFT and renal function at presentation and then weekly. PlGF testing once if there is a suspicion for PET.	Measure FBC, LFT and renal function at presentation and then weekly. PlGF testing once if there is a suspicion for PET.
Fetal assessment	Offer fetal heart auscultation at every antenatal appointment. Carry out US of the fetus at diagnosis and, if normal, repeat every 2–4 weeks, if clinically indicated. Carry out a CTG only if clinically indicated.	Offer fetal heart auscultation at every antenatal appointment. Carry out US of the fetus at diagnosis and, if normal, repeat every 2 weeks, if severe hypertension persists. Carry out a CTG at diagnosis and then only if clinically indicated.

CTG, cardiotocography; PET, pre-eclamptic toxaemia; PlGF, placental growth factor.
Adapted from

Treatment

- Anti-hypertensive agents include labetalol, nifedipine or methyldopa.
- Uncontrolled hypertension is an indication for delivery. Corticosteroids (e.g. betamethasone) should be given prior to delivery to promote fetal lung maturation.
- After delivery, BP should be monitored and treatment adjusted. Women who require anti-hypertensive medication at postnatal review (6–8 weeks) should be referred to a medical specialist for a hypertension review.
- Low dose aspirin (an oral dose of 75 mg) is given to women in subsequent pregnancies to reduce the risk of PIH and pre-eclampsia.

Pre-eclampsia and eclampsia

Pathogenesis

Immune maladaptation is implicated in the beginnings of pre-eclamptic toxaemia (PET) with a type 2 immune reaction to paternal antigens in sperm. Subsequently, abnormal integration of cytotrophoblasts into the spiral artery walls of the placental bed causes endothelial dysfunction, driving hypertension later in pregnancy. Pathogenesis involves a complex cascade of immune and vascular factors, which may explain the range of organs that can be affected.

Clinical features

Women with PET can have minimal symptomology or may present with ≥1 of the following features:

- Headache.
- Visual disturbance, e.g. blurring or flashing before the eyes.
- Oedema of legs, feet, hands or face.
- Nausea and vomiting.
- Abdominal pain (usually subcostal).
- Clinical findings may include hypertension, papilloedema and clonus ≥3 beats.

Diagnosis

Historically a diagnosis of PET has been based on findings of:

- New-onset hypertension (>140 mmHg systolic and/or >90 mmHg diastolic) after 20 weeks gestation together with
- significant proteinuria (>0.3 g protein in a 24-hour urine collection, or >30 mg/mmol on a spot urinary protein:creatinine ratio).

In recent years, the International Society for the Study of Hypertension in Pregnancy have recommended that a diagnosis of PET can also be made if a pregnant woman has new onset hypertension after 20 weeks gestation with any of the following findings:

- Doubling of creatinine levels, or creatinine >90 μmol/L.
- Neurological complications (e.g. severe headache, hyperreflexia).
- Liver involvement (raised transaminases [≥twice the upper limit of normal] ± abdominal pain).
- Haematological complications (DIC, haemolysis, thrombocytopenia).
- Fetal growth restriction.

Women with PIH are at risk of progressing to pre-eclampsia warranting increased maternal and fetal surveillance. Eclampsia is defined as grand mal seizure in a woman with PET and may be the first presentation of PET.

Poor prognostic indicators

- Diagnosis of PET at <34 weeks gestation.
- Severe hypertension – systolic BP >160mmHg and/or diastolic >110 mmHg.
- Proteinuria >5 g over a 24-hour urine collection.
- Progressive renal impairment or oliguria (urine output <500 mL/24 hours).
- Any of the features of HELLP syndrome (➲ see HELLP syndrome, p. 813).
- Cerebral or visual symptoms.
- Pulmonary oedema or cyanosis.

Complications of PET

Maternal complications

- Seizures (eclampsia).
- Haemorrhagic or thrombotic stroke.
- Pulmonary oedema.
- Pulmonary embolus.
- Deep vein thrombosis.
- Renal failure.
- Liver failure.
- Retinal injury.
- Placental abruption.
- Bleeding due to DIC or thrombocytopenia.

Fetal complications

- IUGR.
- Pre-term delivery.
- Neonatal respiratory distress syndrome.
- Intrauterine death/stillbirth.

Management

- Specialist-led care is recommended due to the high morbidity and mortality, with close monitoring as patients with PET may deteriorate rapidly. Specific management is required for the range of presentations.
- The fetus requires increased surveillance with frequent cardiotocography, US and clinical assessment.
- It is delivery of the placenta, rather than any medical therapy that will lead to resolution of PET. For management of hypertension in women with PET, see Table 23.6.

Table 23.6 Management of hypertension in women with PET*

	Mild hypertension	**Moderate or severe hypertension**
Frequency of BP monitoring	Four times a day.	Four times a day.
Medical management and blood tests	Test kidney function, electrolytes, FBC, transaminases, bilirubin twice a week.	Treat with first-line oral labetalol to maintain BP <150/80–100 mmHg. Test kidney function, electrolytes, FBC, transaminases, bilirubin 3 times a week.

* ➲ For further details of second line therapies see Management of gestational hypertension, p. 810 and Table 23.5.
Adapted from © NICE (2019) CG133 Hypertension in pregnancy: the management of hypertensive disorders during pregnancy. Available from https://www.nice.org.uk/guidance/cg133.

- Thromboprophylaxis should be commenced with a low threshold due to the significant thrombotic risk.
- Strict fluid balance monitoring is required due to the risks of renal failure, volume overload and pulmonary oedema.
- Headache should be managed with appropriate analgesia.

- Abdominal pain can be the first sign of fulminating pre-eclampsia with liver dysfunction or placental abruption, and should prompt an urgent medical review.
- The timing of delivery is vital. Early delivery can lead to neonatal complications, but delaying delivery may result in deterioration in maternal health and risk of eclampsia. Delivery should be delayed until 34 weeks gestation if possible; women with severe PET are usually delivered between 34 and 37 weeks gestation. Women with mild or moderate PET reaching ≥37 weeks gestation are usually delivered within 24–48 hours.

Eclampsia

Eclampsia affects 1–2% of women with PET with half of all seizures occurring in the postnatal period and only a third preceding hypertension and proteinuria.

Management

- IV magnesium (loading dose of 4 g given IV over 5 minutes, followed by infusion of 1 g/hour for 24 hours). Magnesium can be given pre-emptively to a woman with a history of eclampsia or evidence of severe PET necessitating delivery within 24 hours. Magnesium levels should be monitored every 2–4 hours particularly in women with impaired renal function, where toxicity can occur.
- If onset is during pregnancy urgent plans should be made for delivery.
- Cerebral imaging is indicated to exclude other pathology, particularly intracerebral bleed, especially if seizures continue.

HELLP syndrome

Haemolysis (H), elevated liver (EL) transaminases and thrombocytopenia (low platelets [LP]) can constitute HELLP syndrome; women with some, but not all of these features are considered to have partial HELLP syndrome. The syndrome can develop rapidly and is now broadly regarded as a severe form of PET with high morbidity and mortality affecting approximately 0.5% of all pregnancies.

Management

- The management principles of PET outlined above apply (➲ see Management, p. 812 and Table 23.6).
- Consideration of urgent delivery should be made in women >34 weeks gestation; those <34 weeks may need to be delivered promptly (e.g. 24–48 hours after receiving corticosteroids to promote fetal lung maturation).
- Hepatic haematoma is a rare, but well recognised complication of the syndrome.

Diagnostic tools in pre-eclamptic toxaemia

Soluble fms-like tyrosine kinase 1 (sFlt1) receptor and placental growth factors (PIGF) levels can be useful diagnostic tools in PET. sFlt1 is a marker of pre-eclampsia, which may have a potential role to identify women at risk of developing severe PET. Low PIGF levels (<5% centile) indicate a low risk of pre-eclampsia in the following 14 days.

Prevention of pre-eclamptic toxaemia in future pregnancies

- Low dose aspirin (oral dose 75mg) reduces the risk of developing PET. It should be prescribed to women who are at high risk of developing PET late in the first trimester, which include those with more than two of the following characteristics:
  - age ≥40 years;
  - pregnancy interval >10 years;
  - BMI of ≥35 kg/m^2 at first antenatal visit;
  - family history of PET;

  or one of the following characteristics:
  - GH and/or PET during a previous pregnancy;
  - chronic (pre-existing) hypertension;

- ◆ chronic kidney disease;
- ◆ autoimmune disease such as SLE or antiphospholipid syndrome;
- ◆ type 1 DM or type 2 DM.
- Calcium supplementation may reduce the risk of PET in women with a low calcium diet.

Further reading

1. Brown MA, Magee LA, Kenny LC, et al. Hypertensive disorders of pregnancy: ISSHP classification, diagnosis, and management recommendations for international practice. *Hypertension*. 2018; 72(1):24–43.

Thrombocytopenia

Platelet count of 100–150 × 10^9/L is common in pregnancy and is not associated with an increased risk to mother or fetus, including during childbirth.

- Immune thrombocytopenic purpura is sometimes diagnosed in pregnancy and may require treatment with a combination of IVIG and/or steroids.
- Thrombocytopenia is also associated with:
  - ◆ PET, eclampsia and HELLP.
  - ◆ Obstetric complications, which can cause DIC (e.g. placental abruption, amniotic fluid embolism and retention of a dead fetus).

Low platelet levels are particularly important in the third trimester when plans for delivery may require consultation with haematologists (see Table 23.7). Sequential changes in platelet count and coagulation may affect bleeding risk (particularly in the context of altered liver function) and close monitoring is therefore required.

Table 23.7 Platelet thresholds for obstetric interventions

Intervention/procedure	**Platelet threshold (×10^9/L)**
Normal vaginal delivery	50
Caesarean section	50
Epidural insertion	80
Epidural removal	100

Venous thromboembolism and pulmonary embolism

The risk of VTE during pregnancy is increased four-fold with an incidence of approximately 1 in 1000 pregnancies; the incidence is higher and continues for 6 weeks in the post-partum period. Pulmonary embolism is a leading cause of death in pregnancy in developed countries, including the UK. A tendency towards thrombosis during pregnancy and the post-partum period may have had an evolutionary advantage in preventing death through haemorrhage.

Pathogenesis

- Physiological changes increasing thrombotic risk (see Table 23.1).
- Decreased venous flow velocity, hormonally (progesterone)-induced decreased vascular capacitance, 'mechanical' compression from the uterus and decreased mobility are all thought to play a role in increasing the risk of VTE.
- Endothelial injury may occur during delivery or in high risk conditions, such as pre-eclampsia due to turbulent blood flow.

Risk factors for thrombosis

- Not related to pregnancy; see Table 9.12.
- Pregnancy risk factors include multiple gestation, hyperemesis, pre-eclampsia, caesarean section, prolonged labour (>24 hours), rotational operative delivery, preterm delivery (<37 weeks), stillbirth and post-partum haemorrhage >1 L.

Clinical features

- For clinical features of VTE ➲ see Chapter 11, Clinical features, p. 367.
- Pregnancy is notable for predominantly left-sided deep-vein thrombosis (85% versus 55% in the non-pregnant state) and higher rates of ilio-femoral disease (72% versus 9%).

Diagnosis

- D-dimer testing does not have a role in diagnosing VTE in pregnancy, as false positive results are more common.
- Other investigations for suspected PE (➲ see Chapter 11, Diagnosis, p. 367 and Table 11.4).
- The risks (to the fetus and mother) of each imaging modality vary with gestational age.
- Compression duplex US should be performed in all women where there is clinical suspicion of VTE.
- Perfusion scans have increased risk to the early stage fetus.
- 2015 British (Royal College of Obstetricians and Gynaecologists [RCOG]) guidelines recommend CTPA in preference to V/Q scanning for diagnosing PE.
    - CTPA (modified/shielded to reduce fetus exposure) is associated with a lower degree of radiation exposure to the fetus, but a higher degree of radiation exposure to breast tissue, with an associated small increase in absolute risk in breast cancer.

Complications

➲ See Chapter 11, Complications, p. 368.

Management

Women are anticoagulated in pregnancy and the post-partum period according to guidelines published by the RCOG (1). Management depends on a total score, derived from a number of risk factors, as follows:

- ≥4 antenatally, consider thromboprophylaxis from the first trimester.
- 3 antenatally, consider thromboprophylaxis from 28 weeks.
- ≥2 postnatally, consider thromboprophylaxis for at least 10 days.

Thromboprophylaxis should also be considered in women admitted to hospital antenatally, particularly if the admission is prolonged (≥3 days), and in those readmitted to hospital within the puerperium.

For patients with an identified bleeding risk, the balance of risks of bleeding and thrombosis should be discussed in consultation with a haematologist with expertise in thrombosis and bleeding in pregnancy.

- Pharmacologic agents (low molecular weight heparin, e.g. enoxaparin, dalteparin, tinzaparin, and unfractionated heparin) are most commonly used. LMWH does not cross the placenta.
- Fondaparinux can be considered and may be useful in women suffering from allergic cutaneous reactions to LMWH. Fondaparinux and danaparoid should only be given in conjunction with a haematologist with expertise in thrombosis.
- The novel oral anticoagulants are not advised as there is no current data during pregnancy.
- Warfarin is teratogenic in the first trimester and has an increased risk of CNS abnormalities in any trimester. It is therefore only rarely given with appropriate counselling in pregnancy.
- Low dose aspirin has no role in prophylaxis or treatment of VTE in pregnancy.
- Mechanical methods (e.g. mobilisation, compression stockings, calf stimulation or intermittent pneumatic compression) can be used when medication is contraindicated or in lower risk individuals.

Treatment of venous thromboembolism

➲ See Chapter 9, Therapeutic anticoagulation, p. 290.

- If VTE is suspected, therapeutic anti-coagulation should be commenced expeditiously without waiting for investigations to be completed.
- Anti-Xa monitoring is increasingly used in women with very high thrombotic conditions in pregnancy, most notably for women on LMWH:
  - who have mechanical heart valves;
  - if body weight is <50 kg or >90 kg;
  - if there is renal impairment.
- Platelet monitoring is not recommended for LMWH, but is suggested if unfractionated heparin is used.
- Treatment should be continued until 6 weeks post-partum or for at least 6 months with regular medical review. The need for long-term anticoagulation treatment should be considered post-partum in a specialist maternal medicine clinic.

Treatment of massive pulmonary embolism

➲ See Chapter 11, Management, p. 368. Specific considerations during pregnancy:

- Immediate care should be provided by a senior-led MDT (physicians, obstetricians, junior medical staff, nurses/midwives, radiologists and surgeons as required).
- There should be preparation to perform maternal resuscitation with left lateral tilt if required.
  - A perimortem caesarean section should be performed within 5 minutes if resuscitation is unsuccessful and gestation is beyond 20 weeks.

References

1. RCOG. Reducing the Risk of VTE during pregnancy and the puerperium. Green-top Guideline No.37a April 2015. https://www.rcog.org.uk/en/guidelines-research-services/guidelines/gtg37a/.

Further reading

- NICE Guideline (CG92). Venous thromboembolism: reducing the risk for patients in hospital, Jan 2010 updated Jun 2015. https://www.nice.org.uk/guidance/cg92.

Radiology in pregnancy

On determining whether to perform a radiological investigation during pregnancy, the risks and benefits of an imaging modality, alternative tests and its absolute necessity should all be taken into account.

Ultrasound

- There are no known adverse effects for the fetus of US imaging.

Magnetic resonance imaging

- There are no known adverse effects of MRI below 1.5 Tesla magnetic field strengths. In clinical practice, MRI is usually avoided during the first trimester.
- Gadolinium (the common contrast agent used in MRI imaging) crosses the placenta to the amniotic circulation so its use is generally not recommended. At standard doses, gadolinium is not thought to be teratogenic, although animal studies have shown that, at higher doses, it may be associated with adverse effects.

X-ray, computed tomography, nuclear imaging and ionising radiation

- During the first 2 weeks after conception the embryo is sensitive to radiation, the embryo is either resorbed on exposure or it survives unharmed.

- It is exposure after 2 weeks that is associated with adverse effects, such as malformations, mental retardation and grow restriction.
- Exposure of <5 rad (<50 mSv) is not associated with fetal malformations, although there may be an increased risk of future childhood leukaemia. Exposure between 5–10 rad (50–100 mSv) may result in an increased risk of malformations, exposure >10 rad (>100 mSv) is considered a highly significant risk.

Imaging technique and radiation exposure

➲ See Table 5.1.

Further reading

1. Bentur Y. Ionizing and nonionizing radiation in pregnancy. In: Koren G (ed.) *Maternal-fetal Toxicology*, 2nd edn. New York: Marcel Dekker, 1994.

Multiple choice questions

Questions

1. A woman who has a history of pre-eclampsia in a prior pregnancy is now planning a second pregnancy. What should be prescribed?
   A. 300 mg aspirin once pregnancy is confirmed.
   B. 300 mg aspirin from late in the first trimester.
   C. 75 mg aspirin from late in the first trimester.
   D. 1.5 mg/kg subcutaneous LMWH from late in the first trimester.
   E. 500 mg Vitamin E daily once pregnancy is confirmed.
2. Five women have recorded the following pairs of BPs. In which patient could a diagnosis of gestational hypertension be made?
   A. 139/86 mmHg at 16 weeks gestation, 125/75 mmHg at first antenatal visit.
   B. 139/86 mmHg at 24 weeks gestation, 139/75 mmHg at first antenatal visit at 14 weeks gestation.
   C. 145/83 mmHg at 24 weeks gestation, 145/75 mmHg at first antenatal visit at 14 weeks gestation.
   D. 145/83 mmHg at 16 weeks gestation, 135/75 mmHg at first antenatal visit at 14 weeks gestation.
   E. 145/83 mmHg at 24 weeks gestation, 135/75 mmHg at first antenatal visit at 14 weeks gestation.
3. The first-line medication for a women diagnosed with gestational hypertension is:
   A. Labetalol.
   B. Methyldopa.
   C. Ramipril.
   D. Metoprolol.
   E. Hydralazine.
4. The key driver in the development of gestational diabetes is:
   A. Increased insulin resistance.
   B. Diminished pancreatic beta cell function.
   C. Maternal weight gain.
   D. Broad shift from Th2 to Th1 immune response.
   E. Placental dysfunction.

5. Which of the following is least commonly indicated in the management of a patient with hyperemesis gravidarum?
   A. Assessment of fluid status and rehydration.
   B. Correction of electrolyte abnormalities.
   C. Vitamin supplementation.
   D. Providing psychosocial support.
   E. Delivery at 32 weeks gestation.

Answers

1. C. Low dose aspirin has been demonstrated to reduce the risk of PET by 24% in high risk individuals. There is no evidence that a higher dose (A or B) or Vitamin E is of benefit. LMWH is prescribed during pregnancy to women at high risk of venous thromboembolism. ➲ See Prevention of pre-eclamptic toxaemia in future pregnancies, p. 813.
2. E. Pregnancy induced or gestational hypertension is defined as an elevated BP >140 mmHg systolic and/or 90 mmHg diastolic recorded for the first time after 20 weeks gestation. Patient (C) arguably has pre-existing hypertension at first antenatal visit. ➲ See Gestational hypertension, p. 808.
3. A. Alternative treatments include methyldopa, nifedipine and hydralazine. ACE-i (e.g. rampiril) should not be used during pregnancy as they can cause a range of adverse effects on the fetus including renal, cardiac, lung and limb defects. There is conflicting research regarding atenolol with some studies demonstrating and others refuting a link with increased rates of growth retardation. ➲ See Treatment, p. 810 and Table 23.5.
4. A. Women who develop GDM have insufficient increase in insulin production to meet demand in the context of hormonal and weight changes which increase insulin resistance. The Th2 to Th1 immune system responses are not responsible for the development of GDM. Placental dysfunction is associated with the development of PET. ➲ See Gestational diabetes, Pathophysiology, p. 799.
5. E. Delivery at 32 weeks is a rare step in the management of HG. Sequelae from prematurity are evident up to term deliveries, therefore, every effort should be made to manage the mother's condition and symptoms. In rare instances, where symptoms are intolerable and the mother's health is at risk, early delivery is indicated. ➲ See Hyperemesis gravidarum, Management, p. 808.

Chapter 24 **Environmental Medicine**

Mike Stacey, Lucy Lamb and David R. Woods

Basic physiology

Human performance and survival are dependent upon successful cellular respiration, which requires exchange of materials with the external physical environment (gases, water, fuel). The human body has evolved to ensure adequate exchange across a range of environmental conditions.

Acclimatisation describes the series of adjustments made by the body in response to a new environment. More complete adaptation occurs in populations that permanently reside in a given environment.

Cardiovascular and respiratory responses are critical to the challenges posed during physical exercise, and throughout acclimatisation and adaptation.

Cardiac output, blood pressure and physical exercise

The cardiovascular system functions to provide oxygen (O_2) and nutrients to the tissues of the body and to remove waste products, including carbon dioxide (CO_2). Cardiac output (CO) is the principal determinant of circulatory blood flow. CO may be expressed as:

$$CO = Heart\,rate \times Stroke\,volume$$

Key factors that influence stroke volume are displayed in Table 24.1.

Table 24.1 Key determinants of cardiac stroke output

Determinant	Definition
Preload	The haemodynamic conditions that determine the end-diastolic volume of the ventricle.
Afterload	A measure of the intraventricular pressure that must be developed to eject blood from the heart.
Contractility	A measure of the force of isovolumetric contraction when afterload and preload are constant.

Systemic blood pressure is the product of CO and systemic vascular resistance (SVR):

$$Systemic\ BP = CO \times SVR$$

The average of systemic BP during a single cardiac cycle is known as the mean arterial blood pressure (MAP) and may be calculated from the diastolic BP and the pulse pressure (the difference between systolic and diastolic BP):

$$MAP = Diastolic\ BP + 1/3\left(Systolic\ BP - Diastolic\ BP\right)$$

Physical exercise increases CO, via stimulation of brainstem centres, causing systolic BP to rise. Meanwhile, massive arteriolar vasodilatation associated with exercising muscle causes a drop in SVR, and diastolic BP often also falls. The net result is a small rise in MAP. In elite athletes, maximal exercise can be accompanied by a 6-fold increase in CO, from 5 L/min at rest, to 30 L/min or greater. Haemodynamic changes at these higher workloads are mediated by rapid vagal withdrawal at the onset of exercise, followed by increased activity of the sympathetic nervous system and other hormonal/metabolic responses as exercise progresses.

Oxygen delivery and uptake

The *oxygen-transport cascade* describes the movement of O_2 from the atmosphere to cellular mitochondria, where respiration takes place. O_2 diffuses from the atmosphere across the alveolar-capillary membrane into the bloodstream. The O_2 content of the blood consists of that which is physically dissolved and O_2 that has been bound by haemoglobin. The rate of O_2 delivery to the tissues (D O_2) may be expressed as:

$$DO_2 = O_2\ content\ of\ blood \times CO$$

The amount of O_2 dissolved in the blood is directly proportional to the tension (or partial pressure, P) of O_2. Variation in PO_2 at each step of the oxygen-transport cascade is shown in Table 24.2. The higher PO_2 in the alveolar capillaries favours loading of the haemoglobin molecule, whereas the low tensions of the tissues favour O_2 release. The presence of 2,3-diphosphoglycerate in red blood cells contributes to this effect, by binding to haemoglobin as O_2 is unloaded and so decreasing the relative affinity.

Table 24.2 Partial pressure of oxygen during near-maximal exercise at sea level

Location	Partial pressure (mmHg)
Atmospheric air	150 mmHg
Alveolus	110 mmHg
Arterial blood	80 mmHg
Venous blood	20 mmHg
Mitochondria	0–1 mmHg

The rate of O_2 uptake into the tissues (VO_2) reflects O_2 consumption. In peak human performers, muscular VO_2 may increase 80-fold during maximal physical exercise. Whole body O_2 may be calculated from measurement of the concentration of O_2 in inhaled and exhaled gases. When this is undertaken during incremental exercise, a measure of capacity to transport and use O_2 known as the maximal O_2 uptake (VO_2max) is derived. This is taken to reflect the subject's endurance capacity.

Heat

Because cell and tissue functions require a relatively constant internal temperature, core body temperature is tightly regulated. *Heat stress* describes conditions that increase body temperature and may be environmental (e.g. solar radiation) or metabolic (e.g. skeletal muscle contraction during exercise). In health, heat stress is limited by negative feedback from sensory neurons in the skin, viscera and spinal cord. These act at the hypothalamus to evoke counter-regulatory autonomic and behavioural responses. *Heat strain* describes the physiological burden of heat stress, to which acclimatisation may occur over days to weeks (Table 24.3). A *heat wave* is defined as >3 consecutive days of environmental temperature >32.2°C (90°F).

Table 24.3 Physiological responses that mitigate heat stress

Organ system	Acute response	Effect	Nature of heat loss	Acclimatisation response
Cardiovascular	Increased cardiac output. Regulation of arteriovenous anastomoses (redirects blood flow).	Skin blood flow increased up to 10-fold. Warm blood shunted from core to skin surfaces. Reduced blood flow to other viscera, e.g. gut.	Convective.	Increased cardiovascular efficiencies. Lower threshold and higher rate of blood flow diversion to skin.
Respiratory	Hyperventilation.	Increased gas exchange.	Evaporative.	
Skin	Thermal sweating. Vasodilatation.	Heat loss maximised by co-ordinated response.	Evaporative.	Earlier onset and increased rate of thermal sweating. Reduced concentration of sodium in secreted sweat.
Renal/ endocrine/ metabolic				Retention of fluid to increase total body and plasma volume. Increased action of aldosterone to conserve total body sodium. Reduction in metabolic rate.

Heat-related illnesses

When thermoregulatory processes fail, body temperature rises and *heat illness* may result (1). Heat illness describes a spectrum of clinical entities and a continuum of symptoms is seen from muscular weakness, headache and disproportionate fatigue through to collapse, coma and death. Heat illness during exertion is a leading cause of death in young athletes (2). The incidence varies by sport or activity, with American football and military training posing high risk of heat illness. Predisposing factors are displayed in Box 24.1.

Box 24.1 Factors that predispose to heat illness

- Obesity.
- Poor physical fitness.
- Increasing age.
- Dehydration.
- Acute infectious illness.
- Cardiovascular disease.
- Sickle cell trait.
- Prescription drug use (β-blockers, antihistamines, antidepressants).
- Prior use of alcohol and illicit drugs (e.g. amphetamines).
- High environmental temperature.
- High humidity.
- Activity during a heat wave.
- Lack of acclimatisation.

Heat cramps often follow prolonged or strenuous exercise, and are sometimes associated with elevated environmental temperature. The aetiology is unclear, but has been ascribed to loss of water and electrolytes, or reflex neurological disturbance with prolonged exercise.

Heat exhaustion describes fatigue and the inability to complete a physical task in a hot environment. Insufficient cardiac output may result in collapse and progression to severe forms of heat illness.

Heat injury is defined as a moderate to severe illness associated with high body temperature and characterised by injury to organs (e.g. liver and kidney) and tissues (e.g. GI and muscle).

Heat stroke is the most serious of the syndromes associated with excess body heat, in which a syndrome of multiple organ dysfunction develops, predominated by encephalopathy.

Classic heat stroke occurs at rest in conditions of elevated environmental temperature. In North America, the incidence during heat waves is 1–2 cases per 1000 residents. Onset may be insidious with a variety of non-specific symptoms, such as apathy, headache and delirium.

Exertional heat stroke affects individuals performing strenuous activities in a range of climatic conditions and results from failure to dissipate heat released by muscle. Heat damages viscera and tissues, including the gut and its epithelial surface, causing a systemic inflammatory response and release of endotoxin (3). Shock and DIC are commonly seen. Physical examination may demonstrate hyperventilation, ataxia and CNS irritability. Rectal temperature should be elevated >40°C for prehospital diagnosis, but may have fallen by the time of presentation to secondary care, or if medical assessment is delayed. It is important to consider other causes of fever and CNS dysfunction in the differential diagnosis of heat stroke (Box 24.2).

Box 24.2 Differential diagnosis of heat stroke

- Infectious disease, e.g. encephalitis.
- Endocrine disease (thyrotoxicosis, phaeochromocytoma).
- Drug intoxication or reaction (e.g. neuroleptic malignant syndrome).

Prevention of heat illness

Heat waves are increasing in frequency, in line with forecasts of higher global mean temperatures. Access to air conditioning and being able to remain indoors are factors that protect against classical heat stroke. Education and awareness of exertional heat stroke amongst athletes, coaches and other at-risk professionals (e.g. soldiers) is important and may prevent deaths.

Management of heat illness and allied disorders

Once heat illness has been recognised, cessation of unnecessary physical activity and removal to a cool environment are central to the management. For heat cramps, stretching, and replacement of fluid and electrolytes may help, with full recovery expected after 24 hours rest. In heat exhaustion, IV saline may provide rapid symptomatic relief. Cooling can be achieved by water spraying or sponging the skin in combination with electrical fanning, in order to encourage evaporative heat loss. Immediate cooling is recommended in heat stroke and cold water immersion may reduce morbidity and mortality in affected athletes. The use of drugs to lower body temperature (e.g. dantrolene, antipyretics) has not been shown to improve clinical outcomes. A structured approach to resuscitation is required concurrent to cooling efforts. Supportive care is often undertaken in a high dependency or critical care environment.

Screening for exertional rhabdomyolysis should be undertaken in all heat casualties, with urinalysis (for myoglobinuria) and measurement of serum creatine kinase (CK). Suspected cases may be treated with forced diuresis concurrent with volume expansion.

References

1. Leon LR, Kenefick RW. The pathophysiology of heat-related illnesses. In: Auerbach PS (Ed.) *Wilderness Medicine*, 6th edn. Philadelphia: Elsevier Mosby, 2012.
2. Armstrong LE, Casa DJ, Millard-Stafford M, et al. American College of Sports Medicine position stand. Exertional heat illness during training and competition. *Med Sci Sports Exerc.* 2007;30(3):556–72.
3. Bouchama A, Knochel JM. Heat stroke. *N Engl J Med.* 2002;346:1978–88.

Cold

Cold stress occurs upon exposure to any environment that is cooler than the human body. Below an ambient temperature of 30°C, cold sensors in the skin are activated and trigger the sensation of cold in the brain, via C-type and smaller myelinated fibres. Thermo-sensitive neurons in the hypothalamus also contribute. Other central stimuli that result in the feeling of cold include hypoglycaemia and increased osmolality from dehydration.

The ability to maintain body temperature is dependent upon adequate thermoregulatory responses. *Hypothermia* may be defined as a relative 2°C decrease in body temperature and is classified as mild, moderate or severe on the basis of absolute *core temperature* (Tc), which reflects the temperature of the brain, lungs and heart (1) and may be measured in the pulmonary artery. The body's responses to cooling and the pathological effects of hypothermia are summarised in Table 24.4. Risk factors for more rapid onset of hypothermia during cooling are displayed in Box 24.3.

Table 24.4 Adaptive and pathophysiological responses to cold stress, according to core temperature (Tc)

System	Early responses during cold exposure (maximal at core temperature of 34–36°C)	Pathophysiology manifesting with progressive fall in Tc
Cardiovascular	Regulation of arteriovenous anastomoses to re-direct blood flow from periphery to core. Increase in blood pressure and tachycardia.	Cardiac output diminishes. Cardiac arrhythmias (Tc <30°C).
Respiratory	Central respiratory stimulation.	Tachypnoea, then falling minute ventilation.
Skin	Erythema, cyanosis, pallor.	Bruising, oedema, frostbite.
Renal	Cold-induced diuresis.	Oligo/anuria and renal failure.
Endocrine/ metabolic	Increase in metabolic rate. Uncoupling of cellular respiration for thermogenesis.	Fall in cellular oxygen uptake. Protective effects on cell membrane function. Profound acid-base disturbance at Tc <26°C.
Central nervous system	Behavioural modification (e.g. personal extraction to a warmer environment, donning extra clothing, taking hot beverages).	Disruption of higher functions. Visual and auditory hallucinations. Maladaptive behaviours, e.g. paradoxical undressing. Loss of consciousness (typically at Tc of 28–30°C).
Musculoskeletal	Increased muscle tone. Shivering thermogenesis.	Reduced motor co-ordination (decreased nerve conduction). Cessation of shivering at Tc <31°C.

Cold injuries

Cold injuries share many risk factors with hypothermia. They may be classified on the basis of whether tissue freezes (*frostbite*) or otherwise (*non-freezing cold injury*).

Box 24.3 Factors that predispose to hypothermia

- Anorexia nervosa, malnutrition, alcoholism.
- CNS dysfunction (e.g. stroke, Parkinson's disease, autonomic neuropathy).
- Endocrine failure (hypoadrenalism, hypothyroidism, diabetic ketoacidosis).
- Extreme physical exertion.
- Serious multisystem disease (infectious illnesses, polytrauma).
- Burns.

Pathophysiology of cold injuries

Increased sympathetic nervous outflow from cold exposure can result in prolonged vasoconstriction and so compromise the blood supply to peripheral tissues. Inflammation of the capillary endothelium itself leads to tissue ischaemia and hypoxia of nerves, muscle and fat. Local injury occurs at tissue temperatures below 10°C. If freezing occurs, further damage is caused by the formation of ice crystals.

Re-warming is associated with hyperaemia and characteristic changes in the appearances of tissues: from white/yellow/waxy to reddish or purple discolouration, with brief cyanosis sometimes intervening. Upon re-perfusion, further damage and cellular apoptosis may be caused by reactive oxygen species. Release of prostaglandins and thromboxane A2 from re-perfusion injury exacerbates the thrombotic tendency seen in cooling. The final common pathway to tissue necrosis is summarised in Figure 24.1.

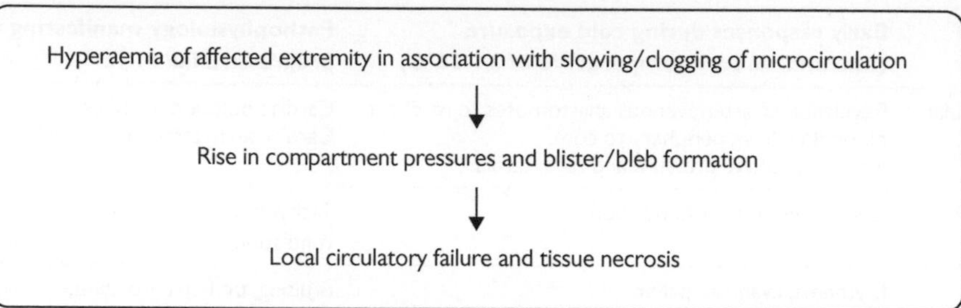

Figure 24.1 Final common pathway to tissue necrosis from frostbite

Non-freezing cold injury

Non-freezing cold injury (NFCI) is a clinical syndrome that occurs in distinct stages (Box 24.4). It more commonly results from exposure to cold-wet conditions, the environmental temperature typically being 0–20°C. Rates and prevalence vary; in military populations, individuals of African and Afro-American ethnicity appear to be at increased risk. Other vulnerable populations include hikers, the elderly, alcoholics and individuals 'sleeping rough'. Diagnosis can be difficult in less severe cases, where examination findings are often lacking. Symptoms may include a general feeling of coldness in the affected limbs, numbness, tingling and burning sensations. Responses to a cold stress test can be assessed by infra-red thermography, but results are variable and no gold-standard investigation is presently available. There is emerging evidence of reduced intraepithelial nerve fibre density. Gangrene can develop in the most severe cases of NFCI, and tissue that remains neuropathic is susceptible to trauma and its complications, including infections of soft tissue and bone (2).

Box 24.4 Clinical stages of non-freezing cold injury in affected extremities

Intense vasoconstriction during cold exposure

Yellowish-white or mottled colour; reduced pulses; loss of sensation and proprioceptive gait disturbance.

Hyperaemia during and after re-warming

Fleeting cyanosis during early re-warming may be seen, then:

- Impaired microcirculation (delayed capillary refill despite bounding pulses), petechial haemorrhages.
- Return of sensation and severe neuropathic pain (peaks on the day following injury).
- Inflammation, oedema and blister formation, which may be haemorrhagic.

Post-hyperaemia

- Abnormal responses to cold, including sweating and cold sensitivity.
- Increased risk of fungal infections, trauma, ulceration and osteomyelitis.
- Phase may last for weeks to months and can fail to resolve fully.

Frostbite

The extent and nature of injury varies according to the severity of exposure. The vast majority of cases involve the feet and/or hands. Initially, appearances are often deceptive and classification is based upon the final outcome (Box 24.5).

Box 24.5 Classification of frostbite by extremity effect

Superficial

- 1st degree: partial skin freezing: hyperaemia and oedema, erythema without blistering.
- 2nd degree: full thickness skin freezing: blistering, gangrene (black eschar) and desquamation.

Deep

- 3rd degree: SC tissues freeze: haemorrhagic blisters, skin necrosis, blue-grey colouration.
- 4th degree: muscle, tendon and bone affected: little swelling, mottled or dusky appearance, becoming 'mummified' and black.

Prevention of hypothermia and cold injuries

Where possible, avoidance of prolonged exposure to cold environments and known precipitants is best. In a cold environment, physical activity can increase peripheral blood flow and metabolic heat production, but sweat accumulation in clothing should be avoided. Wearing layered garments and well-designed equipment can serve to reduce heat loss from the body. Footwear that is comfortable, rather than painful or tight, may reduce sympathetic vasoconstriction and limit circulatory compromise. Education of at-risk individuals is key.

Management of hypothermia and cold-related injuries

General measures include urgent removal from the cold environment and efforts to dry and insulate the casualty. In minor hypothermia, shivering may be augmented by passive re-warming (*full body insulation*). Moderate to severe hypothermia may benefit from truncal application of chemical heat packs. In cases of major hypothermia, the risks of dysrrhythmia, circulatory arrest and collapse should be minimised by immobilisation in a horizontal position with ECG monitoring and careful casualty handling. *Osborn* or *'J' waves* – seen as a hump elevation in the terminal portion of the QRS complex on ECG – can be present and their size may correlate with the severity of hypothermia.

The initiation of active re-warming is best achieved in a hospital environment and transport of the casualty from a field setting should not be delayed. Active re-warming may be external (forced air, e.g. under a specialised blanket, warmed IV fluids) or internal (oesophageal delivery of warm humidified gases, lavage of body cavities, e.g. peritoneal, extracorporeal circulatory methods). Large quantities of warmed fluids may need to be given IV. Hypothermic patients in cardiac arrest require cardiopulmonary resuscitation (CPR) and modification of management protocols to allow for the slower metabolism of drugs and for cold tissues being refractory to intended treatment effects. Alternative or contributory causes of cardiac arrest should be excluded (e.g. drug overdose, myxoedema coma).

In hypothermia, strategies to elevate Tc are paramount but may run counter to the optimal treatment of co-existing cold injuries (3). Rewarming of frozen tissue is undesirable if refreezing is likely (e.g. due to delayed evacuation). NFCI may benefit initially from exposure to a cool stream of air (e.g. electric fan). More rapid rewarming of frostbitten extremities is preferred, using warm water over a period of 15 minutes to 1 hour (e.g. whirlpool basin). *Aloe vera* can be applied to thawed tissue and oral ibuprofen may also be indicated. Opiate analgesia may be required for symptom relief during thawing. Elevation may diminish reperfusion oedema when a limb is warmed, allied to splintage. Where tissue necrosis has occurred, tetanus prophylaxis should be ensured and antibiotics may be required to treat associated infection. In frostbite victims presenting less than 24 hours after injury, outcome may be improved by thrombolysis (e.g. with tissue plasminogen activator). The vasodilator iloprost may be of benefit in subjects who present later. Emergency fasciotomy is indicated for compartment syndrome, whereas amputation should be delayed for up to 3 months, to allow time for healthy tissues to demarcate from those that are truly necrotic.

Prognosis of cold-related illnesses

The decrease in metabolic rate associated with hypothermia can allow survival in very cold and hypoxic states and individuals may recover fully from a cold-associated insult, including cardiac arrest, without residual debility. There is increased susceptibility to future cold injury in frostbitten tissues, so the importance of secondary prevention must be stressed. Persistent pain is a feature after NFCI and chronic neuropathic-type pain is a recognised complication, treated by agents such as amitriptyline and gabapentin.

References

1. Brown DJA, Brugger H, Boyd J, et al. Accidental hypothermia. *N Engl J Med*. 2013;367:1932–8.
2. Imray CHE, Richards P, Greeves J, et al. Nonfreezing cold-induced injuries. *J R Army Med Corps Sp Edn*. 2011;157(1):79–84.
3. Grieve AW, Davis P, Dhillon S, et al. Medicine and physiology at high altitude A clinical review of the management of frostbite. *J Roy Army Med Corps Sp Edn*. 2011;157(1):73–7.

High altitude

High altitude describes the environment 2500 m elevation above sea-level (high altitude: 2500–3500 m; very high altitude 3500–5800 m; extremely high altitude: >5800 m) (1). It is characterised by the combination of decreased barometric pressure and diminished availability of O_2, known as hypobaric hypoxia. Although the percentage of O_2 in the atmosphere remains a constant 21% with increasing altitude, the fall in barometric pressure exponentially reduces the PO_2 and thus the molecular O_2 content of each unit of inspired air (Figure 24.2).

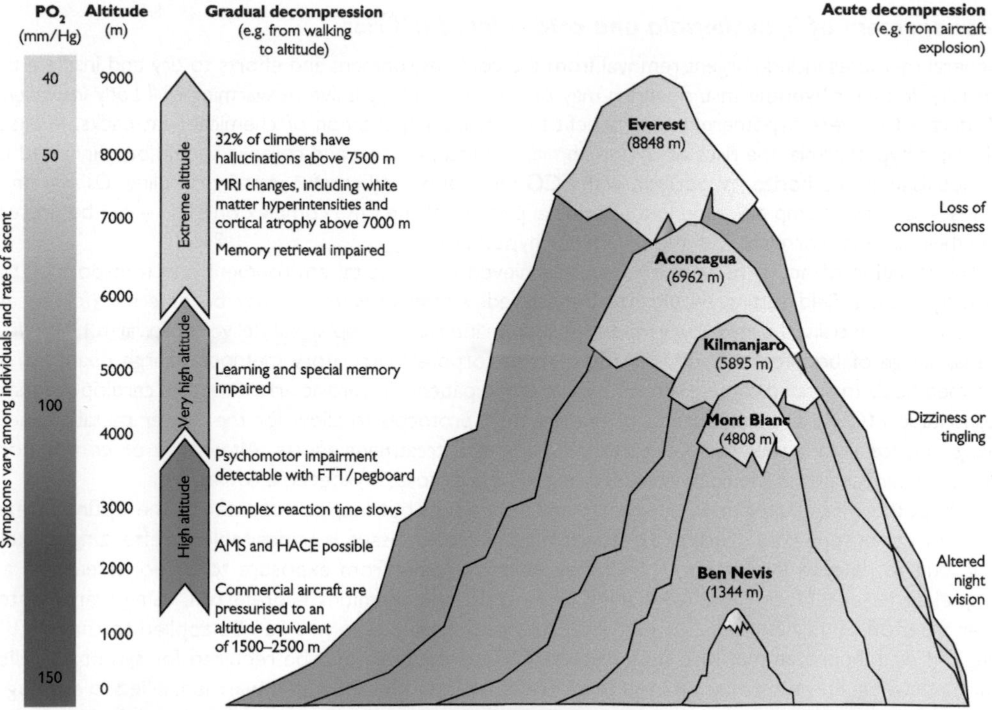

Figure 24.2 Reduction in barometric pressure with elevation above sea level. Neurological changes associated with gradual and acute exposure to the high altitude environment are displayed; FTT = finger tapping test (used to assess psychomotor changes).

Reprinted from *The Lancet Neurology*, 8, 2, Wilson M.H. et al., The cerebral effects of ascent to high altitude, pp. 175–191. DOI:https://doi.org/10.1016/S1474-4422(09)70014-6.

Altitude acclimatisation encompasses rapid responses to acute exposure and changes that occur over days and months living at high altitude. The responses are phased, such that acute adjustments are replaced by biologically sustainable long-term alterations in physiology. Effective acclimatisation maintains tissue oxygen delivery in the face of plummeting atmospheric O_2 levels, but this can no longer be maintained at extreme altitudes. Table 24.5 summarises the acclimatisation responses to high altitude by organ system.

Table 24.5 Acclimatisation changes by organ system

Organ system	Responses to altitude	Physiological consequences	Time course
Central nervous system	Hypoxic stimulus from carotid body chemoreceptors to medullary respiratory centres.	Hyperventilation.	Immediate.
Respiratory	Hyperventilation.	Hypoxic ventilatory drive blunted. Respiratory alkalosis.	First hour.
Renal	Urinary loss of bicarbonate ions.	Increase in CSF H^+. Hypercapnic ventilatory drive sensitised.	Initial hours and days.
Endocrine	Suppression of aldosterone and arginine vasopressin. Increased secretion of BNP and ANP.	Diuresis and natriuresis. Reduction in circulating plasma volume. Increased haemoglobin concentration and haematocrit.	Predominate in first 2–3 weeks.
Haematological	Hypoxia-driven renal and hepatic production of erythropoietin.	Increased red cell mass and haemoglobin concentration. Increase in 2,3-DPG.	Predominate after first 2–3 weeks.
Cardiovascular	Increased heart rate. Decreased stroke volume during exercise (mechanism unknown).	Increased cardiac output. Heart rate elevated during exercise to maintain cardiac output.	Immediate. Persists beyond acclimatisation period.

CSF = cerebrospinal fluid; 2,3-DPG = 2,3-diphosphoglycerate; BNP = brain natriuretic peptide; ANP = atrial natriuretic peptide.

Acute exposure to high altitude

Should an unacclimatised individual undergo hyperacute exposure to the hypobaric hypoxia of 6000 m elevation (by sudden decompression in an aircraft or chamber simulation), the time before unconsciousness supervenes may be 10 minutes or less and will be closely related to the fall in central venous O_2 tension observed. More commonly, individuals attain high altitude by trekking and, in this setting, most altitude-related illnesses occur above 2500–3000 m. Failure to allow sufficient time to acclimatise, by graded exposure to progressively increasing altitude over days and weeks, increases the risk of illness. Pronounced falls in arterial and tissue oxygenation, aberrant body fluid homeostasis and exaggerated hypoxic pulmonary vasoconstriction have been implicated in the pathophysiology of altitude-related illnesses. A failure of the usual diuresis that occurs with high altitude exposure contributes to fluid retention and may be evident as peripheral oedema sometimes seen with acute mountain sickness (AMS).

Acute mountain sickness is a common syndrome that occurs in up to 60% of those who ascend to 4500 m above sea level. It presents within 6–12 hours of arrival at high altitude and frequently results from a rapid ascent profile. It is characterised by headache and at least one further symptom (loss of appetite, nausea/vomiting, fatigue, dizziness, disturbed sleep). Disturbed sleep is commonly associated with *periodic breathing*, which closely resembles Cheyne–Stokes respiration (cycles of hyperpnoea alternating with apnoea) and results from hyperventilation-induced hypocapnia. If no further ascent is undertaken, AMS typically resolves within 24–72 hours. The Lake Louise consensus criteria define AMS using a self-reported questionnaire format, by scoring the number and severity of symptoms (2). Symptoms of AMS (headache, GI symptoms, fatigue/weakness, dizziness/light-headedness, difficulty sleeping) are allocated a score of 0–3 (symptom not present to severe). A total score of >3, in the presence of headache and recent ascent, is diagnostic. Serial evaluations are used to determine progression/improvement in the condition. An alternative scoring system, using the AMS-C score of the Environmental Symptom Questionnaire (ESQ) is composed of 11 questions graded from 0–5 with each symptom given a factorial weighting; the resultant scores are then totalled and multiplied by 0.1927 to give a score in the range 0–5. AMS is then defined as a score ≥0.70.

High altitude cerebral oedema (HACE) is rare and usually occurs above 4000 m. The incidence is 1–2% among those who ascend rapidly to 4500 m. There is evidence of vasogenic brain swelling with intracranial hypertension and extracellular oedema due to the breakdown of the blood–brain barrier. HACE is usually preceded by AMS-type symptoms and traditionally was thought to represent the extreme manifestation of a disease continuum, with a common pathophysiology shared with AMS. Recently, however, there has been debate as to whether HACE represents a separate entity. Whatever the cause, altered mental status and ataxia are usually superimposed upon AMS-type symptoms with progression of HACE, followed by hallucinations and coma. Death, due to brainstem herniation, may ensue within 24 hours of the onset of symptoms. The mountain-side diagnosis is a clinical one. In survivors, ataxia may persist for several days and cases of permanent neurological deficit have been reported from presentations compatible with HACE. There is no evidence that superior physical fitness is protective.

High altitude pulmonary oedema (HAPE) is a non-cardiogenic form of pulmonary oedema that may occur in isolation, without preceding AMS. *De novo* manifestation or worsening of existing pulmonary hypertension is thought likely to contribute to the development of HAPE with impaired alveolar fluid clearance, local hypoxia-mediated inflammation and an exaggerated hypoxic pulmonary vasoconstrictor response with resultant capillary stress being implicated as potential mechanisms. The incidence of HAPE varies according to the rate of ascent and susceptibility of the individual (Box 24.6), but is approximately 1–2% in the general population trekking to high altitude. Exertional dyspnoea heralds the onset of the condition, usually within 2 to 5 days of arrival at high altitude. It is disproportionate to the altitude, degree of exercise and experience of fellow trekkers/mountaineers. Progression to dyspnoea at rest, which is worse at night, can be accompanied by a dry cough that becomes bubbly, wet and may yield blood-stained sputum. Clinical signs include tachycardia, tachypnoea and low-grade fever. Hypoxaemia, crackles on auscultation of the lungs and evidence of raised pulmonary artery pressure may be identified, but are also seen in unaffected individuals. For those cases where chest radiography is available locally, clinical diagnosis in the field may be later confirmed by appearances of patchy peripheral oedema in the lung fields, becoming widespread over time. HAPE is thought to be the leading cause of all deaths at high altitude.

Box 24.6 Factors that increase susceptibility to high altitude pulmonary oedema (HAPE) on ascent to high altitude

- Rapid rate of ascent.
- High level of physical exertion.
- Cold exposure.
- Previous episode of HAPE.
- Existing pulmonary hypertension.
- Structural circulatory abnormalities.

Prevention of high altitude illness

Slow ascent is thought to be the best of all prophylactic approaches to AMS at high altitude (less than 500 m increase in sleeping elevation per day above 3000 m and a rest day, with no ascent to higher sleeping elevation, every 3–4 days) (3).

In general, prophylaxis is not required on first ascent to altitude, but may be recommended in those who have previously suffered an altitude-related illness or who, for occupational or other reasons, are forced to ascend more rapidly than is usually advised. Acetazolamide, a carbonic anhydrase inhibitor, is the preferred prophylaxis for individuals at moderate or high risk of AMS (based on previous susceptibility and ascent profile). It should be started at least 24 hours before ascent and continued until descent has begun. It is recommended that acetazolamide is trialled at sea level for tolerability, because of its potentially unpleasant side effects (metallic taste on drinking carbonated beverages, paraesthesia, diuretic action). An alternative is the glucocorticoid dexamethasone. Limited evidence also exists for the use of ibuprofen or sumatriptan in preventing AMS.

The dihydropyridine calcium antagonist nifedipine (by causing pulmonary vasodilatation) offers some prophylaxis against HAPE, as do the phosphodiesterase inhibitors tadalafil and sildenafil (also by reducing pulmonary hypertension).

Treatment of high altitude illnesses

Descent is the most effective treatment for high altitude illnesses (4). Reducing altitude exposure by as little as 300 m can produce a dramatic clinical improvement, although 1000 m or more may be necessary and descent to an altitude below that where symptoms began is ideal.

Although AMS is not in itself life-threatening, the prospect of progression to HACE mandates stopping further ascent in all but the mildest cases of AMS. Rest and hydration at the altitude gained are appropriate for mild AMS (Lake Louise score 3–4). Simple analgesia (paracetamol, ibuprofen) and anti-emetics may provide symptomatic relief. Acetazolamide may also be considered, and dexamethasone may be co-administered with acetazolamide if symptoms of AMS progress to moderate severity (Lake Louise score >5). Severe symptoms of AMS indicate descent to a lower altitude and affected individuals must be accompanied because of the risk of unrecognised nascent HACE. If circumstances (weather, terrain, debility) temporarily prevent movement, a portable hyperbaric chamber can be employed to simulate descent. Other means of delivering supplementary oxygen to raise arterial O_2 saturation and improve symptoms include a Hudson-type mask or continuous positive airway pressure (CPAP).

O_2 and hyperbaric treatment can also be employed in HACE and HAPE, but only as temporising measures to facilitate descent, which is the mainstay of treatment. The patient with HACE or HAPE will need to be carried down or transferred using mechanised transport. In the evaluation of a patient with suspected HACE, it is important to consider the possibility of hypothermia, hypoglycaemia, migraine or alcohol intoxication/hangover. Any suspicion of HACE mandates immediate descent and these alternate differentials must be treated or excluded in parallel with planning/attempting descent.

Dexamethasone is also a recommended treatment, auxiliary to descent, in the management of HACE. It may be administered by IV or IM routes in obtunded patients. Nifedipine is used as an adjunct to O_2/descent in HAPE, or as monotherapy where these approaches are not possible. Because nifedipine is not selective for the pulmonary circulation, a test dose (10 mg) can be given sublingually to assess for a concurrent fall in systemic BP, which may prohibit use of longer-acting formulations. Diuretics are not recommended in the treatment of HAPE.

References

1. Mellor A (Ed). Medicine and physiology at high altitude. *J Roy Army Med Corps Sp Edn*. 2011;157(1):5–126.
2. Roach RC, Bartsch P, Oelz O, et al. The Lake Louise AMS Scoring Consensus Committee. The Lake Louise Acute Mountain Sickness Scoring System. In: Sutton JR, Houston CS, Coates G (Eds). *Hypoxia and Molecular Medicine*. Burlington: Charles S Houston, 1993.
3. Luks AM, McIntosh SE, Grissom CK, et al. Wilderness Medical Society Practice Guidelines for the Prevention and Treatment of Acute Altitude Illness: 2014 Update. *Wilderness Environ Med*. 2014;25:S4–14.
4. Imray C, Booth A, Wright A, Bradwell A. Acute altitude illnesses. *Br Med J*. 2011;343:411–17.

Decompression

Pathophysiology

Decompression describes a reduction in environmental pressure. Underwater divers are subject to decompression when they ascend towards the surface. Pilots and their passengers can also experience decompression in aircraft that attain high altitude, although cabin space is often pressurised. At sea level, nitrogen is dissolved in the blood at a partial pressure of 570 mmHg. With rapid ascent, bubbles of gas form in the tissues and blood vessels as local pressure is exceeded by the sum of dissolved gas and water vapour tension. Divers inspire high pressure inert nitrogen (or helium) in an environment that is itself hyperbaric. This may lead to supersaturation of the body if the rate of washout of gases from the tissues is exceeded by the rate of decompression (1).

Aviators and divers suffer decompression illness when gas bubbles embolise from the venous circulation or alveoli, via pulmonary blood vessels or cardiac shunts, to the arterial system (arterial gas embolism), or when bubbles form within tissues (decompression sickness). The incidence of decompression illness from both diving and aviation is held to be less than 0.1% per exposure and arterial gas embolism is mostly seen in the hyperbaric (i.e. underwater) setting. Venous gas bubbles may form with underwater descent to just 3 m depth, whereas tissue bubbles tend to form below a threshold of 6m and require 1–3 days of saturation diving. Likewise, the threshold on rapid ascent to high altitude is less for intravascular bubbles (around 3600 m up from sea level) than for extravascular (5500 m ascent).

Decompression sickness can manifest as pruritus and pain affecting the soft tissues and joints. Neurological effects may mimic stroke and ischaemia-reperfusion injury is possible. The brain is the organ most commonly affected by arterial gas embolism and patent foramen ovale, which is present in up to a quarter of the general population, increases the risk of neurological sequelae. Cardiovascular collapse may occur from direct endothelial effects and from gas embolisation to the coronary arteries, which may be fatal. Arterial gas embolism may also be seen iatrogenically, e.g. in relation to vascular catheters.

Treatment of decompression illness

Symptoms may develop up to 24 hours after surfacing from a dive and it is recommended that treatment is sought as early as possible. IV fluids will be required in cases of shock or dehydration. O_2 is delivered to all affected individuals for several hours, regardless of symptom resolution, in order to wash out inert gases (nitrogen, helium) from the lungs. This increases the tissue-alveolus gradient for the gas and increases the rate of removal of bubbles, in addition to diminishing tissue hypoxia caused by bubble formation. 100% O_2 is continued during recompression, which is the definitive treatment. This is conducted in a hyperbaric oxygen facility, to which the casualty should be transported as soon as possible, taking care to maintain ambient pressure in transit (e.g. cabin pressure at 1 surface atmosphere in-flight). Cases that appear milder on initial presentation may not require immediate recompression, but should be observed closely for deterioration. Several recompression cycles may be required in more severe cases and residual neurological deficit may persist. Overall, outcome for treated cases is good.

Reference

1. Vann RD, Butler FK, Mitchell SJ, Moon RE. Decompression illness. *Lancet*. 2011;8(377):153.

Electrical injuries and drowning

Younger adults are at greater risk of accidental injuries such as electrocution and drowning.

Electrical injuries

Electrical injuries tend to occur in the workplace, although around 1000 deaths a year are caused by lightning strikes. The pattern of injury relates to the tissues affected (Table 24.6) and nature of the electrical current, which may be either direct current (DC) or alternating current (AC).

Electrical shocks may be classified as high voltage (>1000 V) or low voltage (<1000 V). Electrical energy is converted to heat as it passes through the body, resulting in burns to tissues and thermal injury to cells (1). Cellular injury also occurs from the creation of a high strength electrical field, with the formation of pores in the cell wall (*electroporation*). Wet skin has less resistance to electrical current than dry skin, increasing the risk of injury. Tetany can result from AC and may 'lock' the victim to the electrical source for an extended period. In high-voltage electrical injury, respiratory arrest from temporary muscular paralysis is more likely. A transthoracic current ('hand-to-hand' pathway) traverses the mediastinum and is more often fatal than a hand-to-foot pathway. Where an explosive shock is delivered, such as in a lightning strike (DC), traumatic injuries may also occur.

Table 24.6 Electrical injuries by affected organ/tissue

Affected organ/tissues	Effects
Heart	Asystolic arrest (more common from DC, e.g. lightning strike). 'R-on-T'-type phenomenon and VF arrest. Ventricular arrhythmias (up to 12 hours after shock). Conduction abnormalities (temporary and long-term). Takotsubo cardiomyopathy (one case report).
Chest wall	Respiratory arrest (tetany from alternating current, paralysis).
Brain	Haemorrhage, oedema, neuronal injury. Respiratory arrest (suppression of respiratory centre in medulla). Neuropsychological impairment (may be long-term).
Sympathoadrenal system	Tachycardia, hypertension, dysrrhythmias and MI (catecholamine release).
Musculoskeletal	Rhabdomyolysis, muscle stricture (including sphincters). Large joint dislocations. Bony fractures (due to loss of consciousness and collapse or explosive force of lightning strike).
Deep soft tissues	Compartment syndrome.

DC = Direct Current; VF = ventricular fibrillation; MI = myocardial infarction.

Lightning strike victims do not carry residual electrical charge and can be resuscitated immediately if the scene is safe (2). Victims of other electrical injuries should be isolated from ongoing electrical threat and moved to a safe environment. Casualties may have fixed and dilated pupils due to autonomic dysfunction, so this sign should not guide decisions to attempt/continue resuscitation. Resuscitation proceeds in a standard format, with the following caveats:

1. Early intubation may be required if airway burns are suspected.
2. Ventilatory support may be required for several hours until muscular paralysis resolves.
3. A secondary, trauma-focused survey should be conducted after explosive shocks.
4. Give IV fluids to maintain a good urine output in extensive tissue injury.
5. If the pathway of current was long (e.g. shoulder-to-foot), there should be a high index of suspicion for severe deep tissue injuries, even if wounds appear relatively minor at the skin.
6. Early surgical intervention, including fasciotomy, should be considered in severe injuries.

In those patients with elevated CK, higher levels are associated with increased requirement for extremity amputation. Mortality is increased in patients who have suffered primary organ damage (myocardial necrosis, significant CNS injury, severe burns) or develop secondary multi-organ failure.

Drowning

Drowning is a more common cause of accidental death (3). It has been defined as respiratory impairment due to submersion/immersion in a liquid medium, covering the face and airway. Alcohol or drug abuse is implicated in up to half of all adult cases. Existing medical problems such as syncope, epilepsy and cardiovascular disease may be contributory. Initial breath holding is usually followed by gulping of liquid. Aspiration then occurs with a period of uncontrolled respiration. Salt water collects in the alveolar space and impairs O_2 transfer, while fresh water crosses the lung membrane, flushing surfactant with it and leading to alveolar collapse. The resulting hypoxia eventually causes a cardiac arrest. Other complications, sequelae and associated conditions are shown in Box 24.7.

The duration of hypoxia and the temperature of the liquid medium are the key determinants of outcome; although cases of survival with full neurological recovery have been reported in children and petite females despite submersion for an hour or longer. Prehospital resuscitation is started/continued if known submersion time is less than 90 minutes, unless futility is clearly evident (e.g. unsurvivable trauma, rigor mortis) (4). Prompt initiation of ventilation improves survival, in association with standard resuscitation protocols, which may be modified to account for hypothermia.

Box 24.7 Complications of drowning

- Pulmonary oedema.
- Pneumonia.
- Acute respiratory distress syndrome (ARDS).
- Raised intracranial pressure and cerebral oedema.
- Hypothermia.

Regurgitated water/material will need to be suctioned from the airway where ventilation is impeded. Spinal immobilisation is required if trauma is suspected. High flow O_2 should be administered and may be augmented with non-invasive or mechanical ventilation if improvement in oxygenation is not demonstrated. Prophylactic antibiotics may be considered if the victim was submerged in grossly contaminated liquid, e.g. sewage. Survivors should be assessed for family history of sudden cardiac death and screened for arrhythmias and other causes of syncope.

References

1. Spies C, Trohman RG. Narrative review: electrocution and life threatening injuries. *Ann Intern Med*. 2006;145:531–7.
2. Wilderness Medical society practice guideline on prevention and treatment of lightning injuries: 2014 update. *Wilderness Environ Med*. 2014;25(4 Suppl):S86–95.
3. Szpilman D, Bierens JJ, Handley AJ, Orlowski JP. Drowning. *N Engl J Med*. 2014;366(22):2102–10.
4. Joint Royal Colleges Ambulance Liaison Committee. *UK Ambulance Services Clinical Practice Guidelines* 2013.

Bites and stings

Venomous bites and stings are rare in the UK. In certain areas of the world, they are a common cause of death and morbidity (1).

Snake bite

A large proportion of bites by venomous snakes fail to inject enough venom to cause clinical envenoming (so called 'dry bites'). Systemic envenomation caused by a snake bite can present in different ways depending on the species involved (2) and the clinical features can be divided according to the system involved:

Musculoskeletal

- Evidence of envenomation by swelling of more than half of the bitten limb and myotoxicity.
- Clinical effects include pain in the bitten limb, swelling, painful lymph nodes, wound blistering, necrosis and myotoxicity (with myalgia, trismus and myoglobinuria).
- Examples of species include: Viperadae, Elapidae, sea snakes and spider bites.

Haematological

- Envenomation leads to systemic bleeding.
- Clinically, patients may bleed from bite or wound sites, and/or present with gingival bleeding, haemoptysis or haematuria.
- Typically caused by Viperidae.

Neurological

- Envenomation causes neurotoxicity shown by a descending paralysis leading to bilateral ptosis, bulbar palsy and descending weakness.
- Commonly caused by Elapidae.

Renal

- Patients present with acute kidney injury.
- Occurs following sea snake and spider bites.

Autonomic nervous system

- Cholinergic effects, including hypersalivation, sweating, lacrimation, vomiting and diarrhoea.
- Adrenergic effects, including tachycardia, hyperglycaemia, hypertension.
- Often caused by scorpion stings and spider bites.

Cardiological

- Envenomation causes myocarditis with arrhythmias, cardiac failure and/or pulmonary oedema.
- Often due to scorpion stings and spider bites.

Scorpion stings

Stings from scorpions tend to occur at night and systemic envenomation is more common in children. The most striking symptom is severe local pain associated with the sting with minimal local signs such as swelling. Features of autonomic stimulation occur with early cholinergic effects (including hypersalivation, sweating, lacrimation, vomiting, hyperthermia) and later adrenergic effects (tachycardias, hyperglycaemia, toxic myocarditis with arrhythmias).

Spider bites

- More common in children.
- May cause local swelling and necrosis of the bitten area (like the recluse spider) or minimal signs of the initial bite.
- Systemic effects include automonic effects like hypersalivation, sweating, nausea and vomiting; cardiovascular effects and renal failure.

Marine envenomation

- Rare.
- Patients present with mixed symptoms and signs including:
    - Local effects of swelling, necrosis.
    - Systemic effects, including cardiovascular disturbance, renal failure.

Management of bites and stings

- Prevention by avoiding unnecessary contact with snakes, scorpions (3) or spiders (4).
- First aid involving (5):
    - Reassuring the patient.
    - Immobilising the patient and the bitten area.
    - Administering pressure immobilisation when appropriate (recommended particularly for Elapid bites).
    - Evacuation to hospital for an initial ABCDE assessment and resuscitation if required.
- In patients with suspected envenomation, a whole-blood clotting test (WBCT) (6) should be taken to assess for systemic bleeding. Following assessment, patients with symptoms or signs of envenomation (bleeding, shock, rhabdomyolysis, neurotoxicity, renal failure, bruising or swelling of more than half a limb) should be given antivenom specific to the species involved in the area where bitten. Antivenom specific to the likely species involved should be administered in a safe environment, monitoring for signs of anaphylaxis. Prophylactic adrenaline should be administered to prevent against the acute adverse reactions which occur when antivenom is given following a snake bite (7).

References

1. Warrell DA. Treatment of bites by adders and exotic venomous snakes. *Br Med J*. 2005;331:1244–7.
2. Wilkins D, et al. Snakebites in Africa and Europe: a military perspective and update for contemporary operations. *J R Army Med Corps*. 2018;164(5):370–9.
3. Chippaux JP. Emerging options for the management of scorpion stings. *Drug Des Devel Ther*. 2012;6:165–73.
4. Isbister GK, Fan HW. Spider bite. *Lancet*. 2011;378(9808):2039–47.
5. Sutherland SK, Coulter AR, Harris RD. Rationalisation of first-aid measures for elapid snakebite. *Lancet*. 1979;1(8109):183–5.
6. de Silva HA, Pathmeswaran A, Ranasinha CD, et al. Low-dose adrenaline, promethazine, and hydrocortisone in the prevention of acute adverse reactions to antivenom following snakebite: a randomised, double-blind, placebo-controlled trial. *PLoS Med*. 2011;8(5):e1000435.

Bioterrorism and epidemics

Anthrax

Anthrax is a zoonotic disease caused by spore-forming *Bacillus anthracis*. It is of concern as an agent of bioterrorism owing to the durability of infective spores in the environment and high mortality rates of inhalational disease despite treatment. Anthrax has three main clinical forms related to entry site of spores: cutaneous, inhalational and GI, although a fourth syndrome related to severe skin and soft tissue infections of IV drug users is emerging. Cutaneous disease accounts for 95% of naturally occurring cases via animal contact.

Diagnosis is defined by clinical presentation compatible with anthrax, isolation of *B. anthracis* and confirmation using serology or another supportive test like PCR.

Management of cases includes instigating appropriate infection control protocols and giving antimicrobial treatment (Table 24.7) (1). Adjunct therapies include anti-toxin immune-based therapies or drugs against toxin binding, processing or assembly. Post-exposure prophylaxis with ciprofloxacin or doxycycline is recommended if there is a risk of exposure to anthrax. There is an anthrax vaccine available in the UK that is administered, on occupational health grounds, to select laboratory, veterinary and military personnel.

Table 24.7 Anthrax clinical syndromes

Syndrome	Entry site	Clinical presentation	Management
Cutaneous anthrax	Spores enter skin.	Swelling, oedema, bullae formation, haemorrhagic vesicles and eschar. Fever and lymphadenopathy.	Ciprofloxacin 500 mg BD or doxycycline 100 mg BD for 60 days.
Gastrointestinal anthrax	Spores are ingested from contaminated meat.	Leads to oropharygneal (ulcers, fever and lymphadenopathy) and intestinal disease (nausea and vomiting, ulcers, shock, ascites).	Ciprofloxacin 400 mg TDS or doxycycline 100 mg BD or benzylpenicillin G 4 MU QDS or rifampicin 300 mg BD ≥60 days therapy. Antitoxin (recombinant monoclonal antibody or human polyclonal serum). Steroids for meningitis or severe oedema.
Inhalational anthrax	Spores inhaled (animal workers/ bioterrorism).	Fever, cough, pleural effusions and widened mediastinum on chest X-ray. Raised haematocrit (particularly in sepsis).	
Injectional anthrax	SC drug injection.	Oedema. Eschar rarely seen. Local soft tissue infection.	

Plague

- Natural infection of rodents, and less commonly other wild and domesticated mammals, caused by *Yersina pestis*.
- Endemic in globally distributed rural areas with 3000 cases reported per year.

- Most commonly transmitted to humans by rodent flea bites (oriental rat flea, *Xenopyslla cheopis*); direct contact and aerosol transmission from both infected animals and humans are also recognised.
- May be used as a biothreat agent.
- Four main clinical forms: bubonic, pneumonic, meningitic and septicaemic:
  - Pneumonic plague is rare, but highly transmissible with 50% mortality rate despite appropriate antimicrobial therapy within the first 24 hours.
  - Bubonic plague consists of fever and acute lymphadenitis.
- Diagnosis is made by culture of the organism, serology or by PCR methods.
- Management involves barrier nursing, respiratory isolation of patients and administration of antimicrobials (2).
- Gentamicin or streptomycin monotherapy represents first line treatment; ciprofloxacin or doxycycline are alternative agents; chloramphenicol is indicated for meningitis as it readily crosses the blood–brain barrier.
- Currently, no vaccine exists, but there are promising preclinical data.
- Post-exposure prophylaxis of face-to-face contacts is warranted.

Emerging diseases

Pandemic flu

Pandemic or 'swine' flu caused by influenza H1N1 emerged in Mexico in 2009. The virus was highly transmissible and within a month had spread globally to Europe and Asia and a pandemic was declared on 11 June 2009. Flu is diagnosed using molecular methods by real-time PCR. Treatment with neuraminidase inhibitors, oseltamivir (Tamiflu®) and zanamivir (Relenza™) is recommended. A vaccine has been produced for at-risk groups (elderly, pregnancy and people with chronic diseases) and is included in seasonal flu vaccines. The WHO declared the end of the pandemic in August 2010, and fortunately the virus was less virulent than expected and overall mortality rates were lower than anticipated.

Severe adult respiratory syndrome

Severe adult respiratory syndrome (SARS) was first reported in China in 2003 (3). It is caused by a novel coronavirus, SARS-CoV-1. SARS is a life-threatening atypical pneumonia, and its clinical course including progression and laboratory features are summarised in Table 24.8. The guidelines produced by the British Thoracic Society, British Infection Association and Public Health England on the management of patients with suspected SARS advocate steroids in patients with respiratory compromise and comment on the lack of evidence for the use of ribavirin and interferon (4). Current research is aimed at vaccine production, and the use of other agents like monoclonal antibodies and enzyme inhibitors.

Table 24.8 Clinical course, progression and laboratory features of SARS

Time	Clinical features	Laboratory findings
Onset	Fever, chills, dry cough, diarrhoea.	Lymphopenia. Raised LDH. Normal chest X-ray.
Week 1	Pneumonia.	Respiratory secretions, urine and stool positive for CoV-SARS (real time PCR). Consolidation on chest X-ray and CT.
Week 2	Improvement (75%) or reoccurrence of fever and deterioration (25%) leading to death.	Severe immunopathology leading to lung damage leads to death with acute respiratory distress syndrome (ARDS) on chest X-ray and CT.
Week 3 onwards	Gradual recovery (>80%) or death (8–15%).	SARS-CoV-1 can be detected in respiratory secretions, stool and urine even after recovery.

Middle East respiratory syndrome

This lethal respiratory disease was first isolated from a patient who died from a severe respiratory illness in 2012 in Saudi Arabia. It causes a range of clinical features from asymptomatic or mild disease to acute respiratory distress syndrome and multi-organ failure (5). Most cases have occurred in Saudi Arabia and the United Arab Emirates, but there have been cases in Europe, the USA and Asia. Dromedary camels are hosts and implicated in direct or indirect transmission to human beings. There is no specific drug treatment; infection prevention and control measures are crucial to prevent spread. Mutation increases its pandemic potential (5).

West African Ebola epidemic

The 2014 Ebola epidemic is the largest and most devastating in history, affecting multiple countries in West Africa particularly Sierra Leone, Liberia and New Guinea. Previously reported in sub-Saharan Africa in 1976, this recent outbreak has case fatality rates of nearly 70% in certain areas. This is the first outbreak to reach epidemic proportions, affecting global health security and involved a worldwide response, and was declared in August 2014 as a public health emergency of international concern (6). Although rates of infection have decreased dramatically, Ebola virus disease has not disappeared and communities throughout West Africa continue to report new cases (➲ see Chapter 8, Viral haemorrhagic fevers, p. 266 and Table 8.31).

COVID-19

At the end of 2019 a novel disease emerged in Wuhan, China. This was shown to represent infection by a coronavirus sharing 79.6% of its genome and a common portal of cell entry (the ACE2 receptor) with SARS-CoV-1 (7). The second coronavirus known to cause SARS in humans, SARS-CoV-2 causes the clinical illness COVID-19 and has spread rapidly across the globe, with widespread transmission occurring in many countries. A pandemic was declared on 11 March 2020. The novelty of this virus meant that, at the time of writing, knowledge of its transmission, clinical features, treatment and long-term consequences is incomplete.

Typical symptoms used for the purposes of dynamic case identification have included fever, cough, shortness of breath and anosmia. Select other features may be shared with those reported in the 2003 SARS outbreak (see Table 24.8). Increased tendency to VTE has been reported with both coronavirus infections, possibly secondary to blood changes in inflammatory and coagulation parameters and/or polyangiitis from direct vessel wall damage (8,9), although many affected patients have additional risk factors for VTE (advanced age, obesity, immobility) and mechanisms specific to SARS-CoV-2 are yet to be elucidated.

Compared with SARS-CoV-1, increased transmissibility may relate to differences in the temporal distribution and load of SARS-CoV-2 in the respiratory tract during early infection. A reduced proportion of infected individuals developing incapacitating illness or death and, therefore, continuing to come into contact with immune-naïve individuals may also account for relatively increased viral spread. Early evidence pointed to asymptomatic infection playing a role in rapid propagation of the infection and undermining counter-measures to track/trace and isolate infective cases (10). As with SARS-CoV-1, there is a general lack of specific treatments and research efforts have been focused on diagnostics, vaccine development and clinical trials of agents with therapeutic potential.

References

1. CDC Anthrax guidance https://wwwnc.cdc.gov/eid/article/20/2/13-0687_article.
2. Bossi P, Tegnell A, Baka A, van Loock F. Bichat guidelines for the clinical management of plague and bioterrorism-related plague. *Euro Surveill*. 2004; 9(12):E5–6.
3. Wong GW, Hui DS. Severe acute respiratory syndrome (SARS): epidemiology, diagnosis and management. *Thorax*. 2003;58(7):558–60.
4. Lange JH. BIS/BTS SARS guidelines. *Thorax*. 2004;59(8):726–7.
5. Zulma A, Hui DS, Perlman S. Middle East respiratory syndrome. *Lancet*. 2015; 386(9997):P997–1007. https://www.thelancet.com/journals/lancet/article/PIIS0140-6736(15)60454-8/fulltext
6. Heymann DL, Chen L, Takemi K. Global Health Security: the wider lessons from the West African Ebola virus disease epidemic. *Lancet*. 2015;385:1884–901.

7. Zhou P, et al. A pneumonia outbreak associated with a new coronavirus of probable bat origin. Nature. 2020;579:270–3.
8. Xiang-hua Yi, et al. Severe acute respiratory syndrome and venous thromboembolism in multiple organs. Am J Respir Crit Care Med. 2010;182:436–7.
9. Ackermann M, et al. Pulmonary vascular endothelialitis, thrombosis and angiogenesis in Covid-19. NEJM 2020; 21 May. doi:10.1056/NEJMoa2015432.
10. Gandhi M, Yokoe DS, Havlir DV. Asymptomatic transmission, the Achilles' heel of current strategies to control Covid-19. NEJM 2020;382:2158–60.

Acknowledgements

The editors and contributors are grateful to Paul Savage (OCE BSc UK Search and Rescue) for his kind commentary on drowning and resuscitation.

Multiple choice questions

Questions

1. You are the expedition doctor for a commercial trek, taking non-mountaineers to Everest base camp. A 42-year-old male member of the party collapses at 4300 m altitude on day 6 of the high altitude section of the trek, in good weather conditions. He has no significant past medication and is taking no regular or prophylactic medication. He was complaining of headache and loss of appetite at breakfast. Rapid structured clinical assessment demonstrates:

   Airway: patent.
   Breathing: laboured, respiratory rate 30, bibasal pulmonary crackles.
   Circulation: pulse rate 120, regular rhythm, good volume on palpation of the radial artery and centrally.
   Disability: GCS 12 (E3,V3,M6), no facial asymmetry or gross sensory/motor deficit elicited.

   Which of the following should *not* be undertaken as part of his further management?

   A. Check of capillary blood glucose with a portable glucometer.
   B. Transfer by stretcher to the medical station at the top of the valley (4400 m elevation, 1 hour away) for further assessment and treatment, including supplementary oxygen.
   C. Intramuscular dexamethasone injection.
   D. Decent to a mountain shelter at 4200 m with access to a helicopter landing site, a 60-minute trek back down the valley.
   E. Assigning a member of the expedition party to observe the casualty and ensure that he is kept warm, while evacuation is co-ordinated in the immediate vicinity by you and the expedition leader.

2. Which of the following is essential to the diagnosis of heat stroke in secondary care?

   A. High environmental temperature.
   B. Elevated rectal temperature.
   C. History of heat cramps.
   D. Eliciting a compatible history and having a low threshold of clinical suspicion.
   E. Patient unacclimatised to environmental conditions.

3. On a recreational walk in the countryside, you encounter a prone casualty, collapsed near overhead power lines. A fishing-rod is on the ground nearby and you suspect high voltage electrical injury. It is safe to approach and you start a primary survey. He is in cardiac arrest. You commence CPR, while your companion arranges emergency transfer to hospital.

Which of the following features should *not* be used to prognosticate during the course of further prehospital and inpatient/specialist care:

A. Extensive severe burns.
B. Fixed dilated pupils during initial resuscitation attempts.
C. Severe brain injury identified on arrival in the Emergency Department.
D. Biochemical and echocardiographic evidence of myocardial necrosis.
E. Development of multiple organ system failure on the Intensive Care Unit.

4. You are a doctor supporting a charity working in a remote area of East Africa with limited medical supplies, but which does include antivenom. A 23-year-old UK student working in a local school comes into your clinic feeling nauseous and weak following a walk to the school through the scrubland, where he feels he may have been bitten by something. He is otherwise fit and well. Initial assessment of the patient includes:

   Airway: patent.
   Breathing: chest clear, RR = 20, sats = 99% on room air.
   Circulation: HR = 100, BP = 110/60, capillary refill time = 2 s.
   Disability: GCS 15/15, PERL bilaterally, no signs of ptosis or opthalmoplegia, BM 5.
   Exposure: small puncture marks at the left ankle; neurological examination reveals global weakness (4+/5).

   Which of the following should *not* be part of your initial management?

   A. Immobilisation of the bitten area including pressure immobilisation.
   B. Evacuation to a hospital.
   C. Antivenom.
   D. WBCT 20 test.
   E. Consideration of tetanus prophylaxis.

5. A young farmer presents with a 3 × 3-cm ulcerating lesion on his left arm with surrounding oedema and cellulitis. He is afebrile and otherwise well. The diagnosis of cutaneous *Bacillus anthracis* is most likely confirmed by:

   A. Repeat blood cultures.
   B. Serology.
   C. Histological examination of a biopsy of the lesion.
   D. Combination of clinical presentation, culture of organism through biopsy and serology or PCR.
   E. Molecular methods like PCR.

Answers

1. B. Descent is imperative in all cases of severe acute altitude illness; 1000 m or more may be necessary and descent to an altitude below that where symptoms began is ideal (➲ see Treatment of high altitude illnesses, p. 829).
2. D. Core body temperature, measured rectally, may have fallen by the time of presentation to secondary care or if medical assessment is delayed, so the history of exposure and high index of clinical suspicion are required for diagnosis (➲ see Heat-related illnesses, p. 821 and Box 24.2).
3. B. Victims may have fixed and dilated pupils due to autonomic dysfunction, so this sign should not guide decisions to attempt/continue resuscitation (➲ see Electrical injuries, p. 830).
4. C. Antivenom should only be administered in an environment with adequate resuscitation facilities (incorporating airway support) to monitor for signs for anaphylaxis treatment and it is recommended that patients are prophylactically treated with adrenaline. Indications for antivenom include systemic bleeding, signs of neurotoxicity, swelling of the bitten limb, renal failure and rhabdomyolysis (➲ see Management of bites and stings, p. 833).
5. D. CDC (Centre for Disease Control, USA) advises that a diagnosis of anthrax is confirmed by a combination of clinical features suggestive of anthrax with culture of the organism and serology/or positive PCR (➲ see Anthrax, p. 834).

Chapter 25 Epidemiology and Public Health

Cordelia E.M. Coltart and Alan Maryon-Davis

Public health

Public health and globalisation

Public health can be defined as 'the science and art of preventing disease, prolonging life and promoting health through the organised efforts and informed choices of society, organisations, public and private communities and individuals' (1). Public health relates to health systems and entire populations, rather than to individual patients or specific disease approaches, which are the day-to-day focus of physicians.

Public health is an interdisciplinary field incorporating epidemiology, biostatistics, health services studies, health economics, public policy, environmental health, community health, behavioural health and occupational health. It encompasses three broad areas:

1. The assessment and monitoring of the health of communities and populations to identify health problems and priorities.
2. The formulation of public policies designed to solve and address identified local and national health problems and priorities.
3. The implementation of policies to ensure that all populations have access to appropriate and cost-effective care, including health promotion and disease prevention services.

Globalisation has led to an increasingly mobile world population importing, exporting and spreading diseases across regions, borders and continents. Both the 2013–2016 Ebola epidemic and the 2009 influenza pandemic demonstrated how the rapid global spread of a disease may pose a real global health risk. Modern travel allows individuals to circumnavigate the world in time periods that are shorter than the incubation period for almost all infectious pathogens. For this reason, most countries rely on the health surveillance, control and reporting of other countries to recognise, report and reduce the spread of diseases. A coordinated international effort through the International Health Regulations (2005) of the WHO has been set up for this particular purpose (2).

References

1. Department of Health. Public health in England (the Acheson report). London: HMSO, 1988.
2. WHO. International Health Regulations. Strengthening health security by implementing the International Health Regulations. Geneva: WHO, 2005. http://www.who.int/ihr/publications/9789241596664/en/.

Global mortality

In recent decades, significant progress has been made in improving the health and survival of the world's population. Overall life expectancy at birth globally has risen from 48 years in 1950–1955 to 68 years in 2005–2010. However, there remains substantial variation in life expectancy, and cause of death at both national and regional levels (Table 25.1). In low-income countries less than one-fifth (17%) of the population live to 70 years. These deaths remain primarily due to infectious diseases: lung infections, diarrhoeal disease, HIV/AIDS, TB and malaria. This is a pattern that was seen in the UK and other developed countries in decades past. However, with advances in medicine, in high-income countries nearly three-quarters (71%) of the population now live beyond 70 and the predominant cause of death is chronic diseases: cardiovascular, chronic lung disease, cancers, dementia and diabetes. The only persisting 'infectious' cause of death is lung infection. In contrast, the newer classification of 'middle-income countries' lie somewhere between these two extremes, where nearly half of the population live to the age of 70, and both chronic diseases and infectious diseases are leading causes of death.

Table 25.1 Variation in the top 10 causes of mortality: globally, in low-income countries and in the UK (male versus female)

World (million deaths/year)*	Low income countries (deaths per 100,000 population/ year)*	UK males (deaths per 100,000 population/ year)**	UK females (deaths per 100,000 population/year)**
Ischaemic heart disease (IHD) (7.4)	Lower respiratory infections (91)	IHD (992)	IHD (434)
Cerebrovascular disease (6.7)	HIV/AIDS (65)	Lung cancer (457)	Dementia (including Alzheimer's) (338)
Lower respiratory infections (3.1)	Diarrhoeal diseases (53)	Cerebrovascular disease (357)	Cerebrovascular disease (331)
COPD (3.1)	Cerebrovascular diseases (52)	Chronic lower respiratory disease (340)	Influenza and pneumonia (217)
Lung cancers (trachea, bronchus or lung) (1.6)	IHD (39)	Dementia (including Alzheimer's) (279)	Lung cancer (298)
Diarrhoeal diseases (1.5)	Malaria (35)	Influenza and pneumonia (273)	Chronic lower respiratory disease (241)
HIV/AIDS (1.5)	Prematurity and low birth weight (33)	Prostate cancer (238)	Breast cancer (244)
Diabetes mellitus (1.3)	Tuberculosis (31)	Colorectal cancer (203)	Colorectal cancer (127)
Road traffic accidents (1.3)	Birth asphyxia and birth trauma (29)	Haematological malignancy (163)	Urinary disease (118)
Hypertensive heart disease (1.1)	Protein energy malnutrition (27)	Liver disease (157)	Haematological malignancy (104)

*WHO. The top 10 causes of death. http://who.int/mediacentre/factsheets/fs310/en.
** ONS. Deaths Registered in England and Wales (Series DR), 2011. http://www.ons.gov.uk/ons/dcp171778_284566.pdf
Data from Global Health Estimates 2016: Deaths by Cause, Age, Sex, by Country and by Region, 2000-2016. Geneva, World Health Organization; 2018. Available at: http://who.int/mediacentre/factsheets/fs310/en/
Data from Office for National Statistics (2012). Deaths registered in England and Wales (series DR) 2011. [online] Available at: http://www.ons.gov.uk/ons/dcp171778_284566.pdf [Accessed 21 Mar. 2019].

These striking disparities also persist in childhood mortality rates (i.e. death before 15 years of age) with 99% occurring in low- and middle-income countries. In low-income countries over one-third of the population (40%) die before their 15th birthday, in stark contrast to 1% in high-income countries.

The differences in morbidity and mortality across countries and regions reflect marked inequities in access to basic human necessities: food, safe drinking water, sanitation and health care. These disparities are compounded by local socioeconomic factors, for example, different health-seeking behaviours between ethnic groups.

International efforts to reduce the morbidity and mortality of the world's poorest populations were targeted in the United Nations (UN) eight Millennium Development Goals, addressing issues including reducing child and maternal mortality, reducing global poverty and hunger, improving water and sanitation, providing universal primary education and promoting gender equality by the target date of 2015. Unfortunately, many of these goals were not met. In recent years, attention has also shifted towards the challenge of non-communicable diseases (such as cardiovascular disease, cancers, respiratory diseases and diabetes).

Further reading

1. WHO. Top ten causes of death: http://who.int/mediacentre/factsheets/fs310/en.
2. United Nations. Millennium Development Goals and Beyond 2015. http://www.un.org/millenniumgoals.

Epidemiology

Epidemiology is defined as 'the study of the distribution and determinants of health-related states or events in specified populations and the application of this study to the control of health problems' (1).

In simpler terms, epidemiology is the study of disease in populations, with the aim of improving disease control.

For why to study epidemiology, see Box 25.1.

Box 25.1 Why study epidemiology?

Epidemiology is used to address the following issues:

- To quantify human health problems:
  - Describe the distribution of diseases, e.g. how much of disease '*x*' is there in the UK?
  - Is the incidence of disease *x* increasing or decreasing?
- To identify the natural history and aetiology of diseases:
  - What are the risk factors for acquiring disease *x*?
  - What happens to people affected by disease *x*?
  - Why do some people get disease *x* more than others?
- To inform clinical and public health recommendations:
  - What is the best test for disease *x*?
  - What is the best treatment for disease *x*?
  - What is the best intervention to prevent disease *x*?

In simpler terms:Who gets disease *x*, when do they get it, where do they get it and why?

References

1. Last JM, (Ed.) *Dictionary of Epidemiology*, 4th edn. New York: Oxford University Press, 2001.

Epidemiological studies

As discussed in ➲ Chapter 26, Research design and sampling, p. 857, Figures 26.1, 26.2, 26.3 and Table 26.1, the choice of study depends on the research question(s), funding, available resources, and what is both ethically and practically possible. Every study has its strengths and limitations, and the resulting data must be interpreted with these in mind and in relation to other existing data, i.e. the totality of evidence.

Epidemiological studies can be descriptive or analytic studies (see Table 25.2). Descriptive studies look at the distribution of diseases: who gets the disease and when they get it. Analytic studies evaluate the determinants of disease acquisition – why people get certain diseases and how they get them. Descriptive studies are often used to formulate a hypothesis that can be later tested by an analytic study.

Table 25.2 Description and examples of each study design

Type of study		Examples	Pros/cons
Descriptive studies			
Correlational study (or ecologic)	Uses population level data to compare disease frequency across populations during a specified time period or within the same population at different times.	The 10-yearly census survey.	Evaluates populations and not individuals. High likelihood of confounding by other variables. Evaluates averages.
Case reports	Detailed report of an individual patient, evaluating factors that could be related to the disease. The most basic type of descriptive study.	Detailed case history of a case of Lassa fever.	No controls/comparison groups.
Case series	As above, but includes a series (>1) of patients.	Comparison of >1 cases of Lassa fever – to compare clinical parameters.	
Cross-sectional studies/survey	Takes simultaneous data on exposure and outcome of individuals assessed, i.e. a snapshot in time.	Framingham study.	Pro: efficient in terms of time and money. No evaluation of the time course of events.
Analytic studies			
Observational			
Case control studies	Selection into the study is based on disease status with retrospective evaluation into past for exposure history.	A study of sauna use and the risk of miscarriage: women who miscarry are compared with women who have a live born infant and all interviewed to assess whether they used saunas during pregnancy.	Pro: Efficient in terms of time and money. Good for long latent periods (as disease already occurred). Can evaluate multiple risk factors for a single disease (e.g. for CVD – smoking, exercise, diet). Cons: Often retrospective, so difficult to get accurate exposure data as rely on patient memory/recall.
Cohort studies	Selection into study is based on exposure status and prospective follow-up to evaluate disease outcome.	Cohort exposed to nuclear radiation and a similar cohort not exposed to radiation are followed up to determine the incidence rate of thyroid cancer.	Pros: Accurate exposure date. Can evaluate temporal relationship. Can evaluate multiple outcomes from a single exposure, e.g. for smoking – CVD, CVA, lung cancer etc. Cons: high cost. Time intensive (especially if a long latent period). High rate of loss-to-follow-up as subjects need to be followed up for a long time.
Interventional studies			
Randomised controlled trials	A type of prospective cohort study where the exposure is allocated by investigator and followed-up to evaluate disease outcome.	Drug trials comparing drug with placebo, where participants are randomly assigned to the two groups with identical follow-up.	Pros: controls for comparison. Can control confounding. Cons: high cost. Difficulty with patient compliance.

Disease patterns and measures of disease frequency

There are many measures to describe diseases within a population. The simplest measure of disease is to state the number of occurrences of a specific condition, e.g. 'there have been 10 reported cases of Creutzfeldt-Jakob disease'. However, this does not specify the period of time over which these cases occurred or the size of the population in which they occurred. It is, therefore, impossible to know if this number of cases is in excess of that which would normally be expected. It is essential to consider the time period and denominator (size of population) when describing disease frequency.

$$\text{Frequency} = \frac{\text{Number of cases of disease 'x' in a specified time period}}{\text{Total population}}$$

Measure of frequency falls into two types:

1. *Prevalence* = the number of cases of disease in a defined population *at a given point in time* (often known as point prevalence).

$$\text{Prevalence} = \frac{\text{Number of people with disease 'x' at a specific time point} \times 100}{\text{Total population (diseased and non-diseased)}}$$

Of note, the point in time can be a specified date, e.g. January 1st, 2020 or a life event (e.g. birth, autopsy, etc.). Therefore, diseases identified by autopsy and birth defects are included in prevalence rates as it is impossible to know when these diseases developed, but they are present at a specific moment in time e.g. autopsy or birth respectively.

2. *Incidence* = the number of *new* cases in a defined population over a *specified period of time* (i.e. are disease-free at baseline, but develop the disease during the reporting period). This includes mortality rates.

There are many terms used to express incidence, e.g. 'cumulative incidence' and 'incidence rate'. The difference is related to how the incidence is calculated due to different ways of calculating the denominator, e.g. in some studies not all individuals are followed for the same time period, but the data obtained before the patient left the study (for example, due to death, or reaching a specified end-point in the study, or loss-to-follow-up) can still be used with more complex calculations.

$$\text{Incidence} = \frac{\text{Number of new cases developing in a specified time period}}{\text{Total individuals at risk}^{1}}$$

Prevalence and incidence are usually expressed in percentage form, but they can be presented in decimal form, e.g. 17.3% or 0.173, or a number of cases per 100, per 1000 or per 100,000 population (depending on the rarity of the disease).

For a worked example, see Box 25.2.

Prevalence is usually described in cross-sectional studies, whereas incidence is the measure in cohort or interventional studies. Incidence can provide an estimate of the probability that an individual will develop a disease over a certain period of time.

Prevalence and incidence are interlinked, and the number of new cases of a disease at any given time (P) depends upon the rate at which new cases of the disease occur (I) and how long the disease lasts (duration, D). Therefore, prevalence is proportional to the incidence and average duration of disease:

$$P \propto ID$$

under steady state, with no epidemics and no new medical breakthroughs.

[1] This may represent the whole population for some diseases, but in other situations patients should be excluded if they are not at risk, e.g. vaccinated individuals are not at risk of polio, and women who have had a hysterectomy are not at risk of endometrial carcinoma and should, therefore, be excluded from the denominator for incidence calculations relating to these respective diseases.

Box 25.2 Worked example

A nuclear power plant in St. Elsewhere has a severe nuclear leak on 1st January 2090. The local public health physician decides to follow-up the children living in St. Elsewhere to see if there is an increased rate of lymphoma (a chronic, non-fatal condition). The children are followed up for 10 years.

On 1st January 2099, 1500 children lived in St. Elsewhere, of which 13 already had lymphoma before the nuclear leak. Between 1st January 2090 and 31st December 2099, 33 children developed lymphoma.

1. What is the prevalence of lymphoma (%) on 1st January 2090?
2. What is the 10-year incidence (%) of lymphoma?
3. What is the prevalence (%) of lymphoma on 31st December 2099 in the children originally exposed?
4. What assumption do you make in order to calculate the answer to number 3 above?

Answers:

1. $13/1500 \times 100 = 0.87\%$.
2. $33/(1500–13) \times 100 = 2.2\%$.
3. $(33 + 13)/1500 \times 100 = 3\%$.
4. Assuming no children die in this 10-year period.

Therefore, if the incidence is high, but people die from the disease quickly, the prevalence will be low, e.g. the influenza pandemic in 1918. However, if the incidence is low but the disease chronic, the prevalence will be high as numbers accumulate e.g. diabetes mellitus or HIV. Similarly, the introduction of a new medication that increases survival but does not cure the disease will lead to an increase in prevalence.

Screening

The UK National Screening Committee defines screening as 'a process of identifying apparently healthy people who may be at increased risk of a disease or condition. They can then be offered information, further tests and appropriate treatment to reduce their risk and/or any complications arising from the disease or condition'.

Screening has the potential to save thousands of lives. The UK has a number of national screening programmes, which differ between the devolved states (England, Scotland and Wales). For current screening programmes in England, see Table 25.3.

There are a number of reasons why it is not possible to screen for every eventuality: there may be no suitable test, there may be no treatment, screening may not be cost effective, and the disease may not be amenable to screening, i.e. there may be no preclinical asymptomatic phase (by definition, screening detects those at risk of developing the disease who are asymptomatic, not those with early symptoms).

For criteria for designing a good screening test, see Box 25.3.

How to counsel a patient on the benefits and risks of screening

As with any medical encounter the screening process involves informed consent. Conceptually, this can be harder for health-care professionals and patients to grasp, as it involves consenting asymptomatic people around potential future threats, which may or may not happen following a positive test. Although the threats may not seem real at the times of screening, people participating in screening need to understand the inherent advantages and disadvantages of the process.

Key issues for counselling a patient for screening are outlined in Box 25.4.

Calculating how good a screening test is

When evaluating a screening test, it is important to know how good it is – how many cases does it miss and how often is the result wrong. There are several measures to evaluate this: sensitivity, specificity, positive predictive value (PPV) and negative predictive value (NPV) (see Box 25.5).

Application of these principles to screening tests

The results from the worked example in Box 25.5 tend towards:

- a high specificity: very few people are incorrectly predicted to have the disease; and
- a high NPV: individuals can be reassured that the result really is negative.

Table 25.3 Current screening programmes in England

Screening programme	Target group(s)
Antenatal and newborn	
Down's syndrome	All pregnant women.
Fetal anomaly ultrasound scan	All pregnant women.
Infectious diseases in pregnancy (HIV, hepatitis B, syphilis and rubella)	All pregnant women.
Antenatal sickle cell and thalassaemia	All pregnant women.
Newborn and infant physical examination	All babies, within 72 hours of birth and repeated at 6–8 weeks.
Newborn blood spot (phenylketonuria, congenital hypothyroidism, sickle cell disease, cystic fibrosis, medium chain acyl-CoA dehydrogenase deficiency)	All infants at 5 days.
Newborn hearing screening	All newborn babies.
Young person and adult	
Abdominal aortic aneurysm	Men >65 years.
Diabetic retinopathy	Diabetics >12 years, retinal photographs yearly.
Breast cancer	Women 50–70 years, every 3 years. Women >70 years can request an appointment.
Cervical cancer	Women 25–49 years, every 3 years. Women 50–64 years, every 5 years.
Bowel cancer	Men and women 60–74 years, every 2 years. Those >74 years can request screening.

Reproduced from: UK Government. Population Screening Programmes. https://www.gov.uk/topic/population-screening-programmes.

Box 25.3 The 10 Wilson and Jungner criteria for designing a good screening test

1. The disease has a serious outcome and is an important health problem.
2. The natural history of the disease is understood.
3. There is a preclinical phase of the disease.
4. Treatment is available and is cost effective, and acceptable to patients, e.g. not too many side effects.
5. Treatment is more effective if started early.
6. The test is inexpensive.
7. The test is easy to administer.
8. The test is well tolerated.
9. The test is ethically acceptable to patients.
10. The test is valid, i.e. has a high sensitivity and specificity, and does what it is supposed to do.

Adapted with permission from Wilson, James Maxwell Glover, Jungner, Gunnar & World Health Organization. (1968). Principles and practice of screening for disease / J. M. G. Wilson, G. Jungner. Geneva : World Health Organization. http://www.who.int/iris/handle/10665/37650. © World Health Organization 1968.

This is useful in situations where the treatment or subsequent diagnostic test is unpleasant or very costly. However, the sensitivity is only 73.5%, meaning that only three-quarters of those with the disease will be correctly detected by the test. In addition, a positive test does not necessarily mean that the subject has the disease as many disease negative women will test positive (low PPV). A high sensitivity is sought in serious diseases with definitive treatment available, infectious diseases and those where the subsequent diagnostic test is cheap and low risk.

Box 25.4 Key issues when consenting a patient for screening

- The purpose of undertaking screening: to find and treat a specific disease (or its risk factors) at an earlier stage.
- The proposed test: the purpose, how it is done, who will do it, any side effects or risks of the test.
- What is being tested for, i.e. the potential results and the likelihood of each option, including uncertainties.
- What happens next if the result is positive, e.g. further investigations.
- Other options available to patient, e.g. for testing or treating if symptoms present.
- An explanation that any screening programme incurs both false positive and false negative results.
- The provision of good-quality educational and advisory materials.

Adapted from General Medical Council. Seeking patients' consent: the ethical considerations. London: General Medical Council; 1999.

Box 25.5 Sensitivity, specificity, positive predictive value and negative predictive value

- Sensitivity = probability that the test is positive, given the patient has the disease.
- Specificity = probability the test is negative, given the patient is disease negative.
- Positive predictive value (PPV) = probability that a patient has the disease, given their test was positive.
- Negative predictive value (NPV) = probability that a patient does not have the disease, given that their test was negative.

Calculating sensitivity, specificity, positive predictive value and negative predictive value:

	Disease present	Disease absent	
Test positive	α	β	$\alpha + \beta$
Test negative	γ	δ	$\gamma + \delta$
	$\alpha + \gamma$	$\beta + \delta$	Total subjects

α = true positive; β = false positive; γ = false negative; δ = true negative.
Sensitivity = $\alpha/(\alpha + \gamma)$, i.e. true positive/all those with the disease.
Specificity = $\delta/(\beta + \delta)$, i.e. true negative/all those without the disease.
PPV = $\alpha/(\alpha + \beta)$, i.e. true positive/all those with a positive test.
NPV = $\delta/(\gamma + \delta)$, i.e. true negative/all those with a negative test.

Worked example

77,139 women were screened for cervical cancer. 83 of the 75,947 women who tested negative were subsequently found to have the disease. In total, 313 women have the disease. What is the sensitivity, specificity, PPV and NPV of the test?

	Disease present	Disease absent	
Test positive	α	β	$\alpha + \beta$
Test negative	83	δ	75,947
	313	$\beta + \delta$	77,139

By simple calculation, you can go on to complete the rest of the table with this information:

	Disease present	Disease absent	
Test positive	230	962	1192
Test negative	83	75,864	75,947
	313	76,826	77,139

Sensitivity = $\alpha/(\alpha + \gamma)$ = 230/313 × 100 = 73.5%.
Specificity = $\delta/(\beta + \delta)$ = 75,864/76,826 × 100 = 98.7%.
PPV = $\alpha/(\alpha + \beta)$ = 230/1192 × 100 = 19.3%.
NPV = $\delta/(\gamma + \delta)$ = 75,864/75,947 = 99.9%.
PPV and NPV are dependent on the prevalence of the disease (or detectable pre-clinical disease) in the screened population.

The cut-off for classifying a test as positive or negative is arbitrary, and altering this cut-off will alter the sensitivity and specificity of a test. For example:

- Increasing the cut-off level so there are less positives will decrease the sensitivity (i.e. more cases missed), but increase the specificity.
- Decreasing the cut-off so more test are positive will increase the sensitivity, but decrease the specificity, so there are more false positives.

The sensitivity and specificity can be traded off against each other to get the best balance for a specific screening test (Figure 25.1).

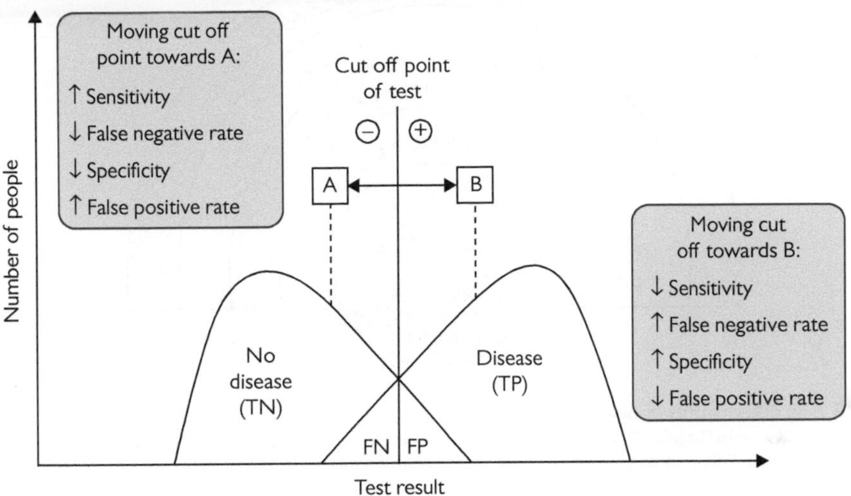

Figure 25.1 Sensitivity versus specificity: the trade off

Key: Disease (true positive TP); no disease (true negative TN); potentially misclassified (FN/FP).

Lead time bias

Lead time bias can occur with screening programmes as patients are detected as 'disease positive' earlier than they would have been based on symptomatic presentation alone. Patients therefore appear to have the disease longer and survive for a longer period of time (they will still die at the same point in time, irrespective of when the disease was detected [unless earlier detection alters the disease prognosis/outcome])(see Figure 25.2).

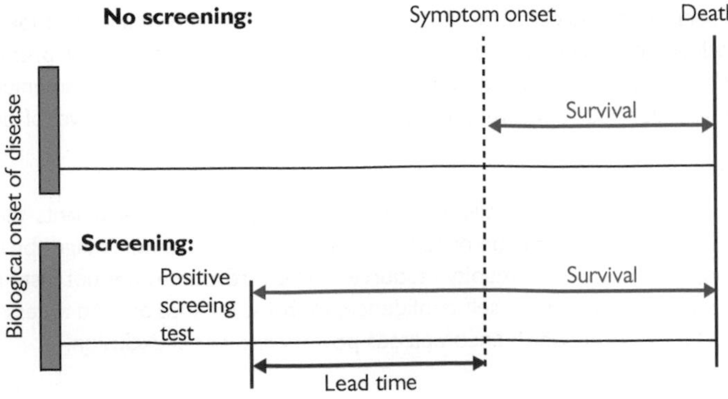

Figure 25.2 Detectable preclinical phase (DPCP) and lead time.

Determinants of health

A fundamental public health concept is that much ill-health is powerfully influenced by factors beyond an individual's age, sex, genes and medical history. Behavioural risk factors, such as smoking and diet, can play an important part. These in turn are influenced by family, friends and the way people live, work, play and engage with their local community and society at large. A useful way to depict the various types of determinants is the 'rainbow' diagram shown in Figure 25.3.

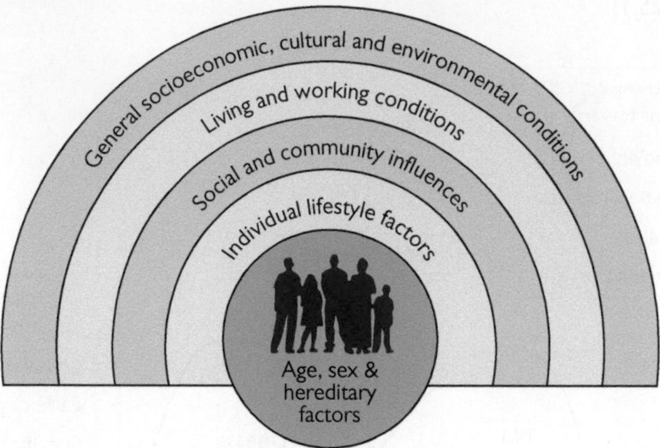

Figure 25.3 The determinants of health 'rainbow'.

Adapted with permission from Dahlgren G., and Whitehead M. Policies and Strategies to Promote Social Equity in Health. Stockholm, Sweden: IFFS. Copyright © 1991 Institute for Futures Studies. https://www.iffs.se/policies-and-strategies/

Intrinsic determinants

Each individual has various in-built or 'intrinsic' biological factors, which are likely to affect or 'determine' their state of health now and in the future. These may include their age, sex, genetic make-up, current health and intelligence. Broadly speaking little can be done to modify these intrinsic factors in order to prevent disease or improve health, although new opportunities to manipulate the genome are being rapidly developed. Identifying these factors can be useful to ensure scarce health-care resources are targeted at those most at risk or likely to benefit.

Extrinsic determinants

Each individual also displays various behavioural factors, sometimes referred to as 'lifestyle factors'. In contrast to intrinsic factors, these are open to change and modification through health promotion and other strategies.

Wider social, environmental and economic factors may influence an individual's attitudes, behaviour and health. These may include beliefs and habits of family and friends, religious or cultural pressures, peer pressure, fashion ('what's cool'), home environment, school, workplace, travel, local amenities and services, commercial marketing, wider economy, welfare support, disposable income and level of deprivation.

Social deprivation

Health and ill-health may be profoundly influenced by a range of wider determinants that contribute to social deprivation. Social deprivation can be broadly defined as 'a set of disadvantages brought about by a relative lack of individual, family or community resources'. These resources are not just financial and may extend to knowledge, literacy, numeracy, self-confidence, mobility, lay support and access to key services. Social deprivation is a broad term, which encompasses poverty and social exclusion.

Poverty

Poverty can be regarded as 'absolute poverty' or 'relative poverty'.

According to the UN (1995) (1), *absolute poverty* is:

> A condition characterised by severe deprivation of basic human needs, including food, safe drinking water, sanitation facilities, health, shelter, education and information. It depends not only on income but also on access to services.

In the developed world, poverty is usually considered in relative terms. For example, in the UK, a widely accepted definition of *relative poverty* put forward by Townsend in 1979 (2) is:

> Individuals, families and groups (whose) resources are so seriously below those commanded by the average individual or family that they are, in effect, excluded from ordinary patterns, customs and activities.

Deprivation indices

Deprivation has many dimensions and can be measured in many ways. For a defined population, such as a local authority area, a hospital catchment population or a workforce, this involves quantifying a range of socio-economic factors to arrive at a composite 'index' of deprivation for that population. In England, the standard index used is the Index of Multiple Deprivation, which incorporates the following appropriately weighted population parameters: income, employment, health/disability, housing, educational level, crime and environment.

Health inequalities

Health inequalities are differences in health and illness largely determined by variations in the effects of social deprivation, exclusion and/or poverty (also referred to as 'social variations'). Comparisons are most often made according to socio-economic status (for example, using the Index of Multiple Deprivation), but differences due to gender, age, ethnicity, mental state, physical state, educational level and domicile should also be considered. Geographical areas can be compared using population data derived from the National Census or other periodic surveys conducted by the Office for National Statistics.

In the UK there are marked differences in the health of many different populations and groups, for example in:

- Life expectancy between local authority populations.
- Age-specific mortality rates between socioeconomic groups.
- Cause-specific hospital admission rates between men and women.
- Smoking prevalence rates between ethnic groups.
- HIV diagnoses between different groups of drug users.
- Suicide rates between different occupational groups.

The term 'health inequalities' is commonly used to imply relatively negative effects on mortality, morbidity, risk factors, well-being and/or quality of life between a particular group or population, and the average or general population. It usually, but not necessarily, relates to some measure of social deprivation or disadvantage.

Lifestyle factors

These are modifiable behavioural risk factors also known as 'health behaviours', which have been shown to influence an individual's risk of developing various diseases. The most commonly encountered lifestyle factors in the UK population by this definition are 'everyday' habits, such as consuming an unhealthy diet, a lack of exercise (and excess sedentary behaviour), alcohol and drug misuse, practising unsafe sex and smoking. Some lifestyle factors, such as smoking, increase the risk of a wide range of diseases, including heart disease, stroke, chronic lung disease and a number of cancers. Others, such as practising unsafe sex, have an impact on a narrower range of diseases.

Unhealthy lifestyles are often linked closely with social disadvantage and/or deprivation. For example, Figure 25.4 demonstrates the correlation (or 'social gradient') between smoking and socio-economic classification. Similar social gradients are also seen with consumption of foods high in fat, sugar and salt, or in lack of leisure-time physical activity, plotted against socioeconomic classification.

Individual and community health

Communities are composed of individuals, each with their own set of determinants. Many characteristics are common to whole families and neighbourhoods. Environmental factors, such as type of housing, transport links, proximity to shops and services, play-space, air quality, community safety and availability of jobs may have an

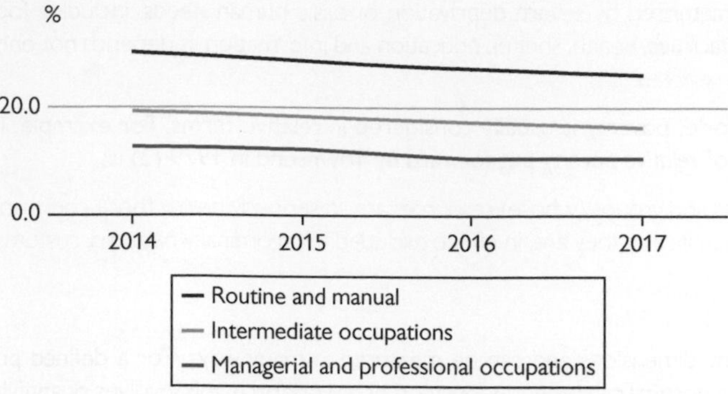

Figure 25.4 Prevalence of cigarette smoking in Great Britain, by socio-economic classification, 2012/2013 (percentages).

Reproduced from Office for National Statistics. Contains public sector information licensed under the Open Government Licence v3.0. http://www.nationalarchives.gov.uk/doc/open-government-licence/version/3/

important influence on the health and well-being of individuals and communities. Many of these factors are determined by local government, and subject to both national and local policies. The physician is well placed to act as advocate for policies likely to have a health-enhancing effect on the patient population and local community.

References

1. United Nations. Report of the World Summit for Social Development, March 6-12,1995.
2. Townsend P. (1979) *Poverty in the United Kingdom*. London, Allen Lane and Penguin Books.

Further reading

1. WHO. European strategies for tackling social inequities in health: Levelling up Part 2. Copenhagen: WHO: 2007. http://www.euro.who.int/__data/assets/pdf_file/0018/103824/E89384.pdf.

Health promotion

Principles of health promotion

An early definition of health promotion, dating from the late 1970s, is 'the science and art of helping people change their lifestyle to move toward a state of optimal health'. This has since been broadened to take in efforts to influence the wider determinants of health. According to the WHO, health promotion (also known as 'health improvement') is 'the process of enabling people to increase control over, and to improve, their health'. This definition moves beyond a focus on individual behaviour towards a wide range of social and environmental interventions and can be represented by the following three theoretical models of health promotion:

1. *The medical model:*
   - Aims to prevent particular illnesses, diseases or disabilities by encouraging, supporting and promoting healthy individual behaviours to reduce specific *risk factors*.
   - Is the form of health promotion most familiar to clinicians and is used primarily in the one-to-one clinical context, e.g. advice to cut down salt intake to help control hypertension and prevent stroke.
   - May be more broadly applied as the basis of a media campaign, e.g. advice to practise safe sex to help prevent HIV/AIDS.
2. *The educational model:*
   - Aims to empower individuals and communities to make healthier choices by shaping knowledge, attitudes, skills and confidence.
   - Example: sex and relationships education as part of personal, social and health education in schools.
3. *The socio-environmental model*
   - Aims to shape the physical, psychological, social, cultural and economic environments in which people live, work, play, travel and connect with each other in ways that are more conducive to health.

- Encompasses national or local policies either intended to 'nudge' people to make healthier choices (e.g. using excise duty to raise the price of cigarettes as a disincentive to smoke) or more forcefully through legislation (e.g. smoke-free workplaces and public places).
- Examples: healthy choices for school meals; the age-threshold for purchasing alcohol; standardised front-of-pack nutritional labelling; separate cycle lanes, lower speed limits in town centres; provision of affordable local exercise and leisure facilities.

These differing approaches are most effective when all three are used in a coordinated way, conveying consistent messages based on reliable scientific evidence.

Health promotion work can be undertaken in a variety of settings:

- Clinical settings such as general practice or hospital (e.g. advice on smoking cessation).
- Community groups (e.g. exercise classes for older people in care homes).
- The home (e.g. by health visitors advising on infant feeding).
- School (e.g. sex education; sports, exercise and games; cooking skills).
- The workplace (e.g. healthy choices in canteens or incentives to cycle to work).
- The high street (e.g. healthy eating promotions in supermarkets).
- The media (e.g. physical activity campaigns).

Behaviour change

At the core of health promotion is behaviour change – helping people to help themselves to better health by encouraging and facilitating healthier habits and ways of living. For a person to change behaviour they have to have the capability, opportunity and motivation to do so:

- Capability: physical and psychological.
- Opportunity: to take advantage of healthier choices and overcome barriers such as unaffordability or lack of access.
- Motivation: to make and maintain the behaviour change.

Doctors are generally held in high regard by patients and their advice is usually trusted. Clinicians are therefore particularly well-placed to encourage, empower and support their patients in adopting and maintaining healthy behaviours. For example, a patient's motivation to give up smoking is increased in the context of a consultation about respiratory symptoms such as cough or wheeze.

Behaviour change motivational techniques

According to the UK's National Institute for Health and Clinical Excellence (NICE)[1], effective behaviour change techniques involve working jointly with the client/patient and include:

- Goals and planning
  - Agree goals for behaviour and the resulting outcomes.
  - Develop action plans and prioritise actions.
  - Develop coping plans to prevent and manage relapses.
  - Consider achievement of outcomes and further goals and plans.
- Feedback and monitoring:
  - Encourage and support self-monitoring of behaviour and its outcomes.
  - Provide feedback on behaviour and its outcomes.
- Social support:
  - If appropriate advise on, and arrange for, friends, relatives, colleagues or 'buddies' to provide practical help, emotional support, praise or reward.

[1] Adapted from © NICE (2014) PH49 Behaviour change: individual approaches. Available from https://www.nice.org.uk/guidance/ph49 All rights reserved. Subject to Notice of rights. NICE guidance is prepared for the National Health Service in England. All NICE guidance is subject to regular review and may be updated or withdrawn. NICE accepts no responsibility for the use of its content in this product/publication.

Health promotion (behaviour change) in clinical practice: some specific examples

Behaviour change is often an important element in standard clinical pathways, particularly with regard to such common conditions as heart disease, hypertension, diabetes, stroke, chronic lung disease, chronic kidney disease, sexually transmitted infections and psychiatric illnesses. By way of example, to illustrate how the above principles are applied in practice, the following sections outline clinical approaches to tackling smoking, alcohol misuse and obesity within a wider context of health promotion.

Example 1: smoking

Smoking is the leading cause of preventable illness and premature death (under age 75) in the UK. It accounts for about one in five of all deaths over the age of 35 – more than the total deaths from alcohol misuse, drug misuse, accidents, falls, suicide and preventable diabetes combined. On average, life-long cigarette smokers die 10 years younger than never-smokers.

Smoking causes about 35% of all respiratory deaths (mainly chronic obstructive pulmonary disease; around 30% of all cancer deaths (mainly lung cancer); and around 15% of deaths from circulatory diseases (mainly heart attack and stroke). Smoking also contributes to a wide range of other illnesses and is particularly harmful for patients with certain pre-existing conditions, notably hypertension, diabetes, peripheral vascular disease, ischaemic heart disease, cerebrovascular disease, chronic lung disease and chronic kidney disease. Smoking in pregnancy is potentially harmful to the unborn child. Second-hand smoke also poses health risks, particularly for small children in enclosed spaces such as in a car or home.

Currently in the UK about one adult in five is a cigarette smoker, men and women equally. The marked social gradient in smoking accounts for about half the excess premature mortality seen in manual workers.

Tackling smoking

The main approaches are through the promotion of a non-smoking culture and encouraging smokers to cut down or stop (smoking cessation).

Promoting non-smoking

This can be achieved through a range of measures:

- *Tobacco-control policies* such as smoke-free workplaces and public spaces; restrictions on advertising, promotion and marketing of tobacco products; age-restrictions on purchase of tobacco products; deterrent pricing and taxation.
- *Educational programmes* in schools, workplaces and other settings about the risks of smoking.
- *Mass media campaigns* to discourage smoking.

Encouraging smoking cessation

Health professionals are well-placed to use every opportunity to encourage and support smokers in cutting down or giving up their habit. There are two main approaches:

- By providing *brief motivational advice* with or without medication such as nicotine replacement therapy (NRT) and follow-up. NRT increases the success of quitting smoking by 50–70%. The efficacy and safety of e-cigarettes are not yet clearly established, although they are likely to be considerably safer than tobacco cigarettes and a useful aid to cutting down.
- By referring patients to *specialist smoking cessation support*. Clinical trials show that one-to-one support or group-based sessions can double the rate of successful quitting.

Example 2: alcohol

Alcohol misuse creates a massive health, social and economic burden across the UK and much of the world. The main health impacts can be divided into:

- *Acute intoxication:* injury (from accidents and violence), coma.
- *Chronic mental and physical harm:* fetal alcohol syndrome, depression, hypertension, liver disease (e.g. fatty liver, hepatitis, cirrhosis), cancers (e.g. oral, pharyngeal, oesophageal, breast in women), cardiomyopathy.
- *Dependency* and its consequences.

In the UK, alcohol-related deaths have doubled over the past 15 years. Deaths from cirrhosis are still rising rapidly. One in 20 hospital admissions is alcohol related. Currently, for a typical district general hospital catchment population of 300,000, there are estimated to be:

- ~65,000 regularly drinking above the government's lower-risk levels.
- >9000 showing some signs of alcohol dependence.
- >1500 moderately or severely dependent on alcohol.
- ~3000 victims of alcohol-related violent crime per year.
- ~6000 admitted to hospital with an alcohol-related condition per year.

For units of alcohol, see Box 25.6.

Box 25.6 Units of alcohol

In the UK, 1 unit represents 10 ml (or about 8 g) of *pure* alcohol, approximately the amount in:

- 1 small glass (125 ml) of average strength wine (10% abv*).
- 1 half-pint of ordinary strength (3.5% abv) beer, lager or cider.
- 1 single pub measure of average strength spirits (40% abv).

*abv: alcohol by volume.

Drinking guidelines

In January 2016, the UK Chief Medical Officers issued the following new weekly guideline for men and women who drink regularly or frequently, i.e. most weeks[2]:

- You are safest not to regularly drink more than 14 units per week, to keep health risks from drinking alcohol to a low level.
- If you do drink as much as 14 units per week, it is best to spread this evenly over 3 days or more. If you have one or two heavy drinking sessions, you increase your risk of death from long-term illnesses and from accidents and injuries.
- The risk of developing a range of illnesses (including, for example, cancers of the mouth, throat and breast) increases with any amount you drink on a regular basis.
- If you wish to cut down the amount you drink, a good way to help achieve this is to have several drink-free days each week.

Tackling alcohol misuse

The main approaches are:

- *Public education* about the potential risks of misuse and how to drink sensibly; through mass media, schools, workplaces and other means.
- *Government policies* around price, availability and marketing.
- *Identification of those most at risk*, offering brief advice and signposting them to appropriate services.
- *Care and support* for those with ongoing alcohol problems.

Clinical approaches

Identification and brief intervention (identification and brief advice [IBA]).

There is strong evidence that identifying alcohol misuse at an early stage and giving simple advice can be effective in reducing people's drinking to lower risk levels. Overall, about 1 in 8 people will respond positively; a higher proportion than for smoking cessation advice. The characteristics of this approach are:

- Opportunistic.
- Brief, up to 10 minutes in duration.

[2] UK CMOs' low-risk drinking guideline: https://assets.publishing.service.gov.uk/government/uploads/system/uploads/attachment_data/file/545937/UK_CMOs__report.pdf

- Based on advice, with or without formal follow-up.
- Usually includes self-help materials.

IBA involves an initial screening test using a standard tool such as the WHO Alcohol Use Disorders Identification Test (AUDIT) followed by brief advice for those in the increasing-risk or higher-risk brackets. However, brief advice is unlikely to be enough for those with marked or prolonged dependence. It may be necessary to refer these patients to appropriate specialist services.

Alcohol dependence

Alcohol dependence is characterised by a strong desire to drink alcohol, with little or no self-control, despite detrimental impacts on personal/work relationships, and mental and physical health. The individual finds it difficult or impossible to function without alcohol. Dependence commonly leads to the need for hospital attendance and care. Full clinical assessment requires a multidisciplinary approach. A number of standardised assessment tools are available (e.g. AUDIT, Severity of Alcohol Dependence Questionnaire [SADQ], Alcohol Problems Questionnaire [APQ]).

The combination of physical, mental and social problems associated with dependence is often challenging for the physician. Prevention and management of acute alcohol withdrawal may also be difficult. Different criteria will be needed for women, older people, children and young people, and for patients with established disease (e.g. liver dysfunction). Guidelines are available from NICE and the RCP.

Example 3: overweight/obesity management

According to NICE, everyone should aim to maintain or achieve a healthy weight to improve their health and reduce the risk of diseases associated with obesity and being overweight, such as coronary heart disease, type 2 diabetes, osteoarthritis and some cancers. The aim is to achieve the right balance between 'calories in' (from food and drink) and 'calories out' (from being physically active).

The clinician's contribution comprises two basic steps:

- Identify patients who are overweight or obese and have associated risk factors.
- Provide lifestyle advice and/or refer to a specialist service in accordance with a standard weight management pathway.

Counselling the overweight or obese patient

This is focused on helping the patient to:

- Understand the risks involved in being overweight or obese.
- Cutting down on energy-dense food and drink: foods high in fats and sugars, and drinks high in sugars and alcohol.
- Avoid very-low-calorie diets, or fad diets that are not scientifically proven.
- Become more physically active, e.g. walk, cycle or swim more.
- Weigh themself regularly, once a week.
- Be patient: losing weight can be frustrating and requires perseverance.
- Even modest weight loss can bring significant health benefits.

The basic principle is to aim at modest reductions in weight over extended periods of time. This means that changes have to be realistic and easy to incorporate into the patient's daily living. Diet sheets from a qualified dietitian can be helpful, but the patient also needs to understand the basic principles of healthy eating as provided in national guidelines.

Likewise, any increase in exercise should be tailored to the patient's clinical condition and individual motivation, aiming at regular enjoyable frequent activity. The essential message is 'Move a little more – Eat a little less'. In patients in whom obesity is linked to a co-morbidity, referral to a supervised 'exercise referral programme' may be appropriate. Most hospitals have access to programmes specifically designed for cardiac or pulmonary patients or for those with back problems, diabetes or hypertension.

Occupational health

Occupational health (OH) is a discipline of medicine focusing on enhancing and maintaining the health and safety of people at work. The health and safety system in the UK was established in 1974 by the Health and Safety at Work Act. This act has significant modifications with the current strategy, 'Be part of the solution' (1), introduced in 2009 in order to provide a unified institutional structure and legal framework for health and safety regulation. The act places responsibility for the health and safety of employees on those who create the risk (i.e. the employer) to do everything 'reasonably practicable' to protect the workforce from harm. This law is primarily enforced by the Health and Safety Executive (HSE) or local authorities (2).

OH teams include doctors, nurses and sometimes allied health professionals.

The role of the occupational health physician

For the duties of an occupational health physician, see Box 25.7.

Box 25.7 The duties of an OH physician

- Workplace visits to advise on health and safety conditions.
- Assessment of the work environment: physical and psychological aspects.
- Development of policies and practices to foster, promote and maintain the physical and mental well-being of workers.
- Assessment of the workforce for fitness to work.
- Recommendations of personal adjustments to optimise individual performance.
- Analysis of surveillance data.
- Monitoring the health of any workers who are exposed to potential hazards.
- Assessment of cases of occupational injuries.
- Helping prevent sick leave and with return to work programmes.
- Health promotion and healthy workforce campaigns.

Adapted from British Medical Association (2018). The occupational physician. [online] Bma.org.uk. Available at: https://www.bma.org.uk/advice/employment/occupational-health/the-occupational-physician [Accessed 21 Mar. 2019]

References

1. HSE. Be part of the solution. http://www.hse.gov.uk/aboutus/strategiesandplans/strategy09.pdf.
2. HSE. A guide to health and safety regulation in Great Britain. http://www.hse.gov.uk/pubns/hse49.pdf.

Multiple choice questions

Questions

1. Which of the following is not a routine screening test in the UK?
   A. Aortic aneurysm screening.
   B. Fetal anomaly screening.
   C. Diabetic neuropathy screening.
   D. Newborn hearing screening.
   E. Bowel cancer screening.

2. What is the leading cause of mortality worldwide?
   A. Ischaemic heart disease (IHD).
   B. Cerebrovascular disease.
   C. Lung cancer.
   D. HIV/AIDS.
   E. Lower respiratory tract infections.

3. Polymerase chain reaction (PCR) is the current gold standard test for diagnosing Ebola virus. A new rapid diagnostic test (RDT) for Ebola is being trialled on 200 patients, 100 of these patients were Ebola PCR positive and 100 Ebola PCR negative. Eighty patients with Ebola had a positive RDT, as did five without Ebola.
   What is the negative predictive value of the RDT test?
   A. 15%.
   B. 17%.
   C. 80%.
   D. 83%.
   E. 85%.
4. Which of the following is an advantage of case control studies?
   A. They can evaluate temporal relationships.
   B. They can evaluate multiple outcomes from a single exposure.
   C. They are good for long latent periods.
   D. They are good for short latent periods.
   E. There are low rates of loss-to-follow-up.
5. Which of the following is not an intrinsic determinant of health?
   A. Age.
   B. Sex.
   C. Genetic make-up.
   D. Religion.
   E. Intelligence.

Answers

1. C. The NHS offers a range of screening tests to different sections of the population in the UK. For adults these include: aortic aneurysm, diabetic retinopathy, and cancer screening for cervical, breast and bowel (see Table 25.3).
2. A. IHD is the leading cause of mortality worldwide (see Table 25.1).
3. D. See Table 25.4 and Box 25.5.
   Negative predictive value (NPV) = True negative/all those with a negative test
   $$NPV = 95 / 115 \times 100 = 83\%.$$
4. C. Advantages of case control studies include that they are efficient in terms of time and money, good for long latent periods (as the disease has already occurred) and they can evaluate multiple risk factors for a single disease. However, they are often retrospective, making accurate exposure data more difficult to collect. See Table 25.2.

Table 25.4

	Disease present	Disease absent
Test positive	80	5
Test negative	20	95

5. D. Individuals have various in-built or 'intrinsic' biological factors, likely to affect or 'determine' their state of health, e.g. age, sex, genetic make-up, current health and intelligence. ➲ See Intrinsic determinants, p. 848.

Chapter 26 **Statistics**

John Whitaker and Anthony C. Brooms

Introduction

Medical research generates large volumes of data. If interpreted correctly, such data allows physicians to reflect the best current evidence in their practice. Guidelines are produced by many specialist societies that are helpful for understanding how research should be interpreted and inform practice. However, new data emerges at a fast rate and is published before it is incorporated into guidelines. Therefore, physicians require an understanding of statistics in order to interpret new literature and maintain practice in line with most recent evidence.

This chapter discusses aspects of experimental design and sampling used for generating data, the distribution theory underpinning many of the commonly used statistical tests and the conditions considered necessary to infer causation in clinical research.

Research design and sampling

Experimental studies

An experimental study attempts to characterise the effect of variation in a defined set of intervention(s) (or *independent variable[s])* on a predetermined outcome (or *dependent variable)*. Each group of participants receives one of the various interventions being tested and the outcome of interest is measured to establish what effect the different interventions have on the outcome. Randomised controlled trials are amongst the most powerful experimental studies in clinical research. RCTs compare the outcome in a group receiving an experimental treatment with the outcome in a group receiving the current best available treatment. In cases where no proven treatment exists, a placebo may be used in the control group. Ethical considerations, as well as the goal of demonstrating an additional benefit over the current best available treatment dictate that, where it exists, the control group should receive the current best treatment, rather than sub-optimal treatment with a placebo.

An experimental study is designed with the aims of:

- *Establishing causation*: if an outcome (the *dependent variable*) is shown to depend upon the choice of intervention (the *independent variable*) delivered during an experimental study, it can offer compelling evidence for causation – the inference that the choice of intervention is responsible for the observed difference in outcome.

- *Controlling for confounding factors*: a well-designed experimental study minimises the likelihood that observed differences in outcome are due to factors other than the independent variables explicitly being tested.
- *Minimising variability within treatment groups*: by reducing the amount of variablity within groups receiving the various interventions being assessed, the likelihood of identifying differences in outcome due to the delivered intervention is maximised. This can be seen as optimising the efficiency of data generated by an experimental study. Rigorously conducted research that generates a negative result may be of equal value to positive results. Such results may be used to reduce unnecessary investigations or treatments, which offer no additional benefit.

The AVERROES (1) trial comparing apixaban (an oral factor Xa inhibitor) with aspirin for prophylaxis against thromboembolism in patients with atrial fibrillation is an example of a high-quality experimental study, which will be used to illustrate important aspects of experimental study design.

Primary outcome

The primary outcome of a trial is defined as the outcome of greatest interest in the trial. The sample size will be calculated on the basis of an estimate of the expected difference in outcome between treatment groups in the primary outcome being assessed. The primary efficacy outcome for an experimental study is required to be specified in the study protocol prior to the recruitment of patients. In the AVERROES trial, the primary efficacy outcome was the rate of stroke or systemic embolism in patients with the characteristics described above. In the setting of novel interventions (including drug treatments) in addition to primary efficacy outcomes, primary safety outcomes are prespecified. In the AVERROES trial the primary safety outcome was the rate of major bleeding.

Secondary outcomes

Any other outcome(s) for which a significant difference is expected (or possible) between treatment groups must also be prespecified. In the AVERROES trial a secondary outcome was the rate of major vascular events (including stroke, systemic embolism, myocardial infarction and vascular death).

Subgroup analyses

Large scale studies (such as the AVERROES trial) generate a vast amount of data relating to the study participants. While the data is collected and analysed primarily to assess for the primary outcome, further analysis may provide important additional information. Subgroup analysis is the practice of considering the data relating to participants with a particular characteristic only (e.g. a certain age or sex). Subgroup analysis may be specified a priori (those analyses specified prior to data collection) or post hoc – the search for patterns after the data has been collected. In general, the conclusions drawn from post hoc subgroup analyses are less robust than prespecified outcomes and should be interpreted with caution. However, post hoc analysis remains an important step used for the identification of unexpected patterns in data, allowing for their subsequent prospective, controlled investigation.

Intention to treat analysis

The practice of analysing outcomes between groups defined by the original treatment to which the participant was assigned. Intention to treat is designed to avoid compromising the original random assignment of participants to treatment groups caused by *cross-over* (➲ see Chapter 4, Parallel and cross-over trial design, p. 107 and Figure 4.3) or *dropout* (when a participant stops the treatment to which they were originally assigned).

Interim analyses

Analysis of the data prior to completion of the study. This procedure may be incorporated into the design of blinded experimental studies to identify potential adverse outcomes in a treatment group, or triggered in response to the earlier than expected demonstration of a clinically (and statistically) significant difference in outcomes between treatment groups, or a suspicion of excess adverse events. Interim analyses are important to avoid prolonging the unnecessary exposure of participants to either harmful or inferior treatments. A prespecified interim analysis of the AVERROES trial identified a statistically significant difference in the rate of the primary outcome between treatment groups. The study was terminated after analysis confirmed that apixaban offered superior prophylaxis against stroke and systemic embolism than aspirin.

Observational studies

An observational study differs from an experimental study in that the investigators do not manipulate the intervention or treatment under investigation. Data is collected that reflects outcomes *independent of the investigation*. Although observational studies are of key importance in the identification of epidemiological patterns, the lack of control and randomisation limits the conclusions that can be drawn from them regarding causation. Established models for conducting observational studies include:

- *Case control*: the 'cases' are defined as participants with a particular outcome of interest (to form one group) and 'controls' are identified without the outcome of interest. A comparison is then made between the groups on the basis of a putative causative factor, or 'categorical variable'. Case-control observational studies are of particular importance in epidemiological research, the classic example of which identified the link between smoking and lung cancer (2). In this study, the authors identified cases (patients with carcinoma of the lung) and compared with controls (general medical and surgical patients without the outcome of interest) who were selected to be exactly matched according to age and sex. As the authors explicitly stated, this report did not provide direct evidence of a causative link between smoking and lung cancer. This link was established later by subsequent investigators inspired by these original observations.
- *Cross-sectional*: the data is collected from a representative sample taken from the population of interest at a *single point in time*. The sample is selected to be representative of a (defined) general population (rather than confined to those with a particular condition) enabling cross-sectional studies to make estimates of the prevalence of a condition within the population of interest. Data from cross-sectional studies may also be used to estimate the absolute and relative risk of particular outcomes within that population and to calculate odds ratios (➲ see Odds ratio, p. 875). A variable (e.g. obesity defined as body mass index [BMI] >30) may be observed as part of the study and compared with an outcome of interest (e.g. the use of continuous positive airway pressure [CPAP] treatment for obstructive sleep apnoea [OSA]). In this example the observation that a BMI >30 is associated with the use of CPAP for OSA does not prove that obesity causes OSA. An alternative explanation would be that the use of CPAP for OSA leads to obesity.
- *Longitudinal studies* collect data at multiple points in time. This allows an observation of the temporal relationship between independent variables and outcome. As such, there is a form of internal control inherent in the design of a longitudinal study. Returning to the example of OSA and obesity, the categorical variable (BMI >30) may develop during the study and the outcome of interest (the use of CPAP) may be observed in the same subject when this categorical variable is present and absent. Longitudinal studies may be used to draw initial conclusions about causation, although these are typically less robust than conclusions drawn from RCTs. The temporal relationship between the development of obesity and the use of CPAP may give more weight to a conclusion about the causative chain in this case.
  - *Cohort studies* are a form of longitudinal study in which a group of participants, the 'cohort', are selected on the basis of a particular set of characteristics. Data is collected longitudinally in order to draw conclusions about the effect of observed characteristics within the cohort (*independent variables*) and outcomes (*dependent variables*). Cohort studies may be prospective or retrospective.
  - *Ecological studies* are a form of longitudinal study in which the outcome of interest is the rate of an outcome *within a population*, rather than in an individual. Ecological studies may be conducted from published statistics regarding rates of an outcome derived from cross-sectional or longitudinal studies, and therefore may be less expensive to conduct.

Sampling

Study population and sample

The majority of statistical exercises are based on the mathematical assumption of an infinitely sized 'population' from which a 'sample' is drawn. An experimental study should be designed to select this sample in such a way that it can be assumed to be representative of the population of interest. If successful in doing so, it allows inferences about the population to be made on the basis of observed events in the sample. In the AVERROES trial, the investigators defined the population of interest as patients over the age of 50 in whom at least one episode of AF had been documented in the preceding 6 months, had at least one risk factor for stroke and who were unsuitable for vitamin K antagonist treatment. A total of 5599 patients were recruited from 522 centres in 36 countries. Carrying out studies across multiple sites and, in this case, across multiple continents, maximises the generalisability of conclusions that can be drawn from the data collected.

Treatment groups

Each treatment group is defined to test the impact on a *dependent variable* of assigning a particular value (or *treatment)* to an *independent variable* under investigation. In the AVERROES trial, the treatment groups consisted of participants with AF at increased risk of stroke who were either prescribed aspirin or apixaban. This design was chosen to allow conclusions to be drawn about the benefit of apixaban over aspirin (but not, in this trial, over warfarin). In an example of a *completely randomised design*, participants meeting the inclusion criteria were assigned to receive one of the two treatments in a *random* fashion (➲ See Chapter 4, Randomisation, p. 107). Balance is the process of assigning the same total number of participants to each intervention. The assumption that the baseline characteristics of the patients in each treatment group were similar (an example of *control*) can be tested by assessing the prevalence of either characteristics or *confounders*, which are known to be relevant to the outcomes of interest between groups. In this trial, clinical characteristics, including age, BP, left ventricular function and classification of AF, were compared between the treatment groups after assignment had taken place. Prior to commencing treatment, the clinical characteristics were found to be similar between the patients assigned to aspirin and those assigned to apixaban. If similar characteristics are found between *known* confounders, the inference may be extended that an even distribution is also likely to be present with *unknown* confounders (i.e. other unmeasured or unknown clinical characteristics on which the outcome of interest may depend). A larger sample will more likely result in the homogeneous distribution of both known and unknown confounders across the groups receiving the different interventions.

In some situations modifications to the completely randomised design are employed. Such modifications include the *randomised block design,* in which participants entering a study are assigned to groups on the basis of a single measurable characteristic. The aim is to ensure that the presence of this particular characteristic is accounted for within each treatment group, thereby explicitly controlling for this factor as a possible cause for any observed differences between the treatment groups. For example, a randomised block design may mandate that males and females are equally represented in each of two intervention groups. The rationale for this is to prevent the known physiological differences between males and females contributing to different outcomes in the treatment groups. As such, the design has *explicitly* controlled for the effect of sex on outcome.

A more sophisticated strategy designed to control for multiple potential confounders is the *matched pairs* design. This may be used when two treatments are being compared. Two participants are matched on the basis of a >1 characteristic (e.g. sex and systolic BP). Having been matched, each element of the pair is assigned to a different treatment group. In the matched pair design, *all* the factors considered in the pairing process are *explicitly* controlled for. Such a design may permit a smaller sample size to demonstrate a difference between treatments by more formally controlling for confounders.

Descriptive statistics

A variable may be defined as an observable characteristic whose value may vary across members of the population of interest. Variables may be *numerical* (in which case they may be continuous or discrete [taking particular values only]) or *categorical*, in which the outcome of interest is a non-numerical value (e.g. disease classification: localised, metastatic, recurrent). Descriptive statistics describe, organise and provide a relevant summary of data collected to allow health professionals to interpret and apply results from a trial. The data may be presented in the form of numerical values, tabulated data or graphically. For example, in the

AVERROES trial, the descriptive statistics chosen to represent the age of each subject enrolled were *sample mean* (representing the 'location' or 'central tendency' of the data) and *sample standard deviation* (representing the 'variabililty', or 'spread', of the data). Other descriptive statistics commonly used to describe the central tendency of data are *median* and *mode*, and the variability of data are *sample variance* and *interquartile range*. Descriptive statistics summarise the characteristics of the sample considered, but do *not* allow for conclusions to be drawn beyond the immediate sample examined. The process of drawing generalised conclusions about population characteristics from a given sample is the process of *inference*. The area of *inferential statistics* involves the formulation of conclusions about population characteristics based on the observed sample data in combination with certain assumptions about the underlying distributional properties of the population.

Distributions

Discrete variables of interest (both independent and dependent) may be described according to their *probability mass function* (PMF). Continuous variables may be described according to their *probability density function* (PDF).

- PDFs may be used to calculate the probability of observing a value of the variable under consideration within a specified range by calculating the area under the PDF curve in the specified range.
- Mathematically, this is the *integral* of the PDF across that interval. In many cases, assumptions may justifiably be made about the underlying PDF of an observed variable (➲ see Parametric statistics, p. 864 and Non-parametric statistics, p. 865).
- There are a number of particularly useful distributions that are central to statistical inference.

Normal distribution

Normal distribution describes a symmetric, unimodal distribution, centred around a mean value (3). A normal distribution is specified jointly by its *mean* and *standard deviation* (SD [a measure of the spread of the variable]). The PDF of a number of normal distributions is illustrated in Figure 26.1 with different means and standard deviations. A population variable is frequently distributed normally around a mean value. For large samples, extension of conclusions based on mathematical manipulation of the normal distribution to populations with distributions other than normal, can provide an approximation of:

- The true distribution of certain types of aggregate quantities (usually handled through one of the various central limit theorems).
- Distributions under particular parameter regimes (e.g. the Poisson distribution).

Standard normal distribution

A standard normal distribution (Figure 26.1A) is a normal distribution with a mean of 0 and a standard deviation of 1. It is frequently helpful to *transform* data to a standard normal distribution to facilitate data processing. 95% of the outcome values lie within 1.96 SD either side of the mean value (this is important for the calculation of confidence intervals). Further helpful proportions of the population of values may also be calculated as required.

Student's t-distribution

The Student's *t*-distribution is related to a standard normal distribution. It is similar in shape to the normal distribution having a unimodal peak at the mean value (zero in a *t*-distribution) with symmetrical tails (Figure 26.2). The height of the peak is lower than the standard normal distribution and the tails are fatter. The *t*-distribution is used for making inferences about the unknown mean parameter for populations assumed to have an underlying normal distribution, but *unknown* SD which is *estimated* from the sample data. This applies to the majority of experiments involving observed phenomena. Estimation of parameters introduces uncertainty into inferences made about the population. Since the *t*-distribution pushes more of its mass into the tails relative to the standard normal, it introduces greater uncertainty into inferences based on the former (as compared with the latter). The *t*-distribution is parameterised by the number of 'degrees of freedom'. As the sample size increases, the number of degrees of freedom associated with the *t*-distribution increases, and thus more closely approximates the standard normal distribution. The relationship between a standard normal and a t-distribution is illustrated in Figure 26.3.

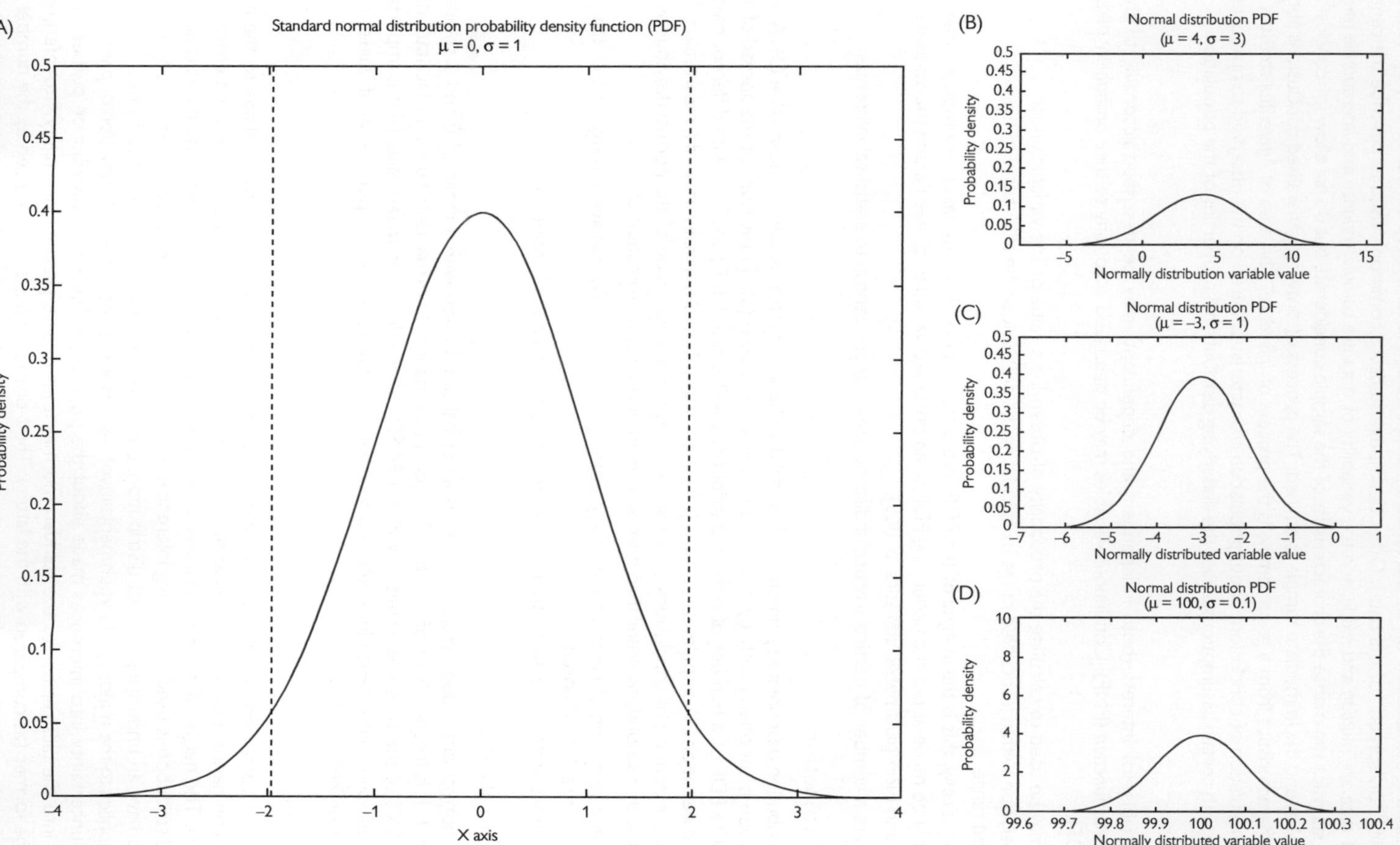

Figure 26.1 (A) Standard normal distribution (i.e. mean $\mu = 0$, standard deviation $\sigma=1$). Dashed lines at $x = 1.96$, $x = -1.96$. These lines indicate boundary within which 95% of the probability lies. (B) Normal distribution with mean 4, SD = 3. (C) Normal distribution with mean –3, SD = 1. (D) Normal distribution with mean 100, SD = 0.1.

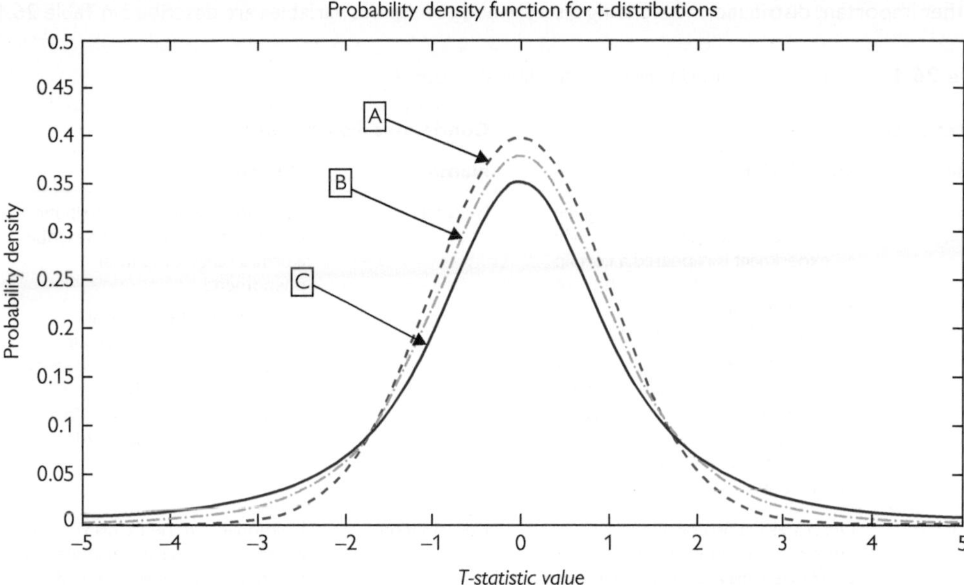

Figure 26.2 *T*-distributions with various degrees of freedom: Line C: 5; line B: 25; line A: 50. It is clear from these PDFs that as the number of degrees of freedom increases there is more probability mass centred around the mean, which will give rise to narrower confidence intervals.

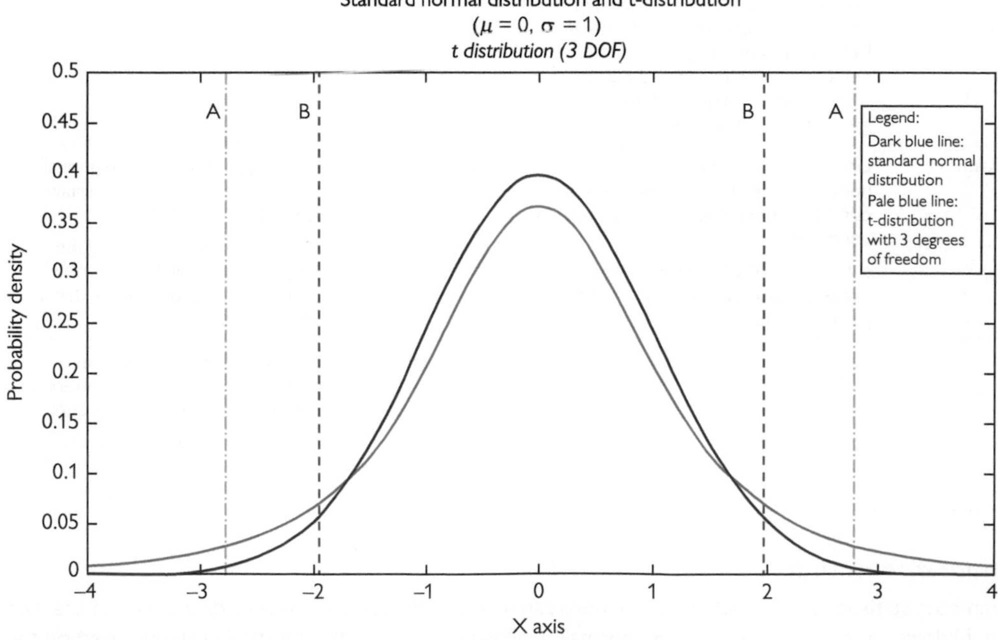

Figure 26.3 Probability density function for a standard normal distribution and a *t*-distribution with 3 degrees of freedom. 95% confidence intervals are indicated for standard normal distribution (B, dashed lines) and *t*-distribution (A, dash-dot lines). Note the wider interval for the *t*-distribution compared with the standard normal distribution.

Other important distributions describing discrete and continuous variables are described in Table 26.1.

Table 26.1 Common distributions relevant to clinical evidence

Discrete distributions		**Continuous distributions**	
Name	**Description**	**Name**	**Description**
Binomial	Describes the probability of a given number of *successful* outcomes when an experiment is repeated a certain number of times. Assumes the same probability of success with each repetition of the experiment, e.g. if each person has a probability of 0.01 of having a particular condition, independently of everybody else, then the number who have the condition in a group of 5000 has a Bin (5000,0.01) distribution.	Normal	Unimodal, symmetric distribution that may be assumed to describe a broad range of natural phenomena, e.g. consider the binomial example. Since size of group, n = 5000, is large and probability of condition, $p = 0.01$, is not too small, then can approximate using Normal (np, np[1 −p]) distribution.
Geometric	Describes the probability of a given number of repetitions until the first success is achieved, or, in the case of the *shifted geometric*, the number of failures prior to the first success, e.g. if each person is examined sequentially, each having a particular condition with probability $p = 0.01$ independently, then number of persons that would need to be examined in order to find somebody with condition follows a geometric (p) distribution; number seen before finding person with condition follows a shifted geometric (p) distribution.	*t*-distribution	Unimodal, symmetric distribution important for statistical inference based on sample estimates of population parameters, e.g. used for constructing *t*-tests.
Poisson	Used to model the probability of the number of events occurring in a given period of time (or space) under certain conditions, e.g. number of patients who visit casualty department during a certain period of time.	Uniform	Describes a distribution where all of the outcomes within a certain interval are equally likely, e.g. position of a fault along the length of a long fibre optic cable connecting two locations within a large hospital.
		Exponential	May be used to describe the probability of a given time interval passing before an 'event' occurs, e.g. length of time that elapses between two consecutive arrivals to a casualty department.

Parametric statistics

Parametric statistics are used when assumptions can be made about the underlying distribution of the data (e.g. biological variables are distributed normally), allowing for powerful statistical analyses based on the mathematical properties of this distribution. The validity of the conclusions drawn based on estimates of the population parameters from the sample statistics is dependent on any assumptions made regarding the underlying distribution of data. The assumptions should be tested using a variety of available procedures if there is doubt as to their validity (e.g. for *tests of normality*). Parametric statistical tests include:

- *T-tests*: the test statistic is assumed to follow the *t*-distribution and is commonly used to assess for differences in parameter values between two groups.
- *Simple and multiple linear regression*: assumes normally distributed error terms along with some systematic relationship between independent variable(s) and a dependent variable. It may be used to identify the quantitative relationship between independent and dependent variables.

Non-parametric statistics

Non-parametric statistics make no assumptions about the underlying distribution of the data. Although non-parametric statistics do not rely on having to make appropriate distributional assumptions, they often do not allow as powerful inferences to be made about the population of interest from a given sample. Non-parametric tests include:

- *Wilcoxon signed rank test*: used to assess the likelihood of a hypothesised treatment effect in a single set of data and may be considered as an alternative to the one sample or two sample paired *t*-test for non-parametric statistics (4). This test estimates the likelihood of a significant difference between the observed data and the null hypothesis (most commonly of no effect on the outcome of interest given a treatment) but does not estimate the magnitude of any effect.
- *Mann–Whitney test*: used to test for a difference between a variable of interest between two independent groups. The Mann–Whitney test may be considered analogous to an unpaired *t*-test for non-parametric data.
- *Kaplan–Meier survival analysis*: represents the 'survival curve' or the proportion of subjects without any other outcome of interest with respect to time. Groups can be defined and compared according to an independent variable of interest. A log rank test is used to assess the differences between the survival curves which gives a *p-value* reflecting the likelihood of the null hypothesis of no difference in the survival curves between the groups (5).
    - *Cox proportional hazards ratio*: allows more detailed analysis of continued absence of the outcome variable including a proportional asessment of the contribution of different potential explanatory variables to the outcome of interest. This test is frequently used to identify predictors of an outcome of interest within a group.

Graphical representation

Graphical methods often represent the most helpful way to conduct an initial exploration of data and to summarise data, and an intuitive way to communicate important results. Box plot charts explore relationships between a categorical explanatory variable (for instance, drug versus placebo in a drug trial) and may give an indication whether a significant difference between outcomes will be found (Figure 26.4A). Scatter plots (Figure 26.4B) investigate the possibility of a relationship between two continuous variables that can be quantified using a regression analysis (➲ see Correlation and regression, p. 871).

Graphical methods are particularly useful in communicating important outcomes to the consumers of research. Very often the outcome of interest in a clinical trial is the time until an event occurs. This type of analysis is called a 'survival analysis' used to compare time to any defined event of interest and is not restricted to an outcome of 'alive' or 'dead' (e.g. Kaplan–Meier plots [Figure 26.4C]; see Kaplan–Meier survival analysis, p.000). Non-parametric data may also be displayed graphically, e.g. pie charts and bar charts.

References

1. Connolly SJ, Eikelboom J, Campbell Joyner BS, et al. Apixaban in patients with atrial fibrillation. *N Engl J Med*. 2011;364:2362–3; author reply 2363–4.
2. Doll R, Hill AB. Smoking and carcinoma of the lung: preliminary report. *Br Med J*. 1950;77:84–93.
3. Whitley E, Ball J. Statistics review 2: samples and populations. *Crit Care*. 2002;6:143–8.
4. Whitley E, Ball J. Statistics review 6: Nonparametric methods. *Crit Care*. 2002;6:509–13.
5. Bewick V, Cheek L, Ball J. Statistics review 12: survival analysis. *Crit Care*. 2004;8:389–94.

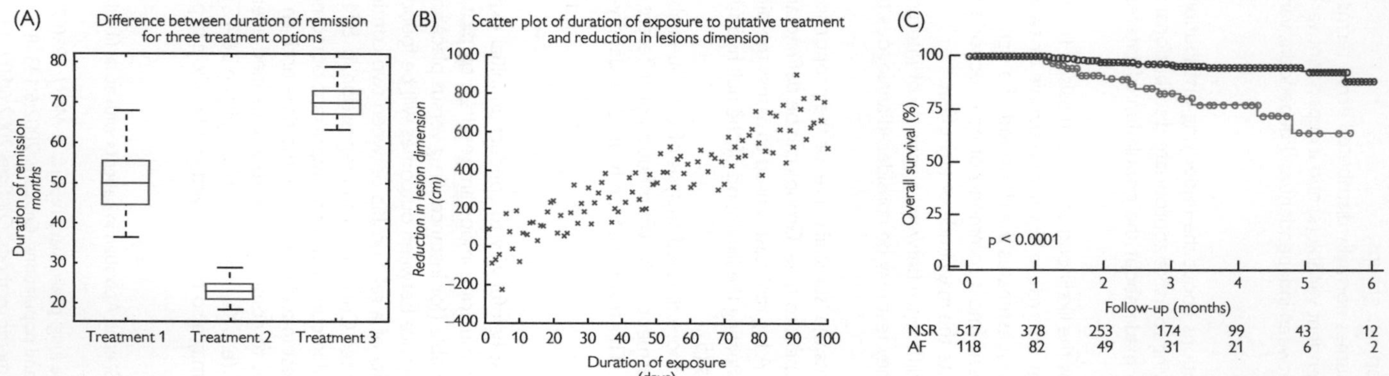

Figure 26.4 (A) Box plot demonstrating (hypothetical) difference in duration of remission of disease for three separate treatment options. Bar indicates median value, box contains *25th and 75th* percentiles, whiskers extend to outer boundaries of data. (B) Scatter plot demonstrating (hypothetical) relationship between the observed reduction in a measured lesion dimension and duration of exposure to a putative treatment. (C) Example of Kaplan–Meier curve demonstrating the effect on mortality of maintaining normal sinus rhythm (NSR) after catheter ablation on mortality (dark blue).

Reprinted from *Journal of the American College of Cardiology*, 51, 8, Nademanee K., et al., Clinical Outcomes of Catheter Substrate Ablation for High-Risk Patients With Atrial Fibrillation, pp. 843–849. https://doi.org/10.1016/j.jacc.2007.10.044.

Significance testing and confidence intervals

Large-scale studies are carried out to comprehensively answer clearly defined, prespecified questions. Clinical trials are implemented with the goal of establishing the optimal intervention to offer patients. Trials are designed to provide significant evidence for or against their original hypothesis without recruiting more participants than required.

Null hypothesis significance testing

Frequently, the aim of clinical studies is to make estimates of unknown population parameters, based on an observed sample. An estimator of a population parameter is a statistic that makes a 'guess' about the value of an unknown population parameter based on some kind of aggregation of the sample data, ideally one that is 'unbiased' i.e. the expected value of the estimator equates to the true value of the population parameter.

The conventional framework for designing a statistical test, based on appropriate estimators, is to define a pair of hypotheses in the following way.

The null hypothesis

Conventionally defined as H_0: The parameter of interest, θ, (which, for example, may refer to the expected value of some measurement for a single group, or to the difference in expected values between two groups) is equal to a specified value, θ_0, (e.g. frequently 0 [corresponding to no difference between groups])

The alternative hypothesis

Conventionally defined as H_1: The parameter of interest does *not* equal the value specified under H_0. The definition chosen for H_1 is important for the subsequent analysis:

- If H_1 specifies simply that $\theta \neq \theta_0$ then a *two-sided test* is usually required.
- If H_1 specifies that $\theta >$ (or alternatively $<$) θ_0 a *one-sided test* will be required.

Test statistics

Having set up the pair of hypotheses to be tested, an appropriate *test statistic* is established. A test statistic is a statistic (calculated from the observed sample) whose value decides whether we reject H_0 (in favour of H_1) or do not reject H_0. Test statistics are selected so that their distribution may be defined and, as such, the probability of observing any particular value (given our assumptions about the underlying distribution of the data) may be specified. The set of values of the test statistic(s) that would lead us to reject H_0 is known as the *rejection region*. The rejection region is chosen on the basis of a prespecified (low) probability of observing a particular set of values for the test statistic if the null hypothesis were true. The selection of the appropriate test statistics for a data set depends on the pair of hypotheses being tested and the distribution(s) of the data being considered: these test statistics are not necessarily unique (for, e.g, a two-sided *t*-test could either be carried out using the actual *t*-statistic or instead squared up to be compared with the *F*-distribution). Depending on the distributional characteristics of the test statistic (specifically the particular distribution and its associated degrees of freedom), the corresponding *p* value may be established from standardised tables of 'critical values' or, more commonly, calculated directly using numerical methods within statistical software packages. Rejection regions from some commonly used test statistic distributions are illustrated in Figure 26.5.

P value

The *p* value is the most familiar quantity used to report the statistical significance of results in clinical trials. It is defined as the probability of seeing the observed value of the test statistic or something more extreme in the direction of H_1 under the assumption that the null hypothesis is true. A lower *p* value gives a greater certitude that the null hypothesis can be rejected. It is important to appreciate that rejecting H_0 on the basis of a small *p* value does not indicate anything about the magnitude of a treatment effect or difference between the groups. Commonly accepted *p* values that are considered to represent adequate statistical significance are 0.05, 0.01 and 0.001. These correspond to a 5%, 1% and 0.1% chance of incorrectly rejecting the null hypothesis.

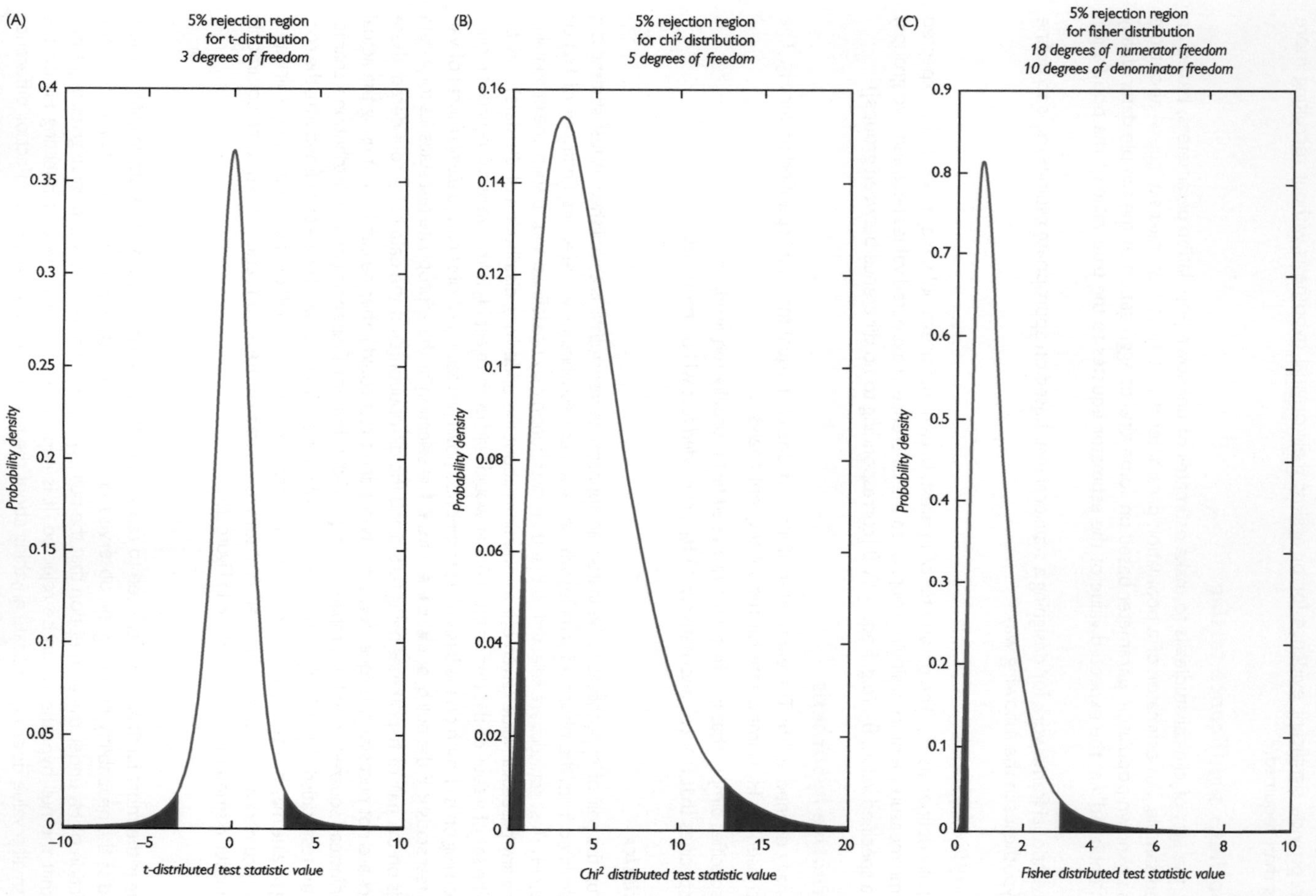

Figure 26.5 Rejection regions: shaded area represents 'rejection region' for three different distributions. If the value of the test statistic falls within the shaded region then this implies rejection at the 5% level of significance. (A) Student's *t*-distribution with 3 degrees of freedom. (B) χ^2 (chi-squared) distribution with 5 degrees of freedom. (C) Fisher distribution with 18 degrees of numerator freedom and 10 degrees of denominator freedom.

The concepts above are illustrated with a small number of selected examples. These are chosen on the basis of the most commonly encountered statistical tests and are not intended to be exhaustive.

Estimating population mean

Data that are drawn or generated from the same population may be used to show (under reasonable assumptions) that the sample mean is an unbiased estimator of the population mean and it may be used in subsequent calculations to make inferences about the population parameters. Further, under the assumption of a normal distribution, the range within which there is a 95% probability of including the true population mean may be calculated (the 95% confidence interval, ➲ see Confidence intervals, p. 870). The width of this confidence interval decreases (that is, the estimate becomes more statistically precise), with increasing sample size in the case of the sample standard deviation being fixed.

t-tests

A *t*-test is any test in which the test statistic follows a *Student's t-distribution*. Selected examples are briefly discussed here.

Tests on sample means

Frequently, comparisons are made between:

- A sample mean and a hypothesised value (a *one-sample t-test*).
- The sample means of two groups with the intention of establishing whether there is a difference in the parameter of interest between the groups (a *two sample t-test*).

Two sample t-test

The particular form that this will take will depend upon the assumptions made about the two samples being compared, specifically, whether:

- The samples contain an equal number of measurements.
- They are assumed to have an equal variance.
- They are independent samples (e.g. not repeated measurements taken from the same subject). The nature of the sampling determines whether it will be considered a *paired* or *unpaired t*-test.

Selected example of t-test

A statistic is presented below to compare the (population) means associated with two independent samples, group X (with sample mean $\bar{X}$, *M* sample points) and group Y (with sample mean $\bar{Y}$, *N* sample points). The statistic is used to test the *null hypothesis* that there is no difference between the (population) means. The overall sample SD for the pooled data is represented by $\hat{S}$. If an underlying normal distribution may be assumed for the variable of interest in each group, and the population variances are asssumed to be equal (but unknown), the *test statistic*, denoted by *T*, is calculated as follows:

$$T = \frac{\hat{X} - \hat{Y}}{\hat{S}\sqrt{\frac{1}{M} + \frac{1}{N}}}.$$

The observed value of *T* may then be used to calculate the associated *p* value for the test, either through direct calculation or by working with standardised tables. Most statistical software packages will conduct *t*-tests and calculate their corresponding *p* values directly. The assumptions on which such tests are based are important to consider when deciding if the test is appropriate.

Example

The mean BP following treatment with two different anti-hypertensive regimes was compared in an early clinical trial of ramipril (1). In this study, mean BP measurements (systolic and diastolic, standing and supine) were compared using a *t*-test (therefore, on the assumption of an underlying normal distribution of the BP readings in each group). The standing systolic blood pressure following 4 weeks of treatment with 5 mg ramipril was compared with placebo. A *t*-test generated a test statistic associated with a *p*-value of <0.001, indicating a less than 0.1% chance of observing this value of the test statistic or some other value further into the tails of the distribution in the case of the null hypothesis being true.

Analysis of variance

The analysis of variance (ANOVA) refers to a suite of statistical methods used for testing whether there is any effect of particular explanatory variables (whether discrete or continuous [e.g. lipid level]) upon some dependent variable (iscahemic heart disease [IHD]). The valid use of ANOVA will be contingent on certain model assumptions pertaining to the underlying linear statistical model holding true for the data set under consideration (e.g. data collected through the use of randomisation). Sometimes reference to the term ANOVA (or ANOVA model) is a conflation of both the statistical methods used to analyse the data, as well as the techniques used to garner the data. The basic idea of ANOVA is that a measure of the overall variation in the data, most commonly the sum of squared deviations of the observed values of the dependent variable from its sample mean, is constructed and this is then disaggregated into the sources of variation attributable to the different factors which are of interest. The significance of a particular (set of) factor(s) can be determined by calculating the relative sizes of the sources of variation and assessing their statistical significance.

Confidence intervals

In addition to making *point estimates* of population parameters, which represent 'best guesses' of the value of the scalar population parameter of interest, it is often helpful to identify a range within which it can be predicted. Such a range should ideally be as narrow as possible and with a suitably high probability that the true population parameter value will be contained within it. These intervals are known as *confidence intervals* and the percentage associated with the interval indicates the probability that the true value lies within this interval. As above, assumptions are made about the distribution of a suitable test statistic. From the PDF of the test statistic, the interval between which a certain proportion of values lie may be calculated directly and visualised graphically. There exists a 'duality' between the rejection region based on a 5% significance level for the observed test statistic and the 95% confidence interval, for the population parameter of interest.

Power and sample size calculation

The demonstration of a statistically significant result depends on an appropriate sample being collected from a population of interest. The size of a sample required to demonstrate a significant result will depend on:

- The magnitude of the effect that is under investigation.
- The confidence which is required for a result to be considered significant (the required *p value*).
- The power that a study has to detect a significant effect.

There is an ethical imperative to reach any conclusion quickly in order to expose the minimum possible number of patients to whichever the sub-optimal treatment strategy under investigation is, as well as maximising the efficiency of resources invested in answering the clinical question.

Power calculations are estimates of the sample size required to demonstrate a genuine difference in a parameter between two populations. The magnitude of the expected effect should be based on the existing literature regarding the subject under investigation. It may be a rough estimate or a more accurate estimate, depending on the available evidence. The duality between *p* values (prespecified) and confidence intervals means that the *p* value relates directly to the confidence interval that will *not* contain the parameter variables for the null hypothesis in the event of the predicted population differences. The power of a study represents the likelihood that a study will demonstrate a significant result if a difference between the populations of the estimated magnitude exists: this is usually reported in terms of a percentage which may be interpreted as the number of times a significant result would be produced if the trial were repeated a hundred times (2).

Simple power calculations may be carried out numerically or by using graphical methods that employ established nomograms (3), from which sample sizes may be read after establishing standardised values regarding expected differences between groups. More complex methods may also be employed to include estimates of lost data to account for incomplete follow-up.

Example

In the AVERROES trial the magnitude of the effect was estimated by predicting a relative risk reduction (➲ see Relative risk reduction, p. 876) of 35% with the use of apixaban when compared with aspirin. The prespecified *p* value of 0.025 was chosen as the threshold to be considered statistically significant (in this case for a one-sided test because the aim was to demonstrate an equal or greater relative risk reduction with apixaban compared with aspirin). The study required a power of 90%, that is, if the trial were repeated 100 times, then in 90 of those trials it would demonstrate a significant result in the event of a difference greater than or equal to the predicted value. This power calculation estimated that 5600 patients would be required to demonstrate the predicted difference in primary outcomes between the groups. In fact, there was a greater than predicted difference in the rate of the primary outcome than was predicted on the basis of this power calculation, although in this case the outcome was, in fact, reported as a Hazard Ratio (indicating an instantaneous risk of the event at any time) of 0.45 with the use of apixaban when compared with aspirin. The power calculation in this case was conservative and the trial demonstrated a statistically significant difference earlier than had been anticipated.

References

1. Villamil AS, Cairns V, Witte PU, Bertolasi CA. A double-blind study to compare the efficacy, tolerance and safety of two doses of the angiotensin converting enzyme inhibitor ramipril with placebo. *Am J Cardiol*. 1987;59:110D–4D.
2. Dos Santos Silva, I. *Cancer Epidemiology: Principles and Methods*. Geneva: WHO, 1999.
3. Whitley E, Ball J. Statistics review 4: sample size calculations. *Crit Care* 2002;6(4):335–41.

Correlation and regression

It is often helpful to establish the nature of the relationship between two continuous variables. This is of particular importance when:

- Comparing quantitative diagnostic tests; for example, when trying to establish whether a test that is easier or safer to conduct provides equivalent results to an established 'gold standard' (e.g. when assessing whether partial pressure of oxygen or pH is comparable between capillary and arterial blood samples).
- One easily determinable variable is shown to predict the magnitude of a clinically significant outcome (e.g. age, which is easy to establish, may be predictive of mortality rates in some conditions).

The first step in establishing the nature of a relationship between variables is to visualise the data graphically (e.g. using a scatter diagram), which will provide an initial indication of whether a relationship between the two variables will be found.

To further investigate this relationship the process of *regression* may be employed. Regression uses a statistical model that aims to quantify the relationship between continuous variables.

Simple linear regression is based on a model whose systematic component is a linear relationship between a continuous *response variable* and a continuous *explanatory variable* of the form:

$$Y_i = \beta_0 + \beta_1 x_i$$

where Y_i is the response variable, x_i the explanatory variable (with each set of measurements indexed by i, i = 1, 2, … ,n), β_0 the intercept of the regression line and β_1 the slope of the regression line.

The model assumes that measurement of the response variable is subject to an error in measurement that has a mean of 0, some fixed (but unknown) variance and is normally distributed, while the explanatory variable is regarded as fixed and without error. These assumptions are important for the subsequent tests applied to the data to establish the significance of any identified relationship.

The *correlation* between two continuous variables expresses the strength of the linear association between the variables. This may be expressed in terms of the *sample correlation coefficient,* r, which varies between –1 and 1. A value of –1 or 1 defines a perfect correlation (in the postiive or negative direction).

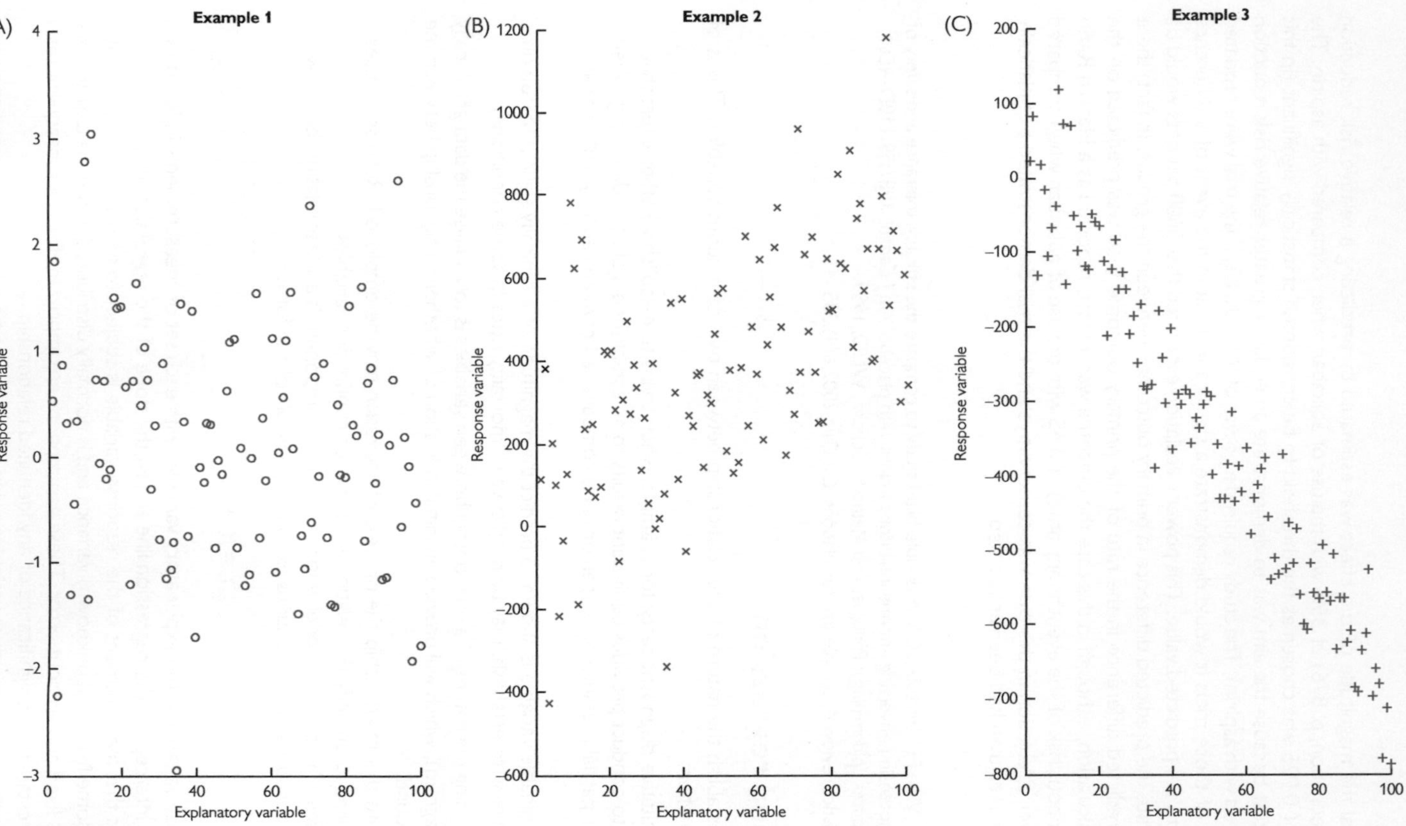

Figure 26.6 Scatter plots demonstrating different levels of correlation. (A) No obvious correlation on initial inspection. (B) Visual suggestion of correlation between explanatory variable and response variable. (C) Visual suggestion of correlation between explanatory variable and response variable. Note that the scatter plot in (C), which demonstrates the strongest correlation has a negative gradient. In this case the coefficient of determination (R^2) remains positive, while the correlation coefficient (also called Pearson's correlation coefficient) would be negative.

Mathematically, it is often more appropriate to use the *coefficient of determination*, denoted by R^2, which varies between 0 and 1. R^2 may be thought of as the proportion of the total variation of the response variable that may be explained by the relevant linear model.

By applying appropriate statistical techniques related to those used for generating point estimates, confidence intervals for estimates of the regression coefficients may be generated. Figure 26.6 illustrates the appearance of scatter plots with different values of R^2.

The relationship between an explanatory and a response variable is investigated in order for predictions to be made regarding the response variable. Making predictions on the basis of observed data introduces an additional error into calculations (that of the uncertainty, or error, associated with the coefficients of regression and the additional error associated with the response variable itself). As a consequence the prediction intervals for the response variable are wider than confidence intervals for estimates of the mean of the response variable.

In reality, a response variable of interest may be expected to depend upon more than one explanatory variable. In such cases, a *multiple linear regression model* may be developed, which is based on similar assumptions to the simple linear regression model but includes *k* explanatory variables:

$$Y_i = \beta_0 + \beta_1 x_{i1} + \beta_2 x_{i2} + \ldots + \beta_k x_{ik}$$

It is often helpful to initially develop simple regression models for potential explanatory variables, which give the greatest opportunity to identify a relationship. Subsequently, multiple linear regression models can include those explanatory variables demonstrated to contribute to the 'goodness of fit' of a regression line.

Further tests applied to multiple linear regression models can identify *redundant explanatory variables* (those whose inclusion in the model does not improve the goodness of fit of the models being tested). The order in which explanatory variables are added or removed from the model may impact upon those that are ultimately identified as significant.

Explanatory variables that are strongly correlated with each other introduce *multicollinearity*, and thereafter instability, into a statistical model. Small differences in the observations can therefore result in dramatic changes in the estimates obtained for the regression coefficients. Intuitively, it should be possible to use explanatory variables that are highly correlated with each other as *alternatives* to each other in the regression model. The choice of which explanatory variable to remove from the regression model depends on multiple situation-specific considerations. Interpreting of evidence based on multiple regression models should consider why particular explanatory variables were included or excluded from the final reported model, and whether or not this was justified.

The above models can be used to test only for a linear relationship between explanatory and response variables in the sense that the *regression parameters* $(\beta_0 \ldots \beta_k)$ appear linearly. Other types of multiple linear regression model can be handled by setting $x_{ij} = f_j(x_i)$, $i = 1, \ldots, n$; $j = 1, \ldots, k$, for suitably defined $f_j(\cdot)$ (e.g. $f_j(x_i) = x_i^j$, in the case of a polynomial relationship).

Meta-analysis

Meta-analysis is the process of combining data from multiple, independent studies to formulate conclusions that comprehensively reflect the available evidence. Meta-analysis involves the systematic identification, appraisal and abstraction of data from all identified literature relating to a well-defined question that the meta-analysis is set up to answer. The complexity of such a process is reflected by the fact that different conclusions may be drawn from various meta-analyses of the same data. Both simple and more complex statistical techniques may be employed in order to analyse combined data. Familiar measures of statistical significance such as confidence intervals and p values are often reported in meta-analysis. Guidelines exist that should be referenced when designing and conducting meta-analysis (1) and offers a helpful approach to the review of meta-analysis, as well as an introduction to some specific statistical methods used (2).

References

1. Moher D, Cook DJ, Eastwood S, et al. Improving the quality of reports of meta-analyses of randomised controlled trials: the QUOROM statement. *Lancet*. 1999;354:1896–900.
2. Russo MW. How to review a meta-analysis. *Gastroenterol Hepatol* (NY). 2007;3:637–42.

Association and causation

A key challenge in clinical studies is identifying causation. In 1965, Sir Austin Bradford Hill proposed nine considerations prior to concluding that an observed association was most likely the result of causation (1). The validity of such considerations depends crucially on the definition of causality, which represents a complex field of philosophical considerations beyond the scope of this text (2). Of key importance is to decide whether an observed association is the result of chance, bias or confounding within the sample considered, or as a direct effect of the differences in explanatory variable tested in the experimental design. While ongoing work continues to refine the strategy for testing and concluding causation, Bradford Hill's considerations are a helpful framework for assessing whether a causal relationship can explain an observed association. These criteria can be summarised as follows:

1. *Strength of association*: the stronger the relationship between an outcome and the explanatory factor the more likely the relationship is to be causal.
2. *Consistency of results*: the result has been demonstrated multiple times across different studies.
3. *Specificity of the association*: a factor specifically influences a particular outcome.
4. *Temporality*: exposure to the putative causative factor must precede the outcome of interest.
5. *Biological gradient*: the outcome increases with increasing exposure to the putative causative factor or follows a function predicted by substantive theory.
6. *Plausibility*: there is a plausible biological mechanism to account for causation.
7. *Coherence*: the explanation should not contradict current, substantive knowledge.
8. *Experiment*: causation is more likely if the association is demonstrated in randomised experiments.
9. *Analogy*: for analogous outcomes and exposures an effect has previously been demonstrated.

Example

In the AVERROES trial similar patients enrolled into the study were randomly assigned to receive either aspirin or apixaban as prophylaxis against stroke or systemic embolisation. The random assignment meant that any significant differences in predisposition to the primary outcome between the two groups would be down to chance. With increasing sample size the chance of significant differences emerging between groups as a result of such extraneous factors was small, but the differences were assessed between potentially confounding variables after randomisation. This data is important to consider when interpreting experimental studies (commonly reported in the first table in a study). No such differences were found in any of the potential confounding factors considered and therefore the identification of a significant difference in the rate of the primary outcome between the two groups could be attributed to the intervention that each group received. This study demonstrates a strong and specific association, satisfying the consideration of temporality with a plausible biological explanation that did not contradict current knowledge of the benefits of apixaban in the context of a randomised experimental design, which was consistent with other trials demonstrating a reduced rate of stroke and systemic embolisation using alternative novel oral anticoagulant drugs (NOACs). As such, considerations 1, 3, 4, 6, 7, 8 and 9 are met by this trial. In order to comprehensively meet Bradford Hill's criteria, further studies would need to demonstrate a consistent result (consideration 2) and a biological gradient (e.g. a dose–response change in outcome, consideration 5).

References

1. Hill AB. The environment and disease: association or causation. *Proc R Soc Med*. 1965;58:295–300.
2. Höfler M. The Bradford Hill considerations on causality: a counterfactual perspective. *Emerg Themes Epidemiol*. 2005;2:11.

Risk and probability

An estimate of the variation in chance (or 'risk') of an outcome of interest conferred by an explanatory variable can be quanitified in several ways. To define these, a simple factor with 2 levels of exposure (exposed and unexposed) and the calculation of risk associated with a binary outcome should be considered, as shown in Table 26.2.

Table 26.2 Incidence of an outcome subdivided according to exposure or otherwise to a factor, which may be used to estimate risk of the outcome relative to exposure to that factor

	Outcome 1	Outcome 2	Total
Exposure to factor	a	b	a + b
No exposure to factor	c	d	c + d
Total	a + c	b + d	Total subjects (= a + b + c + d) = n

Relative risk

Relative risk is the ratio of risk of an outcome in an experimental group when compared with an unexposed group.

$$\text{Relative risk of outcome 1} = \frac{\text{Estimated risk in exposed group}}{\text{Estimated risk in unexposed group}} = \frac{\frac{a}{a+b}}{\frac{c}{c+d}}$$

Relative risk can be calculated by statistical packages (which allow calculation of a 95% confidence interval) and also directly from the raw data (1).

Odds ratio

Odds ratio (OR) is an alternative measure that enables patients and physicians to understand the impact for individuals of the presence or absence of exposure to a risk factor associated with an outcome of interest. The *OR* is the ratio between the odds of having an outcome of interest within a group exposed to a potential risk factor as compared with the odds of having an outcome of interest within a group not exposed to the same potential risk factor.

$$\text{Odds ratio for outcome 1} = \frac{\text{Estimated odds for exposed group}}{\text{Estimated odds for unexposed group}} = \frac{\frac{a}{b}}{\frac{c}{d}}$$

Attributable risk

Attributable risk is the proportion of the outcomes of interest that can be attributed to the explanatory factor under consideration. This is calculated by estimating the number of outcomes of interest that would occur if the entire sample had the same risk as the unexposed group and comparing that with the actual number of outcomes of interest. In the example above, the *expected number of cases of outcome 1 in the entire sample if subjected to the same risk as the unexposed group* could be estimated by:

$$\text{Expected number of cases} = \text{total number of subjects} \times \text{risk in the unexposed group}$$

$$= n \times \frac{c}{c+d}$$

The *attributable risk* of outcome 1 that can be assigned to exposure to this risk factor can be calculated as:

$$\text{Attributable risk} = \frac{(\text{Total number of outcome 1} - \text{expected number of outcome 1 if risk is equal to that of unexposed group})}{(\text{Total number of outcome 1})}$$

Very often, the absolute difference between the chance of the outcome of interest between groups with different exposures needs to be assessed. The *absolute risk reduction* may be calculated as the difference in risk when there has and has not been exposure to the factor under investigation, i.e. the difference between two proportions. When the absolute risk reduction is negative it indicates an increased chance in the outcome of interest arising with exposure to the factor. Absolute risk reduction may also be expressed as a change in percentage points.

$$\text{Absolute risk reduction} = \text{Risk in unexposed group} - \text{risk in exposed group} = \frac{c}{c+d} - \frac{a}{a+b}$$

Relative risk reduction

Relative risk reduction is the absolute risk reduction relative to the risk in the unexposed group:

$$\text{Relative risk reduction} = \frac{\text{Absolute risk reduction}}{\text{Risk in unexposed group}} = \frac{\left(\frac{c}{c+d} - \frac{a}{a+b}\right)}{\frac{c}{c+d}}$$

Absolute risk reduction may be transformed to express the *number needed to treat* (NNT). This measure reflects the number of patients who would need to be exposed to a factor under consideration to prevent one *adverse* outcome of interest.

$$\text{Number needed to treat} = \frac{1}{\text{Absolute risk reduction}}$$

When NNT is negative it indicates an increased number of *adverse* outcomes with exposure to the factor. The sign reversed gives the *number needed to harm*.

Reference

1. Bewick V, Cheek L, Ball J. Statistics review 11: assessing risk. *Crit Care*. 2004;8:287–91.

Diagnostic test accuracy

Diagnostic tests should be assessed in a sample of subjects representative of the clinical group the test will be applied in, and compared against a reference (or 'Gold') standard for making the diagnosis that was obtained without reference to the diagnostic test under consideration (1). The data generated formulates the meaning of a particular test result in a given population and can be quantified in different ways. A hypothetical diagnostic test for a condition of interest is shown in Table 26.3. The presence or absence of the condition was established using the reference standard investigation. The letters represent the number of patients as specified:

- α: a *positive* test result in whom the condition was confirmed ('true positive' result);
- β: a *positive* test result in whom the condition was excluded ('false positive' result);
- γ: a *negative* test result in whom the condition was confirmed ('false negative' result);
- δ: a *negative* result in whom the condition was excluded ('true negative' result).

Table 26.3 Incidence of a positive or negative test result subdivided according to presence or absence of the condition being tested for, which may be used to estimate the sensitivity and specificity of a diagnostic test

	Condition present	**Condition absent**	***Total***
Positive test result	α	β	$\alpha + \beta$
Negative test result	γ	δ	$\gamma + \delta$
Total	$\alpha + \gamma$	$\beta + \delta$	Total subjects (= $\alpha + \beta + \gamma + \delta$) = n

The *sensitivity* of a test is the proportion of patients with the condition who are correctly identified by the test.

$$\textit{Sensitivity} = \frac{\alpha}{\alpha + \gamma}$$

The *specificity* of a test is the proportion of patients who do not have the condition that are correctly identified by the test.

$$\textit{Specificity} = \frac{\delta}{\beta + \delta}$$

An ideal diagnostic test would have a sensitivity of 1 (or 100%) and a specificity of 1 (or 100%), although in practice this is very difficult to achieve. A diagnostic test can be evaluated by the probability of a given condition existing in the context of a positive or negative test result, using the *positive* and *negative predictive value* associated with a test. As well as reflecting the discriminatory value of the test, these parameters are affected by the overall prevalence of a condition. The positive predictive value of a test is the proportion of patients with a positive test result that have the condition as diagnosed by the reference standard and, similarly, the negative predictive value the proportion of patients with a negative test result that do not have the condition.

$$\text{Positive predictive value} = \frac{\alpha}{\alpha + \beta}$$

$$\text{Negative predictive value} = \frac{\delta}{\gamma + \delta}$$

The sensitivity and specificity of a diagnostic test may be combined and reported as *likelihood ratios*:

$$\text{The likelihood ratio of a positive test result} = \frac{\text{sensitivity}}{(1 - \text{specificity})}$$

$$\text{The likelihood ratio of a negative test result} = \frac{(1 - \text{sensitivity})}{\text{specificity}}$$

High likelihood ratios for positive test results and low likelihood ratios for negative test results indicate a more useful diagnostic test.

Diagnostic tests often measure a continuous variable and the threshold at which that continuous variable indicates the presence or absence of a condition is sought, e.g. the serum level of troponin-T that indicates myocardial infarction. By increasing the threshold considered to be diagnostic, the sensitivity of a test will decrease and the specificity will increase. Such results are displayed graphically using a receiver-operator characteristic (ROC) graph in which *1–specificity* is plotted on the abscissa against *sensitivity* on the ordinate. The predictive value of the test may then be estimated by calculating the area under the ROC (AUROC) curve.

Reference

1. Straus SE, Richardson WS, Glasziou P, Haynes, RB. *Evidence Based Medicine. How to Practice and Teach EBM*. Oxford: Elsevier, 2005.

Acknowledgements

The editors and contributors are grateful to Dr Thomas Rossor for proofreading and feedback during the drafting of this chapter.

Multiple choice questions

Questions

1. As part of a trial, 100 patients with left ventricular systolic dysfunction following myocardial infarction were randomised to receive the I_f channel blocking drug ivabradine or placebo. They were followed-up for 1 year and major adverse cardiac events (MACE) were recorded. What will be the most helpful analysis to use in order to identify whether there is any impact on the rate of MACE attributable to the ivabradine?
   A. Kaplan–Meier survival curve.
   B. Two-sample paired student's *t*-test.
   C. Pearson's correlation co-efficient.
   D. Chi-squared test.
   E. Cox proportional hazards analysis.
2. A new drug for pulmonary fibrosis was tested in a randomised controlled trial. The 1-year mortality with the treatment was 7.5% compared with 15% without (a difference that was tested and confirmed to be statistically significant). The absolute risk reduction is:
   A. 0.001%.
   B. 2.5%.
   C. 7.5%.
   D. 15%.
   E. 50%.
3. Each of 209 randomly selected patients was classified according to their smoking history and incidence of bladder cancer. Among the 105 smokers, 22 developed bladder cancer and among the 104 non-smokers, one developed bladder cancer. What is the relative risk of bladder cancer in smokers in this study when compared with non-smokers?
   A. $\frac{22}{105}$.
   B. $\frac{22/83}{1/103}$.
   C. $\frac{22/(22+83)}{1/(1+103)}$.
   D. $\frac{22}{22+83}-\frac{1}{1+103}$.
   E. $\frac{22/22+1}{209}$.
4. In comparing the mean arterial blood pressure (MABP) in two independent populations of patients, a random sample was drawn from each population and a two-sample *t*-test was applied. The *p*-value for this test is:
   A. A measure of the absolute difference between each group's mean BP.
   B. A measure of the relative difference between each group's mean BP.
   C. The probability, under the null hypothesis, of incorrectly rejecting the null hypothesis (of there being no difference in MABP between the two groups).
   D. The number of populations (and, correspondingly, samples) whose MABP is being compared using this test.
   E. The relative frequency with which MABP measurements were drawn from each population.

5. Which of the following is a non-parametric test?
   A. One-sided student's *t*-test.
   B. Kaplan–Meier survival analysis.
   C. Simple linear regression analysis.
   D. Multiple linear regression analysis.
   E. Paired sample *t*-test.

Answers

1. E. A Cox proportional hazards analysis is a test that estimates the proportional assessment of the contribution of different potential explanatory variables to the outcome of interest.
   ➲ See Non-parametric statistics, p. 865.
2. C. The *absolute risk reduction* may be calculated as the difference in risk when there has and has not been exposure to the factor under investigation. In this example:

   Absolute risk reduction = 15%–7.5% = 7.5%.

   ➲ See Attributable risk, p. 875.
3. C. See Table 26.4.

Table 26.4

	Bladder cancer	No bladder cancer	Total
Smokers	22 (=a)	83 (=b)	105 (=a + b)
Non-smokers	1 (=c)	103 (=d)	104 (=c + d)
Total	23 (=a + c)	186 (=b + d)	Total subjects = 209 (= a + b + c + d)

The relative risk of bladder cancer in smokers compared with non-smokers = $\frac{\frac{a}{(a+b)}}{\frac{c}{(c+d)}} = 21.79$ (to 2 d.p.)
➲ See Relative risk, p. 875.

4. C. The *p* value is the most familiar quantity used to report the statistical significance of results in clinical trials. It is defined as the probability of seeing the observed value of the test statistic (or something more extreme in the direction of H_1), under the assumption that the null hypothesis is true.
   ➲ See Test statistics, p. 867.
5. B. One-sided Student's *t*-test, simple linear regression analysis, multiple linear regression analysis and Fisher's exact test all depend on assumptions about the underlying distribution of the data (e.g. biological variables are distributed normally), allowing for powerful statistical analyses based on the mathematical properties of this distribution, and are therefore *parametric* statistical tests. Kaplan–Meier survival analysis does not make any such assumptions about the underlying distribution of the data and is, therefore, a *non-parametric* statistical test.
   ➲ See Parametric statistics, p. 864 and Non-parametric statistics, p. 865.

Chapter 27 **Medical Law and Ethics**

Benjamin Glickstein, Michael Fertleman and Philip Howard

Introduction

In this chapter, we will discuss some of the ethical principles and law relevant to all three parts of the MRCP examination. Scenarios and multiple choice questions have been selected to illustrate the use of important ethical frameworks for dealing with challenging clinical situations. Relevant legal imperatives are outlined.

Four principles are described by Beauchamp and Childress (1): autonomy, beneficence, non-maleficence and justice. These principles provide a widely used framework to help understand and approach complex ethical situations. The four principles are:

- *Respect for autonomy*: autonomy can be thought of as the right of competent adults to make informed decisions about their own medical care. Autonomy relies on the patient being fully informed before giving consent to a procedure. Patients must be protected from coercion, which could infringe upon their autonomy. Treatment decisions made by a capacious patient should normally be respected unless the well-being of others could be affected. For example, a competent patient with a new diagnosis of epilepsy can refuse anti-epileptic medications, but they can be impelled to stop driving, when they risk the safety of others.
- *Beneficence*: medical treatment should be of overall benefit to patients.
- *Non-maleficence*: we should, where possible, avoid causing harm to our patients or inflict the least harm possible to reach a beneficial outcome. For example, when starting a course of treatment, negative side effects, such as pain and discomfort should be outweighed by the overall benefit gained. The nature of the benefit is specific to that clinical situation. It may extend beyond the patient to a wider group, such as for family members when genetic testing is considered.
- *Justice*: justice addresses the distribution of medical care. To ensure justice in medical treatment demands patients with similar conditions are treated equally regardless of socioeconomic status or race. It includes equitable access to health care, and respect for the rights of patients in the provision of care and treatment. The right to life, and freedom from inhumane and degrading treatment are enshrined in the European Convention of Human Rights.

References

1. Beauchamp TL, Childress JF. *Principles of Biomedical Ethics*, 7th edn. New York: Oxford University Press, 2013.

Capacity

Scenario 1

Mr P is a 59-year-old man who attends his GP with intermittent chest pains associated with shortness of breath. A clinical assessment and changes on the ECG raise the strong possibility of acute coronary syndrome.

She warns Mr P of the risks of a heart attack and recommends Mr P to stay seated in the consultation room while she organises an ambulance to take him to the local A&E department. On hearing this, Mr P becomes upset, as he is self-employed and has clients relying on him that afternoon. He declines to stay in the clinic or to be transferred to hospital.

At this point the GP explains the findings to Mr P, and explains her concerns that he may be suffering from acute coronary syndrome. She explains that she wants him to be reviewed in hospital urgently, and emphasises that if untreated his condition could lead to a heart attack, which could be fatal. Mr P understands what the GP has said, but feels she is overreacting; he feels this may just be heartburn, which he has had before. He explains if things get worse, he will go to hospital himself. He says he feels better now and wants to just 'get on with it'.

The GP feels that Mr P has understood and retained the information she has explained to him. He does not appear anxious, and, when questioned does understand the GP's concerns. What are the ethical and legal rules that pertain to this situation, and how could they guide your next steps?

Summary

Mr P has capacity to refuse medical advice and necessary, possibly life-saving, treatment. Self-discharge might lead, at worst, to the sudden death of Mr P. If he drives home there is also a risk to others in the event of a cardiac dysrhythmia, hypotension or arrest.

Autonomy

> A mentally competent patient has an absolute right to refuse consent to medical treatment for any reason, rational or irrational, or for no reason at all, even where that decision might lead to his or her own death.
>
> Lady Justice Elizabeth Butler-Sloss in Re MB (1997)

The only situation in which it is lawful for the doctors to intervene is if it believed that the adult patient lacked the capacity to decide and the treatment was in the patient's best interests. Mr P has given no cause to doubt that he has capacity. He has listened to the GP and understood the concerns regarding his heart, including suffering a heart attack. Having retained and weighed the information from the consultation he has made the decision that he wants to leave.

A doctor might intervene if the patient lacked capacity and the treatment was in their best interests. However, the Mental Capacity Act presumes that a person has capacity until it is demonstrated that he/she lacks it. In this scenario, Mr P's refusal of investigation or treatment must be respected.

Mr P is potentially at risk of a fatal myocardial infarction as he refuses to take medical advice. It would therefore be good practice, but not a legal requirement, to seek the help of a colleague in trying to persuade Mr P to accept medical treatment and to act as a witness to what has been explained. Mr P should be asked to sign a statement that he is refusing treatment against medical advice. The assessment and explanations should be carefully recorded in the clinical notes.

If Mr P were to go home, and present later to hospital with further chest pains and cardiac failure, medical investigation and appropriate treatment should be undertaken even if his ability to communicate becomes compromised. The previous decision to refuse management should be reviewed in the light of the changed clinical situation. If Mr P was to present for urgent life-saving treatment there would be an underlying positive duty of care to take such steps as are reasonable to keep him alive

However, we should consider situations in which capacity has been lost and the implication that this has for clinical decision making. If Mr P were to collapse and become unconscious, he should be resuscitated, as his previous refusal of treatment would no longer be applicable. In this case, there would be grounds for believing that Mr P did not anticipate these events at the time of his decision to leave against advice. It would be reasonable to believe his decision would have been different had he anticipated them.

Beneficence and non-maleficence

For Mr P, treatment of what appears to be an incipient myocardial infarction would be overwhelmingly in Mr P's favour, not only to prevent the imminent risk of death, but also to reduce the risk of long-term myocardial damage. A therapeutic angiogram could treat a blocked coronary artery and prevent fatal arrhythmias or irreversible myocardial damage. The risks from therapeutic angiography, such as contrast-induced kidney injury or coronary thrombosis are outweighed by the potential benefits to Mr P.

Other issues

In this scenario there would be a risk to Mr P and to others if he were to drive home. It is not uncommon for patients to present with medical conditions that make driving unsafe. The risk to fellow road users should be considered if Mr P decides to drive home. The current General Medical Council (GMC) advice is to inform the patient of the risks in driving and their legal duty to inform the DVLA of their medical condition. If the patient fails to take medical advice, the doctor may inform the DVLA and disclose the relevant details in confidence to the medical adviser, having first informed the patient of the intention to refer. In this case, the immediate risks of Mr P driving are so high, immediate disclosure to the authorities may well be warranted.

Scenario 2

Mr K is a 79-year-old man with a past medical history of hypertension, congestive cardiac failure and chronic kidney disease. Four weeks prior to the admission he was prescribed bumetanide 2 mg OD for increased leg swelling by a doctor who did not have access to his medical records. Since that consultation, he has been taking bumetanide in addition to his prior medication of furosemide 80 mg OD, bisoprolol 5 mg OD, ramipril 5 mg OD and aspirin 75 mg OD. His daughters called an ambulance on a Saturday afternoon, as he was acting bizarrely.

On arrival in A&E he is unsteady on his feet and aggressively paranoid, combative and refusing treatment. A junior doctor manages to get a venous blood sample. which shows a sodium level of 109 mmol/L. The doctor discusses Mr K's very low sodium level with him and his family, explaining the life-threatening risk of seizures and death, and also discusses the need for urgent IV access and slow IV fluids to correct a potentially life-threatening hyponatraemia. At this point Mr K accuses the doctor of wanting to poison him and says he 'doesn't want any more of it'. Although unsteady, Mr K manages to walk towards to the door of the A&E department. Mr K's daughters are tearful, but he shouts and lashes out at them when they try and convince him to stay.

The doctor asks Mr K to explain what his medical problems are, and asks if he recognises how serious his low sodium levels could be. Mr K lashes out at the doctor and fails to recall any of the previous discussions. He keeps repeating 'doctors and their poisons, I want to leave'.

Autonomy

The Mental Capacity Act 2005 provides the legal basis to treat Mr K who appears to lack capacity in his best interests. Mental capacity is assessed on the 'balance of probabilities'. In this case it is more likely than not that the patient lacks capacity. Mr K's failure to answer questions, or retain information presented to him puts his capacity into question. This is likely to be caused by the acute electrolyte disturbance.

In order to demonstrate that a patient has capacity to make decisions a patient must be able to:

- understand the information relevant to a decision;
- retain that information;
- use or weigh up the information as part of the process of making a decision; and
- communicate the decision by language or any other means.

Capacity is decision specific. Although the doctor has explained the rationale for treating his life-threatening condition, Mr K is demonstrating no clear understanding of these facts or the ability to retain them. Unlike Mr P, Mr K is not evaluating the information in order to make a decision; neither is he communicating any clear rationale behind what he wants to do.

Multiple choice question

Mr K is refusing treatment; given this, the best course of action would be:

A. Apply to appoint an independent mental capacity advocate (IMCA).
B. Allow Mr K to leave with urgent follow-up from his GP.
C. Treat in his best interests and without his consent. Reasonable measures may be taken to detain him to facilitate this.
D. Psychiatric evaluation (urgent) to determine capacity.
E. Seek advice from the trust legal team.

Answer

C. Mr K's lack of capacity is likely to be due to a metabolic disturbance. It could be permanent if central pontine myelinolysis occurs. Given the serious consequences of not investigating and treating him, treatment can be started immediately and in his best interests. The Mental Capacity Act suggests delaying decisions where possible, in order to allow the patient to regain capacity. In this situation treatment of his underlying condition should not be postponed as he needs urgent correction of hyponatraemia to prevent the possibility of seizures and death. This treatment would not only be in his best interests, but also enhance his decision-making capacity. There is no time for a second, psychiatric opinion on capacity, or for an IMCA. Letting him leave hospital would not be justified, given his lack of capacity.

In deciding a patient's best interests the person must:

- Consider 'all the relevant circumstances', including 'whether it is likely that the person will at some time have capacity' and 'improve his ability to participate, as fully as possible in any act done and any decision affecting him'.
- Have regard to the person's 'past and present wishes and feelings, the beliefs and values that would be likely to influence his decision if he had capacity, and other factors he would be likely to consider'.
- Take into account (if practicable and appropriate) 'any named person to be consulted, those engaged in caring for the person or interested in their welfare', including anyone with lasting power of attorney or who is a court appointed deputy.

When in an emergency medical situation, however, the 'best interests' of a patient will be determined on clinical grounds.

Article 5 of the Human Rights Act requires that persons can only be deprived of their liberty under specified circumstances with appropriate legal procedures in place to ensure the protection of the individual's rights and freedoms. The doctor should pursue the least restrictive method of keeping Mr K safe, and instituting treatment. Keeping Mr K in hospital and omitting the diuretics, while performing neurological observations may be sufficient at this stage. However, if the treatment is prolonged and Mr K continues to lack capacity, the hospital can use an Urgent Authorisation to provide life-sustaining treatment under the Deprivation of Liberty Safeguards (section 4B of the Mental Capacity Act 2005), while a direction is sought from the court.

Mr K is 79 years of age, and it is possible that his paranoia relates to underlying dementia and mental illness. In a chronic situation, compulsory treatment under the Mental Health Act 1983 would take precedence. However, this would not be considered in the current instance unless his medical treatment failed to restore his mental state. The mental health act is covered in more detail in ➲ Chapter 22, Mental Capacity Act and Mental Health Act, p. 795 and Table 22.9.

Confidentiality

Whatever, in connection with my professional practice or not in connection with it, I see or hear in the life of men, which ought not to be spoken of abroad, I will not divulge, reckoning that all such should be kept secret.

Hippocratic Oath

Introduction

Confidentiality is central to the relationship of trust and confidence between doctors and patients. Without strict confidentiality, patients would be reluctant to reveal personal and sensitive information, which is necessary for their medical care. Personal information about patients should not normally be divulged without the patient's consent (or that of a parent, guardian or legal representative) unless the disclosure can be justified on the basis of preventing harm to the patient or others.

The patient's right to confidentiality is protected by the common law and various statutes, including the Human Rights Act 1998 and the European Convention on Human Rights.

However, Article 8 of the European Convention on Human Rights allows restrictions regarding the right to confidentiality when it is necessary 'in the interests of national security, public safety or the economic well-being of the country, the prevention of disorder or crime, the protection of health, or the protection of the rights and freedom of others'.

Scenario 3

Sean is a 48-year-old bus driver who was reviewed in the stroke clinic. He was diagnosed with a left homonymous hemianopia due to a lacunar infarct secondary to hypertension. He had no motor deficit. His secondary risk factors including hypertension were addressed, and he was advised to present himself to the occupational health physician as his residual hemianopia could have serious implications for his work as a bus driver.

He feels he has 'got used to things now' and is planning to go back to work the following week. He told his workplace that he had the flu and has not informed them of his stroke and the resultant visual deficit.

Multiple choice question

On leaving the stroke unit, Sean had been informed not to drive until he had had an assessment by the DVLA. Although it had been made clear to him that disclosure to his employer and the DVLA is essential, he was still insisting that he was safe on the road and not willing to inform the DVLA. The best course of action would be:

A. Explain again how serious driving with his condition could be. Urge him to reconsider and inform the GP.
B. Seek advice from a medical defence organisation as to the best way forward.
C. Ask for a second opinion from another colleague in the hospital.
D. Immediately ring the DVLA to inform them of the situation, be clear with Sean that you are doing this, document clearly and notify his GP.
E. Provide him with a letter detailing your concerns and inform him he must show this to his employers.

Answer

D. Sean has had sufficient warning that his professional driving may be impaired and has not acted on this. The risks to others are great in this situation and, if he continues to drive, or the clinician suspects he is still driving, an immediate and transparent disclosure should be made to the medical advisor of the DVLA regarding the medical situation.

Disclosure in relation to fitness to drive

Where a patient continues to drive against medical advice, the GMC has issued guidelines that include informing the DVLA where necessary (see Box 27.1).

Box 27.1 Confidentiality

1. The *driver is legally responsible for informing the DVLA or DVA* about such a condition or treatment. However, if a patient has such a condition, you should explain to the patient:
   (a) that the condition may affect their ability to drive (if the patient is incapable of understanding this advice, for example, because of dementia, you should inform the DVLA or DVA immediately); and
   (b) that they have a legal duty to inform the DVLA or DVA about the condition.
2. If a patient refuses to accept the diagnosis, or the effect of the condition on their ability to drive, you can suggest that they *seek a second opinion*, and help arrange for them to do so. You should advise the patient not to drive in the meantime.
3. If a patient continues to drive when they may not be fit to do so, you should *make every reasonable effort to persuade them to stop*. As long as the patient agrees, you may discuss your concerns with their relatives, friends or carers.
4. If you do not manage to persuade the patient to stop driving, or you discover that they are continuing to drive against your advice, you should *contact the DVLA or DVA immediately* and disclose any relevant medical information, in confidence, to the medical adviser.
5. Before contacting the DVLA or DVA you should try to *inform the patient of your decision to disclose personal information*. You should then also inform the patient in writing once you have done so.

General Medical Council. (2019). Patients' fitness to drive and reporting concerns to the DVLA or DVA. [online] Available at: https://www.gmc-uk.org/ethical-guidance/ethical-guidance-for-doctors/confidentiality---patients-fitness-to-drive-and-reporting-concerns-to-the-dvla-or-dva/patients-fitness-to-drive-and-reporting-concerns-to-the-dvla-or-dva [Accessed 6 Mar. 2019].

Scenario 3 (continued)

Four weeks later, Sean fails to attend for follow-up. He was involved in an accident in which he drove his bus off the road, mounted the pavement and killed a man standing at a bus stop. The police wish to examine his medical records having found his clinic appointment card after Sean had been arrested for dangerous driving. The case has been referred to the Coroner.

Sean's failure to inform the DVLA has resulted in a tragedy. In this instance, the Inquest must ensure a full examination of the circumstances that led to the person's death. Reports and medical records can be ordered by the Coroner. In an Inquest, the consent of patients is not required for doctors to provide written or verbal statements about their medical problems and treatment.

Scenario 4

Mr H is a 36-year-old fast-food restaurant owner. He presents to A&E acutely jaundiced and is reviewed by the registrar on call. His LFTs and hepatitis screen indicate an acute infection with hepatitis A. Given the significant derangement in his liver enzymes he is advised to stay in for repeat LFTs in 24 hours. He thanks the registrar for his advice, but says that he has to leave immediately to open his shop as there is 'no one else to do it for me'. He is directly involved in food preparation and supply.

Multiple choice question

Mr H is adamant about leaving hospital to open his shop and resume business. In this situation, the best course of action would be:

A. Inform the GP of his diagnosis and advise that he presents to his practice in a weeks' time to re-check his LFTs.
B. Advise Mr H not to engage in food preparation while he is actively unwell with symptoms of diarrhoea.
C. Ask for a second opinion on Mr H's capacity to make this decision.
D. Make clear written notes to explain your advice to him and document the discussion in his discharge summary.
E. Make it clear verbally and in writing what risks his disease poses in terms of risk to others, then inform local health protection team of his diagnosis verbally.

Answer

E. Mr H can choose to leave hospital. He needs to be fully informed to make this decision, which would include a discussion of the small risk of liver failure and death. However, once he understands the risks to himself, he is at liberty to leave hospital. Hepatitis A infection is a notifiable disease. He is, therefore, not at liberty to continue working as he poses risks to other peoples' health as he is involved in food preparation and supply. The health protection team should be contacted verbally. They will make contact with him to obtain contact tracing. There is a duty not only to inform about his hepatitis, but also that he is planning on returning to work.

Notifications in the case of infectious diseases

Notification of certain infectious diseases is required under the Health Protection (Notification) Regulations 2010 made under the Public Health (Control of Diseases) Act 1984 (➲ see Chapter 8, Notifiable disease, p. 236).

Scenario 5

Miss M is a 27-year-old woman admitted to hospital with a history of chronic cough and unintentional weight loss over the past 3 months. She has been a sex worker and has consented for a HIV test. She is cachexic and febrile. Her chest X-ray shows consolidation. Sputum analysis shows acid- and alcohol-fast bacilli (AAFB) on microscopy and later cultures grow acid-fast bacilli. A diagnosis of tuberculosis is made and subsequently confirmed. Her HIV test comes back positive. She is informed of both positive tests, and advised to stay in hospital to start treatment for TB and meet with the infectious disease team to discuss anti-retroviral therapy. After 48 hours, she feels much better and tells the Registrar that she wants to go home. She has heard bad things about long-term TB treatment and does not want to start it.

On discussion with her GP, it transpires that she has been diagnosed previously with multidrug-resistant TB, and on two occasions failed to comply with directly observed treatment (DOT) regimens. The respiratory consultant and TB specialist nurse feel she is at high risk of transmitting tuberculosis to others.

Multiple choice question

Miss M feels better and you find her packing her bags to go home. Despite explaining the rationale for treatment, you cannot persuade her to stay for treatment. The best course of action would be:

A. Prescribe the relevant TB medications and organise outpatient follow-up.
B. Re-refer her to DOT clinic.
C. Ask her to fill in an 'Against Medical Advice' form prior to her departure.
D. Consider applying to a Magistrate for a compulsory detention order.
E. Ring her GP, advise them of the situation, and ask if they can meet with her to discuss re-engaging with treatment.

Answer

D. Miss M has demonstrated a 'track record' of non-compliance with DOT (recommended for patients with TB at high risk of non-compliance). She is suffering from multidrug-resistant tuberculosis, which poses a significant risk to the general public. High-risk patients are considered as those with a history of non-compliance with treatment, or those living on the streets or in sheltered accommodation. NICE advises that the individual's barriers to compliance should be addressed and support be provided to the patient.

However, sections 37 and 38 of the Public Health (Control of Diseases) Act 1984 allow a local authority to apply to a Justice of the Peace for removal and detention in hospital of a person suffering from certain infectious diseases who poses a serious risk of spread to others. In practice, detention is required because of poor compliance with treatment, and thus her continuing infectious state. Nevertheless, proper treatment might reduce the risk of contagion and, hence, the need for isolation. Detention amounts to a deprivation of liberty that might be subject to legal challenge. Any detention under the 1984 Act would have to satisfy the criterion of being a last resort, where lesser measures had been shown to be insufficient to reduce the risk of disease transmission.

Non-compliant patients may be subject to compulsory examination and even detention. but compulsory treatment is not permitted under the Public Health Act. Patients who lack capacity may be treated under the Mental Capacity Act 2005 if it is their best interests.

Provisions for sexually transmitted disease

Although Miss M's diagnosis of TB is notifiable, her HIV status is not. There are a number of sexually transmitted diseases, including HIV/AIDS that are not notifiable. However, various aspects of the management of HIV/AIDS are governed by statute (➲ see Chapter 7, Legal aspects of HIV infection, p. 222).

The National Health Service (NHS) (Venereal Diseases) Regulations of 1974 and NHS Trusts and Primary Care Trusts (Sexually Transmitted Diseases) Directions 2000 place a duty on health authorities to ensure that information on individuals suffering from sexually transmitted disease should not be disclosed, unless it is necessary to communicate with a medical practitioner who is treating the patient or to prevent the spread of the disease. This clearly helps to maintain the confidentiality of patients who might not otherwise present for treatment at all, thereby posing a greater risk to others.

Other situations where disclosure may be legally required

- *Disclosures in relation to safeguarding children or vulnerable adults.* Disclosures may be necessary in the case of safeguarding to protect children and vulnerable adults. The GMC guidance requires practitioners to be aware of the policies and procedures of organisations involved in protecting children.
- *Disclosures in relation to serious crime, judicial or statutory proceedings.* Section 9 of the Police and Criminal Evidence Act 1984 allows access to personal medical records and to human tissue 'which has been taken for the purposes of diagnosis and treatment' in the course of criminal investigations.
- *Disclosures in relation to court proceedings.* Information must be disclosed under the direction of a judge in court proceedings, to a Coroner in relation to an inquest, and to an official request from a statutory regulatory body, such as the GMC. Where there is doubt about disclosures, legal advice should be sought.

Other statutory requirements include providing information to the police, where it may identify a driver alleged to have committed a traffic offence under the Road Traffic Act 1988, and helping to apprehend or prosecute a terrorist under the Terrorism Act 2000, or prevent acts of terrorism.

Confidentiality and the Data Protection Act

A doctors' duty to maintain confidentiality

A doctor has a common law duty to maintain confidentiality and ensure the protection of personal data. This duty is reinforced by contracts of employment within the NHS, professional standards issued by the GMC, and various statutory codes of practice and principles, such as the Data Protection Act principles and later Caldicott Principles. However, the GMC recognises that there are circumstances when it is reasonable, or even necessary, to disclose or share information with others. Clearly, identifiable personal information may be shared in correspondence with other members of the health-care team.

Under the Data Protection Act 1998 patients have the right to view their personal data through a subject access request and to have errors corrected. It is not permitted for the data to be used in a way that might cause harm or distress, or for direct marketing. The Data Protection Act 1998 applies to manual and electronic records (see Box 27.2).

Under the Access to Health Records Act 1990, individuals have a right of access to their own medical records. When a patient has died the personal representative has a right of access, which is important in relation to an inquest and to any claim arising out of the patient's death.

Box 27.2 The Data Protection Act principles

- Data must be processed fairly and lawfully.
- Personal data shall be obtained only for one or more specific and lawful purposes.
- Personal data shall be adequate, relevant and not excessive in relation to the purpose(s) for which they are processed.
- Personal data shall be accurate and, where necessary, kept up to date.
- Personal data processed for any purpose(s) shall not be kept for longer than is necessary for that purpose.
- Personal data shall be processed in accordance with the rights of data subjects under the 1998 Data Protection Act.
- Appropriate technical and organisational measures shall be taken against unauthorised or unlawful processing of personal data and against accidental loss or destruction of, or damage to, personal data.
- Personal data shall not be transferred to a country outside the European Economic Area, unless that country or territory ensures an adequate level of protection for the rights and freedoms of data subjects in relation to the processing of personal data.

Caldicott guardians and principles

In 1997, Dame Fiona Caldicott examined the ways in which patient information was being used and the best ways to ensure that confidentiality is not undermined. This was particularly necessary in view of increased use of electronic data. The subsequent Caldicott Report initially highlighted six key principles, to which a seventh principle was added in recognition of circumstances when it is important to share information for the benefit of patients. She detailed principles to guide the management of confidential data.

Caldicott principles

1. Justify the purpose(s) of the use of identifiable patient information.
2. Do not use patient identifiable information unless it is absolutely necessary.
3. Use the minimum necessary patient-identifiable information.
4. Access to patient-identifiable information should be on a strict need-to-know basis.
5. Everyone with access to patient-identifiable information should be aware of their responsibilities.
6. Understand and comply with the law.
7. The duty to share information can be as important as the duty to protect patient confidentiality.

Anonymised data

Anonymised data may be used for a range of purposes including education, audit, public health surveillance, and for health-care planning and administration. Disclosures may indirectly benefit patients through drug safety monitoring, e.g. the Yellow Card Scheme, confidential enquiries (e.g. into maternal mortality and perioperative deaths) and epidemiological surveys (e.g. of communicable diseases).

In certain circumstances doctors have clear contractual obligations to disclose data to third parties, including those doctors working for occupational health services and insurance companies (with explicit consent of the patient), or agencies that assess claims or benefits, the police, the armed forces and the prison service.

Breaking bad news/do not attempt cardiopulmonary resuscitation

Telling patients and their families the truth, no matter how bleak, is important. The process of breaking bad news has four objectives:

- To find out what information the patient is aware of and understanding what their expectations from the clinical encounter are.
- To provide clear and coherent information for the patient and family.
- To provide support to reduce the emotional impact of the news being given to both the patient and their relatives.
- To provide a clear treatment plan.

The 'SPIKES' method allows for a structured way to deal with this challenging medical situation. If breaking the news goes badly, it can have an effect on future clinical interactions with the patient or family.

Scenario 6

Miss A was found in her house fitting and unresponsive by her teenage son. She was transferred to hospital by ambulance. On arrival the seizure was terminated. However, her GCS was less than 8, and her airway unstable. She had a CT scan, which showed a grade 4 subarachnoid haemorrhage. She was intubated and ventilated by the ITU team. The images were transferred to the neurosurgical team, with whom her case was discussed. The neurosurgical consultant felt that surgical intervention would be futile, based on the severity of the bleed and degree of cerebral oedema. They recommend palliative treatment at the regional hospital. Her son and husband are waiting for you in the family room.

A second ITU opinion was sought to help confirm a diagnosis of brain death. Brainstem death was confirmed and there was a discussion about withdrawing ventilation. As part of this discussion it was explained that if Miss A's heart and breathing stopped when she was taken off the ventilator, cardiopulmonary resuscitation will not be attempted to restart them.

See Box 27.3 for SPIKES approach to breaking bad news.

Multiple choice question

Following discussion with the clinical team, the husband is adamant that he wants everything to be done for his wife and insists on full resuscitation in the event of a respiratory arrest (arising from the brainstem damage). He states that she has 'always been a fighter' and he does not want you to give up on her. What would be the most appropriate response?

A. Inform him that the ultimate decision for or against cardiopulmonary resuscitation (CPR) rests with the consultant, and that a 'do not attempt cardiopulmonary resuscitation' (DNACPR) will be completed.
B. Ask for a second opinion from another consultant and discuss things with the family after this.
C. Ask the nurse to spend some time with the family to let things settle down and try to discuss it again later.
D. Ask the son his opinions, as he is 15 and seems mature enough to take part in the discussion.
E. Document your discussion, delay any completion of DNACPR forms given the family's wishes.

Answer

B. Although A is legally correct, as the patient cannot be involved in decision-making, and there is no nominated power of attorney, it is not the best way forward. While the decision rests with the doctors responsible for the care of the patient, it would be appropriate to obtain a second opinion before making a final decision, if time and circumstances permit.

Do not attempt resuscitation decisions

DNACPR decisions made by health professionals when the patient lacks capacity:

1. In order to make a fully informed decision, where it is both practicable and appropriate, they must discuss the patient's situation and the decision with those close to the patient (subject to any confidentiality restrictions expressed if, and when, the patient had capacity).
2. Where both practicable and appropriate, they should not delay contacting those close to the patient in order to do this. Of note, in a recent judgment it was stated by the judge that 'a telephone

Box 27.3 SPIKES approach to breaking bad news

Step 1 'S' (setting)

Setting up

Review the plan for breaking bad news. Make sure that the family is in an appropriate location. In this scenario, the family room in A&E is the best place to talk. Reduce the likelihood of interruptions. Hand over bleeps and ensure the privacy of the setting that you are in. Ensure all those members of the family who want to be involved in the discussion are present. Sit down with the patient and family while discussing the bad news. Ensuring the correct set-up will help in developing rapport with the family and allow them to feel listened to and central to what is happening.

Step 2 'P' (perception)

Assessing the family's perception of the situation is vital. What do they understand about what has happened so far? Before discussing clinical events, it is vital to understand what the family know. *Do not* assume a certain level of understanding. Do they know the patient has had an intracerebral bleed? Do they understand why the patient was fitting?

Step 3 'I' (invitation)

The invitation to give information about a clinical situation is important. Some patients may not want to hear all the details of their illness, some relatives may wish to pass on the responsibility of hearing the news to other members of the family. In this case, should the child be present to hear what's being said, does the husband feel that the right members of the family are present to discuss what is going on? Empower the patient and family to decide what they want to know and who should know it. For example, 'Would you like me to go through what we know so far about your wife's condition?'

Step 4 'K' (knowledge)

Giving knowledge

This can be preceded by a warning. 'Unfortunately your wife's medical condition is very serious, and I am sorry to tell you . . .'. When imparting bad news try to use simple language. The clinician should be aware of the tendency to 'shut down' when people are told devastating news. Information should be limited to the most relevant clinical facts, and how they affect the situation the patient is in. There will be further chances to give more detailed information later.

Step 5 'E' (empathy)

Address the patient or family's emotions. Try and identify what emotions they are feeling and try to connect with this. Empathy goes beyond sympathy. Try not to rush past this point; patients and their families need this time to express what they are feeling.

Step 6 'S' (strategy and summary)

Reiterate what has been said, be as clear as possible. Try to make it clear what the next steps are. In this case, a second opinion to confirm brainstem death may be needed, prior to a discussion of withdrawal of ventilation.

Adapted with permission Baile, W. F. et al. SPIKES- A Six-step Protocol for delivering Bad News: Application to the Patient with Cancer. *The Oncologist*, 5(4); 302–311. doi: 10.1634/theoncologist.5-4-302. The oncologist by Society for Translational Oncology Adapted with permission of ALPHAMED PRESS in the format Book via Copyright Clearance Center.

call at 3.00 am may be less than convenient or desirable than a meeting in working hours, but that is not the same as whether it is practicable'.

3. When it is not possible to contact those close to the patient immediately and an anticipatory decision about CPR is needed in order to deliver high-quality care, the decision should be made in accordance with the relevant legislation

These recommendations apply when a decision is being considered because attempting CPR would not succeed in preventing a patient's death or when a decision about CPR is being considered on a balance of risk and benefit in a patient's individual situation at that time.

(Resuscitation Council, November 2015)

If a patient has the capacity to discuss resuscitation then it should be discussed with them, giving the reasons why resuscitation may or may not be appropriate. When a patient lacks capacity it is important to establish if there is an advance directive, or a legally appointed deputy, who has the ability to make such decisions. Advance directives are only applicable to refusals of specified treatment, positive advance directives are not recognised by the law. Court-appointed deputies can help with decision-making, but are not empowered to refuse life-sustaining treatment under the Mental Capacity Act.

Legal challenges to DNACPR decisions have led to the judgment in the Court of Appeal in the case of Tracey *(2014)* in which Lord Dyson, Master of the Rolls stated:

Since a DNACPR decision is one which will potentially deprive the patient of life-saving treatment, there should be a presumption in favour of patient involvement. There need to be convincing reasons not to involve the patient.... There can be little doubt that it is inappropriate to involve the patient in the process if the clinician considers that to do so is likely to cause them to suffer physical or psychological harm .... In my view, doctors should be wary of being too ready to exclude patients from the process on the grounds that their involvement is likely to distress them.

Lord Dyson rejected the view that if the doctor regards CPR as futile he is under no obligation to discuss it with the patient, even if it would cause no harm because:

The patient is entitled to know that such an important decision has been taken and should not be deprived of the opportunity to seek a second opinion.

Organ donation

The Human Tissue Act 2004 governs cadaveric organ donation in England and the Human Tissue Act 2006 applies in Scotland. Both Acts applied the principle of 'opting in'. However, the Organ Donation (Deemed Consent) Act 2019 has instituted an 'opt out' system in England from May 2020. The decision to be a donor rests with the individual. If the wishes of the individual to be a donor are known, there is no provision for the families to block this. Therefore, it is important to check the donor register before discussing donation with the family. If the views of the patient are not known, authority for the decision passes to the nominated or appropriate representatives.

For the decision-making hierarchy for organ donation, see Table 27.1.

In Wales, presumed consent would normally apply for adult donors, unless the person had 'opted out'. However, if the potential donor was a child, those in an ongoing relationship (e.g. parent/foster carer) would be approached to give consent.

Medical errors

According to the National Patient Safety Agency around 10% of patients admitted to NHS hospitals have been involved in a patent safety incident (NPSA, 2018) (1). Events that have led to at least moderate harm should be reported to the patient and where appropriate to the family. The NPSA defines moderate harm as anything that has resulted in a moderate increase in the patient's treatment, causing significant, but not permanent, harm to the patient.

Table 27.1 Decision-making hierarchy for organ donation

Human Tissue Act 2004 England Wales (and Northern Ireland)	Human Tissue Act Scotland 2006
Spouse or partner.	Spouse or partner.
Parent or child.	Person living with the adult as husband/wife, or as a civil partner for not less than 6 months.
Brother or sister.	Child.
Grandparent or grandchild.	Parent.
Niece or nephew.	Brother or sister.
Stepfather or stepmother.	Grandparent.
Half-brother or half-sister.	Grandchild.
Friend of long standing.	Uncle or aunt.
	Cousin.
	Niece or nephew.
	Friend of long standing.

Adapted from https://www.odt.nhs.uk/

According to the GMC, doctors have a duty to be 'open and honest with patients if things have gone wrong' (2). If a patient has suffered harm or distress under your care you should:

- Put matters right (if that is possible).
- Offer an apology.
- Explain fully and promptly what has happened, and explain the short- and long-term effects.

Scenario 7

Mrs M is an 88-year-old woman who was admitted to A&E with abdominal pain. She arrived in the department at 7 p.m., and was reviewed by an A&E senior house officer (SHO) at around midnight. She was confused and agitated. Her WCC was 6 and her CRP was 20; she was afebrile. Her urine dip showed blood 2+, ketones 2+, Leuk 1+, nitrates negative. A diagnosis of urosepsis was made and she was given a dose of gentamicin, a medical review was awaited following discussion with the medical registrar on call.

The medical registrar discussed the case with the A&E SHO and advised that given the presentation with abdominal pain a surgical review should be requested. This information was misunderstood; the patient was not put on the medical list and not reviewed by the medical or surgical teams that night.

At the handover meeting the following morning the nurse in charge queried what was happening with her care. On assessment Mrs M was drowsy and had a grade 2 sacral sore. The A&E consultant rang the daytime medical specialist registrar (SpR). The patient was not on the list and they did not know anything about her. They agreed to come and review the patient urgently.

On assessment she was found to have a diffusely tender abdomen. Repeat bloods showed a lactate of 4 and a new acute kidney injury. A CT abdomen was requested and the patient was reviewed by the surgical team. A diagnosis of a perforated diverticulum was eventually made. Given her co-morbidities, conservative management with IV fluids and antibiotics was recommended. The surgical team suggested she stay under the medical team with daily surgical review, given her multiple medical problems.

That afternoon Mrs M's son arrived in the hospital, having flown back from Germany where he lived and worked. He was furious. He demanded to see the consultant to explain how his mother had 'ended up in such a mess'. She was delirious and in pain, her pressure sore was breaking down. As far as he could see 'nothing has been done'. As the ward doctor, you are asked to come and talk with him, as the consultant is off site.

When patients are harmed it is usually due to a combination of individual and organisational failures. In this instance, we do not know why there was a breakdown of communication, a prolonged wait in A&E in breach of the 4-hour target, and failures in the handover and senior clinical review. We were not told about the bed state, possible staff shortages or the number of admissions that night.

Multiple choice question

In response to the request to speak with the son, the ward doctor should:

A. Meet with the son, explain the sequence of events, establish the son's main concerns and apologise.
B. Explain they cannot comment on care given prior to the patient's arrival on the ward.
C. Refer the patient to the Patient Advice and Liaison Service (PALS), who can help establish facts and begin an investigation.
D. Suggest the son makes an appointment with the consultant to discuss his concerns.
E. Leave a message on the consultant's mobile phone and avoid speaking with the son at this stage.

Answer

A. The doctor speaking to the son must be open and honest about what has happened to his mother during her admission. Offering an appointment with the consultant to discuss the issues further would also be reasonable, especially as the doctor does not have first-hand experience of all the events. Ultimately, the consultant does have responsibility for the patient.

Meeting with the son early, discussing what has happened and offering an apology can make future engagement with the patient and family easier. It will help to build a relationship of trust, which is essential for caring for patients and their families. An apology does not constitute an admission of liability or of unprofessional conduct or performance, per se. In civil proceedings, questions of negligence are for the Court to decide. Protection from liability does not extend to circumstances in which the apology also includes an admission of fault.

The doctor should explain the future management plan in relation to the treatment of sepsis, why the treatment is conservative rather than surgical in view of her co-morbidities, and the management of her pressure sore with the appropriate pressure-relieving mattress, in conjunction with the tissue viability team.

Duty of candour

There is a professional duty of candour for doctors and nurses, and a legal duty of candour for organisations where mistakes have occurred. The doctor offering an explanation to patients or relatives may not possess all the relevant facts. On the available evidence, it would appear that Mrs M has come to at least moderate harm, although the final outcome is unclear. Lying on a trolley for 14 hours overnight in A&E without fluids may not only have resulted in a grade 2 pressure ulcer, but may also have contributed to her acute kidney injury. She did not receive the appropriate antibiotics in a timely manner for intra-abdominal infection according to the Trust's guidelines. There was a delay in senior medical and surgical review, which has impacted on her treatment and chances of recovery. Although the statutory duty of candour is directed towards institutions, the individuals involved in adverse events should complete a clinical incident report in order to understand what has happened and so that lessons can be learned.

References

1. National Patients Safety Incident Reports. http://improvement.nhs.uk/national-patient-safety-incident-reports-21-march-2018/.
2. https://www.gmc-uk.org/ethical-guidance/ethical-guidance-for-doctors/good-medical-practice.

Acknowledgements

The editors and contributors are grateful to the late Professor Mitchell Glickstein (Professor Emeritus of Neurosciences at University College London), for his advice throughout the writing of this medical law chapter.

Index

Note: tables, figures, and boxes are indicated by an italic *t*, *f*, and *b* following the page number.

B

D

H

J

M

O

Q

R

S

U